Davidson's Principles and Practice of Medicine

*The Editor*

JOHN MACLEOD
M.B., Ch.B., F.R.C.P.Edin

*Formerly: Chairman of University Department of Medicine, Western General Hospital, Edinburgh*
*Consultant Physician, Western General Hospital, Edinburgh*
*Consultant Physician, Royal Edinburgh Hospital*
*Consultant Physician, Clinic for Rheumatic Diseases, Royal Infirmary, Edinburgh*

*The Contributors*

Primarily from the Departments of Medicine and
Therapeutics, University of Edinburgh, but also
from other University Departments in Britain,
Africa and Australia

# Davidson's Principles and Practice of Medicine

A TEXTBOOK FOR STUDENTS AND DOCTORS

EDITED BY

**John Macleod**

THIRTEENTH EDITION

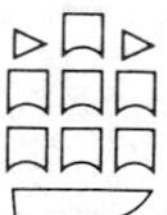

CHURCHILL LIVINGSTONE
EDINBURGH LONDON MELBOURNE AND NEW YORK 1981

CHURCHILL LIVINGSTONE
Medical Division of Longman Group Limited

Distributed in the United States of America by Churchill Livingstone Inc., 1560 Broadway, New York, N.Y. 10036, and by associated companies, branches and representatives throughout the world.

© E. & S. Livingstone, 1952
© Longman Group Limited, 1981

All rights reserved. No part of this publication may be reproduced, stored in a retrieval system, or transmitted in any form or by any means, electronic, mechanical, photocopying, recording or otherwise, without the prior permission of the publishers (Churchill Livingstone, Robert Stevenson House, 1–3 Baxter's Place, Leith Walk, Edinburgh, EH1 3AF).

First Edition 1952
Second Edition 1954
Third Edition 1956
Fourth Edition 1958
Fifth Edition 1960
Sixth Edition 1962
Seventh Edition 1964
First ELBS Edition published 1965
Eighth Edition 1966
ELBS Edition of Eighth Edition 1967
Ninth Edition 1968
ELBS Edition of Ninth Edition 1968
Tenth Edition 1971
ELBS Edition of Tenth Edition 1971
Eleventh Edition 1974
ELBS Edition of Eleventh Edition 1974
Twelfth Edition (including Tropical Diseases) 1977
ELBS Edition of Twelfth Edition 1977
Thirteenth Edition 1981
ELBS Edition of Thirteenth Edition 1981
ELBS Edition reprinted 1982
Thirteenth Edition reprinted 1983

ISBN 0 443 02487 1 (Cased)
ISBN 0 443 02489 8 (Limp)

**British Library Cataloguing in Publication Data**
Davidson, *Sir* Stanley
Davidson's principles and practice of medicine. –
13th ed.
1. Pathology
2. Medicine
I. Title II. Macleod, John
616 RD111

Printed and bound in Great Britain
at The Pitman Press, Bath

# Preface to the Thirteenth Edition

With this new production, *Davidson's Principles and Practice of Medicine* will have appeared in 13 editions and more than 20 reprints since it was first published over a quarter of a century ago. The book has established an international reputation; it is used extensively throughout the English speaking world and has also been translated into Spanish, Italian, Greek and Croato-serbian. Since 1965 it has been published in Africa and Asia in a paperback edition under the auspices of the English Language Book Society. This continuing success is a remarkable tribute to the genius and vision of Sir Stanley Davidson and the editorial policy he instituted, but we are acutely aware that, if the book is to retain its unique place in the field of medical education, it must be kept completely up to date in terms of both content and approach. This objective has, we hope, been achieved by consensus support for a progressive editorial policy and by the regular recruitment of younger authors.

There are more changes in this than in any previous edition of 'Davidson'. Sections entirely rewritten include diseases of the blood, connective tissues, joints and bones, acute poisoning (including ionising radiation), infections of the respiratory system and tuberculosis. Extensive changes have also been made throughout the remainder of the text to keep pace with new developments in rapidly advancing disciplines, notably in regard to immunology, alimentary disease, diabetes mellitus and the treatment of tropical diseases. The end result, we believe, is a textbook of medicine which will meet the needs of the 1980s.

Although much new material has been included, it has nevertheless proved possible to contain the book to a manageable size, slightly smaller than its predecessor, mainly by discarding what has been superseded. The price has been kept at a modest level despite increasing costs at every stage of production.

A close interrelationship has been maintained with the 5th edition of *Clinical Examination** in which several of the contributors and the editor participate. In addition, for the reader who wishes to test his or her understanding of the material included in both these books, an M.C.Q. Companion† is now available.

The opening chapters of the 13th edition deal with fundamental general factors in disease such as genetics, immunology, infection, nutrition and electrolyte balance. These are followed by accounts of diseases of the various systems and by outlines of psychiatry and acute poisoning. A chapter on tropical disease and helminthic infections is included to meet the needs of readers in Asia and Africa and so that Western readers will have at least some knowledge of medical problems and human needs in countries other than their own and be alerted to the dangers of imported disease. A final short chapter deals with the promotion of health and prevention of disease, re-emphasising the prominence given to prophylaxis throughout the book. In recognition of the fact that education must be a continuing process, many of the chapters conclude with brief comments on prospects for the immediate future.

The task of preparing the 13th edition has been made easier for the editor and

* Macleod, J. (ed.) (1979) *Clinical Examination*, 5th edn. Edinburgh: Churchill Livingstone.
† Fleming, P. R. (ed.) (1980) *1200 MCQs in Medicine*. Edinburgh: Churchill Livingstone.

contributors by the pleasure and satisfaction derived from working as a team, by the stimulus provided by new authors and by the challenge of constructive criticism from students and doctors all over the world. Our primary objective, as before, has been to ensure that the book provides a *rational and easily comprehensible basis for the practice of medicine*. We hope that it will continue to make as substantial a contribution to the education of medical students, both undergraduate and postgraduate, in the future as it has done in the past.

Edinburgh, 1981 *John Macleod*

# Acknowledgments

We have had generous help from many colleagues and we would like to express our thanks especially to Dr R. T. Thin (sexually transmitted disease), Dr John Peutherer (viral hepatitis), Dr R. Hay (tropical medicine), Dr D. H. Cummack (radiographs of alimentary tract), Dr J. F. Cullen (diabetic retinopathy), Mr J. E. Pizer (line drawings), Dr Moira Aitken (proof reading) and Greta Proven (preparation of manuscript). Other acknowledgments are made in the text.

To Graham Birnie we are particularly indebted for maintaining efficient and harmonious relationships between publishers, printers and editor.

# List of Contributors

ALLAN, N.C., M.B., Ch.B., F.R.C.P.Edin., F.R.C.P. Path.
*Senior Lecturer, University Department of Medicine, Western General Hospital, Edinburgh and formerly of University of Ibadan, Nigeria. Consultant Haematologist, Western General Hospital, Edinburgh.*
Diseases of the Blood and Blood Forming Organs. Exposure to Ionising Radiation.

BAIRD, JOYCE D., M.A., M.B., Ch.B.Aberd., F.R.C.P.Edin.
*Senior Lecturer, University Department of Medicine, Western General Hospital, Edinburgh and Hon. Consultant Physician, Western General Hospital, Edinburgh.*
Diabetes Mellitus and other Metabolic Disorders. Obesity.

BRYCESON, A. D. M., M.D., F.R.C.P.Edin., D.T.M. and H.
*Senior Lecturer, London School of Hygiene and Tropical Medicine. Consulting Physician, Hospital for Tropical Diseases. Consultant in Tropical Dermatology, St John's Hospital for Diseases of the Skin, London.*
Tropical Diseases and Helminthic Infections.

CREAN, GERARD P., Ph.D., F.R.C.P. Edin., F.R.C.P G.
*Hon. Lecturer in Medicine, University of Glasgow (Western Infirmary). Consultant Physician, Southern General Hospital, Glasgow. Physician-in-charge, The Gastrointestinal Centre, Southern General Hospital, Glasgow.*
Diseases of the Alimentary Tract and Pancreas.

EMERY, A.E.H., M.D., Ph.D (Johns Hopkins), D.Sc., F.R.C.P.Edin., M.F.C.M., F.R.S.Edin.
*Professor of Human Genetics (Western General Hospital), University of Edinburgh. Consultant in Medical Genetics, Lothian Health Board, Scotland.*
Genetic Factors in Disease.

FINLAYSON, N.D.C., Ph.D., M.B., Ch.B., F.R.C.P.Edin., M.R.C.P.Lond.
*Physician, Gastrointestinal and Liver Service, The Royal Infirmary, Edinburgh.*
Diseases of the Liver and Biliary Tract.

GEDDES, A. M., M.B., Ch.B., F.R.C.P.Edin., M.R.C.P.Lond.
*Senior Clinical Lecturer and Tutor in Infectious Diseases, University of Birmingham. Consultant Physician, Department of Communicable and Tropical Diseases, East Birmingham Hospital, Birmingham.*
Infection and Disease.

Girdwood, R. H., M.D., Ph.D., F.R.C.P.Edin., F.R.C.P.Lond., F.R.C.Path., F.R.S.Edin.
*Professor of Therapeutics and Clinical Pharmacology, University of Edinburgh. Hon. Consultant Physician, Royal Infirmary, Edinburgh.*
Diseases of the Blood and Blood-forming Organs.

Grant, I. W. B., M.B., Ch.B., F.R.C.P.Edin.
*Senior Lecturer, University Department of Medicine, Western General Hospital, Edinburgh. Consultant Physician, Respiratory Unit, Northern General Hospital, Edinburgh.*
Diseases of the Respiratory System.

Horne, N. W., M.B., Ch.B., F.R.C.P.Edin.
*Senior Lecturer, Department of Respiratory Medicine, University of Edinburgh. Consultant Physician, Chest Unit, City Hospital, Edinburgh.*
Diseases of the Respiratory System.

Irvine, W. J., D.Sc., M.B., Ch.B., F.R.C.P.E., M.R.C.Path.
*Reader, Department of Medicine, University of Edinburgh. Consultant Physician, Royal Infirmary, Edinburgh.*
Immunological Factors in Disease. Diseases of the Endocrine System.

Julian, D. G., M.A., M.D., F.R.C.P.Edin., F.R.C.P.Lond., F.R.A.C.P.
*British Heart Foundation Professor of Cardiology, University of Newcastle-upon-Tyne. Consultant Cardiologist, Freeman Hospital, Newcastle-upon-Tyne.*
Diseases of the Cardiovascular System.

Lawson, A. A. H., M.D., F.R.C.P.Edin.
*Hon. Senior Lecturer in Medicine, University of Edinburgh. Consultant Physician, Milesmark Hospital, Dunfermline and to associated hospitals in West Fife District, Fife. Postgraduate Tutor for West Fife Postgraduate Board for Medicine, University of Edinburgh.*
Acute Poisoning.

McCormick, J. N., M.B., Ch.B., M.R.C.P.Edin.
*Hon. Senior Lecturer, Departments of Medicine and Bacteriology, University of Edinburgh. Consultant Physician, Rheumatic Diseases Unit, Northern General Hospital, Edinburgh.*
Diseases of Connective Tissues, Joints and Bones.

McHardy, G. J. R., M.A., B.Sc., B.M., F.R.C.P.Edin., F.R.C.P.Lond.
*Senior Lecturer, Department of Respiratory Medicine, University of Edinburgh. Consultant Physician, Chest Unit, City Hospital, Edinburgh. Consultant Clinical Respiratory Physiologist, City Hospital and Western General Hospital, Edinburgh.*
Diseases of the Respiratory System.

Matthews, M. B., M.A., M.D.Cantab., F.R.C.P.Edin., F.R.C.P.Lond.
*Chairman, University Department of Medicine, Western General Hospital, Edinburgh. Consultant Cardiologist, Western General Hospital, Edinburgh,*
Diseases of the Cardiovascular System.

MAWDSLEY, C., M.D., F.R.C.P.Edin., F.R.C.P.Lond.
*Senior Lecturer in Medical Neurology, University of Edinburgh. Hon. Consultant Neurologist, Royal Infirmary and Northern General Hospital, Edinburgh.*
Diseases of the Nervous System.

NUKI, GEORGE, M.B., B.S., F.R.C.P.Edin., F.R.C.P.Lond.
*Professor of Rheumatology, University of Edinburgh. Hon. Consultant Physician Northern General Hospital and Royal Infirmary, Edinburgh.*
Diseases of Connective Tissues, Joints and Bones.

RICHMOND, JOHN, M.D., F.R.C.P.Edin., F.R.C.P.Lond.
*Professor of Medicine, University of Sheffield. Hon. Consultant Physician, Sheffield Area Health Authority (Teaching).*
Diseases of the Liver and Biliary Tract.

ROBSON, J. S., M.D., F.R.C.P. Edin.
*Professor of Medicine, University of Edinburgh. Hon. Consultant Physician, Royal Infirmary, Edinburgh.*
Disturbances in Water and Electrolyte Balance and in Hydrogen Ion Concentration.
Diseases of the Kidney and Urinary System.

SHEARMAN, D. J. C., Ph.D., M.B., Ch.B., F.R.C.P. Edin., F.R.A.C.P.
*Mortlock Professor of Medicine, University of Adelaide and Head of the Professorial Medical Unit, Royal Adelaide Hospital, Australia.*
Diseases of the Alimentary Tract and Pancreas.

SIMPSON, J. A., M.D.Glasg., F.R.C.P.Edin., F.R.C.P.Lond., F.R.C.P.Glasg., F.R.S.Edin.
*Professor of Neurology, University of Glasgow. Senior Neurologist, Institute of Neurological Sciences, Southern General Hospital and Consultant Neurologist, Western Infirmary, Glasgow.*
Diseases of the Nervous System.

SMALL, W.P., V.R.D., M.B., Ch.B., Ch.M., F.R.C.S.Edin., F.R.C.P.Edin.
*Consultant Surgeon, Gastrointestinal Unit, Western General Hospital, Edinburgh.*
Diseases of the Alimentary Tract and Pancreas.

TRUSWELL, A. S., M.D., F.R.C.P.Lond., F.F.C.M.
*Boden Professor of Human Nutrition, Sydney University, Australia. Head of Nutrition Section, School of Public Health and Tropical Medicine, Sydney. Honorary Consultant in Nutrition, Royal Prince Alfred Hospital, Sydney.*
Nutritional Factors in Disease. Promotion of Health and Prevention of Disease.

WALTON, H. J., Ph.D., M.D., F.R.C.P.Edin., D.P.M.
*Professor of Psychiatry, University of Edinburgh. Director, University Department of Psychiatry, Western General Hospital. Hon. Consultant Psychiatrist, Royal Edinburgh Hospital.*
Psychiatry.

WRIGHT, F. J., M.A., M.D.Cantab., F.R.C.P.Edin., F.R.C.P.Lond., D.T.M. & H. Eng.
*Lately Head of Medical Department, Kilimanjaro Christian Medical Centre, Moshi, Tanzania. Hon. Senior Lecturer in Medicine, University of Dar es Salaam, Tanzania. Formerly Senior Lecturer in Diseases of Tropical Climates, University of Edinburgh and Government Medical Specialist, Kenya.*
Tropical Diseases and Helminthic Infections. Promotion of Health and Prevention of Disease.

# Contents

# 1. Genetic Factors in Disease

Nowadays there is an increasing awareness of the importance of genetic factors in the aetiology and pathogenesis of many disorders affecting man. Perhaps of more importance is that this knowledge has also led to possible means of prevention of such disorders through genetic counselling and antenatal diagnosis.

At the turn of the century morbidity and mortality in infancy and childhood could largely be attributed to environmental factors such as infections and nutritional deficiencies. With advances in medicine these problems are decreasing, at least in the developed countries, while others, in which genetic factors are largely or even entirely responsible, are becoming more obvious. In a survey carried out in Newcastle in 1970, no less than 42% of childhood deaths could be attributed to diseases which are genetic in causation. The contribution of genetic factors to mortality and morbidity in adults is more difficult to assess but is also increasing.

It is useful to consider human disease as forming a spectrum at one end of which we have those diseases which are entirely genetic in origin and in which environmental factors play little if any part. This group of disorders includes *chromosomal abnormalities* and so-called *unifactorial disorders*. The latter are due to single gene defects (Mendelian factors); though individually rare there are over a thousand of them. They are usually serious disorders; they often present at birth or in childhood, though notable exceptions are Huntington's chorea, myotonic dystrophy and polyposis coli. The mode of inheritance is straightforward and follows Mendelian principles, and the risks of occurrence in relatives are high. For the vast majority of these unifactorial disorders there is as yet no effective treatment and prevention is the main approach to the problem.

At the other end of the spectrum are those diseases such as infections and nutritional deficiences which are entirely environmental in aetiology. In the middle of the spectrum are many common conditions which are partly genetic and partly environmental in causation, so-called *multifactorial disorders*. These include many congenital malformations (such as congenital dislocation of the hip, club foot, congenital pyloric stenosis, congenital heart disease, anencephaly and spina bifida), 'diseases of modern society' (diabetes mellitus, essential hypertension, coronary artery disease) and possibly certain psychiatric disorders (such as schizophrenia and manic-depressive psychosis). In multifactorial disorders the genetic component is complex, probably involving in each case many genes. The risks to relatives are usually low.

In this chapter, after a review of the chemical basis of inheritance, an outline is given of chromosomal abnormalities, unifactorial and multifactorial disorders and the prevention of genetic disease.

## Chemical Basis of Inheritance

In the nucleus of every cell are the chromosomes containing the genes composed of deoxyribonucleic acid (DNA) within which genetic information is stored.

DNA is composed of two polynucleotide chains, twisted together to form a double helix (Fig. 1.1). Each nucleotide is composed of a nitrogenous base, a sugar molecule

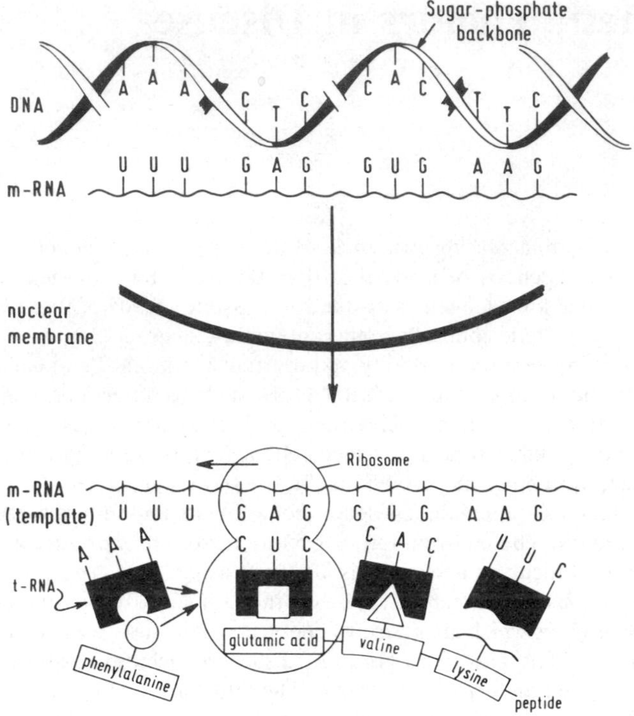


Fig. 1.1 Translation of genetic information into protein synthesis. Guanine (G) pairs with cytosine (C) and adenine (A) with thymine (T) or uracil (U).

(deoxyribose) and a phosphate molecule. The nitrogenous bases in DNA are adenine and guanine (purines) and cytosine and thymine (pyrimidines). The arrangement of the bases is not random: a purine in one chain always pairs with a pyrimidine on the other chain. There is also specific base pairing: guanine in one chain always pairs with cytosine in the other chain and adenine always pairs with thymine. This is the Watson-Crick model of DNA. It is postulated that at nuclear division the two strands of the DNA molecule separate and as a result of specific base pairing each chain then builds its complement. In this way, when a cell divides, genetic information is conserved and transmitted to each daughter cell.

The primary action of the gene is to synthesise protein by various combinations of 20 different amino acids. Genetic information is stored within the DNA molecule in the form of a triplet code such that a sequence of three bases specifies the structure of one amino acid.

Whereas DNA is found mainly in the chromosomes, ribonucleic acid (RNA) is found mainly in the nucleolus and the cytoplasm. RNA has a structure similar to DNA (Fig. 1.1): both nucleic acids contain adenine, guanine and cytosine but thymine is replaced by uracil in RNA and the latter contains the sugar ribose. The information stored in the DNA code of the gene is transmitted to a particular type of RNA, so-called messenger-RNA (m-RNA). Each m-RNA is formed by a particular gene, such that every base in the m-RNA molecule is complementary to a corresponding base in the DNA of the gene: cytosine with guanine, thymine with adenine but adenine with uracil since the latter replaces thymine in RNA. The m-RNA then migrates out of the nucleus into the cytoplasm where it becomes associated with the ribosomes which are the site of protein synthesis. In the ribosomes the m-RNA forms the template or mould for arranging particular amino acids in sequence. In the cytoplasm there is yet another form of RNA referred to as transfer-RNA (t-RNA). Each amino acid in the cytoplasm becomes attached to a particular t-RNA. The other end of the t-RNA molecule consists of three bases which combine with complementary bases on the m-RNA. Thus a particular triplet in the m-RNA is related through t-RNA to a specific amino acid. The ribosome moves along the m-RNA in a zipper-like fashion, the assembled amino acids linking up to form a polypeptide chain.

There are essentially two types of genes: structural genes which are responsible for the synthesis of specific proteins such as haemoglobin, collagen and enzymes, and control genes which are thought to modify the action of structural genes.

A change (mutation) of a base pair of the DNA molecule may result in any one of a number of possible effects. If the altered triplet codes for the same amino acid then of course the change will go undetected. Possibly 20 to 25% of all possible single base changes are of this type. Alternatively a single base mutation may result in a triplet which codes for a different amino acid resulting in an altered protein. The latter may retain its biological activity (e.g. enzyme activity) but have altered physico-chemical properties such as electrophoretic mobility or stability so that it is more rapidly broken down. This is the case in many of the abnormal haemoglobinopathies in which the aberrant haemoglobin may be detected by its altered electrophoretic mobility. However the substitution of a different amino acid may result in reduced or even absent biological activity. In inborn errors of metabolism therefore the level of a particular enzyme may be reduced because it is not synthesised, or it is synthesised but has reduced activity or because of its instability it is more rapidly broken down.

## Chromosomes and Chromosomal Disorders

**Chromosome Structure and Number**. Among higher animals each species bears within the nucleus of its cells a set of chromosomes which is characteristic both in number and in morphology for that species. Each nucleus in the somatic cells of man contains a set of 46 chromosomes. Two of these chromosomes determine the sex of the individual and are therefore known as *sex chromosomes*; the remaining 44 chromosomes are known as *autosomes*.

The DNA of higher organisms is coated with histone and non-histone proteins. This produces a deoxyribonucleoprotein fibre (chromatin) which forms the basic unit of chromosome structure. Chromsomes are in a suitable state for detailed study only during specific intervals within the period of cell division, for it is during these periods that the chromosomes become contracted, thicker and more readily stained. Chromosomes in the resting nucleus do not take up most stains in a satisfactory way.

Each chromosome has a point along its length, a constriction, known as the *centromere* which divides the chromosomes into two arms which are usually unequal in length. The chromosomes also differ in their overall length. Further by using certain stains each chromosome can be shown to have a specific banding pattern. By these criteria it is now possible to identify individual chromosomes.

The chromosomal complement of any nucleus is composed of two sets of chromosomes which are arranged in pairs. Because the two members of any given pair (with the exception of the sex chromosomes) resemble one another they are said to be *homologous*. One homologue of any pair is derived from one parent and its partner from the other parent. Thus man has 22 pairs of homologous chromosomes (autosomes) and one pair of sex chromosomes.

During gametogenesis the number of chromosomes is halved in order that the number of chromosomes remains constant and is not doubled at each conception. Thus somatic cell nuclei contain twice as many chromosomes as gametes and with respect to their chromosome complement are said to be *diploid*, whereas gametes are said to be *haploid*.

The two sex chromosomes of the female are identical and are referred to as *X chromosomes*. The sex chromosomes of the male, however, are not identical. One of the pair resembles the X chromosomes seen in females while the other is much smaller, differs considerably in morphology and is referred to as a *Y chromosome*. Thus the sex chromosome constitution is XX in a female and XY in a male. In the female each ovum bears one or other of the X chromosomes, whereas in the male the sperms bear either an X or a Y chromosome. At fertilisation an ovum therefore has an equal chance of being fertilised by either an X or a Y bearing sperm. It is for this reason that the sex ratio is approximately (not exactly) unity at birth.

**Mitosis**. Unlike highly differentiated cells such as neurones, the cells of many tissues in the body repeatedly undergo division. In fact some cells, such as those of the intestinal tract and bone marrow, continue to divide throughout the life of an individual. For the error rate in cell division to remain as low as it is, nuclear division must be extremely well regulated. The process by which nuclei divide to produce two identical daughter nuclei is known as mitosis. During mitosis each chromosome divides into two so that the number of chromosomes in each daughter nucleus is the same as in the parent cell. Though mitosis is a continuous process, one step merging imperceptibly into the next, it can be divided into stages for ease of description. These stages are known as interphase, prophase, metaphase, anaphase and telophase (Fig. 1.2).

*Interphase* is the resting stage between nuclear divisions when the chromosomes are loosely coiled and difficult to visualise. By the end of interphase each chromosome has divided longitudinally into two daughter chromosomes, or *chromatids*, which remain attached to each other at the centromere.

During *prophase*, the chromosomes take up stains more readily and therefore become easier to visualise. By the end of phophase the nucleoli are no longer visible and each chromatid is a tightly coiled structure which is closely aligned to its partner.

*Metaphase* begins with the disappearance of the nuclear membrane and the formation of the spindle apparatus, which consists of a number of minute 'threads' which run from one pole of the nucleus to the other. The chromosomes become orientated around the centre of the nucleus in the equatorial plane. Each chromosome is attached to the spindle by means of its centromere. The spindle is responsible for the movement of the chromosomes during mitosis.

During *anaphase* the centromere of each chromosome divides into two, each half 'repels' the other and the chromatids move apart towards opposite poles of the spindle. When the chromatids reach the poles they form two separate but identical groups.

*Telophase* begins as the daughter chromosomes arrive at the poles of the spindle. The two groups of chromosomes become surrounded by a new nuclear membrane and gradually become less visible. Cell division is completed by cleavage of the cytoplasm. New cell membranes develop and the nuclei of the two daughter cells re-enter the interphase stage. Thus at the end of mitosis a cell has divided into two daughter cells each with an identical genetic constitution.

**Meiosis**. The process by which the chromosome number is halved during gameto-

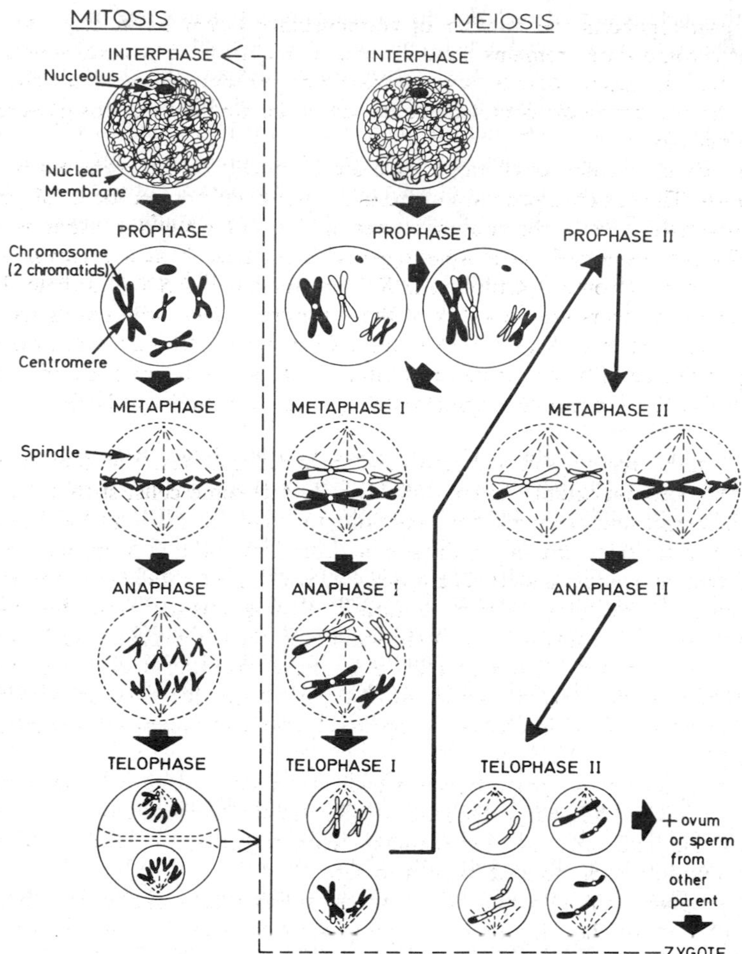


Fig. 1.2 Stages of mitosis and meiosis

genesis is known as meiosis. Although meiosis involves two division stages, the chromosomes divide only once, each gamete normally receiving either of a pair of homologous chromosomes.

Each of the two steps in meiosis has a phophase, metaphase, anaphase and telophase stage as in mitosis (Fig. 1.2). The prophase of the first stage is very long. It is thought that DNA replication has already taken place by the onset of this stage, although each chromosome still appears morphologically to be a single thread. During prophase the chromosomes become more contracted, as a result of tighter coiling, and homologous chromosomes come together and pair along their length. Then a process known as *crossing-over* may occur in which there is an exchange of genetic material between chromatids of homologous chromosomes.

Following prophase the sequence of events is essentially similar to that occuring in mitosis, except that during this first meiotic division the centromere does not divide. Instead the members of each pair of homologous chromosomes migrate to opposite poles of the nucleus so that each daughter nucleus receives only one member of each pair and therefore bears a haploid chromosome complement.

In the second stage of meiosis the centromere divides and the chromatids of each chromosome separate and migrate into different nuclei. Thus each daughter cell from the first meiotic division has in turn divided to form two identical cells. Meiosis therefore results in each gamete having a haploid number of chromosomes and receiving one or the other member of each homologous pair of chromosomes and the genes it bears. This forms the cytological basis for Mendelian inheritance.

**Methods of Studying Chromosomes**. There are a variety of ways in which the study of chromosomes can be approached. Broadly these fall into two categories: those techniques which are used to study the complete chromosome complement of an individual, or those which enable information to be gained about the sex chromosome constitution of a person without having to do a complete chromosome analysis.

Since it is only during critical stages of the mitotic or meiotic cycle that the chromosomes are in a suitable state to study, chromosome analysis requires the provision of a large number of cells which are actively dividing. Meiotic studies can of course be done only on specimens of tissue obtained from the gonads. Mitotic studies, on the other hand, can be made on a variety of different and more easily available tissues, e.g. directly from cells which are rapidly dividing *in vivo*, as in bone marrow. More commonly, however, specimens are obtained from tissues which are not rapidly dividing *in vivo* but are much more accessible to study, such as skin and blood leucocytes, and the cells are stimulated to divide *in vitro* by the addition of phytohaemagglutinin. The addition of colchicine arrests cell division at the metaphase stage when the chromosomes are most suitable for study. The use of hypotonic solutions causes the cells to swell, disperses the chromosomes and makes them easier to study and count (Fig. 1.3). Finally the material is stained (e.g. with Giemsa) to demonstrate the banding patterns of the chromosomes. A suitable metaphase spread is then photographed through a high power microscope and the individual chromosomes are cut out from the photograph. The chromosomes are then arranged in an orderly fashion, in homologous pairs, to produce a standard arrangement known as a *karyotype*.

Methods are available for studying the sex chromosome constitution of an individual without having to resort to the costly and time-consuming process of preparing and analysing the complete karyotype. These include the study of sex-chromatin and fluorescent bodies in buccal smears and 'drumsticks' in polymorphonuclear leucocytes.

Female nuclei contain a distinctive mass of nuclear chromatin characteristically situated close to the nuclear membrane, the *sex chromatin* or "Barr-body', which represents a genetically inactive X chromosome. In the female inactivation of one X chromosome in normal cells is a random process so that either the paternal or maternal X chromosome can be inactivated in any particular cell of the same person. The cell nuclei of all the tissues in a human female contain a sex-chromatin body, but for convenience the most suitable cells for study are those of the buccal mucosa. The inside of the cheek is gently scraped with a spatula and the cells obtained spread onto a glass slide (*buccal smear*). These cells are then fixed and stained and can be examined for the presence of sex-chromatin bodies which are seen in 30 to 60% of nuclei of a normal female. Since only one X chromosome is active per cell, then the number of sex-chromatin bodies (inactivated X chromosomes) is one less than the total number of X chromosomes. Thus a normal female has one sex chromatin body, a patient with XO Turner's syndrome (p. 11) has no sex-chromatin bodies (chromatin negative) and a patient who has Klinefelter's syndrome (p. 11) with three X chro-

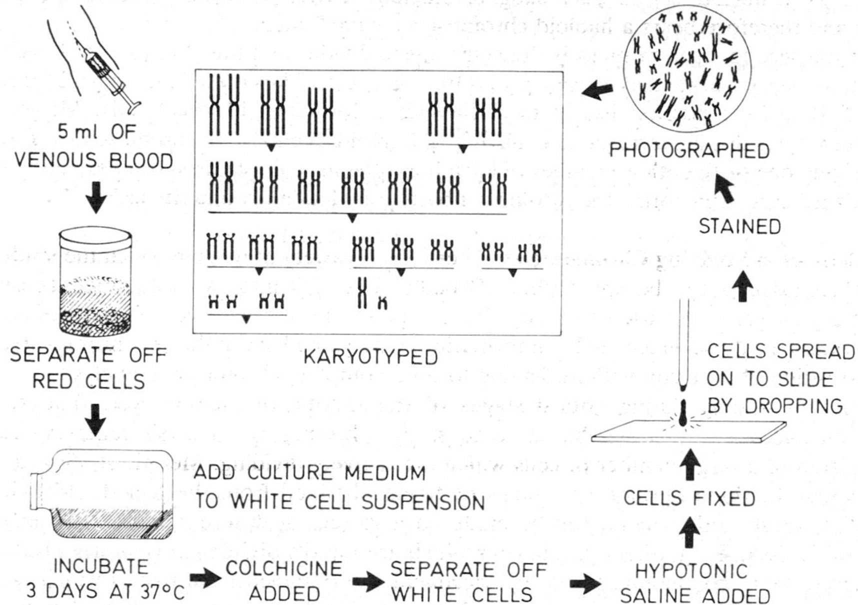


Fig. 1.3 Preparation of a karyotype

mosomes (XXXY) has two sex chromatin bodies.

In suitably stained smears of peripheral blood about 3% of the polymorphonuclear leucocytes of females show a small accessory nuclear lobule, which resembles a drumstick and projects from the main mass of the nuclear lobes. This is not seen in polymorphs from normal males, or females with an XO sex-chromosome constitution. The number of drumsticks is not, however, related to the number of X chromosomes.

Interphase nuclei of cells from males exhibit a fluorescent spot called the F body (or Y-chromatin) when stained with quinacrine; the number of F bodies represents the number of Y chromosomes. The technique can be adapted for use with buccal smears and so provides a method of assessing the number of Y chromosomes comparable with the sex-chromatin method of studying X chromosomes.

It can be seen, therefore, that these techniques are complementary and by combining them the sex chromosome constitution of an individual can be determined with ease, speed and accuracy. This is extremely useful clinically in the investigation of patients with abnormalities of sexual development or infertility, or for use in large-scale population surveys. Apart from these more common applications these techniques are also being used in new fields involving the separation of X and Y bearing sperm (half of human sperms contain an F body and are presumably Y bearing) and the determination of the sex of an unborn child.

**Chromosome Nomenclature**. A shorthand notation is used to describe a karyotype in the simplest way. This consists first of the total number of chromosomes (in numerals), followed by the sex chromosome constitution, and finally by any abnormalities that are present. Thus a normal male is 46, XY; a normal female is 46, XX. A girl with Turner's syndrome may be 45, XO and a boy with Klinefelter's syndrome, 47, XXY. The short and long arms of any chromosome are designated 'p' and 'q' respectively. A (+) or (–) sign is placed before an appropriate symbol where it means an additional or missing whole chromosome, but after a symbol when it refers only to part of a chromosome. Thus a boy with Down's syndrome is 47,XY,+21 and a boy with part of the short arm of chromosome 5 missing is 46,XY,5p–.

## Chromosomal Disorders

Specific chromosomal abnormalities are associated with recognised diseases or clinical syndromes in man. These include Down's syndrome (mongolism), abnormalities of sexual development (Turner's and Klinefelter's syndromes), syndromes of multiple congenital malformations (13- and 18-trisomies), spontaneous abortions, personality disorders (XYY and XXX etc.), chronic myeloid leukaemia and ataxia telangiectasia.

It has been found that 1 in every 200 live-born babies has a gross abnormality of chromosome number or structure. High as this figure is, it does not indicate fully the frequency with which chromosomal anomalies occur at fertilisation, for in a study of early spontaneous abortions chromosomal aberrations occurred in over 50%. Many of these chromosomal anomalies are rarely found in live-born babies and are therefore presumably lethal and the cause of a significant number of early abortions.

Chromosomal abnormalities can be divided into those which involve the autosomes and those which involve the sex chromosomes. These can be further divided into abnormalities of number and of structure. Numerical abnormalities arise when one or more chromosomes are either lost or gained, a phenomenon referred to as *aneuploidy*. When a whole set of chromosomes is gained the phenomenon is known as *polyploidy* and is not compatible with survival in man. The loss of a whole autosome, *monosomy*, also appears to be lethal in man. The addition of an extra chromosome, so resulting in three chromosomes instead of two (*trisomy*), seems, however, to result in less severe effects.

**Autosomal abnormalities.** Trisomy of a number of different autosomes have now been reported in man; the most common is trisomy-21 which results in Down's syndrome. The two other well-recognised syndromes (trisomy-13 and trisomy-18) occur far less frequently than Down's syndrome. They are both more severe in effect and usually result in death within the infant period.

DOWN'S SYNDROME occurs in about 1 in 700 live-births and is characterised by a flat face with widely spaced and upward slanting eyes, epicanthic folds, brachycephaly, malformed ears, broad and/or short neck, and a single, transverse palmar crease. They are invariably mentally retarded, but have a pleasant, quiet personality and show a great fondness for music. This condition is also associated with an increased frequency of both congenital visceral anomalies, particularly congenital heart disease, and acute leukaemia. Although the mortality rate of these patients is high within the first year of life, many now survive into adulthood and there are several reports of women with Down's syndrome having children; on average half their offspring are normal and half have Down's syndrome.

About 95% of cases of Down's syndrome are due to regular trisomy-21 which arises as a result of non-disjunction during meiosis. Normally during meiosis the two homologous chromosomes of any pair separate and pass into different gametes. Occasionally an accident occurs and the chromosomes fail to separate, both members of the pair passing into the same gamete. If such a gamete is then fertilised by a normal gamete the resulting zygote will possess an additional chromosome. All the trisomy syndromes are found to have a significant relationship to maternal age, the frequency of trisomic births increasing with increasing maternal age. It is thought that perhaps some effect of ageing in the ova of older mothers makes them more prone to non-disjunction. There have been reports, however, of trisomy-21 recurring in some families, which suggests that the phenomenon of non-disjunction may be under genetic control at least in these rare families.

About 1% of cases of Down's syndrome are *mosaics*, that is, they possess two different cell lines, one of which has a normal chromosome constitution, the other an extra chromosome 21. This arises as a result of non-disjunction occurring at or after the first zygotic division and is very rarely inherited. The clinical picture may often be considerably modified in some of these cases.

About 4% of cases of Down's syndrome result from a phenomenon known as *translocation*, in which there is an exchange of segments between different chromosomes. The mechanism is thought to be that two chromosomes lying close to one another suffer simultaneous breaks followed by an exchange of chromosomal material. For example, in Down's syndrome a large part of chromosome 21 may be united with part of chromosome 15. A carrier of such a translocation (who has only 45 chromosomes) produces four types of gametes. A gamete may contain a normal chromosome 15 and a normal chromosome 21, in which case the resulting offspring will be normal. Or a gamete may contain a translocation (15/21), in which case the resulting offspring will have only 45 chromosomes and will be a carrier like the parent. Or a gamete may contain the translocation and a normal chromosome 21, in which case the offspring will have 46 chromosomes but in effect will be trisomic for chromosome 21 and will therefore have Down's syndrome. Finally a gamete may contain a chromosome 15 but no chromosome 21; this would produce a zygote monosomic for chromosome 21 which is lethal and would presumably result in an abortion. Theoretically, therefore, a carrier of such a translocation has a 1 in 3 chance of having a child with Down's syndrome, but for reasons which are not clear, the actual risk is much less. In Down's syndrome the translocation usually involves an exchange of material between chromosomes 13, 14 or 15 and chromosome 21. Rarely there may be an exchange between chromosomes 21 and 22 or even between two 21s.

OTHER AUTOSOMAL ABNORMALITIES. *Deletions* arise when a segment of a chromosome has been lost. New techniques have led to the demonstration of deletions involving a number of autosomes and an increasing number of these are being associated with clinically recognisable syndromes, examples of which are summarised in Table 1.1. Other rarer forms of chromosomal abnormalities are *ring chromosomes* and *isochromosomes*. Ring chromosomes involving both autosomes and sex chromosomes have been described; they are thought to be formed when two ends of a chromosome have been deleted and the broken (more 'sticky') ends fuse to form a ring. In effect ring chromosomes are manifest as deletions and in shorthand they are represented as an 'r'. An isochromosome is formed when the centromere divides horizontally instead of longitudinally resulting in a chromosome consisting of either two long arms or of two short arms.

The *Philadelphia chromosome* (Ph[1]) is an *acquired* chromosomal abnormality associated with chronic myeloid leukaemia. The long arm of chromosome 22 is translocated to another autosome, usually chromosome 9.

**Sex Chromosome Abnormalities.** Numerical abnormalities of the sex chromosomes are more common than with the autosomes, and in general they produce less severe effects. They are brought about by the same phenomenon of non-disjunction. As

Table 1.1 Autosomal abnormalities associated with recognised clinical syndromes

| Chromosome abnormality | Syndrome | Clinical features |
|---|---|---|
| trisomy-21<br>translocation 13–15/21<br>translocation 22/21<br>translocation 21/21 | Down's | characteristic facies<br>mental retardation<br>hypotonia<br>congenital heart disease<br>Simian palmar crease |
| trisomy-8 | —— | moderate mental retardation<br>concomitant strabismus<br>clinodactyly<br>other skeletal defects |
| trisomy-9 | —— | abnormal facies<br>skeletal abnormalities<br>hypoplastic genitalia<br>congenital heart disease |
| trisomy-13 | Patau's | motor and mental retardation<br>microcephaly<br>microphthalmia<br>cleft palate/hare lip<br>polydactyly<br>congenital heart disease |
| trisomy-18 | Edwards' | motor and mental retardation<br>flexion deformities of fingers<br>micrognathia<br>'rocker-bottom' feet<br>congenital heart disease |
| trisomy-22 | —— | mental and motor retardation<br>microcephaly<br>abnormal facies and ears |
| trisomy-4p | —— | abnormal facies<br>digital anomalies<br>foot deformities |
| trisomy-9p | —— | abnormal facies<br>large, low-set ears<br>mental retardation<br>incurved and short V digit |
| 4p – | —— | mental retardation<br>abnormal facies<br>cleft palate<br>coloboma<br>epilepsy<br>hypospadias<br>scalp defects |
| 5p – | Cri du chat | mental retardation<br>microcephaly<br>hypertelorism<br>characteristic cry |
| 13q –<br>13r | —— | mental and motor retardation<br>abnormal facies<br>microcephaly<br>abnormal thumbs<br>abnormal ears |
| 18q – | De Grouchy's | mental retardation<br>'carp-mouth'<br>abnormal ears<br>tapering fingers |
| 18p – | De Grouchy's | mental retardation<br>ocular abnormalities<br>abnormal ears |

Table 1.1 (*continued*)

| Chromosome abnormality | Syndrome | Clinical features |
|---|---|---|
| | | dental decay<br>CNS abnormalities |
| 18r | —— | combination of 18p – and 18q – features |
| 21 q –<br>(G deletion syndrome I) | 'anti-mongolism' | antimongoloid slant of eyes<br>hypertonia<br>micrognathia<br>growth retardation<br>skeletal malformations |
| 22q –<br>(G deletion syndrome II) | —— | epicanthic folds<br>hypotonia<br>syndactyly<br>retarded development |

with the autosomes, abnormalities of structure also occur although they are far less common than the numerical anomalies.

KLINEFELTER'S SYNDROME was the first sex chromosome aneuploidy to be demonstrated in man. Affected males have an extra X chromosome resulting in an XXY sex chromosome constitution or as many as four X chromosomes may be present; an extra Y chromosome may also be present on occasions resulting in an XXYY sex chromosome constitution. The main clinical features are eunuchoid body proportions, sterility (due to azoospermia), hypogonadism, gynaecomastia and often mental retardation. There appears to be a relationship between mental retardation and the number of X chromosomes in both males and females. In Klinefelter's syndrome all individuals with an XXXY sex chromosome constitution are mentally retarded, whereas this is so in only about one-quarter of those with XXY sex chromosome constitution. Like the autosomal trisomies, Klinefelter's syndrome is found to occur more frequently in the sons of older mothers.

THE XYY CONSTITUTION is another sex chromosome aneuploidy in the male. Such men are reported to occur with increased frequency amongst inmates of institutions for the mentally retarded with criminal tendencies. It has been shown by various surveys that between two and five per cent of such populations may be XYY. However, the exact relationship of this chromosomal anomaly with either mental retardation or criminal tendencies is uncertain especially as XYY individuals have been found amongst the normal general population.

TURNER'S SYNDROME was the first aneuploidy to be described in females. An XO sex chromosome constitution is the commonest abnormality, but clinical features of Turner's syndrome may also result from iso-chromosomes, deletions, and rings involving the X chromosome. This abnormality must arise by non-disjunction, but unlike Klinefelter's syndrome, Turner's syndrome does not show a relationship with maternal age. The main clinical features are shortness of stature, primary amenorrhoea, lack of secondary sex characteristics and a variety of congenital abnormalities such as webbing of the neck, increased carrying-angle of the forearm (cubitus valgus) and coarctation of the aorta. Although, overall, patients with Turner's syndrome have a significantly lower I.Q. than normal, marked retardation is uncommon and the discrepancy is mainly in the performance aspect of their I.Q.

Females have also been described with three or even four X-chromosomes (XXX, XXXX); they may occasionally be mentally subnormal or have psychiatric disorders, but in all other respects appear to be healthy. Usually children born to XXX females are normal.

## Unifactorial Inheritance

These disorders are due to defects of a single gene, i.e. to a primary error in the DNA code. They are inherited in a simple fashion, following Mendelian laws. The risk of their recurring in a family may therefore be accurately predicted on theoretical grounds making genetic counselling more straightforward.

These disorders may be subdivided according to the chromosome on which the abnormal (or mutant) gene is situated and also by the nature of the trait itself. Thus a trait which is determined by a gene situated on an autosome is said to be inherited as an *autosomal* trait, and this may be either *dominant* or *recessive*. A trait determined by a gene situated on one of the sex chromosomes is said to be *sex-linked* and may also be either dominant or recessive.

**Autosomal Dominant Inheritance.** A dominant trait is one which is manifested in the *heterozygote*. In other words a person exhibiting an autosomal dominant trait possesses both the mutant gene and the normal gene, the presence of only one mutant gene being necessary for the trait to be manifested in the carrier. If the disorder is common, then some affected individuals could be *homozygotes* (i.e. have a 'double dose' of the mutant gene), but if the disorder is rare (as is usually the case), then affected individuals are almost always heterozygotes. It should be noted that the normal and abnormal genes are known as *alleles*, i.e. they are alternative forms of the same gene.

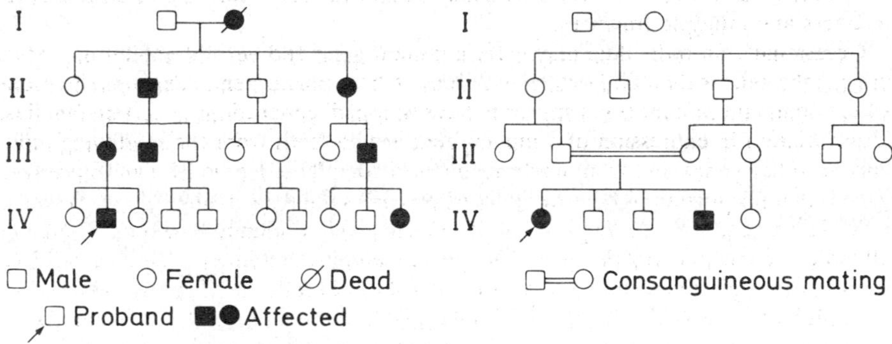


Fig. 1.4 Characteristic pedigree: autosomal dominant trait.

Fig. 1.5 Characteristic pedigree: autosomal recessive trait.

Usually persons affected with an autosomal dominant trait are found to have an affected parent, the trait being transmitted from one generation to the next in a family, as illustrated in Figure 1.4. This is not always the case, however; sometimes the disorder may appear suddenly in a family when no members of previous generations have been affected. This may be due to illegitimacy, to one parent being minimally affected and passed unnoticed, or more commonly to the occurrence of a new mutation. This may complicate genetic counselling and is a problem which arises particularly in conditions inherited in a dominant fashion. In diseases which are severe, affected individuals seldom have children because they are either infertile or do not survive to reach reproductive age. In such conditions the disease will eventually become extinct in affected families and is maintained in the population only by fresh mutations. Achondroplasia is one of the forms of short-limbed dwarfism and is inherited as an autosomal dominant trait. In one large study it was shown that affected individuals exhibited a marked reduction in reproductive fitness. It is not surprising, therefore, that a high proportion of cases are the result of new mutations.

In conditions which do not have a marked effect on survival it is often possible to trace the conditions through many generations of a family. Such a condition is the adult form of polycystic disease of the kidneys. Although affected individuals may eventually die from chronic renal failure, they often show no symptoms or signs of the disease until early middle life when they have already had their family and run the risk of transmitting the trait to their children.

In autosomal dominant conditions, if an affected individual marries a normal person, then on average half their children will be similarly affected. This arises because the affected individual produces gametes, half of which contain the normal gene and the other half contain the mutant gene. The normal partner produces gametes all of which contain the normal gene. Thus at fertilisation the normal partner's gametes have an equal chance of uniting with a gamete carrying either a normal or an abnormal gene with the result that at conception there is a 1 in 2 chance of producing an affected individual. Because of the smaller size of modern families, by chance all the children of an affected individual may be normal, or similarly by chance again all his children may be affected. It is on average that half the offspring of an affected individual will be affected.

Some autosomal dominant traits are extremely variable in severity, this variability in clinical manifestation being referred to as *expressivity*. Osteogenesis imperfecta, for example, is an autosomal dominant condition in which affected individuals may have only blue sclerae, whereas others may exhibit the full syndrome of blue sclerae, deafness and multiple fractures.

Occasionally an individual may carry a mutant gene and yet not exhibit any of its effects; the gene is then said to be *non-penetrant*. This phenomenon explains situations where dominant mutant traits appear to have 'skipped' generations in certain families. This variation in expression of a mutant gene results both from the modifying influence of other genes and from environmental factors. The degree of penetrance of a gene is that proportion of heterozygotes who express the gene in any degree, however mild. For a gene to be *fully penetrant* its effects must be manifest to some degree in all individuals who carry the gene. The phenomenon of varying penetrance can give rise to problems when estimating recurrence risks in order to give genetic advice. For example, tuberous sclerosis (epiloia) is inherited as a dominant trait but is not always penetrant. This condition is characterised by adenoma sebaceum (small papules over the cheeks and nose), epilepsy and mental retardation of varying severity. Some individuals carrying the gene may be so mildly affected as to pass as normal and so produce an apparently 'skipped' generation. However, it is unusual to find a proven carrier (e.g. with an affected child and an affected parent) who does not show at least some evidence of the disease, such as a few typical papules on the face.

**Autosomal Recessive Inheritance.** Autosomal recessive traits also affect both males and females. Unlike dominant traits, recessive traits are manifest only in the homozygous state, that is, in those individuals who possess a double dose of the mutant gene. Heterozygotes who possess only one mutant gene are usually perfectly healthy.

Similarly the offspring of an affected person are usually normal, because most recessive conditions are so rare that it would be most unlikely that an affected person would marry a person heterozygous for the same mutant gene. In the even more unlikely event of two persons homozygous for the same recessive trait marrying, all their children would be affected. In general, however, both parents and offspring of a person homozygous for a rare recessive gene will be healthy. Characteristically in recessive traits affected individuals cannot be traced from one generation to the next and if more than one member of a family is affected they are usually sibs, i.e. brothers and sisters. The pedigree of an autosomal recessive trait (Fig. 1.5), therefore, differs from that of a dominant trait.

At conception there is a 1 in 4 chance that any child of two heterozygous parents will be affected. Each parent produces gametes of two types, one bearing the normal gene and the other bearing the mutant gene. At conception, therefore, one-quarter of the offspring will be normal, one-half will be healthy heterozygotes and one-quarter will be affected. These are average figures; by chance all the offspring of such a couple might be affected, or similarly all their offspring might be normal. It has been calculated theoretically that in marriages between two heterozygotes, in 75% of families with only one child that child will be unaffected, in 56% of families with two children both children will be unaffected, but in only 32% of families with four children will all four children be unaffected.

When dealing with rare recessive diseases the parents of affected individuals are often found to be related, because such individuals are more likely to have inherited the same mutant gene from an ancestor they have in common. The chance that first cousins will carry the same recessive gene is 1 in 8, but the chance that two unrelated individuals will carry the same recessive gene is very much lower and depends on the frequency of the particular gene in the population. In general the rarer the gene the greater the frequency of consanguinity amongst the parents of affected individuals.

At present roughly 1 in 200 marriages in Britain is between first cousins, so that giving advice on the genetic consequences of cousin marriages is a problem with which geneticists are frequently faced. Several extensive studies have shown that among the offspring of consanguineous matings there is an increased perinatal mortality rate together with an increased frequency of both congenital abnormalities and mental retardation, but the actual risks are small and in fact only slightly greater than in the general population. The situation is quite different, however, if there is a family history of a recessive disorder, when the risks will be greatly increased.

Many conditions show an autosomal recessive mode of inheritance and include, for example, many inborn errors of metabolism, some types of deaf-mutism and some types of congenital blindness. The commonest autosomal recessive trait known in Western Europe is cystic fibrosis which affects one in every 2000 births.

**Sex-linked Inheritance.** Conditions determined by genes situated on either of the sex chromosomes are said to be inherited as sex-linked traits. Genes carried on the X chromosome are said to be X-linked, those on the Y chromosome being Y-linked.

Y-linkage of a gene implies that only males would be affected and that all the sons of an affected male would inherit the gene. With the possible exception of hairy ears, there are no proven examples of Y-linked single gene disorders in man. Thus all known sex-linked conditions are due to genes on the X chromosome. As with autosomal traits these conditions may be either dominant or recessive.

*X-linked dominant conditions* are manifest both in females who are heterozygous for the mutant gene and in males who carry the mutant gene on their single X chromosome. The pedigree of an X-linked dominant trait (Fig. 1.6) can superficially resemble that of an autosomal dominant trait, but there is a fundamental difference. Although an affected female will transmit the trait to half her offspring of either sex, an affected male will transmit the trait to all of his daughters but to none of his sons. There will therefore be an excess of females in families exhibiting such conditions. There are few X-linked dominant disorders but a notable example is one form of vitamin D resistant rickets.

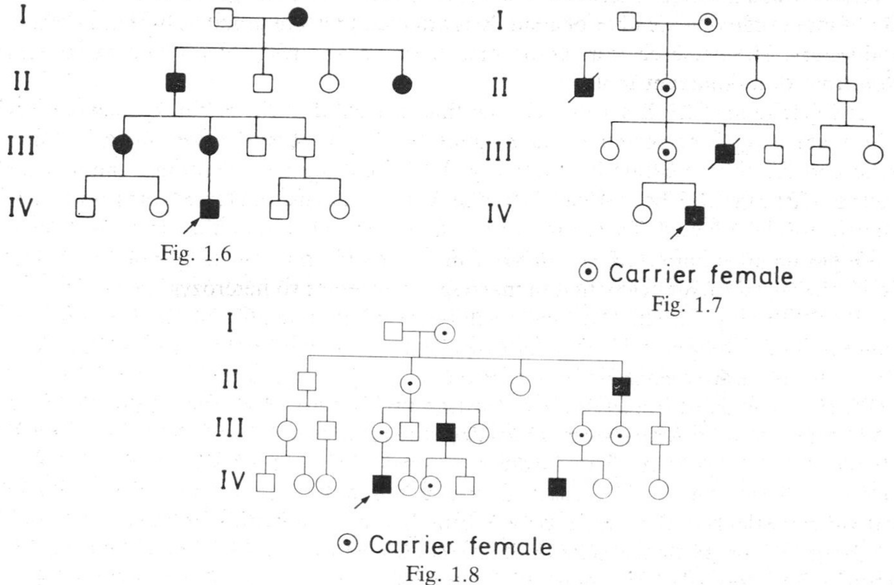


Fig. 1.6 Characteristic pedigree: X-linked dominant trait.
Fig. 1.7 Characteristic pedigree: X-linked recessive trait when affected males do not reproduce (e.g. Duchenne muscular dystrophy).
Fig. 1.8 Characteristic pedigree: X-linked recessive trait when affected males do reproduce (e.g. haemophilia).

An *X-linked recessive condition* is caused by a gene carried on the X chromosome and is manifest in females only when the gene is in the homozygous state. In males, a mutant gene present on the single X chromosome is always manifest because it is unopposed by the modifying effect of a normal gene on the second X chromosome, as happens in females. As with autosomal recessive conditions, the heterozygous carrier is usually healthy. Conditions inherited in this way therefore predominantly affect males and are transmitted by healthy female carriers (Fig. 1.7). In those conditions where affected males may survive to have children, the condition will also be transmitted by affected males (Fig. 1.8).

Haemophilia is the best known example of an X-linked recessive trait. Whereas in the past most boys with this disease died at an early age, with improvements in treatment most now survive. If an affected man marries a normal woman, then all his daughters will be carriers but none of his sons will be affected. An X-linked trait is never transmitted from father to son. This is because a man transmits his only X-chromosome (which if he is affected bears the mutant gene) to each of his daughters but his Y chromosome to each of his sons.

If a woman carrying an X-linked recessive trait marries a normal man, then half of her sons will be affected and half of her daughters will be carriers because each of her children has an equal chance of inheriting from her either the normal X chromosome or the one bearing the mutant gene.

Duchenne muscular dystrophy is inherited as an X-linked recessive trait and because affected boys die young, it is transmitted solely by healthy female carriers.

Very rarely a female may exhibit an X-linked recessive trait. This situation may arise in several different ways. Firstly, she may have an abnormal chromosomal constitution resulting in her only having one X chromosome, such as in Turner's syndrome (XO). Secondly, she may be homozygous for the mutant gene, but this is very unlikely with rare recessive disorders because she would have to have inherited the disorder from both her parents. The third possibility is that she may be a 'manifesting heterozygote'. If, by chance, in the majority of her cells it is the normal X chromosome which is inactivated, then a female heterozygote may exhibit the trait. Careful examination of carriers of Duchenne muscular dystrophy sometimes reveals varying degrees of weakness in the same groups of muscles that are weak in affected boys.

The modes of inheritance for some unifactorial disorders are given in Table 1.2.

Table 1.2 Mode of inheritance of some unifactorial disorders

| Autosomal dominant | Autosomal recessive | X-linked recessive |
|---|---|---|
| Achondroplasia | Albinism | Christmas disease |
| Facioscapulohumeral muscular dystrophy | Ataxia telangiectasia | Duchenne muscular dystrophy |
| Gilbert's syndrome | Congenital adrenal hyperplasia | Glucose-6-phosphate dehydrogenase deficiency |
| Haemoglobinopathies | Congenital goitrous cretinism | Haemophilia |
| Hereditary spherocytosis | Crigler–Najjar syndrome Type I | Hunter's syndrome |
| Huntington's chorea | Cystic fibrosis | Lesch–Nyhan syndrome |
| Hyperlipoproteinaemia Type II | Dubin–Johnson syndrome | Nephrogenic diabetes insipidus |
| Marfan's syndrome | Fançoni's syndrome | |
| Myotonia congenita | Friedreich's ataxia | |
| Myotonic dystrophy | Galactosaemia | |
| Neurofibromatosis | Gaucher's disease | |
| Osteogenesis imperfecta | Glycogen storage diseases | |
| Polycystic disease of kidneys (adult form) | Hepatolenticular degeneration | |
| Polyposis of colon | Hurler's syndrome | |
| Porphyria, acute intermittent | Limb girdle muscular dystrophy (Erb) | |
| Rotor syndrome | Niemann–Pick disease | |
| Tuberous sclerosis | Phenylketonuria | |
| von Willebrand's disease | Pendred's syndrome | |
| | Tay–Sachs disease | |

## Multifactorial Inheritance

Many human characteristics can be measured and if the values are plotted against the number of individuals in the population with each particular value then a bell-shaped or normal frequency distribution curve is found (Fig. 1.9). This applies to such characteristics as intelligence, stature, weight, skin colour and blood pressure. Some of these traits may be largely environmentally determined, such as weight, whereas others are largely genetically determined, such as stature and intelligence. In each case many genes are probably involved. Characteristics which are due to many genes plus the effects of environment are said to be inherited on a multifactorial basis.

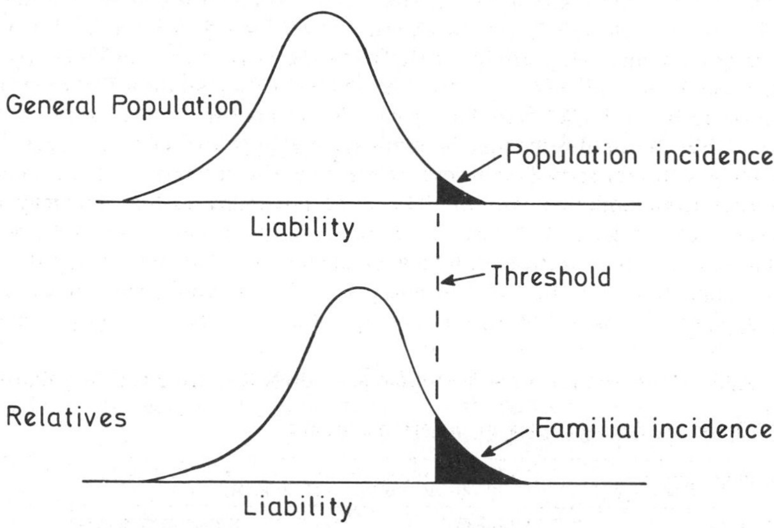


Fig. 1.9 Hypothetical curve of liability in the general population and in relatives for a hereditary disorder in which the genetic predisposition is multifactorial.

It is now believed that many common disorders are inherited in this way. In such conditions it is assumed that there is some underlying graded attribute which is related to causation. This is referred to as the individuals' *liability*, which includes not only their genetic predisposition but also the environmental factors which render them more or less likely to develop the disease. It is assumed that the curve of liability has a normal distribution in the general population. In one simple model (Fig. 1.9), it is believed that there is a *threshold* value such that all affected individuals have a liability above this value and all unaffected individuals have a liability below this value. Relatives of affected individuals have a higher average liability than the population average so the curve of liability for relatives is shifted to the right. In the general population the proportion above the threshold is the population incidence and among relatives the proportion above the threshold is the familial incidence. Such a model can be used to explain the familial incidence of such disorders as essential hypertension, coronary artery disease, peptic ulceration and many of the commoner congenital malformations.

There are several consequences of such a model. Familial incidence will be greater among the relatives of more severely affected individuals because presumably they are more extreme deviants along the curve of liability and the number of abnormal genes segregating in such families is greater than in families in which individuals are less severely affected. Thus in hare lip with or without cleft palate the proportion of affected sibs and children is roughtly 6% when the index patient has double hare lip and cleft palate, but only 2·5% if the index patient has a single hare lip. By similar reasoning it would be expected that the incidence among sibs born subsequent to the index patient would be greater the more affected relatives there were in the family. In spina bifida, for example, the incidence of this condition, or the related disorder anencephaly, in sibs born after one affected child is roughly 5%, but the incidence rises to 10% after the birth of two affected children. This is quite different from the situation in unifactorial disorders where the risk to subsequent sibs remains constant irrespective of the number of affected individuals in the family (e.g. 1 in 4 for an autosomal recessive trait). Finally as a consequence of this model it might be expected that when there is a sex difference in the population incidence, the relatives of the less frequently affected sex would be more often affected. The reason for this is that in the less frequently affected sex, when individuals are affected they are presumably more extreme deviants along the curve of liability and possess more abnormal genes. Thus in congenital pyloric stenosis, which is 5 times commoner in boys than girls, the proportions of affected relatives of male index patients are roughly 5·5% for sons and 2·4% for daughters, but 19·4% for sons and 7·3% for daughters when the index patient is a female.

Though it is not possible to measure liability to a particular disease it is possible to estimate how much of the aetiology can be ascribed to genetic factors as opposed to environmental factors. This is referred to as the *heritability* which is calculated from the known incidences of the disorder in the general population and in relatives. Some estimates of heritability are given in Table 1.3. The values, though approximate, do indicate that genetic factors are of more importance in aetiology in asthma and schizophrenia than in, for example, peptic ulcer.

Table 1.3 Estimates for heritability for various multifactorial disorders

| Disorder | Incidence (%) | Heritability (%) |
|---|---|---|
| Schizophrenia | 1 | 85 |
| Asthma | 4 | 80 |
| Cleft lip ± cleft palate | 0·1 | 76 |
| Pyloric stenosis (congenital) | 0·3 | 75 |
| Ankylosing spondylitis | 0·2 | 70 |
| Club foot (congenital) | 0·1 | 68 |
| Coronary artery disease | 3 | 65 |
| Hypertension (essential) | 5 | 62 |
| Dislocation of hip (congenital) | 0·1 | 60 |
| Anencephaly and spina bifida | 0·5 | 60 |
| Peptic ulcer | 4 | 37 |
| Congenital heart disease (all types) | 0·5 | 35 |

## Prevention of Genetic Disease

Since there is at present no effective treatment for most genetic disorders the role of the medical practitioner lies mainly in the prevention of such conditions through genetic counselling. This involves providing advice on the chances of recurrence of a genetic disorder in the children of either healthy parents who already have an affected child, or when one of the parents or a near relative is affected with a disease which is known to be inherited.

**In chromosomal disorders** if the parents have normal karyotypes, i.e. do not carry a translocation which in the unbalanced state would cause abnormality, then the chances of recurrence are usually low. The most important chromosomal disorder from this point of view is Down's syndrome. The risk of having a child with Down's syndrome is about 1 in 100 in women who have previously had an affected child, and at least 1 in 50 in women over the age of 40. However, the risks are higher if one of the parents carries a chromosome translocation (Table 1.4).

Table 1.4 Recurrence risks of Down's syndrome due to various chromosome aberrations. C = Carrier, N = Normal

| Karyotypes | | | |
|---|---|---|---|
| Patient | Father | Mother | Recurrence risk (%) |
| *Translocation:* | | | |
| 21/13–15 | N | C | 10–15 |
| | C | N | 5 |
| 21/22 | N | C | 10–15 |
| | C | N | 5 |
| 21/21 | N | C | 100 |
| | C | N | 100 |
| *Trisomy 21* | N | N | 1 |
| *Translocation or mosaic* | N | N | 1 |

**In unifactorial disorders** the chances of recurrence are based on Mendelian principles. As we have seen, for example, for a fully penetrant autosomal dominant disorder there is a 1 in 2 chance of recurrence in any child of an affected parent. However, if both parents are healthy an affected child must be the result of a new mutation and the chances of recurrence in subsequent children are negligible. If parents have had a child with an autosomal recessive disorder the chance of recurrence in subsequent children is 1 in 4. Should such a child survive there is very little chance of its having affected children. Finally, with X-linked recessive disorders there is a 1 in 2 chance that any son of a known carrier will be affected and a 1 in 2 chance that any daughter will be a carrier. All the daughters of an affected male will be carriers.

In recent years the most important advance in the prevention of X-linked disorders has been the development of tests for detecting healthy female carriers of such disorders as Duchenne muscular dystrophy and haemophilia. An urgent problem at present is the need for reliable methods of detecting symptomless, preclinical cases of autosomal dominant disorders such as Huntington's chorea, polyposis coli, polycystic kidney disease and myotonic dystrophy in which symptoms often do not develop until the third or fourth decade of life. If such tests should become available it would be possible for individuals likely to become affected, and therefore transmit the disease to their children, to receive advice before they had a family.

**In multifactorial disorders** risks of recurrence cannot be predicted from Mendelian principles but have to be determined by studying the frequency of the condition among the relatives of affected individuals. Examples of risk figures, derived in this way (so-called *empiric* risks), for some relatively common conditions are given in Table 1.5.

## Genetic Advice

The first step in giving genetic advice is to establish a precise diagnosis, secondly to be certain that the disorder in question is genetic and thirdly to verify the presence or absence of the disease in relatives. Without a precise diagnosis it is not possible to give reliable genetic counselling since certain disorders though superficially similar may be inherited differently. For example Hunter's syndrome and Hurler's syndrome both present similar clinical features of 'gargoylism' but whereas clouding of the cornea does not occur in the former condition it is present in the latter. Further,

Table 1.5 Empiric risks (in %) for some common disorders

| Disorder | Incidence | Sex ratio M:F | Normal parents having a second affected child | Affected parent having an affected child | Affected parent having a second affected child |
|---|---|---|---|---|---|
| Anencephaly | 0·20 | 1:2 | 5* | — | — |
| Cleft palate only | 0·04 | 2:3 | 2 | 7 | 15 |
| Cleft lip ± cleft palate | 0·10 | 3:2 | 4 | 4 | 10 |
| Club foot | 0·10 | 2:1 | 3 | 3 | 10 |
| Cong. heart disease (all types) | 0·50 | — | 1–4 | 1–4 | — |
| Dislocation of hip | 0·07 | 1:6 | 4 | 4 | 10 |
| Epilepsy ('idiopathic') | 0·50 | 1:1 | 5 | 5 | 10 |
| Hirschsprung's disease | 0·02 | 4:1 | | | |
| male index | | | 2 | — | — |
| female index | | | 8 | — | — |
| Hypospadias | 0·20 | — | 10 | — | — |
| Manic-depressive psychosis | 0·40 | 2:3 | — | 10–15 | — |
| Mental retardation ('idiopathic') | 0·30–0·50 | 1:1 | 3–5 | — | — |
| Profound childhood deafness | 0·10 | 1:1 | 10 | 8 | — |
| Pyloric stenosis | 0·30 | 5:1 | | | |
| male index | | | 2 | 4 | 13 |
| female index | | | 10 | 17 | 38 |
| Renal agenesis (bilat.) | 0·01 | 3:1 | | | |
| male index | | | 3 | — | — |
| female index | | | 7 | — | — |
| Schizophrenia | 1–2 | 1:1 | — | 16 | — |
| Scoliosis (idiopathic, adolescent) | 0·22 | 1:6 | 7 | 5 | — |
| Spina bifida | 0·30 | 2:3 | 5* | 3* | — |

* Anencephaly or spina bifida

Hunter's syndrome is an X-linked recessive trait and therefore the unaffected sister of an affected boy may be at risk of having affected children. Hurler's syndrome on the other hand is an autosomal recessive disorder and only affects sibs. In this condition there is therefore no chance of an unaffected sister having affected children, provided she does not marry a near relative who might also carry the mutant gene.

It is always advisable to check that the disease in question is in fact genetic and not due to some environmental factor (i.e. a *phenocopy*). For example congenital deafness is often due to a rare recessive gene but it may also result from intrauterine infection with rubella during the first three months of pregnancy which may also cause other abnormalities in the fetus such as congenital heart disease and eye defects. If it can be shown in a particular case that congenital deafness was due to maternal rubella then there would be no chance of recurrence in subsequent children. It is therefore important before giving genetic advice to ask about the possibility of maternal exposure to radiation, drugs or infections during pregnancy and details of any birth trauma which might possibly account for the disorder in question.

Factors which influence the parents' decision whether or not they will accept a risk of having an affected child include the severity of the abnormality, whether or not there is an effective treatment, the actual risk, their religious attitude and possibly their socioeconomic status. In general, however, parents usually accept the risk of having an affected child if this is less than one in 20 but do not accept a risk of greater than one in 10 if the disease is serious.

**Antenatal Diagnosis.** Family limitation is not the only course of action open to parents who are found to be at high risk of having a child with a serious genetic disorder. Other possibilities include artificial insemination by donor (if the father is affected with a dominant disorder, or if both parents are heterozygous for a rare recessive gene) and antenatal diagnosis with selective abortion of affected fetuses. This is possible by studying cells present in amniotic fluid or the amniotic fluid itself. About 5 to 10 ml of fluid is removed by transabdominal amniocentesis around the 16th week of gestation. The specimen is centrifuged and the uncultured cells (which are derived largely from the fetal skin) may be studied to determine the sex of the fetus by fluorescent (F-body) and sex-chromatin studies, though it is advisable to confirm the sex of the fetus by also culturing the cells for full karyotype analysis. This is valuable in X-linked disorders which cannot yet be diagnosed *in utero* (e.g. Duchenne muscular dystrophy). In this way a known carrier mother can be guaranteed a daughter who will not be affected (though she might be a carrier), for if the fetus is a male the parents may decide on termination since there is a one in two chance the fetus could be affected. Amniotic fluid cells can also be cultured and from the study of this material it is possible not only to sex the fetus but also to diagnose cytogenetic abnormalities and certain inborn errors of metabolism in the fetus. At present the main application of such studies is in the antenatal diagnosis of Down's syndrome and many centres now offer amniocentesis to all pregnant women over the age of 40 because of their increased risk of having a child with this disorder. Finally anencephaly and open spina bifida are associated with raised levels of alpha-fetoprotein in amniotic fluid and these disorders may therefore also be diagnosed *in utero*.

**Conclusion.** The main contribution which genetics can make to medicine is in understanding more about the aetiology of certain disorders and in preventing such disorders through genetic counselling. But it is not sufficient merely to quote risk figures. As far as possible the nature and cause of the disease should be explained to parents and any feelings of guilt should be removed. Since genetic counselling may have profound long-term effects on a family such advice must never be given without careful appraisal of all the factors involved if the needs of the individual are to be met. Genetic counselling, like many other aspects of medicine, is as much an art as a science.

## Prospects in Genetics

With regard to the future, the most exciting developments in medical genetics are likely to be in molecular biology, by helping us to understand more about the molecular basis of human disease, and in prevention through advances in antenatal diagnosis. We are also likely to see the development of presymptomatic treatments for those who are healthy but would otherwise develop a genetic disorder. In the case of congenital defects it may one day be possible to treat the affected fetus before birth.

A. E. H. Emery

*Further reading:*

Emery, A. E. H. (1973) *Antenatal Diagnosis of Genetic Disease*, Edinburgh: Churchill Livingstone.
Emery, A. E. H. (1979) *Elements of Medical Genetics*, 5th edn. Edinburgh: Churchill Livingstone.
Emery, A. E. H. (1976) *Methodology in Medical Genetics*. Edinburgh: Churchill Livingstone.

# 2. Immunological Factors in Disease

The science of immunology arose from the study of man's resistance to infection. The most striking feature of this resistance is the specific nature of its enhancement in individuals following infection. Thus, antigenic stimulation and antibody production began to be elucidated in the context of infectious disease and immunity to it. Terms such as 'immunology', 'immunisation' and 'specific immune response' are derived from these origins.

It soon appeared that such specific 'immune' responses might also confer unpleasant and sometimes dangerous hypersensitivity to subsequent exposure to the provoking antigen. Resistance to infection is not an essential feature of the immune response; for example, bacteria may induce antibodies which have no obvious protective value and immune reponses are often evoked by injection of intrinsically harmless non-living organic substances, such as serum protein from another individual or species. After exposure to antigen the individual develops a changed reactivity or *allergy*, a term which originally included immunity and hypersensitivity but which is now restricted to the latter. The ability to develop specific immunity to infection is only one consequence of a wider capacity in the individual to recognise and to respond specifically to the foreignness of a wide range of biological substances that are not normally present. Immunology is the study of what this 'changed reactivity' is in terms of cellular biochemistry, how it is brought about, and how it is regulated both quantitively and qualitatively. In the present chapter an account of current concepts of the physiology of the immune system is given in order that the clinical application of immunology may be understood in such diverse conditions as infection, asthma, drug reactions and certain endocrine, gastrointestinal, haematological, connective tissue and neurological disorders.

## The Immune System

### The Lymphocytes

The antigenicity of a substance (i.e. its ability to induce an immune response) is determined by one or more specific molecular groups on its structure known as *antigenic determinants*. When immunocompetent lymphocytes recognise a foreign substance (antigen) they respond by transforming into lymphoblasts and then into antibody-producing plasma cells or lymphocytes as indicated in Figure 2.1.

If antigenic material (either part of self or a foreign substance) comes into contact with the cells of the antibody-forming system at the stage before the cells have reached maturity, e.g. in fetal life, the result is a failure of response rather than stimulation of antibody formation or other form of immune reaction against the antigen concerned. This is referred to as *immune tolerance* to the antigen. Probably for this reason an individual does not normally show a significant immune response against components of his own tissues. In the abnormal situation where an immune reaction does occur, the reaction is referred to as *autoimmune*.

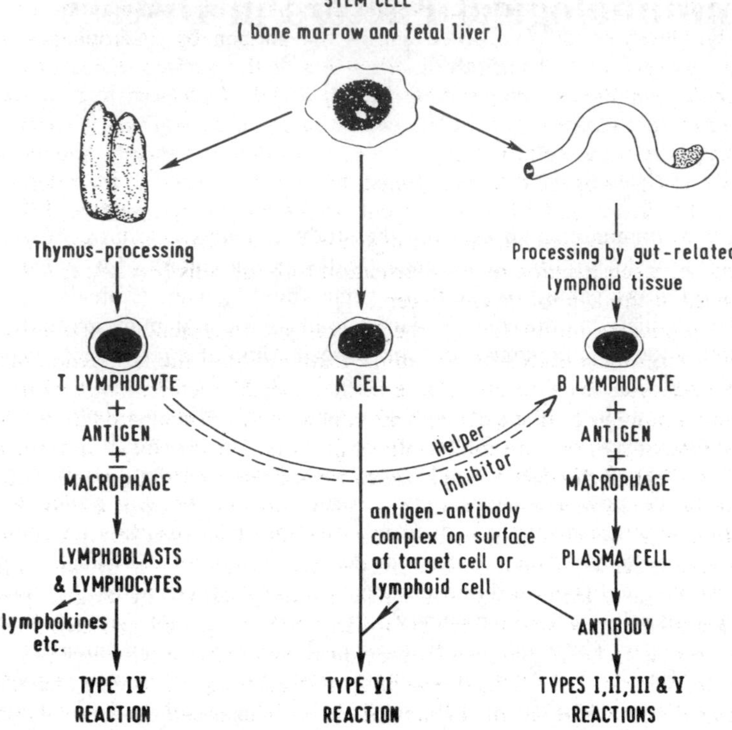


Fig. 2.1 Role of T lymphocytes, B lymphocytes and K cells in immunological responses. Many of these events involve active cell proliferation, but for simplicity this has not been shown.

Immune reactions are mediated by *humoral* or *cellular mechanisms*. Included among the humoral factors is antibody (immunoglobulin) secreted by plasma cells. The cellular component is made up of lymphocytes sensitised to specific antigens and reactive with those antigens without the presence of free antibody. Stem-cells originating in the bone marrow differentiate to form two main lymphocyte populations known as T and B lymphocytes or cells. *T lymphocytes* are dependent upon a hormone or factor produced by the epithelial cells of the thymus for becoming immunologically competent from non-competent predecessors originating in the bone marrow. T lymphocytes cause cell-mediated hypersensitivity (p. 33).

*B lymphocytes* are independent of the thymus but are dependent on the bursa of Fabricius in birds; its equivalents in man are probably the tonsils and the lymphoid tissue of the gut. B lymphocytes are responsible for the synthesis of humoral antibody.

The recognition of antigen by B lymphocytes is believed to be mediated by antibody synthesised in the cell and bound into the surface membrane, the specificity of the antibody being determined by the genetic characteristics (programming) of the individual lymphocyte. T lymphocytes, on the other hand, do not have detectable antibody on their surface but have antibody-like receptors for antigens, the exact nature of which is not clear. In both instances combination with the appropriate antigen then triggers off the immunological response.

The *induction of mitosis* in T lymphocytes and their transformation to larger 'blast' cells may be effected both by specific antigens and by non-specific mitogens which include agents such as phytohaemagglutinin. It is likely that stimulation of mitosis in some T lymphocytes involves processing of the antigen by macrophages, possibly leading to presentation of antigen determinants at the surface of the macrophage. For example, lymphocyte preparations largely freed of phagocytic cells are unresponsive to certain antigens but activity can be restored by addition of macrophages. Lymphocytes in tissue-culture can be seen to wander incessantly and presumably identify the antigens of the cells over which they move in terms of their degree of 'fit' with the antibody or antibody-like receptor on the lymphocyte surface. Likewise, in the body the lymphocytes migrate through the tissues (*immunological surveillance*) permitting their sensitisation or transformation to blast cells by contact with antigen with or without the help of macrophages.

The T lymphocyte sensitised to a specific antigen undergoes blast transformation and proliferation on contact with the antigen. In addition, the interaction of antigen with T lymphocytes leads to the release of non specific factors, *lymphokines*, which bring about a number of tissue changes associated with cell-mediated hypersensitivity reactions. One of these factors inhibits the migration of macrophages in tissue culture. *In vivo* the effect of this factor would be to immobilise randomly wandering macrophages at the site of reaction with antigen, where they might exert a cytotoxic action or merely act as scavengers of cells already damaged by lymphocytes. Other lymphokines can increase vascular permeability or cause inhibition of growth or death of tissue cells. Transfer factor is a dialysable substance produced by normal lympocytes and can apparently pass the 'information' necessary for specific cell-mediated hypersensitivity reponses to be mounted by previously unsensitised lymphocytes. Another lymphokine, interferon (p. 79), blocks the reproduction of viruses. The release of lymphokines is an example of an amplification mechanism, like the complement system, that augments the specific response initiated by relatively few cells. In addition to lymphokines, specific macrophage arming factor is released which renders macrophages cytostatic to cells bearing that particular antigen.

How B lymphocytes are stimulated to become the antibody-forming cells of the plasma cell line is not yet fully understood. A possible sequence of events is shown diagrammatically in Figure 2.2. Certain antigens are apparently capable of reacting directly with the corresponding antibody on the surface of a B lymphocyte to induce it to transform and proliferate into active antibody-producing plasma cells. Such antigens generally have many antigenic determinants of the same specificity so that they can simultaneously trigger a number of receptors on the surface of the same B lymphocyte. Other antigens, or small doses of antigen, may have to be taken on to the surface of a macrophage, as mentioned in relation to T lymphocytes, thus being more readily available for stimulating a B lymphocyte either directly or through the co-operation of a helper T lymphocyte. In this way a high local concentration of antigen is achieved during cell to cell contact with the B lymphocyte, thereby stimulating a greater number of receptor sites in a given cell than if the antigen were uniformly dispersed throughout the body fluids. Once stimulated, the cell undergoes division and produces the antibody that it is genetically programmed to do.

There is evidence for negative in addition to positive control of immunological mechanisms as indicated in Figure 2.2. A sub-population of T lymphocytes (*suppressor T cells*) exists which can exert an inhibitory effect on the synthesis of antibody by B cells. Relaxation of this control may play an important role in the development of autoimmunity.

T and B lymphocytes differ in their distribution and probably in their life span. T lymphocytes constitute a greater part of the pool of small lymphocytes that circulate in the blood, interstitial spaces and lymph and most of them have a relatively long

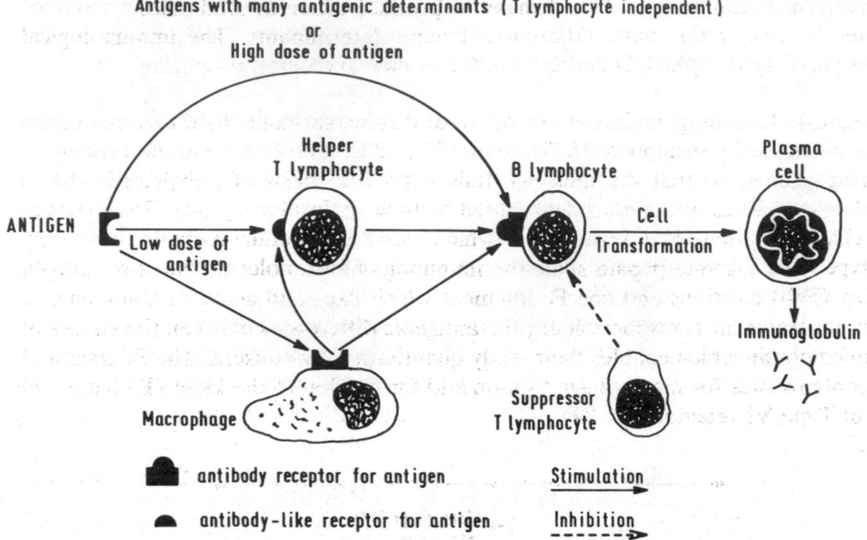


Fig. 2.2 Possible sequence of events in humoral antibody formation, illustrating co-operation between T lymphocytes, B lymphocytes and macrophages and the role of suppressor T lymphocytes.

life (months or years in man) while the B lymphocytes are more restricted to lymphoid tissue and most of them appear to be short-lived (several weeks). There is evidence for the existence of sub-classes, presumably with differing functions, within these main classes; e.g. short-lived T lymphocytes and long-lived B lymphocytes. Thus *immunological memory* is achieved by the existence of long-lived T and B cells.

Certain lymphoid cells and monocytes, although not themselves specifically sensitised, can gain specificity in the presence of antibody or antigen-antibody complexes on the surface of the target cells or on their own surface. This is known as antibody-dependent cell-mediated cytotoxicity (p. 34). The lymphoid cells involved are referred to as *killer* or *K cells*. Natural killer cells are mononuclear cells that rapidly lyse certain tumour cell lines *in vivo* and *in vitro*, without prior sensitisation to the target.

The lymphocyte population is therefore a heterogeneous group of morphologically similar cells. About 70% of lymphocytes in the peripheral blood are T cells, some of which are cytotoxic and others either helper or suppressor cells. About 20% are B cells producing immunoglobulin. The remaining 10% comprise K cells and 'null cells' whose function has not yet been clearly defined.

## Immunoglobulin

It is considered that the population of antibody-producing cells arises by random mutation and that a single cell will then react to produce a family of cells (*clone*) with a specific function. Essential to this concept is that random mutation of lymphocytes allows the genesis of cells that are capable of responding to all antigens, although a single cell can react to only one antigen. Antibody production is a special example of protein synthesis, i.e. the putting together of amino acids to form protein molecules, in this instance, immunoglobulins, and the replication of this process according to a pattern. It can be varied on demand to produce different antibodies capable of reacting to any of the many different antigenic determinants. The immunological classes (IgG, IgM, IgA, IgD and IgE) differ in their biological properties.

**Structure**. Immunoglobulins are made up of distinct sub-units held together in the whole molecule by disulphide (S–S) bonds (Fig. 2.3). The bonds can be broken by reducing agents, so that the molecule falls apart into pairs of polypeptide chains called light and heavy chains as determined by their molecular weights. Two types of light chain exist, kappa and lambda, of which individual immunoglobulins have only one type. The enzyme papain splits the immunoglobulin molecule into two antigen binding (Fab) fractions and one Fc fragment which fixes and activates complement. The latter fragment is responsible for the antigenic differences between the classes of immunoglobulin which enables their ready quantitation by antisera. The Fc fragment also contains sites for macrophage fixation and for fixation to the killer (K) lymphoid cells of Type VI reactions (p. 34).

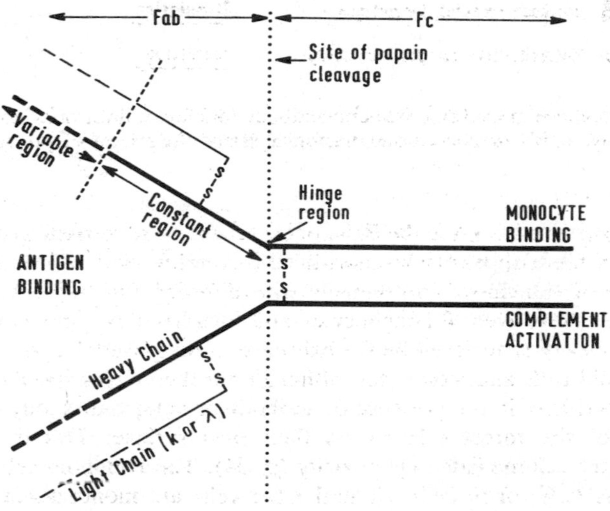


Fig. 2.3 Structure of immunoglobulin IgG. Disulphide bond cleavage produces two light chains and two heavy chains. Papain cleavage produces two Fab portions and one Fc portion. The amino acids that vary in sequence for different antibodies are shown as interrupted ends of the light and heavy chains.

**Classification and Functions.** *IgG*. In healthy adults, the total IgG accounts for 73% of the immunoglobulins in normal serum and is distributed equally between the blood and interstitial fluids, about a quarter passing across the capillary walls each day and the same amount returning via the thoracic duct. In man, IgG is the only immunoglobulin that is transported across the placenta to reach the fetal circulation and provide the baby with passive immunisation during its early life. IgG antibody is particularly suited to neutralising soluble toxin such as that of *C. diphtheriae*.

*IgM*. The macro-molecular IgM is predominantly intravascular. It constitutes only 7% of the serum immunoglobulins and is made up of five immunoglobulin units linked with disulphide bonds to provide ten identical combining-sites instead of the two of IgG. IgM is especially effective in activating complement to produce immune lysis of foreign cells by digesting holes in the cell membranes at the sites where antibody has reacted. IgM antibodies are much more efficient than IgG antibodies in linking particulate antigens together for agglutination and phagocytosis and would seem to be specially adapted for dealing with cell debris or bacteria in the bloodstream.

*IgA* accounts for 19% of the total serum immunoglobulins and is preferentially secreted into colostrum, saliva, intestinal juice and respiratory secretions. The major sites of IgA synthesis are the laminae propriae underlying the mucous membranes throughout the respiratory tract and the gut. The monomer produced locally by plasma cells is taken up as a dimer by the epithelial cells of the gut, and a secretory piece is added which protects the immunoglobulin from digestive enzymes. Secretory IgA is available right through to the colon and these antibodies are vital in the defence of the gut against enteroviruses, e.g. poliomyelitis. In general, IgA plays a major role as part of an antiseptic secretion over the mucous surfaces of the body.

*IgD* have some of the properties of the IgG globulins, although little is known of their exact role.

*IgE* have a very low serum level and a distinctive affinity for cell surfaces. They are an integral part of immediate hypersensitivity reactions such as occur in hay fever (p. 265). The physiological function of IgE antibodies is obscure but they may possibly have a role in the defence against helminths.

## Complement System

Complement belongs to the group of plasma systems termed 'triggered enzyme cascades', which also include the coagulation, fibrinolytic and kinin generating systems. They are all effector mechanisms which can produce a rapid and amplified response to a trigger stimulus. They are complex both in their reaction pathways and in the homeostatic mechanisms which have been evolved to control them. The complement system is activated characteristically by antigen-antibody interactions; the

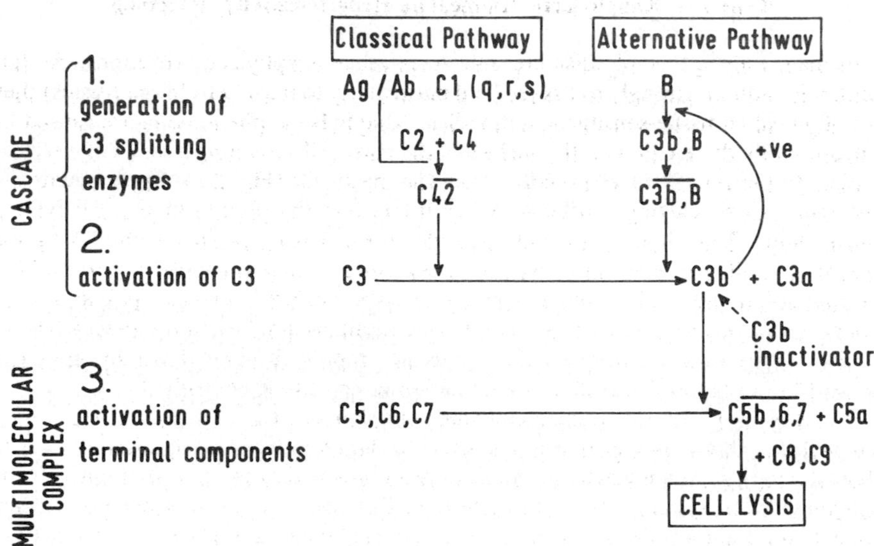


Fig. 2.4 The complement system. The bar over a component represents an activated state, usually enzymatic, generated during the complement sequence. B represents a factor of unknown nature which activates the alternative pathway.

sequence of events involved consists of three stages (Fig. 2.4): 1. The generation of C3 splitting enzymes by the classical and by the alternative pathways.

2. The activation of C3, which is the central event of the complement sequence and its bulk reaction, analogous to the conversion of fibrinogen to fibrin in blood coagulation. The fixation of C3 at complement fixation sites (e.g. the Fc component of IgG after reaction with antigen) is probably the system's most important activity. Bound C3 reacts with various receptors on phagocytic cells, platelets, erythrocytes and certain lymphocytes and retention of cells at complement fixation sites contributes largely to the activity of the complement system in inflammation. The generation of C3b leads to the activation of a self-amplifying positive feedback cycle which is damped by the action of the C3b inactivator (Fig. 2.4).

3. The activation of the terminal components is initiated by the activation of C5 and is the last enzymic reaction in the complement sequence. Thereafter the remaining components (C6–C9) combine to form a multimolecular complex which mediates the most characteristic *in vitro* event of the complement system: the generation of membrane lesions leading to cell lysis.

## Types of Immune Reaction and their Relation to Human Disease

There are six types of immune reaction (Fig. 2.5).

Type I — anaphylactic (immediate hypersensitivity)
Type II — cytotoxic
Type III — immune complex
Type IV — T cell-mediated (delayed hypersensitivity)
Type V — stimulating antibody
Type VI — antibody-dependent cell-mediated cytotoxicity (ADCC).

### Type I — Anaphylactic (Immediate Hypersensitivity) Reactions

In man, only IgE antibodies are able to produce anaphylactic reactions. As IgE antibodies adhere strongly to tissues (and particularly to mast-cells in the tissues) they are often called tissue-sensitising antibodies. Anaphylactic phenomena are caused by antigen-antibody reaction on the surface of the mast cell activating a series of enzymes leading to the release of vasodilators from the mast cells (Fig. 2.5). These agents are histamine, slow reacting substance-A, serotonin and the plasma kinins, bradykinin and kallidin. The kinins are simple peptides formed from plasma globulins by the enzymes, kallikrein, plasmin or trypsin. They cause increased capillary permeability, vasodilatation and a fall in blood pressure. Another effect is to cause polymorphonuclear leucocytes to migrate from blood vessels and accumulate in the tissues (chemotaxis). Once they are formed the kinins are rapidly broken down by kininases present in the blood. Thus their accumulation at any site is controlled.

Previous usage of the term anaphylaxis emphasised the clinically severe form, anaphylactic shock, but current usage refers to the underlying mechanism and not to clinical severity. Anaphylactic reactions depend on whether the portal of entry of the antigen is local, systemic or via the intestine. Relatively mild symptoms occur when antigen-antibody reactions take place on an exposed mucosal surface. These reactions occur most commonly to pollens or animal dander and the symptoms may be limited to rhinorrhoea and conjunctivitis. However, intense bronchospasm may be produced as a result of inhalation of the antigen. Patients with asthma induced by contact with

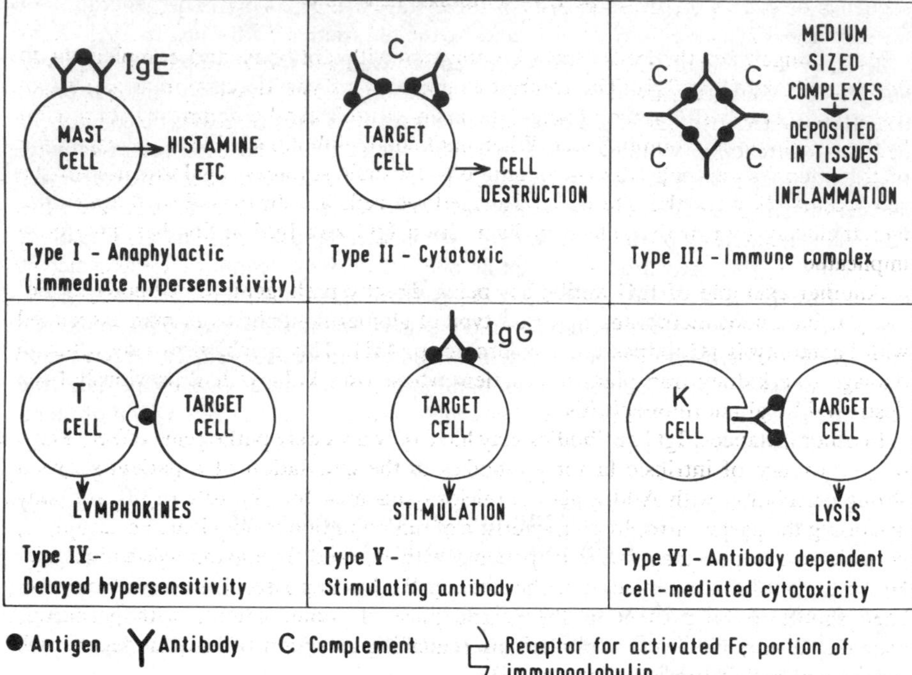


Fig. 2.5 Immune reactions which may be harmful to the tissues.

antigens in this manner have levels of IgE immunoglobulin that may be much higher than those found in patients with asthma that is not induced in this way.

*Systemic anaphylaxis* consists of a group of much more severe reactions which may occur rapidly if the antigen is injected parenterally, as in the case of a drug such as penicillin, foreign sera, or the sting of an insect. The features are bronchospasm, laryngeal oedema resulting in extreme dyspnoea and cyanosis and a marked fall in blood pressure (anaphylactic shock). There may also be nausea, vomiting and diarrhoea. Systemic anaphylaxis is a potentially fatal condition if not treated promptly with adrenaline, hydrocortisone and an antihistamine.

*Urticaria*, the formation of weal and flare lesions in the skin, is an anaphylactic phenomenon which can develop as a result of absorption of antigen through the intestinal tract. Common allergens are present in strawberries, nuts, egg and shellfish. Urticaria often occurs alone, but may be associated with other signs of anaphylaxis. Not all urticaria is caused by an immune reaction; the pharmacological agents which cause urticaria can be released by other means, especially physical agents such as trauma or cold.

**Diagnostic Methods.** Intradermal testing in sensitised individuals is the most convenient *in vivo* method for the detection of specific IgE antibodies. A simple, rapid, radioallergosorbent test is available for the *in vitro* detection and quantitation of antigen specific IgE.

## Type II — Cytotoxic Reactions

Here antigen on the cell's surface combines with antibody and complement to destroy the cell (Fig. 2.5). The clearest example of a Type II reaction as a cause of disease occurs in autoimmune haemolytic anaemia; this can be demonstrated *in vitro* by the antiglobulin (Coombs') test. When antihuman globulin is added to a suspension of the patient's red cells that have antibody on their surfaces, agglutination of the cells occurs. *In vivo*, the altered or damaged red cells are destroyed by the reticulo-endothelial system in the spleen or liver. Both IgG and IgM antibodies have been implicated.

Another example of IgG antibodies being directly pathogenic is antibody to glomerular basement membrane in a rare type of glomerulonephritis in man associated with haemoptysis (Goodpasture's syndrome, p. 431). This mechanism may result in damage to a kidney transplant in a patient whose own kidneys had previously been destroyed by glomerulonephritis.

In other instances, IgG antibodies may have only a weakly pathogenic effect. Thus, the occurrence of intrinsic factor antibodies in the circulation of a patient shows a strong correlation with Addisonian pernicious anaemia, but the role of the antibody in causing the gastric atrophy characteristic of this condition is not clear. For example, pernicious anaemia may occur in patients with marked hypogammaglobulinaemia. However, antibody reactive with the vitamin $B_{12}$ binding site of intrinsic factor has been shown to be present in the gastric juice of some patients with pernicious anaemia: it may block the action of any remaining secretion of intrinsic factor with consequent malabsorption of vitamin $B_{12}$.

There are circumstances in which IgG antibodies may be pathogenic only when combined with cell-mediated hypersensitivity or other forms of tissue damage. Thus complement-fixing IgG antibodies to thyroid secretory epithelium are a frequent occurrence in autoimmune thyroid disease but they seem to have little or no pathogenic role by themselves. These antibodies can be transmitted across the placenta with no evidence of damage to the fetal thyroid. Although at least one of these antibodies can bring about rapid destruction of trypsinised human thyroid cells *in vitro* in the presence of complement, *in vivo* it seems to have difficulty in reaching the intracellular antigens in the absence of some other damaging agent.

Finally, in other situations, antibodies detectable in the serum and often useful diagnostically, seem to have no discernible pathogenic role when acting on their own. For example, antibody to thyroglobulin is harmless to thyroid cells in tissue culture and infusion into animals produces at most a weak granulomatous reaction in the thyroid. However, antibody to thyroglobulin may play an important role in pathogenesis when part of a type VI reaction (p. 34). A second example is the mitochondrial antibodies with no tissue specificity which occur most commonly in patients with primary biliary cirrhosis.

**Diagnostic methods.** *The indirect immunofluorescence technique* is used to detect autoantibodies to nuclei, to the cytoplasm of thyroid, gastric parietal, adrenal cortical, steroid-producing ovarian and pancreatic islet cells and to glomerular basement membrane. Cryostat sections of the appropriate tissue are incubated with serum and, after thorough washing, with fluorescein labelled antihuman Ig serum. They are then examined by fluorescence microscopy.

*Complement Fixation Tests*. Certain antigen-antibody reactions fix complement and the occurrence of such a reaction *in vitro* can be detected by determining whether complement, which had been added in a critical amount, is still present in the free form. An indicator system is used consisting of sheep red cells coated with horse or rabbit antibodies against the red cells. If complement has been fixed before the addition of the indicator system, it is no longer available to permit lysis of the sheep red cells. This technique forms the basis of the Wassermann reaction for syphilis; it is also used in the demonstration of antibodies against certain viruses and also for thyroid and gastric autoantibodies in serum.

*Precipitation testing* may be used, for example, in the detection of antibodies to thyroglobulin in the differential diagnosis of thyroid disorders.

*Tanned Red Cell or Latex Particle Agglutination*. Sheep red cells are treated with tannic acid so that they can be coated with antigens (e.g. thyroglobulin). In the presence of the corresponding antibody the cells undergo agglutination. This provides a very sensitive and semi-quantitative method for the detection of certain serum antibodies, e.g. to thyroglobulin. Latex particles coated with human γ-globulin are used to detect the presence of the rheumatoid factor in patients' serum (p. 609).

## Type III — Immune Complex Reactions

Immune complex reactions are induced by deposition of antigen and antibody in the tissues, causing the activation of complement; this results in a polymorphonuclear inflammatory response and also damage to the cell membranes of adjacent tissues (Fig. 2.6). Hydrolytic enzymes released from the granules of the leucocytes also contribute to the vascular damage which is the hallmark of this type of immune reaction.

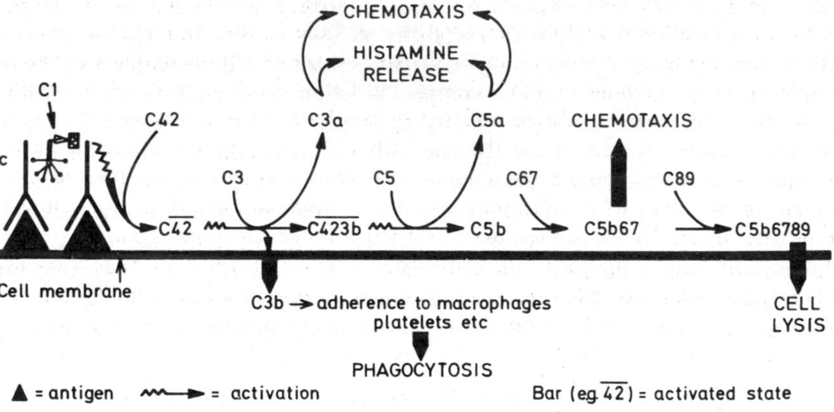


Fig. 2.6 The role of components of the complement system in the production of inflammation. Amplification of the immune response is achieved by the action of the complement system as an enzyme cascade. Thus one C1 complex generates many C42 complexes which in turn activate many molecules of C3b and so on to cell lysis. When the antigen is not part of an intact cell wall the biological effects are the same apart from cell lysis.

The immune complex reaction can be induced in man by the intradermal injection of antigens if there is a high level of circulating IgG antibodies, for example in pulmonary aspergillosis (p. 275) and 'farmer's lung' (p. 275). Red and oedematous changes reaching maximum intensity between 4–12 hours appear at the site of injection of the antigen. This is known as the *Arthus reaction*.

The systemic syndrome known as *chronic serum sickness* is based on an immune complex reaction and can be produced by a wide range of different antigens, such as antitetanus serum and especially drugs such as penicillin and streptomycin. It consists of rashes, fever, joint pains and often swelling of the regional lymph nodes. The duration of symptoms varies greatly. The illness is seldom serious, though it may give rise to much discomfort.

*Glomerulonephritis* can also be caused by an immune complex reaction. Thus, in the clinical entity of glomerulonephritis, there are at least two immune pathogenic mechanisms and, in all probability, numerous aetiological factors capable of initiating each. As described on page 31, in the rare glomerulonephritis produced by a Type II immune reaction, antibodies react with glomerular basement membrane. In glomerulonephritis produced by an immune complex reaction the specificity of the antibodies is irrelevant; what is important is that antigen-antibody complexes of appropriate size are present in the circulation and are deposited in the glomerular capillary walls.

The only property of antigen-antibody complexes presently known to affect the localisation in vessels is size and this depends on the ratio of antigen and antibody in the complexes. Small complexes in great antigen excess tend to remain in the circulation whereas frank precipitates formed at equivalence or at antibody excess are rapidly taken up and disposed of by phagocytes. The intermediate-sized complexes formed in moderate antigen excess are still soluble but large enough to react with complement and are the most likely to be deposited in vessel walls and so induce inflammation. The vessel walls of the renal glomeruli are particularly vulnerable. Morphologically the trapped antigen-antibody complexes appear under the electron microscope as heaped-up lesions on the glomerular basement membrane (p. 431).

Immune complex reactions may or may not be related to autoimmunity. The antigen involved may be foreign to the body or it may be autogenous. Thus, post-streptococcal proliferative glomerulonephritis, at least as seen in children, is caused by the deposition of circulating non-glomerular antigen-antibody complexes. The best example of an autogenous immune complex reaction causing glomerulonephritis in man is that occurring in systemic lupus erythematosus. It is associated with the formation of antinuclear antibodies (particularly to DNA) and the deposition of these antibodies, nuclear antigens and complement in the renal glomerulus (p. 629).

*Other conditions* in which lesions occur due to immune complexes include rheumatoid arthritis (p. 605), polyarteritis, viral hepatitis, the renal manifestations of infective endocarditis, the nephrotic syndrome in children with *P. malariae* infections and lepromatous leprosy. Immune complex reactions thus occur in response to diverse antigens related particularly to micro-organisms, drugs and autogenous sources.

### Type IV — Cell-mediated (Delayed) Hypersensitivity Reactions

Type IV reactions are those mediated by T lymphocytes and in which free antibody plays no part (Fig. 2.5). Antigen stimulates the T cell to produce lymphokines (p. 25). Type IV reactions are characteristically induced by infectious agents which are predominantly intracellular in the infected host, e.g. many viral infections and some bacterial infections such as tuberculosis, brucellosis, pertussis, and syphilis. The classical example of this reaction is the tuberculin test (p. 254). Homograft rejection is believed to be predominantly produced by cell-mediated hypersensitivity.

Type IV reactions can also occur by skin contact with a variety of substances notably drugs, including penicillin. These substances are not themselves antigenic but become antigenic by co-valent binding to proteins in the skin. The hypersensitivity of the skin is generalised and may be detected by the application of a small patch test containing the substance anywhere on the body.

*Autoimmune Disease*. Evidence suggesting the importance of cell-mediated hypersensitivity as a main factor in autoimmune disease can be summarised as follows: 1. The histology of the affected organs shows lymphocytic infiltration and atrophy, e.g. in Hashimoto thyroiditis, atrophic gastritis of Addisonian pernicious anaemia and idiopathic (autoimmune) adrenal failure. 2. Similar histological changes can be produced in animals by sterile methods that cause cell-mediated hypersensitivity. 3. When such diseases have been induced immunologically in experimental animals they can be transferred to normal animals by means of lymphocytes alone. 4. Positive *in vitro* tests supposedly for cell-mediated hypersensitivity have been obtained with the lymphocytes from the peripheral blood of patients or of experimental animals with certain autoimmune diseases. These tests include the leucocyte migration inhibition test, transformation and cytotoxicity tests.

### Type V — Stimulating Antibody Reaction

Certain IgG antibodies have the ability to stimulate their target cells rather than to inhibit or kill them (Fig. 2.5). Human specific TSH receptor antibodies are the likely cause of thyrotoxicosis when there is diffuse involvement of the thyroid (Graves's disease p. 467). The transfer across the placenta of these thyroid stimulating antibodies is the most probable explanation for neonatal hyperthyroidism.

### Type VI — Antibody Dependent Cell-Mediated Cytotoxicity (ADCC)

K cells may be defined as belonging to a subpopulation of lymphoid cells or monocytes which *in vitro* are able to lyse target cells coated with antibody. The cytotoxic reaction is complement-independent and is initiated through contact of the K cell with the Fc portion of the antibody molecule complexed with antigen on the surface of the target cells (Fig. 2.5). K cells may also be 'armed' through the Fc receptor with antigen-antibody complex which, if present in antibody excess, will be cytotoxic to target cells coated with that specific antigen. Should immune complexes be produced in the presence of excess antigen, there would be no free combining sites left on the antibody moiety to react with antigen on target surfaces so that this type of K cell would be ineffective (blocked). K cell mediated cytotoxic mechanisms may be important in the pathogenesis of autoimmune disease and in tumour rejection. K cells are also involved in the defence against helminthic infections such as schistosomiasis where the size of the parasite is too large for effective phagocytosis.

### Autoimmune Disease

Immune mechanisms may simply be part of a chain of events that leads to the final end product, the clinical manifestation of disease. Thus a viral infection may initiate tissue damage or combine with a cell constituent to act as a hapten and thereby engender an autoimmune response in a susceptible individual. This may occur for example in insulin-dependent diabetes. The interactions of immune mechanisms in the production of autoimmune disease are shown in Figure 2.7.

**Aetiology.** *Defect in immunological tolerance*. Normally a person or animal does not mount a significant immune response against its own body constituents because intricate controlling and suppressor mechanisms exist to prevent this happening. For example, it has been suggested that clones of immunocompetent cells capable of

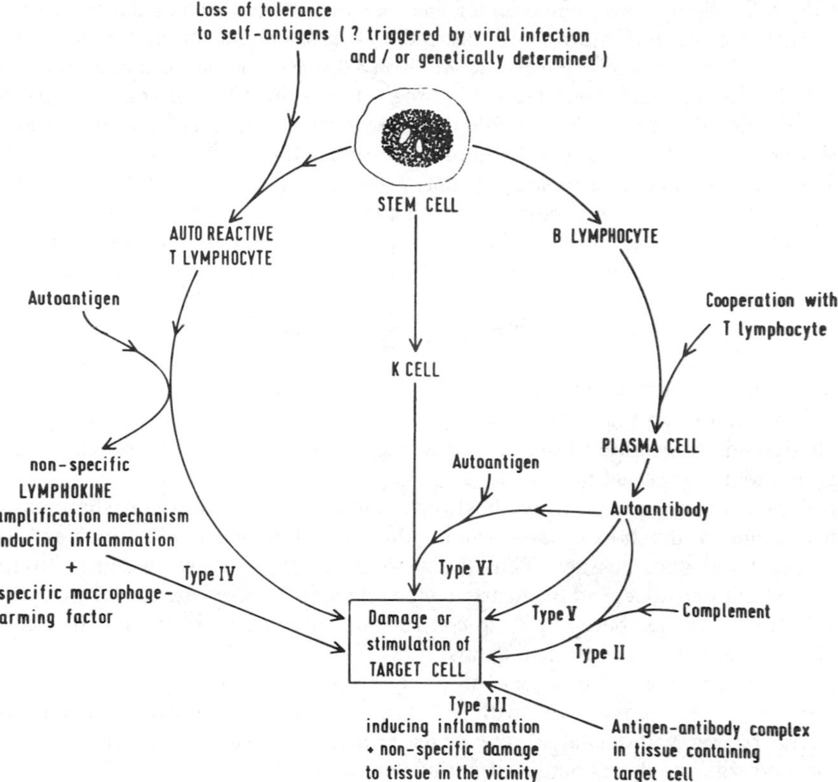


Fig. 2.7 Diagram representing the interactions of immune mechanisms types II–VI in the production of autoimmune disease. The different mechanisms may have greater importance in some diseases than in others. Thus type II reactions are predominant in autoimmune haemolytic anaemia, while types II, IV and VI are predominant in Hashimoto's thyroiditis, and type V in thyrotoxicosis.

reacting with self-antigens are either eliminated or rendered unresponsive by early and continued exposure to antigen (p. 23). Unresponsiveness may exist either at the level of the helper T lymphocyte or at the level of the antibody-producing B lymphocyte or at both. If unresponsiveness exists only at the level of the helper T cell, autoantibody synthesis will occur when the requirement for T cell help is bypassed. As discussed on page 25 it has also been suggested that a subpopulation of T lymphocytes can suppress the synthesis of antibody by B cells. The dose of antigen presented to the immune system is also relevant to the breakdown of control (tolerance). In spite of these intricate control mechanisms, however, man can and does synthesise antibodies against body components and these are frequently associated with disease (clinical or subclinical) mediated by one or more of the mechanisms illustrated in Figure 2.7.

A defect in immunological tolerance may either occur spontaneously or be induced by some exogenous factor. It could be argued that the intricate and precise system whereby foreign substances are normally distinguished from the body's own constituents must be liable to breakdown so that errors are made as to what is part of the body and what is not. On the present evidence it would seem that the bulk of the autoimmune diseases may come under this category. At one end of the spectrum are the organ-specific, but interrelated, disorders — autoimmune thyroid disease, Addisonian pernicious anaemia, idiopathic Addison's disease, idiopathic hypoparathyroidism and autoimmune ovarian failure. At the other end of the spectrum are the non-organ-specific diseases such as systemic lupus erythematosus and Sjögren's disease. The autoimmune liver diseases perhaps come somewhere in between.

There is some evidence to suggest that, at least in the organ-specific autoimmune diseases, there is a loss of suppressor T cell control on the function of the B lymphocytes. The observation that T cell function diminishes with age provides an attractive explanation for the rising incidence of subclinical and clinical organ-specific autoimmune disease with advancing years.

*Sequestrated Antigen*. There are some antigens that do not normally come into contact with the immunological system so that there has been no opportunity for immunological tolerance of self-recognition to develop. For example, sperm, if extravasated following unilateral blockage of the vas deferens, may induce antibody formation and contribute to sterility. Sperm antibodies may also be produced following vasectomy in normal men.

*Infection*. In the hypersensitive host, invading micro-organisms may share antigen with certain of the host's tissues and induce the formation of antibodies which cross-react with these tissues. Thus the sharing of antigen between some Group A haemolytic streptococci and the heart may be relevant to rheumatic carditis. Likewise, the sharing of antigen between *Esch. coli* 014 and colonic epithelium may be relevant to the pathogenesis of ulcerative colitis.

*Drugs* such as methyldopa seem to alter the immunological system so that antibodies develop that are reactive with red cells producing a haemolytic anaemia which is reversible on withdrawal of the drug. Other drugs such as procainamide are associated with the development of antinuclear antibodies.

*Genetic factors* operate in the autoimmune diseases, but the exact mode of inheritance escapes clear definition. A characteristic feature of the autoimmune diseases is that the autoantibodies are formed continually, at least over a period of years. By contrast, if a tissue is damaged by some other means — such as occurs in myocardial infarction or burns — in general the corresponding antibodies appear only temporarily.

The genetic factor could operate as a built-in defect in the immune system so that, usually later rather than sooner, tolerance breaks down according to a certain pattern. Alternatively, what may be genetically determined is susceptibility to an exogenous agent such as a virus, for which there is some evidence in a special strain of mice. However, there is as yet no convincing evidence that genetic susceptibility to a viral infection is the basis of autoimmune disease in man except possibly in insulin-dependent diabetes. Whether or not there is an exogenous factor operating in man is a question that remains unanswered. Also unanswered is why immunological tolerance should break down according to patterns that clinicians recognise as interrelated diseases in which immune mechanisms play an important part.

## HLA and Disease

Organ transplantation gave a great impetus to the study of tolerance. The antigens causing the immune response that results in rejection of a tissue allograft are known as histocompatibility antigens. They are genetically determined and situated on chromosome 6. The major histocompatibility system is known as HLA (Human Lymphocyte Antigen). Histocompatibility antigens are found in most tissues, but differ

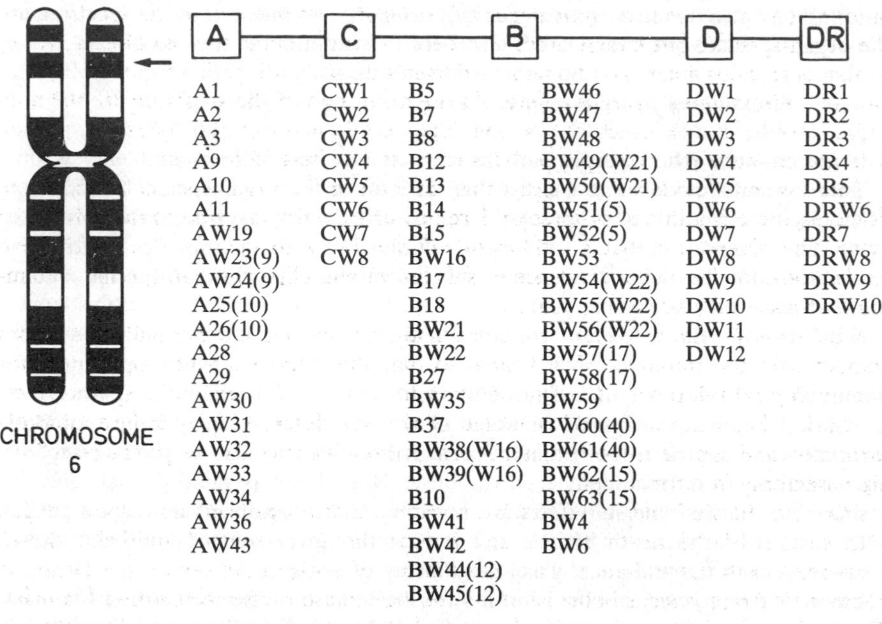


Fig. 2.8 The HLA System

quantitatively in their distribution on these tissues; they can be detected either by serological techniques or in lymphocyte culture.

The antigens which are detected serologically can be divided into four series, HLA-A, HLA-B, HLA-C and HLA-DR (D related) (Fig 2.8). Another series of antigens, HLA-D, can be determined by their ability to stimulate lymphocytes in culture. The D and DR antigens may be the same. Well-defined antigens in each series are given a number, e.g. HLA-A1, HLA-A2, etc., while less well defined antigens are given the letter W, e.g. HLA-AW19. The possible number of combinations of alleles on a chromosome (this being known as a haplotype) is enormous, although certain alleles tend to occur together on the chromosome, e.g. HLA-A1 and HLA-B8. Nevertheless the chance of two unrelated people being identical for HLA is very low.

Skin grafts between HLA identical siblings show a marked prolongation of survival, while renal allografts between HLA identical siblings have very few rejection episodes and a 95% survival at three years. However, in unrelated cadaver renal transplantation, true HLA identity is rare and a partial matching for HLA can offer only a modest improvement in survival figures.

Some very strong associations between HLA and susceptibility to certain diseases have been described, especially the autoimmune diseases and certain other conditions with a probable allergic basis, e.g. ankylosing spondylitis (B27); rheumatoid arthritis (DR4); idiopathic Addison's disease (B8, DW3); insulin-dependent diabetes (B8, DR3, B15, DR4); thyrotoxicosis (B8, DR3); myasthenia gravis (B8); and haemochromatosis (A3).

Certain HLA antigens occur together more commonly than would be expected by chance (*linkage disequilibrium*); e.g. A1, B8, DW3 and DR3; A2, CW3, B15, DW4 and DR4; A3, B7, DW2 and DR2. In some instances the presence of an HLA antigen (or group of antigens in linkage disequilibrium) are protective or confer resistance to acquiring the disease (e.g. B7, DW2 and DR2 in insulin-dependent diabetes).

## Suppression of Immune Reactions or of their Effects

*Antihistamines.* When anaphylaxis presents as an acute clinical problem the immediate aim is to give drugs which antagonise the effects of the mediators. These antagonists are the antihistamines and various drugs which have opposite actions to the mediators.

The antihistamines occupy the same tissue receptors as histamine without providing any stimulus to the effector cells. In man, the intravenous injection of an antihistamine quickly produces adequate tissue concentrations. The weal, the erythema and the itch of acute urticaria are reduced but there is no consistent improvement in lung function in acute bronchial asthma. The failure of the antihistamines to relieve airway obstruction caused by an anaphylactic reaction has been attributed to high concentrations of histamine close to the smooth muscle cells. It may also be due to the presence of other mediators of the anaphylactic response. Bradykinin is rapidly inactivated in plasma by a kininase but its effects are not inhibited by antihistamines. No specific antagonists of bradykinin or SRS-A are known, although salicylates have been shown to suppress experimental anaphylaxis in guinea-pigs.

*Sodium cromoglycate* is believed to inhibit the release of the mediators from mast cells following the interaction of antigens with IgE antibodies. It is partially effective in preventing the induction of asthma by specific antigens. If inhaled by an asthmatic subject before exposure to the antigen, protection may last for several hours, but if given after exposure to the antigen it has little effect.

*Adrenaline and related drugs* act by producing effects which oppose the mediators and are more effective in emergencies than the antihistamines. Adrenaline, isoprenaline and aminophylline are efficient bronchodilators in bronchial asthma. Urticaria is relieved and where oedema threatens the airway, the risk of asphyxia is lessened. Despite their effectiveness these non-specific antagonists have serious disadvantages. They are antagonists in their own right, acting on receptors which differ from those occupied by the mediators, and their effects never precisely counteract those of the mediators. The dose of a sympathomimetic amine which relieves airways obstruction may produce tachycardia and palpitations even when the amine is administered as an aerosol. Salbutamol does not have these disadvantages as it is more specific in its action on β-adrenergic receptors in the bronchi.

*Corticosteroids.* Hydrocortisone or prednisolone produce improvement in status asthmaticus in a few hours. The mechanism is not known but is probably related to their anti-inflammatory actions and not to selective interference with any particular stage in the development of the anaphylactic response. Their use in Types II, III and IV immune reactions is discussed below.

*Hyposensitisation.* Anaphylactic individuals can be made less sensitive by multiple subcutaneous injections of antigen in gradually increasing dosage. Pollen antigens can be used to prevent the development of hay fever and asthma in some patients. The patient develops IgG antibodies against the antigen; these antibodies have a higher avidity for the antigen than do IgE antibodies and are able to compete successfully for the antigen sites on the pollen, or whatever has induced the anaphylactic response. As reactions with the IgG antibodies do not take place at cell surfaces, anaphylactic phenomena are not produced and there is no harmful effect as the amount of IgG antibodies produced is not sufficient to cause an immune complex reaction. In this context the IgG antibodies are referred to as blocking antibodies.

*Immunosuppressive Drugs*. The production of immunoglobulins and the cellular immune response are dependent upon the division of lymphoid cells. Drugs which interfere with dividing cells are therefore all potentially immunosuppressive. Such drugs were originally developed as antitumour agents and are referred to as cytotoxic drugs. Of these azathioprine, cyclophosphamide and methotrexate have been used for immunosuppression. In organ transplantation the use of azathioprine has become almost universal and it is under trial in the treatment of other diseases such as systemic lupus erythematosus, rheumatoid arthritis and ulcerative colitis. Immunosuppression drugs may have serious adverse effects, including bone marrow suppression and the promotion of tuberculous, viral or fungal infection.

*Cyclosporin A* is a potent immunosuppressive drug which is toxic for human lymphoblasts of both T and B cell origin, but not for resting lymphocytes or cells of myeloid or other origin. Its role in organ transplantation is at present limited on account of nephrotoxicity.

*Antilymphocyte serum* is a potent agent for the suppression of cell-mediated immunity. It is prepared by immunising another species, usually the horse, with human lymphocytes. The precise mode of action is debatable but it interferes with the function of T lymphocytes while not affecting antibody formation to previously encountered antigens. Its main application has been in relation to organ transplantation. The major side-effects are the development of anaphylactic reactions to the injection of serum of another species and the development of antibodies to the antilymphocyte serum with deposition of immune complexes in the kidney and consequent renal damage. A further possible hazard, shared by other immunosuppressive agents, is an increased incidence of malignant tumours, such as lymphomas, possibly on account of the suppression of immunological surveillance of the body tissues which is part of the normal mechanism for the control of spontaneous tumours (see below).

*Anti-D Immunoglobulin*. The clearest example of interference with a specific immune response is the use of human anti-D immunoglobulin to prevent haemolytic disease of the newborn (p. 564).

*Anti-inflammatory Agents*. Drugs which interfere with the unwanted consequences of Types II, III and IV immune reactions include the corticosteroids and, to a lesser extent, salicylates. The corticosteroids may also partially suppress the development of immune responses, but in high dosage they have serious side-effects. Use is therefore being made of other anti-inflammatory drugs such as indomethacin or phenylbutazone, sometimes in combination with an immunosuppressive drug.

*Plasmaphoresis*. The technique of plasma exchange has been used beneficially in myasthenia gravis and Goodpasture's syndrome, removing acetylcholine-receptor and glomerular basement membrane antibodies respectively. It is used in conjunction with cytotoxic drugs and steroids in order to check the rate of resynthesis of antibody. Controlled trials are required in relation to the immune complex diseases such as rheumatoid arthritis and systemic lupus erythematosus.

*Thymectomy* as a treatment for autoimmune diseases other than myasthenia gravis may be effective only in childhood when the influence of the thymus on the immunological system is particularly important.

*Cancer Immunology*. Cancer cells lose some of the normal tissue-specific antigens and appear to gain some tumour-associated antigens which were not previously present in the cells from which they were derived. It used to be thought that the process of immunological surveillance destroys many early cancers by virtue of the recognition by the normal immune system of the 'foreignness' of tumour-associated antigens. However, immunodeficiency, either primary or induced by immunosuppressive drugs is mainly associated with lymphomas and not with cancer generally. It is more likely that the immune system is important in relation to the control of oncogenic viruses, rather than immune surveillance *per se*. Attempts have been made to augment the normal immune response so as to help ablate malignant growth after the bulk of the tumour has been removed or killed by conventional means. Thus allogeneic irradiated malignant cells may be beneficial in acute myeloid leukaemia (p. 574).

In the presence of continued antigenic stimulation, macrophages, previously coated with specific macrophage arming factor, may become activated so that they are cytolytic to rapidly dividing (e.g. malignant) as opposed to normal cells. Also antigens from malignant tumours may be released into the circulation in excess of the amount of antibody produced against the tumour; this situation of antigen excess would block Type VI cytotoxic reactions and thereby overcome one of the body's defences. It is also likely that nonimmunological toxic factors may induce a state of relative immunodeficiency in cancer patients.

Although positive claims have been made, as yet there is no convincing evidence for an immunological test in relation to a common cancer antigen. Certain tumour associated macromolecules are, however, potentially useful as indicators of the presence or, in certain defined situations, the amount of tumour in a patient, e.g. cancer embryonic antigen (CEA) in colorectal cancer.

## Immunodeficiency Disorders

So important are the immunological mechanisms for survival that it is not surprising that patients are rarely seen suffering from major defects. Deficiences of the humoral and cellular components of the immunological system may occur separately or together. Figure 2.9 shows the probable sites of the primary defects in the immune system for a number of clinical patterns that have been recognised.

### Combined Deficiency States

A block in the development of the stem-cell leads to deficiency in both the T and B lymphocyte systems and therefore to impairment of cell-mediated hypersensitivity and of synthesis of humoral antibody (Fig. 2.9, lesion 1). A failure of stem-cell development at an even earlier stage leads to the additional feature of agranulocytosis although the red cells and platelets are normal. About half the infants with the autosomal recessive form of severe combined immunodeficiency have a concomitant deficiency of adenosine deaminase which has enabled prenatal diagnosis by finding the enzyme deficiency in cultured amnion cells. Infants with either the autosomal or the X-linked types are incapable of limiting the most benign viral infections. Death has resulted from generalised chickenpox, or measles or from cytomegalic or other viral infections. Vaccination results in progressive, ultimately fatal vaccinia infection.

### Deficiency of Humoral Immunity

**Primary Immunodeficiency**. Selective deficiency of the B lymphocyte system occurs in X linked recessive hypo- or a-gammaglobulinaemia (Fig. 2.9, lesion 2). The lack of immunoglobulins is not absolute but the patient fails to respond to antigenic stimuli. However, cell mediated hypersensitivity is normal. It is not incompatible with survival for many years, though the patient is very susceptible to bacterial infections, particularly to pyogenic cocci.

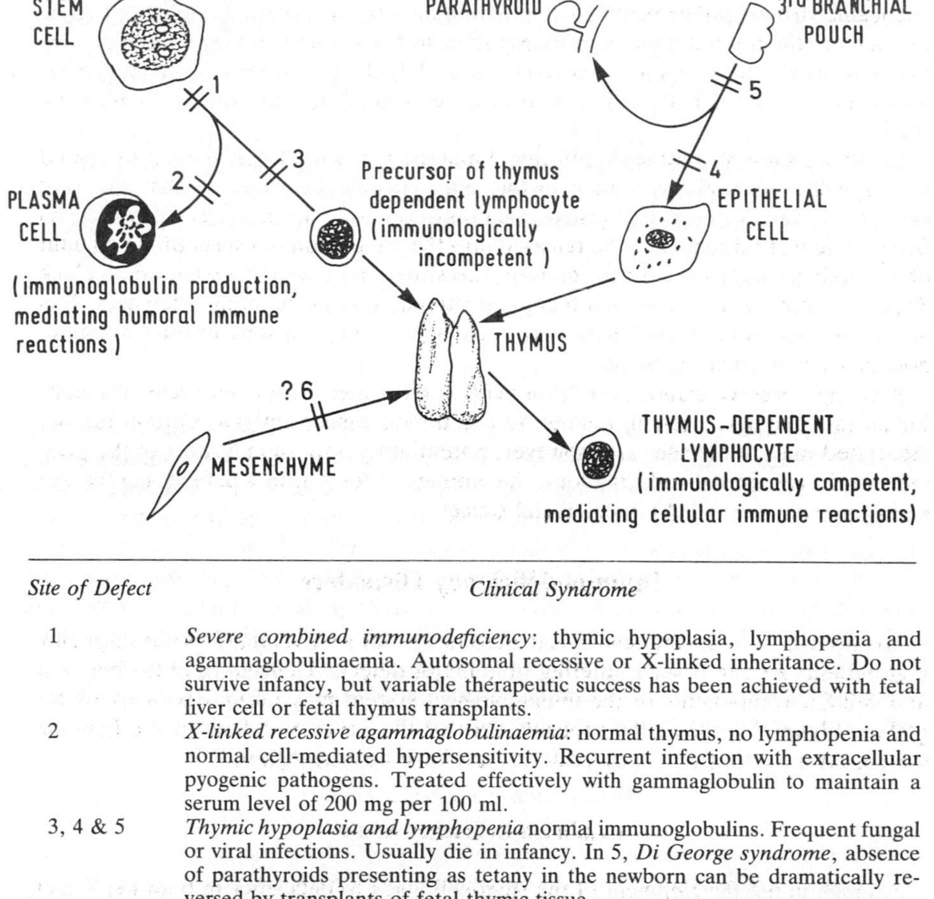


| *Site of Defect* | *Clinical Syndrome* |
|---|---|
| 1 | *Severe combined immunodeficiency*: thymic hypoplasia, lymphopenia and agammaglobulinaemia. Autosomal recessive or X-linked inheritance. Do not survive infancy, but variable therapeutic success has been achieved with fetal liver cell or fetal thymus transplants. |
| 2 | *X-linked recessive agammaglobulinaemia*: normal thymus, no lymphopenia and normal cell-mediated hypersensitivity. Recurrent infection with extracellular pyogenic pathogens. Treated effectively with gammaglobulin to maintain a serum level of 200 mg per 100 ml. |
| 3, 4 & 5 | *Thymic hypoplasia and lymphopenia* normal immunoglobulins. Frequent fungal or viral infections. Usually die in infancy. In 5, *Di George syndrome*, absence of parathyroids presenting as tetany in the newborn can be dramatically reversed by transplants of fetal thymic tissue. |
| | *Wiskott-Aldrich syndrome* difficult to classify X-linked eczema, thrombocytopenia and recurrent infections survival rare beyond first decade. There appears to be a progressive deterioration of thymus-dependent cellular immunity with concomitant changes in the lymph nodes. Serum IgM usually low IgG and IgA normal or elevated. No unifying hypothesis explains the disparate elements of this syndrome yet most aspects have been ameliorated by the administration of transfer factor obtained from dialysis of normal donor lymphocytes (p. 25). |
| 6 | *Thymic hypoplasia-ataxia telangiectasia*. May be part of a more widespread mesenchyne deficiency. Thymas fails to develop. Autosomal recessive inheritance. Difficult to classify. |

Fig. 2.9 The sites of developmental defects which lead to some of the immunodeficiency syndromes observed clinically.

Most patients with immunodeficiency have 'acquired' or 'late onset' agammaglobulinaemia known as *'common, variable, unclassifiable immunodeficiency'*. B lymphocytes are usually, but not always present in contrast to their absence in the X-linked form of agammaglobulinaemia. Deterioration of T cell function may also be observed. Primary acquired agammaglobulinaemia is associated with an unusually high incidence of autoimmune disease, such as pernicious anaemia or haemolytic anaemia. A prominent and frequent complication is a sprue-like syndrome and *Giardia intestinalis* infection (p. 814) is common. Another distinguishing feature of the acquired form is the frequent occurrence of non-caseating granulomas, e.g. in lungs, liver, and skin.

As the different immunoglobulins have different functions, deficiencies might be expected to produce different clinical pictures. Thus IgM deficiency is possibly associated with meningococcal meningitis and lack of IgA with gastrointestinal or respiratory tract infections. In the absence of IgA the lowered resistance permits invasion of the normally sterile upper gut by bacteria, some of which would produce decomposition of bile salts and thus affect the absorption of fat.

Immunoglobulin injections (300 mg/kg body weight) consisting mainly of IgG can provide effective protection against severe, recurrent pyogenic infections in patients with various types of hypo- or a-gammaglobulinaemia. Since the half-life of the gamma globulin injected is 30 days or more, these patients must receive minimally a monthly injection of 100 mg per kg to maintain the desired level of approximately 200 mg per 100 ml. Smaller doses are ineffective.

**Secondary Immunodeficiency.** Maternal IgG is transferred across the placenta by active secretion to the fetus during the third trimester of pregnancy. Premature babies may thus have some degree of hypogammaglobulinaemia and prophylactic IgG treatment may reduce the incidence of infections. The production of immunoglobulins in the early years of life is well below that of adults and this may well explain the greatly increased susceptibility of the young to infection, particularly gastrointestinal and respiratory tract infection in relation to IgA deficiency. IgA is present in colostrum and there is evidence that breast feeding provides the infant with intestinal immunity.

Immunoglobulin deficiency may arise also in adults as a result of abnormal metabolism of serum proteins as occurs in uraemic patients in whom susceptibility to infection is increased. Drugs may also depress the immune system.

### Deficiency of Cellular Immunity

This condition is a selective primary deficiency of T lymphocytes (Fig. 2.9, lesions 3, 4 and 5). There is severe lymphocytopenia and a predominance of reticulum cells in the lymphoid tissue. The patient's lymphocytes are unable to respond by transformation into lymphoblasts following stimulation with antigens. On account of the deficiency in cell-mediated hypersensitivity, affected children do not respond in the normal way to antigens such as monilia. Infants with thymic aplasia in whom the cell-mediated aspect is completely lacking are highly susceptible to viral infections, which usually prove fatal.

The fact that there are deficient humoral antibody responses to some antigens in conditions associated with lesions at sites 3, 4 and 5 of Figure 2.9 exemplifies the existence of co-operation between T and B lymphocytes in relation to certain antigens. Diseases such as sarcoidosis and Hodgkin's lymphoma are associated with a depression mainly of cell-mediated hypersensitivity.

The transplantation of fragments of human fetal thymus has been effective in replacing the cellular immune deficiency in congenital thymic aplasia and transfer factor (p. 25) has been used in the Wiskott-Aldrich syndrome (Fig. 2.9).

### Deficiency of Complement

Study of complement deficiency indicates that the principal activities of the complement system are related to protection against infectious disease. In the case of failure of C3 activation, syndromes are produced that are basically very similar to those of the antibody deficiency syndrome. Absence of the components of the classical pathway C3 convertase seem to cause a more subtle immunity deficiency where infection with essentially non-virulent organisms may give rise to immune complex disease. Deficiency of the late-acting complement components may be associated with an increased susceptibility to certain forms of bacterial infection, particularly *Neisseria*.

## Prospects in Immunology

The most significant disease added to the list of disorders in which autoimmunity may have a pathogenic role is the type of diabetes mellitus with insulin-dependency as its end stage. This condition may also exemplify the possible interaction between viral infection and autoimmunity, each depending on genetic factors. Among the genetic markers so far recognised, HLA has had the greatest impact. Other genetic markers should be discovered which will give more information as to the risk of an individual developing certain diseases and about the natural history of these diseases.

In order to prevent autoimmune disease a better understanding is needed of how self-recognition is achieved and how self-reactivity is normally controlled. Thereafter, what is required are methods of manipulating the immune response, not in a blunderbuss fashion as at present, but in relation to its many different components.

W. J. IRVINE

*Further reading:*

Irvine, W. J. (ed.) (1979) *Medical Immunology*. Edinburgh: Teviot Scientific Publications. New York: McGraw Hill.
Irvine, W. J. (ed.) (1980) *Immunology of Diabetes*. Edinburgh: Teviot Scientific Publications.
Roitt, I. M. (1977) *Essential Immunology*, 3rd edn. Oxford: Blackwell.
Weir, D. M. (1977) *Immunology. An outline for students of medicine and biology,* 4th edn. Edinburgh: Churchill Livingstone.

*More detailed texts:*

Parker, C. W. (ed.) (1980) *Clinical Immunology*. Vols I and II. Philadelphia: Saunders.
Samter, M. (ed.) (1978) *Immunological Diseases*, 3rd edn. Boston: Little, Brown.

# 3. Infection and Disease

During the past 50 years there has been a dramatic fall in the incidence of infectious diseases, particularly in developed countries. This is due to several factors, including immunisation, antimicrobial chemotherapy, improved nutrition, and better sanitation and housing. In less developed countries, however, especially in the tropics, infection continues to be one of the commonest causes of death, particularly in children. In contrast, many recent advances in medicine and surgery such as cancer chemotherapy and organ transplantation have been complicated by infection, often causing the death of the patient.

The control of infection depends on a knowledge of microbiology (the infecting organism and its sensitivity to chemotherapeutic agents), epidemiology (source and spread of infection) and immunology (host defences against infection).

## The Micro-organism

Virtually all micro-organisms can cause infection in man although some are more virulent than others. However, less pathogenic bacteria such as *Staphylococcus epidermidis*, a commensal organism which is a common inhabitant of the skin of healthy persons, can cause infection in patients with abnormal defence mechanisms against infection (compromised hosts). Certain bacteria such as *Staphylococcus aureus* cause disease by the local action of the organism on tissues such as bone. Others, notably those causing diphtheria and tetanus, produce potent toxins which circulate in the blood and damage organs at some distance from the primary site of infection.

Some organisms are inherently resistant to certain antibiotics but can also develop resistance to others. For example, *Mycobacterium tuberculosis* is invariably resistant to penicillin but frequently sensitive to streptomycin. Resistance to streptomycin can however develop during treatment with the antibiotic. Gram-negative bacilli such as *Escherichia coli* can readily become resistant to antibiotics and it is therefore necessary to have an up-to-date knowledge of the current sensitivity patterns of common bacteria. This can vary between different hospitals and is related to the use of antibiotics in a particular environment.

## Source and Spread of Infection

Infection may originate from the patient (autogenous) usually from the skin, nasopharynx or colon, or from outside sources (exogenous), commonly from another person who may either be suffering from an infection or carrying a pathogenic micro-organism. Carriers are usually healthy and may harbour the organism in throat (diphtheria) or stool (salmonella infection). Non-human sources of infection include animals (rabies), soil (tetanus) and water (typhoid fever). Fomites is the term used to describe inanimate articles such as blankets, furniture and crockery which can be reservoirs of infection.

Micro-organisms may be transmitted by several routes. Autogenous infection may develop as a result of local spread e.g. from bowel to peritoneum, or by the blood stream. An example of the latter is infective endocarditis caused by *Strep. viridans* originating in the patient's mouth and entering the blood during dental procedures. Exogenous infection may be acquired directly or indirectly by one of the following routes:

1. *Direct contact.* Venereal and skin infections are transmitted by contact between body surfaces.
2. *Airborne transmission.* This includes transmission by airborne droplets and dust particles. Infected droplets originate in the nasopharynx and mouth and are expelled during talking, breathing and sneezing carrying micro-organisms with them. Respiratory tract infections and many of the common infectious diseases of childhood such as measles are spread by this route.
3. *Faecal-oral spread.* Infections transmitted by this route are usually acquired by the ingestion of food or drink contaminated by human faeces. This often occurs during preparation of meals as a result of a low standard of personal hygiene in kitchen workers. Large outbreaks of hepatitis or cholera may follow pollution of domestic water supplies. Other diseases spread by the faecal-oral route include dysentery and enterovirus infections such as poliomyelitis. Hand washing is the vital factor in the prevention of infection transmitted by this route.
4. *Animal, bird or insect borne.* Animals and birds may transmit infection directly (rabies and psittacosis) or indirectly via food and drink (salmonella infection and brucellosis). Blood sucking insects are important vectors in the transmission of many important infections such as malaria, yellow fever, plague and rickettsial diseases.
5. *Transmission by medical and nursing procedures.* Infection may be transmitted by inadequately sterilized instruments, faulty nursing techniques or contamination of transfused fluid or blood.

**Incubation period** is the period of time which elapses between the invasion of the tissues by pathogens and the appearance of clinical symptoms and signs of infection.

## Defence of the Human Host

**Susceptibility to Infection.** Both man and animals show group or individual differences in their liability to infection. Resistance to infection is also affected by age, environment and illness and its treatment. Thus infants during the first six months of life are relatively insusceptible to infection owing to transplacental-derived immunity (p. 27) and this may be augmented by breast feeding. An unfavourable environment may lower resistance to infection and pathogenic or saprophytic organisms harboured by the individual may precipitate disease. Medical or surgical treatment may interfere with resistance to infection by reducing immunity, e.g. by the use of cytotoxic drugs or irradiation, or by destroying the physical barriers to invasion, e.g. by surgical operation or instrumentation.

**First Line of Defence.** The surface barrier presented by the intact skin, the mucosa of the respiratory and alimentary tracts and of the conjunctival sac is augmented by chemical defences in the secretions. Mucus acts mechanically but along with other secretions contains low concentrations of antibody and enzymes which inactivate and kill microbes which are not adapted to a commensal existence.

The ciliated epithelium of the respiratory tract collects micro-organisms trapped in the mucus and carries them upwards eventually to be swallowed and killed by acid in the stomach. The alimentary tract is also protected from contaminating pathogens by the defence barrier of the commensal microflora. Removal of these commensals by chemotherapy can allow minority populations such as *Candida albicans* to flourish and cause thrush.

**Second Line of Defence.** The first stage of infection is invasion of the tissues. Factors related to the pathogenicity of the micro-organism or accidental or surgical wounding allow penetration of the surfaces into the underlying tissues. Contamination of deeper tissues may occur directly after wounding and this bypasses the surface defences so that the deep or tissue defences are immediately called on. These defences are cellular, humoral and mechanical.

*Cellular Defence.* Immediately after invasion of the tissues, micro-organisms are phagocytosed by reticulo-endothelial cells, both wandering and tissue macrophages and polymorphonuclear leucocytes (p. 536); these deal successfully with the great majority of incidents, but if the organism is virulent and multiplies faster than the rate of phagocytosis, it will dominate.

*Humoral Defence.* The role of antibodies has been described in the preceding chapter.

*Mechanical Defence.* In many infections a mechanical barrier forms against the spread of infection, e.g. the fibrin from the acute inflammatory reaction of a pyogenic infection, or the fibrous tissue around a tuberculous focus or a hydatid cyst. It should be remembered however that some organisms elaborate substances which weaken this defensive barrier, e.g. $\beta$-haemolytic streptococci may produce a fibrinolysin which dissolves fibrin, and hyaluronidase, a substance which enables the organisms or their products to spread more rapidly through the tissues.

**Reactions of the Host to Specific Infections.** The nature of the responses of the body and their intensity depend upon the type of infecting agent, its quantity and its virulence. Viral infections tend to excite a local lymphocytic reaction and a polymorph leucopenia with relative lymphocytosis in the blood. Rarely there is an initial polymorph leucocytosis. Many worm infections are associated with an eosinophilia. When the infection is bacterial, the character of the ensuing reaction varies. Pyogenic organisms (staphylococci, streptococci, pneumococci, meningococci, gonococci and *Esch. coli*) give rise to an acute local inflammation with the outpouring of neutrophil polymorphonunuclear leucocytes, serum and fibrin and a general reaction of abrupt onset with pyrexia and polymorph leucocytosis. Typhoid and paratyphoid infections cause a local monocyte response, a polymorph leucopenia and a gradual increase of fever over several days. Whooping-cough induces a lymphocytosis.

## Diagnosis of Infectious Disease

A knowledge of infections prevailing in the locality may be a valuable guide to diagnosis, e.g. when mumps is prevalent, the occurrence, without apparent cause, of acute epididymo-orchitis in an adult may be attributed to mumps with some confidence, a diagnosis which could not be made on clinical evidence alone. It is wise to enquire about contacts among the family, friends and workmates. Persons following certain occupations may be exposed to infection, e.g. leptospirosis occurs in coal miners, pig farmers, sewer-workers and fish cleaners; anthrax occurs in tanners and in handlers of imported bone meal.

A recent history of laporotomy or of obscure abdominal pain should suggest subphrenic or intrahepatic abscess.

Residence or travel abroad within the previous year or two raises the possibility of malaria, amoebic abscess of the liver or other exotic disease.

In many infections a diagnosis beyond all reasonable doubt may be made on clinical grounds, e.g. measles or chickenpox. In others there may be doubt about the identity of the causal organism and demonstration of its presence is essential for diagnosis.

**The Laboratory Diagnosis of Infection.** The causal organism may be identified in some instances microscopically in tissue, exudate or excreta, e.g. *N. gonorrhoeae* in urethral exudates, or *Myco. tuberculosis* in sputum. In the majority, however, it is necessary to isolate the organism in artificial culture, or more rarely in laboratory animals. In cases where these methods are inapplicable or unavailing, e.g. in many viral diseases or in the convalescent stages of infection, indirect means must be used to demonstrate specific antibody in the patient's serum.

Antibody is present in significant amounts from about 7 days after the onset of infection. The demonstration of specific antibody is of value in the diagnosis of toxoplasmosis, brucellosis, leptospirosis, syphilis, infectious mononucleosis and certain types of streptococcal and staphylococcal disease. The clinical value of serological tests is limited in most viral infections by the fact that recovery has often occurred before the result has been obtained.

As the normal range of antibody values is wide, at least two specimens should be examined at an interval of not less than 7 days so that a change in titre may be measured. In all cases the results of serological tests must be interpreted with a knowledge of the patient's occupation, history and clinical findings, previous immunisation and residence in endemic areas.

**Differential Diagnosis of Infection.** Most febrile illnesses are due to infection and often the diagnosis can be made by clinical examination alone. In other instances a diagnosis may require confirmation by haematological examination, radiography, scanning, bacteriological investigation of blood or other body fluids, discharges or excreta. Often detection of specific antibodies in the serum may have to be undertaken before the diagnostic problems may be solved. Occasionally the cause of a febrile illness remains uncertain in spite of investigation and such a case is categorised PUO (pyrexia of unknown origin). In order to establish the diagnosis the following measures should be undertaken:

1. Retake the history; a symptom may have been overlooked or misinterpreted; enquire whether the patient has lived or travelled overseas.
2. Repeat the examination of the patient; new signs may have appeared while others could have been missed or their significance not appreciated.
3. Examine the urine repeatedly for protein, white and red blood cells and micro-organisms.
4. Inspect the temperature charts for evidence of some characteristic appearance such as the undulations seen in some cases of lymphoma or the periodicity of malaria.
5. Review the results of laboratory investigations, thoroughly rescrutinise any radiographs and repeat such examinations as may seem necessary.

If the diagnosis is still uncertain, further tests will be required. These will be indicated by any new information obtained as a result of the clinical reassessment. It should be borne in mind that most problematic fevers are due to a common disorder with an unusual presentation. In Britain the more common causes of PUO are tumours (such as carcinoma with or without metastases, or Hodgkin's disease), infections (among which tuberculosis is important), connective tissue disorders and drug hypersensitivity. In the tropics and elsewhere a wide variety of infections must be considered, as a glance at the map on page 795 will demonstrate.

Mysterious fevers, particularly in patients who have some knowledge of medicine or nursing, may be due to deceit (factitious fever). Doubts should be raised if the skin of a supposedly febrile patient does not feel hot or if the general health does not deteriorate in spite of persistant fever. The occurrence of some bizarre symptom or sign may arouse suspicion that the temperature is being falsified. There are both subtle and simple techniques for doing this. The latter include holding the thermometer close to a hot water bottle or other source of heat, dipping it into a hot drink, applying friction to the bulb, or shaking it in a retrograde manner.

If the diagnosis remains obscure another opinion should be obtained, as reconsideration of the evidence by an unbiased observer may throw new light on the problem.

When a diagnosis still cannot be established and the patient's condition is deteriorating, various remedies, e.g. antibiotics, may be tried empirically in the hope of influencing the course of the disease. A therapeutic trial should not be regarded as a satisfactory diagnostic test and it can further obscure the diagnosis by suppressing but not curing the infection. It is most useful in suspected tuberculosis.

## The Prevention of Infection

The prevention of infection depends on three concepts which may be inter-related:

1. *Elimination of the source of infection.* Examples of this include the eradication of tuberculosis and brucellosis from cattle in many countries and the world-wide elimination of smallpox. The laboratory screening of donated blood for syphilis and hepatitis B virus has virtually eliminated these sources of infection.
2. *Prevention of transmission of infection.* This may be accomplished by the isolation of infected patients (source isolation) and of those such as the immunosuppressed who are particularly susceptible to infection (protective isolation). Strict antisepsis in operating theatres and good nursing practices in wards are essential if transmission of infection is to be prevented. Hand-washing is of paramount importance.

   Insect control by the elimination of breeding grounds and the use of insecticides, is a major factor in malaria prevention programmes. Individuals who have been in close contact with serious infectious diseases such as diphtheria or Lassa fever are placed in quarantine — a term derived from the period of 40 days of compulsory isolation of ships after leaving a port where life-threatening infections such as plague were rife. The duration of quarantine depends on the incubation period of the disease. For the common infectious diseases of childhood strict quarantine is not necessary although the child should normally be kept away from school until non-infectious.
3. *Protection of susceptible persons.* This involves the judicious use of prophylactic antibiotics (p. 80) and of active or passive immunization.

**Active Immunisation.** In Britan parents should be advised to have their children immunised against whooping-cough, diphtheria, tetanus, measles and poliomyelitis (Table 3.1). Because of the risk of damage to the developing embryo or fetus if rubella should occur during pregnancy, it is recommended that rubella vaccine be given to all girls between 11 and 14 years and to non-pregnant women of child-bearing age who are found to be serologically negative for this antigen. Similarly, immunisation against tuberculosis should be given to all non-reactors to tuberculin during adolescence.

The indications for vaccination against influenza, enteric fevers, cholera, plague, typhus, yellow fever and rabies depend upon the likelihood of exposure or international health regulations (p. 893). Acute demyelinating encephalomyelitis (p. 715) is a rare complication of vaccination.

**Passive Immunisation.** An injection of immunoglobulin will provide temporary protection against certain infectious diseases. Human normal immunglobulin (pooled) is indicated for prevention of measles (p. 68)and virus A hepatitis (p. 396), and human specific immunoglobulin for chickenpox (p. 70), virus B hepatitis and tetanus (p. 62).

Table 3.1. Immunisation schedule generally followed in Britain

| Age | Visits | Vaccine | Intervals |
|---|---|---|---|
| 4–12 months | 3 | Three administrations of DTP + OPV | 6–8 weeks and 4–6 months |
| 12–24 months | 1 | Measles vaccination | |
| First year at school | 1 | Booster DT + OPV | |
| 10–13 years | 1 | BCG for the tuberculin negative | |
| Girls: 11–13 years | 1 | Rubella vaccination | |
| 15–19 years or on leaving school | 1 | TT + OPV | |

DTP = Diphtheria, tetanus, pertussis ('triple') vaccine.
OPV = Oral poliomyelitis vaccine.
DT = Diphtheria, tetanus vaccine.
TT = Tetanus toxoid.

## DISEASES DUE TO INFECTION

Diseases due to infection are the commonest cause of ill health throughout the world. Organisms involved include bacteria, mycoplasmas, rickettsiae, viruses, protozoa, metazoa and fungi. The term infestation is now limited to ectoparasites, usually arthropods such as lice and fleas, which remain on the surface of the body but which may transmit a systemic infection. Protozoal infections such as malaria, amoebic dysentery, sleeping sickness and leishmaniasis and helminthiasis (worms) are of great importance in the tropics. Fungi causing ringworm and thrush occur all over the world but systemic infections with other fungi, such as coccidioidomycosis, histoplasmosis and the blastomycoses, are rare except in certain geographical locations.

The range of diseases caused by bacteria is large; streptococci and staphylococci are widespread and produce similar diseases throughout the world. Others such as the cholera vibrio and plague bacillus are locally endemic but may produce epidemics from time to time. Some bacterial infections may be acute such as diphtheria and tetanus, others chronic such as tuberculosis, syphilis and leprosy.

Organisms smaller than true bacteria, the rickettsiae which cause typhus fevers, the mycoplasmas of atypical pneumonia and the chlamydia of psittacosis, lymphogranuloma and trachoma are now recognised to be widespread and are susceptible to chemotherapy. Thus most bacterial, protozoal and fungal infections can be successfully treated with antibiotics and chemotherapeutic agents provided that the appropriate drug is prescribed early in the disease. This emphasises the need for rapid and accurate diagnosis supplemented where necessary by specific tests to indicate the most effective therapeutic agent.

As yet few specific therapeutic measures are available for viral diseases, among which are the exanthemata—chickenpox, smallpox, measles and rubella; mumps and glandular fever; respiratory illnesses such as the common cold, pharyngitis and influenza; diseases of the nervous system such as rabies and other forms of encephalitis, poliomyelitis and choriomeningitis, and liver disorders such as infective hepatitis and yellow fever. The problem of chemotherapy is to control the growth and propagation of the virus without damage to the host cell on which it is dependent. The number of viral infections for which prophylaxis is available is increasing in parallel with modern advances in virology and now there is preventative treatment for smallpox, rabies, yellow fever, poliomyelitis, measles and rubella. Several viral infections may be prevented temporarily by passive immunisation with human gammaglobulin.

Diseases due to infection which involve one system predominantly are described in the appropriate chapters in this book. Those infectious diseases which are limited to the tropics or are commoner there than in temperate regions are described in the section 'Tropical Diseases and Helminthic Infections'. The infectious diseases described here are:

*Bacterial:* Streptococcal infections, Staphylococcal infections, Whooping cough, Diphtheria, Typhoid and paratyphoid fevers, Bacterial food poisoning, Bacillary dysentry, Tetanus, Brucellosis, Meningococcal infections, Gonorrhoea, Syphilis, Leptospirosis.

*Viral:* Measles, Rubella, Mumps, Chickenpox, Smallpox.

## Streptococcal Infections

A number of different streptococci cause disease in man. These include *Strep. pyogenes* (scarlet fever, impetigo and erysipelas), *Strep. faecalis* (pylonephritis and endocarditis), *Strep. viridans* (endocarditis) and anaerobic streptococci (liver abscess and pulmonary infections). All can cause septicaemia which may be rapidly fatal. The present section describes infections caused by Group A haemolytic streptococci (*Strep. pyogenes*).

Haemolytic streptococcal infection results in features which vary with the invasiveness of the organism, its capacity to produce toxins, the site involved and the reaction of the host. If the resistance is low and the invasive properties of the haemolytic streptococcus are high, a rapidly spreading erysipelas, or cellulitis, lymphangitis or bacteraemia, may result. The haemolytic streptococcus may produce a specific exotoxin causing a widespread punctate erythema. When the infection is associated with such a rash the syndrome is known as scarlet fever. The same type of streptococcus may produce in one person acute tonsillitis, in another scarlet fever and in a third erysipelas.

### Scarlet Fever

Although scarlet fever is at present a mild disease, it may not necessarily remain so, as fluctuations in its severity have been recorded for the past two or three hundred years. The primary site of infection in scarlet fever is usually the pharynx or the tonsils but the disease may follow haemolytic streptococcal infection in other sites, e.g. in the genital tract after childbirth resulting in 'puerperal' scarlet fever or in wounds resulting in 'surgical' scarlet fever. It is transmitted by airborne infection, or more rarely by milk or ice-cream contaminated by streptococci. The disease is notifiable. The incubation period is about two to four days. Quarantine is not necessary.

**Clinical Features.** Scarlet fever occurs most commonly in children. It has a sudden onset and the more severe cases present with a sore throat, shivering, pyrexia, headache and vomiting. There is inflammation of the fauces; the tonsils are enlarged and may be covered with a follicular exudate. The exudate may be distinguished from the membrane seen in diphtheria by its yellow appearance and the ease with which it is wiped off. There is tender enlargement of the tonsillar lymph nodes. The rash, which usually appears first behind the ears on the second day, rapidly becomes a generalised punctate erythema. It is most intense in the flexures of the arms and legs. The face is not affected by the rash, though it is usually flushed due to fever, and the region round the mouth is pale. The tongue is initially furred but shows prominent red papillae, an appearance known as the 'white strawberry' tongue. In two or three days the fur peels leaving the 'red strawberry' tongue.The rash fades in about one week and is succeeded by desquamation.

A profuse growth of haemolytic streptococci can usually be obtained from a throat swab. A high antistreptolysin O titre (ASO) may be demonstrated in the serum.

The complications are less common than formerly as a result of the mild form of the disease and the introduction of effective chemotherapy. Extension of infection along the Eustachian tubes may lead to acute suppurative otitis media. Suppurative cervical adenitis and sinusitis also occur. Rheumatic fever and nephritis are rare sequelae which develop two or three weeks after the onset of any haemolytic streptococcal infection.

**Treatment and Prevention.** The treatment of scarlet fever is the same as for streptococcal sore throat. Most cases respond rapidly to phenoxymethylpenicillin (250 mg for children and 500 mg for adults t.i.d. for 7 days). An institutional epidemic calls for chemoprophylaxis with penicillin.

## Erysipelas

Erysipelas is an acute haemolytic streptococcal infection of the skin. It occurs in both sexes and is much commoner in the elderly than in the young. The disease is notifiable. A quarantine period is not necessary.

The onset is abrupt with heat and pain in the infected skin together with a systemic upset. There is a rapidly spreading red patch of inflamed skin with underlying oedema of the subcutaneous tissues. The edge of the patch is palpably raised and clearly defined and the lymph nodes draining the area become enlarged and tender. As the oedema subsides vesicles and bullae appear in the central part of the affected area. The face is involved in at least 80% of all cases of erysipelas as a result of the spread of streptococci from the nose.

Erysipelas is usually brought under complete control within 48 hours of treatment with penicillin; hence the prognosis is now excellent for a disease which used to be very serious.

## Staphylococcal Infections

*Staph. aureus* is responsible for a wide variety of suppurative conditions such as infected lacerations, styes, boils, carbuncles, abscesses, osteomyelitis, pneumonia, endocarditis, umbilical cord sepsis, enterocolitis and bacteraemia with pyaemic abscesses. Many infections, particularly boils, carbuncles and abscesses, are due to autogenous infection as the organisms can be grown from the nasopharynx and skin of up to 30% of healthy persons. The staphylococcus is readily spread from these sites and from clothing to contaminate the dust in which it survives in the dry state for weeks or months. In hospital this organism is an important cause of wound infection, pneumonia and neonatal sepsis. Under suitable conditions it multiplies freely in food and milk and so is an important cause of food poisoning.

When the severity of the disease warrants antibiotic therapy, the choice depends on whether the infection has been acquired inside or outside hospital. In the latter case the organism may be sensitive to penicillin. If the illness is severe treatment should be commenced with the cloxacillins (p. 73), unless the patient is known to be allergic to the penicillins when erythromycin should be given.

## Whooping Cough

Whooping cough (pertussis) is a highly infectious disease caused by *Bordetella pertussis*. It is spread by droplet infection. Clinical diagnosis in the early and most infectious stage is virtually impossible so that epidemics occur. The disease is notifiable. The incubation period is 7 to 14 days to the catarrhal stage. A quarantine period is not necessary. Whooping cough occurs at all ages but approximately 90% of cases are children under 5 years of age.

**Clinical Features.** The first stage of whooping cough consists of a highly infectious upper respiratory catarrh lasting about one week during which conjunctivitis, rhinitis and an unproductive cough are present. The distinctive paroxysmal stage follows and is characterised by severe bouts of coughing. The number of such paroxysms in 24 hours varies from an occasional attack to 40 or 50 and they are more severe at night. Each paroxysm consists of a succession of short sharp coughs, gathering in speed and duration and ending in a deep inspiration during which the characteristic whoop may be heard. It may be absent in older children and in adults because the air passages are so much wider. The last paroxysm of a series frequently ends with vomiting. The paroxysmal stage lasts from one to several weeks and is followed by the stage of convalescence during which the cough becomes less frequent and the sputum less tenacious. After the illness there is usually a lasting immunity.

The most important complications of whooping cough are pneumonia and segmental or lobar collapse which may be followed by bronchiectasis. Fits may be induced by cerebral anoxia. Subconjunctival or periorbital haemorrhage, ulceration of the frenum of the tongue, and prolapse of the rectum are relatively umimportant results of the stress of coughing. Neonates are highly susceptible and the mortality is greatest in the first year of life.

The diagnosis of whooping cough is very difficult in the catarrhal stage when the disease is most infectious. It can be confirmed in the laboratory by the isolation of *Bord. pertussis* taken from the posterior wall of the nasopharynx on small swabs passed along the floor of the nose. Examination of the blood shows a lymphocytosis which, however, may not develop until the disease is well established. The diagnosis is easy in the paroxysmal stage when the whoop has developed, but by this time the danger of transmission of infection has largely disappeared.

**Treatment.** Erythromycin may reduce the severity of the infection if given during the catarrhal stage. Antibiotics are of no value if the spasmodic stage has been reached and they should not be used unless secondary infection occurs. The milder case need not be kept in bed, and is better out of doors. A cough suppressant such as linctus methadone may be helpful in controlling the severity of paroxysms. When the illness is of long duration and vomiting is frequent, skilled nursing will be required to maintain nutrition, especially in infants and young children. Feeds are usually accepted and retained if they are given immediately after the vomiting which frequently follows a paroxysm of coughing.

**Prevention.** Active immunisation (p. 49) can occasionally cause convulsions or rarely neurological damage and adverse publicity regarding this has led to a marked decrease in the number of children who are immunised against the disease. However, the adverse effects of the vaccine have to be balanced against the risk of contracting a potentially serious disease, especially in young children. Many of the deaths from whooping cough occur in the first three months of life and hence very special care must be taken to avoid exposure of infants to the risk of contracting the disease.

## Diphtheria

By 1946 diphtheria, which was formerly a common and lethal disease in Britain, became so rare as a result of prophylactic inoculation that many doctors have never seen it. Yet in many parts of the world diphtheria is still an important cause of illness.

Infection with *Corynebacterium diphtheriae* occurs most commonly in the upper respiratory tract and sore throat is frequently the presenting feature. The disease is usually spread by droplet infection from cases or carriers. The organisms remain localised at the site of infection and the serious consequences result from the absorption of a soluble exotoxin which damages the heart muscle and the nervous system.

The infection may occur rarely on the conjunctiva or the genital tract, or it may complicate wounds, abrasions or diseases of the skin.

The disease is notifiable. The average incubation period is two to four days. Cases are isolated until cultures from six daily nose and throat swabs are negative.

**Clinical Features.** The diagnostic feature is the 'wash-leather' elevated membrane of variable extent on the tonsils with a well-defined edge and surrounded by a zone of inflammation. The membrane is firm and adherent. There may be swelling of the neck and tender enlargement of the lymph nodes. In the mildest infections, especially in the presence of a high degree of immunity, a membrane may never appear and the throat is merely slightly infected.

The disease begins insidiously. The temperature is seldom much raised although tachycardia is usually marked. The infection may remain mild if the membrane is confined to the anterior nares or the larynx or the tonsils. With anterior nasal infection there is also nasal discharge often tinged with blood. In laryngeal diphtheria there is a husky voice, a high-pitched cough, and a danger of respiratory obstruction which can be fatal if tracheostomy is not carried out. Tonsillar diphtheria usually causes a sore throat. When the infection spreads towards the uvula, to the fauces and then to the nasopharynx, the patient is often gravely ill and apathetic. The complexion is pale, the pulse rapid and of poor volume and the blood pressure low. Death from peripheral circulatory failure may occur within the first 10 days. Those who survive the earlier toxaemia may later develop arrhythmias or cardiac failure. Electrocardiographic changes are common and are due to myocarditis. These are reversible and there is no permanent damage to the heart in those who survive.

Involvement of the nervous system sometimes occurs, and after tonsillar or pharyngeal diphtheria it usually commences with palatal palsy on about the tenth day of the illness. The voice assumes a nasal quality, while regurgitation of fluids through the nose and sluggishness of palatal movements may be observed. Paralysis of accommodation soon follows and may be inferred from the patient's complaint of difficulty in reading small print.

A week or two later, though somewhat rarely, weakness and parasthaesia in the limbs due to polyneuritis may develop. In exceptional cases paralysis of the respiratory muscles may necessitate the use of a mechanical respirator. Recovery from such neuritis is always ultimately complete.

**Treatment.** Upon making a clinical diagnosis of diphtheria, the case should be notified to the community medical authorities and sent urgently to a hospital for infectious diseases. Antitoxin should be injected intramuscularly without awaiting the report on a throat swab. Every moment of delay increases the danger to the patient, because toxin, once fixed to the tissues, can no longer be neutralised by antitoxin. However, horse serum, in which antitoxin is contained, being a foreign protein, is liable to cause undesirable reactions. Firstly, there may be an immediate anaphylactic reaction with dyspnoea, pallor and collapse or even death. Secondly, within 7 to 12 days serum sickness, with fever, urticaria and joint pains may occur. If there is a previous history of inoculation of horse serum, the symptoms commonly appear in three or four days. As anaphylaxis is potentially lethal, every patient must be asked whether they have ever had antiserum before and whether they suffer from any allergic disorder. In all cases a small test injection of serum should be given half an hour before the full dose.

When a reaction does occur after the test dose in an allergic subject, rapid desensitisation must be undertaken with extreme caution. In all cases an ampoule of $^{1}/_{1000}$ adrenaline solution must be close at hand to deal with any immediate type of reaction (0·5–1·0 ml i.m.). An antihistamine is also given.

In a very severe case the risk of anaphylactic shock is outweighed by the mortal danger of diphtheritic toxaemia and up to 100 000 units of antitoxin should be injected intravenously if the test dose has not given rise to symptoms. For cases of moderate severity 16 000–32 000 units i.m. will suffice, and for mild cases 4000–8000 units.

Penicillin should be administered for one week to eliminate *C. diphtheriae*. Patients allergic to penicillin can be given erythromycin.

**Prevention.** The mortality in diphtheria, combined with the fact that the risks and cost of treatment are considerable, emphasise the necessity for active immunisation. This should be given in accordance with the instructions on page 49.

If diphtheria occurs in a closed community, a daily examination of the throat of all contacts should be made during the incubation period and swabs taken for the detection of carriers and potential cases. Those with positive throat swabs or with the slightest suspicion of clinical diphtheria should be isolated and given erythromycin which is more effective than penicillin in eradicating the organism in carriers. All contacts should also be advised to have active immunisation or a booster dose of toxoid.

Cases, convalescents and healthy carriers are isolated until six daily throat swabs are negative on culture.

## Salmonella Infections

There are more than 1200 Salmonella serotypes. The large majority originates in animals or poultry and is transmitted to man either directly or in food. The exception is *Salmonella typhi* which invariably has a human source.

Salmonellae can cause a number of different conditions:

1. Typhoid and paratyphoid fevers.
2. Food poisoning producing gastroenteritis, sometimes associated with septicaemia which may lead to metastatic abscess formation or endocarditis.
3. An asymptomatic carrier state which may follow 1. or 2.

### Typhoid and Paratyphoid (Enteric) Fevers

In many countries where sanitation is primitive, typhoid and paratyphoid fevers, which are transmitted by the faecal–oral route, are an important cause of illness. Elsewhere they are relatively rare. Nevertheless, outbreaks occur from time to time and the infection may be contracted by persons travelling abroad.

**Aetiology.** The enteric fevers are caused by infection with *S. typhi* and *paratyphi* which are specific human pathogens. Other members of the Salmonella group, many of which cause infection in animals, produce disease in man ranging from mild food poisoning to more serious infection which may simulate many of the features of paratyphoid fever including bacteraemia. Typhoid and paratyphoid infections have a world-wide distribution and occur endemically wherever sanitation is poor and the water supply is liable to be contaminated by human excreta. In Britain spread is usually by carriers, often food handlers, through the contamination of food, milk or water; infected shell fish are occasionally responsible for an outbreak. In carriers the bacilli may live in the gallbladder for months or years after clinical recovery and pass intermittently in the stools and less commonly in the urine.

**Pathogenesis.** After a few days of bacteraemia, the bacilli localise mainly in the lymphoid tissue of the small intestine. The typical lesion is in the Peyer's patches and follicles. These swell at first, then ulcerate and ultimately heal, but during this sequence they may perforate or bleed.

The incubation period of typhoid fever is about 10 to 14 days; that of paratyphoid is somewhat shorter. The diseases are notifiable. Quarantine is not necessary, but contacts are kept under surveillance for three weeks.

**Clinical Features.** *Typhoid Fever.* The onset may be insidious. The temperature rises in a step-ladder fashion for 4 or 5 days. There is malaise, with increasing headache, drowsiness and aching in the limbs. Cough and epistaxis are not uncommon; constipation may be present although in children diarrhoea and vomiting may be prominent early in the illness. The pulse is often slower than would be expected from the height of the temperature. At the end of the first week the typical rash may appear on the upper abdomen and on the back as sparse slightly raised, rose-red spots which fade on pressure. It is usually not visible on non-white skin. About the seventh to tenth day of illness the spleen becomes palpable. Often about this time constipation is succeeded by diarrhoea and generalised abdominal distension with tenderness in the right iliac fossa. Bronchitis may develop and there may be delirium. By the end of the second week the patient may be profoundly ill unless the disease is modified by antibiotic treatment. In the third week toxaemia increases and the patient may pass into coma and die. The prognosis may worsen at this stage due to haemorrhage from or perforation of the ulcerated Peyer's patches. In those who recover the temperature falls by lysis, the appetite returns, distension disappears, and strength improves. After an initial recovery recrudescence of the disease may occur.

*Paratyphoid Fever.* The most common variety in Britain is due to *S. paratyphi B*. The course tends to be shorter and milder than that of typhoid fever but the onset is often more abrupt with acute enteritis. The rash may be more abundant and the intestinal complications less frequent.

**Complications.** Haemorrhage and perforation may occur at the end of the second week or during the third week of the illness. The bleeding may be sudden and severe. The features of shock suggesting that a haemorrhage has occurred are described on page 331. Perforation usually occurs from ulcers near the ileocaecal valve. Additional complications may involve almost any viscus or system as a result of the septicaemia which is present during the first week. Pneumonia, thrombophlebitis, myocarditis, myositis, arthritis, periostitis, osteomyelitis, meningitis and cholecystitis are all recognised complications.

**Investigation.** In the first week of the disease the diagnosis may be difficult as in this invasive stage with bacteraemia the symptoms are those of a generalised infection without localising features. A white blood count may be helpful as there is typically a leucopenia. In a suspected case, blood culture is the most important diagnostic method, particularly during the first week of the disease. During this period the organism may not grow from the stool and urine using selective media. The faeces will contain the organism more frequently during the second and third weeks. Agglutinating antibodies to the causative organisms form after the second week of the disease (*Widal reaction*), but their detection is of limited value.

**Treatment.** The patient should be treated in bed and preferably in isolation. A high standard of nursing is required with special attention to the maintenance of nutrition and fluid intake, care of the mouth and the prevention of pressure sores. Scrupulous precautions must be taken against the spread of infection by the provision of special gowns and adequate washing facilities by the bed-side, and sterilisation of excreta and of articles used by the patient.

Chloramphenicol should be given for 14 days initially in a dose of 3 g daily, reducing to 2 g daily as the patient responds. Co-trimoxazole (or amoxycillin) is an alternative to chloramphenicol in typhoid fever and is the drug of choice for paratyphoid fever. Pyrexia may persist for up to five days after the start of antibiotic therapy. Even with effective chemotherapy there is still a danger of complications, of recrudescence of the disease and of the development of a carrier state. For the first few days a semifluid diet should be given, followed by a low roughage diet. A second course of chemotherapy must be given in the event of a relapse and this usually produces good results. The chronic carrier should be treated for several weeks with co-trimoxazole, as chloramphenicol has proved ineffective. In some cases cholecystectomy may be necessary.

The treatment of haemorrhage is described on page 331. Prior to the introduction of chloramphenicol the treatment of perforation was by immediate recourse to surgery, which carried a high mortality in the seriously ill. Such patients can be treated conservatively while chloramphenicol is continued, but advice from a surgeon should be sought as laparotomy may be indicated.

The patient should be considered as infective until six consecutive stools and urines are found to be negative on culture.

**Prevention.** Those who propose to travel to or live in countries where enteric infections are endemic should be inoculated with vaccine containing killed *S. typhi* and *S. paratyphi* A and B(TAB) (p. 894). The monovalent typhoid vaccine is probably more effective and is less likely to cause reactions.

## Bacterial Food Poisoning

Food poisoning includes a number of disorders presenting with diarrhoea and vomiting due to acute gastroenteritis developing up to 48 hours after the consumption of food or drink. It is customary not to include under this term the enteric fevers (p. 55), dysenteries (p. 59) and cholera (p. 830) which are also spread by infected food and drink. In contrast to enteric fever which is relatively uncommon and cholera which has been almost unknown in Britain for the past 100 years, there is an increase in the reported incidence of bacterial food poisoning.

Food poisoning may also be due to intestinal allergy, e.g. to shell fish, or to children eating unripe fruit or other unsuitable foods. Rarely a poisonous substance may be eaten, e.g. *Amanita phalloides*, in mistake for a mushroom or a chemical poison in food may be unwittingly consumed, an extreme example being arsenic administered murderously in the tradition of the Borgias. Food which has been placed in a container previously used for holding a chemical poison may be contaminated. Placing acid fruit juices in cheap enamel or zinc vessels may result in the liberation of antimony or zinc.

**Aetiology.** Bacterial food poisoning is usually divided into the infection and toxin types.

*Infection Type.* The organisms mainly responsible belong to the Salmonella group whose source is certain birds, rodents, cattle and less frequently reptiles, such as pet tortoises. The domestic fowl is one of the commonest sources and modern methods of poultry husbandry involving battery-rearing and deep-freezing of carcasses encourage the spread and transmission of infection. *Salmonella typhimurium* causes at least three-quarters of the cases of food poisoning of the 'infection' type in Britain. Food may be contaminated with infected excreta of mice or rats, or infection may be transferred by flies or by human carriers employed in the handling of food. The size of the infecting dose of bacteria bears a close relationship to the speed of onset of symptoms and to the severity of the illness. This indicates the dangers of bacterial multiplication which may take place when food is contaminated and thereafter remains warm for many hours or days. The types of food which are particularly likely to be affected are twice-cooked meat dishes, stews, soups, milk and synthetic cream. The danger of food poisoning is greatly reduced if such foods are kept in a refrigerator. Ducks tend to be carriers of salmonella organisms in the oviduct and alimentary tract, and ducks' eggs are not suitable for the preparation of lightly cooked foods. Hens' eggs are rarely affected.

Gastroenteritis caused by Campylobacter species is a common form of bacterial food poisoning. Sources of this infection include poultry and dogs.

*Toxin Type*. Such poisoning is most commonly caused by the enterotoxin of *Staph. aureus*. This frequently originates from a food handler suffering from a septic lesion. Incubation at a suitable temperature leads to growth of the organism and production of toxin which is relatively heat resistant and may not be destroyed by cooking. Strains of *Clostridium welchii*, many of them relatively resistant to heat, may contaminate certain foods, particularly meat. Pre-cooking of stews and pies may not destroy all the spores and the keeping of such food will lead to the formation of heat-stable toxins which can give rise to gastroenteritis, sometimes severe.

Outbreaks of food poisoning affecting large numbers of persons occur in canteens, restaurants, hospitals and other institutions.

**Clinical Features.** The simultaneous occurrence of symptoms in more than one member of a household or institution often simplifies diagnosis. The incubation period is a useful pointer to the aetiology. If vomiting starts within 30 minutes of the ingestion of suspected food, it is likely to be due to a chemical poison; if it arises 12 to 48 hours later, it is probably due to a Salmonella infection. The incubation periods of staphylococcal and clostridial food poisoning are usually intermediate between these extremes being from 1 to 12 hours.

The principal symptoms are nausea, vomiting, diarrhoea and abdominal colic. Staphylococcal food poisoning may be associated only with vomiting while diarrhoea and abdominal pain are more prominent with *Cl. welchii* toxins. In severe cases there may be prostration, collapse and dehydration. In the chemical and toxin types of food poisoning the onset tends to be sudden and severe and the patient may rapidly become shocked. Recovery however usually occurs within 24 hours. In the infection type, symptoms develop more slowly and there is usually pyrexia and toxicity. The patient may be ill for several days. The stools are watery and offensive, and may contain blood and some mucus, in contrast to bacillary dysentery where there is also pus. Salmonella septicaemia may be associated with osteomyelitis, septic arthritis, endocarditis or meningitis.

*Botulism* is a rare form of bacterial food poisoning due to the ingestion of one of the most potent poisons known to man, namely the toxin produced by *Cl. botulinum*. Imperfectly treated tinned food or preserved fish may be contaminated with the organism and be the source of the toxin. The clinical features differ from all other types of bacterial food poisoning and consist chiefly of vomiting and pareses of skeletal, ocular, pharyngeal and respiratory muscles. The mortality can be high.

**Investigation.** A specimen of the patient's stool or vomit together with the suspected food, if available, should be sent for culture. Organisms of the Salmonella group can usually be readily isolated. In more severe cases blood should be sent for culture. Notification of Salmonella infection and other types of food poisoning is compulsory in Britain.

**Treatment.** Most cases are mild and can be treated at home. Solid food should be withheld and the patient instructed to take fluids only. A pinch of salt added to one pint of water flavoured with a small quantity of fruit juice provides a satisfactory oral replacement solution. Patients who are severely ill, collapsed or dehydrated require intravenous fluid therapy.

Symptoms normally pass off spontaneously in a day or two. When acute symptoms cease, a semi-fluid low-roughage diet may be taken containing bread, butter, eggs, fish, soft puddings and jellies. Codeine phosphate or loperamide is useful in controlling diarrhoea.

Antibiotics should not be given for acute diarrhoea and vomiting as they are ineffective and frequently exacerbate symptoms. If salmonella bacteraemia is suspected or confirmed, ampicillin, 1 g every six hours should be given by intramuscular injection. Co-trimoxazole is a satisfactory alternative. Campylobacter infection is treated with erythromycin.

If the poisoning is thought to be due to a chemical or a poisonous food, the patient's stomach should be washed out with tepid water, using the technique described on page 785.

**Prevention.** In Salmonella food poisoning the carrier state persists on the average for about 14 days after infection but may be much longer, and the patient must not be allowed to handle food until he has stopped excreting the organism. A reduction in the high incidence of food poisoning can best be achieved by improving the standards of personal hygiene, especially in those handling food, and by stressing the importance of hand-washing after using the lavatory. Increasing facilities for low temperature storage of food which has to be kept for some hours or days before being consumed is of the greatest importance. It is essential to keep frozen poultry at room temperature for at least eight hours before cooking or pathogens at the centre may survive unharmed.

## Dysentery

Dysentery is an acute inflammation of the large intestine characterised by diarrhoea with blood and mucus in stools. Its causes are bacillary or protozoal infection. Amoebic dysentery is described on page 812.

### Bacillary Dysentery

The bacilli belong to the genus *Shigella* of which there are three main pathogenic groups, *Shiga*, *Flexner* and *Sonnei* the last two having numerous strains. In Britain the majority of cases of bacillary dysentery in recent years have been caused by *Shigella sonnei*.

**Epidemiology.** Bacillary dysentery in endemic form is found all over the world. It occurs in epidemic form wherever there is a crowded population with poor sanitation, and thus has been a constant accompaniment of wars and natural catastrophies. Spread may occur by contaminated food or flies but contact through unwashed hands after defaecation is by far the most important factor. Hence the modern provision of plenty of handbasins, disposable towels and hot air driers goes a long way towards the prevention of the faecal–oral spread of disease. Outbreaks are not uncommon in mental hospitals, residential schools and other closed institutions. The disease is notifiable.

**Pathology.** There is generalised inflammation of the large bowel which may extend to involve the lower part of the small intestine. Sigmoidoscopy shows that the mucosa is red and swollen, the submucous veins are obscured and mucopus is seen on the surface. Bleeding points appear readily at the touch of the endoscope. Ulcers may form.

**Clinical Features.** There is great variation in severity. Sonne infections may be so mild as to escape detection and the patient remains ambulant with a few loose stools and perhaps a little colic. Flexner infections are usually more severe while Shiga dysentery may be fulminating and cause death within 48 hours.

In a moderately severe illness, the patient complains of diarrhoea, colicky hypogastric pain and tenesmus. The stools are usually small, and after the first few evacuations, contain blood and purulent exudate with little faecal material. There is frequently fever, with dehydration and weakness if the diarrhoea persists. On physical examination there will be tenderness over the colon more easily elicited in the left iliac fossa. In Sonne infection the patient may develop a febrile illness and diarrhoea may be mild or even absent; there is usually some headache and muscular aching. Arthritis, encephalitis or iritis may occasionally complicate bacillary dysentery.

Diagnosis depends on culture of faeces. Amoebic infections usually have a less acute onset than bacillary dysentery.

**Treatment and Prevention.** Diarrhoea may be controlled by codeine or loperamide. A fluid or semifluid low-roughage diet should be given depending on the severity of the diarrhoea but if this is severe, it will be necessary to replace the water and electrolyte loss by intravenous therapy.

Bacillary dysentery is usually a self-limiting disease and antibiotics or sulphonamides are not indicated in most cases. In severe infections, especially those caused by Shiga or Flexner strains, ampicillin 500 mg 6 hourly or co-trimoxazole two tablets twice daily should be given. In Britain the majority of shigellae are now sulphonamide-resistant although in tropical countries sulphonamides are still of value in severe bacillary dysentery. When they are used, an ample intake of fluids must be ensured in order to guard against anuria due to the precipitation of crystals in the kidneys.

The prevention of faecal contamination of food and milk, the isolation of cases, and the identification of carriers, are methods which are theoretically important but may be difficult to apply except in limited outbreaks. Hand-washing is very important.

### Travellers' Diarrhoea

A short attack of diarrhoea commonly affects travellers, especially in the tropics. The attack is usually acute, with watery stools and sometimes vomiting. It lasts 2 to 5 days and is self-limiting. Enterotoxigenic *Esch. coli* has been implicated in many attacks. Specific antimicrobial treatment is not indicated but fluid balance should be maintained by adequate drinking or, rarely, intravenous fluids. Symptoms may be controlled by codeine phosphate or loperamide. If diarrhoea persists stools should be examined microscopically for *Giardia intestinalis* and *Entamoeba histolytica*, and cultured for salmonella and shigella. Persistence of mild diarrhoea after travel is a feature of giardiasis (p. 814) and amoebiasis (p. 812).

## Tetanus

This disease results from infection with *Clostridium tetani*, which exists as a commensal in the gut of man and domestic animals and is found in soils. Infection enters the body through wounds, often trivial, such as those caused by a splinter, a nail in the boot or a garden fork or following septic infection such as a dirty abrasion. The disease is thus most commonly found in agricultural workers and gardeners. If childbirth takes place in an unhygienic environment *tetanus neonatorum* may result from infection of the umbilical stump or the mother may develop the disease.

In circumstances unfavourable to the growth of the organism, spores are formed and these may remain dormant for years. Spores germinate and bacilli multiply only in the anaerobic conditions which occur in areas of tissue necrosis or if the oxygen tension is low as a result of the presence of other organisms, particularly aerobic ones. The bacilli remain localised but produce an exotoxin with an affinity for motor nerve endings and motor nerve cells. Involvement of the former by direct spread causes local tetanus. The anterior horn cells are affected after the exotoxin has passed into the blood stream and their involvement results in rigidity and convulsions. Symptoms first appear from two days to several weeks after injury — the shorter the incubation period, the more severe the attacks and the outcome may well be fatal with an incubation period of only a few days.

**Clinical Features.** Much the most important early symptom is trismus — spasm of the masseter muscles which causes difficulty in opening the mouth and in masticating, hence the name, 'lockjaw'. This tonic rigidity spreads to involve the muscles of the face, neck and trunk. Contraction of the frontalis and the muscles at the angles of the mouth gives rise to the 'risus sardonicus'. There is rigidity of the muscles of the neck and trunk of varying degree. The back is usually slightly arched and the board-like abdominal wall resembles that seen a few hours after the perforation of a peptic ulcer, but there is little or no tenderness. In the more severe cases sudden violent spasms lasting for a few seconds to 3 or 4 minutes occur spontaneously or may be induced by stimuli such as moving the patient, knocking the bed or making a noise. These convulsions are painful, exhausting and of very serious significance, especially if they appear soon after the onset of symptoms. They gradually increase in frequency and severity for about one week and the patient may die from exhaustion, asphyxia or aspiration pneumonia. In less severe cases convulsions may not commence for about a week after the first sign of rigidity and in very mild infections they may never appear.

Rarely the only manifestation of the disease may be *local tetanus* — stiffness or spasm of the muscles near the infected wound — and the prognosis is good if treatment is commenced at this stage. If local tetanus follows wounds of the head and neck, the resulting irritation or paralysis of cranial nerves may resemble tuberculous meningitis or polioencephalitis and in cases of doubt the cerebrospinal fluid should be examined; in tetanus it is normal. Lumbar punctures should be avoided except in cases of real doubt.

The diagnosis is made on clinical grounds. It is rarely possible to isolate the infecting organism from the original locus of entry. Spasm of the masseters due to dental abscess, septic throat or other causes is painful, in contradistinction to tetanus.

Tetanus is still one of the major killers of adults, children and neonates in the tropics; the mortality is nearly 100% in the newborn and around 40% in others.

**Treatment.** This should be begun as soon as possible. The essentials are as follows:

1. *Prevention of further Absorption of Toxin from the Wound.* A single intravenous injection of immune serum containing 10 000 i.u. of antitoxin should be given immediately the diagnosis is suspected. Whenever possible *human* antitetanus globulin should be used. The wound requires to be thoroughly cleaned and drained if there is evidence of necrotic tissue, foreign body or sepsis. Surgery should not be undertaken until 1 hour after the injection of antitoxin. Benzylpenicillin should be administered in doses of 300 mg 6 hourly.

2. *Control of Spasms.* The patient should lie in a quiet darkened room on a flat comfortable bed, with the bedclothes supported by a cradle. A notice should be put outside the door requesting silence. All necessary manipulation of the patient should be done gently and with due warning, for unexpected stimuli are particularly liable to provoke spasms. Expert nursing is of supreme importance.

In most cases spasms may be prevented by diazepam. In more serious cases curare should be given, but only when facilities for assisted respiration are available. The aim of such measures is to control spasms which are terrifying, exhausting and occasionally fatal.

3. *General Measures.* Nutrition and fluids are of vital importance to enable the patient to survive an ordeal which may be prolonged. In milder cases it may be possible for the patient to swallow fluids or to tolerate a stomach tube left *in situ*. If oral treatment is impossible, intravenous feeding should be commenced without delay. Aspiration of bronchial secretions and antibiotic treatment of pneumonia may be necessary.

**Prevention.** Active immunisation should be given (p. 49). Contaminated injuries must be treated by debridement. The immediate danger of tetanus can be greatly reduced by the injection of a dose of a long-acting preparation of penicillin followed by a 7-day course of oral penicillin. When the risk of tetanus is judged to be present, further protection may be given by a subcutaneous injection of 250 units of human tetanus antitoxin, and an intramuscular injection of toxoid which should be repeated one month and six months later. For those already protected only a booster dose of toxoid is required.

## Brucellosis

*(Undulant Fever; Malta Fever; Abortus Fever)*

Brucellosis is caused in Britain by infection with *Brucella abortus* which is usually spread to man by the ingestion of raw milk from infected cattle. It is also an occupational hazard of veterinary surgeons, laboratory personnel, slaughterhouse workers and others. In Malta and many other countries the disease is frequently due to *Br. melitensis* and is transmitted by infected goat's milk. In the USA and the Far East *Br. suis* acquired from pigs may be the causative organism. The disease is not notifiable. The incubation period is about 3 weeks.

**Clinical Features.** The disease commences as a blood stream infection and the clinical manifestations are gradual in onset and variable. The symptoms in order of frequency are sweating, weakness, headache, anorexia, pain in limbs and back, constipation, rigors, and joint pains. The spleen may be palpable. The temperature characteristically shows undulations, during which febrile and afebrile periods alternate over periods of a week or so. In other cases the pyrexia may be continuous and sweating profuse. Arthritis, spondylitis, bursitis and osteomyelitis may occur (p. 626). Untreated, the disease may last for a few days or continue for many months, and in the latter case the patient often becomes extremely depressed. Neutropenia and lymphocytosis usually occur in the more severe cases.

The diagnosis of brucellosis is most readily confirmed by agglutination and complement-fixation tests. Blood culture in special media should be attempted but it is rarely positive in *Br. abortus* infections in man. Other conditions causing prolonged fever must be considered in differential diagnosis (p. 47).

**Treatment and Prevention.** Tetracycline 500 mg 6 hourly or co-trimoxazole 2 tablets twice a day for 21 days is usually effective. The spread of brucellosis by milk is prevented by pasteurisation or boiling. Veterinary surgeons and others handling infected animals need to exercise scrupulous hygiene.

## Meningococcal Infections

Infections caused by the Gram-negative diplococcus, *Neisseria meningitidis*, are serious and not infrequently fatal. In the Sudan savanna belt of Africa special climatic conditions predispose to annual outbreaks of 10 000 to 100 000 cases. Spread is by the airborne route and epidemics occur, particularly in cramped living conditions or when the climate is hot and dry. The organism invades through the nasopharynx producing bacteraemia and usually also pyogenic meningitis. The meningococcus is the commonest cause of bacterial meningitis in Britain where an increasing proportion of meningococci have become sulphonamide-resistant; fortunately, all strains remain sensitive to penicillin.

**Clinical Features**. The disease may present in a fulminating form with abrupt onset and prostration associated with shock and a widespread purpuric rash. The progression of the infection may be relentless even with chemotherapy and the patient can die within hours of the first symptom. Disseminated intravascular coagulation (p. 601) can also occur in the course of meningococcal infections.

Meningitis (p. 702) is a much commoner presentation. Upper respiratory symptoms for 1 to 2 days are followed by fever, vomiting, headache and usually a petechial rash. This frequently starts with a few lesions on the buttocks spreading to involve limbs and trunk. The spots can remain petechial but occasionally large purpuric areas may form. The patient, often a child, is febrile and toxic, and signs of meningeal irritation are common. Convulsions may occur, especially in babies.

Chronic meningococcaemia is a rare condition in which the patient can be unwell for weeks or even months with recurrent fever, sweating, joint pains (p. 626) and transient rash.

**Investigation**. There is a polymorph leucocytosis. The CSF is turbid due to the presence of many polymorphs, the protein content is raised and the glucose reduced. The diagnosis is confirmed bacteriologically by culture of *N. meningitidis* from blood or CSF. Microscopic examination of CSF may show Gram-negative kidney-shaped diplococci in the polymorphs. However, in a proportion of cases, particularly if the patient has been treated with an antibiotic prior to admission to hospital, Gram stain and culture of CSF may be unhelpful and an early clinical diagnosis is therefore of the utmost importance in a disease which can be so rapidly fatal.

**Treatment and Prevention**. Benzylpenicillin, given initially by intravenous injection, is the antibiotic of choice for meningococcal infection. Because of superior penetration of the 'blood-brain barrier' sulphadimidine is frequently given as well as penicillin, but this is not necessary. An intravenous infusion should be set up and shock treated (p. 167). Intravascular coagulation may be an indication for heparin therapy (p. 601).

Close contacts of patients with meningococcal infections, especially children, should be given a 5 day course of minocycline or rifampicin. Vaccines are available for the prevention of disease caused by meningococci of Groups A and C but not Group B which is the commonest serogroup isolated in many countries including Britain.

## Sexually Transmitted Disease

Venereal diseases are almost invariably contracted during coitus. Gonorrhoea and non-gonococcal urethritis are common in Britain, but syphilis is relatively rare. Chancroid (p. 835), granuloma inguinale (p. 823), and lymphogranuloma venereum (p. 851) are very rare in Britain but are frequent in parts of the tropics. About half of the cases of syphilis and a quarter of the cases of gonorrhoea in British men occur in homosexuals.

### Gonorrhoea

Gonorrhoea, a major epidemic disease in the world today, is due to infection of the mucous membrane of the genitourinary tract with *Neisseria gonorrhoeae*. The eyes, rectum and throat may also be infected. The incubation period is about 2 to 10 days.

**Clinical Features**. In the male the infection starts in the anterior urethra and tends to spread to the posterior urethra and epididymes. There is dysuria and a white or yellow discharge from the urethra. If untreated or inadequately treated, the discharge becomes less or intermittent and may be observed only on waking.

In females the infection starts in the lower cervical canal, the urethra or the rectum. At the onset there may be dysuria and vaginal discharge but in about half the women there are no symptoms. Upward spread leads to pelvic involvement in a few cases. Infection of the conjunctiva of infants born of infected mothers causes purulent discharge and damage to sight. This condition, known as *ophthalmia neonatorum*, is now very rare in Britain, but remains an important cause of blindness in many tropical areas. Systemic spread of gonorrhoea is rare and usually takes the form of bacteraemia characterised by fever, joint pains and a rash — commonly peripheral haemorrhagic pustules surrounded by a zone of erythema, though other lesions may occur. Gonococcal arthritis (p. 626) is now rare. Gonorrhoea may be suspected clinically but the diagnosis depends on results of laboratory tests. Gram-negative intracellular diplococci can be seen in pus from infected tracts, but this finding must be confirmed by culture of exudate on an appropriate medium.

**Treatment**. A single i.m. injection of 2·4g (2·4 million units) of procaine penicillin plus 1 g of probenecid by mouth or ampicillin (2 g) plus probenecid (1 g) together by mouth are usually sufficient to cure most infections in Britain. For refractory infections or those in which the gonococci have been shown to be relatively resistant to penicillin, the dose of procaine penicillin may be increased to 4·8 million units and that of ampicillin to 3·5 g but probenecid must also be given. Co-trimoxazole or spectinomycin are effective alternatives for patients allergic to penicillin and these two preparations or cefoxitin may be given when penicillin resistant gonococci are involved. Gonococcal conjunctivitis responds to intramuscular penicillin and local chloramphenicol. It is essential to establish that cure of gonorrhoea and any accompanying infection is complete by repeating cultures of secretions from infected tracts. Syphilis acquired at the same time as gonorrhoea may be missed because of its long incubation period or it may be obscured by chemotherapy. It is obligatory that serological tests for syphilis are repeated after three months.

**Trichomoniasis**. Infection with *Trichomonas vaginalis* is commonly present in women with gonorrhoea and requires treatment with metronidazole 2 g in a single oral dose or 200 mg thrice daily for 7 days.

**Non-Gonococcal Urethritis.** In Britain, urethritis in males is more commonly due to organisms other than the gonococcus. About half of these cases are due to chlamydiae and some are due to ureaplasmas. Treatment is with tetracycline. Non-gonococcal urethritis also occurs in Reiter's syndrome (p. 620).

## Syphilis

This is a chronic infection due to *Treponema pallidum*. It may be acquired by the patient during sexual intercourse or a fetus may be infected *in utero* — the congenital form of the infection. Acquired and congenital syphilis are conveniently divided into early infectious and late non-infectious phases.

Early acquired syphilis may be sub-divided into primary and secondary stages, while late acquired syphilis may be sub-divided into tertiary or benign gummatous syphilis, neurosyphilis (p. 704) and cardiovascular syphilis (p. 214). During the early and late phases of both acquired and congenital syphilis, latent periods occur and the disease may be latent throughout its long course. It must be realised that the disease is systemic from the beginning and is continuous.

### Clinical Features

**1. Acquired Syphilis.** PRIMARY STAGE. The primary lesion (chancre) develops at the site of infection after an incubation period of 9 to 90 days. The chancre usually occurs on the genitalia but it may occasionally be found at the anus or elsewhere. A small pink macule appears which soon becomes papular and ulcerates. The regional lymph nodes are enlarged, rubbery and painless but not tender.

SECONDARY STAGE. The primary lesion tends to heal and 6 to 8 weeks after its appearance evidence of generalised infection appears with malaise, headache and low irregular fever. Four cardinal signs must be remembered though any of them may be absent.

*1. A rash* is present in 75% of patients. This starts as a faint macular eruption and develops into a papular rash which is characteristically polymorphic, symmetrical, dull red and does not itch; it may become scaly.

*2. Condylomata lata* are large flat papules that develop in warm moist areas such as the perineum. They contain many treponemes and are highly infectious.

*3. Lymphadenopathy* is found in 50% of patients and is widespread. Lymph nodes become moderately enlarged, but are not tender.

*4. Mucous patches*, occurring in 30% of patients, are superfical ulcers on the mucous membranes of the genitalia, mouth and throat. They may have a characteristic white base and narrow red margin and may coalesce to form so-called snail track ulcers. They are highly infectious.

In over 30% of cases changes occur in the cerebrospinal fluid, indicating involvement of the central nervous system; the clinical features of low-grade meningitis may rarely be present, accompanied sometimes by cranial nerve palsies. Rarely there may also be disease of the eyes, bones or abdominal viscera. After several months the secondary changes gradually disappear to be followed by a latent period.

TERTIARY STAGE. This takes ten or more years to develop and mainly affects skin and subcutaneous tissues, mucous membranes and sub-mucosa, and the long bones. Lesions run a long but benign course. The characteristic pathological lesion is a granuloma called a gumma.

NEUROSYPHILIS AND CARDIOVASCULAR SYPHILIS. Neurosyphilis (p. 704) and cardiovascular syphilis (p. 214) take longer to develop characteristic features and may lead to the patient's death.

**2. Congenital Syphilis**. The fetus may contract syphilis from an infected mother. There is then no primary stage. The disease may be so severe that the child is born dead, or skin eruptions may be present at birth. The child may appear to be normal at birth but fails to thrive, and within a few months develops a rash, and signs of syphilitic disease of bone, liver, kidneys and other organs. In a third group of cases the overt manifestations may be delayed for years until such features appear as deformities of bones and teeth, iritis, keratitis, lesions of the eighth cranial nerve, juvenile tabes or general paralysis.

Congenital syphilis is now rare in Western countries as screening in antenatal clinics and treatment of a syphilitic woman during pregnancy usually ensures the birth of a normal baby.

**Diagnosis**. In the primary and secondary stages, treponemes may be demonstrated in serum from the chancre, papular rash, condylomata or mucous patches. The serological tests for syphilis become positive from about the fourth week of the disease and are invariably strongly positive in the secondary stage in untreated cases. It should be realised that non-specific antigen is used in the usual serological screening tests – Wassermann (WR), Kahn and Venereal Disease Research Laboratory (VDRL) tests. Hence the specificity and sensitivity of such tests is variable. False positive results may be found in glandular fever, systemic lupus erythematosus and other generalised diseases, while negative results may be observed in some patients with late syphilis. For conclusive results additional tests which use specific treponemal antigen, e.g. fluorescent treponemal antibody (FTA-ABS), *T. pallidum* haemagglutination (TPHA) and treponemal immobilisation (TPI) tests, are required.

**Treatment.** *T. pallidum*, though very sensitive to benzylpenicillin, needs exposure to it for longer periods than most micro-organisms. Hence longer acting forms such as procaine penicillin are used. A patient with primary syphilis requires 600 mg procaine penicillin daily for 10 to 12 consecutive days. For secondary, tertiary or latent syphilis the course should be continued for 14 to 15 days, and for neurosyphilis and cardiovascular syphilis it should be prolonged for 21 days. In large patients the dose should be increased to 900 mg or even 1·2 g procaine penicillin. Tetracycline should be given to patients allergic to penicillin. All patients must be followed up to ensure cure.

## Leptospirosis

Although over 100 serotypes of leptospires have been identified only *Leptospira icterohaemorrhagiae* and *L. canicola* have been shown to cause human disease in Britain.

The natural host of *Weil's disease,* caused by *L. icterohaemorrhagiae*, is the rat. An infected rat's urine contains the organisms which can penetrate the skin or mucosa of a man. Fish cleaners, farm workers, veterinarians, and vagrants are those most at risk. Immersion in canals or stagnant water may also result in sporadic infection. In patients dying from Weil's disease, there is a combination of hepatic, renal and cardiac failure.

Infection by *L. canicola*, which is contracted from dogs and pigs, usually presents as aseptic meningitis or pyrexia of unknown origin. It is not often associated with jaundice and is less severe than Weil's disease.

**Clinical Features**. The average incubation period is 10 days, the range being 4 to 21 days. A high proportion of infections are subclinical or cause a mild undiagnosed fever. In the more severe infections the illness begins abruptly with headache, severe myalgia, pyrexia, conjunctival suffusion, anorexia and vomiting. Infrequently, there are rashes or petechiae and enlargement of the liver and spleen.

After about a week leptospiral antibodies appear in the blood. The temperature falls by lysis and is usually normal for 2 or 3 days. In the majority of patients, there is further pyrexia for a few days and transient meningism (p. 702) followed by prompt recovery. In other cases, especially those caused by *L. icterohaemorrhagiae*, during this phase, hepatitis, renal tubular necrosis, myocarditis and meningitis may occur. The condition may progress to acute liver necrosis (p. 397). Renal tubular necrosis may lead to acute renal failure (p. 447). Myocarditis is suggested by tachycardia, fall in blood pressure and cardiac enlargement. The development of profound hypotension, arrhythmias and cardiac failure are ominous signs. Meningitis causes severe headache, neck stiffness and a positive Kernig's sign (p. 702) and is the usual clinical picture in *L. canicola* infections.

By the third and fourth week of the illness, the majority of patients enter the convalescent phase. When there has been serious involvement of the liver, kidneys and heart, mortality in Weil's disease is in the region of 15 to 20%. Those who recover do so completely.

**Investigation**. Most patients with leptospirosis show a polymorphonuclear leucocytosis. When there is liver involvement, liver function tests indicate a mild hepatocellular jaundice with an intrahepatic obstructive element; bilirubin and urobilinogen are present in the urine. In patients with renal failure the urine contains protein, red blood cells and cellular and granular casts; in severe cases the rise in blood urea is progressive. Meningitis is characterised by an increase of lymphocytes in the cerebrospinal fluid with little or no rise in protein; xanthochromia may be observed in the jaundiced patient.

The diagnosis is made by culturing the organism from the blood in the first week or from the urine in the second and third weeks. Alternatively, blood or urine specimens may be inoculated into a guinea-pig. From the second week onwards, a rising titre of specific leptospiral antibodies is found. The titre may not reach diagnostic levels in those cases treated promptly.

**Treatment.** Leptospires are sensitive to penicillin *in vitro*. Benzylpenicillin, 600 mg (1 million units) 6 hourly for 7 days is effective provided it is given early enough and in adequate doses; it shortens the average illness and reduces the incidence of complications. Penicillin is of doubtful value if treatment is initiated late in the infection. Appropriate fluid replacement is important during the period of acute illness. In severely affected patients supportive treatment for acute liver necrosis, acute renal failure, arrhythmias and cardiac failure may be required.

## Measles

Measles is a viral disease which spreads by droplet infection. One attack confers a high degree of immunity. Most people suffer from measles in childhood, and a mother who has had the disease confers passive immunity on her infant for the first six months of life. Measles is very severe with a high mortality in many tropical countries. The incubation period is about 10 days to the commencement of the catarrhal stage. A quarantine period is not necessary.

**Clinical Features.** *Catarrhal Stage.* Measles commences in much the same way as a common cold. There is an acute febrile onset, with nasal catarrh, sneezing, redness of the conjunctivae, swelling of the eyelids and watering of the eyes. In addition a cough, hoarseness of the voice due to laryngitis, and photophobia usually appear by the second day. At this stage, a diagnosis of measles may be made from the presence of Koplik's spots on the mucous membrane of the mouth. These are small white spots surrounded by a narrow zone of inflammation. Though often numerous on the inside of the cheeks, they may be sparse and confined to the region around the opening of the parotid duct. The disease is highly infectious during the catarrhal stage and the child is miserable and irritable.

*Exanthematous Stage.* After 3 or 4 days of the catarrhal stage, the diagnostic Koplik's spots disappear while the dark red macular or maculopapular rash develops. The rash is first seen at the back of the ears and at the junction of the forehead and the hair. Within a few hours there is invasion of the whole skin area, and there is usually some accentuation of fever. As the spots rapidly become more numerous they fuse to form the characteristic blotchy appearance of measles. The face is ordinarily the most densely covered area. When the rash is fully erupted in 2 or 3 days, it tends to deepen in colour and then fade into a faint brown staining followed by a fine desquamation of the skin. The malaise and the fever subside as the rash fades.

**Complications.** Convulsions occur in young children and are commonest as the rash is appearing. Secondary infection by haemolytic streptococci, pneumococci or staphylococci may cause otitis media or pneumonia. Persistent conjunctivitis may be followed by corneal ulceration which, if neglected, may result in impairment of vision. Stomatitis, gastroenteritis, appendicitis and encephalitis may also occur.

**Treatment.** The patient should be isolated if possible and excluded from school for 10 days from the appearance of the rash. Most cases of measles, in spite of the high temperature, remain uncomplicated, and antibiotics should be prescribed only for unequivocal bacterial complications.

**Prevention.** ACTIVE IMMUNISATION. One injection of live attenuated measles virus should be given subcutaneously in children over one year old who have not had the disease. The protection lasts for over 12 years.

PASSIVE IMMUNISATION. Human immunoglobulin, given intramuscularly, is recommended for the prevention or attenuation of measles, particularly for contacts under 18 months of age and for debilitated children. The dose is 250 mg for children under one year old and 500 mg for those over this age.

## Rubella (German Measles)

Rubella is a viral disease which spreads by droplet infection. One attack confers a high degree of immunity. It tends to affect older children, adolescents and young adults and spreads less readily than measles. The disease in children is trivial. In adults the illness may be more severe, but of short duration and of little importance except when it develops in a woman during the first four months of pregnancy. In such cases the child may be born with a congenital malformation such as a cardiac or mental defect, cataract or deafness. The risk of damage to the fetus by the rubella virus varies from over 70% during the first 4 weeks of pregnancy to virtually zero after the end of the fourth month. The disease is not notifiable. The incubation period is usually about 18 days. A quarantine period is not necessary.

**Clinical Features.** In children the constitutional symptoms are so slight that the illness is rarely suspected until the rash is seen. The spots are pink macules which appear first behind the ears and on the forehead. The rash spreads rapidly, first to the trunk and then to the limbs. A minor degree of conjunctival suffusion is common. Tender enlargement of the suboccipital lymph nodes is usual. Sometimes many groups of lymph nodes are affected and the tip of the spleen may be palpable. In adolescents and adults the onset may be acute with fever and generalised aches, but even then the illness lasts for only 2 or 3 days.

Polyarthritis, is the commonest complication. Encephalomyelitis and thrombocytopenic purpura are very rare. Complete recovery from all of them is the rule.

The diagnosis can be confirmed by isolation of the virus from the throat or by demonstration of a rising titre of antibody in the blood.

**Treatment and Prevention.** No treatment is available. If infection is known to have occurred during the first 16 weeks of pregnancy there is such a high chance of fetal abnormality that termination should be recommended. It is therefore advisable to vaccinate all girls between their 11th and 13th birthdays who have not had the disease. Women of child-bearing age who are found to be serologically negative should also be offered vaccine provided that they are not pregnant and are willing to avoid pregnancy for eight weeks after vaccination.

## Mumps

Mumps is caused by a virus which spreads by droplet infection and affects mainly children of school age and young adults. The infectivity rate is not high and there is serological evidence that 30–40% of infections are clinically inapparent. The incubation period is about 18 days. A quarantine period is not necessary.

**Clinical Features.** Malaise, fever, trismus and pain near the angle of the jaw is soon followed by tender swelling of one or both parotid glands. Indeed, parotid swelling alone is often the first feature. The submandibular salivary glands may also be involved. The swollen glands subside in a few days, and may be succeeded by swelling of a previously unaffected gland. Orchitis occurs in about one in four males who develop mumps after puberty; it is usually on one side only, but if it is bilateral, sterility may be a sequel. Obscure abdominal pain may be due to pancreatitis or oöphoritis. Acute lymphocytic meningitis is another mode of presentation. Encephalomyelitis is rare.

Most cases of mumps can be diagnosed on clinical grounds alone, but the diagnosis can be confirmed in doubtful cases by the demonstration of specific antibodies, or the virus may be cultured from the saliva, or from the cerebrospinal fluid in meningitis.

**Treatment.** Oral hygiene is important when the mouth is very dry due to lack of saliva. Apart from the relief of symptoms as they appear, no other treatment is necessary. Orchitis can be relieved by prednisolone (40 mg daily for 4 days). Cases of mumps should be isolated until the gland last affected has subsided.

## Chickenpox

Chickenpox (varicella) is a viral infection which spreads by droplets from the upper respiratory tract or by contamination from the discharge from ruptured lesions of the skin or through contact with herpes zoster (p. 711). Herpes zoster is due to reactivation of infection with chickenpox virus and may be accompanied by a varicelliform rash. Chickenpox is highly infectious and chiefly affects children under 10 years of age. Most children are little incommoded by this disease but, as often happens with viral infections, adults may develop a more severe illness including a prodromal rash. Second attacks are very rare. In patients on long-term steroid therapy the disease may be severe or even fatal. Most recorded fatalities have been suffering from leukaemia and it is probable that the blood disorder has been the major factor in reducing resistance to the virus. The disease is not notifiable. The incubation period is 14 – 21 days.

**Clinical Features.** Constitutional symptoms are usually brief and mild, and the first sign of the disease is often the appearance of the rash. Lesions are sometimes present on the palate before the characteristic rash appears on the trunk on the second day of the illness. Then the face and finally the limbs are involved. The spots reach their maximum density upon the trunk, and are more sparse on the periphery of the limbs. Macules appear first and within a few hours the lesions become papular and then vesicular. The vesicles are unilocular, very superficial and thin-walled. The shape is elliptical rather than spherical. Within 24 hours the lesions become pustular. The vesicles and pustules are so fragile that they may be ruptured by the chafing of garments. Damage from scratching is also frequent, since itching may be troublesome. Whether or not the pustules rupture, they dry up in a few days to form scabs. The spots appear in crops, so that lesions at all stages of development are seen in any area at the same time.

The course of the disease is usually uneventful but secondary infection may occur. Serious complications, which are rare, include chickenpox pneumonia (p. 244), proliferative glomerulonephritis (p. 430), and acute demyelinating encephalomyelitis (p. 715).

**Treatment.** No treatment is required in the majority of cases. At the first sign of secondary infection a local antiseptic should be applied to the skin, e.g. chlorhexidine. If bacterial infection progresses, an antibiotic should be prescribed. Children who lack natural immunity owing to leukaemia, immunological deficiency, or treatment with corticosteroid or cytotoxic drugs, and who have been in contact with chickenpox should be given an injection of human anti-varicella gammaglobulin.

Spread of infection can be prevented by isolation of the patient and the sterilisation of all soiled articles, but the disease is usually so mild that in domiciliary practice these precautions are not normally required.

### Smallpox

As a result of an intensive WHO programme of case detection and vaccination, it is confidently believed that smallpox has been eradicated. Apart from two laboratory-acquired infections in 1978, the last known case occurred in Somalia in 1977. Major smallpox produces a severe constitutional disturbance associated with a peripherally distributed rash with lesions which, in any one area, progress in unison from macules through papules to pustules. The mortality rate may be as high as 40%.

A similar virus causes *monkeypox* in primates in jungle areas of Central Africa, with lesions resembling those of smallpox. Some human cases have occurred in those in contact with infected primates but inter-human spread is exceptional.

The virus of smallpox is being maintained in a few designated laboratories, particularly in order to be able to differentiate such diseases as monkeypox from smallpox. Only staff employed in the vicinity of these designated laboratories now require to be vaccinated against smallpox. Limited stocks of smallpox vaccine are available for this purpose and in case, contrary to all expectation, the disease should reappear.

## CHEMOTHERAPY OF INFECTIONS

The ability of one micro-organism to interfere with the growth of another is called antibiosis and is due to specific diffusible metabolic products termed *antibiotics*. Since the introduction of penicillin in 1940, research has produced a wide range of antibiotics. A variety of chemotherapeutic agents such as metronidazole, trimethoprim, dapsone and isoniazid has also followed the demonstration of the therapeutic effect of sulphanilamide in 1935. A general term for all of these substances is *antimicrobial agent*. Effective chemotherapy is now available against all known bacteria, rickettsiae, mycoplasmas and chlamydia. Specific antiprotozoal compounds are used in the treatment of diseases such as sleeping sickness, kala azar, malaria and amoebic dysentery. Topical antifungal agents are widely prescribed, but fully effective, non-toxic, antifungal drugs have not yet been found for use in systemic infection. Antimicrobial agents active against viruses have also been discovered but few have been successful therapeutically.

### The Sulphonamides

Although the sulphonamides have been superseded in many countries by antibiotics, their usefulness has been greatly extended by the introduction of co-trimoxazole, a combination of a sulphonamide and trimethoprim. The preparations most suitable for clinical use are the short-acting sulphonamides, e.g. sulphadimidine. It is rapidly absorbed and quickly excreted in the urine in a soluble form. Administration is every 4 to 8 hours, by mouth; a preparation is also available for intravenous or intramuscular administration.

The most common indication for the use of sulphonamides is cystitis. A dose of 1 g, 8 hourly is adequate since the drugs give high concentrations in the urine. Sulphonamides have long been used in the treatment of meningococcal infection, particularly meningitis; unfortunately the incidence of resistant strains is increasing and therefore penicillin is now used in treating this condition.

**Adverse Effects.** Sulphonamides have a wide range of potential hazards including rashes, fever, agranulocytosis, haematuria and anuria. The risks of haematuria and anuria can be decreased by ensuring an adequate output of alkaline urine. Serious but rare complications are haemolytic anaemia, purpura and pancytopenia. Glucose-6-phosphate dehydrogenase deficiency (p. 556) is a contraindication to the use of sulphonamides, as haemolysis may be induced. The Stevens–Johnson syndrome (erythema multiforme and ulceration of mucous membranes) may be induced by sulphonamide and can be fatal. When any of the above complications develop the drug must be stopped immediately.

Sulphonamides can detach protein-bound drugs such as warfarin and sulphonylurea antidiabetic agents and thereby cause overdosage.

Sulphonamide preparations applied to the skin are liable to cause light sensitivity which may persist for a number of years; they should not be used topically.

**Co-trimoxazole.** The two components of this compound, trimethoprim and sulphamethoxazole, act by inhibiting enzymes at two successive stages in the synthesis of para-aminobenzoic acid to folic acid and DNA. Co-trimoxazole is particularly useful in exacerbations of chronic bronchitis and infections of the urinary tract. It is also effective in the treatment of invasive Salmonella infections and typhoid carriers. The adult dose is 2 tablets twice daily and there is a preparation for injection.

The adverse effects are those of the sulphonamides but the clinician must also be on the alert for possible haematological reactions to trimethoprim including thrombocytopenia and megaloblastic anaemia due to folate deficiency (p. 552).

*Trimethoprim* alone is now available for the treatment of urinary tract infection for which it is given in a dose of 200 mg twice a day, or 100 mg each evening for long-term chemoprophylaxis. Side-effects are less than with co-trimoxazole.

## The Beta-Lactam Antibiotics

These are the *penicillins* and *cephalosporins* and are so-called because of the 4 membered beta-lactam ring which forms part of their basic structure. Resistance is commonly due to bacterial enzymes called beta-lactamases (penicillinases and cephalosporinases) which can inactivate the antibiotics by opening the beta-lactam ring. The plasmids which code for these enzymes are transmissable between bacteria.

### The Penicillins

All penicillins are bactericidal and the range of activity of the group is wide as both Gram-positive and certain Gram-negative organisms are sensitive to individual penicillins. The outstanding adverse effect is the risk of inducing a hypersensitivity reaction. Even so the penicillins are the most useful antibiotics at present available. The principal penicillins are:

1. *Benzylpenicillin*, which is the original and most active penicillin; it must be given by injection. Its action can be prolonged by combining it with procaine — *procaine penicillin* and an even longer-acting form is *benzathine penicillin*.
2. *Phenoxymethylpenicillin* is absorbed when administered by mouth.
3. *Cloxacillin* is not inactivated by staphylococcal penicillinase and is reserved for the treatment of severe staphylococcal infections resistant to benzylpenicillin. *Flucloxacillin* is better absorbed than cloxacillin when given by mouth.
4. *Ampicillin* and its analogue *amoxycillin* are effective against Gram-negative bacilli, in contrast to the other penicillins whose activity is largely limited to Gram-positive organisms and Gram-negative cocci.

5. *Carbenicillin*, *ticarcillin* and *mezlocillin* are used in pseudomonas infections.

**Benzylpenicillin** is rapidly absorbed following intramuscular injection and is excreted by the kidneys within a few hours. A dose of 300 mg (half a million units) 6– or 8–hourly will suffice for most infections due to sensitive organisms. Large intramuscular or intravenous doses (up to 12 million units daily) may be required to achieve therapeutic concentrations within deep-seated or walled-off foci of infection, as occurs in infective endocarditis or lung abscess. The intramuscular injection of large doses is painful. Probenecid, 2 g daily by mouth will raise the blood level of penicillin by delaying its excretion by the kidney and allow smaller doses to be used.

Benzylpenicillin remains the antibiotic of choice for the treatment of pneumococcal, meningococcal and streptococcal infections, gonorrhoea and syphilis, yaws, diphtheria, tetanus, gas gangrene, anthrax and actinomycosis. It is also indicated for infections caused by penicillin-sensitive strains of *Staph. aureus*.

Penicillin is also used prophylactically. Benzylpenicillin is given to patients with valvular heart disease before a dental extraction to reduce the risk of infective endocarditis (p. 182). It is also given to prevent gas gangrene and tetanus after high amputations of ischaemic legs and for wounds containing dirt and devitalised tissue.

Benzylpenicillin passes in very small quantities into cerebrospinal fluid or pleural, pericardial or joint spaces. In the presence of inflammation its diffusion to these sites is greater. Benzylpenicillin may be given by local injection when treating severe infections of the joints, pleura or pericardium.

**Procaine Penicillin and Benzathine Penicillin.** These are long-acting penicillins given by injection and used in the treatment of gonorrhoea and the treponemal diseases, syphilis and yaws. *Procaine penicillin* in aqueous suspension, in a dose of 600 mg (600 000 units) intramuscularly once daily, is relatively painless and will maintain an adequate blood level for 24 hours. *Benzathine penicillin* has a duration of action of 3 to 4 weeks. A single injection of 600 000 units has proved to be an effective cure for yaws, but the blood levels are inadequate for acute infections such as pneumonia. It can be used for the prophylaxis of rheumatic fever in patients who cannot be relied upon to take oral penicillin.

**Phenoxymethylpenicillin** is incompletely absorbed from the stomach and frequent oral administration will produce reasonable blood levels. The usual dose is 500 mg every 4 to 6 hours, taken half an hour before meals to ensure maximum absorption. In patients who are ill or vomiting, intramuscular benzylpenicillin is essential because of uncertainties in absorption. During recovery oral therapy may be substituted in such patients. Phenoxymethylpenicillin is indicated for minor streptococcal infections and for pneumococcal pneumonia after initial therapy with benzylpenicillin. It is used prophylactically on a long-term basis following an attack of rheumatic fever to prevent recurrences.

**Cloxacillin.** Unlike benzylpenicillin, this semisynthetic penicillin is unaffected by staphylococcal penicillinase. Cloxacillin should be kept in reserve for the treatment of severe infection caused by staphylococci resistant to benzylpenicillin. It can be given orally in a dose of 500 mg 6-hourly, but for seriously ill patients treatment should be initiated by the injection of 1 g every 4 hours. Cloxacillin cannot be prescribed if the patient is allergic to benzylpenicillin. In these circumstances erythromycin or clindamycin should be used.

*Flucloxacillin* has an identical antibacterial range to cloxacillin. It is preferable for oral therapy as its absorption is more reliable.

**Ampicillin.** This is a semisynthetic penicillin which is effective by mouth and which has a bactericidal action against Gram-positive organisms and also a variety of Gram-negative organisms, including salmonellae, shigellae, *H. influenzae* and certain strains of *Esch. coli* and *Proteus*. It is inactivated by staphylococcal penicillinase. Ampicillin is of value in urinary tract infections due to *Esch. coli* and *Proteus* and in exacerbations of chronic bronchitis. The dose is 250 mg to 1 g, 4– to 8–hourly by mouth. Preparations for injection are also available. Maculopapular rashes occur in approximately 5% of all patients given ampicillin and in over 90% of patients with infectious mononucleosis; this antibiotic should not therefore be prescribed for sore throats which may be due to glandular fever.

*Amoxycillin* is an analogue of ampicillin which has a similar antibacterial range but is better absorbed from the gastrointestinal tract. It is effective in typhoid fever.

*Clavulanic acid* is a new beta-lactam agent with only weak antibacterial activity. It is, however, a potent inhibitor of many beta-lactamases and can protect beta-lactamase-susceptible antibiotics, such as amoxycillin, from inactivation by these enzymes.

**Carbenicillin, Ticarcillin and Mezlocillin.** Carbenicillin was initially the only penicillin with activity against *Ps. aeruginosa*. This organism, however, is only moderately sensitive to carbenicillin which has been replaced by its more active analogue ticarcillin. A further development has been the introduction of the ureidopenicillins, mezlocillin and azlocillin. These are derivatives of ampicillin with a broader spectrum than the parent compound and also significant activity against *Ps. aeruginosa*. Azlocillin is more effective than mezlocillin against this organism. The ureidopenicillins, like ampicillin, are inactivated by beta-lactamases.

*Ps. aeruginosa* is usually of relatively low virulence but it is an important cause of disease in patients with impaired defence mechanisms. Treatment is with either ticarcillin or a ureidopenicillin but in pseudomonas septicaemia a combination of an aminoglycoside with a penicillin is required; tobramycin plus ticarcillin (5 grams t.i.d.) is probably the best choice.

### Adverse Effects of the Penicillins

An increasing number of patients have acquired hypersensitivity to the systemic administration of the penicillins. This takes the form of urticaria and pyrexia or of an acute anaphylactic reaction which has occasionally proved fatal. Ampicillin commonly produces a maculopapular rash which differs from penicillin-induced urticaria and is specific for ampicillin alone. It is almost certainly unrelated to true penicillin allergy and is therefore not a contraindication to future treatment with other penicillins. The patient should always be asked about previous allergy to any form of penicillin before treatment is commenced as a severe reaction may be provoked by the administration of only a few milligrams. Patients who suffer from bronchial asthma or are hypersensitive to other drugs are particularly liable to become allergic to penicillin.

Skin sensitisation may result from topical applications of any antibiotic, but is so frequent with penicillin that it should never be applied locally.

Although penicillin is otherwise a safe antibiotic, its accumulation in patients with renal failure may lead to encephalopathy, so that dosage in these circumstances must be guided by the blood levels. The injectable preparations of all penicillins are formulated as sodium or potassium salts and hypernatraemia or hyperkalaemia can also result if large doses are given to patients with renal failure. Great care should be taken with the intrathecal administration of penicillin as fatal encephalopathy can occur if the dose is excessive.

It is important to avoid accidental intravenous administration when injecting procaine penicillin intramuscularly as this may result in a very severe reaction consisting of a sensation of impending death, paraesthesiae and confusion lasting up to an hour and followed by exhaustion and anxiety.

### The Cephalosporins

The cephalosporins have a wide range of activity against many, but not all, important Gram-positive and Gram-negative bacteria and are therefore of value for the initial 'blind' therapy of undiagnosed infections. *Cephalexin* and *cephradine* are both absorbed from the gut but the other available cephalosporins such as *cefuroxime* and *cephazolin* must be given by injection. *Cefoxitin*, also known as a cephamycin antibiotic, has the additional advantage of activity against the anaerobic organism *Bacteroides fragilis*, a common pathogen in intra-abdominal infections. Cefuroxime and cefoxitin are very resistant to degradation by beta-lactamases.

The dose of the cephalosporins ranges from 250–1000 mg 6 hourly depending on the size of the patient, renal function, and severity of infection. For abdominal sepsis the dose of cefoxitin is 2 g.

Adverse reactions are similar to those of the penicillins. A small number of penicillin-sensitive patients may also be allergic to the cephalosporins which should be avoided if there is a history of significant hypersensitivity to the penicillins. Nephrotoxicity is discussed on page 454.

## Erythromycin

Erythromycin has a fairly wide range of antibacterial activity but its main indication is in the treatment of streptococcal and pneumococcal infections in patients hypersensitive to penicillin. Its use in hospital is limited by the development of resistant organisms. Erythromycin is prescribed in a dosage of 250–500 mg by mouth every 6 hours. A parenteral preparation is also available. Jaundice occasionally occurs with erythromycin estolate but clears on withdrawal of the antibiotic. Allergic reactions to erythromycin are rare. Being well tolerated and easily administered it is useful for the treatment of respiratory infections in children in domiciliary practice. It is the best antibiotic for diphtheria carriers. Erythromycin is also effective in whooping cough, campylobacter enteritis and Legionnaires' disease, provided it is given early enough in the course of the illness.

## The Tetracyclines

*Tetracycline*, *oxytetracycline* and *chlortetracycline* are very closely related bacteriostatic agents which for practical purposes have an identical range of activity. The adult dose is 250–500 mg 6 hourly before meals. *Doxycycline* has the advantage that it is given only once daily, 200–300 mg on the first day and 100–200 mg thereafter.

The tetracyclines inhibit the growth of a wide range of Gram-positive and Gram-negative bacteria and are particularly useful in the treatment of exacerbations of chronic bronchitis, but their value is limited by an increase in tetracycline-resistant pneumococci and *H.influenzae*. The tetracyclines are also active against rickettsiae (typhus fevers), *Coxiella burneti* (Q-fever), *Mycoplasma pneumoniae* and chlamydia (lymphogranuloma venereum, psittacosis, non-gonococcal urethritis) and are effective in brucellosis.

The tetracyclines are employed systemically in the treatment of acne vulgaris and rosacea where their beneficial effect is almost certainly not due solely to their antibacterial action. Chlortetracycline is used for the local treatment of skin infections as it does not cause cutaneous sensitisation.

**Adverse Effects.** The tetracyclines are safe antibiotics with few side-effects. The commonest is diarrhoea which usually stops when the antibiotic is discontinued. Tetracyclines chelate with calcium and are deposited in developing bone and teeth causing a brown discoloration. They should not therefore be given to children or pregnant women. With the exception of doxycycline, the tetracyclines can exacerbate renal failure and should not be given to patients with kidney disease.

## Chloramphenicol

Chloramphenicol has a range of activity similar to that of the tetracyclines with the important difference that it is effective in enteric fever. It is more active than the tetracyclines against *H. influenzae* and is the antibiotic of choice in meningitis due to this organism. The daily dose for an adult is 1–3 g. Preparations for parenteral administration are also available. Chloramphenicol eye drops and ointment are indicated for purulent conjunctivitis.

**Adverse Effects.** Chloramphenicol has in its chemical structure a benzene ring of the type known to cause bone marrow aplasia. Although pancytopenia due to chloramphenicol is very uncommon, it is almost invariably fatal; this antibiotic should be used systemically only for the treatment of typhoid fever and *H. influenzae* infections and in other conditions if there is no alternative therapy.

Chloramphenicol should never be given to premature infants and very rarely to the newborn because of the risk of the development of the frequently fatal '*grey syndrome*'. This is a state of peripheral circulatory failure caused by the very high blood levels of chloramphenicol due to its inadequate conjugation in the liver at this age.

## Clindamycin

Clindamycin (7-chlorolincomycin) has a similar antibacterial spectrum to penicillin against most Gram-positive organisms and is also stable to staphylococcal beta-lactamases. It penetrates well into bone and is therefore useful for osteomyelitis caused by *Staph. aureus*. The other principal indication is for the treatment of infections caused by *Bacteroides fragilis*. The dose is 300 mg 6 hourly, orally or by injection.

Clindamycin is the commonest cause of *antibiotic-associated pseudomembranous colitis*. This adverse reaction, which can also complicate treatment with other antibiotics, especially ampicillin, is due to selective overgrowth of *Clostridium difficile* which produces a toxin detectable in the faeces and is the direct cause of the disease. Treatment is with metronidazole or vancomycin.

## Sodium Fusidate

This sodium salt of fusidic acid is highly bactericidal against staphylococci and is useful in infections caused by penicillin-resistant organisms. Like the lincomycins it is well concentrated in bone. Sodium fusidate is given orally in doses of 250–500 mg thrice daily, is rapidly absorbed, attains high tissue levels and is reasonably well tolerated, although nausea and vomiting are not uncommon during therapy. An intravenous preparation is available. This antibiotic is expensive and is principally indicated for bone infections due to staphylococci.

## The Aminoglycoside Antibiotics

**Streptomycin, Kanamycin, Gentamicin, Tobramycin, Amikacin and Neomycin**

These have similar chemical structures, pharmacological actions and adverse effects. They are not absorbed and for systemic treatment must be given by injection.

The outstanding property of *streptomycin* is its bactericidal effect on the tubercle bacillus. It is given in conjunction with two other antituberculous drugs and this triple therapy prevents the emergence of resistant strains (p. 259). For long-term therapy the daily dose of streptomycin should not exceed 1 g. Its use in other infections due to Gram-negative bacilli is restricted by the rapid development of bacterial resistance. When infective endocarditis is due to an organism relatively resistant to penicillin, such as *Strep. faecalis*, good results may be obtained by combining streptomycin with large doses of benzylpenicillin or ampicillin.

*Spectinomycin* is an aminocyclitol compound with certain structural similarity to streptomycin although it is not an aminoglycoside. Its only clinical use is for the treatment of uncomplicated gonorrhoea if penicillin is contraindicted.

*Kanamycin* is active against many Gram-negative bacilli and resistance develops much more slowly than with streptomycin. It has been mainly replaced by gentamicin for infections caused by Gram-negative bacilli.

*Gentamicin* has a range of activity similar to kanamycin but has the very important additional advantage of being effective against *Ps. aeruginosa*. It is also active against penicillin-resistant staphylococci but inactive against streptococci and anaerobic organisms. The dose depends on renal function and the age and weight of the patient. Up to 7·5 mg per kilogram body weight per 24 hours in divided doses is required for serious infections but 2 mg per kg is sufficient for uncomplicated urinary tract infections. *Tobramycin* is more active than gentamicin against *Ps. aeruginosa* but has no other advantage.

*Amikacin* has less intrinsic antibacterial activity than gentamicin, but has the advantage of being stable to eight of the nine characterised aminoglycoside-inactivating enzymes, in contrast to gentamicin which is susceptible to six of the nine. For this reason amikacin is active against many gentamicin-resistant Gram-negative bacilli and should be reserved for the treatment of infections caused by these organisms. The dose is 500 mg 12 hourly — this may have to be increased for serious infections.

*Neomycin* is too toxic to be given parenterally but local applications containing neomycin are used in infections of the skin and eye. Neomycin is used in hepatic encephalopathy to reduce the numbers of colonic bacteria.

**Adverse Effects.** The outstanding toxic effect of all the aminoglycosides is on the eighth cranial nerve. With streptomycin and gentamicin the vestibular division is initially affected with resultant vertigo and incoordination. Later, deafness may also occur. Kanamycin tends to cause deafness first. Aminoglycosides, especially gentamicin, should not be administered together with the diuretics frusemide or ethacrynic acid, as both can cause eighth nerve damage and additive ototoxicity may result from the combination. The ototoxicity of the aminoglycosides is related to the age of the patient, the serum level of the antibiotic and the duration of administration. The aminoglycosides are principally excreted from the body by the kidneys and the risk of toxicity is increased when there is impairment of renal function. In such cases serum levels of the antibiotic must be monitored and the frequency of dosage adjusted accordingly. The aminoglycosides can also cause kidney damage, occasionally leading to renal failure. Application of neomycin to the skin may cause hypersensitivity.

## Metronidazole

This imidazole compound has high activity against anaerobic bacteria and protozoa but none against aerobic organisms. It is the drug of choice for infections due to *Trichomonas vaginalis* and *Entamoeba histolytica* (p. 812) and is widely used for the treatment and prophylaxis of infections caused by anaerobic bacteria, notably *Bacteroides fragilis*. It is a non-toxic drug but should not be given to women during the first trimester of pregnancy as fetal abnormalities have been reported in animals given high doses for prolonged periods. Alcohol should be avoided during therapy with metronidazole which has a similar action to disulfiram (p. 776). The oral dose varies from 200–400 mg given 3 or 4 times a day. Up to 800 mg 3 times a day is required for amoebic infections. There is a preparation for intravenous infusion.

## Antifungal Agents

For therapeutic purposes, fungal infections are classified as superficial (skin or mucous membranes) and systemic. The former are commonly caused by *Candida albicans* and usually respond readily to topical applications of an anti-fungal agent. Systemic fungal infections often occur in a compromised host and can be extremely difficult to cure.

*Nystatin* is the most commonly prescribed agent for the treatment of Candida infections of skin and mucous membranes (thrush). It is not absorbed when given by mouth and cannot be administered parenterally because of its low solubility and toxicity. A suspension, tablets and pessaries are available for the treatment of oral, intestinal and vaginal thrush.

*Miconazole* and *econazole* are imidazole antifungal agents which can be administered topically for superficial infections. Miconazole is incompletely absorbed from the gut but there is an intravenous preparation for the treatment of invasive fungal infections.

*Amphotericin* remains the most important antibiotic for the treatment of systemic fungal infections. It is a moderately toxic drug and side-effects are relatively common. These include fever, vomiting, thrombophlebitis and nephrotoxicity. The antibiotic is given by i.v. infusion in gradually increasing daily doses commencing with 1 mg.

*Flucytosine* is well absorbed from the gut and side-effects are relatively uncommon. *C. albicans* can, however, develop resistance.

*Griseofulvin* is selectively concentrated in keratin and is the drug of choice for widespread or chronic dermatophyte infections such as ringworm. It is well absorbed from the gut and is given in a daily dose of 250 mg (child) and 500 mg (adult). Skin lesions respond quickly but infection of the nails requires several months of therapy.

Localised and minor ringworm lesions usually respond to topical application of Whitfield's ointment or miconazole.

## Antiviral Agents

The main problem with antiviral chemotherapy is to find an agent which will arrest the replication of the virus without interfering with the metabolism of the host cell. Another difficulty is that by the time a viral infection has been diagnosed much of the damage has already been done to the host tissues. The following is an outline of the present position.

*Idoxuridine* is effective in herpes infections of the skin (shingles) and cornea (*H. simplex* keratitis) if applied early; it is too toxic for parenteral administration. *Acyclovir*, which is under clinical trial, is more active than idoxuridine against herpes viruses and is apparently not toxic. *Vidarabine* (adenine arabinoside) has been used for *H. simplex* encephalitis with variable effect.

*Interferon* is a lymphokine produced by T cells in response to viral infections (p. 25). It is effective in the treatment of experimental viral infections and has been used in humans. Interferon is species-specific and only small quantities have been available to date; it is undergoing critical appraisal.

## Selection of Antimicrobial Agent

In addition to knowledge about the properties of the available antimicrobial agents, important considerations in the choice of effective chemotherapy are the nature and site of the infection, adverse effects and cost.

**The Nature and Site of the Infection.** In instances where the nature of the infection can usually be predicted from the clinical features of the illness, treatment can proceed without isolation of the causative organism. For example, acute follicular tonsillitis and lobar pneumonia are sufficiently characteristic on clinical examination to allow the causative organism and its antibiotic sensitivity to be assumed with a high degree of probability and the appropriate antibiotic (penicillin) given. In exacerbations of chronic bronchitis the causative organisms are almost always pneumococci and *H. influenzae* and the use of ampicillin or co-trimoxazole is indicated without specific laboratory diagnosis.

Where there is uncertainty about the nature of the infection a bacteriological diagnosis should be made so that the appropriate antibiotic can be given. If the organism is one such as *Strep. pyogenes*, which has a predictable susceptibility to the generally used antimicrobial agents, no further laboratory sensitivity tests are necessary.

Sensitivity tests will be required for bacteria known to vary in their susceptibility to antimicrobial agents. The acquisition of resistance occurs particularly with staphylococci, Gram-negative bacilli and tubercle bacilli. Once the sensitivity of the organism has been determined, it is relatively rare for this to change in the course of treatment. However, there is not a complete correlation between the results of sensitivity tests and the response to chemotherapy and sometimes clinical judgement may indicate a different drug from that recommended by the bacteriologist.

When sensitivity tests indicate that several antimicrobial agents are effective it is advisable in the first instance to select one that is bactericidal in order that the organisms are killed rapidly; bacteriostatic drugs suppress the growth of the organism while the natural defence mechanisms of the body dispose of it. The choice is probably of no great significance in the majority of infections but may be important in the treatment of bacteraemia and in patients with deficient defence mechanisms.

The use of two or more antibacterial drugs is only occasionally of proven value. Thus in tuberculosis three agents are prescribed, at least initially, so as to reduce the emergence of resistant strains. Combinations of antibiotics with differing ranges of activity may also be used to treat infections due to more than one species of micro-organism or where it is believed that the effect of the combination of drugs is more potent than an equivalent amount of any one of the compounds acting alone. This has been described as 'synergy'; an example of this is co-trimoxazole. Unfortunately there have been relatively few clinical trials which have compared the efficacy of combinations of antibiotics with single drugs so that the use of combinations remains somewhat empirical. Whenever possible their choice should be specifically directed by bacteriological diagnosis and accompanying sensitivity tests.

The selection of an antimicrobial agent is also determined by the site of the infection. This is discussed with the treatment of individual diseases and in the management of bacteraemia (p. 81).

**Selection of Antimicrobial Agents in Relation to Adverse Effects.** Before prescribing an antimicrobial agent enquiry should be made about any previous allergic reactions. Pregnant women and children should not be given tetracyclines. Co-trimoxazole is also best avoided in pregnancy and this compound, together with other sulphonamides, must not be given to patients with glucose-6-phosphate dehydrogenase deficiency as haemolysis may be precipitated (p. 556). Chloramphenicol should be prescribed only in the circumstances described on page 76 and is contraindicated in the neonate. Ampicillin must not be given to patients suffering from glandular fever and the aminoglycoside antibiotics should be used with caution in patients with renal disease and in the elderly. Clindamycin should not be used for trivial infection because of the risk of colitis (p. 76).

**Prophylactic Use of Antibiotics.** The indications for this are limited. They include the prevention of meningococcal infections (p. 63) and diphtheria (p. 54) in susceptible contacts. Chemoprophylaxis is also indicated in patients with heart valve lesions undergoing dental or urological procedures (p. 182), for the prevention of tetanus (p. 62) and gas gangrene, and to prevent infective complications following gastrointestinal and gynaecological surgery.

**Cost.** The chemotherapy of infections can be very expensive, especially when newly introduced preparations are used. Unusual antibiotics should not be prescribed without good reason as the difference in cost can be over a hundred-fold.

### Bacteraemia, Septicaemia and Bacteraemic (Septic) Shock

Spread of infection to the blood stream is known as *bacteraemia* and, if the organisms multiply there, as *septicaemia*. Further dissemination may result in 'metastatic' foci of infection in bone, liver, brain or heart valves. The primary infection varies but can be diverticulitis, cholecystitis, or infection of the urinary tract, especially in the compromised host. Many organisms, and Gram-negative bacteria in particular, produce toxins which cause an increase in capillary permeability leading to bacteraemic shock. These toxins may also cause disseminated thrombosis (disseminated intra-vascular coagulation, D.I.C. p. 601) and depress the myocardium.

**Clinical Features.** The pyrexia of the infection may be overtaken by the hypothermia of shock. Hypotension is usually followed by a fall in cardiac output. Leukopenia, thrombocytopenia and a prolonged bleeding time point to D.I.C. Progressive impairment of blood flow may then lead to organ failure, particularly of the brain, kidneys, liver and lungs (shock lung). Mortality can be over 60% in Gram-negative sepsis causing severe hypotension and a low cardiac output.

**Treatment.** Antibiotic therapy must be commenced immediately with a combination such as gentamicin and an agent active against Gram-positive cocci plus possibly a third against anaerobes. This is adjusted when the nature of the infection has been determined. Two pulsed doses of corticosteroid (e.g. dexamethasone 1·5 mg/kg) may be beneficial. Shock (p. 167) and D.I.C. (p. 601) must also be treated.

Where Gram-positive cocci are the cause of the infection, benzylpenicillin should be given if the organism is known to be sensitive to penicillin. Flucloxacillin is indicated if penicillinase-producing staphylococci are responsible for the infection. If the patient is allergic to penicillin or the organism is resistant to cloxacillin, the next choice is clindamycin. Metronidazole is indicated for anaerobic infections. Gentamicin alone will suffice for other Gram-negative infections but not for pseudomonas (p. 74). Amikacin is reserved for gentamicin-resistant organisms.

## Conclusion

### General Principles in the Use of Antimicrobial Agents

1. Antimicrobial agents should be prescribed only if there is a specific indication for their use and then only for limited periods. They should not be given for trivial infections such as minor skin sepsis or gastroenteritis and, with very few exceptions (p. 79), they are ineffective in viral disease.

2. Serious infections should be treated whenever possible with bactericidal as opposed to bacteriostatic preparations and initially with parenteral agents. Although the average recommended dose of an antibiotic is sufficient for the treatment of the majority of infections, higher dosage may be necessary when the condition is serious.

3. Many acute infections such as streptococcal tonsillitis and pneumococcal pneumonia which are caused by organisms of predictable sensitivity can be treated without assistance from the laboratory. Laboratory aid is however required for bacteraemia, recurrent infections and those caused by less common pathogens.

4. Well established and usually cheaper antibiotics are preferable to new and generally more expensive preparations unless there is some commanding reason to choose otherwise.

5. Antibiotics with a relatively limited range of activity such as benzylpenicillin are preferable to broad-spectrum compounds like tetracycline, so as to reduce the danger of superinfection.

6. There are very few indications for combinations of antibiotics (p. 80) or prophylactic antibiotics (p. 80).

7. Many adverse effects and even death may result from the use of antibiotics, and their careless prescription is to be deplored.

A. M. Geddes

*Further reading:*

Christie, A. B. (1981) *Infectious Diseases: Epidemiology and Clinical Practice*, 3rd edn. Edinburgh: Churchill Livingstone.

Cruickshank, R. (1973) *Medical Microbiology*, 12th edn. Edinburgh: Churchill Livingstone.

Garrod, L. P., O'Grady, F. & Lambert, H. P. (1981) *Antibiotic and Chemotherapy,* 5th edn. Edinburgh: Churchill Livingstone.

Kucers, A. & Bennett, N. McK. (1979) *The Use of Antibiotics,* 3rd edn. London: Heinemann.

# 4. Nutritional Factors in Disease

Although man has used foods for ritual purposes and attributed magical properties to some of them since the beginning of history, the science of nutrition has nearly all originated in the twentieth century. The concept of vitamins was introduced around 1912; the cure of human rickets with vitamin D was established in 1922; nicotinamide was first used to treat pellagra in 1938. Kwashiorkor was originally reported in 1932 from an obscure African hospital, but medical science did not become aware of its importance until 1952. Human zinc deficiency was not established until 1972.

The world's population is estimated to have reached about 4 300 000 000 and presents the greatest threat to mankind. This explosive growth in population is due not to increased fertility but to the remarkable reduction in the death rate that has been achieved in recent decades. The most obvious effects of overpopulation are actual shortage of food for many poor people in under developed communities and ever rising food costs in industrial countries. Some 450 million people are undernourished, many of them children. Famines are occurring most of the time in one part of the world or another. Agricultural production is hampered by bad climates, soil erosion, lack of fertilisers, antiquated farming methods, political upheavals and war. The situation will deteriorate unless national programmes of population control and family planning based on modern contraceptive techniques are effectively put into operation. Food production can be further increased by the application of science to peasant agriculture but nothing will be gained if machines displace people from the land and increase the numbers of unemployed in the developing countries.

A knowledge of nutrition has three uses in clinical medicine:

1. Elsewhere in this book diseases are described the multiple causes of which may include what or how people eat over long periods; among these are dental caries, coronary heart disease, diabetes mellitus, and even some of the carcinomas, e.g. of the liver and of the colon. These diseases take a long time to develop and the precise importance of one factor such as diet involves discussion and sometimes controversy. Details are not appropriate to a clinical primer and may be sought in a textbook of nutrition (p. 125).

2. For some diseases, modification of the diet is valuable treatment. In gluten enteropathy and phenylketonuria the correct diet is of crucial importance. For other diseases like chronic renal failure and diabetes mellitus appropriate adjustment of the diet forms a major aspect of the management. Principles of therapeutic diets are discussed with the diseases concerned. Space does not allow inclusion of a full set of diet sheets; those for obesity and diabetes appear on pages 900–904. For other diet sheets the reader is referred to a textbook of nutrition (p. 125).

3. There are diseases which result primarily from disturbed nutrition; these are described in this chapter. It should be stressed that these primary nutritional diseases seldom present in pure form. Where food is short in quantity or defective in quality all the members of a community are not equally affected. People with physical (or mental) diseases are likely to succumb first. Nutritional diseases thus often have a predisposing illness and when this is prominent the resulting malnutrition is spoken

of as conditioned or secondary. Furthermore someone who has one type of malnutrition is likely to have another; sometimes it is possible to find clinical or biochemical signs of six or more nutrient deficiencies in the same patient. For this reason treatment should never be confined to large intakes of the nutrient whose deficiency is the most prominent clinical feature. Lastly malnourished patients are liable to complications, particularly certain infections. These may be the presenting illness or they may occur in modified form because the malnutrition has suppressed some of their characteristic features. Complications must be sought out and treated.

Much of the skill in diagnosing patients with malnutrition consists in being aware of and disentangling predisposing illnesses, other types of malnutrition and complicating illnesses. Only when this is done can treatment be fully effective.

## Classification and Aetiology of Nutritional Disorders

**Classification.** There are five essential types of nutritional disorders:

1. *Quantitative Dietary Deficiency*. Not enough food results in undernutrition or when more severe, frank starvation.

2. *Qualitative Dietary Deficiency*. Wrong food results in malnutrition. The term 'malnutrition' should be restricted to those nutritional disorders, e.g. rickets and scurvy, which are due to lack of protein or other essential nutrients.

3. *Quantitative Overnutrition*. Too much food results in obesity.

4. *Qualitative Overnutrition*. This is due to too much of one food component, e.g. hypervitaminosis D and siderosis. High intakes of saturated fat raise the plasma cholesterol and predispose to coronary heart disease; high salt intake may be a factor in essential hypertension.

5. *Effects of Natural Toxins in Foods*. Some foods contain small amounts of toxic substances which can lead to disease if a person or community has to rely too heavily on a single foodstuff, e.g. lathyrism.

**Social and Economic Causes of Nutritional Disorders**. Even in countries where the overall food supply is adequate, cases of malnutrition may occur because of unequal distribution of income or because of ignorance or social disorganization. The old, the solitary and the children are most often affected.

**Pathological Causes of Nutritional Disorders.** CONDITIONED MALNUTRITION. Even with an ample income, an adequate home and some knowledge of dietetics, a patient may develop a nutritional disorder secondary to disease which 'conditions' (facilitates) it in one or more of the following ways.

1. DEFECTIVE INTAKE OF FOOD. *(a) Loss of appetite* may be an important symptom of organic disease, e.g. cancer of the stomach, and also of psychogenic disease, e.g. anxiety, depression and anorexia nervosa. *(b) Persistent vomiting* from any cause. *(c) Food fads*, e.g. in very strict vegetarians (vegans). *(d) Alcohol* provides calories but no essential nutrients. Chronic alcoholics suffer from malnutrition more often than undernutrition. *(e) Unbalanced therapeutic diets*, e.g. diets for digestive diseases may lack ascorbic acid unless care is taken to provide it. *(f) Prolonged intravenous fluids* with glucose and saline solutions only may precipitate acute deficiencies of the vitamin B complex.

2. DEFECTIVE DIGESTION AND ABSORPTION. *(a) Achlorhydria* is a factor in the causation of iron deficiency anaemia. *(b) Steatorrhoea* leads to malabsorption, *(c) Intestinal*

*hurry* due to surgical short circuits, etc. may impair digestion. In starving people the ingestion of unsuitable foods often causes intestinal hurry and intensifies their plight. *(d) Antibiotics*, if their administration is prolonged, may interfere with the synthesis of certain vitamins by intestinal bacteria e.g. vitamin K.

3. DEFECTIVE UTILISATION. *(a) Cirrhosis* of the liver may interfere with the utilisation of ingested nutrients, e.g. of protein and vitamin K. *(b) Malignancy*, in some unknown ways, may produce a state of undernutrition despite an adequate diet. The same may be true of tuberculosis and other prolonged infections. *(c)* In *renal failure* vitamin D is not converted to the active metabolite (p. 101). *(d)* Some *drugs*, e.g. anticonvulsants, are antagonists of folate and of vitamin D. *(e) Inborn errors of metabolism* may interfere with nutrients, e.g. Hartnup disease leads to pellagrous signs on ordinary diets (p. 114).

4. LOSS OF NUTRIENTS FROM THE BODY. *(a)* In the *nephrotic syndrome* protein is lost in the urine. *(b)* In *diabetes mellitus* uncontrolled glycosuria causes undernutrition. *(c)* In *excessive menstrual bleeding* (menorrhagia) secondary iron deficiency anaemia is common. *(d)* In severe or chronic *diarrhoea* potassium is lost.

5. INCREASED NUTRITIONAL NEEDS. *(a)* In *pregnancy, lactation* and *adolescence* (especially after an illness in the last named), and for those engaged in hard physical work, particularly in cold climates, the usual diet may be insufficient. *(b)* In *fevers* and *hyperthyroidism* the increased metabolism calls for more calories. *(c)* After *burns, trauma* and major *surgery*, there is an increased catabolism of protein and ascorbic acid.

**Nutrients can be sub-divided into three groups:**

1. Energy-yielding nutrients (carbohydrates, fats and proteins)
2. Water, electrolytes and minerals
3. Vitamins

In this chapter the related disorders will be described under these headings and thereafter overnutrition will be considered.

## ENERGY-YIELDING NUTRIENTS

**Carbohydrates** usually provide the greater part of the energy in a normal diet, but no individual carbohydrate is an essential nutrient in the sense that the body needs it but cannot make it for itself from other nutrients. If the carbohydrate intake is less than 100 g per day ketosis is likely to occur.

**Fats.** With their high caloric value, fats are useful to people with a large energy expenditure; moreover they are helpful in cooking and making food appetising. Though rats need linoleic or arachidonic acids in their diet, *essential fatty acid deficiency* is rare in man. It has been demonstrated in patients who have been fed intravenously for long periods without fat emulsions. They develop a scaly dermatitis and eicosatrienoic acid accumulates in plasma lipids. Essential fatty acids are precursors for the synthesis of prostaglandins.

**Proteins** provide some 20 amino acids, of which eight are essential for normal protein synthesis and for maintaining nitrogen balance in adults. These *essential amino acids* are methionine, lysine, tryptophan, phenylalanine, leucine, isoleucine, threonine, and valine. Histidine and perhaps arginine are also needed for growth in infants.

The 'biological value' of different proteins depends on the relative proportions of essential amino acids they contain. Proteins of animal origin, particularly from eggs, milk and meat, are generally of higher biological value than the proteins of vegetable origin which are deficient in one or more of the essential amino acids. However it is possible to have a diet of mixed vegetable proteins with high biological value if the principle of *supplementation* is used. For example cereals, e.g. wheat, contain about 10% protein and are relatively deficient in lysine. Legumes contain around 20% of protein which is relatively deficient in methionine. If two parts of wheat are mixed (or eaten) with one part of legume, a food results which contains 13% of a protein of high biological value. This happens because cereals contain enough methionine and legumes enough lysine to supplement the other component of the mixture.

The usual recommended allowance for an adequate protein intake is 10% of the total calories i.e. about 65 g for the average adult. The minimum requirement is less, around 40 g per day of good biological value protein for an adult.

### Energy Requirements

Requirements for energy (calories) vary widely, even among apparently similar individuals. 'Recommended Allowances' provide only an approximation for an individual. WHO recommended in 1974 that 3000 kcal is adequate for a moderately active man and 2200 kcal for a moderately active woman. Slightly lower figures are suitable in the affluent countries where most people are sedentary.

The population of Britain, including infants, children and adults, probably needs an average *intake* of 2500 kcal/head/day. In order that the population may actually consume this amount, the food retailed must provide more to allow for household wastage, pets, tourists etc. The food supplies of Britain ordinarily provide around 3000 kcal/head/day. It is this gross value of our food supplies that is sometimes discussed in the Press and Parliament and often confused with average physiological requirements.

There are two units in use for energy: calories and joules. Though both are metric, joules are SI units and are gradually replacing calories in scientific usage.

1 kcal = 4·184 kJ.

## Undernutrition and Starvation

Starvation may conveniently be defined as undernutrition of sufficient severity to warrant in-patient treatment in hospital; the body weight is reduced to less than 75% of normal.

**Aetiology**. Undernutrition and starvation arise (1) when there is not enough food to eat, for instance in times of famine, (2) when there is severe disease of the digestive tract, preventing the absorption of nutrients, as in the malabsorption syndrome and cancer of the oesophagus or (3) when there is a condition which prevents normal metabolism of nutrients by the tissues, e.g. in renal or hepatic failure or protracted infections. In all these circumstances there is wasting of the body with much loss of both muscle and fat.

**Clinical Features**. When the caloric value of the diet is inadequate, adults lose weight, and children cease to grow or even lose weight. The loss may be rapid at first, but tends to slow down and stabilize at a lower level because the body is able to adapt itself, at least partly, to an insufficient intake of food. This is possible because *(a)* the bulk of the muscles and glands is reduced in size, requiring less energy for their maintenance, *(b)* the basal metabolism is reduced, *(c)* the lighter body requires less work to move it about, and *(d)* unnecessary voluntary movements are curtailed.

The patient becomes thin and the skin lax, most noticeably over the upper arm and abdomen. The skin is thin, dry, inelastic and often cyanosed at the extremities. The hair becomes dull, dry and inflexible ('staring' hair). The eyes are dull and sunken, yet the wasting of orbital tissues may give them an unusual prominence. The heart is reduced in size and there is often bradycardia and a reduced systolic blood pressure. Atrophy of the small intestine is present and may be severe, in which case the inability to digest and absorb nutrients requires great care during refeeding. In severe cases, once diarrhoea has begun, the loss in the stools causes disturbances in water and electrolyte balance.

Loss of 2–4 kg of body water in the urine is a characteristic immediate response to severe calorie or carbohydrate restriction. It is probably related to depletion of glycogen which has water-holding properties. This phenomenon explains why reducing diets for obesity can be so successful for the first few days. After prolonged intake of insufficient food, dependent 'famine' oedema begins to appear. It is often preceded by a period of nocturnal polyuria. Famine oedema is not necessarily associated with any fall in the level of plasma proteins, but is due rather to wasting of tissues without a corresponding loss of body water. Mild normocytic, normochromic anaemia is common, due to a reduction in the red cell population without corresponding alteration in the plasma volume.

Seriously underfed patients are weak and sometimes suffer from attacks of syncope. Hypothermia should be looked for with a low-reading thermometer. Psychological symptoms frequently occur in starving people. Mental restlessness, irritability and indifference to the troubles of others may be combined with physical apathy. Undernourished individuals are susceptible to infections. With respiratory muscles weakened by wasting, bronchopneumonia carries an increased mortality. Diarrhoea is very common and starving groups in famines have often had high mortalities from epidemics, e.g. of typhus or cholera.

The severity of the starvation can be assessed by working out the patient's weight for height as a percentage of the estimated normal for the population (Table 18.2, p. 905). Starvation is severe and dangerous when weight is less than 70% of normal.

**Treatment**. In mild undernutrition, all that is needed is suitable food. Management is more an administrative than a medical problem. When the patient is seriously ill treatment must depend on the facilities available.

Most famine victims, because of alimentary dysfunction, cannot deal with large quantities of food. The patient's appetite may be immense and no guide to digestive capacities. Limitation of the food intake is essential if there is diarrhoea or a severe degree of cachexia.

The choice of food needs care. In advanced cases only bland food can be tolerated by the thin-walled intestines lacking essential digestive enzymes. Skimmed milk may not be well tolerated if the patient has deficient intestinal lactase activity. It is advisable to give foods with which the patient is familiar.

The ideal diet to start with is one based on the patient's staple cereal and some sucrose or glucose together with moderate amounts of bland, protein-rich food, e.g. milk powder, and some fat or oil. Small feeds should be given at frequent intervals and new foods added one at a time to see that they do not increase diarrhoea. It is advisable to give a multivitamin preparation. With refeeding there may be some increase in oedema, unless the supply of salt is restricted.

There may come a time when a patient with severe starvation refuses all food, although fully rational. Feeding of milk and other fluids through a nasogastric tube then provides the only hope.

Physical and psychological recovery is usually complete if sufficient calories are provided for cases of primary undernutrition. When irreversible changes have developed in the heart and small intestine in severe starvation, the prognosis is poor.

**Prevention** rests with legislators and administrators. Famines from crop failure can be greatly alleviated by advanced contingency planning. Those caused by a natural disaster like an earthquake are unexpected: the outcome depends on how well the country's administration stands up to the strain. Famines resulting from war are the most difficult. The problems of prevention and relief of famine are discussed in a book published by the Swedish Nutrition Foundation (p. 126).

## Protein Energy (Calorie) Malnutrition

**Aetiology and Classification**. Protein energy malnutrition (PEM) in early childhood is a spectrum of disease. At one end there is *kwashiorkor* in which the essential feature is deficiency of protein with relatively adequate energy intake. At the other end is *nutritional marasmus* which is total inanition of the infant, usually under 1 year of age, and which is due to a severe and prolonged restriction of all food, i.e. energy and protein as well as other nutrients. In the middle of the spectrum is *marasmic kwashiorkor* in which there are clinical features of both disorders.

Some children adapt to prolonged energy and/or protein shortage by *nutritional dwarfism*. The most prevalent of all the varieties of PEM is *mild to moderate PEM* or the underweight child (Table 4.1). Children with one form of PEM often shift to another form. Thus a child with mild to moderate PEM may develop kwashiorkor after an infection. Such a child when treated loses oedema and may look marasmic.

The incidence of PEM in its various forms is high in India and Southeast Asia, in most parts of Africa and the Middle East, in the Caribbean Islands and in South and Central America. PEM is the most important dietary deficiency disease in the world. Severe forms affect around 2% and mild to moderate PEM affects around 20% of young children in the Third World; hence it will be described in detail.

### Kwashiorkor

Cicely Williams in 1933 was the first to record that 'some amino acid or protein deficiency' might be an aetiological factor in kwashiorkor, the name given to this disease by the Ga tribe living in and around Accra, the capital of Ghana.

**Aetiology.** Kwashiorkor typically arises when, after prolonged breast feeding, the child is weaned on to a traditional family diet, which is low in protein, such as cassava, plantain or yam, or a cereal that has been refined and diluted (Fig. 4.1, p. 93). There is little or no milk and custom, sometimes reinforced by taboos, determines that the limited supply of foods of animal origin is given to the men of the family, or the small amount of high protein food is in a sauce, which is made with hot peppers or spices and unsuitable for young children. In many rural areas, where kwashiorkor is endemic, the food supply becomes scarce each year before the harvest; at this

Table 4.1 Classification of PEM

| | Body weight as percentage of international standard for age | Oedema | Deficit in weight for height |
|---|---|---|---|
| Kwashiorkor | 80–60 | + | + |
| Marasmic kwashiorkor | <60 | + | + + |
| Marasmus | <60 | 0 | + + |
| Nutritional dwarfing | <60 | 0 | minimal |
| Underweight child | 80–60 | 0 | + |

Based on Joint FAO/WHO Committee on Nutrition. 8th Report, 1971 (with modifications in weight/height column).

'hungry season' the incidence of kwashiorkor and other nutritional diseases increases.

If the customary diet of a population is limited in protein and in calories to around the levels of minimum requirements, a child may be in moderate health until the protein requirements are raised by an infection. Gastroenteritis, measles and malaria are all notorious precipitating causes of kwashiorkor.

**Pathology.** The insufficient supply of amino acids leads to inadequate protein synthesis, which impairs tissue replacement and development of organs and reduces synthesis of enzymes and plasma proteins. Some enzymes and tissues, particularly those with a rapid turnover, are more severely affected than others.

The total protein content of the body may be as low as 60% of normal for height, while the water content is increased. The failure to synthesise plasma albumin reduces the concentration to around 15 g/*l*. By contrast the plasma gammaglobulin is usually well maintained. Synthesis of digestive enzymes is usually impaired, including those secreted by the pancreas and the mucosa of the small intestine (especially lactase). This may be partially responsible for the gastrointestinal upsets and diarrhoea which are so commonly present and which lead to loss of potassium and magnesium in the stools. The protein content of the liver is greatly reduced, while its lipid content is much increased. Subnormal cell-mediated immunity makes the child susceptible to infections like measles, tuberculosis and herpes.

**Clinical Features.** *Failure of Growth.* The child's weight is usually well below standard for the age (Table 18.1, p. 904) but the deficit may be masked by *oedema* from hypoalbuminaemia. This usually affects the feet but may also be found in the hands and face. Ascites and pleural effusions are usually slight and, if detected clinically, suggest the presence of an infection such as tuberculosis.

*Muscles and Fat.* The muscles are wasted. This is particularly noticeable around the chest and the upper arm; the wasting of the legs and around the hips is frequently concealed by oedema. Subcutaneous fat is often plentiful in children whose diets have provided ample energy but little protein. If the disease has resulted from a restriction of both calories and protein, an almost complete lack of subcutaneous fat and muscle wasting are the most striking features, but the feet are oedematous ('marasmic kwashiorkor').

*Mental Changes.* The child is apathetic and miserable.

*Hair.* This is nearly always affected in African children; in Asiatics the changes are less frequent. The hair becomes fine, straight and is often sparse. The hair of African children may show a variety of pigmentary changes from brown and reddish to grey, blond or even white. Children with long straight black hair may show a pale band across the hair, corresponding to an earlier episode of kwashiorkor, the 'flag sign'. The extent of these changes in the hair is an indication of the duration rather than the severity of the disease.

*Skin.* Alterations in the skin are usually present, especially in severe cases. These include pigmentation, desquamation and ulceration. In moderate cases the dermatosis resembles crazy paving. A severe case may look like an extensive burn. The legs, buttocks and perineum are most frequently involved, but any region may be affected. This is in contrast to pellagra in which the dermatosis occurs mainly on the exposed surfaces. The skin lesions are determined in part by associated vitamin deficiencies and in part by infections and trauma.

*Mucous Membranes.* Angular stomatitis, cheilosis and a smooth tongue are commonly seen, as is ulceration around the anus.

*Liver.* This may be enlarged and extend to the umbilicus but the liver can be fatty without being clinically abnormal. Hepatosplenomegaly from malaria and other causes is common in the tropics.

*Gastrointestinal System.* Anorexia is usually present and sometimes vomiting. There is usually diarrhoea, with the passage of stools containing undigested food. This feature may be secondary to failure to secrete digestive enzymes, to intestinal mucosal atrophy or to an associated gastroenteritis.

*Anaemia.* Some degree of anaemia is frequently present. It often becomes worse during treatment. The degree of anaemia and its nature are largely determined by associated infections and other dietary deficiencies.

*Associated Vitamin Deficiencies.* Vitamin A deficiency with xerophthalmia and keratomalacia (p. 100) occurs in from one to 70% of severe cases of PEM. It is a major cause of preventable blindness in developing countries. Biochemical signs of thiamin and niacin deficiencies are commonly associated with kwashiorkor in countries where rice and maize respectively are the staple weaning foods. Folate deficiency is also fairly frequent. Children with PEM have often been indoors out of the sun for weeks and a minority of cases have signs of rickets (p. 102). Deficiency of vitamin K may result in purpura or bleeding.

**Treatment.** GENERAL MEASURES. An easily digested diet which provides adequate amounts of protein, minerals and vitamins with extra calories for 'catch-up growth' is essential. Milk is a good base, and the most convenient locally available form may be used. If skimmed milk is given, however, it is necessary to include additional fat. Plant protein mixtures, such as corn-soya-dried milk, may also be used.

Severely ill children may be unable to maintain their body temperature even in the tropics, especially where there is a large fall of atmospheric temperature at night. Heated rooms or electric blankets are essential for such cases.

If dermatosis is severe the skin should be cleaned and carefully protected. The child's weight tends to fall during the first days of treatment due to loss of oedema fluid. Initiation of cure is indicated by increasing appetite, improvement in general condition, loss of oedema and rise of plasma albumin.

*Diets for Acute Cases.* All the major units with research experience of kwashiorkor have evolved somewhat different therapeutic diets, depending on local availability of and preferences for weaning foods. The principle of all the regimes is to work up to protein intakes of 3 to 4 g/kg/d and energy intakes of 150 kcal/kg/d or more. For the first day or two, if the child is unable to feed from a spoon, nasogastric intubation will be necessary. A recipe successfully used in Jamaica is: dried, skimmed milk 60 g, flour 20 g, butter 15 g, and water to make 250 ml. This is offered freely in five to six feeds daily. The mixture contains 22 g protein and 250 kcal per 250 ml. A child recovering from kwashiorkor, unless progress is retarded by infection, will accept very high calorie intakes until the weight approaches the normal value for height.

Anorexia may be serious, but often can be overcome by feeding the child very slowly in the mother's lap and by giving frequent feeds. Food may be taken better cold than hot. If the diarrhoea appears to be made worse on feeds containing skimmed milk, lactose intolerance may be present (p. 351). Such a child should respond to a mixture such as Casilan, cream, glucose and cereal.

As the clinical condition improves and the child attains normal weight for height, the local diet should be given in frequent feeds, care being taken to introduce a variety of plant and animal protein foods and maintain the fat content of the diet.

SUPPLEMENTS. Vitamins A and D, B complex and C and therapeutic doses of iron should be given routinely. If there is any suspicion of xerophthalmia 30 mg vitamin A should be given for 3 days.

Infants may lose 1–4 g of potassium chloride in the stools in one day if there is severe diarrhoea. The effect of the resulting potassium depletion on the myocardium may cause sudden death. Potassium should be given by mouth as a routine to all infants admitted with kwashiorkor. Depending on the age and weight of the child and the severity of the diarrhoea, the dose should be from 0·5 to 1 g of potassium chloride dissolved in water and added to three or four feeds each day. There is little or no danger of potassium intoxication when the mixture is given by mouth in these doses. Some centres also give magnesium.

PARENTERAL THERAPY. For very ill patients in a well-equipped and well-staffed hospital, who are suffering from marked dehydration, hypoglycaemia, acid-base disturbance or electrolyte imbalance, parenteral therapy with solutions such as half isotonic Darrow's solution with 2·5% dextrose may be a life-saving measure which should be started before dietetic treatment. Likewise, for severe anaemia from any cause, small slow transfusions of packed erythrocytes are of great value. In developing countries facilities for these measures are not available for the majority of severe cases of PEM.

COMPLICATIONS. Early recognition and prompt specific treatment of infection is crucial. Patients with PEM have increased susceptibility to (i) gastrointestinal infections and Gram-negative bacteraemia (ii) respiratory infections (iii) certain viral diseases, especially measles and herpes simplex (iv) tuberculosis (v) streptococcal and staphylococcal skin diseases (vi) helminthic infections. The usual signs of pyrexia and leucocytosis may not appear. The possibility of tuberculosis must always be considered, particularly if the child does not make the expected progress to recovery.

Antimalarial drugs are well tolerated whereas all anthelmintics are potentially toxic and must be used with due care in patients who are seriously ill. If anaemia from hookworm is so severe as to endanger life, small transfusions with packed cells should be given and will probably restore the child's condition sufficiently to permit appropriate treatment later. Iron-deficiency anaemia, which is frequently present due to associated dietary deficiency of iron and as a consequence of infections, requires appropriate treatment. Less commonly a megaloblastic anaemia is present which responds to folic acid.

CONVALESCENCE. When a child who has had severe kwashiorkor comes to be discharged from hospital he is still usually well below normal weight and height for his age. At this stage 'catch-up' (supernormal) growth is possible and obviously desirable, but it will not occur unless the child is in a favourable environment and getting all the food he will eat. If home conditions are difficult some simple convalescent home or nutritional rehabilitation centre would be ideal where available. In any case follow up should be arranged to see that the child does not deteriorate.

MILD KWASHIORKOR AND FOLLOW-UP CASES. Most cases have to be treated outside hospital. Dried skimmed milk sprinkled over the food is recommended if available or a local protein-rich food mixture. Mothers should be given instruction in regard to hygiene and methods of feeding. The doctor should try to arrange help for socio-economic problems where possible. A well-run nutrition rehabilitation centre can be very effective in treating these children at modest cost.

**Prognosis.** Severe kwashiorkor has a mortality of around 20% even in a well equipped hospital. Most deaths occur in the first 10 days. Jaundice, petechiae and stupor are bad signs. The usual causes of death are intercurrent infections and severe malnutrition, including potassium deficiency. The availability of medical care is another factor influencing prognosis.

In the long term, follow-up studies have shown that the fatty liver of acute kwashiorkor does not progress to cirrhosis. Physical growth of the brain is retarded in children who suffer from severe PEM in the first two years of life. There is circumstantial evidence that intelligence may be impaired, particularly if the child goes home to an environment in which catch-up growth cannot occur. Hence the great importance of trying to arrange the best possible conditions for a child's nutrition and mental development after leaving hospital.

**Prevention.** Poverty and ignorance are two main factors responsible for kwashiorkor. Every effort should be made to alleviate these causes. Education in nutrition, the introduction of improved farming methods and measures to reduce infections in young children, are all important. In each country careful thought must be given to the provision of protein-rich foods made from local crops which are suitable both for infant feeding and for supplementing diets low in protein. Cameron and Hofvander (p. 125) recommend over a hundred weaning recipes from many developing countries.

Even small amounts of food of animal origin, such as dried milk, egg, a little meat or concentrates of fish protein, are of great value when mixed with high protein vegetable foods. Although milk powder is a convenient source of protein it is only essential for treating severe kwashiorkor. The disease can, and often has to be prevented by appropriate combinations of local foods, e.g. cereals and legumes or groundnuts.

Education of parents, particularly mothers, in regard to the value of foods and best methods of preparing them, especially at the time of weaning, is invaluable. Much is being done by the establishment or extension of Child Welfare Clinics and Health Centres where free or subsidised skimmed milk powder or a protein food mixture is supplied, advice on diet given, and diseases liable to lead to kwashiorkor are prevented or treated. At the same time the advantages to mother and child of wider spacing of births should be explained and contraceptives provided.

## Nutritional Marasmus

In some developing countries marasmus is of greater clinical importance than kwashiorkor. It affects principally infants under 1 year of age in contrast to kwashiorkor which is chiefly encountered between 1 and 4 years of age. Marasmus is more likely to occur in poor people in underdeveloped countries who live in cities, while kwashiorkor occurs more frequently in those living in rural areas. The factors which predispose to marasmus are a rapid succession of pregnancies, and early and often abrupt weaning, followed by dirty artificial feeding of the infants with very dilute milk or milk products given in inadequate amounts to avoid expense. Thus the diet is low in both calories and protein. In addition unsatisfactory home conditions make the preparation of uncontaminated feeds almost impossible. Repeated infections therefore develop, especially of the gastrointestinal tract, which the mother often treats with water, rice water or some other non-nutritious fluid (Fig. 4.1).

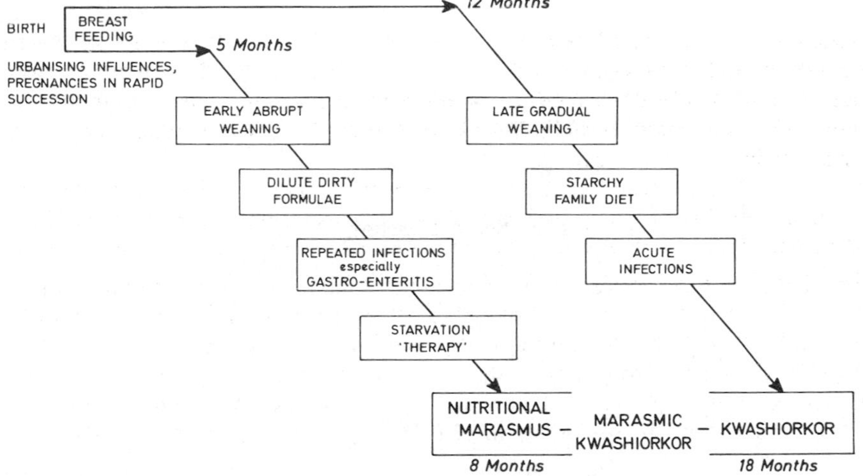


Fig. 4.1 Paths leading from early weaning to nutritional marasmus and from protracted breast feeding to kwashiorkor. (By courtesy of Dr D. S. McLaren and the editor of the *Lancet*.)

The most important cause of marasmus, early weaning, is in contrast to the late weaning, often extending over two years, which is characteristic of kwashiorkor. The mother may be induced to stop breast feeding for various reasons, including the presence of infection in herself or in the infant. She may have been influenced by advertisements which advocate the advantages of artificial food products. One reason for stopping breast feeding is economic pressure on the mother to go out and work. Another reason is pregnancy; there is widespread belief among uneducated women in developing countries that the milk of a pregnant woman is bad for her child.

**Clinical Features.** The two constant features of marasmus are: (1) retardation of growth and reduction of weight which is much more marked than that of length, and (2) wasting of subcutaneous fat and muscles which gives the infant a wizened, old appearance. There is usually watery diarrhoea or semi-solid, bulky, acid stools. In contrast to kwashiorkor, oedema is absent and the characteristic changes in the hair and skin, apathy and anorexia are seldom encountered. The abdomen may be distended with gas but the liver is not fatty. A careful search must be made for chronic infection like tuberculosis which predisposes to marasmus. The features of associated vitamin disorders such as angular stomatitis or keratomalacia, may develop, as may a deficiency of minerals, especially potassium and magnesium. Dehydration frequently occurs as a consequence of gastrointestinal infection.

**Treatment and Prevention.** In the acute stage of marasmus survival depends primarily on the efficiency with which measures can be applied to combat dehydration and restore electrolyte balance. In addition the child must be given a satisfactory diet along similar lines to those described for kwashiorkor. A longer refeeding period is usually required because the marasmic child is more severely wasted. The mortality rate during treatment is similar to that of kwashiorkor.

Prevention is a complex and difficult problem. A more equal distribution of land and wealth in developing countries and employment for all who can work is the ideal solution. Failing or pending that, education of mothers about birth spacing and about continuing breast feeding for as long as possible is of great importance. Further research is urgently needed into improved methods of feeding both healthy and ill infants in developing countries. It is probable that in the future marasmus will become of increasing clinical importance in developing countries as a consequence of a continuing decline in breast feeding and the urbanisation of uneducated families, socially insecure and living in poor, insanitary houses and with insufficient money to buy adequate supplements of milk or milk substitutes.

### Nutritional Dwarfing

Some children adapt to very prolonged mild to moderate calorie and/or protein deficiency by a proportional failure of growth. They are light in weight and short in stature but have superficially normal body proportions and subcutaneous fat. Such children are more prone to infections than normal. Unless the weight for age of such a child is checked against normal standards (Table 18.1, p. 904) it is easy for the doctor in a busy clinic to miss this form of PEM.

### Mild to Moderate PEM (The Underweight Child)

For every florid case of kwashiorkor or marasmus there are several children in the community with mild to moderate PEM. The situation is like an iceberg. There is more malnutrition below the surface than is recognisable on clinical inspection. The children with subclinical PEM can however be detected by their weight for age, which is less than 80% of the international standard (Table 18.1). In areas where kwashiorkor is the predominant florid form of PEM, subclinical cases have reduced plasma albumin and sometimes other biochemical signs of protein deficiency ('prekwashiorkor'). In parts of many developing countries surveys may show up to 5% of children under 5 years with signs and symptoms of kwashiorkor or marasmus while up to 50% are underweight.

The great importance of mild to moderate PEM is that these children are growing up smaller than their potential and they are very susceptible to gastroenteritis and respiratory infections, which in turn can precipitate frank malnutrition. Mild to moderate PEM is probably the major underlying reason why the one to four year mortality in a developing country can be 30 to 40 times higher than in Europe or North America. Official statistics record most of these deaths as due simply to infections.

## WATER, ELECTROLYTES AND MINERALS

The normal distribution of water and electrolytes in the body and the disturbances which result when their intake or output is diminished or increased are discussed in detail on pages 128 to 138.

Twelve or more elements are essential for man, as they are for other animals; deficiency disease is known for each but may not always result from an inadequate diet but from other causes such as excessive losses. The elements are sodium (p. 128), potassium (p. 131), magnesium (p. 134), calcium, phosphorus, iron, sulphur, iodine, zinc, copper, chromium and selenium. Fluoride appears to be essential for rats and optimal intakes reduce dental caries in man. Cobalt is physiologically active only in the form of vitamin $B_{12}$.

In addition manganese, tin, vanadium, molybdenum, nickel and silicon have been shown, by highly artificial isolator systems, to be essential for animals. Human deficiency disease is not known for any of these minor trace elements.

### Elements of Importance in Human Nutrition

**Calcium.** The body of an adult normally contains about 1200 g of calcium. At least 99% of this is present in the skeleton, where calcium salts (chiefly hydroxyapatite), held in a cellular matrix provide the hard structure of the bones and teeth. Obviously all of this calcium comes from the diet. Among common foods, the calcium-containing protein of milk (caseinogen) is much the richest source, which is one reason why milk and cheese are especially valuable for growing children. Half a litre of cow's milk contains about 0·6 g of calcium. Most other foods contribute much smaller amounts. However, peas, beans, other vegetables and particularly cereal grains are frequently the chief contributors because of the large amounts eaten.

Drinking water can provide significant amounts of calcium. In Britain the average intake from this source is about 75 mg Ca/day; but the variations are large: from none in water from peaty, acidic hill lochs in Scotland to 200 mg or even more in water obtained from wells sunk in chalk or limestone.

*Absorption.* 70 to 80% of the calcium in the food is normally excreted in the faeces. Calcium absorption may be impaired either by lack of vitamin D, by any conditions causing small intestinal hurry, by the combination of calcium with excess fatty acids to form insoluble soaps in steatorrhoea, or by certain substances in the diet which can form insoluble salts with calcium. These include foods rich in oxalic acid (e.g. spinach) and phytic acid which is present in the outer layers of cereal grains. Hence 'wholemeal' bread contains more phytic acid than white. To overcome the influence of phytic acid, calcium carbonate has been added to flour in Britain.

*Recommended Intakes of Calcium.* WHO (1974) recommends a daily intake of 500 mg for adult men and women, rising to 1200 mg during pregnancy and lactation. For adolescent boys and girls the recommended intake is 600 to 700 mg daily.

In many parts of Africa and Asia children develop healthy bones and adults remain in calcium balance despite calcium intakes which may be no more than half the above recommendations. Abundant sunshine possibly produces this effect. However a daily intake of 1000 mg should be taken during pregnancy and lactation.

Deficiency of calcium and vitamin D go hand in hand and are best considered together (p. 101).

**Phosphorus.** Eighty-five per cent of the phosphorus is normally present in the bones in combination with calcium. The remainder is chiefly in the cells. Phosphorus is essential for most metabolic processes.

Phosphorus is present in all natural foods, though in refined and processed foods the content may be greatly reduced. Primary dietary deficiency is not known to occur in man. Phosphorus depletion can occur from prolonged and excessive intake of aluminium hydroxide antacids which bind dietary phosphate in the gut. The features are weakness, anorexia, malaise and bone pains. Plasma inorganic phosphorus and urinary phosphate are very low.

**Iron.** A good mixed diet with average amounts of meat and vegetable contains about 12–15 mg of iron. Cheap monotonous high carbohydrate diets based on refined wheat flour contain much less. Foods which are particularly rich in iron are meat, liver, eggs, wholemeal cereals, oatmeal, peas, beans and lentils. The availability of the iron varies in different foods. Tests in man with $^{59}$Fe incorporated into foods have shown that iron is absorbed well from meat, haemoglobin and wine, moderately from pulses and poorly from eggs. Absorption is enhanced in iron deficient individuals. An account of the measures for the prevention and treatment of iron deficiency anaemia is given on page 546. Next to obesity this is probably the most important nutritional cause of ill-health in Britain and other prosperous countries.

*Siderosis.* Dietary iron overload is seen in South African Bantu men who cook and brew beer in iron pots. They may ingest as much as 100 mg of iron per day. Iron accumulates in the liver and when severe can lead to cirrhosis. A similar condition has been described in other countries following excessive indulgence in cheap wines which can contain 30 mg of iron per litre.

**Iodine.** Simple enlargement of the thyroid gland attributed to lack of iodine in the food occurs particularly in mountainous regions far from the sea. Other factors may also contribute to the causation of simple goitre (p. 478).

*Sources.* Iodine in small amounts is widely distributed in living matter. Seafoods are the only rich source in the diet. Vegetables and milk may contain useful amounts.

*Prophylactic Uses.* The prophylactic requirement is around 150 μg/day. The Medical Research Council recommended the addition of potassium iodide to all table salt in Britain as this has been proved to be highly successful in reducing the incidence of simple goitre in Switzerland, the USA and other parts of the world. The legislation required to enforce this recommendation in Britain has not yet been enacted.

**Fluoride.** The regular presence of fluoride in minute amounts in human bones and teeth and its influence on the prevention of dental caries justifies its inclusion as an element of importance in human nutrition.

*Sources.* Most adults ingest between 1 and 3 mg of fluoride daily. The chief source is usually drinking water, which, if it contains 1 part per million (p.p.m.) of fluoride, will supply 1–2 mg/day. Soft waters usually contain no fluoride, whilst very hard waters may contain over 10 p.p.m. Compared with this source, the fluoride in food-stuffs is of little importance. Very few contain more than 1 p.p.m.; the exceptions are sea-fish which may contain 5–10 p.p.m. and tea. In Britain, Australia and China, where people drink tea frequently, the adult intake from this source may be as much as 3 mg daily.

*Use of Fluoride in the Prevention of Dental Caries.* Epidemiological studies in many parts of the world have established that where the natural water supply contains fluoride in amounts of 1 p.p.m. or more, the incidence of dental caries is lower than in comparable areas where the water contains only traces of the element.

Fluoride becomes deposited in the enamel surface of the developing teeth of children. Such teeth are unusually resistant to caries. It may be that traces of fluoride in the enamel discourage the growth of acid-forming bacteria; alternatively, the calcium hydroxyapatite of the enamel may be rendered more resistant to organic acids by combination with traces of the element. It should be noted that fluoride is not deposited in fully developed adult teeth, so that little benefit to adults can be expected when they begin for the first time to drink water containing traces of fluoride.

The deliberate addition of traces of fluoride to those public water supplies which are deficient is now a widespread practice throughout North America where about 100 million people are now drinking fluoridated water. In at least 30 other countries similar projects have been started. In Britain regrettably some local authorities are not yet adding fluoride to their water supplies in those areas in which the element is lacking.

*Fluorosis*. In parts of the world where the water fluoride is high (over 3 to 5 p.p.m.) *mottling of the teeth* is common. The enamel loses its lustre and becomes rough, pigmented and pitted. The effect is purely cosmetic; fluorotic teeth are resistant to caries and not usually associated with any evidence of skeletal fluorosis, or any impairment of health.

*Chronic fluoride poisoning* occurs in several localities in India, China, Argentina, East and South Africa, where the water supply contains over 10 p.p.m. fluoride. Fluorine poisoning has also occurred as an industrial hazard among workers handling fluorine-containing minerals such as cryolite, used in smelting aluminium. The main clinical features are referable to the skeleton which shows sclerosis of bone, especially of the spine, pelvis and limbs, and calcification of ligaments and tendinous insertions of muscles.

**Sulphur** is mainly supplied by the S-containing amino acids in the diet—methionine and cysteine; effects of its deficiency are therefore inseparable from those of protein.

**Zinc** deficiency may impair maturation and immunocompetence. A syndrome has been described in Egypt and Iran of dwarfism and hypogonadism in late teenage boys. Serum zinc was low and prolonged treatment with zinc sulphate accelerated growth and sexual maturation. The cause is thought to be interference with zinc absorption by phytate in unleavened bread, which is the staple diet. Zinc deficiency in malnourished children causes thymic atrophy.

**Other Minerals.** *Copper* deficiency occasionally occurs in young children; the main features are anaemia, neutropenia, retarded growth and skeletal rarefaction. *Chromium* facilitates the action of insulin. Deficiency has been reported in some children with protein calorie malnutrition. The roles of sodium, potassium and magnesium are discussed in the next chapter.

## THE VITAMINS

Disorders due to vitamin deficiency are still widespread in many parts of the world. Even in industrial countries certain types of people are known to be at risk of developing some vitamin deficiency. Doctors should be ready to diagnose these treatable conditions in their early stages.

Vitamins are organic substances in food which are required in small amounts but which cannot be synthesised in adequate quantities. 12 vitamins have, so far, been demonstrated to have clinical effects in man. These are:

| Fat-soluble | Water-soluble | |
|---|---|---|
| Vitamin A | Vitamin C—Ascorbic acid | |
| Vitamin D | Vitamin B complex | Thiamin ($B_1$) |
| Vitamin E | | Niacin |
| Vitamin K | | Riboflavin |
| | | Pyridoxine ($B_6$) |
| | | Biotin |
| | | Cobalamins ($B_{12}$) |
| | | Folate |

Pantothenic acid, a major component of coenzyme A, also appears to be essential, but human deficiency disease has not been reported, perhaps because the vitamin is widely distributed in foods, as its name implies.

### Factors influencing the Utilisation of Vitamins

*Availability.* Fat-soluble vitamins may be deficient if dietary fat is not eaten or absorbed. Not all of a vitamin may be in absorbable form. For instance niacin in maize is bound in such a way that it is not absorbed from the gut.

*Antivitamins* are known to be present in some natural foods, e.g. thiaminase in raw fish. Some synthetic antagonists of the vitamins are used as drugs in the therapy of neoplasms (e.g. methotrexate p. 552) or of infections (e.g. pyrimethamine, p. 811). Neoplastic cells and micro-organisms are much more sensitive than normal cells but with high doses of the antivitamin a conditioned vitamin deficiency can occur.

*Provitamins.* Substances occur in foods which are not themselves vitamins but are capable of conversion into vitamins in the course of digestion. Thus some of the carotenes are provitamins of vitamin A and, to some extent at least, the amino acid tryptophan can be converted to niacin.

*Bacteria in the Gut.* The normal bacterial flora of the gut is capable of synthesising significant amounts of vitamin K. Bacteria are also capable of extracting vitamins from the ingested food and retaining them until excreted in the faeces. Except for vitamin K and probably biotin, bacteria are more likely to reduce than to increase the amounts of vitamins available for absorption, as is demonstrated in bacterial colonisation of the small intestine (p. 348).

*Biosynthesis in the Skin.* Vitamin D need not be provided in the diet if the skin is regularly exposed to adequate sunshine (p. 102).

*Interactions of Nutrients.* If the diet is rich in carbohydrates or alcohol more thiamin is needed for their metabolism. The requirement for vitamin E is increased when the intake of polyunsaturated fats is high.

These considerations indicate how difficult it may be in practice to define the nutritive value of a diet simply from chemical analysis of its vitamin content.

## Vitamin A (Retinol)

On the world scale vitamin A deficiency is one of the seven most common causes of blindness (the others being trachoma, onchocerciasis, gonococcal ophthalmia, accidents, cataract and glaucoma). FAO estimates that 50 to 100 thousand children become blind every year from keratomalacia.

Retinol is found only in foods of animal origin. Herbivores obtain the vitamin from its precursors or provitamins—some of the carotenoid pigments in plants. The conversion of even the best of these, $\beta$ carotene, into retinol in the human small intestinal wall is only 30% efficient. The absorption of both retinol and carotene is facilitated by fats and bile salts. Retinol has a place in the function of the retina and of epithelial and probably other cells.

**Dietary Sources.** Retinol is chiefly found in milk, butter, cheese, egg yolk, liver and some of the fatty fish. The liver oils of fish are the richest natural sources but these are used as nutritional supplements rather than foods.

Carotene is found chiefly in green vegetables in association with chlorophyll; the green outer leaves of cabbage and lettuce are good sources. Other useful sources are yellow and red fruits and vegetables. Vegetable oils are devoid of vitamin A activity except red palm oil which is a rich source of carotene. In Britain and some other countries retinol is added artificially to margarine to provide the same concentration as in good quality summer butter. Both retinol and carotene are stable to ordinary cooking methods, though some loss may occur at temperatures above 100°C.

Recommended daily intakes of retinol are 300 $\mu$g for infants and young children, 500–750 $\mu$g for children of 9 to 15 years, 750 $\mu$g for adolescents and adults, and 1200 $\mu$g for lactating women (1 $\mu$g retinol = 3 of the old i.u.). In many parts of the world most or all of the requirements are obtained from carotenoids in vegetable foods. Because only approximately $^1/_3$ of $\beta$ carotene is absorbed into the intestinal wall and then only ½ of this is converted into retinol, 1 $\mu$g retinol equivalent (=1 $\mu$g retinol) is now taken as = 6 $\mu$g $\beta$ carotene. Healthy adults in Britain have large stores of retinol in their livers.

**Pathology.** Deficiency of the vitamin results in morphological changes in the epithelial surfaces of all parts of the body. The cells undergo squamous metaplasia whereby they become flattened and heaped one upon another. The sebaceous glands and hair follicles of the skin and the tear glands of the eye become blocked with horny plugs of keratin so that their secretions diminish. The lack of tears and the heaping up of epithelium on the scleral conjunctiva and cornea produce xerophthalmia. When softening, ulceration and necrosis of the cornea develop, the condition is referred to as keratomalacia.

### Night Blindness

Retinol is an essential component of the pigment rhodopsin (visual purple) on which vision in dim light depends. Hence lack of retinol may result in impairment of 'dark adaptation' which can be measured by means of an adaptometer. Night blindness is common, as also is vitamin A deficiency, in poor people living in underdeveloped countries; it can occur in the malabsorption syndrome in affluent countries. Fatigue and anxiety states may cause persons to complain of night blindness. It may also result from organic disease of the eye such as retinitis pigmentosa. The diagnosis of vitamin A deficiency is supported by low plasma vitamin A concentration and is confirmed by marked improvement in dark adaptation following therapeutic doses of retinol.

### Xerosis Conjunctivae, Bitôt's Spots and Xerophthalmia

The earliest sign of xerosis conjunctivae is a dry, thickened and pigmented bulbar conjunctiva with a peculiar smoky appearance. Bitôt's spots are glistening white plaques formed of desquamated thickened conjunctival epithelium, usually triangular in shape and firmly adherent to the underlying conjunctiva. Xerosis conjunctivae and Bitôt's spots are certainly common in children whose diet is deficient in vitamin A but they can also occur in children whose intake of the vitamin is satisfactory. When dryness spreads to the cornea it takes on a dull, hazy, lacklustre appearance due to keratinisation, and xerophthalmia is said to be present.

In young children, xerophthalmia is almost always attributable to recent vitamin A deficiency and is usually associated with PEM. In older children and in adults its interpretation is less simple. Exposure to dust and glare may produce similar changes. They should, however, always call attention to the diet. Xerophthalmia is very important in young children because once the cornea is involved the process can rapidly progress to keratomalacia.

### Keratomalacia

This disease causes blindness among Indians, Indonesians and other rice-eating people of Asia; it also occurs in parts of Africa, the Middle East and Latin America. In Europe and North America it is very rare. Children between the ages of 1 and 5 years are most commonly affected. It occurs only in persons who have been living for a long period on diets almost entirely devoid of vitamin A. The disease is frequently associated with PEM.

The earliest manifestations are night blindness and xerophthalmia. Later the cornea undergoes necrosis and ulceration. Unless early and adequate treatment is given, there is a grave risk of blindness or death from associated diseases.

**Treatment.** A good mixed diet and attention to any associated infection are essential for the treatment of the above disorders. In xerophthalmia or severe adult cases of night blindness the administration of vitamin A in a dose of 30 mg retinol daily for three days should be started immediately. It is recommended that half the dose should be given orally in the form of halibut or similar rich fish oil and half intramuscularly as retinol acetate or palmitate, in order to ensure that the patient is actually getting the vitamin. During convalescence 9 mg of retinol daily in the form of fish-liver oil orally is adequate.

For the secondary bacterial infection, antibiotics are of value. Local treatment of the eye will be required only if disorganisation is already present, in which case the services of an ophthalmic surgeon should be obtained.

**Prevention.** Doctors and nurses working in the tropics, who may have been trained in Europe or North America, should make sure they are familiar with the appearances of xerophthalmia. If in doubt it is better to give a short course of vitamin A treatment. Pregnant women should be advised to eat dark green leafy vegetables. This helps to build up stores of retinol in the fetal liver. They should also be taught to give such vegetables or locally available yellow or orange fruits to their babies. In some countries where keratomalacia is a major cause of blindness, e.g. in India, single prophylactic oral doses of 60 mg retinol are being tried in young children.

### Follicular Keratosis

In this condition the hair follicles are blocked with horny plugs of keratin, rendering the skin surface rough and dry like the skin of a toad. The typical distribution is over the backs of the upper arms and the fronts of the thighs. Therapeutic trials in Africa have shown a striking clinical improvement in follicular keratosis when patients are given halibut liver oil or red palm oil. Nevertheless, it is not a specific sign of vitamin A deficiency, since it occurs not uncommonly in people who, by every other criterion, are adequately nourished in respect of vitamin A.

## Vitamin D

The material originally described as *vitamin* $D_1$ was subsequently found to be an impure mixture of sterols. *Vitamin* $D_2$ (*ergocalciferol*) is manufactured by the action of ultraviolet light on ergosterol, a sterol found in fungi and yeasts. When the term 'calciferol' is used in clinical practice it refers to ergocalciferol. Although widely used in therapeutics, it occurs very rarely in nature. *Vitamin* $D_3$ (*cholecalciferol*) is the natural form of the vitamin which occurs in man and other animals. It is formed in the skin by the action of ultraviolet light on 7-dehydrocholesterol.

Cholecalciferol is not the active form of the vitamin. It is converted in the liver to 25-hydroxycholecalciferol (25-OH-D) which is further hydroxylated in the kidney, mainly to 1,25 dihydroxycholecalciferol (1,25 (OH) D). Most of the hydroxylated forms of vitamin D in human plasma are based on vitamin $D_3$ (cholecalciferol) derived from synthesis in the skin or from fish liver oils. A smaller proportion is based on vitamin $D_2$ (ergocalciferol) from calciferol tablets or fortified milk (e.g. in USA). Though plasma 25-OH-$D_3$ and 25-OH-$D_2$ can be distinguished by immunoassay, they and their corresponding derivatives appear to have identical activities. 1,25 (OH) D is many times more potent than cholecalciferol and can be regarded as a hormone rather than a vitamin which requires further metabolic transformation to become biologically active. It is transported in the blood to target organs, notably gut and bone and is regulated by a complex feedback system. The main function of 1,25(OH)D is to increase calcium absorption to meet the demands of growth, pregnancy and lactation. An adequate concentration of calcium is thus ensured for the formation of calcium phosphate in bone where calcium comes in contact with inorganic phosphates, liberated from organic phosphates under the influence of phosphatase produced by osteoblasts.

$1\alpha$ hydroxycholecalciferol ($1\alpha$ OH-D) is a synthetic analogue which is converted into 1,25 (OH) D in the liver without the need for hydroxylation in the kidney. It is used in renal disease (p. 439).

The main reasons for impaired production of 1,25 (OH) D are: (1) deficiency of 25-OH-D due to lack of sunlight, an inadequate diet or malabsorption; (2) disturbed metabolism in liver or renal disease, notably chronic renal failure and (3) depression of the feedback system as in hypoparathyroidism.

**Dietary Sources**. The richest sources are fatty fish and their liver oils, some of which contain thousands of micrograms of vitamin D per 100 g. Vitamin D is also present in much smaller quantities in dairy products such as butter and eggs. In Britain vitaminised margarine is the most reliable food source of the vitamin for adults: 28 g (1 oz) contains nearly the daily requirement. Milk has a very small content of vitamin D; meat and white fish have insignificant amounts and cereals, vegetables and fruit have none. Unlike vitamin A, stores of vitamin D in the body are not large; only a little is stored in the liver and moderate amounts in adipose tissue.

The recommended daily intake (WHO) for infants and children up to 5 years of age and for pregnant or lactating women is 10 μg. For older children and adults about 2·5 μg is adequate (1 μg = 40 i.u.). People who regularly have adequate exposure of their skin to sunlight do not normally need vitamin D in their diet.

## Rickets

Rickets is a disease of calcium and phosphorus metabolism which occurs when infants or children obtain insufficient vitamin D. It is still an important clinical problem in some developing countries, especially in large towns and cities. Infants in their first year are mainly affected due to an inadequate intake of vitamin D because of the low content of this vitamin in both human and animal milk and the failure to provide them with a supplement of vitamin D in any form. In addition, for various social and cultural reasons, their mothers wrap them up in clothes which prevents their exposure to sunlight. By the second year the infant is able to crawl about in the sunshine and spontaneous healing usually occurs. The disease is now uncommon in countries where vitamin D is freely available. In Britain clinical rickets occurs in Asian immigrant children, often of schoolgoing age, from a combination of little exposure of the skin to sunlight and very low dietary intakes of vitamin D. High phytate intake in chapatti flour may contribute by inhibiting calcium absorption. The disease is also liable to occur in premature babies.

Epileptic patients on long-term anticonvulsants are liable to develop rickets in childhood or osteomalacia in adult life; these drugs induce changes in liver microsomal enzymes which lead to the conversion of vitamin D to inactive metabolites.

**Clinical Features.** The infant with rickets has often received sufficient calories and may appear well nourished, but is restless, fretful and pale, with flabby muscles. Sweating of the head is common. The abdomen is distended. The infant is prone to respiratory infections and gastrointestinal upsets. Development is delayed; the teeth often erupt late and there is failure to sit, stand, crawl and walk at the normal ages.

The bony changes are the most characteristic signs of rickets. The earliest lesion is often craniotabies — small round unossified areas in the membranous bones of the skull, yielding to the pressure of the finger, with a crackling feeling. This sign is of particular value in the diagnosis of rickets in developing countries where the disease is common in infants under 1 year of age. It usually disappears within 12 months of birth. Two other early signs are enlargement of the epiphyses at the lower end of the radius and at the costochondral junctions of the ribs, the latter known as the 'rickety rosary'. Later there may be 'bossing' of the frontal and parietal bones and delayed closure of the anterior fontanelle. Later still, there may be deformities of the chest such as pigeon chest and Harrison's sulcus.

If rickets continues into the second or third year of life, deformities such as kyphosis develop as a result of the new gravitational and muscular strains, caused by sitting up and crawling. At the same time there may be enlargement of the epiphyses at the lower ends of the femur, tibia and fibula. When the rachitic child begins to walk, deformities of the shafts of the leg bones develop, so that 'knock knees' or 'bow legs' are seen. Pelvic deformities may follow and lead later to serious difficulties at childbirth.

When there is a reduction in ionised plasma calcium, infantile tetany may result, with spasm of the hands and feet and of the vocal cords. The latter causes a high-pitched distressing cry and great difficulty in breathing. Epileptic fits may also occur.

**Investigation.** Radiological examination of the wrist will show characteristic changes at the epiphyses; the outline of the joint is blurred and hazy, and the epiphyseal zone becomes broadened. In older children, the classical concave 'saucer' deformity is shown.

*Chemical Pathology*. Plasma calcium tends to fall from its normal level (p. 906). More commonly the serum phosphate falls due to the parathyroid glands responding to a slight reduction in calcium by increasing the excretion of phosphorus in the urine.

Clinical rickets may occur when the levels of calcium and phosphorus in the plasma are still within normal limits. A diagnostic change is an increase in alkaline phosphatase. This enzyme is formed by the osteoblasts which, unable to make bone without a sufficient supply of calcium, liberate into the circulation the excess of this enzyme which they cannot use. Plasma 25-hydroxycholecalciferol is the main circulating form of vitamin D and is very low or zero in rickets.

**Treatment.** The two essentials of treatment are the provision of a supplement of vitamin D and an ample intake of calcium.

A therapeutic dose of vitamin D varies from 25 to 125 μg (1000–5000 i.u.) daily, depending on the severity of the disease and age of the child. In contrast, the prophylactic dose is 10 μg or less daily depending on the sunlight. Children can be given halibut-liver oil in a very small dose (1 ml) since it contains 30 times the vitamin D concentrations of cod-liver oil. For severe cases needing 125 μg or more daily, synthetic calciferol is useful.

In times of social upheaval, such as may be occasioned by war or disasters, when a young child may be seen once by an emergency medical service and perhaps not again for months, a single massive dose of vitamin D, e.g. 3·75 mg, can be given by mouth with reasonable safety and curative effects. The daily administration of small doses is the method recommended for normal practice, because of the danger of overdosage (p. 104).

In addition to vitamin D, rachitic infants and children require an ample supply of calcium, the best source of which is milk. At least half a litre should be taken daily by a young child with rickets. For a severe case a supplement of calcium tablets should also be given such as calcium gluconate.

Treatment of tetany is described on page 483.

PROGRESS. The earliest evidence of healing in rickets is provided by radiological examination of the growing ends of the bones. The levels of calcium and phosphorus in the serum provide an unreliable guide. Decrease in the raised serum alkaline phosphatase does not usually occur for several weeks after treatment is initiated. The therapeutic dose of vitamin D should be continued so long as the phosphatase level remains elevated; thereafter it may gradually be reduced to the prophylactic dose of 10 μg daily.

Rickets is not a fatal disease *per se*, but the untreated rachitic child is always at risk of infections, notably bronchopneumonia. The skeletal changes, if mild in degree, usually tend to heal spontaneously as the child gets older, but in severe cases pigeon chest, spinal curvature, knock knees, bow legs or contracted pelvis persist.

VITAMIN D RESISTANT RICKETS. Occasionally cases of rickets are encountered which are resistant to ordinary therapeutic doses of vitamin D. The disease persists into late childhood ('late rickets') or even adult life, producing the clinical appearance of osteomalacia, unless adequately treated. One cause is defective reabsorption of phosphate as occurs in uncommon congenital disorders of the renal tubules e.g. the Fanconi syndrome (p. 423). A similar state may sometimes arise as a conditioned deficiency resulting from malabsorption of vitamin D or from chronic renal failure in which renal formation of 1,25 di OH cholecalciferol is impaired. Whatever the cause, treatment consists in giving large doses of vitamin D by mouth together with calcium salts. The initial dose of calciferol may be 1·25–3·75 mg daily but it should be reduced at the first suspicion of toxic symptoms.

HYPERVITAMINOSIS D. In the case of vitamin D it is possible to have too much of a good thing. Large doses are toxic and cause hypercalcaemia. The symptoms include nausea, vomiting, constipation, drowsiness and signs of renal failure; metastatic calcification in the arteries, kidneys and other tissues may occur. Since renal damage may develop before clinical signs of toxicity appear, all patients on large doses of vitamin D should have their serum calcium level checked regularly at three-monthly intervals and if this is found to be above 2·6 mmol/*l* (10·5 mg/100 ml) it is an early indication of overdosage.

**Prevention.** The provision of adequate milk for children, the clearing of slums, the building of new housing estates and smoke abatement schemes are basic prophylactic measures which must be continued. In addition mothers must be educated in the need to keep their infants and children in the sunshine as much as possible. Nevertheless, in northern countries, the supply of the vitamin from this source is uncertain and attention must be paid to the dietary supply. None of the common foods in a child's diet is a good source of vitamin D and children may benefit from a daily supplement of about 10 $\mu$g of cod-liver oil, continued at least in the winter for the first 5 years of life or more.

It is necessary to consider how much vitamin D an infant is getting from other sources. Some proprietary cereal foods for infants are 'fortified' with vitamin D by the manufacturers, as in margarine (p. 102). Not only is there no advantage in giving infants and young children more than 10 $\mu$g of vitamin D daily from *all sources* for prophylactic purposes, but higher doses given over a long period could predispose to infantile hypercalcaemia, a form of hypervitaminosis D. The prophylactic dose of vitamin D for premature infants should be twice that for full-term infants and it should be started within 2 weeks of birth.

## Osteomalacia and Osteoporosis

Osteomalacia, which means softening of bone, is primarily due to a deficiency of vitamin D, and to a lesser extent of calcium, or both. This results in a failure to replace the turnover of calcium and phosphorus in the organic matrix of bone. Hence the calcium phosphate content is reduced and bony substance becomes replaced by soft osteoid tissue.

Osteoporosis, which is atrophy of bone, is believed to be due to defective formation of bone matrix which leads to a reduction in the total mass of bone. In other words osteoporosis is too little bone of normal mineral content. In contrast to osteomalacia the ratio of calcium phosphate to matrix is normal.

## Osteomalacia

**Aetiology**. Osteomalacia is the adult counterpart of rickets. It was formerly common in women in purdah in oriental countries, living on poor cereal diets devoid of milk, kept indoors and seldom seeing the sun. Symptoms occurred with pregnancy.

In Scotland and in other countries where osteomalacia is a relatively common disease in old people, especially women, the disease may be due to malabsorption from any cause, including operations like partial gastrectomy, or to direct dietary deficiency of vitamin D. Chronic renal disorders are a less important cause. Adult epileptics who have to take anticonvulsants for years are likely to develop osteomalacia (p. 102).

**Clinical Features.** Skeletal pain is usually present and persistent and ranges from backache to severe pain. Bone tenderness on pressure is common. Muscular weakness is often present and the patient may find difficulty in climbing stairs or getting out of a chair. A waddling gait is not unusual. Tetany may be manifested by carpopedal spasm and facial twitching. Spontaneous fractures may occur, independent of the pseudo-fractures described below. The biochemical changes in the blood are the same as in rickets.

Radiological examination shows rarefaction of bone and commonly translucent bands (pseudo-fractures, Looser's zones), often symmetrical, at points submitted to stress. Common sites are the ribs, the axillary border of the scapula, the pubic rami and the medial cortex of the upper femur. Looser's zones are pathognomonic when well-developed.

Histological examination of stained undecalcified sections of bone obtained by biopsy may be required as this shows unequivocally the presence of excess osteoid tissue.

**Treatment**. When osteomalacia is primarily due to defective intake, treatment is essentially the same as for rickets, namely 25 to 125 $\mu$g vitamin D daily. The response is usually dramatic. If there is evidence of malabsorption the dose should be 1·25 mg daily and it may have to be given intramuscularly at weekly intervals. If the disease is secondary to renal disorders double or treble this dose may be necessary. Maintenance treatment with vitamin D will be required for all cases of osteomalacia in which the cause cannot be removed. In addition a good diet should be given which includes milk. A supplement of calcium should be given orally, namely one to two tablets of calcium gluconate thrice daily. Within 4 to 8 weeks of starting treatment the pain and weakness have usually disappeared. The decision to reduce or discontinue the dose of vitamin D and calcium is based on the improvement in the clinical features and the disappearance of biochemical and radiological abnormalities. The dangers of vitamin D intoxication should be kept in mind.

**Prevention.** With improved education and better standards of living the disease is now much rarer in many Asian towns where previously it was common. Free access to sunshine and an adequate intake of dairy produce, supplemented when necessary with fish-liver oil, will prevent nutritional osteomalacia. Particular attention to these prophylactic measures should be given to inmates of geriatric and mental hospitals and to old people living alone whose exposure to sunshine is limited and also to those who have had gastric surgery. Epileptic patients on long-term anticonvulsant therapy should be given prophylactic doses of vitamin D.

### Osteoporosis

Osteoporosis is the commonest metabolic disease of bone and is found most frequently in elderly women when it is known as postmenopausal osteoporosis. It may occur in elderly men (senile osteoporosis) and rarely in younger people (idiopathic osteoporosis). There is a wide variation in the geographical and racial incidence of generalised osteoporosis. For example, in the United States it is more prevalent in Caucasians than in Negroes.

**Aetiology and Pathology.** A physiological decrease in skeletal mass occurs in all persons from the age of 40 to 50 onwards; the process is more marked in women, and in some individuals it would appear to be accelerated by factors which are largely unknown. In postmenopausal women there is a failure of oestrogen secretion and in men diminished androgen formation may contribute. It would appear unlikely that simple dietary deficiency has a primary role in the aetiology.

Inadequate physical activity promotes generalised osteoporosis and may, in part at least, account for the high incidence of this condition in affluent societies. Immobilisation by splinting, inflammation or pain is the main cause of local osteoporosis.

Generalised osteoporosis may be secondary to prolonged treatment with adrenal corticosteroids; it occurs in various endocrine disorders, notably Cushing's syndrome and hypogonadism, and also in severe malnutrition and chronic renal disease. Osteoporosis, like anaemia, may therefore be the end result of a number of diverse processes.

The histological appearances are in keeping with Albright's original conception of a primary osteoblastic hypoplasia. The bone is deficient in quantity but there is no abnormality of its quality or architecture, in contrast to osteomalacia where there are abnormally large amounts of osteoid tissue.

**Clinical Features.** The patient is usually an elderly woman who is otherwise healthy. There may be no disability despite obvious radiological abnormality. In others there are episodes of severe pain usually due to fractures of the brittle bones often occurring after minimal trauma. The lumbar and thoracic vertebrae, the neck of the femur, the upper end of the humerus and the lower end of the radius are the commonest sites of fracture. Healing is not impaired and as it occurs pain usually subsides. More persistent backache is a later feature of osteoporosis due to progressive compression or collapse of several vertebrae. This may result in loss of stature and in kyphosis. Persistent pain elsewhere is not a feature of osteoporosis but is more characteristic of osteomalacia, Paget's disease or skeletal metastases. In contrast to these conditions there is also a tendency for spontaneous improvement to occur in osteoporosis. Idiopathic osteoporosis is occasionally found in younger persons in whom it also tends to be self-limiting.

The radiological changes are more marked in the bones of the axial skeleton than in the limbs; they consist of loss of bone density, reduction in the number and size of trabeculae and thinning of the cortex. The upper and lower surfaces of the lumbar and thoracic vertebral bodies become biconcave, and later compression or collapse causes anterior wedging.

The calcium, phosphorus and alkaline phosphatase levels in the blood are normal in contrast to osteomalacia.

**Treatment.** Any primary factor such as excessive corticosteroid therapy or endocrine disease should be corrected if possible. The physiological decline in skeletal mass, the obscure aetiology of idiopathic osteoporosis and its tendency to remission, together with the need for long-term assessment, make therapeutic measures very difficult to evaluate.

The patient should know that the natural history of the disease is characterised by spontaneous improvement and that suitable regular exercise is beneficial. The patient should remain ambulant if symptoms permit. The use of spinal supports is undesirable. Immobilisation following a fracture should be limited to the part involved and accompanied by graduated remedial exercises. It should be borne in mind that osteomalacia can coexist with osteoporosis especially in patients with a fracture of the neck of the femur.

Cyclical oestrogen therapy (p. 500) may be prescribed for otherwise healthy postmenopausal women. On general principles, at least an adequate intake of vitamin D and calcium should be ensured. Cows' milk is the best source of the latter, half a litre providing about 20 g of protein and 600 mg of calcium, but obesity must be avoided and, if present, corrected. There is evidence that calcium supplements are beneficial and possibly also 1$\alpha$ OH-D combined with oestrogens.

## Vitamin E

Alpha-tocopherol is the most potent of eight related substances with vitamin E activity. It is found in vegetable oils, eggs, butter, wholemeal cereals and broccoli and peas.

Vitamin E prevents oxidation of polyunsaturated fatty acids in cell membranes. The main feature of human deficiency is a mild haemolytic anaemia. This has been described only in premature infants and in a few cases of malabsorption.

There is no scientific justification for self-medication with vitamin E in the belief that this will increase energy or virility.

## Vitamin K

Vitamin K is required for the formation in the liver of factor II (prothrombin) and factors VII, IX and X, which are necessary for the normal clotting of blood. It exists in nature in two forms, vitamin $K_1$ and vitamin $K_2$. Vitamin $K_1$ (phytomenadione) is soluble in fat solvents but only slightly in water. It is found in leafy vegetables and is available for oral and parenteral use.

Foods of animal origin, including fish-liver oils, are poor sources unless they have undergone extensive bacterial putrefaction, with formation of one of the vitamin $K_2$ series. Adequate amounts are normally supplied in the average diet and bacterial synthesis occurs within the colon.

Vitamin K deficiency is discussed on page 598.

## Vitamin C (Ascorbic Acid)

Ascorbic acid is a simple sugar. It is the most active reducing agent found in living tissues and is easily and reversibly oxidised to dehydro-ascorbic acid. Its highest concentrations are in the adrenal cortex and in the eye. Stress and corticotrophin lead to a loss of ascorbic acid from the adrenal cortex. The presumption, therefore, is that ascorbic acid is intimately concerned in bodily reactions to stress. Man is one of the few animals that cannot synthesise ascorbic acid from glucose.

**Dietary Sources**. Blackcurrants, guavas, citrus fruits, berries and green vegetables are the richest sources. Foods of animal origin contain very little except for liver and glandular tissue. Dried cereals and pulses contain no ascorbic acid.

Ascorbic acid is very easily destroyed by heat, alkalis such as sodium bicarbonate, traces of copper or by an oxidase liberated by damage to plant tissues. Ascorbic acid is very soluble in water. For these reasons many traditional methods of cooking reduce or eliminate it from the diet. A satisfactory daily intake is 30 mg (WHO). Body stores last for about 2½ to 3 months on a deficient diet.

### Scurvy

**Aetiology**. In 1497 when Vasco da Gama sailed round the Cape of Good Hope 100 out of his 160 men died of scurvy. For the next 300 years scurvy was a major factor determining the success or failure of all sea ventures even after it was recognised by Lind (1753) and by Cook (1755) that it results from the prolonged consumption of a diet devoid of fresh fruit and vegetables. Final proof and isolation of vitamin C were not possible until the guinea pig was found to provide a suitable animal model (1907).

Sporadic cases of scurvy continue to arise in infants as a result of ignorance, poverty and maternal neglect and also amongst old people, especially men living alone who are not feeding themselves properly. Scurvy appears to be rare in most tropical countries but is more likely to occur in arid regions in times of drought.

**Pathology**. Ascorbic acid deficiency results in defective formation of collagen in connective tissue because of failure of hydroxylation of proline to hydroxyproline, the characteristic amino acid of collagen. There is in consequence delayed healing of wounds. There are also capillary haemorrhages and subnormal platelet stickiness.

**Clinical Features**. ADULT SCURVY. The pathognomic sign is the swollen and spongy gums particularly of the papillae between the teeth, sometimes producing the appearance of 'scurvy buds'. These are livid in colour and bleed easily. The teeth may become loose and even fall out in severe cases. There is always some infection; indeed this seems necessary for the production of the scorbutic gingival appearances since volunteers suffering from experimental deficiency did not develop it if their gums were previously healthy. Associated with the infection there is an offensive fetor. In patients without teeth the gums appear normal.

The first sign of cutaneous bleeding is often found on the lower thighs. These are perifollicular haemorrhages—tiny points of bleeding around the orifice of a hair follicle. There is a heaping-up of keratin-like material on the surface around the mouth of the follicle, through which a deformed 'corkscrew' hair characteristically projects. Perifollicular haemorrhages are often followed by petechial haemorrhages, developing independently of the hair follicles, which are usually first seen on the feet and ankles. Thereafter large spontaneous bruises (ecchymoses) may arise almost anywhere in the body, but usually first in the lower extremities, producing the characteristic 'woody leg'. Haemorrhage may occur into joints, into a nerve sheath, under the nails or conjunctiva or into the gastrointestinal tract; there may be epistaxis. Scurvy can present with any of these features. By the time the disease is fully developed the patient is usually anaemic.

Before the changes in the gums and skin appear, the patient has usually felt feeble and listless for some weeks. A patient with scurvy may die suddenly and without warning apparently from cardiac failure. Another characteristic of scurvy is that fresh wounds fail to heal—a feature that the surgeon has to bear in mind.

The dietary and social history is helpful in doubtful cases. Old, solitary people may insist that they fend very well for themselves, but careful questioning will reveal that they do not bother to purchase fresh fruit or vegetables. In other instances the proper foods may be purchased but they are so badly cooked that the diet loses all its vitamin C.

Plasma ascorbate is very low (p. 119); a fresh sample of plasma is needed because the vitamin can decompose in a few hours at warm room temperatures. Probably a better index of tissue reserves of the vitamin is its concentration in the buffy layer or the platelets.

INFANTILE SCURVY The main clinical features are lassitude, anaemia, painful limbs and enlargement of the costochondral junctions. Until the teeth have erupted, scorbutic infants do not develop gingivitis. The first sign of bleeding is usually a large subperiosteal haemorrhage in one of the long bones. This gives rise to intense pain, especially on movement.

**Treatment**. Because of the danger of sudden death, ascorbic acid should be given at once in adequate amounts. Parenteral treatment has no advantage over oral administration. The aim should be to saturate the body quickly with ascorbic acid. The normal body contains about 1·5g of the vitamin, so that a dose of 250 mg by mouth four times daily should achieve this within a few days, despite a considerable loss in the urine which quickly follows each dose.

Attention should be paid to correcting the general deficiencies of the patient's former diet. A liberal mixed diet should be given. If the patient is anaemic iron and sometimes folic acid are indicated.

With adequate treatment no patient dies of scurvy and recovery is usually rapid and complete.

**Prevention**. Fruit juice should be given for the first 2 years of life, especially to bottle-fed infants.

No simple administrative means has been found of preventing scurvy among the old and solitary, who are largely unresponsive to education. Should the physician be unable to persuade such a person to eat fruit or vegetables, one 25 mg tablet of synthetic ascorbic acid should be taken daily. Alternatively a massive dose can be given at longer intervals—say, 500 mg every month.

Trauma, surgery and burns, infections, smoking and certain drugs—adrenocortical steroids, aspirin, indomethacin and tetracycline—all increase the requirement for vitamin C. Consequently any sick patients in hospital require considerably more than the recommended allowance of 30 mg/d.

ASCORBIC ACID AND THE COMMON COLD. It has been claimed that ascorbic acid in doses of 1–2 g daily will prevent the common cold. If it does, this is a pharmacological and not a vitamin effect as coryza is not a manifestation of scurvy. In the largest controlled trial, in Toronto, two placebo groups were included. One of these had fewer colds than those taking 1/4, 1 or 2 g vitamin C per day prophylactically. It is inadvisable for people to dose themselves with large quantities of ascorbic acid as this favours the formation of oxalate stones in the urinary tract.

## Thiamin (Vitamin $B_1$)

Thiamin salts are readily soluble in water but not in fat. Thiamin pyrophosphate (TPP) is an essential coenzyme for the decarboxylation of pyruvate to acetyl coenzyme A. This is the bridge between anaerobic glycolysis and the tricarboxylic acid (Krebs) cycle. TPP is also the coenzyme for transketolase in the hexose monophosphate shunt pathway and for decarboxylation of α-ketoglutarate to succinate in the Krebs cycle. Consequently when thiamin is deficient (*a*) the cells cannot utilise glucose aerobically; this is likely to affect the nervous system first, since it depends entirely on glucose for its energy requirements; (*b*) there is accumulation of pyruvic acid and of lactic acid derived from it, which produce vasodilatation and increase cardiac output. High carbohydrate diets predispose to and aggravate thiamin deficiency.

In man thiamin deficiency can produce cardiomyopathy and/or peripheral neuropathy and/or encephalopathy. These occur in various combinations in wet and dry beriberi, infantile beriberi and Wernicke's encephalopathy.

**Dietary Sources**. Legumes, pork, liver, nuts, the germ of cereals and yeast, are the only rich sources. Green vegetables, roots, fruits, flesh foods and dairy produce (except butter) contain small amounts of the vitamin. It is not found in fats or refined oils. In refined sugar and many cereal products (wheat, rice) nearly all the naturally occurring vitamin may be removed; there is little or none in most alcoholic drinks.

As thiamin is readily soluble in water, considerable amounts may be lost when vegetables are cooked in an excess of water which is afterwards discarded. It is relatively stable below 100°C provided that the medium is slightly acid, as in baking with yeast. But if baking powder is used, or if soda is added in cooking vegetables, almost all the vitamin may be destroyed. The loss of thiamin in cooking an ordinary mixed diet is usually around 25%. Modern processes for freezing, canning and dehydrating food result in only small losses. Thiamin is not stored in the body to any appreciable extent; hence symptoms due to deficiency may develop within a few weeks.

The recommended daily intake is 0·4 mg/1000 kcal or about 1·2 mg in an adult man.

### Beriberi

Beriberi is a nutritional disorder formerly widespread in South and East Asia. The word comes from the Singhalese language and means 'I cannot', signifying that the patient is too ill to do anything. It has almost disappeared from prosperous Asian countries such as Japan, Taiwan and Malaysia and from big cities such as Hong Kong, Manila and Singapore. Oriental beriberi is usually caused by eating diets in which most of the calories are derived from polished, i.e. highly milled, rice. The disorder is often precipitated by infections, hard physical labour or pregnancy and lactation. In Britain and North America occasional cases of beriberi heart disease are seen, usually in alcoholics who have been consuming little but alcohol for some weeks.

**Chemical and Pathological Findings**. Owing to a lack of thiamin, carbohydrates are incompletely metabolised and lactic and pyruvic acids accumulate in the tissues and body fluids. These metabolites cause dilatation of peripheral blood vessels, as in normal exercise. In beriberi this vasodilatation may be extreme, so that fluid leaks out through the capillaries, producing oedema. At the same time the blood flows rapidly through the dilated peripheral circulation. There is a high cardiac output and as the disease progresses the heart dilates because the myocardium is both overworked and unable to use glucose efficiently as an energy substrate. Cardiac failure accentuates the oedema. Sudden death may result. Microscopic examination usually shows loss of striation of myocardial fibres, which are also finely vacuolated and often fragmented and separated by oedema.

In dry beriberi there is severe wasting of muscles. In long-standing cases there is degeneration and demyelination of both sensory and motor nerves. The vagus and other autonomic nerves may be affected. In dry beriberi the level of blood pyruvate is usually within normal limits.

In Wernicke's encephalopathy there are foci of congestion and petechial haemorrhage in the upper part of the mid-brain, the hypothalamus, and the walls of the third ventricle. The mamillary bodies are always involved and this is believed to account for defects of memory.

**Clinical Features**. The *early* symptoms and signs are common to wet and dry beriberi. The onset is usually insidious, though sometimes precipitated by unaccustomed exertion or a febrile illness. There is anorexia and malaise, associated with heaviness and weakness of the legs. There may be a little oedema of the legs or face and the patient may complain of precordial pain and palpitations. The pulse is usually full and moderately increased in rate. There may be complaints of 'pins and needles' and numbness in the legs. The tendon jerks are usually reduced and the calf muscles may be tender on pressure. Hypoaesthesia or anaesthesia of the skin, especially over the tibiae, is common. In areas where beriberi is endemic such a condition may persist for months or even years with only minor alterations in the symptoms. The patients are only mildly incapacitated and many continue to earn their living even as manual labourers, but at a very low level of efficiency. At any time this chronic malady may develop into either of the severe forms.

WET BERIBERI. Oedema is the most notable feature and may develop rapidly to involve not only the legs but also the face, trunk and serous cavities. Palpitations are marked and there may be pain in the legs after walking, probably due to the accumulation of lactic acid. The neck veins become distended and pulsate freely. The heart is enlarged. There is usually tachycardia and an increase in pulse pressure. While the circulation is well maintained, the skin is typically warm owing to the vasodilatation; as heart failure advances, the skin of the extremities becomes cold and cyanotic. The mind is usually clear. Electrocardiograms often show no changes except sinus tachycardia but in some cases there are inverted T waves or evidence of disturbed conduction.

DRY BERIBERI. The essential feature is a polyneuropathy (p. 734). The muscles become progressively weak and wasted, and walking becomes increasingly difficult. The thin, even emaciated patient needs at first one stick, then two, and may finally become bedridden. The disease is essentially a chronic one, which may be arrested at any stage by improving the diet. Bedridden patients and those with severe cachexia are very susceptible to infections. Patients with dry beriberi are always liable to a sudden onset of oedema which may be due to a variety of dietary causes, e.g. lack of thiamin, protein or calories.

INFANTILE BERIBERI. This is seen in areas where adult beriberi is endemic. It occurs in breast-fed infants, usually between the second and fifth months. Although the mothers of such infants must have been eating a diet and secreting milk with a low thiamin content, classical signs of beriberi are stated to be absent in 50% of them. The illness usually starts acutely and is rapidly fatal, if not promptly treated. The mother may have noticed that the infant is restless, often cries, is passing less urine than normal and shows signs of puffiness. The infant then may suddenly become cyanosed with dyspnoea and tachycardia and die within 24 to 48 hours. Other serious signs are convulsions and coma. In severe cases partial to complete aphonia is characteristic and is usually preceded by the infant's cry becoming thin with a plaintive whine. Infantile beriberi was formerly the chief cause of death between 2 to 6 months of age in rice-eating rural areas in S.E. Asia, and it may still occur in isolated areas.

WERNICKE'S ENCEPHALOPATHY AND KORSAKOFF'S PSYCHOSIS. This cerebral form of thiamin deficiency occurs in Europe and North Ameria. It often presents acutely, usually in an alcoholic but it is sometimes seen in people with malnutrition, e.g. persistent vomiting; it occurred in prisoners of war on small rations of polished rice. The patient is quietly confused and the most valuable clinical sign is some form of bilateral, symmetrical ophthalmoplegia. This may be in one or more than one direction and accompanied by abnormal pupillary reflexes and/or nystagmus. Ataxia is also present. The confusion is liable soon to progress to stupor or death if treatment is delayed. There may be permanent memory defect, *Korsakoff's psychosis*, the characteristic bedside feature of which is confabulation. The patient is disorientated and psychological tests show a severe defect of memorising, i.e. storing new information.

Wernicke's encephalopathy and Korsakoff's psychosis are often associated with polyneuropathy but it is surprising how uncommon these cerebral forms are in S.E. Asia and that beriberi cardiomyopathy is seldom seen with Wernicke/Korsakoff disease.

**Investigation**. Plasma pyruvic or lactic acids are not elevated in the more chronic forms of beriberi and if they are increased are not specific. The best laboratory test is measurement of transketolase activity in red cells with and without added thiamin pyrophosphate *in vitro*. The test requires fresh red cells and heparinized whole blood must be taken before thiamin treatment is started. A grossly abnormal result appears to be specific for beriberi or Wernicke's encephalopathy.

**Treatment.** *Wet Beriberi*. Treatment must be started as soon as the diagnosis is made, because fatal heart failure may occur suddenly. Complete rest is essential and 50 mg thiamin should be given intramuscularly for three days. Thereafter 10 mg three times a day should be continued by mouth until convalescence is established.

The response of a patient with beriberi to thiamin is one of the most dramatic events of medicine. Within a few hours the breathing is easier, the pulse rate slower, the extremities cooler and a rapid diuresis begins to dispose of the oedema. In a few days the size of the heart is restored to normal. Muscular pain and tenderness are also dramatically improved. The ECG may show characteristic paradoxical changes while the patient improves. In a typical case the tracing is normal while heart failure is severe, then as recovery starts T wave inversions appear over the right ventricle for a few days.

*Dry Beriberi*. The treatment is that of a nutritional polyneuropathy as described on page 736.

*Wernicke's encephalopathy* should be treated without delay with 50 mg thiamin hydrochloride by slow intravenous injection followed by 50 mg thiamin intramuscularly daily for a week.

*Infantile Beriberi.* The simplest way to treat infantile beriberi is via the mother's milk. The mother should receive 10 mg thiamin hydrochloride twice daily—in severe cases by injection. In addition the infant must be given thiamin starting with 20 mg intramuscularly.

*Associated Deficiencies.* Other deficiencies in the patient's diet may include protein, vitamin A, nicotinic acid and riboflavin. In the early stages the other B vitamins should be supplied, e.g. as tablets, and a good protein intake given. Thereafter a mixed diet with less emphasis on rice is needed.

**Prevention.** In principle all that is necessary in endemic areas is to prevent the production of over-milled rice or wheat. In practice, however, there are many difficulties in the control of milling processes and in persuading people to change their customary diet.

It is desirable to try to reduce the proportion of rice in the diet and encourage the growing of alternative crops and the consumption of other foods. Much can sometimes be done with small gardens properly cultivated. The substitution of parboiled rice for highly milled rice also greatly reduces the incidence of beriberi. Parboiling is the term used to indicate that unhusked rice has been steamed or boiled after preliminary soaking. If this is done before the rice is milled the greater portion of the vitamin B complex is conserved.

In Western countries the prevention of beriberi and Wernicke's encephalopathy is related to the control of alcoholism.

## Niacin

*(Nicotinic Acid and Nicotinamide)*

Nicotinamide is an essential part of the two important pyridine nucleotides, NAD and NADP which are hydrogen-accepting coenzymes for dehydrogenases at many steps in the pathways of glucose oxidation. NAD is also the coenzyme for alcohol dehydrogenase. Nicotinic acid (niacin) is readily converted in the body into the amide. For nutritional purposes the two have equal biological activity and are considered together in foods under the generic term 'niacin'. Both are water-soluble and resistant to heat.

**Dietary Sources.** Niacin is widely distributed in plant and animal foods, but only in relatively small amounts, except in meat (especially the organs), fish, wholemeal cereals and pulses. Removal of the bran in milling cereals reduces their niacin to low levels. A cup of good coffee provides about 1 mg of niacin. In a normal Western European diet about half the nicotinic acid content is provided by meat and fish.

Cooking causes little destruction of niacin but considerable amounts may be lost in the cooking water and 'drippings' from cooked meat if these are discarded. In a mixed diet, from 15 to 25% of the niacin of the cooked foodstuffs may be lost in this way. Commercial processing and storage of foodstuffs cause little loss.

A special feature of this vitamin is that it is normally synthesised in the body in limited amounts from the amino acid tryptophan; 60 mg of tryptophan yields 1 mg of nicotinamide. For this reason niacin equivalents in a diet are calculated by adding together the niacin plus $^{1}/_{60}$ of the trypotophan intake (in mg). The recommended daily intake is 18 mg of niacin equivalents in adult men.

## Pellagra

Pellagra is a nutritional disease endemic among poor peasants who subsist chiefly on maize (American corn). The greater part of the niacin in maize is in a bound form, niacytin, which is unavailable to the consumer. Moreover the principal protein of maize, zein, is deficient in the essential amino acid tryptophan, the alternative source of niacin.

Pellagra is a relatively new disease, unknown to classical and mediaeval physicians. It has occurred all over the world, wherever maize is the staple cereal. e.g. the southern states of the USA, Africa and Southern Europe and also in certain regions in India, Asia and Latin America. In recent years pellagra has disappeared from many countries where it was once endemic; in areas where it remains the incidence is much less than formerly. An exception is southern Africa where big outbreaks occur in the spring and summer in certain Bantu areas.

Isolated cases of pellagra occur among people who are not dependent on maize. It is occasionally seen in alcoholics and in the malabsorption syndrome. Pellagra has been reported as a complication of very low protein diets used in patients with renal failure if supplementary B vitamins are forgotten. In the rare inborn error of metabolism, *Hartnup disease*, tryptophan absorption is impaired and there is a pellagrous dermatitis with neurological abnormalities which respond to nicotinamide.

**Pathology**. There is dermatitis and the mucous membranes of the alimentary tract and vagina usually show abnormal epithelium with underlying inflammation. Small mucous cysts are seen in the colon and sometimes ulcers. In the nervous system there may be chromatolysis of ganglion cells and patchy demyelination in the spinal cord.

**Clinical Features.** *General*. Pellagra can develop in only 6 to 8 weeks on diets very deficient in niacin and tryptophan. The patient is often underweight, and presents the general features of poor nutrition. Pellagra has been called the disease of the three D's: dermatitis, diarrhoea and dementia.

*Skin*. The diagnosis is generally first suggested by the appearance of the skin. Characteristically, there is an erythema resembling severe sunburn, appearing symmetrically over the parts of the body exposed to sunlight. Local trauma or irritation of the skin may also determine the site of the lesion. The affected areas are well demarcated from normal skin. They are at first red and slightly swollen; they may itch and burn. In acute cases the skin lesions may progress to vesiculation, cracking, exudation and crusting with ulceration and sometimes secondary infection; but in chronic cases the dermatitis occurs as a roughening and thickening of the skin with dryness, scaling and a brown pigmentation. Dermatitis of the vulva, perineum and perianal area is usually present. Nasolabial seborrhoea is sometimes seen (p. 116).

Pellagra may sometimes occur without skin lesions if the patient has been confined indoors. This variety has been called 'pellagra sine pellagra' and should be remembered if unexplained delirium or dementia is found in a housebound person who has been taking a poor diet for a prolonged period.

*Alimentary Tract*. Diarrhoea is common but not always present. There may be anorexia, nausea, dysphagia and dyspepsia. The tongue characteristically has a 'raw beef' appearance — red, swollen and painful. Glossitis is an early symptom and may precede the skin lesions. The mouth is sore and often shows angular stomatitis and cheilosis (p. 116). It is probable that a non-infective inflammation extends throughout the gastrointestinal tract and accounts for the diarrhoea which is usually watery, sometimes with blood and mucus in the stools.

*Nervous System*. In the milder cases the symptoms consist chiefly of weakness, anxiety, depression, irritability and failure of concentration; in severe cases delirium is the most common mental disturbance in the acute form of the disease and dementia in the chronic form. Because of these changes, chronic pellagrins may be admitted to mental hospitals.

**Treatment**. Nicotinamide is given in a dose of 100 mg every 4 to 6 hours by mouth, although a smaller dose is likely to be effective. The vitamin is rapidly absorbed from the stomach, despite severe digestive disorders. There is therefore no indication for giving it parenterally. The response to nicotinamide is usually rapid; within 24 hours the erythema of the skin diminishes, the tongue becomes paler and less painful and the diarrhoea ceases. Often there is also striking improvement in the patient's behaviour and mental attitude.

Nicotinamide alone is usually insufficient to restore health. Some of the features found in pellagra are clearly the result of associated nutritional deficiences. First, a relatively low intake of protein including tryptophan is an essential condition for development of the disease, and hypoalbuminaemia is common. Secondly, anaemia may coexist, either of iron or folate deficiency type. Thirdly, deficiences of other B complex vitamins are to be expected. Peripheral neuropathy may be caused by thiamin or pyridoxine deficiency, nasolabial seborrhoea and angular stomatitis by riboflavin deficiency and spinal cord lesions, when present, by vitamin $B_{12}$ deficiency. Lastly the patient has usually lost weight. Nicotinamide treatment should therefore be supplemented with a nutritious diet, high in protein. Vitamin B complex tablets should be given and iron, folic acid and vitamin $B_{12}$ may be necessary in addition for some cases. Alcohol should be forbidden.

Rest in bed and sedation are necessary for severely ill pellagrins. If mental symptoms are marked they can sometimes be troublesome to nurse. If the dermatitis is associated with much crusting or secondary infection, gentle washing with a bland solution is indicated. If the diarrhoea is severe enough to cause electrolyte disturbances parenteral fluids may be needed. Infection may well be present and require appropriate treatment.

**Prognosis**. In endemic areas most cases are mild, improving in the winter and relapsing with the increased sunshine in the spring. In long-standing cases there may be persistent mental, spinal cord and digestive disorders.

Occasionally a fulminating form develops, with fever and prostration, and may be fatal. In the past, most of the deaths arose from secondary infections, or from emaciation due to PEM intensified by the diarrhoea.

**Prevention**. The disappearance from the southern states of America of pellagra which before the Second World War afflicted tens of thousands of poor country folk, demonstrates that the disease is preventable. Fortification of bread and maize meal with nicotinic acid, is only one of several factors which have produced this satisfactory result. General improvement in the economic state, education and nutrition of the population appears to have had more effect.

In Central America the peasants eat a staple diet of maize but pellagra is unusual. This is because of the traditional method of boiling the maize in lime water (dilute calcium hydroxide) before they make tortillas. It has been found that the indigestible niacytin is hydrolysed to free niacin in dilute alkali.

From the standpoint of agricultural policy, it is clearly wise to avoid too much dependence on a single cereal crop, such as maize, or to devote too great an acreage of fertile land to the cultivation of cash-crops, such as cotton or tobacco. Animal husbandry and cultivation of legumes should be encouraged in all areas where pellagra is endemic.

For the medical practitioner in such an area, without direct influence on agricultural policy, the best advice that he can give to people is to take as many animal products and legumes as they can afford. He will also do well to prescribe tablets of vitamin B complex for patients with a poor dietary history or skin signs suggesting early pellagra.

## Riboflavin

Riboflavin is a constituent of the flavoproteins which are concerned with tissue oxidation. It is a yellow-green fluorescent compound soluble in water. Though stable to boiling in acid solution, in alkaline solution it is decomposed by heat. It is also destroyed by exposure to light.

**Dietary Sources**. The best sources of riboflavin are liver, kidney, milk, meat, cheese and eggs. Green vegetables contain moderate amounts. It differs from other components of the vitamin B complex in that it occurs in good amounts in dairy produce, but is relatively lacking in cereal grains, especially when highly milled. It is also present in beer. Ordinary methods of cooking do not destroy the vitamin apart from losses that occur when the water in which vegetables have been boiled is discarded. If foods, especially milk, are left exposed to sunshine, large losses may occur. The recommended daily intake is 1·7 mg in adult men.

### Disorders due to Riboflavin Deficiency

When human volunteers have been given diets very low in riboflavin, the most consistent clinical manifestations were angular stomatitis, cheilosis and nasolabial seborrhoea; these responded to the addition of pure riboflavin in the deficient diet.

*Angular stomatitis* is not specific for riboflavin deficiency. Deficiences of niacin, pyridoxine and iron can all produce it. It can follow herpes febrilis at the angle of the mouth. A common cause is ill-fitting dentures, associated with candidiasis.

*Cheilosis* is the name given to a zone of red, denuded epithelium at the line of closure of the lips. It has occurred in experimental pure niacin deficiency. It is often associated with angular stomatitis and frequently seen in pellagrins.

*Nasolabial seborrhoea or dyssebacea* is the term given to enlarged follicles around the sides of the nose which are plugged with dry sebaceous material. It is seen in some patients with pellagra.

*Other Abnormalities*. Vascularisation of the cornea, scrotal dermatitis, a magenta-coloured tongue and anaemia have been attributed to riboflavin deficiency but its place in their causation in man is controversial.

Riboflavin clearly plays a vital role in cellular oxidation and there are communities and individuals who have both minimal dietary intakes and very low concentrations in urine or blood. Yet it is surprising that the clinical effects of riboflavin deficiency are trivial and mostly non-specific. Features of riboflavin deficiency are most likely to be found in pellagrins and in malnourished rice-eaters in Southeast Asia. In the first situation they are overshadowed by niacin deficiency and in the second by thiamin or protein deficiency.

**Treatment**. The therapeutic dose of riboflavin is 5 mg three times a day by mouth. It gives the patient's urine a green fluorescence. As discussed above, other B complex vitamins should also be given.

## Pyridoxine (Vitamin $B_6$)

Pyridoxine, pyridoxal and pyridoxamine are three closely related compounds with similar physiological actions. The active form of the vitamin in man is pyridoxal phosphate, the coenzyme for over 60 different enzyme systems, including aminotransferases, involved in the metabolism of all the amino acids. Vitamin $B_6$ is widely distributed in plants and animal tissues. Liver, whole grain cereals, peanuts and bananas are good sources. The normal adult requirement is 2 mg per day.

### Disorders due to Pyridoxine Deficiency

Although a series of pathological changes in the skin, liver, blood vessels, nervous tissue and bone marrow have been produced experimentally in various animals, disorders due to deficiency of pyridoxine rarely occur in man, and then very seldom as a result of dietary deficiency.

Convulsions, which respond to pyridoxine, have been reported to occur in infants on artificial feeds of powdered milk deficient in pyridoxine. In adults dermatitis, cheilosis, glossitis and angular stomatitis have been produced by means of the pyridoxine inhibitor, 4-desoxy-pyridoxine. The peripheral neuropathy associated with isoniazid therapy is due to a conditioned pyridoxine deficiency. Some cases of sideroblastic anaemia respond to treatment with pyridoxine (p. 547).

Biochemical features of pyridoxine deficiency can occur in women taking oral contraceptives, and the mild depression which affects a small proportion of such women may be relieved by pyridoxine.

## Biotin

Biotin functions as coenzyme for several carboxylases. It is present in a number of different foods; the requirement is small (about 100 $\mu$g/day) and it can be synthesised by intestinal bacteria. Human deficiency is rare; it has occurred in adults who have taken for long periods large amounts of raw egg which contain the antagonist avidin. The clinical features include dermatitis. A form of seborrhoeic dermatitis of infants responds to biotin.

## Vitamin $B_{12}$ and Folate

These vitamins and disorders due to their deficiency are discussed on page 548 and page 551.

## Biochemical Diagnosis and Subclinical Vitamin Deficiencies

Biochemical methods are an integral part of modern medical diagnosis. For example, plasma sodium and potassium concentrations are essential for the diagnosis and treatment of difficult electrolyte problems and plasma or red cell folate and vitamin $B_{12}$ concentrations are desirable before treating a patient with megaloblastic anaemia. Likewise with the other vitamins, biochemical tests have been developed which are more or less valuable, *(a)* for confirming the diagnosis of a deficiency disease in places where it is uncommonly seen or if the clinical picture is complicated or *(b)* in community surveys, for identifying individuals with subclinical vitamin deficiencies.

The tests which can be used for the major nutrients are listed in Table 4.2. As with other tests in chemical pathology there can be false positives and false negatives. Each result needs to be evaluated with critical understanding; for example, serum vitamin $B_{12}$ is increased in acute hepatitis and alkaline phosphatase may not be elevated if rickets is accompanied by PEM.

In general when the dietary intake of a nutrient is inadequate the individual goes through three stages. The first stage is that of adaptation to the low intake. For example, urine excretion falls but there is no evidence of abnormal function or of depletion of the cells.

In the second stage there are in addition biochemical changes indicating either impaired function, e.g. reduced red cell transketolase activity in thiamin deficiency, or cellular depletion, e.g. reduced white cell ascorbic acid. But clinical manifestations of deficiency are absent or non-specific.

The third stage is that of clinical deficiency disease.

Most clinical biochemistry laboratories provide only some of the methods as a routine but others might be provided in special circumstances or, alternatively, specimens could be sent to a laboratory specialising in nutrition research.

## Prevention of Nutritional Deficiencies

There are broadly three ways of approaching prevention:

1. *Increasing food consumption per head.* This requires increased production of food in the country or increased export earnings with which to import food. However, an overall increase of food in a country will be of little value unless the majority of people have jobs which provide sufficient money to buy the food they need. In addition effective national programmes of population control must be implemented in many countries. Doctors are likely to have more of a role to play in helping with birth control than with agricultural or economic planning.

2. *Nutrition education and food enrichment.* Education in nutrition consists of teaching and motivating people to make a healthy choice of foods. It ranges from advising agricultural planners on which crops should be encouraged to teaching mothers how to feed their children and distribute food sensibly in the family, using what is available to them.

Where vitamin or mineral deficiencies occur, or could occur, food enrichment is one possible solution. This is used mostly in industrial countries; it is difficult to organise in developing countries where there are many small farmers who grow their own food. To be effective the enriched food should reach the potentially deficient segment of the population, so the choice of which staple food to enrich needs careful consideration. Addition of vitamins A and D to margarine and iodization of salt are good examples of useful food enrichment. The use of nutrients which are toxic in large amounts must be limited. Food enrichment should be supervised and monitored by the appropriate government ministry. It is not the answer to every nutritional deficiency even in industrial countries; for example, further enrichment of bread with

Table 4.2. Biochemical methods for diagnosing nutritional status (protein, major vitamins and minerals)

| Nutrient | Principal Methods: Indicating Reduced Intake | Principal Methods: Indicating Impaired Function (IF) or Cell Depletion (CD) | Supplementary Methods |
|---|---|---|---|
| Protein | Urinary nitrogen | Plasma albumin (IF) | Fasting plasma amino acid pattern |
| Vitamin A | Plasma vitamin A (retinol) and plasma carotene | | |
| Thiamin | Urinary thiamin | RBC transketolase and TTP effect* (IF) | Plasma pyruvate and lactate* |
| Riboflavin | Urinary riboflavin | RBC glutathione reductase and FAD effect (IF)* | RBC riboflavin |
| Niacin | Urine N'methyl nicotinamide and 2–pyridone | | Fasting plasma tryptophan |
| Pyridoxine | Urinary 4-pyridoxic acid | RBC glutamic oxal-acetic transaminase and PP effect (IF)* | Urinary xanthurenic acid after tryptophan load* |
| Folic Acid | Plasma folate *(Lactobacillus casei)* | Red cell folate (CD) Haemoglobin, PCV and smear (IF) | Urinary FIGLU after histidine load*. Bone marrow morphology |
| Vitamin $B_{12}$ | Plasma vitamin $B_{12}$ *(Euglena gracilis)* | Haemoglobin PCV and smear (IF) | Schilling test. Bone marrow morphology |
| Ascorbic Acid | Plasma ascorbic acid | Leucocyte ascorbic acid (CD) | Urinary ascorbic acid |
| Vitamin D | Plasma 25-hydroxy-cholecalciferol | Plasma alkaline phosphatase (IF)* | Serum calcium and inorganic phosphorus |
| Vitamin E | Plasma tocopherol | RBC haemolysis with $H_2O_2$ *in vitro* | |
| Vitamin K | | Plasma prothrombin (IF) | |
| Sodium | Urinary sodium | Plasma sodium | |
| Potassium | Urinary potassium | Plasma potassium | Total body potassium by $^{40}K$ |
| Iron | Plasma iron and transferrin | Haemoglobin, PCV and smear (IF) | Plasma ferritin (CD) |
| Iodine | Urinary (stable) iodine | Plasma thyroxine and $T_3$(IF) | |

Asterisk(*) indicates value *increased* in deficiency.

iron will not solve the problem of iron deficiency anaemia. It is better dealt with by the third strategy.

3. *Health and medical action for vulnerable groups*. Many countries provide nutritious lunches for school children. Pregnant mothers should be given prophylactic doses of iron and folate; young childrens' mothers should expose them to sunlight regularly or they should be given small prophylactic doses of Vitamin D. Women with menorrhagia and patients who have had gastric surgery should be given iron tablets periodically. The housebound elderly should be given prophylactic amounts

of vitamin D and sometimes other nutrients. Patients receiving diuretics should have a good intake of potassium. Doctors should be trained to anticipate the possibility of certain types of malnutrition in association with particular diseases.

In developing countries where most people do not have direct access to a doctor, maternal and child health clinics provide a centre for therapeutic, preventive and educational services at moderate cost, aimed at the most vulnerable sections of the community. In this setting nutrition and infection must be treated in an integrated way and can often be combined with family planning.

A. S. TRUSWELL

## Obesity

Obesity is the most common nutritional disorder in affluent societies. Its significance requires constant emphasis because it is associated with increased mortality, predisposes to the development of important diseases and diminishes the efficiency and happiness of those affected.

Obesity may be defined as a condition in which there is an excessive amount of body fat. This simple definition gives rise to two questions: how can body fat be measured, and what is 'excessive'? All methods of measuring the fat content in the living subject are, to a greater or lesser degree, indirect. The simplest, but also the least direct, is the measurement of body weight and this is the method almost exclusively used in clinical practice. In the clinical context the 'desirable' or 'ideal' weight (p. 905) is that associated with the lowest mortality in actuarial terms and excessive weight that associated with increased mortality.

**Aetiology.** Excess fat accumulates because there is imbalance between energy intake and expenditure. This can arise in different ways and obesity is a clinical sign with several possible causes. There is no satisfactory aetiological classification of obesity, but a number of factors are known to be associated with its development.

*Age.* Obesity is most prevalent in middle-age, but can occur at any stage of life. Obesity in childhood and adolescence is likely to be followed by obesity in adult life.

*Socio-economic.* In affluent countries obesity is more common in the lower socio-economic groups. In developing countries it can occur only in the prosperous elite. Some occupations predispose to obesity, e.g. cooks and barmen, whilst jockeys, fashion models and airline pilots have to keep themselves slim. In some societies fat men are respected and fat women considered beautiful; in others they are not.

*Heredity.* A familial tendency exists in many cases, but it is difficult to disentangle environmental and genetic components. Patterns of eating and activity are influenced by social, cultural and economic factors which may be handed on from one generation to another. However, studies involving twins and adopted children indicate the importance of genetic factors in influencing both total body fat and its distribution. There is no evidence in man of obesity produced by a single gene, as in the genetically obese strains of rodents.

*Endocrine Factors.* An endocrine influence on body fat is seen both in normal physiological situations and in pathological states. The normal fat content of young adult women is about twice that of young men and pregnancy is characterised by an increase in body fat. Obesity in women commonly begins at puberty, during pregnancy or at the menopause. Obesity frequently, but not invariably, accompanies hypothyroidism, hypogonadism, hypopituitarism and Cushing's syndrome. However, the overwhelming majority of obese patients show no clinical evidence of an endocrine disorder. The plasma concentration of insulin and cortisol is commonly raised and that of growth hormone reduced in obese subjects, but these changes probably result from, rather than cause the obesity, since they disappear when weight is lost.

*Energy Intake.* A very small excess of calories, if habitual, can lead eventually to a large accumulation of fat. If a person eats a slice (20 g) of bread that is not needed each day or goes by car instead of walking for 20 minutes, the daily extra 48 kcal (200 kJ) will build up over 10 years to 20 kg of fat deposited. Social factors, such as advertising and business lunches, may contribute to overeating and some people overeat because they are unhappy. There is some evidence that in obese people eating is determined less by 'internal cues', i.e. hunger and satiety, than by external influences like the availability, appearance and taste of food or the environment in which the food is served. However, while some obese subjects, for one reason or another eat more than those who are not obese, undoubtedly many do not and the presumption must be that many obese subjects have an unusually low energy expenditure.

*Energy Expenditure.* Physical inactivity has an important role in the development of obesity. Affluence is commonly associated with reduced energy expenditure. It is well recognised that physical activity is less in the obese than in the lean, but this may result from, rather than cause, the obesity. Moreover, the amount of energy expended by an obese person on most tasks is likely to be more because of the extra weight to be moved.

Little is understood about the control of energy balance in man, but there can be no doubt that some individuals gain weight more readily than others. Apart from possible alterations in the efficiency of basal metabolism there is some evidence that the thermic response to food may be less than normal in obese subjects leading to greater conservation of energy. The possible roles of brown adipose tissue and of the sodium pump are being investigated.

*Drugs.* The use of steroids, oral contraceptives, phenothiazines and insulin is commonly followed by obesity, mainly because appetite is stimulated.

**Clinical Features.** In most cases the diagnosis will be apparent from the patient's appearance but the degree of obesity should also be assessed, usually by measurement of height and weight and reference to the table on page 905 where the weight of the patient can be compared with that of an 'ideal' subject of the same sex, height and frame. In addition, the skinfold thickness over the triceps muscle can be measured using special spring-loaded calipers. Obesity is indicated by a reading above 20 mm in a man, and above 28 mm in a woman.

This very common disorder is frequently overlooked because the doctor is preoccupied by one of its many complications or ignores it because it is so familiar.

Obesity must be distinguished from a gain in weight due to fluid retention associated with cardiac, renal or hepatic disease, bearing in mind the fact that oedema does not become manifest clinically until the extracellular fluid has increased by about 15%.

**Complications.** *Psychological.* Obese patients are often psychologically disturbed, but it is difficult to distinguish between cause and effect. Depressed or anxious patients or the emotionally deprived may seek solace in food. Many obese people, especially younger adult females, are ashamed of their unattractive appearance and develop psychosocial and sexual problems.

*Mechanical Disabilities.* Flat feet and osteoarthrosis of the knees, hips and lumbar spine are more common in obese people. The abdominal muscles supporting the viscera and the leg muscles, whose contractions promote venous return, are less efficient, predisposing to the development of abdominal and diaphragmatic hernias and varicose veins. Adipose tissue round the trunk interferes with the mechanics of respiration resulting in exertional dyspnoea and increased susceptibility to respiratory infection.

*Metabolic Disorders.* Hyperlipidaemia (with elevation of both cholesterol and triglyceride), gallstones, hyperuricaemia and gout and non-insulin dependent diabetes mellitus are all more common among the obese than in the general population.

*Cardiovascular Disorders.* Obesity increases the work done by the heart, which enlarges with rising body weight. The cardiac output, stroke volume, and blood volume all increase. Hypertension is common but, in the obese, blood pressure recorded with a standard sphygmomanometer cuff may be higher than direct intra-arterial measurements. The major source of error is failure of the blood pressure cuff completely to encircle the arm. The contribution which obesity alone makes to the aetiology of ischaemic heart disease is controversial. There is little doubt that obesity is associated with this disease, but it is difficult to separate the contribution of obesity from that of other risk factors which may be causally associated, such as diabetes and hyperlipidaemia, or from that of independent risk factors, such as smoking. Special mention should also be made of physical inactivity, which may be both a cause and an effect of obesity and also plays an important role in the genesis of ischaemic heart disease.

*Life Expectancy.* With all these possible complications it is not surprising that overweight is associated with an increased rate of mortality at all ages. The level of excess mortality varies more or less in proportion to the degree of obesity. Thus subjects 30% overweight incur a 30% increase in mortality and for those 35 to 40% overweight the increase rises to 50%. There is also evidence that a substantial reduction of the body weight of overweight people is alone sufficient to diminish the greater death rate. In the Society of Actuaries Build and Blood Pressure Study of 1959, the mortality was reduced to normal in those who successfully lost and maintained weight within the desirable range. Thus the diagnosis and effective treatment of obesity is literally of vital importance, and recording the patient's height and weight must be just as much a routine part of clinical examination as taking the blood pressure or testing the urine.

**Treatment.** Whatever the ultimate cause of obesity in the individual case the immediate cause is energy imbalance, and weight reduction can be achieved only by reducing energy intake or by increasing output, or by a combination of the two. This involves change in the individual's life-style. Thus treatment is difficult and the patient needs motivation. Rewards must be seen ahead and psychological understanding and behavioural advice are essential weapons. It is most important for success that patients should be educated and informed about their disorder and misconceptions corrected. There are no 'slimming foods' or 'slimming tablets', which do not depend on a reduced energy intake. Long-term results are best where patients are well motivated and educated, follow structured diets designed to provide 800 to 1600 kcal daily (p. 900) and are being seen and weighed regularly, every one to two weeks initially, by the same person. The number of patients requiring supervision is so great, the need for support is so prolonged and the success of some lay organisations such as 'Weight Watchers' compares so favourably with conventional medical methods, that it is justifiable to take advantage of the facilities provided by these groups. Most refer members to their own doctors at the first suggestion of any untoward developments.

However supervision is arranged, it is most important for success that obese patients should be given precise instructions as to how they should reorganise their dietary and other habits, a target weight to aim for and an indication of the rate of weight loss expected.

Among the important lessons to be learned by obese people is the need to manage the disorder themselves. Unlike many conditions for which patients seek help, success does not depend upon operations, drugs, injections or other manipulations undertaken by the therapist but rather on the ability of the patient to accept advice, to act upon it, and to persist indefinitely with some restriction on dietary freedom.

The physician's role is to provide advice and continuing support. Many doctors find obese people unattractive, have difficulty in sympathising with their problems and fail to establish satisfactory rapport with them. Such attitudes contribute to the frequent lack of success in treatment.

THE CONSTRUCTION OF A WEIGHT REDUCING DIET. A weekly weight loss of 0·5 to 1 kg should be the general aim. An obese middle-aged housewife will usually lose weight satisfactorily on a diet providing 800 to 1000 kcal per day, such as the example on page 900. An obese man engaged in active physical work will not tolerate a diet as low as 1000 kcal per day but a satisfactory weight loss can be expected from a diet containing about 1500 kcal per day.

*Protein.* Dietary protein of 50 g/day is sufficient to maintain nitrogen balance. High protein diets may satisfy appetite more effectively than high carbohydrate diets, but they are expensive, may not be particularly palatable after a time, or may have a high incidental content of fat, and are therefore seldom practicable.

*Carbohydrate.* The intake of foods rich in carbohydrate must be reduced since overindulgence in these is common. Obese people seldom develop more than a trace of ketosis and never sufficient to cause symptoms as long as they consume small amounts of carbohydrate. In a diet of 1000 kcal/day, 100 g of carbohydrate is a suitable allowance and this should be taken as foods providing complex carbohydrates and dietary fibre (such as fruits and vegetables and whole grain cereals) rather than as foods containing glucose and sucrose.

*Fat.* A diet containing 100 g of carbohydrate and 50 g of protein, cannot include more than 40–45 g of fat. This allowance of fat, though small, is sufficient to make the diet palatable.

*Vitamins.* The diet should contain plenty of green vegetables and fruits, since they contain few calories, while their bulk helps to fill the stomach and relieve hunger; they also help to minimise the constipation common with a low food intake. Their vitamin A activity and vitamin C will be sufficient to meet the body's needs. With meat, fish and eggs in the diet and little or no refined cereals and sugar, it is improbable that deficiency of any component of the vitamin B complex will arise.

*Minerals.* The only minerals that need serious consideration are calcium and iron. Provided the diet includes 300 ml of skimmed milk, there is little likelihood of a negative calcium balance developing in an adult. The supply of iron is less sure and may call for the prescription of iron supplements.

*Fluids and Salt.* At one time, patients were often advised to restrict their intake of water, but there is no logical reason for keeping fat patients thirsty. Sweetened 'juices' must be avoided, except those sold for diabetic patients, which have a low caloric content. *Alcoholic drinks* are also a source of calories and hence are best avoided, but if taken, a corresponding reduction in the diet is necessary.

The obese are particularly susceptible to water and salt retention but diuretics must be used with discrimination because potassium depletion is particularly liable to occur while patients are on a reducing regimen. Salt restriction alone may be sufficient to alleviate oedema, but when diuretics are considered essential, potassium supplements should be given.

*General.* This diet is suitable for treatment of obese persons in Britain but it may be unsuitable in other circumstances and in other climates. Dietitians with knowledge of local eating customs can devise diets which are socially acceptable and which provide about 1000 kcal made up from about 100 g carbohydrate, 50–60 g protein and 40–45 g fat.

In the absence of oedema or any endocrine disorder, failure to respond to such a diet nearly always indicates non-compliance, despite protestations to the contrary! In such cases, treatment in hospital under strict supervision for one or two weeks may be beneficial to demonstrate that the prescribed regimen is effective if carefully followed and to allow a period of intensive education.

THERAPEUTIC STARVATION. A period of several weeks of starvation in hospital with only water, non-caloric drinks with vitamin and mineral supplements being allowed, has been recommended for very obese patients who have failed to respond to orthodox treatment. Although the initial loss of weight may be marked, the long-term results are no more satisfactory than other systems since many patients regain most of the weight lost when strict measures are discontinued. Such a regime is contraindicated for older patients, especially if they have cardiovascular complications, since deaths have occasionally occurred. Ketosis may be troublesome in the early stages and hyperuricaemia, sometimes accompanied by gout, may develop.

EXERCISE. Most obese patients lead sedentary lives and benefit from physical activity such as walking, swimming and gardening, provided it does not exceed their cardiovascular capacity. Regular daily exercise is much more valuable than episodic activity.

An hour's walk at 3 miles per hour will expend about 300 kcal (or more for a heavy person). This may seem a small amount, equivalent to about 30 g of fat, but if the daily walk becomes a habit it will add up, other things being equal, to a weight loss of 9 kg in a year. Doctors should suggest, discuss and work out with each patient an increasing programme of exercise which is within the physical capacity and which will add to the quality of life of the individual.

DRUG THERAPY. This is no substitute for a dietary regime but has a limited use as an adjunct in carefully selected patients with refractory obesity. Some of the more effective drugs used in the past, notably amphetamine, are addictive and have been so widely abused that they should not be prescribed for the treatment of obesity.

Amphetamine-like drugs with similar anorectic properties but causing less central nervous stimulation include diethylpropion (25 mg an hour before meals) and phentermine (15–30 mg before breakfast). They may be given intermittently for periods of about a month to help attain a short-term goal. They should not be used in patients with hypertension or coronary heart disease.

Fenfluramine probably acts by stimulating satiety rather than inducing anorexia. It may cause nausea, diarrhoea, lethargy, excessive dreaming and, particularly if suddenly withdrawn, depression. It must be given only under careful medical supervision in a dose of 20 mg b.d., gradually increased to a maximum of 120 mg daily, unless adverse effects intervene. Treatment can be continued as long as weight is being lost.

None of these drugs must be given to a patient with a history of psychiatric illness.

The administration of thyroxine to euthyroid patients is not only useless but is potentially dangerous, especially if heart disease is present. It should be prescribed only if hypothyroidism coexists with obesity.

FIBRE-RICH PRODUCTS. There is evidence that some foods rich in fibre have an effect on satiety. Methylcellulose is an indigestible substance which adds bulk to the diet. It distends the stomach and so may help to allay hunger. In clinical trials it has been shown to have little if any effect in promoting weight loss.

SURGICAL TREATMENT. Operations such as small intestine bypass, aimed at inducing malabsorption, have been undertaken in some centres for the treatment of intractable cases of severe 'morbid' obesity. The side-effects, particularly diarrhoea, have often been distressing. Wiring the jaws together to prevent eating has also been undertaken. It seems unlikely that these experimental techniques will contribute substantially to the management of obesity in more than a very small minority of the most resistant cases.

**Prognosis.** It is easy for an obese person to lose up to 5 kg in weight. This accounts for the temporary successes of numerous popular 'slimming cures'. How difficult it is to achieve further losses is not generally realised. The published records of seven obesity clinics in the USA showed that satisfactory results ranged only from 12 to 28% if the index of success was the loss of 12 kg or more.

Experience in many clinics has also shown that it is difficult for patients to maintain their reduced weight since this requires some restriction of energy intake on a long-term basis.

**Prevention.** This must depend in part on the doctor who discerns when his patients, be they infants, children or adults, are gaining too much weight. For this purpose alone, among the most useful information that a doctor can keep about his patients is a record of body weight, measured at regular intervals. The doctor's responsibility with an overweight patient, at any time, is advisory and educational; the attention of patients must be drawn to the dangers of obesity and to the appropriate methods of correcting it.

All the health agencies available should be mustered to support a steady campaign of education and persuasion of patients and potential patients on the need to avoid obesity. The antenatal services, infant welfare clinics, school health authorities, health visitors and many others to whom the public look for advice when they are in difficulties should contribute to this educational programme. The media also play an increasingly important role.

JOYCE D. BAIRD
A. S. TRUSWELL

*Further reading:*

Alleyne, G.A.O., Hay, R.W., Picou, D.I., Stanfield, J.P. & Whitehead, R.G. (1977) *Protein Energy Malnutrition.* London: Arnold. — The latest monograph by authors with experience in Africa and the W. Indies.

Cameron, M. & Hofvander, Y. (1976) *Manual on Feeding Infants and Young Children (for application in the developing areas of the world with special reference to home-made weaning foods)*, 2nd edn. New York: Protein-Calorie Advisory Group of the United Nations System. — Obtainable free of charge; write to 866 United Nations Plaza, New York, N.Y. 10017, U.S.A. Valuable recipes for nutritious home-made combinations of foods suitable for young children, which come from and can be applied in many different countries.

Davidson, Sir Stanley, Passmore, R., Brock, J.F. & Truswell, A.S. (1979) *Human Nutrition and Dietetics*, 7th edn. Edinburgh: Churchill Livingstone. — The standard textbook. Covers the whole field of nutrition in 64 chapters.

Garrow, J.S. (1978) *Energy Balance and Obesity in Man,* 2nd edn. Amsterdam: North-Holland; New York: American Elsevier.— An admirably balanced book on the physiology of obesity. Thoughtful but readable.

Jelliffe, D.B. (1966) *The Assessment of the Nutritional Status of the Community (with special reference to field surveys in developing regions of the world)*. WHO Monograph Series No. 53. Geneva: World Health Organization.— The best manual on the subject, with some good photographs. Being revised at present.

Munro, J.F. (ed.) (1979) *The Treatment of Obesity*. Lancaster: M.T.P. Press, — eight chapters on different approaches to treatment by experts from Britain, USA and Sweden.

Paul, A.A. & Southgate, D.A.T. (1978) *McCance and Widdowson's the Composition of Foods*, 4th edn. London: HMSO. — British food tables: data on more nutrients than any other available in a single volume at present.

Passmore, R., Nicol, B.M., Rao, M.N., Beaton, G.H. & De Maeyer, E.M. (1974) *Handbook on Human Nutritional Requirements*. Published as either FAO Nutritional Studies No. 28, Rome or WHO Monograph Series No. 61, Geneva.— An international handbook on requirements of the major nutrients.

Report of the Royal College of Physicians (1976) *Fluoride, Teeth and Health*. London: Pitman Medical.— A working party of the College reviews fluoridation of water and concludes that it is safe in a temperate climate.

Research on Obesity: A report of the DHSS/MRC Group (1976) Compiled by James, W.P.T., London: HMSO.

Stuart, R.B. & Davis, B. (1972) *Slim Chance in a Fat World: Behavioural Control of Obesity*. Champaign, Illinois: Research Press.— Details of how to do it by the man who pioneered this type of management.

Swedish Nutrition Foundation (1971) *Famine*. Uppsala: Almqvist and Wiksell.— Report of a symposium with international speakers. Scientific research papers on this topic are rare.

# 5. Disturbances in Water and Electrolyte Balance and in Hydrogen Ion Concentration

The chemical events collectively called metabolism require the concentration of hydrogen ions and electrolytes to remain within narrow limits in the tissue cells and in the fluid which bathes them. Derangement of water and electrolyte balance and disturbances in hydrogen ion concentration occur in a wide variety of clinical conditions which are separately described in the appropriate chapters of this book. It is convenient, however, to summarise here the relevant physiological facts and to describe briefly the more common abnormalities. The kidney plays an important part in maintaining water, electrolyte and acid base balance; the details of the movements of ions that occur in the nephron are given on pages 422 and 424.

## Normal Distribution of Water and Electrolytes

**Water.** The body of a normal man of 65 kg contains approximately 40 litres of water. About 28 litres of this is intracellular, and 12 litres extracellular. The latter is composed of 9–10 litres of interstitial fluid and 2–3 litres of plasma. Water readily passes through almost all membranes of the body and permeates easily into all fluid compartments. Its final distribution between the compartments is determined by osmotic and hydrostatic pressures and under normal conditions the total amount of water in the body is kept remarkably constant.

**Electrolytes.** The inorganic ions dissolved in the body water include sodium, potassium, calcium, magnesium, chloride, phosphate, bicarbonate and sulphate. These are not dispersed in the same concentrations throughout the various body fluid compartments. Sodium and chloride are confined mainly to the extracellular fluids where they are present in average concentrations of 142 mmol/*l* and 100 mmol/*l* respectively. These ions contribute the major part of the total osmolal concentration of the plasma and extracellular fluids. Potassium, magnesium, phosphate, and sulphate are present in highest concentration inside the cells where they maintain the osmolal concentration analogous to that of sodium and chloride in the extracellular fluids. In extracellular fluid potassium is present in a mean concentration of only 4·5 mmol/*l* and magnesium in a concentration of about 1 mmol/*l*. Bicarbonate is found in the fluid outside the cells and in the tissue cells themselves in concentrations of 25 mmol/*l* and 10 mmol/*l* respectively. Hydrogen ions are present in a concentration of only 40 nanomol/*l*. They are present within cells at a higher concentration than in the extracellular fluids.

Because of the permeability of the capillaries, the concentration of electrolytes in the plasma and in the extracellular fluids in the tissue spaces is very similar. Interchange between these extracellular compartments is limited, however, in respect of protein molecules, the concentration of which is many times greater in the plasma than in the interstitial fluid. The volume of the plasma is largely the result of hydrostatic pressure which tends to force water outwards, and the colloid osmotic pressure of the plasma proteins which draws water back into the vascular bed. In spite of the differences in the ionic pattern inside the cells as compared with that of the fluid which bathes them, under normal conditions the osmotic pressure is believed to be identical in extracellular and intracellular fluids. The differences in composition are established and maintained by the activity of ionic pumps within the cell membrane and are essential to life.

## Disturbances in Water and Electrolyte Balance

The complexity of the composition of body fluids is reflected in the variety of disturbances that may occur in them either as a result of disease or as a consequence of therapeutic endeavour and drug administration. Such disturbances not only contribute to the clinical picture of many diseases, but are themselves a hindrance to recovery. For this reason it is important to maintain the chemical composition of the body fluids and correct as far as possible any derangements that may arise. It is also essential that specific disturbances are recognised and appropriately treated. The labelling of such abnormalities in fluid and electrolyte balance simply as 'dehydration' and the indiscriminate use of intravenous isotonic NaCl solution, i.e. 'normal' saline in an attempt to correct them is to be deprecated. The more important disturbances in water and electrolyte balance are depletion or excess of sodium, potassium, magnesium or water, either singly or in combination. The ranges of normal adult values are given on page 906.

### Sodium Depletion

Normal sodium balance depends upon an equality between the amounts of sodium excreted and ingested. In health in temperate climates negligible amounts of sodium are lost in the stools and from the skin. In the absence of renal disease the kidneys possess considerable power to conserve sodium in the face of reduced intake and normal sodium balance may be maintained with a very small daily intake. For these reasons sodium depletion generally occurs because of excessive loss of salt from the body rather than because of inadequate intake.

Because of the intimate relation of salt to water balance, loss of sodium is usually accompanied by a corresponding reduction in the water content of the body. *Pure sodium depletion* unattended by significant water loss is rare and probably occurs only as a result of abnormal loss of salt and water when an unrestricted intake of water has been permitted or encouraged. This may arise, for example, from excessive sweating in unfavourable environments when fluid loss is replenished by salt-free liquids. In these circumstances the change in total body water may be negligible in spite of a considerable deficit of body salt. More commonly, however, conditions giving rise to sodium depletion are attended by some degree of water loss and unless large amounts of salt-free fluids have been given, a *mixed depletion* exists, though the salt loss usually predominates over the water loss.

**Causes of Sodium Depletion.** In temperate regions predominant sodium depletion arises as a result of excessive loss of salt in the urine or because of increased loss of sodium-containing fluids from the gastrointestinal tract.

Failure of the kidney to conserve salt may develop because of intrinsic renal disease or inadequate hormonal control. Examples are found in some patients with pyelonephritis (i.e. 'salt-losing nephritis'), the diuretic phase of acute renal failure of ischaemic origin, Addison's disease and to a lesser extent in hypopituitarism. Excessive loss of salt in the urine together with water loss occurs in the osmotic diuresis of uncontrolled diabetes mellitus and chronic uraemia. If diabetic ketoacidosis develops, urinary sodium loss is further increased as the renal mechanism for hydrogen ion secretion is unable to cope with the severe degree of acidosis. Sodium depletion may also be induced by the excessive or prolonged use of diuretics.

Gastrointestinal causes of sodium depletion include all conditions involving external loss of salt-containing fluids, i.e. acute or chronic diarrhoea, intestinal fistulae, aspiration of gastrointestinal contents and vomiting. Considerable degrees of sodium loss also occur if sodium containing fluid is sequestered in dilated loops of intestine as in ileus or in the peritoneal cavity as in ascites.

Sweating is a well-known cause of sodium depletion in tropical countries and often aggravates the degree of sodium depletion caused by disease (p. 803). Loss of sodium from the skin is also important and occurs in extensive burns, severe generalised dermatitis and in children suffering from cystic fibrosis.

**Consequences of Predominant Sodium Depletion.** As sodium is mainly extracellular, depletion quickly reduces the volume of the extracellular fluids. When proportionately more sodium than water is lost, the extracellular fluids become hypotonic and the plasma sodium concentration falls. This tendency is mitigated by two events, (1) the normal proportion of water relative to solute excreted in the urine is initially increased in order to restore the normal osmolality of the body fluids, and (2) some extracellular water migrates into the cells so that the threatened extracellular dilution is minimised. As a result there is a further diminution in the volume of extracellular fluid, including plasma, while the water content of the cells may even increase. The fact that predominant salt depletion chiefly affects the volume of the extracellular fluid is responsible for many of the clinical features such as loss of elasticity of the skin, diminution of intra-ocular pressure and dryness of the tongue. Thirst is not a prominent complaint, and its absence may be due to the hypotonicity of the body fluids. The decrease in blood volume leads to a fall in blood pressure and in the rate of glomerular filtration; oliguria then occurs. The capacity to excrete urea diminishes and uraemia develops. The pulse rate rises. Selective vasoconstriction diminishes the circulation through the skin so that the extremities become pale and cold. Although the plasma sodium concentration may be within normal limits, it may be reduced to 120 mmol/*l* or less in severe cases or in those in whom the deficit of water has been partly made good; in such patients muscle cramps are common.

**Treatment.** The administration of water or of glucose in water in conditions associated with sodium depletion is fraught with danger because the hypotonicity may be further aggravated. As more salt-free fluid is given, the kidneys respond by excreting dilute urine in an attempt to restore normal osmolal concentrations and the extracellular fluid volume remains low. The ill-effects of such treatment, moreover, are all too easily obscured by the conventional fluid balance chart which records only fluid intake and urine output, without reference to sodium balance. Adequate treatment consists of giving salt and water by mouth or an isotonic NaCl solution intravenously. The latter is required in all but mild cases with normal recumbent blood pressure. In adults with moderately severe depletion two to four litres of isotonic NaCl solution intravenously in 6–12 hours represents the usual requirements. In the severe cases with marked circulatory impairment, deficits equivalent to 4–8 litres of isotonic NaCl solution occur. Such deficits should be repaired largely by isotonic sodium chloride. The first 2–3 litres should be given rapidly within the first 2–3 hours, the remainder being given within 24–48 hours. The best guides to the amount required are the disappearance of the signs of salt depletion and the restoration of normal blood pressure and pulse rate. Plasma sodium determinations are useful in controlling the treatment of severe cases, especially when the causative disease is likely to lead to a continued salt loss, (e.g. severe and persisting diarrhoea) and in regulating the relative amounts of sodium and water to be given. Excessive administration of salt is to be avoided; the bases of the lungs should be frequently examined for crepitations, and the jugular venous pressure assessed. In severe cases it is often helpful to monitor the right atrial (central) venous pressure (p. 167).

Severe sodium depletion is almost invariably associated with water depletion and disturbance in acid-base balance. Frequently potassium balance and occasionally magnesium metabolism are also disturbed. In these circumstances appropriate amounts of other electrolytes need to be added to the intravenous fluid once the circulation has been restored by the isotonic chloride.

## Primary Water Depletion

Pure or predominant water depletion is one of the simplest of chemical disorders. The water content of the body is reduced both absolutely and relatively to the salt content, and the osmolal concentration of the extracellular fluids rises. Between ½–1 litre of water is lost daily from the body in the expired air and by evaporation from the skin. This daily loss continues irrespective of the water intake. The urine is the other main channel of excretion of water but its volume can be reduced if necessary by increasing its concentration up to a limit determined by renal concentrating ability and the amount of solute to be excreted.

**Causes of Water Depletion.** Primary water depletion occurs less commonly in clinical practice than sodium depletion and usually arises because water intake is reduced below an amount necessary to maintain balance. It is liable to occur in patients who suffer from dysphagia or have obstructive lesions of the oesophagus or in those who are comatose, depressed or apathetic, as is common for example, in the aged. Water deficit then occurs because the intake falls below the amount being lost from the lungs, skin and urine. This obligatory daily loss of water from the lungs and skin is increased by hyperpnoea, hyperthyroidism and in conditions associated with pyrexia. Excessive loss of water in the urine is a less common cause of water depletion but occurs in patients in whom the renal power of concentration is restricted, as for example in diabetes insipidus or hyperparathyroidism.

Water deficit may be induced by giving patients excessive protein or salt-containing artificial foods mixed with insufficient water. Newborn infants are especially susceptible to this danger as their power to concentrate the urine is not fully developed.

**Consequences of Water Depletion.** As water is lost from the body the extracellular fluid becomes hypertonic and the concentrations of plasma sodium rises. Water then migrates from the cells in accordance with this increase in osmotic pressure and intracellular dehydration occurs. The overall body water loss is thus shared by the extracellular and intracellular fluids. For this reason the circulatory signs of dehydration are not so obvious as those of salt depletion. Thirst is usual unless the patient is senile or confused. The migration of water from the cells to the extracellular fluids helps to maintain the volume of the extracellular fluid nearly within normal limits for a time, so that the blood pressure, packed cell volume, and plasma and blood concentrations remain unaltered until considerable depletion has occurred. The patient, however, may exhibit mental confusion or complain of vertigo and difficulty in swallowing. In severe cases the skin and tissues acquire a curious 'doughy' consistency. Ultimately renal blood flow is reduced and the blood urea concentration rises. The plasma sodium concentration and the haemoglobin concentration then become elevated.

**Treatment.** Water depletion can often be prevented if the need to maintain an adequate intake is recognised in patients who are unable to swallow or who do not drink enough of their own accord. Established depletion should be treated by giving salt-free fluids. The use of isotonic NaCl solution is contraindicated. If the patient is conscious and is not vomiting, water should be given by mouth until thirst is quenched and thereafter amounts of between 1·2 to 2·5 litres per day are usually sufficient. If the patient is unable to swallow fluids in sufficient amounts, 5% glucose in water should be given by intravenous infusion. The amount required varies with the degree of depletion. In moderately severe cases 2–4 litres of 5% glucose in the course of 24 hours is usually sufficient. In severe water depletion 5–10 litres may be needed. The best guides to the amount of fluid required are the clinical improvement of the patient and the increase in the volume of urine, which should rise to about 1·5 litres per 24 hours. When water depletion is associated with salt loss, isotonic NaCl solution and water are both required and should be given together in amounts determined by clinical assessment of the relative degrees of the two deficiencies.

## Potassium Depletion

Depending upon the daily intake, the healthy individual in potassium balance excretes over 85% of the daily potassium intake in the urine and the remainder in the stools.

**Causes of Potassium Depletion.** Potassium depletion usually occurs as a result of excessive loss of potassium from the gastrointestinal tract or in the urine. Alimentary losses occur as a result of severe, acute or chronic diarrhoea, vomiting, fistulous drainage or gastric aspiration. The chronic use of laxatives is sometimes an underlying cause and is easily missed and a potassium secreting villous adenoma of the rectum is an important but uncommon cause.

Renal wastage of potassium is complex in its origin. Almost all the potassium in the body lies within the cells, and circumstances which encourage its transfer to the extracellular fluid lead to increased urinary losses and ultimately to potassium depletion. Such circumstances include hypoxia, impaired oxidation of carbohydrate, water depletion and acidosis of metabolic or respiratory origin in which the buffering of $H^+$ within cells leads to the loss of $K^+$ from them.

Renal wasting of potassium also occurs in conditions which favour the diffusion of potassium into the lumen of the distal tubules. There are two main categories:

1. Circumstances in which the electrochemical gradient is increased facilitate diffusion. This occurs in primary aldosteronism, Cushing's syndrome and in patients receiving corticosteroids or carbenoxolone. The mechanism is also responsible in secondary aldosteronism due to heart failure, liver disease and the nephrotic syndrome. Diuretics which increase the flow of urine and the delivery of sodium to the most distal tubules also encourage potassium loss in this way.

2. In many circumstances the rate of secretion of potassium is related inversely to the rate of $H^+$ excretion. Since both are secreted by the distal tubular cells it seems

likely that their relative intracellular concentration determines this relationship. In renal tubular acidosis and metabolic alkalosis, in which tubular secretion of $H^+$ is also reduced, the urine is alkaline and potassium loss is increased.

Many elderly people who take a diet inadequate in potassium become mildly potassium-depleted. The precise mechanism is unknown but it is most likely due to continued urinary loss.

**Consequences and Clinical Features of Potassium Depletion.** Significant depletion of potassium may occur without alteration in the plasma potassium concentration and the diagnosis of intracellular potassium deficit is made difficult by the inaccessibility of the intracellular fluid to analysis. Biochemical evidence of potassium lack may be suggested by an elevation in plasma bicarbonate concentration or a diminution in plasma sodium concentration. These effects are believed to be due to the migration of hydrogen and sodium ions from the extracellular into the intracellular fluids.

Symptoms attributable to potassium deficiency include apathy, muscular weakness, mental confusion and abdominal distension. It is clear that such features arise in the course of many diseases. Nevertheless, their occurrence in circumstances which are known to lead to potassium deficiency, and their relief after potassium administration justify the diagnosis. Potassium depletion reduces the ability of the kidney to concentrate urine hence polyuria and thirst commonly occur. Potassium depletion may induce cardiac arrhythmias such as atrial tachycardia; it also gives rise to increased susceptibility to intoxication with digitalis. Severe potassium depletion lowers the cardiac output and this may give rise to oedema.

Potassium deficiency sufficiently severe to be associated with reduction of the plasma concentration is more easily recognised, but is less common than simple intracellular depletion. It may occur in any of the conditions mentioned above if the deficiency is sufficiently severe and is particularly liable to develop in cases of diabetic ketoacidosis which have been vigorously treated with sodium containing solutions or glucose and insulin; this therapy causes a migration of potassium from the extracellular to the intracellular space with resulting hypokalaemia. The clinical picture of extracellular potassium deficit is characterised by generalised muscular weakness with paresis or flaccid paralysis and ileus. Paraesthaesiae are also frequently present and loss of memory, disorientation and mental confusion may occur. The electrocardiogram commonly shows a small T wave and ST depression. Death may occur if potassium depletion is unrelieved or if treatment is inadequate.

**Treatment.** Potassium depletion should be treated by giving a potassium salt orally or intravenously. The former route is more commonly used and is less dangerous than parenteral administration. The normal daily intake of potassium is about 2–3 g.

1. Established deficiencies of moderate severity (about 400 mmol) can be remedied by giving 10–15 g of potassium chloride per day orally, in divided doses for some days in addition to a diet rich in potassium, i.e. containing fruit and fruit juices.

Potassium chloride tablets sometimes cause gastrointestinal ulceration especially if there is delay in intestinal transit. 'Slow release' tablets of potassium chloride are less troublesome in this respect, each tablet containing 600 mg of KCl. Some patients tolerate effervescent potassium tablets more readily as these appear to be less nauseating. Each tablet contains 250 mg of potassium and some also contain chloride. The latter is useful in correcting the metabolic alkalosis which is associated with potassium depletion and which is frequently due to concurrent chloride depletion (p. 142).

2. Intravenous infusions of potassium chloride are needed for patients who are

unable to take potassium by mouth, but should be given only when the existence of hypokalaemia is established by chemical analysis. Such infusions should rarely be given in the presence of anuria or oliguria and only when facilities for repeated chemical analysis are available.

If oliguria is due to associated water and salt depletion these should be treated first. For intravenous administration, potassium chloride (1·5 g in sterile ampoules) can be conveniently added to 500 ml of isotonic NaCl or 5% glucose solution. The solution then contains 40 mmol/*l* and should be given slowly over 2 to 3 hours. Repeated measurements of the plasma potassium are necessary to determine whether further infusions are required. Administration of potassium by mouth should be then started as soon as possible, as the major portion of the deficit can be corrected only by this means. When the depletion of potassium has arisen because of persistent vomiting and is associated with alkalosis due to loss of gastric hydrochloric acid, potassium is conveniently given with sodium and ammonium chloride as described on page 143.

Prophylactic administration of potassium chloride (3–4 g daily) or effervescent potassium tablets should be given to patients who are being treated by drugs known to increase urinary loss of potassium. These include corticosteroids and many diuretics.

### Potassium Excess

**Causes.** Abnormal accumulation of potassium in the blood and extracellular fluid usually occurs in association with severe oliguria or anuria. It is commonly found in conditions leading to acute renal failure, e.g. circulatory failure from blood loss or injury and severe cases of Addison's disease; it may occur in diabetic ketoacidosis prior to adequate treatment with insulin and intravenous solutions. Some patients with severe chronic renal failure develop hyperkalaemia especially if potassium supplements, spironolactone or potassium conserving diuretics (p. 137) are given.

**Consequences of Potassium Excess.** Patients with hyperkalaemia develop muscular weakness which may progress to flaccid paralysis with loss of tendon reflexes. Abdominal distension due to ileus also occurs. These features are indistinguishable from those of hypokalaemia. In addition tingling of the face, hands and feet is common. The pulse becomes irregular and heart block of variable degree occurs. Hyperkalaemia is of considerable clinical importance because of the danger of cardiac arrest with concentrations of plasma potassium above 7·5 mmol/*l*. The diagnosis is made more frequently by knowing the circumstances in which intoxication is likely to arise and confirming the suspicion by plasma potassium analysis than from any specific clinical feature. Typical electrocardiographic changes occur; these include increase in the amplitude of the T wave, atrioventricular and intraventricular conduction defects and ultimately ventricular fibrillation or asystole.

**Treatment.** It is important to prevent the occurrence of potassium intoxication in conditions associated with oliguria and anuria. The recommendations made with regard to the diet in acute renal failure (p. 448) are designed with this aim in view. When dealing with an established case of hyperkalaemia, the following measures are advised:

*(a)* Immediate restriction of foods rich in potassium (e.g. fruit juices) and in protein.

*(b)* The repair of any associated depletion of water or salt with the aim of re-establishing a normal circulation as early as possible and the correction of metabolic or respiratory acidosis by appropriate methods (pp. 141 and 144).

*(c)* The sodium or calcium loaded ionic exchange resin absorbs potassium in the intestine from the blood and intestinal secretions and contents. A suspension of 30 g in a small volume of water should be given by mouth 3 or 4 times per day or as required. In the event of vomiting the resin may be administered as a retention enema.

*(d)* The administration of glucose and insulin in order to encourage migration of potassium from the extracellular fluids into the cells. Ten units of soluble insulin and 50 g glucose as a 50% solution should be given intravenously. This treatment may be repeated every 2–4 hours; an alternative is a slow infusion of 20% glucose with 10 to 12 units insulin over 6–12 hours. At the same time ½ to 1 litre of isotonic sodium bicarbonate is given intravenously.

*(e)* Calcium gluconate (10%), 10 ml given intravenously and repeated in 2 to 3 hours, has been shown to reduce the cardiotoxic effect of potassium.

*(f)* If these methods fail or if the rise of concentration of potassium is rapid, removal of potassium by peritoneal dialysis or by haemodialysis is indicated.

## Magnesium Deficiency and Excess

Disorders of magnesium metabolism are occasionally responsible for otherwise puzzling clinical features and are susceptible to therapeutic control.

**Magnesium Deficiency**. The most frequent cause of magnesium deficiency is prolonged diarrhoea or vomiting, which has been treated with parenteral fluid without magnesium supplements. It is associated with chronic diarrhoea and severe undernutrition, such as occurs in protein-energy malnutrition and the malabsorption syndrome. Uncontrolled diabetes mellitus, aldosteronism, hyperparathyroidism, the diuretic phase of acute renal failure and chronic alcoholism lead to magnesium deficiency from excessive urinary loss. It occasionally follows long continued diuretic therapy.

Clinical features are predominantly neuromuscular, with tremor, choreiform movements and aimless plucking of the bedclothes. Mental depression, confusion, agitation, epileptiform convulsions and hallucinations also occur. The diagnosis can be confirmed by finding the concentration of magnesium in the plasma to be less than 0·75 mmol/*l*.

Magnesium deficiency is best treated parenterally; 50 mmol of magnesium chloride may be added to 1 litre of 5% glucose or other isotonic solution and given over a period of 12 to 24 hours. The infusion should be repeated daily until the plasma concentration remains within the normal range.

**Magnesium excess** mainly occurs in acute and chronic renal disease and contributes to the central nervous features associated with uraemia (p. 437). Its treatment is that of the primary disorder.

## Water Excess

Healthy individuals can safely drink very large volumes of water and respond to this by a vigorous water diuresis. The capacity of the kidney to excrete water when given without electrolytes is dependent upon many factors which include the rate of glomerular filtration and the power of the distal tubules to produce a dilute urine. Many patients who are ill for a variety of reasons have a restricted ability to dilute the urine when given large amounts of water. These include patients suffering from acute and chronic renal disease, severe heart failure, hypopituitarism, adrenocortical insufficiency, severe hypothyroidism and hepatic cirrhosis. Occasionally tumours of the lung, pancreas or ovaries secrete a polypeptide with antidiuretic properties which leads to water intoxication. Post-operative subjects are also incapable of diluting the urine because of the liberation of antidiuretic hormone by the stress of the operation. In addition, a number of drugs induce water retention because of antidiuretic hormone-like effects and can lead to water intoxication. These include the oral hypoglycaemic drug, chlorpropamide phenylbutazone, and morphine.

In all these circumstances even a modest water intake reduces the plasma osmolality and the concentration of sodium and produces symptoms which are primarily those of disordered cerebral function; these are partly due to cerebral oedema and include dizziness, headache, nausea and mental confusion. Severe water intoxication can produce convulsions, coma and death. Diagnosis depends upon being aware of the circumstances in which water intoxication is likely to occur and the demonstration of a plasma sodium concentration below 130 mmol/*l*.

Treatment consists of restricting water intake for a few days. In severe cases 100 ml 5% sodium chloride solution should be given intravenously and repeated in a few hours if there is little or no clinical improvement. The use of fludrocortisone is beneficial in cases of hyponatraemia due to tumours and is also indicated in Addison's disease.

## Sodium and Water Excess

In health, the total amount of sodium in the body is kept within narrow limits in spite of great day-to-day variations in the amount ingested. Positive sodium balance with consequent accumulation of sodium in the body results from a renal excretion that is inadequate in relation to the amount ingested. The accumulation is generally accompanied by the retention of water so that the concentration of sodium in the extracellular space is usually not materially altered. When the distribution of the retained fluid is generalised, the expansion in the volume of the extracellular space does not become clinically detectable until the increase is of the order of 15%.

The primary mechanisms responsible for the accumulation of water and salt which lead to oedema vary with the nature of the disease and they are discussed in the appropriate sections of this book. They include reduction in the osmotic pressure from hypoproteinaemia as occurs in the nephrotic syndrome; an increase in venous hydrostatic pressure with migration of fluid from the vascular space to the tissue spaces is a factor in heart failure and primary renal retention of salt and water is responsible in acute glomerulonephritis. In addition several compensatory reactions occur which promote further retention of water and salt. These include a rise in the levels of circulating antidiuretic hormone and also an increased secretion of aldosterone mediated by the renin angiotensin system (p. 424).

The therapeutic use of corticosteroids, androgens or oral contraceptives with a high oestrogen content may also give rise to water and sodium retention by virtue of their action on the kidney. Other drugs which do so include carbenoxolone and phenylbutazone. Some oedema is not uncommon in normal women during the premenstrual stage of the menstrual cycle. Oedema is commonly present in normal pregnancy but is more severe and is associated with proteinuria in renal disease or pregnancy hypertension. Other disorders associated with generalised oedema include nutritional oedema and thiamin deficiency. In some diseases several mechanisms appear to be operating simultaneously. This is exemplified particularly in the oedema and ascites of hepatic cirrhosis in which portal hypertension, hypoproteinaemia and possibly salt retaining and antidiuretic hormones all contribute.

The clinical feature of water and salt accumulation depend to some extent upon the distribution of the retained fluid. These are described under the various diseases.

**Principles of Treatment**. These are: (1) The use of measures designed to remedy specific factors leading to the oedema, e.g. digitalis in heart failure, corticosteroids in some forms of glomerulonephritis, the intravenous administration of plasma proteins or salt-free albumin in conditions associated with hypoproteinaemia, and a high protein diet in oedema of nutritional origin, hepatic cirrhosis and the nephrotic syndrome. (2) The restriction by dietary means of the raw materials necessary for the formation of extracellular fluid, i.e. water and salt. These dietary restrictions have largely been superseded by (3) Increasing the excretion of salt and water by the use of effective diuretics.

**Diuretic Therapy**. Drugs which block reabsorption of sodium or chloride by the renal tubules also increase the urinary volume because of the osmotic effect of the extra solute. The following are the most important diuretics discussed in order of their potency.

HIGH POTENCY DIURETICS. The diuresis induced by these agents is rapid, intense and of short duration. They include frusemide, bumetanide and ethacrynic acid. They are sometimes called *loop diuretics* because their predominant action reduces the reabsorption of sodium and chloride in the ascending limb of the loop of Henle. As a result they reduce the renal concentrating power and so eliminate a greater volume of water than do other diuretics; because they deliver an increased amount of sodium and water to the distal tubules they also lead to increased potassium loss in the urine.

*Frusemide* may be given orally (40–80 mg) or intravenously (20–40 mg). On a weight basis *bumetanide* is more potent than frusemide, comparable oral doses being 1–2 mg, but is otherwise similar in its action. Frusemide and bumetanide are drugs of great value in the treatment of severe generalised oedema and severe pulmonary oedema. They have few adverse effects but may lead to a rise in plasma urate and precipitate gout.

*Ethacrynic acid* represents a different chemical class of diuretic and can be given orally in doses of 50–200 mg per day. It has similar adverse effects to frusemide but in addition may induce gynaecomastia, tinnitus and deafness, especially if given in a single large intravenous dose.

MEDIUM POTENCY DIURETICS. Thiadiazine (thiazide) diuretics have two separate effects on renal function. They have a variable effect on the activity of carbonic anhydrase and so of sodium bicarbonate reabsorption in the proximal renal tubules, but their main action is to depress tubular reabsorption of sodium and chloride in the distal convoluted tubules. Potassium depletion occurs both because of the reduction of $H^+$ secretion and because of the delivery of increased amounts of sodium to the very distal tubular cells. Chlorothiazide was the prototype but the drugs most commonly used now are *bendrofluazide* (10 mg) and *hydrochlorothiazide* (100 mg). *Chlorthalidone* (100–200 mg) is similar in its action to chlorothiazide and its analogues but it produces a slower and more prolonged diuresis extending over 48 hours. Adverse effects of thiadiazines include allergic reactions; hyperuricaemia and diabetes may also be produced in susceptible patients.

LOW POTENCY DIURETICS. These consist of several agents which are not sufficiently potent by themselves but, because of other properties, are sometimes valuable when combined with more potent diuretics. *Amiloride* (20 mg) and *triamterene* (200 mg) antagonise the effects of aldosterone. Neither has a steroid structure and they do not compete for aldosterone combining sites. Their very mild natriuretic effect is due to inhibition of sodium reabsorption in the distal tubule; potassium secretion is not increased and so they do not lead to potassium deficiency. *Spironolactone* (100–400 mg daily) is a specific antagonist to aldosterone and reverses the renal effect of the hormone. Its important clinical effect is the reduction in the capacity of the kidney to excrete potassium which it shares with the low potency diuretics. These diuretics should not be given with potassium supplements as dangerous hyperkalaemia may develop.

ADVERSE ELECTROLYTE EFFECTS OF DIURETIC THERAPY. *Potassium Depletion.* High potency and thiadiazine diuretics produce potassium depletion, especially when given repeatedly over long periods and when combined with diets low in sodium. Symptoms of potassium deficit may arise before satisfactory loss of oedema has been achieved and are then superimposed upon the clinical features of water and sodium accumulation. This state of affairs is especially prone to develop in the treatment of severe cardiac failure and is particularly serious since it may be responsible for increased sensitivity to digitalis, with the development of toxic manifestations to this drug before adequate digitalisation and control of the heart failure has been attained. In hepatic disease with oedema and ascites the potassium depletion may seriously aggravate or precipitate the neurological features of hepatic insufficiency. Prophylactic administration of potassium is therefore essential when diuretics are being given frequently, e.g. on alternate days. Between 3 and 4 g potassium chloride is required daily given either as slow release or effervescent tablets.

*Sodium depletion.* A 'low salt syndrome' is much less common than potassium deficiency but is more likely to occur when treatment with high potency diuretics is prolonged. These patients exhibit some of the features of sodium depletion although they may still be oedematous. They become apathetic and suffer from anorexia and vomiting. The circulatory characteristic of sodium depletion is present, namely hypotension with an increase in the pulse rate. The blood urea is increased and the plasma sodium is reduced to 130 mmol/*l* or less. Such patients are usually seriously ill and, when the oedema is cardiac in origin, may be in the last stage of their disease. In these circumstances persistent attempts to reduce the oedema leads to further deterioration. Diuretics should be withheld and a diet unrestricted in its salt content permitted. In a few instances the intravenous administration of hypertonic saline may be dramatically successful in relieving the symptoms of the low salt syndrome. Two hundred ml of 5% saline should be given slowly by intravenous infusion, and may be repeated after 24 hours.

### Diagnosis of Disturbances in Water and Electrolyte Balance

It is apparent from this summary of the consequences of body depletion of sodium, water, potassium and magnesium and of potassium and magnesium excess that these disturbances present considerable diagnostic difficulty and are not characterised by pathognomonic signs or symptoms. The neuromuscular abnormalities of potassium depletion are indistinguishable from those of hyperkalaemia; severe sodium depletion is attended in the majority of instances by considerable water deficit so that these cases do not exhibit a clearly defined clinical picture. Furthermore, it is not uncommon for dual electrolytic deficits to develop simultaneously. For example, in diabetic ketoacidosis, potassium depletion may occur in conjunction with predominant sodium depletion. In addition the symptoms of lethargy, apathy and mental confusion are common accompaniments of many diseases in which no significant body fluid distortion exists.

It has also to be recognised that the results obtained from biochemical analysis of blood and urine are of only limited diagnostic value. Potassium or magnesium deficit may occur without significant alteration in their plasma concentrations, and serious sodium depletion commonly develops with plasma sodium concentrations within the recognised limits of normality. A low plasma sodium may not even indicate salt depletion, and hyponatraemia is frequently seen in the late stages of malignant disease, generalised tuberculosis and more rarely in association with vasopressin secreting tumours or other causes of water intoxication.

The measurement of electrolytes in the urine without knowledge of the dietary intake is also obviously of limited value. In the majority of conditions in which there is a reduced blood or ECF volume the urinary loss of sodium is less than 10–20 mmol. However, the presence of larger amounts in the urine of patients who are volume-depleted strongly suggests a renal salt wasting disorder. Urinary potassium determination is also of limited value but is sometimes helpful in patients who are found unexpectedly to have hypokalaemia. Then the finding of a urinary $K^+$ of more than 20 mmol indicates that the kidney is responsible unless extrarenal losses are of recent and sudden onset. In contrast the finding of a urinary $K^+$ of less than 10 mmol/*l* in the presence of hypokalaemia indicates the route of the loss is extrarenal and is usually a gastrointestinal disorder.

Accurate diagnosis largely depends upon a knowledge of the conditions and diseases which may give rise to abnormalities in water and electrolyte balance. In the presence of such diseases, the suspicion that these abnormalities may exist is strengthened by the presence of the clinical features known to occur with them and possibly by the results of appropriate biochemical and electrocardiographic examinations.

By understanding the mechanism by which the economy of the fluids of the body becomes disturbed and by the intelligent use of the reparative fluids which have been described, much can be done to restore the distortions of body fluid balance wrought by disease.

## Hydrogen Ion Concentration

Life is possible only if the blood is kept within a range of alkalinity, and, in health, a physiological hydrogen ion concentration of 36–44 nmol/*l* corresponding to a pH of between 7·37 and 7·45 is maintained by two widely different mechanisms which are closely integrated. Some understanding of these mechanisms is necessary to appreciate the clinical implications of acidosis and alkalosis.

The blood is alkaline because it contains bicarbonate, phosphate and proteins which are quite strong bases. It also contains carbonic acid and the $[H^+]$ of the blood depends principally upon the ratio of the main acid component, carbonic acid and the main base, bicarbonate. The concentration of carbonic acid in the plasma is determined by the partial pressure of carbon dioxide ($P_{CO_2}$) in the alveoli. The latter is normally about 5·3 kPa (p. 222) which gives rise to little over 1 mmol/*l* of carbonic acid in physical solution in the plasma. The alveolar partial pressure of carbon dioxide is itself maintained steady by the equality between its rate of production by the tissues and the rate at which ventilation eliminates it from the body. On the other hand, the concentration of bicarbonate is regulated by the tubular epithelium of the kidneys and in health is kept at about 22–24 mmol/*l* by the mechanism described on page 424.

A great many metabolic processes result in the production of acids and these must be eliminated from the body if the reaction of the tissue and the blood is to remain within the normal range. The route of disposal of acids depends upon whether or not they are capable of being oxidised completely to carbon dioxide and water. Carbon dioxide forms carbonic acid within the body and is eliminated as carbon dioxide by ventilation. Other acids such as acetoacetic acid or sulphuric acid which are derived from the oxidation of fatty acids or sulphur-containing proteins respectively are excreted by the kidneys. At the site of their production in the tissues and during their carriage in the blood all acids increase the hydrogen ion concentration. The extent of this increase is minimised by the stabilising power of the blood and tissues and this in turn depends on the presence of the physiologically important buffers.

Carbonic acid is produced by metabolic reactions in far greater amounts than any other acid. A small part of the carbon dioxide is transported in the blood reversibly bound to haemoglobin as a carbamino compound. A greater part is converted to carbonic acid in the red blood cells which are rich in carbonic anhydrase, and is then buffered by haemoglobin when it gives its oxygen to the tissues and is converted to deoxyhaemoglobin (Fig. 5.1). The hydrogen ions of the carbonic acid are taken up by the haemoglobin in the red cells while the bicarbonate ion moves out from the red cells to the plasma in exchange for chloride ions (chloride shift). Most of the carbonic acid added to the blood therefore appears not as acid but as bicarbonate ion. When the blood passes through the lungs and the haemoglobin is reoxygenated this process is reversed and the carbon dioxide formed is expelled by ventilation.

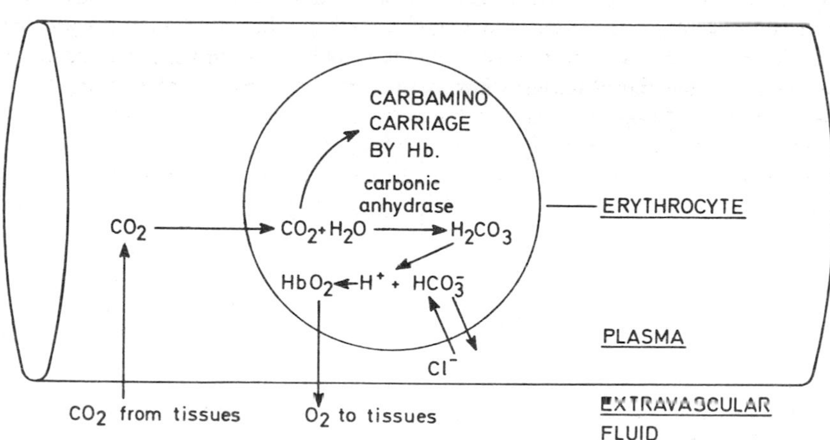


Fig. 5.1 Transport of $CO_2$.

In health, on a normal diet, 40–80 mmol of organic acid are excreted in the urine daily. However in some disorders, notably diabetic ketoacidosis, a large amount of acetoacetic acid is formed. The tissues and blood are buffered against these acids by a different mechanism which involves in particular the sodium bicarbonate and carbonic acid buffer system in the plasma. The addition of acid to the plasma results in a movement of the reactions in the direction indicated by the broad arrow (Fig. 5.2). As a result of this and of a similar reaction on the part of the other buffer systems, many of the hydrogen ions which would otherwise increase the acidity of the plasma are removed to form increased amounts of carbonic acid. There is a corresponding diminution in the concentration of bicarbonate ions. By this means the $[H^+]$ of the plasma rises far less than it would do if the buffers were not present. The rise in $[H^+]$ stimulates ventilation and the excess carbonic acid is removed from the body as carbon dioxide. The anion of the acid (e.g. acetoacetate) and the depleted body bicarbonate are dealt with simultaneously by the kidney. The renal tubules form carbonic acid, much of the hydrogen ion of which is used to form ammonium ions which are then excreted in the urine with the acid anion. The bicarbonate ion generated in this process is returned to the blood and reconstitutes the depleted blood buffer. (p. 424)

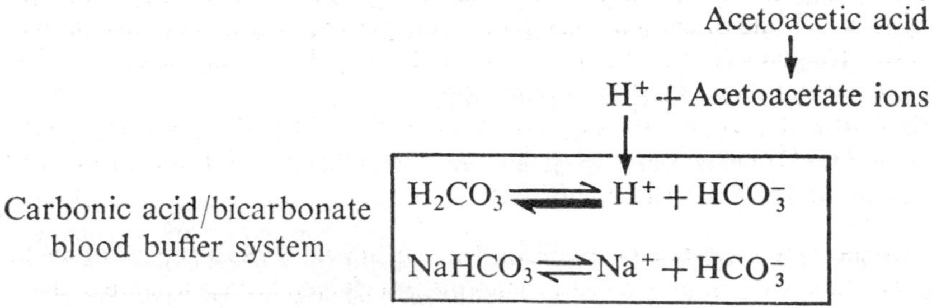


Fig. 5.2 Effect of acid on the blood buffer system.

These buffering and excreting mechanisms are continually in operation in response to the normal production of acids derived from the food and its metabolism. It is clear from this simplified description that the important limiting factor in the buffering power of blood is the available haemoglobin and bicarbonate. The excreting power of the kidneys is the limiting factor in the body's ability to rid itself of anions derived from inorganic and organic acids other than carbonic acid.

## Disturbances in Hydrogen Ion Concentration

Abnormalities in the reaction of the body fluids are reflected in changes in the concentration of carbonic acid (i.e. $Paco_2$) and by alterations in body base, notably that of bicarbonate. The estimation of $Paco_2$ is of particular value in respiratory disorders and its use in these conditions is described on page 227. As there is no entirely satisfactory method available for the determination of $[HCO_3^-]$, it is usually calculated from a knowledge of $Paco_2$ and pH using the Henderson Hasselbach equation or a nomogram based upon it. Since the concentration of bicarbonate is itself influenced by $Paco_2$ it is common practice to express the $[HCO_3^-]$ as the concentration which would exist at a standard value of $Paco_2$ of 5·3 kPa. It is then known as standard bicarbonate and normally ranges between 22 and 26 mmol/*l*.

## Metabolic Acidosis

Metabolic acidosis arises as a result of the production or ingestion of acids other than carbonic acid, or as a consequence of body depletion of the base bicarbonate. The condition is characterised by a rise in $[H^+]$ and a marked reduction in the concentration of bicarbonate in the plasma. The $Paco_2$ is reduced secondarily by the hyperventilation produced by stimulation of respiration; this mitigates to some extent the increased $[H^+]$ which arises from the fall in $[HCO_3^-]$.

The production of large amounts of lactic acid in vigorous exercise is probably the most common cause of acidosis and is to be regarded as physiological. Shock from any cause, notably severe myocardial infarction or cardiac arrest, causes metabolic acidosis because of hypoxia of the tissues and the accumulation of organic acids, particularly lactic acid. Lactic acid acidosis is also a recognised complication of treatment with oral hypoglycaemic biguanides such as phenformin; it is also seen in acute alcoholic intoxication. In all these circumstances the accumulation of lactic acid is related to a rise in the ratio of cellular NADH : NAD. Other important causes of acidosis are diabetic ketoacidosis and renal failure. In the former condition, $\beta$-hydroxybutyric acid and acetoacetic acid are produced in abnormally large amounts, and at a rate which is greater than the capacity of the body for their oxidation. In patients with acute or chronic renal failure, the power of the kidneys to conserve and generate bicarbonate ions and to produce and secrete hydrogen and ammonium ions is impaired and their excretion is diminished.

Depletion of body bicarbonate occurs from direct loss of sodium bicarbonate in the stools in chronic or severe acute diarrhoea or from loss of intestinal contents from fistulae or by intestinal aspiration.

**Consequences of Metabolic Acidosis.** The most obvious consequence of acidosis is the stimulation of respiration by the abnormally high blood concentration of hydrogen ions. In severe cases the respirations become deep and rapid (Kussmaul's respiration). It is clear, however, from the list of causes given above that the clinical picture in the individual case is largely determined by the underlying condition and by the presence of other concomitant disturbances in water and salt balance. By the time acidosis is severe in diabetic ketoacidosis, considerable water and salt depletion has usually occurred. The acidosis of chronic diarrhoea is similarly associated with salt loss and especially with potassium deficit. The failure of ammonium and hydrogen ion production by the kidney in chronic nephritis, which leads to acidosis, is necessarily accompanied by abnormal loss of sodium and potassium in the urine. As in the case of disturbances in water and electrolyte balance, the diagnosis of metabolic acidosis is facilitated by an awareness of those pathological conditions in which it is likely to arise. The diagnosis should be confirmed by the determination of the concentration of bicarbonate in the blood. In acidosis of moderate degree this value is reduced to 15 mmol/*l*, while concentrations below 10 mmol/*l* represent severe degrees of acidosis.

**Treatment.** Since metabolic acidosis is commonly associated with some degree of salt depletion and water deficiency, it is reasonable to correct these disturbances, in the first instance, by the administration of isotonic NaC1 solution (p.129); this is a neutral solution and by itself might be expected to have only a little influence on the reaction of the blood and tissues. In fact, provided the kidneys are not primarily diseased and provided the degree of salt and water depletion is not so severe as to impair renal function seriously, its intravenous administration is usually effective in correcting metabolic acidosis of moderate severity. Its success depends upon the capacity of the kidneys to generate bicarbonate from carbon dioxide and water and to retain this with the infused sodium, rejecting the chloride in the urine (p. 423).

In the presence of renal disease, severe acidosis and severe salt depletion giving rise to uraemia, it is unwise to depend upon the collaboration of the kidney for the alkalising effect of sodium chloride. In these circumstances, isotonic sodium bicarbonate should be given by intravenous infusion in addition to isotonic sodium chloride. The two solutions should be given in a ratio of 1 to 2 and need not be mixed. The total volume of the combined solutions required varies with the severity of the salt depletion and with the degree of acidosis. A moderately severe case of diabetic acidosis, for example, may require as much as 4–6 litres in the first 24 hours, of which 1–2 litres should be the isotonic bicarbonate solution. The latter infusion should be given for as long as there is evidence of acidosis, as determined by the estimation of blood [$H^+$] and of the bicarbonate concentration. When this has returned to normal levels, it may be necessary to continue the intravenous infusion of isotonic sodium chloride alone. This is indicated if there is still evidence of predominant salt depletion.

In severe shock or cardiac arrest, acidosis develops without salt depletion. In these circumstances it is best to give sodium bicarbonate in a small volume of hypertonic concentration, i.e. 200–300 ml 8·4% solution intravenously in the course of 10 to 15 minutes. The treatment of lactic acidosis in diabetes is given on page 522.

### Metabolic Alkalosis

Metabolic alkalosis arises most commonly as a result of the abnormal loss of hydrochloric acid in the course of prolonged or severe vomiting. Chloride deficiency itself also leads to alkalosis because it stimulates the renal tubular reabsorption of bicarbonate. This is especially liable to occur with the use of high potency diuretics which block chloride reabsorption. Potassium depletion also gives rise to alkalosis as this encourages the transfer of hydrogen ions into cells as well as their excretion in urine (p. 131).

**Consequences of Alkalosis**. The sequence of events which occurs when hydrochloric acid is lost from the body as a result of vomiting is shown in Figure 5.3. The loss of hydrogen ions in severe and continuous vomiting lowers the hydrogen ion concentration of the blood and leads to alkalosis. The effect is mitigated by an increase in the ionisation of blood carbonic acid to hydrogen and bicarbonate ions, as indicated by the broad arrow. The former tends to restore the hydrogen ion concentration towards normal, and the latter replaces the chloride in the blood which has also been lost in the gastric contents. For as long as the chloride deficiency persists increased tubular conservation of bicarbonate sustains the alkalosis.

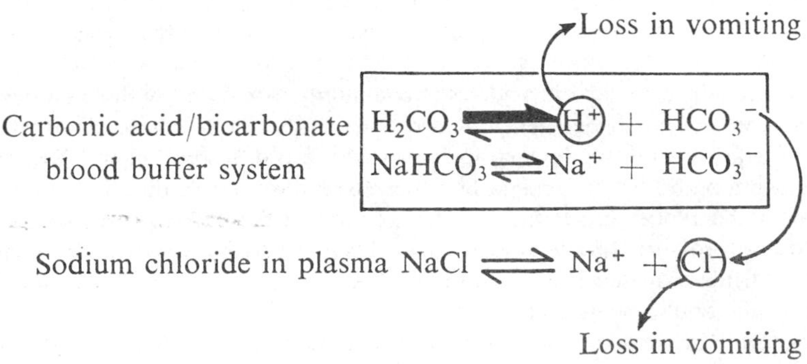


Fig. 5.3 Effect of alkalosis on the blood buffer system.

Alkalosis of some duration is often associated with significant depression of renal function with uraemia. Protein and casts are found in the urine, and the diagnostic error of attributing vomiting due to pyloric stenosis to primary renal disease must be avoided. In spite of the existence of metabolic alkalosis, the urine may remain acid. There are two causes for this paradoxical aciduria. The alkalosis is frequently associated with chloride depletion, and under these circumstances an alkaline urine cannot be elaborated. Secondly, respiratory compensation for the alkalosis results in a rise in $Paco_2$ which is also known to increase renal tubular reabsorption of bicarbonate. Apathy, personality changes, delirium and stupor occur; since the patient usually suffers from associated water and potassium depletion, it is probably wrong to attribute these features solely to the effect of alkalosis. Tetany may occur spontaneously or be induced by the Trousseau manoeuvre and is due to a reduction in the concentration of plasma ionised calcium.

The diagnosis of alkalosis may be made with certainty only by estimation of the concentration of plasma bicarbonate. In moderately severe alkalosis this is elevated to 35 mmol/*l*. The pH of the blood is also elevated.

**Treatment.** In patients with mild or moderate alkalosis in whom the bicarbonate concentration is not elevated above 30 mmol/*l*, it is often possible to correct the abnormality by the intravenous administration of isotonic sodium chloride. This treatment is effective only if there is normal renal function. In this event the chloride is retained and excess bicarbonate in the plasma is excreted in the urine. Two to four litres may be required in the course of 24 hours.

In severe cases the administration of ammonium chloride by intravenous infusion has been found effective and is conveniently prepared in a solution which is designed also to repair the commonly associated potassium deficit. This is called the 'gastric solution'. One litre of a solution containing 63 mmol/*l* of sodium chloride, 17 mmol/*l* of potassium chloride and 70 mmol/*l* of ammonium chloride may be given in 4 to 6 hours and repeated as indicated by blood analysis. The use of this solution is of particular benefit in these patients who are being prepared for operation for relief of gastric outlet obstruction (p. 333) and in whom repeated daily gastric lavage is needed to prevent vomiting and reduce the size of a dilated stomach.

## Ketosis without Acidosis

The excessive production of $\beta$-hydroxybutyric acid and acetoacetic acid in diabetic ketoacidosis has already been described as a cause of acidosis. Abnormal amounts of acetoacetic acid also arise in the body when the carbohydrate in the food is inadequate and increased amounts of fat are being utilised for energy. This is commonly found in cases of cyclical or severe vomiting in children, severe vomiting of pregnancy, starvation, and in postoperative vomiting. Two opposing tendencies are obviously in operation, the ketosis tending to increase, and vomiting tending to decrease the concentration of hydrogen ions in the blood. In these cases it is not uncommon, therefore, to find that metabolic alkalosis coexists with ketosis. Thus, the presence of acetoacetic acid in the urine does not necessarily imply the existence of acidosis, and the existence of metabolic acidosis is established only by the determination of the blood pH or bicarbonate concentration.

Apart from the possible need to treat concomitant acidosis or electrolyte disturbances, ketosis is best remedied by restoring the consumption of carbohydrate to normal. In cases of diabetic ketosis the administration of insulin is essential. In the other forms of ketosis this need not be given. Ample supplies of glucose should be provided; if this cannot be taken by mouth an intravenous infusion of 5% glucose in water may be given. Two to four litres of this solution may be needed in the course of the day.

## Respiratory Acidosis and Alkalosis

Respiratory acidosis arises when the effective alveolar ventilation does not keep pace with the rate of production of carbon dioxide (p. 222). As a result the $Paco_2$ and carbonic acid concentration of the blood increases, and the pH falls. The distinction between respiratory acidosis and metabolic alkalosis is usually easily made from a knowledge of the cause of the disturbance. The reaction of the arterial blood is decisive; in both the $Paco_2$ is increased, but in respiratory acidosis [H+] is increased, whereas in metabolic alkalosis the [H+] is reduced. The kidney responds to an increase in $Paco_2$ by excreting an acid urine and conserving sodium bicarbonate. The causes and consequences of respiratory acidosis are given on page 228.

Respiratory alkalosis occurs when there is excessive loss of carbonic acid by overventilation of the lungs. Most commonly this occurs in hysterical overbreathing or in overventilation during the course of assisted respiration, though it may arise also in the course of meningitis, encephalitis, salicylate intoxication, and liver failure. As a result the $Paco_2$ of the blood falls. Renal compensatory mechanisms result in the excretion of sodium bicarbonate which mitigates the fall in blood [$H^+$]. The distinction between respiratory alkalosis and metabolic acidosis is usually clear from the clinical circumstances. In both, the concentration of plasma bicarbonate is reduced and the reaction of the blood is again decisive. In respiratory alkalosis the plasma [$H^+$] falls while in metabolic alkalosis it rises. Tetany may also ensue.

Electrolyte repair solutions play no part in the treatment of respiratory acidosis or alkalosis, and therapy should be directed to the underlying disorder. The treatment of hypercapnia is described on page 236 and that of respiratory alkalosis due to hysterical overbreathing on page 483. Tetany may be treated by an intravenous injection of 10 ml of 10% calcium gluconate if necessary. The underlying causative factors should receive appropriate attention.

J. S. ROBSON

*Further reading:*

Brenner, B. & Stein, J. H. (1978) (1) *Sodium and Water Homeostasis*, (2) *Acid-base and Potassium Homeostasis*. Edinburgh: Churchill Livingstone.

Lant, A. F. & Wilson, G. M. (1972) Diuretics. In *Renal Disease*, 3rd edn, ed. Black, D. A. K. Ch. 23. Oxford: Blackwell.

Passmore, R. & Robson, J. S. *Companion to Medical Studies*, 2nd edn. Vol. I (1976), Chs 6, 31 & 35; 2nd edn. Vol. II (1980), Ch. 12; Vol. III (1974), Ch. 49. Oxford: Blackwell.

Robinson, J. R. (1975) *Fundamentals of Acid-Base Regulation*, 5th edn. Oxford: Blackwell.

# 6. Diseases of the Cardiovascular System

At all ages and in all countries, diseases of the cardiovascular system are major causes of death and disability. As infections in infancy become less dangerous, congenital heart disease contributes proportionately more to death and disability in early life. Partly because of the success of cardiac surgery more survivors with congenital heart disease now reach the child-bearing years. In Britain acute rheumatic fever is becoming something of a rarity and the incidence of chronic rheumatic heart disease is reducing progressively. In most countries with a high standard of living, coronary and cerebral arterial disease and hypertension are responsible for more than 50% of deaths and of these at least half are due to ischaemic heart disease. Over the last century, not only have coronary attacks become more common, but now it is not unusual for men in their thirties to be admitted to a coronary care unit, particularly heavy cigarette smokers in whom arterial disease of the legs is also common. For those who breathe air polluted by smoke, pulmonary damage may lead to cardiac failure especially in men from the mid-forties onwards.

Patients present not only with breathlessness, swollen ankles and cardiac pain, which are the cardinal symptoms of heart disease, but also with major disabilities due to embolism from thrombus formed within the heart, so that the heart disease may not immediately be recognised. Patients with unexplained fever or anaemia may be found to have infective endocarditis; pericarditis may be the first manifestation of a connective tissue disorder. The presentation of cardiovascular disease is thus protean.

### The Symptoms of Heart Disease

*Dyspnoea.* Awareness of unaccustomed breathlessness on exertion is often the first symptom of heart failure. The breathing is rapid and shallow but is generally not distinguishable by its character from that due to disease of the lungs (p. 226). The anxious patient, however, often has an intermittent sighing dyspnoea which is readily recognisable. *Orthopnoea* is the name given to breathlessness which prevents the patient lying flat. When supine there is increased work in depressing the diaphragm and, in addition, retained fluid is more likely to gravitate towards the lungs. The initial increase in venous return on first adopting the horizontal position is another factor of transient relevance. Redistribution of retained fluid towards the lungs at night may reach a critical level before a patient is wakened by breathlessness and has to sit up to obtain relief. There is often a repetitive cough which, initially at least, is unproductive. This *paroxysmal nocturnal dyspnoea* is an alarming experience causing tachycardia and temporary hypertension, which may make matters worse. Usually the attack subsides in a few minutes. If the breathlessness continues and the cough becomes productive of watery and often blood stained sputum, *pulmonary oedema* has supervened. The patient sits up gasping for breath. Respiration often becomes bubbly; if the breathing is wheezy, this is sometimes called *cardiac asthma*. There is often intense venoconstriction and the skin is cold and cyanosed. *Periodic breathing (Cheyne-Stokes respiration)*, in which there is waxing and waning of ventilation, from hyperventilation to apnoea, is common in cardiac failure due to depression of the medullary centres from decreased blood flow. It also occurs in the elderly, particularly during sleep.

*Oedema* is most commonly found in the feet as its site is mainly determined by gravity; the sacrum and thighs may become oedematous in patients confined to bed. Pressure with the thumb, if sustained, will displace the fluid and leave a pit.

*Pain.* The cardinal symptom of cardiac ischaemia is the pain known as angina pectoris (p. 184). The pain of pericarditis is described on page 203. Precordial catch is the name given to a stabbing pain felt momentarily by normal people but causing undue concern to the anxious; it is often indicated by a finger pointing below the left breast. Hepatic pain is felt in the epigastrium when the liver is rapidly distended by fluid retention. Pleural pain is a feature of pulmonary infarction, which often occurs with heart failure. Occasionally an aneurysm of the aorta or a grossly enlarged left atrium can cause persistent pain in the back of the chest from pressure on the vertebrae.

*Palpitation* is awareness of the heart beat; it is a common result of exercise or anxiety and occurs with increased catecholamine secretion or with sympathomimetic drugs. Patients often feel the thump of an ectopic beat. Palpitation may be the only symptom of paroxysmal tachycardia; often the patient can indicate its rate, and usually is able to say whether the heart beat is regular as in atrial tachycardia, or irregular as in paroxysmal atrial fibrillation.

*Syncope* is usually not due to heart disease. *Simple (vasovagal) syncope* results when the venous return is not maintained, e.g. with prolonged standing, particularly when it is hot or when there is a loss of fluid, as from diarrhoea. It may be reflex as a result of a frightening, unpleasant or painful experience. A feeling of nausea and sometimes a failure of vision and a ringing in the ears may herald its onset. Pallor, sweating and a slow pulse are characteristic.

Syncope can also ensue when a rise in intrathoracic pressure reduces the venous return sufficiently as with the *Valsalva manoeuvre*. It may also occur with prolonged vigorous coughing (*cough syncope*) or when elderly men strain to empty the bladder (*micturition syncope*). Syncope on standing—*postural syncope*—is a feature in some patients with an unusually low blood pressure as in Addison's disease. It also occurs from failure of the normal vasomotor reflexes, e.g. with diabetic neuropathy, or, as a result of the use of some antihypertensive agents. Syncope induced by movement of the neck suggests either a hypersensitive carotid sinus or reduction in the vertebro-basilar blood flow.

Cardiac causes are rare. *Exercise syncope* may occur when the cardiac output is very much restricted on exertion, as with aortic stenosis or pulmonary vascular obstruction. Syncope may result from certain rhythm disturbances, e.g. *Adams-Stokes* attack (p. 164).

*Other Symptoms.* Tiredness is a common complaint with severe heart failure and with myocardial infarction. In those with valvular disease without heart failure it should lead to a suspicion of infective endocarditis. Swelling of the ankles often disappears overnight and the mobilisation of fluid may be responsible for nocturia. Cough is a feature of pulmonary oedema. In severe protracted heart failure, anorexia, nausea and vomiting are all common.

## Physical Examination

While taking the history and before proceeding to the examination of the heart, certain pertinent observations may be made. The presence should be noted of any anaemia, obesity, breathlessness or cyanosis. Peripheral cyanosis is due to an excessive extraction of oxygen from the blood when the circulation is impaired from vasoconstriction, low cardiac output or stasis; it occurs in healthy people when the extremities are cold, and warmth abolishes it. Central cyanosis is due to oxygen undersaturation of the arterial blood from poor gaseous exchange in the lungs in such conditions as emphysema, pulmonary oedema and pneumonia or when there is a right to left shunt, e.g. in congenital heart disease. If the tongue is cyanosed, it may be deduced that the cyanosis is central in origin. A combination of central and peripheral cyanosis may occur and is often seen in cardiac failure.

The temperature of the skin varies with the skin blood flow. In cardiac failure, except in those forms where the cardiac output is increased, the extremities are abnormally cold, even in an equable environment. Unduly moist palms suggest anxiety if they are cold or thyrotoxicosis if they are warm. Clubbing of the fingers occurs in cyanotic congenital heart disease and in advanced infective endocarditis. Subungual or 'splinter' haemorrhages may result from trauma and occur in normal individuals but when numerous suggest infective endocarditis.

**The arterial pulse** should be examined for rate, rhythm, volume and the character of the pulse wave. The radial pulse is traditionally used but the carotid is more reliable partly because it is bigger, but also because the wave form is less altered by transmission. Bradycardia (p. 156) describes a heart rate of 60 per minute or less, and tachycardia (p. 156) a heart rate of 100 or more. In health the pulse is normally regular, but—particularly in children—a slowing of the pulse during expiration is common (sinus arrhythmia, p. 155). The other causes of irregularity are discussed on page 156. A pulse of small volume is a feature of reduced cardiac output, as in shock, major haemorrhage or massive pulmonary embolism, or with severe obstruction to blood flow at a cardiac valve. A pulse of large volume is found when there is a rapid flow of blood out of the arterial system, with peripheral vasodilation, as in fever or hyperthyroidism or with aortic regurgitation. It is also found when arterial run off is abnormally prolonged, as in complete heart block. Elevating the arm increases the run off and pulse volume— the so-called *collapsing pulse*; the sensation conveyed to the palm of the hand placed across the forearm when the arm is elevated under these circumstances has a knocking quality and is sometimes called '*muscle knock*'.

*Pulsus paradoxus*, a variation in volume with breathing, is an exaggerated variety of the normal and is hence misnamed. In health, arterial pressure records show that the arterial and pulse pressure fall in inspiration; with an increased intrathoracic pressure swing, as in asthma, the pulse may disappear in inspiration. Similar variation in the pulse volume is found with a sufficiently large pericardial effusion or with constrictive pericarditis. Minor degrees are best detected by allowing the pressure in a sphygmomanometer cuff to fall slowly; on first appearing the arterial (Korotkov) sounds may be audible only during expiration. Over a range of 5 mmHg or so this is a normal finding.

In *pulsus alternans* the pulse is regular but the amplitude is large and small in alternate beats. It is also best detected with the sphygmomanometer where there may be a difference of 10 to 40 mmHg between the strong and weak beats. It is a sign of left ventricular failure. In aortic stenosis a notch may sometimes be felt on the upstroke of the pulse and the wave may be prolonged and of small amplitude; this is the *anacrotic pulse*. A pulse with a double peak—*pulsus bisferiens*—is suggestive of combined aortic stenosis and regurgitation. In old age arteries lose their elasticity and become thickened. This is due to medial sclerosis which is not related to hypertension or disease of the intima; it is the latter which mainly determines whether or not the arterial lumen is narrowed. Medium-sized arteries, e.g. brachials, frequently show evidence of arterial thickening, tortuosity and undue mobility.

Arterial pulsation in the neck is increased in aortic regurgitation and coarctation of the aorta; in elderly patients, particularly hypertensive women, an arterial pulsation is often seen above the right clavicle due to 'kinking' of the carotid artery. A bruit heard over a major artery with the stethoscope bell is an important sign of partial obstruction. In younger hypertensive patients and in children suspected of having congenital heart disease, the radial and femoral pulse should be palpated simultaneously. With coarctation of the aorta, the femoral pulses are very seldom absent but it is of small volume and delayed after the radial pulse; measurement of the arterial pressure in the legs with a suitably large cuff shows it to be lower than in the arms.

**Jugular Venous Pulse.** With the patient reclining against pillows at about 45° and with the neck muscles relaxed the jugular venous pulse may be examined from movement of the skin overlying the internal jugular vein, although the vein itself is not visible. It is distinguished from an arterial pulse because it is less vigorous and because there are usually *a* and *v* components. The venous pulse is also identified by the fact that the level of filling of the jugular veins alters with the angle of the patient and varies with respiration. It can be abolished by light pressure at the root of the neck. The venous pulse is usually impalpable. When the venous return is increased by pressure on the abdomen the level moves upwards and this can be used to identify the fact that the pulsation is venous. The *a* wave is synchronous with atrial contractions and the *v* peak is immediately prior to the opening of the tricuspid valve (Fig. 6.1).

Where there is abnormal resistance to right atrial discharge, as in tricuspid stenosis, or when the right ventricle is hypertrophied, the *a* wave may be abnormally large. With tricuspid regurgitation a systolic *cv* wave is found. Cannon waves occur in any condition in which the atrium contracts against a closed tricuspid valve, e.g. complete heart block.

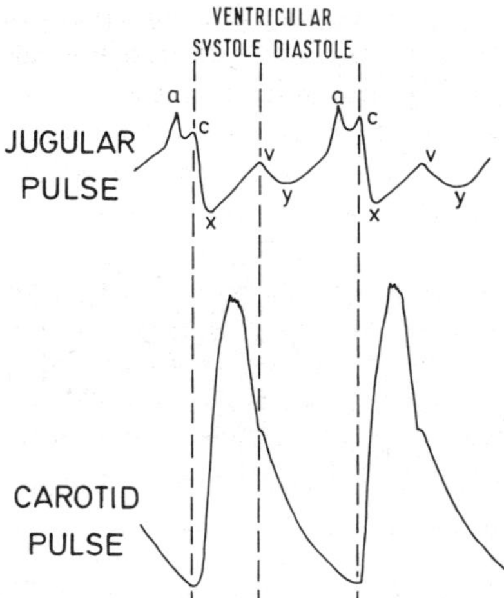


Fig. 6.1 Simultaneous central arterial and venous pulses to demonstrate carotid and jugular pulse wave form. a = atrial contraction, c = onset of ventricular contraction, v = pressure peak immediately prior to opening of tricuspid valve, c–x = x descent, v–y = y descent.

**Jugular Venous Pressure**. The internal jugular veins provide a convenient manometer for the measurement of right atrial pressure. The measurement is made by determining the point of collapse of the vein, i.e. where atmospheric pressure exceeds the venous pressure. Jugular venous pressure is measured in cm of blood by the vertical height of this point of collapse above the sternal angle. Normal jugular venous pressure is not more than 2 or 3 cm, but occasionally it is elevated by anxiety.

**Examination of the Heart**. The methods employed are inspection, palpation, percussion and auscultation and at each stage the intelligent use of one of these methods often makes the deployment of the next easier. Enlargement of the right ventricle during the growing period may show as a prominence to the left of the sternum in children. The apical impulse may be visible in left ventricular hypertrophy and an abnormal pulsation may occasionally be seen over an area of aneurysm of the ventricle. Occasionally an aneurysm of the aortic arch can be seen to move the upper sternum with each systole; when the heart is very much enlarged, as with chronic rheumatic heart disease, the whole chest may move with each heart beat.

Systolic pulsation in the epigastrium due to aortic pulsation is common in health, particularly in those who are thin. In tricuspid regurgitation the liver may produce pulsation in the epigastrium and right hypochondrium; correct interpretation is enabled by recognising the accompanying gross systolic jugular venous pulsation.

PALPATION. The position and the quality of the cardiac apical impulse have next to be assessed. The term *apex beat* is used for the furthest outward and downward point where the finger is lifted during systole; localisation may be impossible if there is obesity or emphysema. In health the apex beat is within the midclavicular line in the fifth intercostal space. Significant displacement of the apex beat to the left is usually a reliable indication of cardiac enlargement, although the evidence is never so good as that provided by a chest radiograph. However, if the mediastinum is displaced, e.g. by fibrosis, collapse, or removal of the lung on the left side or by a pleural effusion on the right the apex beat may be displaced to the left without cardiac enlargement. The quality of the apical impulse should also be noted. In left ventricular hypertrophy it is forceful whereas sharp closure of the mitral valve, either with anxiety or when associated with mitral stenosis, may give it a tapping quality. When the heart is damaged by ischaemic heart disease the apex beat may also be displaced to the left, usually without the apical impulse being forceful.

With right ventricular hypertrophy a pulsation may be imparted to the hand on the chest to the left of the sternum. A pulmonary artery under abnormally high pressure may cause a pulsation in the second left intercostal space beside the sternum. Closure of the semilunar valves under abnormal pressure may give a diastolic shock.

Turbulent blood flow may impart a vibration to the hand; this '*thrill*' is the palpable equivalent of a loud murmur. A systolic thrill at the apex usually indicates mitral regurgitation, a diastolic thrill mitral stenosis. A systolic thrill can often be felt at the lower left sternal edge with a ventricular septal defect and at the base of the heart in aortic or pulmonary stenosis. An aortic diastolic thrill is extremely rare and usually indicates rupture of an aortic valve cusp; pulmonary and tricuspid diastolic thrills are virtually unknown.

PERCUSSION is seldom used except when seeking for abnormal dullness to the right of the sternum in a patient with a suspected pericardial effusion when a radiograph is not available. One of the physical signs of emphysema is a loss of the normal cardiac dullness.

AUSCULTATION. It is essential to employ a satisfactory stethoscope incorporating both a diaphragm and a bell. The diaphragm, firmly pressed against the chest, preferentially conveys high-pitched sounds and murmurs, whereas the bell, lightly applied to the skin, favours the transmission of lower pitched sounds and murmurs.

*Sounds*. The *first heart sound* results particularly from closure of the mitral but also of the tricuspid valve. It is loudest at the apex and may be diminished in the presence of obesity or emphysema. It is accentuated by tachycardia, as in anxiety or thyrotoxicosis, and is sharp, due to abnormal closure of the mitral valve, in mitral stenosis. The first heart sound may be diminished when the valve fails to close properly with mitral regurgitation or from damage to papillary muscles by myocarditis or ischaemic heart disease. It may be obscured by the murmur of mitral regurgitation. Both mitral and tricuspid components may be audible in health, or when contraction of one ventricle is delayed as in bundle branch block (p. 164).

The *second heart sound* is due to closure of the aortic and pulmonary valves. Normally closure is synchronous in expiration; it is asynchronous towards full inspiration because of increased filling of the right ventricle and decreased filling of the left ventricle at this time. Accentuation of the sound of closure of the relevant semilunar valve is a feature of both systemic and pulmonary hypertension but is not a reliable sign. Similarly stenosis of either valve, particularly with calcification of the aortic valve, may impede closure so that the sound is abnormally quiet.

Delay of closure of one of the semilunar valves may result from conduction or mechanical factors. An example of the former is when aortic valve closure is delayed by left bundle branch block. This leads to reversed splitting of the second sound splitting being heard during expiration rather than inspiration. When pulmonary valve closure is delayed by an increased right ventricular stroke volume due to a left to right shunt through an atrial septal defect, there is splitting of the second heart sound throughout the respiratory cycle.

Various added sounds may also be significant. In the young a low-pitched *third heart sound*, at the onset of left ventricular filling, is often heard at the apex. In older patients this sound is associated with abnormal ventricular filling, either from an increased volume as may occur in mitral regurgitation, or from altered left ventricular compliance, as may be found with ischaemic heart disease. A *fourth heart sound* is comparable in its genesis to the *a* wave of the jugular venous pulse and indicates an abnormally forceful left ventricular distension as a result of atrial discharge; it is a feature of long standing hypertension, when left ventricular hypertrophy offers increased resistance to filling. It also results from loss of compliance of the left ventricle soon after a myocardial infarct and may be palpable. The *opening snap* is a feature of mitral stenosis with a pliant mitral valve and when found should lead to a special search for the characteristic mitral diastolic murmur. The opening snap is usually even more high pitched than the second heart sound and is best heard with the diaphragm of the stethoscope to the left of the lower sternum. An early systolic click (*ejection sound*) occurs at the time of opening of the relevant semilunar valve in association with either hypertension or stenosis (p. 177). A systolic click, usually in midsystole, is also a feature of prolapse of the mitral valve.

*Murmurs* are associated with turbulent blood flow. When the cardiac output is increased, as with pregnancy or severe anaemia, the turbulent flow through the pulmonary valve is heard as a systolic murmur at the left sternal edge in the second intercostal space. Murmurs also arise when blood is projected through, or leaks back through, abnormal valves; the murmurs then usually radiate in the direction of the abnormal flow. It is therefore necessary, in coming to a decision as to the cause of a murmur, to note its intensity and also where it is loudest. The murmur has also to be allocated to systole or diastole and to the appropriate part of either. Its quality, pitch and direction of preferential conduction also need to be determined. The characteristics of the main murmurs are shown in Figures 6.20, 6.21, 6.22, 6.28, 6.30 and 6.31. As a general rule, however, a harsh murmur like a saw is almost always systolic, a fact which can be confirmed by simultaneous palpation of the carotid artery or by identifying that the murmur precedes the second heart sound, which is usually best heard at the base of the heart. The murmur of regurgitation through either of the semilunar valves is usually best heard down the left sternal edge. Because of its quality it is easily confused with a breath sound so that when seeking a quiet murmur of this type it is necessary for the patient to stop breathing; it is best heard with the patient leaning forward with the breath held in expiration. The murmur of mitral stenosis, on the other hand, is low-pitched and is most likely to be heard if the bell of the stethoscope is pressed lightly at or near the apex with the patient turned half towards the left side, particularly after exercise.

**Blood Pressure**. The inflatable cuff of a sphygmomanometer is wrapped carefully round the upper arm with the bag over the brachial artery and is connected with a mercury or aneroid manometer. The bell of the stethoscope is applied over the brachial artery and the cuff is inflated to a level well above that which abolishes the Korotkov sounds. The pressure in the cuff is then allowed to fall slowly and the return of the sounds is taken as the systolic pressure. As the pressure falls the sounds become louder, and then usually quite suddenly they become muffled (so-called phase 4) and later disappear (phase 5). Phase 5 is usually closer to the true diastolic pressure and also has the advantage that there is less observer variation. When the blood pressure is to be recorded in the leg the patient should lie prone; a special large cuff should be applied to the thigh and an equivalent procedure followed with the stethoscope diaphragm placed in the popliteal fossa. The *pulse pressure* is the difference between the systolic and diastolic pressures; it tends to be abnormally high in the elderly who have rigid arteries and in patients with conditions that give rise to an increased stroke volume. Arterial pressure may be very difficult to measure in a patient in shock or when there is beat-to-beat variation as in atrial fibrillation.

The blood pressure varies throughout the day, falling to low levels during sleep and rising to high levels with anxiety. Isolated blood pressure records can therefore prove misleading, particularly in those who are unusually anxious. Sometimes this is manifest from tremor, undue sweating or tachycardia. In nervous patients repeated blood pressure readings tend to result in progressively lower figures as boredom replaces anxiety; this is, however, by no means invariable. It would be helpful if normal blood pressure could be clearly defined. This is not feasible, however, because it varies according to circumstances, particularly age. In an infant levels of 60/30 would be normal; in the 20-year-old age group, blood pressure taken at rest in most normal subjects varies between about 140/90 and 95/55. In Britain there is a tendency for blood pressure to rise with advancing years. This affects particularly the systolic pressure and is mainly due to loss of elasticity in the large arteries. In practice, for a man in his third or fourth decade to have a persistent diastolic pressure of 95 or more would be unusual. It has been shown, however, that prognosis may depend as much on systolic pressure; a level persistently above 150 in this age group should be regarded as abnormal.

## Investigation

**Electrocardiography** plays an essential role in the diagnosis and investigation of heart disease. Its main value lies in the elucidation of cardiac arrhythmias and conduction defects, and in the diagnosis and localisation of myocardial infarction. It also provides important information about problems such as digitalis toxicity, electrolyte disturbances and hypertrophy of the various chambers of the heart. However, difficulties with interpretation commonly arise and the electrocardiogram (ECG) must always be viewed in the light of the clinical findings, notably such facts as blood pressure and drug therapy.

The normal resting cell is polarised as a result of an ionic gradient across the cell wall produced by the sodium pump, which reduces the intracellular and increases the extracellular sodium concentration; the ionic balance is preserved by a high intracellular potassium concentration, compared with the extracellular. It is the potassium gradient across the cell membrane which is mainly responsible for the electrical potential difference across it.

When the membrane is electrically stimulated, the pump is inactivated. As a result, there is a sudden inrush of sodium ions, and the cell becomes depolarised. The sodium pump subsequently repolarises the cell but this process is slower. When an exploring electrode is so placed that the depolarisation current flows towards it, there is an upright (positive) deflection; when it is flowing away the deflection is inverted (negative). As currents flow in many directions simultaneously, the electrocardiogram represents the summation of these events.

In the standard (bipolar) leads, the potential difference between two limbs is recorded (lead I: left arm — right arm; lead II: left leg — right arm; lead III: left leg — left arm). Unipolar leads use an exploring electrode placed on a chosen site linked with a central terminal whose potential is close to zero. The central terminal is formed by connecting all three electrodes in the case of V leads or, in the case of augmented (a) unipolar limb leads (aVR, aVL and aVF), by connecting the two limb electrodes to which the exploring electrode is not attached. The chest lead positions are shown in Figure 6.3.

Normally, the impulse starts in the SA node but this cannot be detected by the ECG. The impulse then flows through the atrium producing the P wave. On reaching the AV nodal tissue, through which conduction is comparatively slow, it then goes rapidly through the left and right branches of the bundle of His to the Purkinje fibres of the ventricles. The next part of the ECG — the QRS complex — represents various components of ventricular depolarisation. The septum is first activated by the left bundle branch from left to right producing an initial upward deflection (R) in leads V1 and V2 over the right ventricle and an initial downward deflection (Q) in leads V4–V6 over the left ventricle (Figs. 6.2 and 6.3). The impulse then spreads out simultaneously through both ventricles from endocardial to epicardial surfaces. The amplitude and duration of the QRS complexes depend to some extent on the bulk of the muscle tissue through which the impulse is passing; as the left ventricle is normally much thicker than the right most of the QRS complex is due to activation of the left ventricle, causing for example an S wave in V1 and an R wave in V5. Atrial repolarisation, which is occurring at the same time, cannot normally be visualised. After a short period of inactivity, represented by the ST interval, repolarisation occurs producing the T wave which should normally be upright in all leads except aVR and sometimes leads III and V1. Examples of abnormal ECGs are given in the subsections of this chapter.

**Radiological examination** is indispensable for accurate determination of the size and shape of the heart. Individual chambers and the great vessels can also be studied (Fig. 6.19, p. 175). Characteristic configurations are often to be seen in the various

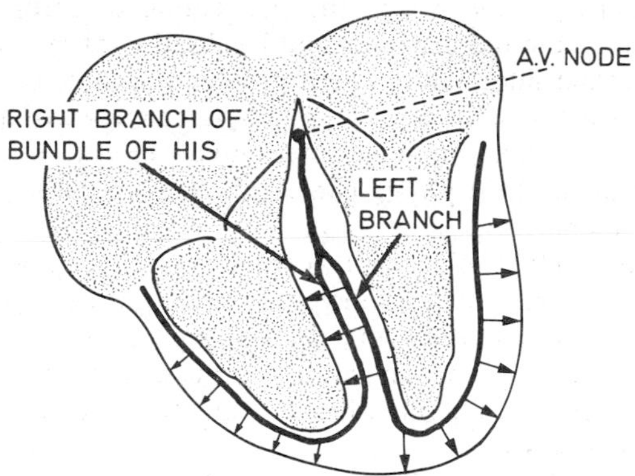


Fig. 6.2 Activation of the septum is from left to right by the left branch of the bundle of His and is followed by spread of the impulse throughout both ventricles.

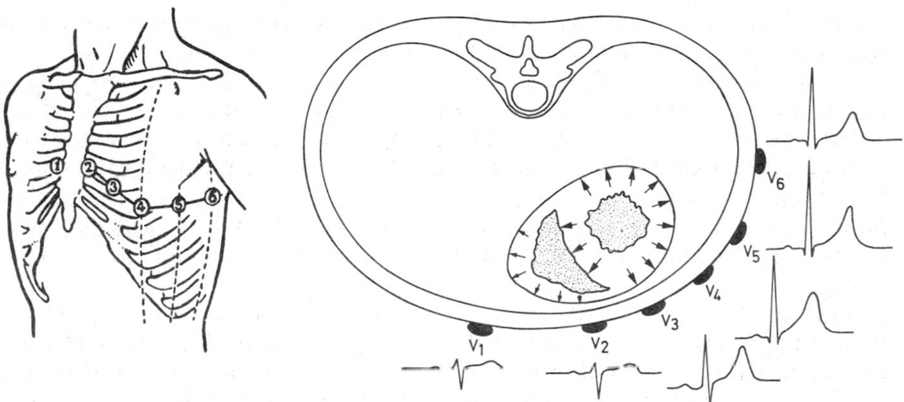


Fig. 6.3 Unipolar chest leads V1–V6.

forms of valvular and congenital heart disease, in syphilitic aortitis and in aneurysm of the heart and aorta. The oesophagus can be visualised by giving the patient barium emulsion to swallow and any backward displacement by the enlarged left atrium in mitral disease can be demonstrated in the lateral view. Serial radiographs provide a useful record of the patient's progress.

The lung fields can also be studied. Congestion and oedema can often be shown radiologically before they can be detected clinically. Congestion is first revealed by dilated pulmonary veins; oedema by thickened septa and dilated lymphatic vessels which result in horizontal lines in the costophrenic angles. More advanced changes are a hazy opacification spreading from the hilar region, and pleural effusion.

*Radioscopy* of the heart, preferably with the aid of an image intensifier, is of value in the detection of abnormal pulsations and of calcification particularly of abnormal valves.

*Angiocardiography*. The individual chambers of the heart and the great vessels may be visualised by the injection of a radio-opaque material into a vein or by catheter directly into the aorta and heart before making a series of radiographs in rapid succession. Such studies are very useful in the differentiation of various congenital cardiac lesions and of vascular from other abnormal mediastinal shadows. Coronary angiography is necessary before surgery for ischaemic heart disease.

**Phonocardiography** records heart sounds and murmurs and may help to elucidate difficult problems of auscultation.

**Echocardiography.** When an ultrasonic beam encounters a boundary between structures of different acoustic densities, some of the waves are reflected. A piezoelectric crystal, which acts as both transmitter and receiver, is used to generate high frequency pulses of very short duration. These travel through body tissues at a known velocity; the reflections which occur from acoustic interfaces are detected by the transducer, amplified and then displayed either on an oscilloscope or on a strip-chart recorder.

Because both bone and lung interfere with the ultrasonic transmission, only a small area of the heart is directly accessible to study. The normal procedure involves placing the transducer in the fourth intercostal space at the left sternal edge. By locating the probe in this position and pointing it directly posteriorly, the investigator can identify the mitral valve by its characteristic pattern of motion. The probe is then angled in different directions so that the movements of the left ventricle, the tricuspid valve, the aortic valve and the left atrium are displayed. In 'real time' echocardiography multiple beams are recorded simultaneously to provide a moving picture of cardiac structures.

Echocardiography has proved particularly valuable in studying disorders of the mitral valve. In the normal valve, the cusps open rapidly in early diastole and quickly return towards the closed position. In mitral stenosis, the downward movement of the cusps may be well preserved but, because of the high pressure in the left atrium, the cusps are held down an abnormally long time in the left ventricular cavity — i.e. the diastolic closure rate is slow. Calcification of the mitral valve results in multiple echoes from the valve leaflets. Mitral regurgitation can be suspected by abnormal movements of the valve leaflets. Regurgitation of blood through the aortic valve produces a characteristic vibration of the anterior mitral cusp.

Echocardiography is also useful in detecting abnormalities in other forms of valve disease, pericardial effusion and most varieties of congenital heart disease.

**Cardiac Catheterisation.** A radio-opaque catheter can be passed from a vein into the right atrium, right ventricle and pulmonary artery; its tip can be wedged in a small pulmonary artery and thus a record of the 'pulmonary arterial wedge' or 'indirect left atrial pressure' can be obtained. A catheter may also be passed retrogradely into the aorta and so into the left ventricle. Pressures can be recorded and the oxygen saturation of extracted blood samples estimated. Valuable information may be obtained in cases of congenital heart disease and in certain types of acquired heart disease. For example, in pulmonary hypertension the pressure in the pulmonary artery and right ventricle is increased; when there is stenosis of the pulmonary valve the systolic pressure is higher in the right ventricle than in the pulmonary artery; with stenosis of the aortic valve it is higher in the left ventricle than in the aorta. In atrial septal defect, because of the left to right shunt, the oxygen content of the blood in the right atrium is higher than that in the venae cavae; in ventricular septal defect the oxygen content of the blood in the right ventricle is higher than that in the right atrium.

If the oxygen content of blood from the pulmonary artery and brachial artery and also the oxygen consumption are known, then the cardiac output can be calculated from the Fick formula:

$$\text{Cardiac output } (l/\text{min}) = \frac{\text{Oxygen consumption (ml/min)}}{\text{Arteriovenous oxygen difference } (\text{ml}/l)}$$

The area of a valve can be calculated if the pressure difference across it, and the forward flow through it are known. Likewise the volume of a shunt can be calculated from measurement of the relevant oxygen saturations, in conjunction with the oxygen uptake. Dye dilution techniques are also used. When a known quantity of dye is injected into a vein, or directly into the heart through a catheter, estimation of its serial concentration in an artery can be used to calculate the cardiac output.

**Radioisotopes** are used for the estimation of cardiac output and ventricular volume and for calculating the ventricular ejection fraction with an intravenous radionuclide bolus usually of technetium. They also provide a method of assessing myocardial blood flow; thallium is used to demonstrate 'cold spots' or zones of decreased radionuclide accumulation in an infarct. Radioisotopes can also demonstrate improved myocardial perfusion after coronary bypass surgery.

## Disorders of Cardiac Rate, Rhythm and Conduction

**The Control of Cardiac Rate.** Cardiac cells have the faculty of self-excitation. The pacemaking of the heart is due to this activity and it is normally controlled by the cells with the fastest natural rate. These are usually in the sinoatrial (SA) node. The SA node has its own intrinsic rate but it is also under nervous control; vagal activity slows it and sympathetic activity accelerates it. The sinus rate may become unduly slowed with increased vagal tone, and lower centres may then take over the pacemaking, e.g. either the AV node — so-called junctional rhythm — or sometimes an ectopic ventricular focus. At other times the natural rate of lower centres may be increased as a result of disturbances of cellular metabolism, such as occur with electrolyte disorders and with digitalis, or as a result of cellular damage from myocardial disease. Sometimes an impulse may be unable to enter a normal pathway if it is refractory; the impulse then has to take a different course. It may arrive when the distal end of the normal pathway is no longer refractory and may then travel through it retrogradely. This short circuit, the so-called re-entry phenomenon, can lead to a rapid circus movement and is one of the causes of paroxysmal tachycardia.

### Sinus Rhythms

**Sinus Arrhythmia** (Fig. 6.4). In breathing there is a phasic variation in the output of the two ventricles, expiration increasing left and inspiration increasing right ventricular filling. The variation in arterial pressure which results triggers baroreceptors in the carotid sinus and elsewhere and the heart rate may then slow in expiration, sinus arrhythmia is particularly common in normal children.

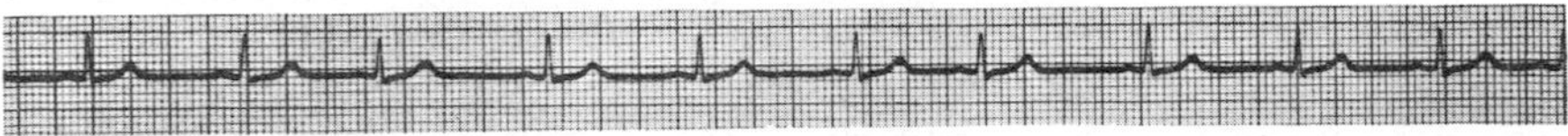

Fig. 6.4 Sinus arrhythmia. PQRST is normal but the interval between successive complexes varies.

**Sinus Bradycardia** (Fig. 6.5). The term is used when the sinus rate is less than 60/min and is a normal finding in many athletes. Sinus bradycardia may also be a feature of myxoedema, jaundice and raised intracranial pressure, and may occur in some patients soon after myocardial infarction. Sinus bradycardia can be caused by beta adrenergic receptor blocking drugs and by digitalis. In *sinoatrial disease* (*sick sinus syndrome*) sinus bradycardia may be so extreme as to lead to syncope. A common feature is liability to atrial tachycardia or fibrillation. An artificial pacemaker may be required to ensure an adequate heart rate and permit the use of anti-arrhythmic drugs such as digitalis.

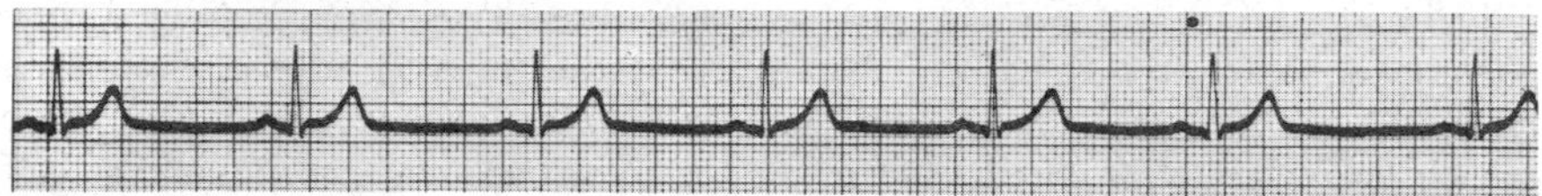

Fig. 6.5 Sinus bradycardia. The rate is 50 per min.

**Sinus tachycardia** (Fig. 6.6) is defined as a sinus rate of more than 100 and is a normal finding with exercise and anxiety. It is also a feature of fever, hyperthyroidism and acute circulatory and cardiac failure. Whatever the cause, the rate rarely exceeds 160, except in infants; the electrocardiogram is otherwise normal.

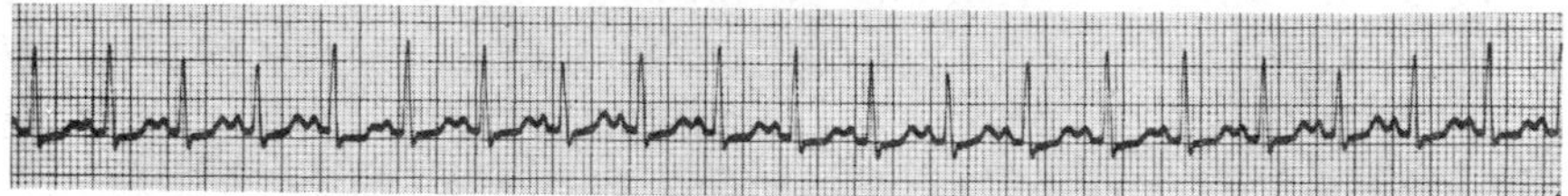

Fig. 6.6 Sinus tachycardia. The rate is about 150 per min. The QRS complexes are normal and each is preceded by a P wave.

## Ectopic Rhythms

When the impulses arise elsewhere than in the SA node the rhythm is known as ectopic; it may be regular or irregular. Ectopic rhythms arise either because of increased automaticity of pacemaker cells in the atria or ventricles or because of re-entry.

### Atrial Ectopic Rhythms

**Ectopic Beats** (*Extrasystoles*, *Premature Beats*). These usually cause no symptoms but can give the sensation of an extra or thumping beat. The rhythm is basically regular, but premature beats may occur either at regular intervals or apparently randomly. If sufficiently premature they may produce no pulse, causing a dropped beat at the wrist, but their presence can usually be detected with the stethoscope. The QRS (Fig. 6.7) is normal but the conformation of the P is often different because the impulse starts at an abnormal site.

**Atrial Tachycardia** (Fig. 6.8). Paroxysmal tachycardia may occur with a rate of between 140 and 220 as a result of re-entry or a rapidly firing ectopic focus. This usually occurs in hearts which are otherwise normal and may last from a few seconds

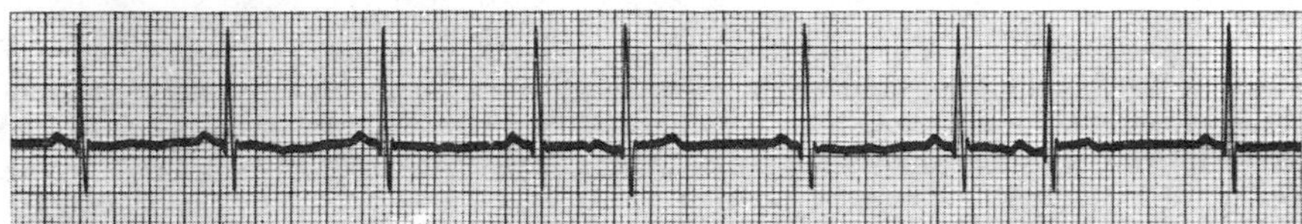

Fig. 6.7 Atrial ectopic beats. The QRS complexes of the two ectopic beats are similar to those of the normal beats and are preceded by a P wave.

to a day or two when untreated. The patient is usually aware that the heart has suddenly started to beat fast and may feel faint or breathless. With prolonged attacks polyuria is sometimes a feature. Particularly if the heart is otherwise abnormal, cardiac pain or left ventricular failure may occur. Coffee, alcohol, tobacco and anxiety can all be precipitating factors but anxiety is of course much more commonly responsible for a sinus tachycardia.

The ECG shows a QRST of normal configuration and confirms the rapid rate. Massage of the carotid sinus on one side for a few seconds may terminate an attack. If it does not do so a sedative and retiring to bed may be all that is required; many patients then awake to find that the attack is over. Atrial tachycardia can usually be terminated by intravenous practolol, digoxin, verapamil or by DC shock. If attacks are frequent or otherwise disabling, propranolol and digoxin used either alone or in combination may be helpful in reducing their frequency or in abolishing them.

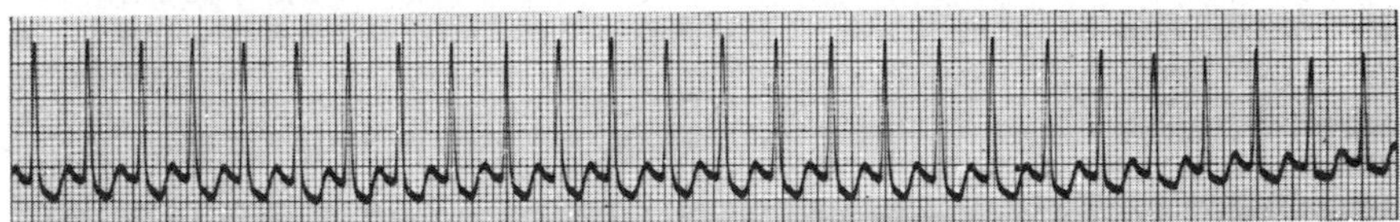

Fig. 6.8 Atrial tachycardia. The rate is 190 per min. The QRS complexes are normal.

**Atrial Tachycardia with Atrioventricular Block.** In this arrhythmia a rapid atrial rate (140–220/min) is also present, but it is accompanied by atrioventricular block of varying degree. If there is first degree block, i.e. only prolongation of the PR interval, the ventricular rate may be rapid, and heart failure may result. Carotid sinus pressure may slow the ventricular rate by increasing the block, but unlike paroxysmal tachycardia without block the attack cannot be terminated. In atrial tachycardia without block, carotid sinus pressure is either ineffective or stops the attack. Atrial tachycardia with block is serious because it seldom occurs in otherwise normal hearts and is frequently a manifestation of digitalis intoxication which can be lethal if digitalis is not stopped. There is nearly always intracellular hypokalia even if the serum potassium is normal and potassium supplements should be given. Practolol intravenously (p. 191) often restores sinus rhythm. When this arrhythmia occurs in those who are not taking digitalis, paradoxical as it may seem, digoxin is the treatment of choice if the ventricular rate is fast.

**Atrial Flutter.** The atrial rate is usually about 300/min; the ventricular rate is commonly 150 per minute or less because of a two, three or four to one atrioventricular block. Atrial flutter may cause or aggravate cardiac failure. The aetiology is the same as for the commoner atrial fibrillation.

Flutter waves can sometimes be detected at about 5/sec in the jugular venous pulse. Carotid sinus massage often increases the atrioventricular block, as from 2:1 to 3:1 for example; the pulse will then still be regular but will be slower. The ECG shows a saw-tooth appearance due to the F (flutter) waves which are usually best seen in leads II, III and aVF. Digitalis is used to increase the AV block and slow the ventricular rate. It either abolishes the arrhythmia or changes the rhythm to that of atrial fibrillation. Digitalis provides a useful prophylactic against recurrence when sinus rhythm returns; patients with mitral stenosis in particular should be protected from the rapid ventricular rate which is liable to be found with atrial flutter in the undigitalised patient.

**Atrial Fibrillation.** The atria beat chaotically and ineffectively; the baseline of the ECG (Fig. 6.9) is disturbed by so-called f (fibrillation) waves. These are obvious in atrial fibrillation of recent onset but may be almost invisible when the arrhythmia is long established, as in patients with chronic rheumatic heart disease; then the diagnosis is made by the totally irregular QRST complexes and the absence of P waves.

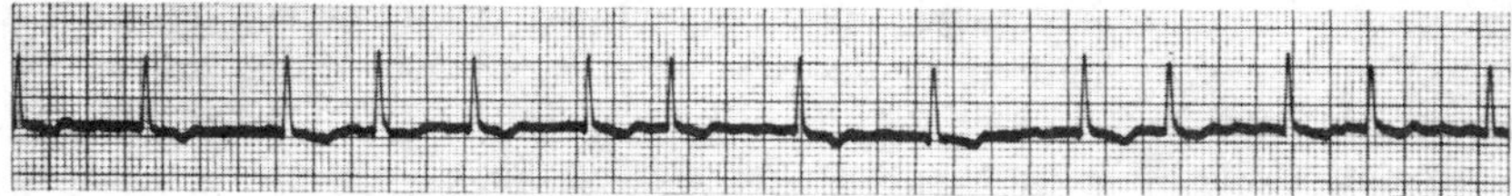

Fig. 6.9 Atrial fibrillation. The ventricular complexes are irregular, there are no P waves and irregular oscillations (f waves) disturb the base line.

Rheumatic mitral valve disease is the commonest cause of atrial fibrillation in young and middle-aged patients; ischaemic heart disease is the usual explanation in older patients in whom thyrotoxicosis is also an important and often undetected cause. Atrial fibrillation may occur temporarily with myocardial infarction. It is rare in congenital and pulmonary heart disease and in isolated disease of the aortic valve. Sometimes it occurs with pericarditis and after thoracic operations. Atrial fibrillation may be found in the absence of any other evidence of heart disease, and then may be intermittent at first but later often permanent. Episodes of atrial fibrillation can be provoked, in those who are prone to it, by alcohol and infections.

Atrial fibrillation may also cause or aggravate heart failure in those with an abnormal heart, particularly with mitral stenosis. Diastole is shortened because of the tachycardia and the left atrial pressure rises. The absence of the contribution of atrial systole to ventricular filling is another adverse factor. Stasis in the atrium favours the formation of thrombus and hence there is an increased danger of embolism particularly for a few days after the change of rhythm.

The pulse is totally irregular. Without digitalis the ventricular rate is usually rapid so that when the interval between heart beats is sufficiently short the ventricle may not fill enough to produce a pulse; the difference between the heart rate and the pulse rate is then called the pulse deficit. There is no 'a' wave to be seen in the jugular venous pulse, and in patients with mitral stenosis the presystolic murmur disappears.

Ectopic beats, if very numerous, may mimic atrial fibrillation well enough to be distinguishable only by an ECG. However, atrial fibrillation is much the more likely diagnosis if the rhythm has suddenly changed and in particular if there is evidence of thyrotoxicosis or of rheumatic heart disease. Exercise tends to eliminate ectopic beats, at least when the heart is otherwise normal.

Prognosis varies with the cause of the arrhythmia. Atrial fibrillation can usually be abolished if thyrotoxicosis is successfully treated. Its development is a milestone on the downward path of chronic rheumatic heart disease, and is often associated with worsening of cardiac failure or the development of embolism. In the elderly, untreated atrial fibrillation is often accompanied by a normal ventricular rate and may be an incidental finding.

Digitalis is used to reduce the ventricular rate and this alone may result in a striking improvement, particularly in patients with mitral stenosis. When atrial fibrillation persists after correction of hyperthyroidism, sinus rhythm can often be restored with DC shock. In chronic rheumatic heart disease such therapy is pointless because the arrhythmia is almost certain to return, unless the valve lesions can be improved by surgery. When atrial fibrillation develops in patients with chronic rheumatic heart disease, treatment with heparin followed by warfarin should be instituted as there is a danger of embolism at that time. There is disagreement about the efficacy of permanent anticoagulant therapy which carries its own risks in the long term management of such patients.

## Ventricular Ectopic Rhythms

**Ectopic Beats**. An ectopic ventricular focus may initiate impulses which activate the ventricles prematurely as a result of ventricular escape, enhanced rate of the ectopic focus, or re-entry. Ectopic beats are fairly frequent in normal people but commoner after myocardial infarction and with digitalis therapy. If an ectopic beat occurs after a normal one it may suppress the next expected normal beat; when this is repetitive, coupling, or pulsus bigeminus, results.

The symptoms and signs are precisely similar to those of atrial ectopic beats from which they can be distinguished only by the ECG (Fig. 6.10). Ventricular extrasystoles have an abnormally widened QRS complex. They are usually of little importance but often digitalis is responsible and the dose should then be reduced. They may, however, be of crucial importance in myocardial infarction, for an unusually premature ventricular extrasystole may fall on the T of a normal beat ('R on T') and initiate ventricular tachycardia (Fig. 6.11) or ventricular fibrillation (Fig. 6.12).

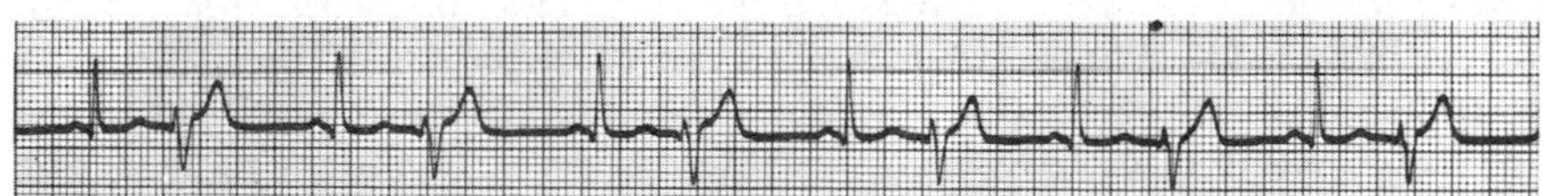

Fig. 6.10 Ventricular ectopic beats. Alternate beats have an abnormally wide QRS complex with no preceding P wave, i.e. coupling of the pulse results.

**Ventricular tachycardia** (Fig. 6.11) generally occurs in patients with serious heart disease and may constitute a clinical emergency. The ventricular rate is of the order of 140 to 220; untreated the tachycardia may last from seconds to days; it may cause heart failure or acute circulatory failure, particularly in patients with myocardial infarction.

The patient may be aware of the tachycardia during an acute phase or may feel faint or become breathless. The independent atrial contractions are sometimes visible in the jugular venous pulse and are responsible for varying ventricular filling, which may be reflected in a variation in the intensity of the first heart sound and in the pulse volume. Carotid sinus pressure is ineffective.

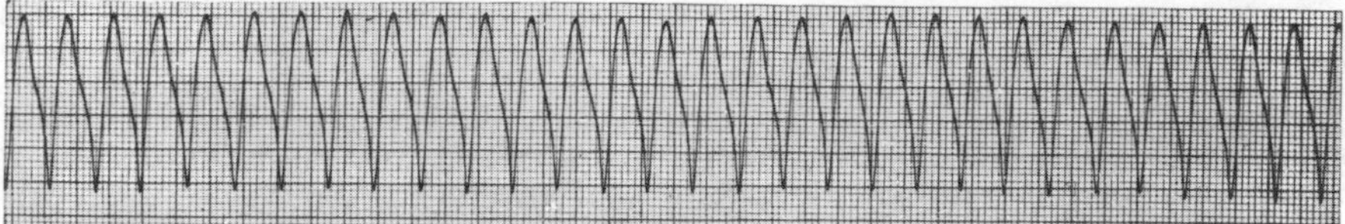

Fig. 6.11 Ventricular tachycardia. The rate is 220 per min. The complexes are broad and abnormal.

If there is no distress, urgent treatment is usually not required, but if there is, particularly immediately after myocardial infarction, lignocaine should be given intravenously (p. 166). Mexiletine or disopyramide (p. 165) may also be effective. If these measures fail, DC shock should be used, unless the patient is digitilised when there would be a danger of producing ventricular fibrillation.

The prophylactic use of oral procainamide can reduce the likelihood of further episodes but should not be continued for more than 6 weeks as it is liable to produce a syndrome resembling SLE (p. 627). Some patients may require long-term prophylaxis with quinidine in a long-acting form or with oral mexiletine or disopyramide.

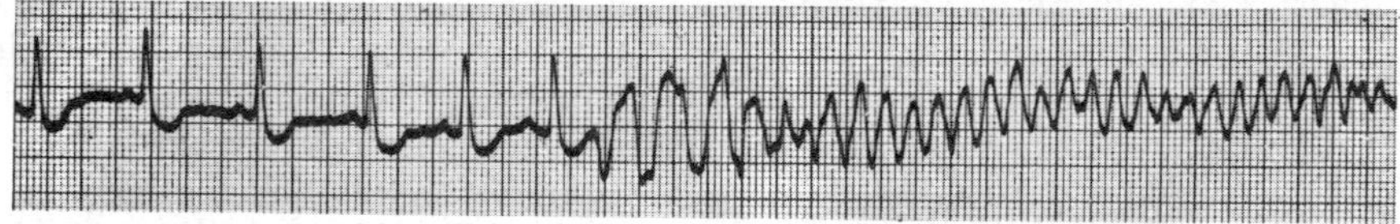

Fig. 6.12 Ventricular fibrillation. The change from sinus rhythm to ventricular fibrillation occurs when a ventricular ectopic beat falls on the T of the previous complex.

**Ventricular fibrillation** is the commonest immediate cause of sudden death. It is generally due to myocardial infarction but it may result from accidents such as electrocution or drowning. The ventricles have a rapid, ineffective, uncoordinated movement which produces no pulse, and the ECG (Fig. 6.12) has broad, bizarre, irregular complexes. Within seconds of the onset of the attack the patient loses consciousness. Respiration ceases, the patient develops a deathly pallor and no pulse is palpable even in a large artery. Without treatment the pupils become dilated and death is virtually inevitable. When this arrhythmia occurs as a complication of myocardial infarction in the coronary care unit, the immediate application of DC shock can restore sinus rhythm within seconds. Under other circumstances the circulation has to be maintained by the resuscitation procedure for cardiac arrest (p. 161). Failure of the circulation causes acidosis and sodium bicarbonate should be given intravenously (p. 142). If sinus rhythm is restored lignocaine should be given to reduce the likelihood of recurrence followed by procainamide or mexiletine orally (p. 165).

**Ventricular asystole** is the more sinister of the two arrhythmias which can cause sudden death. When asystole complicates myocardial infarction the outlook is usually very poor. The treatment, if this is thought appropriate, is that for cardiac arrest, but DC shock is valueless and artificial ventricular pacing is usually either impracticable or unsuccessful. With spontaneously terminated attacks, the Adams-Stokes syndrome

(p. 164), an artificial pacemaker may be required to stimulate the heart and to prevent recurrences. As a result of the use of 24 hour ECG monitoring with miniaturised portable recording equipment, episodes of asystole, e.g. with the sick sinus syndrome, are much more commonly recognised.

## Cardiac Arrest

Cardiac arrest is the sudden and complete loss of cardiac function. It is usually due to ventricular fibrillation and less often to asystole. They can usually be distinguished only by an ECG or during cardiac surgery when the heart is visible. More commonly attempts at resuscitation have to be commenced before an ECG is available. The indication for resuscitation is clearest when the death has occurred as a result of an accident, as with an electric shock or from drowning, or when the cardiac arrest occurs during the course of an investigation such as cardiac catheterisation or even from an intravenous injection.

The development of the technique of closed chest cardiac massage (external cardiac massage), together with mouth-to-mouth ventilation, has improved the outlook immeasurably and now all doctors, nurses, ambulance drivers and attendants should have received instruction in this vitally important form of first aid. One of the problems in hospital practice is to determine when it is inappropriate to attempt resuscitation and to ensure that such attempts are not made, with all the anxiety which they inevitably produce for other patients in the ward, when there is a great likelihood that they will be unsuccessful or that, even if successful, the quality of the life to which the patient returns may not justify the use of the procedure. Inevitably it is sometimes necessary to institute resuscitation until someone familiar with the patient's illness can make the decision as to whether the attempt should continue.

**Treatment.** The brain suffers irreversible damage unless some circulation of oxygenated blood can be achieved within 2 or 3 minutes. A smart blow should be given to the left of the sternum with the hand or fist, and both legs should be elevated to 90 degrees. If the heart does not start immediately, as indicated by the return of the carotid or femoral pulse, closed chest massage and mouth-to-mouth breathing should be instituted.

TECHNIQUE OF CARDIOPULMONARY RESUSCITATION. The patient is laid on the back on the floor, or on boards which are put on the mattress behind the chest. The operator places the hands one on top of the other (Fig. 6.13) on the patient's lower sternum and commences forceful rhythmic compressions at the rate of 60–100/min. The danger of fracturing ribs is reduced if the pressure is transmitted through the ball of the hand on to the sternum. At the same time ventilation must be ensured. The head is extended and the jaw pulled forward. Mouth-to-mouth or mouth-to-nose breathing is employed until a face mask and bag are available. The lungs should be ventilated after every fifth compression of the sternum. Meanwhile an intravenous infusion should be set up containing sodium bicarbonate (50–100 mmol) in order to combat acidosis. Where a defibrillator is available it should be used as soon as possible, for no harm is done if the patient proves to have asystole rather than ventricular fibrillation.

The success rate is best for accidental death or for those who have had a myocardial infarction but without shock or heart failure. If it transpires that the acute circulatory failure was due to cardiac rupture following myocardial infarction, cardiac tamponade or massive pulmonary embolism, resuscitation will be almost certainly unsuccessful.

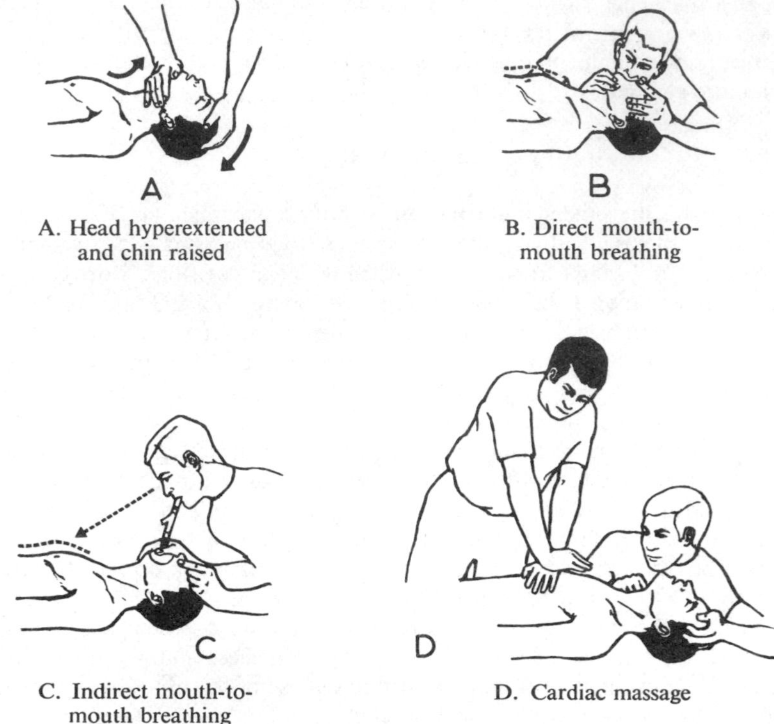


A. Head hyperextended and chin raised

B. Direct mouth-to-mouth breathing

C. Indirect mouth-to-mouth breathing

D. Cardiac massage

Fig. 6.13 Emergency resuscitation.

Such a cause can be suspected from failure to produce a pulse and this evidence should always be sought in every patient having closed chest cardiac massage. Nowadays those who have simple syncope are increasingly at risk of overenthusiastic resuscitation measures.

## Heart Block (SA and AV Block)

**Sinoatrial (SA) Block.** A complete cardiac cycle is missed so that a gap appears in the pulse. The electrocardiogram shows that both atrial and ventricular complexes are absent. This condition is uncommon and of little clinical importance.

**Atrioventricular (AV) Block.** Conduction between the atria and ventricles is impaired.

1. In *first degree heart block* (delayed AV conduction) the PR interval is prolonged beyond the upper limit of normal (0·20 sec) (Fig. 6.14).

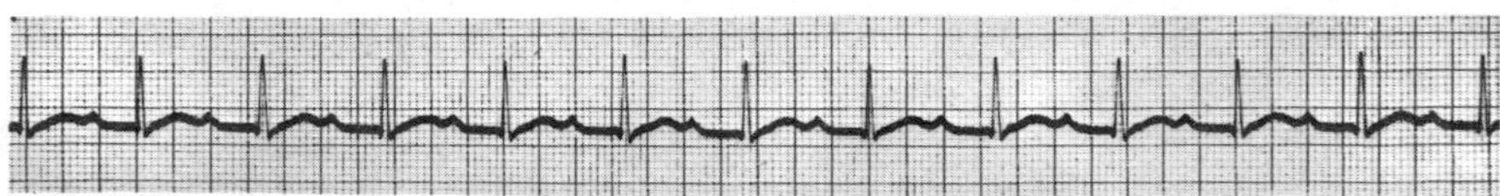

Fig. 6.14 First degree heart block. The PR interval is 0·26 sec.

2. In *second degree heart block* (partial heart block) some impulses from the atria fail to get through to the ventricles, i.e. dropped beats occur. Sometimes there is progressive lengthening of successive PR intervals followed by a dropped beat. This is known as Wenckebach's phenomenon (Fig. 6.15) and is due to progressive fatigue of the AV bundle with recovery following the rest period when the dropped beat occurs.

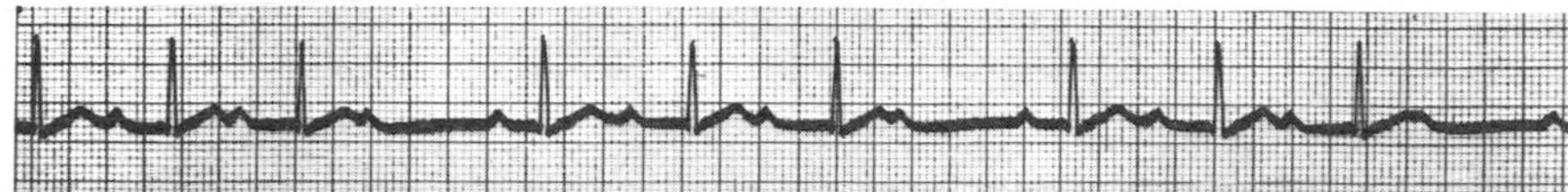

Fig. 6.15 Second degree heart block (Wenckebach's phenomenon). The first beat in the cycle has a PR of 0.28 sec; it lengthens with the next two beats and the fourth P wave is not followed by a QRS — the dropped beat.

3. In *complete heart block* no impulses from the atria reach the ventricles, which beat at their intrinsic rate of about 40 per minute (Fig. 6.16).

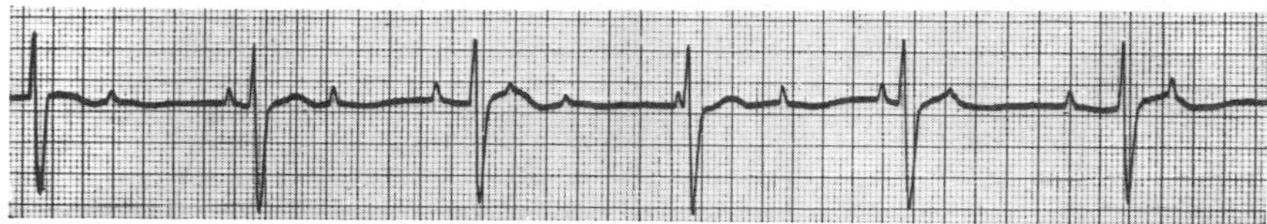

Fig. 6.16 Complete heart block. There is complete dissociation of atrial and ventricular complexes. The atrial rate is 70 and the ventricular rate 40 per min.

**Aetiology.** Depression of conductivity is most commonly due to ischaemia, fibrosis or inflammation of the AV bundle, or to vagal stimulation. Myocardial infarction is the most frequent cause of heart block which develops suddenly. Idiopathic focal fibrosis, strategically situated, is a common cause of chronic heart block, particularly in the elderly. Prolongation of the PR interval is often found in rheumatic fever and digitalis overdosage. Complete heart block may be a late manifestation of digitalis poisoning and occasionally results from a congenital maldevelopment of the bundle. It also occurs as a complication of Chagas' disease (p. 820).

**Clinical Features.** *First degree heart block* can be diagnosed only by ECG.

*Second Degree Heart Block.* When the atrial and ventricular contractions bear a simple ratio to one another such as in 2:1 and 3:1 block, the pulse is slow and regular. Change in the degree of partial heart block may give rise to sudden changes in pulse rate. The degree of block may sometimes be diagnosed by comparing the number of *a* waves in the jugular pulse with the carotid pulse. More complex ratios between atrial and ventricular contractions such as 3:2 or 4:3 block give rise to 'dropped beats'. On auscultation it can be appreciated that there has been no ventricular beat, thus distinguishing the condition from ectopic beats. Partial heart block is usually transient and may occur during an acute infection, from digitalis overdose, or from coronary heart disease.

*Complete heart block* should be suspected when the pulse is slow (30 to 40 min) and regular, and does not vary with exercise. There is complete dissociation between the jugular *a* waves and the carotid pulses. There may be varying intensity of the first heart sound and audible atrial sounds. Venous 'cannon' waves (p. 148) may be seen in the neck. The pulse volume is large but often variable depending on whether ventricular filling has been increased by an appropriately timed atrial contraction.

*Adams-Stokes Syndrome.* When cerebral blood flow ceases as a result of ventricular asystole, tachycardia or fibrillation, syncope rapidly ensues. Convulsions may occur if the heart does not begin to beat again within about 10 seconds, and death will result if the arrest is prolonged. The skin blanches and later cyanosis occurs. When the heart starts beating again there is a characteristic flush as the emptied vessels are filled with blood. The syndrome is a complication of complete heart block or less commonly partial heart block. Patients who have repeated attacks may be aware of the imminence of unconsciousness, but frequently syncope occurs without warning.

**Treatment.** Complete heart block in acute myocardial infarction requires treatment to prevent undue bradycardia or asystole. Isoprenaline, as an intravenous infusion (1–5 mg in 500 ml dextrose) is effective in increasing the ventricular rate, but has the disadvantage of increasing ventricular stroke work. Electrical pacing may be carried out by advancing an electrode from a peripheral vein until its tip lies against the endocardium of the right ventricle. Its proximal end is attached externally to a pulse generator. Pacing is usually required for only a few days.

When chronic heart block is responsible for heart failure or Adams-Stokes attacks, long-acting isoprenaline may be given in a dose of 30 mg or more four times daily, but nearly all cases are better managed with a pacemaker.

### Bundle Branch Block and Hemiblock

Bundle branch block may affect either the right or the left bundle and result in delay in contraction of the right or left ventricle, respectively. Incomplete bundle branch block is the term used when the QRS complex is widened to less than 0.12 seconds. It commonly occurs when the depolarisation pathway is prolonged due to ventricular dilation as in the right bundle branch block associated with an atrial septal defect. In complete bundle branch block the QRS complex is longer than 0.12 seconds and this usually results from ischaemia. The condition may be recognised clinically (p. 150). Examples of the ECG abnormalities are shown in Figures 6.17 and 6.18. The treatment and prognosis are in general those of the underlying disease. Right bundle branch block may be a benign congenital condition.

Damage to the fasicles of the left bundle may cause hemiblock or complicate other forms of block.

### Treatment of Arrhythmia and Bradycardia

**Pharmacological Methods.** These include drugs used to suppress or prevent ectopic rhythms, to block atrioventricular conduction, or to increase a slow heart rate.

1. *Drugs used to suppress or prevent ectopic rhythms*, whether atrial or ventricular, are thought to act mainly on the cell membrane by slowing depolarisation. Quinidine, mexiletine, lignocaine and procainamide act in this way. There may also be slowing of conduction velocity and depression of contraction amplitude. *Quinidine sulphate* is used less widely than when it was the only anti-arrhythmic available, because of its liability to cause nausea, vomiting and diarrhoea and, more importantly, because of its cardiotoxic effects, which include heart block, asystole and ventricular fibrillation.

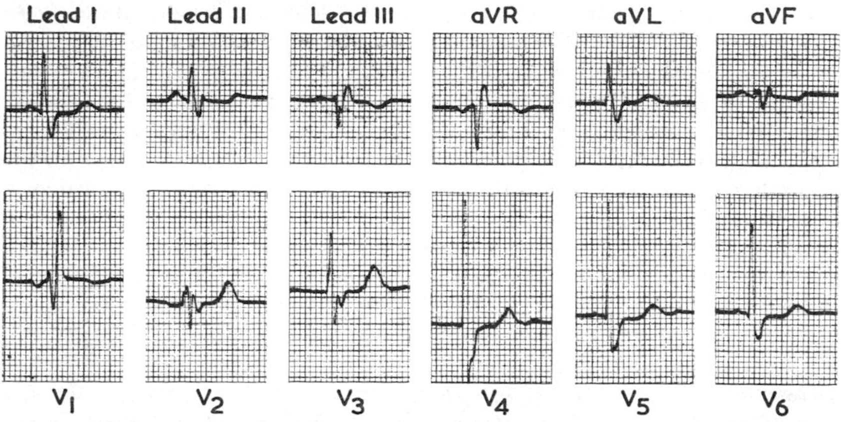


Fig. 6.17 Right bundle branch block. Note that in V1 the late secondary R wave indicates a delay in depolarisation of the right ventricle.

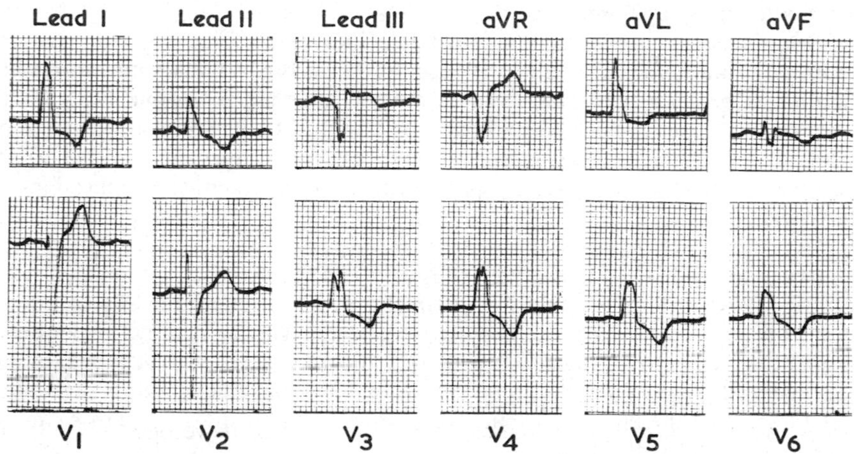


Fig. 6.18 Left bundle branch block. The wide QRS in V6 and aVL indicates a delay in depolarisation of the left ventricle.

A sustained-action preparation is available which is less toxic and may be used if there are no facilities for conversion of atrial arrhythmias by electrical means. When sinus rhythm is restored, a maintenance dose depending on the needs of the individual patient is used; it may be controlled by estimations of blood levels. Conversion to sinus rhythm should be monitored by ECG, watching for widening of the QRS complex, which is a warning of too great a cardiotoxic effect.

*Mexiletine* is effective in the management of increased ventricular excitability associated with myocardial infarction. Toxic effects include nausea and tremor. It may be given intravenously (200 mg over 5–10 minutes), or on a long-term basis (200–250 mg 8 hourly by mouth).

*Disopyramide* resembles quinidine but is probably safer. It usually controls ventricular arrhythmias in a dosage of 100–150 mg three to four times a day. Side-effects, which are mainly anticholinergic, include dry mouth, blurred vision and retention of urine but it may precipitate cardiac failure in those with poor left ventricular function.

*Intravenous lignocaine* is particularly useful in the coronary care unit and is given as a bolus of 5–10 ml of the 1% solution. This is followed by an intravenous infusion at a rate of 4 mg per minute for 30 minutes, subsequently being reduced to 3 mg and then to 2 mg per minute.

*β-adrenoceptor blocking drugs* such as propranolol, oxprenolol and practolol are all of value, but the last can now be used only intravenously in the acute situation in view of the serious side-effects which occasionally follow its long-term use. Propranolol is the longest established and is used in a dose of 10–40 mg 8 hourly. Oxprenolol is similar. Other properties of β blocking drugs are discussed on page 197.

*Phenytoin* is also effective particularly with digitalis-induced arrhythmias either orally or i.v. (max dose 1 g; not faster than 100 mg in 5 minutes).

2. *Drugs used to depress atrioventricular conduction* are digitalis derivatives and β blockers. The former is used particularly in the management of atrial fibrillation and the latter in thyrotoxicosis. *Verapamil* (5–10 mg given slowly i.v.) is also used to terminate supraventricular tachycardia. It has a negative inotropic effect and may lower blood pressure; it should therefore not be used in patients with cardiac failure or soon after myocardial infarction.

3. *Drugs used to increase a slow heart rate* include atropine and isoprenaline. *Atropine* (0·6 mg i.v., s.c. or i.m.) is used for sinus bradycardia with myocardial infarction. *Isoprenaline* in a long-acting form is of value in the treatment of chronic heart block in a dose of 30–60 mg 6 hourly by mouth. The patient may be aware of the 'pounding' of the heart, but in some patients it is sufficiently satisfactory in preventing Adams-Stokes attacks to spare them from the potential complications of an artificial pacemaker.

**Electrical Methods.** 1. *Pacemaking*. The heart can be electrically stimulated if an electrode, attached to a generator, is in contact with the endocardial or epicardial surfaces of an atrium or ventricle. In *temporary* pacemaking an external generator is connected to an electrode which is usually inserted via a subclavian vein with its tip positioned in the right ventricle. In *permanent* pacemaking a generator is implanted under the skin of the chest wall. Such generators can last up to 10 years or more before they require replacement.

2. *Direct current shock* (cardioversion). A large DC shock can be used to produce transient asystole, after which the sinus node usually asserts its dominance over cardiac electrical activity. Such a shock must be timed (synchronised) to avoid delivery during the T wave, because then ventricular fibrillation may be induced. Synchronised DC shock is effective in terminating atrial tachycardia, flutter and fibrillation, and ventricular tachycardia, though these arrhythmias may subsequently recur. DC shock is used for the termination of ventricular fibrillation.

## Acute Circulatory Failure (Shock)

These terms are used for a clinical state which includes pallor, sweating, hypotension and tachycardia. The most usual cause of the shock syndrome is loss of fluid from haemorrhage, severe diarrhoea or vomiting, or from exudation as a result of extensive burns. This is known as *hypovolaemic shock*. Acute circulatory failure may also occur in severe infection, i.e. *bacteraemic* or *septic shock* (p. 80). Shock may result from sudden failure of the heart itself to maintain a satisfactory circulation, as for example in myocardial infarction, and the condition is then known as *cardiogenic shock*. A sudden obstruction of the circulation, such as occurs with massive pulmonary embolism, can also cause acute circulatory failure. *Anaphylactic shock* is discussed on page 30.

When the cardiac output drops suddenly a compensatory differential alteration in the arteriolar resistances occurs which favours perfusion of the heart and brain. In some cases this may fail and oliguria and clouding of consciousness ensue. If tissue hypoxia and resultant acidosis are severe and prolonged, there may be irreversible damage e.g. to the brain or kidneys.

**Treatment** must be directed primarily at the cause, hypovolaemic, cardiac or bacteraemic. Any deficiency in the blood volume must be corrected if possible, as for example, following haemorrhage.

In order to avoid overloading the circulation, intravenous infusions must be monitored by observation of the venous pressure. As these patients have to be nursed lying flat the jugular venous pressure cannot be measured. The central venous pressure (CVP) can be determined and fluid administered through a catheter inserted along the subclavian or basilic vein to the right atrium. This procedure is particularly helpful when large or rapid infusions are required; a rise in CVP indicates an excessive load while a fall in the CVP is a useful early sign of oligaemia, e.g. from further haemorrhage.

In cardiogenic shock there may be predominant failure of the left ventricle; pressure should then be monitored in the pulmonary artery by a catheter of the Swan-Ganz balloon tipped type, if the circumstances permit. Dopamine is a positive inotropic agent which may improve myocardial contractility in cardiogenic shock but it is still under trial. The use of vasodilators is also being assessed. For example, phentolamine may be used to reduce afterload if vaso-constriction and oliguria persist when the systolic blood pressure is 90 mm or higher.

The treatment of bacteraemic shock is described on page 81 and of anaphylatic shock on page 38.

Early recognition of the conditions likely to give rise to acute circulatory failure and prompt treatment can prevent its development in some cases. Examples of this are where haemorrhage can be stopped, where blood or fluid lost can be appropriately replaced or where pain can be relieved with morphine.

## Cardiac Failure

The heart is considered to have failed when it is unable to maintain an output sufficient for the needs of the body, or can do so only at the expense of an abnormally high venous pressure. Cardiac failure is liable to develop in patients with conditions which lead to the heart having too great a load over a long period, or because the function of the heart muscle is inadequate, or from a combination of both factors. Under such circumstances a complicated derangement of cardiovascular, renal and endocrine functions can develop which include abnormal retention of sodium and water in most cases. The increased body fluids tend to accumulate in the lungs when the left ventricle is under an abnormal load, or is itself abnormal, and then the onset of symptoms may be acute, with pulmonary oedema. Gravity is the main determinant of the site of collection of oedema when the right ventricle fails. However, because the disturbance of renal and endocrine function is common to both conditions, the terms left and right heart failure tend to be oversimplifications.

**Pathophysiology.** The heart may fail when overwhelmed by an excessive preload, i.e. the volume which it has to handle, or by increased after-load, i.e. the work done during ejection. Both ventricles may be affected when the cardiac output is increased as in hyperthyroidism, beriberi and severe chronic anaemia. Only one ventricle may be affected, e.g. the left in persistent ductus arteriosus or the right in atrial septal defect. There may be increased afterload as a result of hypertension or aortic valve obstruction. The function of the heart muscle itself may be impaired as in myocarditis or hypoxia or the myocardium may be deficient after infarction. The filling of a ventricle may be restricted by a pericardial effusion or constrictive pericarditis. Often these circumstances may be combined as in the patient with mitral stenosis who has impaired filling of the left ventricle and increased afterload of the right ventricle due to pulmonary arterial hypertension. Similarly in aortic stenosis the left ventricle has an increased afterload which may be combined with impairment of ventricular function due to the coronary flow being less than the hypertrophied ventricle requires.

There are, of course, compensatory responses to an extra load. In increased *preload* the ventricles dilate; over the years this is a feature of a left to right shunt. When the preload develops suddenly, as with ruptured chordae of the mitral valve, there may be flooding of the lungs in the early stages, but with the passage of time the left ventricle may become able to contend with the added load. The effect of dilatation is liable to be self-defeating, for the more a ventricle is stretched the greater is the amount of work required of it to eject a given quantity of blood.

In increased *afterload*, as with aortic stenosis and hypertension, the left ventricle becomes hypertrophied. Ultimately the hypertrophy becomes so great that the cavity of the ventricle is reduced; the diminished compliance puts an added load on the left atrium and the nutrition of the ventricular muscle becomes impaired to such an extent that fibrosis may develop. These factors together contribute to a deterioration which reaches the stage where it is irreversible even if the valvular obstruction is relieved.

After a varied length of time, impairment of myocardial contractility occurs. There may be other contributory factors, such as ventricular work wasted in expanding a myocardial aneurysm. Ultimately such effects lead to chronic congestive cardiac failure. If the situation were simply the direct effect of a failing pump, the output would be expected to fall and the upstream pressures to rise. Although this does occur the situation is more complicated, partly as a result of other mechanisms, such as a reduction in renal blood flow. Vasomotor controls impose a rationing system which becomes evident at first only on exercise. The needs of exercising muscles are met by reduction of blood flow to other areas, apart from the brain and heart, by appropriate differential vasoconstriction. The renal blood flow is reduced and the resultant decrease in glomerular filtration rate is a relatively minor factor in a disadvantageous retention of water and salt. Another important mechanism, which is still not understood, is a disorder of renal tubular function which is the main cause of salt and water retention. It is this process which leads to the increase of total body sodium and water, which is an almost invariable feature of heart failure of all forms. In a small proportion of patients, hyperaldosteronism is induced and is a contributory factor, but the relative inadequacy of aldosterone antagonists in improving cardiac failure helps to confirm that it is not very important. Poor tissue perfusion may also lead to migration of sodium into cells in exchange for potassium which is excreted in the urine. Reduced total body potassium therefore tends to be a feature of cardiac failure even before treatment for the failure is instituted.

In a small proportion of patients in whom the cardiac failure is due to a high metabolic demand (as in hyperthyroidism) or impairment of oxygen transfer at the periphery (as in beriberi) the heart may fail despite a cardiac output higher than in normal persons. This is known as 'high output failure'. Although this form of heart failure constitutes a very small proportion of the whole its importance is that a correct diagnosis may lead to cure rather than palliation, e.g. in hyperthyroidism.

Fluid tends to accumulate where the transcapillary pressure is highest, namely in the lungs when there is obstruction at the mitral valve or an incompetent left ventricle, and in the legs when the right ventricle is mainly involved. However, there is no direct relationship between the height of the relevant venous pressure and the extent of transudation of fluid; for example, in the gradually increasing obstruction of the valve in mitral stenosis there are important compensatory mechanisms, such as thickening of capillary walls and increased lymphatic drainage, which tend to protect the lungs from pulmonary oedema.

Some of the factors responsible for the development of cardiac failure are still not understood and some of the varieties of clinical presentation are still unexplained. It is best to describe the clinical syndrome found in a particular patient, e.g. pulmonary or systemic oedema or ascites, rather than to use the labels of right and left heart failure.

**Clinical Features.** Examination of the heart may contribute information which allows understanding of how the cardiac failure has developed, e.g. by the finding of cardiac enlargement, clinical evidence of hypertrophy of either ventricle, auscultatory evidence of valvular disease or third or fourth heart sounds.

The retention of sodium and water may show itself as oedema particularly in the feet or, in patients confined to bed, in the sacral area or at the backs of the thighs. There may be pleural effusion on one side or on both; sometimes there is evidence of ascites. Other clinical features are those associated with right or left atrial hypertension or restriction of cardiac output.

*Right Atrial Hypertension.* Elevation of jugular venous pressure indicates this but cannot always be measured if the accessory muscles of respiration are in action. In infants enlargement of the liver provides the only, if rather crude, manometer for the detection of right atrial hypertension.

Tricuspid regurgitation is a feature of many forms of heart failure, particularly with rheumatic heart disease and chronic cor pulmonale; the sight of the characteristic systolic wave which often moves the ears in a patient reclining at 45 degrees may allow the recognition of this disorder by the trained eye from the end of the bed. Few physical signs are as important. Rapid distension of the liver commonly gives rise to epigastric pain and then a tender and sometimes pulsatile hepatomegaly may be found.

*Left Atrial Hypertension.* The most reliable evidence of left atrial hypertension is from the chest radiograph which can show dilatation of the pulmonary veins of the upper lobes. If there is interstitial oedema of the lungs there may be horizontal shadows in the costophrenic angles, which indicate engorgement of interlobular septa with excess fluid. With left atrial hypertension the tense pulmonary veins reduce lung compliance and are a cause of breathlessness, which is first experienced on exercise. Later the breathlessness occurs at rest. Paroxysmal nocturnal dyspnoea and pulmonary oedema may ensue (p. 145). These are liable to occur particularly when cardiac failure is due to left ventricular failure or when there is a sudden reduction of mitral valve flow, as when atrial fibrillation and a consequent rapid heart rate develop in a patient with mitral stenosis.

*Restriction of Cardiac Output.* The effects of this may be apparent at first only on effort. Syncope on exertion may be the presenting symptom, for example with aortic stenosis or pulmonary arteriolar hypertension, or exceptionally when normal cardioacceleration is prevented, as in complete heart block. When the cardiac output is seriously restricted even at rest, this, combined with compensatory peripheral vasoconstriction, leads to coldness, pallor and cyanosis of the skin at the periphery. Renal and hepatic function become impaired; cachexia is common in advanced cases. The reduced limb flow is probably a factor in rendering such patients particularly liable to venous thrombosis and pulmonary embolism.

*Precipitating Factors.* Cardiac failure may be precipitated by atrial fibrillation, pulmonary embolism, myocardial infarction, the increased demands imposed by pregnancy, anaemia or infection, or by an increase in salt intake. The patient with cardiac failure who feels weak may take to meat extract with a high salt content which may produce disastrous effects.

**Treatment.** Unfortunately it is only in a small minority of patients that it is possible to eradicate the cause of the heart failure, but this possibility must not be overlooked. Thyrotoxicosis should be appropriately treated and anaemia corrected. Once medical treatment has been used to improve the patient's condition as much as possible, surgical relief of a stenosed valve, replacement of a regurgitant valve or closure of a left to right shunt may allow the patient to return to a normal life.

*Reduction of the Work Load Imposed upon the Heart.* In patients who are ambulant, loss of surplus weight may considerably improve the ability to exercise. Patients in severe heart failure who have not responded to medical treatment when ambulant may gain benefit from a period of complete rest in bed, as serial weight charts in the oedematous patient will show. The breathless patient may find a chair more comfortable than bed. Prolonged bed rest has its own dangers, particularly venous thrombosis. Complicating factors such as a correctable arrhythmia or infection should be treated.

*Salt and water retention* is best treated with diuretics (p. 136). High potency diuretics such as frusemide, bumetanide or ethacrynic acid have a rapid action and are useful in an emergency. They are more costly than diuretics of medium potency such as bendrofluazide, which should be used for maintenance purposes. Potassium supplements must also be prescribed when diuretics are being used frequently. In resistant cases of cardiac failure an antialdosterone drug such as spironolactone (p. 137) may prove helpful.

Excessive use of high potency diuretics may lead to hyponatraemia and uraemia. In these patients the total body sodium may become dangerously low; the dose of the diuretic must be reduced and the salt intake must be unrestricted (p. 129). In contrast hyponatraemia with persistent oedema (dilutional hyponatraemia) is characterised by an increase in total body sodium and water. The appropriate treatment is to restrict sodium, to reduce the intake of water to about 1 *l*/day, to continue diuretics and to give potassium supplements. The other adverse effects of diuretic therapy are described on page 137.

It is not logical to use diuretics, whose action depends on the elimination of salt and water, without also restricting the patient's salt intake, at least to some extent. The amount of salt used is largely a matter of habit, and questioning will reveal that some patients are overindulgent in their use of it. A 'salt-free' diet has been described as 'not prolonging life but making it seem longer', and is not necessary except in very few patients with advanced heart failure. Most such patients can be controlled with high doses of potent diuretics (e.g. frusemide 160 mg/b.d.). Often it is useful to give the evening dose at about 5 p.m. so that the diuresis is over before bedtime.

It is seldom that serous transudates cannot be eliminated with diuretic therapy and salt restriction but occasionally aspiration of a pleural effusion or ascitic fluid may be helpful.

*Pulmonary oedema* presents one of the most alarming crises that a patient can experience and provides an occasion where informed medical aid may be of dramatic benefit. By far the most effective remedy is morphine 10 to 20 mg. preferably intravenously, in a severe attack. Morphine alone transforms the situation by allaying anxiety, reducing catecholamine output and causing systemic venodilatation which allows blood to be sequestrated peripherally. Cyclizine, 50 mg, should also be injected to reduce the risk of vomiting. Morphine should not be employed in patients who are significantly hypotensive, or if there are grounds to suppose that there may be respiratory failure. Aminophylline (0·25–0·5 g i.v.), given slowly, is a useful alternative. Oxygen is helpful and an intravenous diuretic such as frusemide will make a recurrence less probable. Under dire circumstances venous occlusion cuffs on all four limbs may make a contribution though the limb blood flow is so much reduced that their benefit may be slight. Each cuff should be deflated in rotation for 5 minutes in every 15. If all these methods are ineffective venesection may be life-saving. A regular diuretic and usually digoxin should be given to prevent a recurrence.

*Digitalis* after 200 years remains the most powerful inotropic drug. It increases myocardial contractility and thus reduces the diastolic cardiac volume; this in turn promotes the efficiency of cardiac contraction. The better cardiac performance is followed by an improvement in renal function so that there is a secondary diuretic effect. In addition digitalis depresses atrioventricular conduction, which is of particular value in reducing the ventricular rate with atrial fibrillation. With digitalis, however, ventricular ectopic beats are common and alternative ventricular extrasystoles (pulsus bigeminus) are characteristic of over-digitalisation.

Although logic should demand that the first drug to be used in treating heart failure should be one that improves myocardial function, the difficulties in the proper administration of digitalis make it usually wiser to prescribe diuretics in the first instance. Digitalis is the most effective treatment of atrial fibrillation with a rapid ventricular rate. It is used in the treatment of paroxysmal atrial tachycardia or flutter and in the prevention of these conditions. Digitalis is contraindicated in ventricular tachycardia and usually in partial heart block because the degree of block may be increased.

Digoxin is the preparation of choice and is prescribed in an initial dose of 0·5–1 mg. When given by mouth the maximal effect is achieved in about 6 hours or, when given intravenously, in 2 hours. The dose thereafter depends on the weight of the patient; 0·5 mg once daily is usually sufficient, but some patients require double this dose. Digitalis is particularly toxic in the presence of hypokalaemia or renal failure and in the elderly. For a patient in the seventies, 0·0625 mg b.d. is often all that is required.

The main toxic effects consist of anorexia and nausea and the significance of these should be recognised before the onset of vomiting. Digoxin should then be omitted for 2 days and recommenced at a smaller dose. Ectopic beats, ventricular tachycardia, paroxysmal atrial tachycardia with atrioventricular block and, occasionally, complete heart block may result from digitalisation. Beta receptor blocking drugs are particularly valuable in the management of paroxysmal atrial tachycardia induced by digitalis. The adverse effects of digitalis may be precipitated by the use of diuretics and enhanced by potassium depletion.

The measurement of digoxin levels in the blood is helpful in difficult cases. The upper therapeutic level is about 2·6 nmol/*l*.

*Additional Treatment in Cardiac Failure.* Vasodilators are being increasingly used as supplementary therapy in the management of cardiac failure resistant to treatment by the usual methods. It is known that glyceryl trinitrate is effective in the relief of pulmonary oedema and that the principal mechanisms responsible are a reduction in afterload by a decrease in the peripheral vascular resistance and a reduction in preload by pooling of blood in dilated peripheral veins. On a longer term basis in the management of chronic right ventricular failure, isosorbide dinitrate or the $\alpha$–adrenoceptor blocking agent, prazosin may each be useful.

## Rheumatic Fever

Rheumatic fever is predominantly a disease of childhood and adolescence. Rare in Britain now, it remains common in Asia, Africa and Eastern Europe. Recurrences are frequent unless prophylactic treatment is given. Mild and subclinical forms occur and about half the patients who are found to have disease of the heart valves of rheumatic origin give no history of rheumatic fever.

The precise cause of rheumatic fever is unknown. However, there is much evidence that it is related to infection with Group A haemolytic streptococci, possibly on the basis of an antigen common to the heart and the streptococcus. The disease is often preceded by tonsillitis or pharyngitis one to three weeks before.

**Pathology.** The connective tissues of the myocardium, endocardium, pericardium, synovial membranes and tendons are in particular affected. In the exudative stage there is hyperaemia, oedema of the collagen tissue and infiltration with leucocytes. The hallmark of rheumatic fever is the Aschoff nodule, which may be found in the interstitial tissues of any part of the heart, most frequently in relation to small blood vessels, particularly beneath the endocardium of the left ventricle. The microscopic appearance of the Aschoff nodule is of a central area of necrosis surrounded by small round cells, histiocytes and giant cells. The mitral and, to a lesser extent, the aortic valves have pinhead-size warty vegetations. Subsequent scarring leads to the valve changes of chronic rheumatic heart disease.

**Clinical Features.** The onset may be sudden with pain, swelling and stiffness in one or more joints, fever, sweating and tachycardia, or it may be insidious with fatigue, malaise and loss of weight. The large joints are principally affected, e.g. knees, ankles, shoulders and wrists, but almost any joint may be involved. Characteristically there is a migrating polyarthritis, one joint improving as another becomes worse. In severe cases the joints become hot, swollen, red and very tender. The synovium and periarticular tissues are principally involved. Sterile effusions may develop. The joints become normal when the attack is over.

Fever is usual in acute attacks. Sweating may be profuse. Other accompaniments of fever, such as anorexia, furred tongue, constipation and proteinuria, are often present. Tachycardia tends to be out of proportion to the degree of fever and may persist after the latter has settled. The sleeping pulse rate will differentiate tachycardia due to anxiety or excitement, and is useful in deciding when more physical activity can be permitted.

Although pancarditis probably occurs to some extent in all cases of acute rheumatic fever, only about half of them have later evidence of chronic rheumatic heart disease. In the early stages endocarditis may be suspected from diminished intensity of the first heart sound or from the development of a systolic murmur. A transient mitral diastolic murmur may be heard (Carey Coombs murmur). Aortic regurgitation can also occur. Myocarditis may be assumed to be present if there is endocarditis or pericarditis. Its presence is also suggested by undue tachycardia, decreased intensity of the first heart sound, increasing enlargement of the heart, evidence of cardiac failure and abnormalities in the ECG (see below).

Pericarditis may be suspected as a complication when there is a recrudescence of fever with the development of malaise, restlessness and pallor. Retrosternal or precordial pain is common and pericardial friction may be heard. An effusion may develop. Pericarditis is not in itself a serious manifestation of rheumatic fever.

Rheumatic nodules are seen far less frequently than 20 years ago because rheumatic fever is less common and less severe. They occur most often in childhood and their principal importance lies in the almost invariable association with active carditis. They are situated subcutaneously, are painless, not attached to the skin and tend to occur over bony prominences such as elbows, knees, scapulae, occiput and vertebrae or on tendons.

Erythema marginatum (erythema annulare) consists of transient pink patches which appear mainly on the trunk and rapidly enlarge to form irregular crescent shapes which join together to form larger areas. The margins are slightly elevated.

Sydenham's chorea is described on page 720. The majority of children with chorea subsequently develop evidence of rheumatic valvular disease.

A polymorph leucocytosis is common in the acute stage. A raised ESR is usually present and may persist as evidence of activity of the rheumatic process when all other manifestations have subsided. In about a quarter, a group A streptococcus can be grown from the throat. A high ASO (antistreptolysn 'O') titre rising or raised to above 300 units provides evidence of recent streptococcal infection.

The chest radiograph often shows enlargement of the cardiac shadow due to dilatation of the heart, a pericardial effusion or a combination of both. The commoner ECG changes are prolongation of the PR interval and abnormalities of ST segments and T waves or those of pericarditis (p. 203).

**Progress.** Persistent rheumatic activity is suggested by the presence of fever, tachycardia, anaemia, changing cardiac signs, failure to gain weight, a raised blood sedimentation rate and abnormalities in the electrocardiogram. Activity implies progressive damage to the heart by the rheumatic process. It may be followed by a period lasting several years, during which the contraction of fibrous tissue leads to increasing deformity of the involved valves. Thereafter, unless further attacks of rheumatic fever occur, deterioration is due to the mechanical effects of valvular disease combined with myocardial damage as a sequel to the acute pancarditis. The combined effects, in varying proportion, may lead to cardiac failure.

**Treatment.** *Rest in bed* is indicated until symptoms and fever have subsided, the sleeping pulse rate, white count and haemoglobin level have returned to normal, and weight is being regained. Thereafter, the return to activity should be gradual. The ESR is a useful guide to progress.

*Phenoxymethylpenicillin* should be given for 7 to 10 days routinely at the start of treatment with the object of killing haemolytic streptococci in the nose and throat.

*Salicylates* are effective in combating fever and pain. Acetylsalicylic acid (aspirin) is preferable to sodium salicylate because it is better tolerated, has a greater analgesic effect and avoids giving extra sodium to the patient at risk of heart failure. The daily dose of aspirin is 50 mg per kg body weight divided into 4 hourly doses, with a double dose at night to avoid waking the patient. This dosage should be continued until fever and symptoms have been controlled for at least 10 days and then gradually reduced. Should rheumatic manifestations return, larger quantities will have to be resumed. If toxic symptoms develop, the dose must be reduced and then maintained at the highest level which can be tolerated. Nausea, headache, dizziness, tinnitus and deafness are the early toxic symptoms, followed by vomiting, hyperventilation and mental symptoms. Occasionally haemorrhage may occur from hypoprothrombinaemia.

Salicylates relieve symptoms but probably do not influence the cardiac complications, or materially shorten the course of the disease. Steroids such as prednisolone are nearly always effective in controlling both cardiac and other features of the disease but should be reserved for the more severe cases. They do not affect the long-term results. Clinical trials have shown that the combination of prednisolone with salicylates in high dosage is the most effective treatment for severe cases.

*Convalescence* in a suitable environment will be required when the active stage is over and before return to school or work. Its duration will depend on the length of the preceding illness and the presence or absence of cardiac complications.

**Prevention** is important because there is no specific treatment for rheumatic fever and little can be done to mitigate damage to the heart which is liable to be further affected in subsequent attacks. The incidence of relapses diminishes with age; they may be largely prevented in children and adolescents by phenoxymethyl penicillin (125 mg b.d.) or sulphadimidine (0·5 g daily) if the patient is hypersensitive to penicillin. Either should be taken regularly and continued until about 20 years of age. In the United States a monthly injection of benzathine penicillin is advised.

## Diseases of the Heart Valves

The principal cause of valvular disease is rheumatic endocarditis. This most commonly affects the mitral valve, next the aortic valve, comparatively infrequently the tricuspid valve and very rarely the pulmonary valve. Syphilis may cause aortic regurgitation secondary to dilatation of the aorta. Congenital lesions are responsible for most cases of pulmonary valvular disease, some cases of aortic disease and occasionally for tricuspid disease. Infective endocarditis may be superimposed on rheumatic and congenital lesions and cause further damage. Exceptionally a cusp may rupture either spontaneously or as a result of external trauma. A diseased valve may be narrowed (stenosed) or may fail to close adequately and thus permit regurgitation of blood. The term incompetence may be used synonymously with regurgitation but the latter is preferable as a stenosed valve is obviously not 'competent'. Regurgitation may be present without structural changes in the cusps, e.g. from dilatation of the mitral valve ring in left ventricular failure, the tricuspid valve ring in right ventricular failure, the pulmonary valve ring in pulmonary hypertension or the aortic valve ring in aortic aneurysm.

### Mitral Stenosis

In about half the patients there is a history of rheumatic fever or chorea. The gradual scarring process in the heart takes many years to develop fully. The commissures of the mitral valve become adherent and the chordae often become short and deformed. The mitral valve orifice is about 5 $cm^2$ in diastole in health and is reduced in severe mitral stenosis to about 1 $cm^2$. Rheumatic disease also damages heart muscle; the more severe this is the larger the heart tends to be, and the greater the liability to atrial fibrillation and to the formation of thrombus in the left atrium. With the reduction in size of the valve orifice the cardiac output can be maintained only by a rise in left atrial, pulmonary venous and pulmonary capillary pressures with a resultant loss of lung compliance. Thickening of the capillaries and increased pulmonary arteriolar resistance and lymphatic drainage restrict the accumulation of

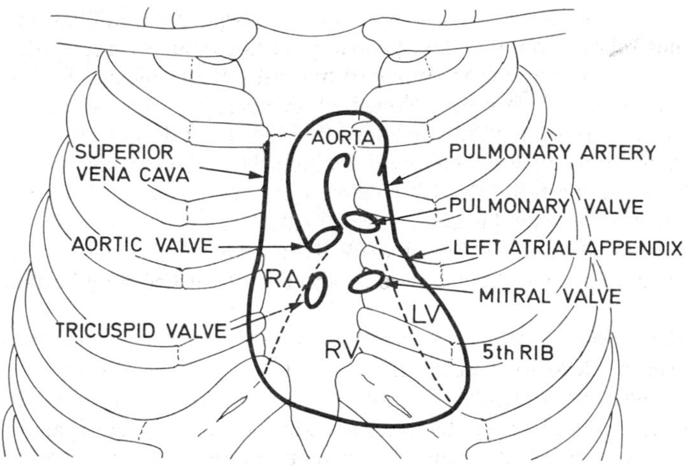


Fig. 6.19 The radiological outline of the heart and the surface projection of its valves.

oedema in the lungs. Some patients develop, for reasons unknown, excessive narrowing of the small pulmonary arteries which leads to severe pulmonary hypertension and right ventricular hypertrophy. There may be concomitant mitral regurgitation or disease of aortic or tricuspid valves.

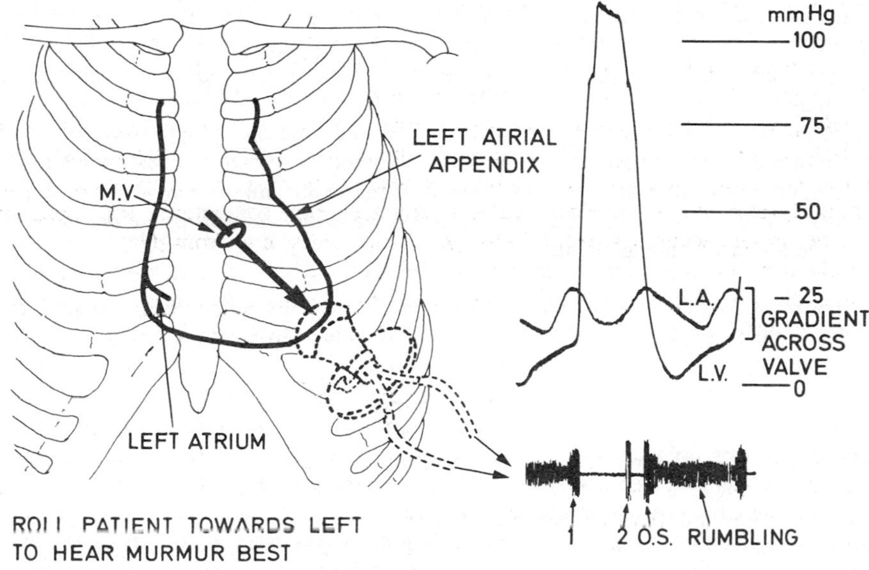


Fig. 6.20 Mitral stenosis. O.S. = opening snap.

**Clinical Features.** The gradual reduction in the mitral valve orifice usually produces breathlessness in about the third decade. The extra demands of pregnancy, of tachycardia, or the loss of left atrial contraction with the onset of atrial fibrillation, are common precipitating factors and may bring on breathlessness even at rest. The elevated pulmonary vascular pressures may also cause cough and haemoptysis. Angina occurs in a few patients. Systemic embolism may cause a hemiplegia and is commoner in patients with atrial fibrillation.

In some patients with mitral stenosis the face may have a 'malar flush'. The specific signs, however, result from the abnormalities of the abnormal mitral valve. It closes with an unusually loud sound which may be palpable — the tapping apex beat. The turbulent flow, which is heralded by the opening snap, causes the murmur and often a thrill (Fig. 6.20). The murmur may be accentuated during atrial contraction. In early and asymptomatic patients a presystolic murmur may be the only auscultatory abnormality, but in patients with symptoms the murmur usually extends from the opening snap to the first heart sound. If the valve is calcified there is usually no snap. With accompanying mitral regurgitation there may be a pansystolic murmur.

There may be an abnormal pulsation to the left of the sternum due to right ventricular hypertrophy or left atrial pulsation. Pulmonary valve closure may be unusually loud. Also with pulmonary hypertension there may be a prominent *a* wave in the jugular venous pulse as evidence of right atrial hypertrophy; with cardiac failure the jugular venous pressure is elevated and with accompanying tricuspid regurgitation there may be a prominent systolic venous pulse (p. 148). If the cardiac output is low the pulse volume may be small.

The ECG may show either the bifid P waves associated with left atrial hypertrophy or atrial fibrillation. There may be evidence of right ventricular hypertrophy. Enlargement of the left atrium and its appendage, and of the main pulmonary artery may be seen in the chest radiograph (Fig. 6.20) in contrast with the normal findings shown in Figure 6.19. There may be enlargement of the upper pulmonary veins, and horizontal shadows in the costophrenic angles as indications of a high left atrial and pulmonary venous pressure. In the lateral and right anterior oblique position an enlarged left atrium causes a characteristic displacement of the barium-filled oesophagus.

The physical signs of mitral stenosis are often found before symptoms develop, or an abnormality in the cardiac outline may be noted in a routine chest radiograph. The finding of the abnormal physical signs is of particular importance in the obstetric department, since the identification of mitral disease allows appropriate decisions to be made about its management.

**Treatment.** When cardiac failure develops in patients with mitral stenosis the medical management is similar to that of heart failure from other causes, with the important difference that surgical relief of mitral stenosis is now a standard form of treatment. Usually operation is not advisable until symptoms develop, but it is often appropriate to recommend mitral valvotomy prophylactically at a time which avoids operation during pregnancy (p. 211). Cardiac catheterisation is often used to confirm the severity of mitral stenosis by measurement of the gradient across the mitral valve by recording pressures simultaneously in the left ventricle and left atrium (or pulmonary arterial wedge position). Echocardiography (p. 154) provides evidence as to the rigidity, calcification and rate of movement of the valve cusps and, with increasing experience, may make invasive investigation unnecessary. Mitral valvotomy may be done with a dilator introduced into the mitral valve through the left ventricle under guidance from a finger inserted into the left atrium, or under direct vision with cardiopulmonary bypass. When the operation is successful, patients can expect 5 to 10 years of benefit in most cases before the stenosis recurs. In some patients traumatic mitral regurgitation is produced which is often slight but may require subsequent mitral valve replacement. The most successful results are in the younger patients with sinus rhythm, relatively small hearts and an uncalcified valve. If there is accompanying mitral regurgitation, or the mitral valve is heavily calcified, mitral valve replacement is usually the better operation. Prosthetic or heterograft valves are used.

### Mitral Regurgitation

This can result from dilatation of the mitral valve ring in association with diseases involving the myocardium such as rheumatic fever, diphtheria, viral myocarditis or cardiomyopathy. It also occurs with damage to the papillary muscles, usually from infarction or from spontaneous rupture of the chordae tendinae. In the last two instances the mitral regurgitation may come on suddenly and lead to acute pulmonary oedema. The valve cusps may be damaged gradually from chronic rheumatic heart disease, in which case there is often associated mitral stenosis, and there may be co-existing abnormalities of the aortic or tricuspid valves. Mitral regurgitation may develop quickly with infective endocarditis. In old age the valve often undergoes myxomatous degeneration which may be accompanied by mitral regurgitation.

**Clinical Features.** The symptoms depend on how suddenly the regurgitation develops. When the valve damage is a slow process the symptoms are similar to those in mitral stenosis. In myocardial disease the mitral regurgitation exacerbates an already serious situation.

The physical signs arise from the regurgitant jet which causes an apical systolic murmur which often radiates into the left axilla and may be accompanied by a thrill. The apex beat is usually displaced to the left as a result of dilatation of the left ventricle. The abnormal valve closure is often associated also with a quiet first heart sound, and the increased forward flow through the mitral valve may give rise to a loud third heart sound or a short mid-diastolic murmur. The radiograph and ECG often give evidence of left atrial or left ventricular hypertrophy.

**Treatment.** If mitral regurgitation is due to myocardial disease, treatment, when available, is directed to the latter. When the valve disease is predominant and the symptoms severe, mitral valve replacement is indicated. Infective endocarditis should, if possible, be brought under control prior to surgery.

### Aortic Stenosis

Stenosis of the aortic valve may be a congenital fault, may arise from fusion of the valve cusps from rheumatic damage, or it may be a late development from an accelerated ageing process in a congenital bicuspid aortic valve. This congenital lesion is found in 0·5% of routine post mortems and accounts for a significant proportion of cases of aortic stenosis in the elderly. Rarely congenital aortic stenosis may be due to a subvalvar diaphragm or more rarely still to a supravalvar stenosis. Except in the congenital forms, aortic stenosis develops slowly; the cardiac output is maintained at the expense of a gradually increasing gradient across the aortic valve. The left ventricle becomes increasingly hypertrophied and fibrotic changes may follow. The coronary blood flow may become inadequate, particularly if there is concomitant coronary atheroma. When hypertrophy involves the interventricular septum there is often reduction in the volume of the right ventricle. By these means both atria may become hypertrophied. Particularly in rheumatic heart disease there is often accompanying aortic regurgitation.

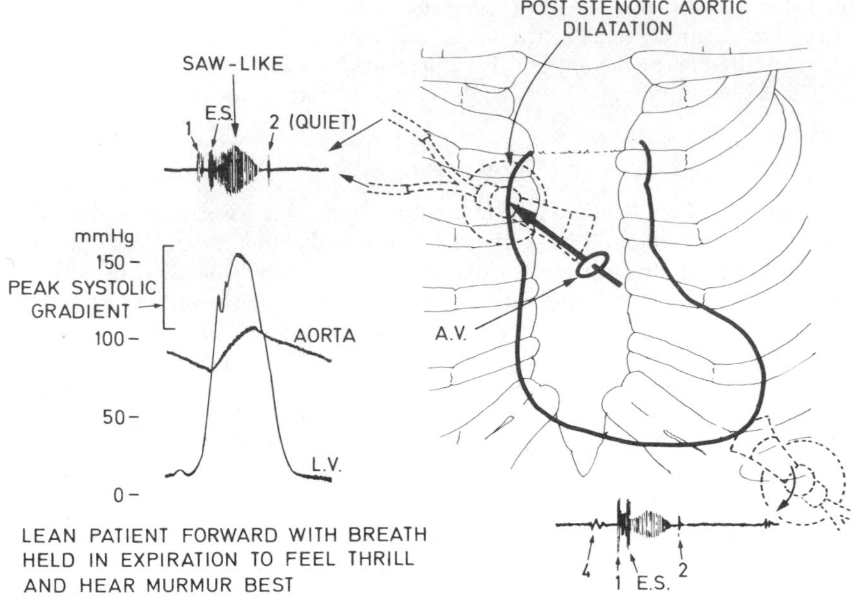


Fig. 6.21 Aortic stenosis. E.S. = ejection sound (p. 150).

**Clinical Features.** The symptoms arise from restriction of the cardiac output on exercise, which may cause syncope, from inadequate coronary blood flow causing angina, or from left ventricular failure giving rise to dyspnoea on exertion or nocturnal dyspnoea. Breathlessness does not develop until left ventricular hypertrophy fails to compensate for the obstruction and is therefore late in the disease. Sudden death is common with severe aortic stenosis.

The physical signs arise from the jet through the aortic valve (Fig. 6.21) which causes a systolic murmur and often a thrill which may be transmitted to the carotid pulse as the so-called 'carotid shudder'. There is commonly an ejection sound from movement of the stenotic aortic valve prior to the onset of the murmur. The thrusting apical impulse of left ventricular hypertrophy is characteristic. Left ventricular distension at the time of left atrial discharge may cause a fourth heart sound unless concomitant mitral stenosis restricts this. Reduction of right ventricular capacity from hypertrophy of the septum may lead to an *a* wave in the jugular venous pulse. The restricted cardiac output is often reflected in a small volume arterial pulse which rises abnormally slowly and the pulse pressure is often lower than the average for the age.

The radiographic changes are shown in Figure 6.21. Under the image intensifier calcification of the aortic valve can usually be demonstrated. The ECG shows left atrial and left ventricular hypertrophy and in advanced cases changes of the latter are gross (Fig. 6.27, p. 195).

**Treatment.** Unlike patients with mitral stenosis it is often necessary to recommend surgical replacement of the valve when symptoms are slight or even absent if the aortic stenosis is severe. To wait too long may result in irreversible damage to the left ventricle. The valve is replaced under cardiopulmonary bypass with a prosthetic or heterograft valve. In this way left ventricular failure may be prevented; postoperatively there is usually ECG evidence of reduction in the left ventricular hypertrophy. In some cases of severe congenital aortic stenosis, valvotomy may be required as an intermediate measure until an adult size valve can be inserted.

## Aortic Regurgitation

This results from abnormal aortic cusps as in congenital bicuspid valves, or when valves have been damaged by rheumatic heart disease or infective endocarditis. Aortic regurgitation may also be due to dilatation of the first part of the aorta in cystic medionecrosis, tertiary syphilis or atheroma. When the leak is large the stroke output may be increased to two- or three-fold. The major arteries are then conspicuously pulsatile; the left ventricle dilates and hypertrophies and initially compensates for the fault in the valve. The left ventricular diastolic pressure rises, at first only with exercise; the pulmonary vascular pressures then also increase and breathlessness develops.

Until the onset of breathlessness the only symptom may be an awareness of the heartbeat, particularly when lying on the left side. Paroxysmal nocturnal dyspnoea may be the first symptom. Peripheral oedema may follow. Angina may occur particularly when there is coexisting coronary atheroma or when the coronary ostia are involved in syphilitic aortitis.

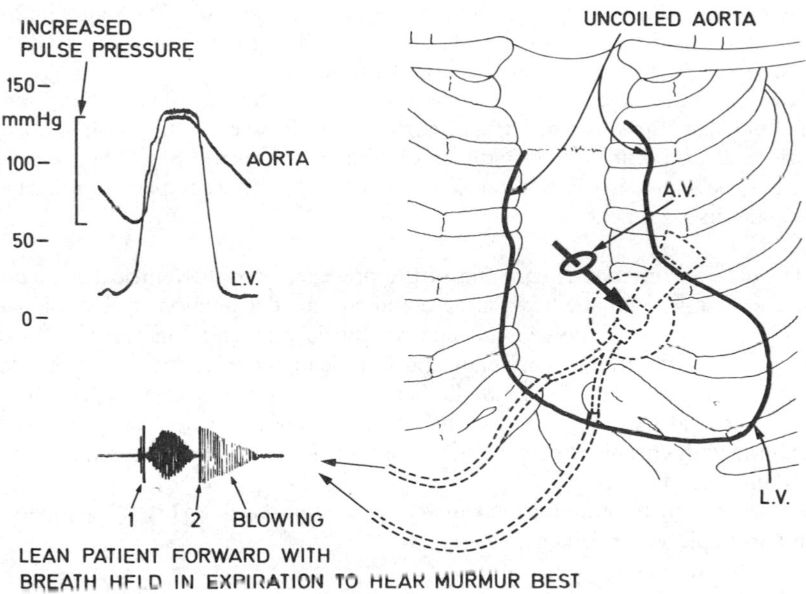


Fig. 6.22 Aortic regurgitation.

The characteristic murmur is illustrated in Figure 6.22; although it is usually best heard to the left of the sternum it is sometimes louder to the right particularly with syphilitic aortitis. A thrill is very rare. When the leak is small the murmur will be heard only if the steps shown in Figure 6.22 are followed; this is of crucial importance in the early detection of infective endocarditis affecting the aortic valve. A systolic murmur due to the increased stroke volume is common and should not be regarded as due to accompanying stenosis without other evidence of the latter. When the leak is large the diagnosis is usually easy, with gross pulsation in the large arteries, a 'muscle knock' (p. 147), a low diastolic and an increased pulse pressure. There is usually a thrusting apex beat and often a presystolic impulse and a fourth heart sound as evidence of left atrial hypertrophy. An example of the change in the radiographic outline is shown diagramatically in Figure 6.22. The ECG usually shows left ventricular hypertrophy (Fig. 6.27).

Replacement of the aortic valve with a prosthesis or a heterograft valve under cardiopulmonary bypass now carries a mortality of less than 5% in skilled hands and is the treatment of choice if there is evidence of increasing left ventricular overload or when symptoms develop.

## Tricuspid Valve Disease

**Tricuspid stenosis** is usually due to chronic rheumatic heart disease and is almost always accompanied by mitral stenosis and often also by aortic valve disease. The symptoms are those of the accompanying mitral valve disease, but if the tricuspid stenosis is severe there is an increased likelihood of the development of ascites and peripheral oedema. With sinus rhythm the *a* wave in the jugular venous pulse is conspicuous and there may be presystolic hepatic pulsation. There may be mid-diastolic and presystolic murmurs similar in timing to those in mitral stenosis but lacking the rumbling quality and often increased by inspiration. The radiograph may show evidence of disproportionate enlargement of the right atrium; in the ECG there may be the peaked P waves of right atrial hypertrophy.

Occasionally tricuspid valve replacement is required, but the operation is often less satisfactory than those for mitral and aortic valve disease, partly because tricuspid stenosis tends to occur in those patients who have had severe rheumatic pancarditis. There may be an added difficulty in assessment because of accompanying mitral valve disease and its treatment.

**Tricuspid regurgitation** is common in the presence of right ventricular dilatation, particularly with rheumatic heart disease and chronic cor pulmonale. Occasionally it results from rheumatic valve or ischaemic myocardial damage. Characteristically there is a large *cv* wave in the jugular venous pulse which may move the ear lobes with the patient reclining at 45 degrees; systolic hepatic pulsation may also be present. With effective medical treatment these signs usually disappear except in those patients, particularly with chronic rheumatic heart disease, in whom there is organic tricuspid valve damage.

Replacement or plication of the valve may be required in a very few patients with organic tricuspid valve damage.

## Pulmonary Valve Disease

**Pulmonary stenosis** is usually congenital and may be isolated or part of Fallot's tetralogy (p. 208). It is recognisable from an ejection systolic murmur to the left of the upper sternum, radiating towards the left shoulder, often accompanied by a thrill which is best appreciated when the patient leans forward and breathes out. The murmur is often preceded by an ejection sound and valve closure is usually quiet. An increased right ventricular thrust, radiographic evidence of poststenotic dilatation of the main pulmonary artery and ECG evidence of right ventricular hypertrophy and right atrial hypertrophy are all to be expected if the stenosis is severe.

Some patients require pulmonary valvotomy, best done with cardiopulmonary bypass.

**Pulmonary regurgitation** is rare and is usually a feature of pulmonary hypertension. The murmur is decrescendo and heard in early diastole at the left sternal edge (Graham Steell murmur); the distinction from aortic regurgitation can generally be made from other evidence.

## Infective Endocarditis

Endocarditis may result from infection by many different microorganisms and by fungi. In the rarer acute form the disease is fulminating, may affect normal valves and if untreated may result in death in a few days, e.g. in staphylococcal septicaemia. At the other end of the spectrum the disease is insidious and may have been present for many months before diagnosis. Abnormal valves such as bicuspid aortic, rheumatic or prosthetic valves, or various forms of congenital heart disease, e.g. ventricular septal defect or persistent ductus arteriosus, are the usual underlying lesions. Regurgitant mitral and aortic valves are the commonest to be affected. It occurs at all ages, but seldom before 20 years; it is now increasingly recognised in the elderly.

**Pathology.** Fibrin and platelets are deposited at the site of closure of normal valves and their absorption into the substance of the valve leads to a gradual thickening of the cusps over the years. This process is exaggerated with abnormal valves, or where an abnormal jet impinges on the endocardium, and colonisation of such deposits of fibrin and platelets by blood-borne organisms may occur and cause infective endocarditis.

*Strep. viridans*, a common cause of periodontal infections, is liable to enter the bloodstream at the time of a dental extraction. Staphylococci and *Strep. faecalis* are other causative organisms; with the latter there may be a history of urethral or pelvic surgery. *Coxiella burneti* endocarditis is more common in, but not peculiar to, those who work with sheep or with carcases.

Affected valves develop vegetations which may be exuberant and a source of embolism; regurgitation may develop or increase due to loss of substance or perforation of a cusp. Weeks or months after the onset mycotic aneurysms may develop in systemic arteries and rupture. Normal valves, particularly the tricuspid valve, are liable to become infected in 'main-line' drug addicts. At postmortem it is common to find infarction of the spleen and the kidneys in particular. Glomerulonephritis is also found, which may be associated with an immune complex reaction (p. 32).

**Clinical Features.** Infective endocarditis should be suspected when a patient known to have congenital or valvular heart disease develops a fever or complains of unusual tiredness. Often, however, infective endocarditis occurs in patients whose heart disease has been hitherto unsuspected and the diagnosis is often dangerously delayed because it has not been considered. Persistent fever, often recognisable from a history of sweating at night, unexplained arterial occlusion, or the discovery of anaemia or splenomegaly may be presenting features. The disease is almost invariably fatal if untreated and even if the infection is controlled there is a high mortality. Delay in diagnosis may result in an embolic stroke, progressive valve damage, heart failure and death.

In the early stages the patient looks well but later pallor may be obvious. Other features commonly listed should nowadays be regarded as evidence of unreasonable delay in diagnosis; these include purpura and petechial haemorrhages in skin and mucous membranes and splinter haemorrhages under the fingernails which, although they occur in health, are more frequent with infective endocarditis. Osler's nodes consist of painful tender swellings at the fingertips and are rare. Clubbing is usually relatively late. The spleen is frequently just palpable. In coxiella infections the spleen and liver may be considerably enlarged, and palmar erythema is usual. Embolism may be revealed only by loss of foot pulses or may be the presenting feature with cerebral, coronary or splenic infarction. Microscopical haematuria is common. The finding of any of these features requires re-examination for hitherto unrecognised heart disease such as trivial aortic regurgitation.

**Investigation.** Elevation of the ESR is usual. Normochromic, normocytic anaemia is common. Thrombocytopenia and disturbed liver function tests, particularly elevation of the alkaline phosphatase, are usual in coxiella infections. Blood culture is the crucial procedure and should be prompt and multiple, e.g. six, preferably paired, blood cultures in the first 6 hours incubated both aerobically and anaerobically. No advantage is gained by waiting for an elevation of temperature. Fungi should normally be detected by standard methods of culture. The administration of antibiotics before taking the blood may prevent laboratory isolation of the causative organism. Q fever endocarditis can be diagnosed by showing high titres to coxiella antigens in complement fixation tests.

**Treatment.** If penicillin sensitive *Strep. viridans* is isolated, benzylpenicillin should initially be given intravenously (2–4 mega units 6 hourly). This needs to be continued for 4 weeks but oral therapy with phenoxymethyl penicillin (0·5 g 4 hourly) and probenecid may be substituted if the infection has been brought quickly under control and provided satisfactory blood levels of penicillin can be maintained. For cases due to *Strep. faecalis*, gentamicin (80 mg 8 hourly) should be given in conjunction with penicillin and probenecid. The dosage of gentamicin must be adjusted on the basis of serum levels and continued for up to 4 weeks. The above regime is also suitable as initial therapy in cases in which no causative organism is found, but it may be necessary to try other antibacterial agents, e.g. co-trimoxazole or the lincomycins, if there is no response to the penicillin and gentamicin. For coxiella endocarditis there have been reports of successful therapy with tetracycline combined with lincomycin.

Any source of infection should be removed if possible; for example, a tooth with an apical abscess should be extracted.

If the valve damage is extensive the valve may need to be replaced, preferably when the infection has been brought under control but sometimes as a matter of urgency, as when perforation of an aortic cusp leads to pulmonary oedema. It often proves impossible to eradicate infection from a prosthetic valve which usually needs to be replaced.

**Prevention**. Every patient with heart disease susceptible to infective endocarditis should be warned of the absolute necessity of taking special care of the teeth and of having antibiotic cover for dental extractions. A single injection of fortified procaine penicillin (300 mg procaine penicillin plus 60 mg benzylpenicillin) given immediately before dental extraction provides both an immediate high level and persistent effect.

However, it is probable that oral amoxycillin will provide adequate cover. Prolonged administration of penicillin before extraction allows selection and subsequent multiplication of resistant strains and should be avoided. For other surgical procedures a 2 day course of penicillin and streptomycin (1 g 12 hourly), started just before the procedure, is appropriate.

## Ischaemic (Coronary) Heart Disease

Atheromatous disease of the coronary arteries is the most important single cause of death in the Western world. Although its global incidence is still increasing there has been a recent marked fall in the United States and elsewhere. Atheroma is the commonest cause of angina pectoris and leads also to myocardial infarction and its complications, to cardiac failure and to sudden death.

*The Coronary Circulation.* The right coronary artery arises from the right sinus of Valsalva and passes in the right atrioventricular groove to supply the right ventricle, part of the interventricular septum and the inferior part of the left ventricle; a branch supplies the AV node. The left coronary artery arises from the left sinus and divides into (1) an anterior descending branch, which supplies part of the septum and the anterior and apical parts of the heart and (2) the circumflex branch, which passes in the left atrioventricular groove and supplies the lateral and posterior surfaces of the heart. In health there are small anastomoses between the coronary arteries; these enlarge under the influence of ischaemia if the flow through a neighbouring coronary artery is compromised. With advancing years an extensive network of anastomotic vessels develops.

**Aetiology.** The cause of ischaemic heart disease is not yet established, but the strong correlations that have been shown between it and smoking, hypertension, diabetes and lipid abnormalities suggest that these may be causal. Other contributory factors may be lack of exercise, soft water, and psychological characteristics but proof of each of these is lacking. Most controversy surrounds the importance of diet in the genesis of atherosclerosis. While there can be little doubt that individuals with high cholesterol and/or low high-density lipoprotein levels in their blood are at relatively high risk of coronary disease, the role of dietary fat is less clear.

**Pathology.** The process of reduction in the lumen of a coronary artery may be due to atheroma affecting the intima, fibrin and platelet deposition on the intima, haemorrhage under the intima, thrombosis, or to a combination of these factors. When angina develops one or more coronary arteries are usually already critically reduced in lumen or even occluded. The anterior descending coronary artery is especially vulnerable to atheroma and sudden occlusion of this vessel is particularly dangerous.

In myocardial infarction, there is usually an occlusion due either to a platelet thrombus or to rupture of an atheromatous plaque. This may result in subendocardial or transmural infarction. During acute infarction there is an inflammatory reaction and if the epicardial surface is affected there is usually overlying pericarditis; if the endocardial surface is affected, there may be intraventricular thrombosis. Over a period of 1 or 2 months the area damaged by infarction is replaced by fibrosis; it may ultimately become difficult to find which area was involved even at postmortem.

### Angina Pectoris

Angina pectoris is the name for a clinical syndrome rather than a disease. The term is used to describe a discomfort due to transient myocardial ischaemia. Characteristically it is a tight sensation in the centre of the chest, provoked by exertion, and lasting only a few minutes. It is likely to occur when the coronary blood flow is less than is required; atherosclerosis is the commonest cause. Factors which increase myocardial oxygen requirement include any which add to the ventricular preload such as exercise, anaemia or hyperthyroidism; additional afterload from hypertension, aortic stenosis or obstructive cardiomyopathy also demands a greater coronary blood flow. Increased tension of the ventricular wall, as occurs in dilatation or hypertrophy, may reduce coronary flow. Tachycardia increases cardiac work and often brings on pain. A rapid arterial run-off during diastole reduces coronary arterial pressure and flow in aortic regurgitation. Coronary artery spasm is increasingly recognised as a cause or exacerbating factor in angina pectoris.

**Clinical Features.** Angina pectoris is usually experienced as a sense of oppression or tightness in the middle of the chest—'like a band round the chest'—and the patient commonly places the hand or clenched fist on the sternum or both hands on the lower chest with the fingers touching at the sternum when describing it. It is usually induced by exertion, particularly out of doors, or by anxiety. Angina is likely to be worse when walking against a wind, uphill, on a cold day and particularly after meals. Some patients find that pain comes when they start walking and that later it does not return despite greater effort. Others can 'walk it off'. Some experience the pain when lying flat (*angina decubitus*), and some are awakened by it (*nocturnal angina*) particularly with 'energetic' or alarming dreams. Rarely pain may come capriciously as a result of coronary arterial spasm, and be accompanied by transient ST elevation in the ECG (*Prinzmetal's angina*).

The pain is often accompanied by discomfort in the arms, more commonly the left, the wrists and sometimes the hands; the patient may describe a feeling of uselessness in the limb. Angina may more rarely be epigastric or interscapular or may radiate to the neck and jaw, or occur at any of these places of reference without chest discomfort. The precipitation by effort or anxiety, and the relief within a few minutes by rest or with the use of glyceryl trinitrate, should allow the cause of the pain to be recognised. There may be accompanying breathlessness. Pain may be induced by a cardiac arrhythmia.

*Physical examination* is frequently negative, but evidence of contributory or concomitant disease should be sought. Aortic valve disease, particularly aortic stenosis, may cause angina. Rarely a quiet early diastolic murmur or calcification of the ascending aorta may betray syphilitic aortitis which can obstruct the coronary ostia. The patient should be examined for anaemia, obesity and thyroid and peripheral vascular disease. Diabetes and hyperlipidaemia, potent causes of premature arterial disease, should also be excluded.

*Electrocardiograms* are normal in most patients at rest between attacks. In some there is evidence of established infarction. In others ischaemic changes (ST depression and T inversion) may be present or be induced by exercise. Although both 'false positive' and 'false negative' ECGs can be recorded immediately after exercise, ST depression of 2 mm or more is in favour of myocardial ischaemia.

*Coronary arteriography* is sometimes performed for diagnostic purposes and is obligatory if surgery is contemplated. This procedure is potentially hazardous, but in good hands, mortality is less than 1 in 1000. It must be emphasised that the demonstration of arterial narrowing does not prove that it is the cause of symptoms as this may also be found in the asymptomatic.

**Differential Diagnosis.** Effort angina has few significant mimics if a careful history is elicited. Musculo-skeletal pains are provoked by specific movements rather than by walking. Asthma, when induced by exercise, may give a sense of tightness in the chest but lasts longer than angina and dyspnoea is more prominent. The pain of pericarditis occasionally comes only with exercise, but its other characteristics (p. 203) should help to make the distinction. Angina occurring at rest may be confused with oesophagitis, with or without a hiatus hernia, but pain due to oesophagitis usually has a burning quality and tends to be exacerbated by hot liquids and to be relieved by alkalis. A small hiatus hernia occurs in about 20% of the population and certainly should not be considered to be the cause of the pain without good evidence.

**Treatment.** Patients usually respond to a careful explanation of the problem, which can be presented as what it is—a mismatch between coronary supply and cardiac needs. The natural process of repair by development of anastomoses should be stressed. Patients can then learn how to help themselves, e.g. by avoiding walking after meals, particularly in the cold or against a wind, and severe unaccustomed exertion. They may need encouragement and support in their endeavours to stop smoking cigarettes or to lose weight. In a few patients hyperlipoproteinaemia requires treatment by diet and other measures (p. 532).

Fresh glyceryl trinitrate (GTN 0·5 mg), allowed to dissolve under the tongue or crunched for more rapid effect and retained in the mouth, usually relieves the pain in 2 to 3 minutes and at about the same time it often produces a slight headache. The best use of GTN is prophylactically before exercise recognised as liable to produce pain. The good effect comes from venous and arterial dilatation which lowers the blood pressure and also dilates the coronary vessels provided their disease does not prevent this. Not more than about two per hour should be used. Patients can be reassured that GTN is not dangerous or habit forming and that it does not lose its effect. If the requirement for it increases significantly the patient should seek medical advice. The appropriate use of GTN allows more exercise to be taken; this should be encouraged for there is evidence that physical activity favours the development of collateral vessels. Long acting nitrates, such as isosorbide dinitrate (10 mg or more, 3–6/d) are of value in some cases.

If these measures do not allow the patient to live a reasonable life, $\beta$–adrenergic blockade should be employed. Propranolol can be prescribed initially in small doses (e.g. 10 mg 6 hourly) with progressive increments until benefit is obtained, which is often not until the resting heart rate has been significantly slowed. There is considerable individual variation and as much as 240 mg 6 hourly or even more may be required. A $\beta$–blocking drug should not be withdrawn abruptly because of the risks of dangerous arrhythmias and myocardial infarction. Other properties of the $\beta$–blocking drugs are described on page 197. In resistant cases perhexilene or nifedipine may prove helpful.

Patients who are severely disabled by angina may be dramatically improved by aorta-coronary bypass surgery, using the saphenous vein as a graft. The best surgeons have an operative mortality of as little as 1%; for patients with multiple coronary arterial obstruction and particularly with a blockage of the left main coronary artery the operation may also improve the prognosis.

**Prevention.** The Joint Working Party of the Royal College of Physicians of London and the British Cardiac Society (p. 218) stressed particularly the advantage of stopping cigarette smoking in reducing the risk of coronary heart disease. This report also made general recommendations in the hope of altering the widespread habits of overeating and inadequate exercise. Only in the relatively young with established hyperlipidaemia did it recommend strict diets in which animal fat intake is reduced and butter replaced by margarine made with polyunsaturated fats, together with considerable replacement of meat with fish, and reduction in the intake of eggs and cream. There is little to suggest that there is potential benefit for those over 50 years of age who have had a heart attack by adopting diets of this kind, and many find them irksome. The advantage of controlling blood pressure is mainly in reducing the liability to stroke and renal failure but it may also lower the risk of coronary disease. Oral contraceptives should preferably not be used by women over 35 years of age, particularly if there are other risk factors whether genetic, or from smoking, hypertension or hyperlipidaemia.

**Prognosis.** When prospective studies of patients with angina pectoris are sufficiently long it is recognised that the outlook is better than used to be thought. More than half live for 5 years and a third for 10 from the time of diagnosis. Spontaneous recovery, which may prove temporary, occurs in as many as a third, a fact which is useful to remember when talking to patients about their disease. Prognosis is worse in the patient who has had multiple cardiac infarcts or who has cardiac failure.

## Unstable Angina

The term 'unstable' is used to describe angina which has become abruptly more prolonged or more severe in the absence of evidence of infarction. Many different factors may be responsible, including the natural progression of coronary atherosclerosis or the development of coronary arterial spasm. Affected patients are often admitted to hospital under suspicion of myocardial infarction. Most patients will respond to rest, mild sedation, nitrates and β–adrenergic blocking drugs. It has been claimed that nifedipine has a special place in the management of coronary arterial spasm. The persistence of symptoms in spite of these measures should lead to consideration of coronary arterial surgery.

## Myocardial Infarction

The diagnosis of myocardial infarction was not widely made until the late 1920s, and then almost exclusively among the prosperous. More than 50 years later it is one of the commonest causes of emergency admission to hospital in affluent societies, affecting patients from all walks of life.

The illness in its mildest form may go unrecognised and only be disclosed subsequently by ECG evidence; at the other end of the spectrum there is permanent severe disability and death. At the onset of the illness sudden death, presumably from ventricular fibrillation or asystole, may occur immediately and most of the patients who die do so within the first hour. If the patient survives this most critical part of the illness, the liability to dangerous arrhythmias remains, but diminishes as each hour goes by. If the damage is sufficiently extensive the cardiac output falls and there is a wide range of consequent effects, from slight reduction in skin perfusion and blood pressure at one end to cardiogenic shock at the other. The latter, if severe and persistent, is almost always fatal. If the left ventricle is sufficiently damaged, upstream pressures may rise and pulmonary oedema ensue.

The precipitating factors leading to an episode of myocardial infarction are still imperfectly understood. In terms of blood flow the mismatch between coronary supply and myocardial demand, which is temporary and reversible in angina, may with reducing supply and/or increased demand lead to irreversible cellular damage. Myocardial infarction is particularly likely to occur in elderly patients admitted to hospital for operations of various kinds, and in many of these the coronary disease goes unrecognised until the development of the infarct.

**Clinical Features.** The cardinal symptom is pain but breathlessness, syncope, vomiting and extreme tiredness are common. The pain occurs in the same sites as for angina but is usually more severe and lasts longer. It is most often described as a tightness, heaviness or constriction in the chest. At its worst the pain is one of the most severe which can be experienced and the patient's expression and pallor may vividly convey the seriousness of the situation. Many patients are breathless and in some this is the only symptom; a few develop pulmonary oedema at the onset. Syncope may occur and the blood pressure falls particularly if the patient is upright, or from the development of a serious arrhythmia or complete heart block. Vomiting is often a feature and is commoner in the more severe cases, particularly in those with cardiogenic shock. The risk of dying in the first few hours is high; death during this time is usually due to ventricular fibrillation. At any time after the first 12 hours or so the patient may recognise that a different pain has developed, even though it is at the same site. It is worse, or only appears, on inspiration and may be altered by a change of position. It is due to pericarditis consequent upon the infarct and is confirmed if a pericardial friction rub is heard. In rare cases the infarct may go unrecognised until endocardial thrombosis resulting from it leads to systemic embolism.

The physical signs may be few in a mild attack but in severe cases there is usually pallor, sweating and breathlessness. The heart rate is usually increased and with shock the pulse volume may be much reduced and the skin perfusion poor. Most patients admitted to hospital with a myocardial infarction have a normal initial blood pressure, but transiently it may be high as a result of pain, anxiety or the unfamiliarity of the environment. The blood pressure gradually falls over the first 3 or 4 days. In the minority who develop cardiogenic shock the blood pressure is, of course, low. The jugular venous pressure is often elevated when the patient is first seen; this may be due to cardiac failure but, just as with the arterial pressure, anxiety may contribute at this stage. Examination of the heart is often relatively uninformative but the first heart sound may be quiet and a third, or more commonly a fourth heart sound, may develop. Pericardial friction is most often heard on the second or third day and is usually transitory. Occasionally it persists for days and exceptionally for weeks. Crepitations, particularly if widespread and persistent after coughing, suggest pulmonary oedema. Oliguria is common if the blood pressure is low. In many cases myocardial necrosis is associated with fever reaching a maximum on the third or fourth day and not much higher than 38°C. A leucocytosis is usually at its peak on the first day and the ESR often becomes raised. A chest radiograph may demonstrate pulmonary oedema which has been undetected clinically.

**Investigation.** ELECTROCARDIOGRAPHY. During the first few hours of the attack the infarct causes an elevation of the ST segment over the affected area. When there has been anteroseptal infarction the changes are found in one or more leads from V1 to

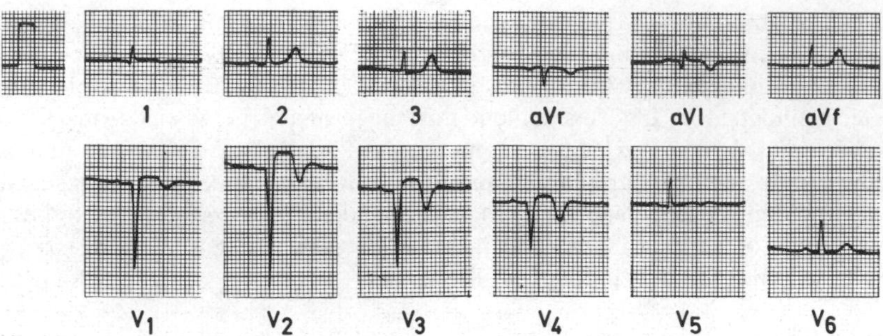


Fig. 6.23 Recent anteroseptal myocardial infarction. In leads V1–V4 there is ST elevation, and in these leads and in aVL inverted T and deep Q waves.

V4 (Fig. 6.23). Anterolateral infarction produces changes in leads V4 to V6, in aVL and hence also in lead I; in strictly anterior infarction the changes may be confined to leads V3 and V4. Inferior infarction is shown in lead aVF and in leads II and III (Fig. 6.24). Infarction of the posterior wall of the left ventricle is not recorded in standard leads by ST elevation but may be detected in V1–V4 by ST depression or a tall R.

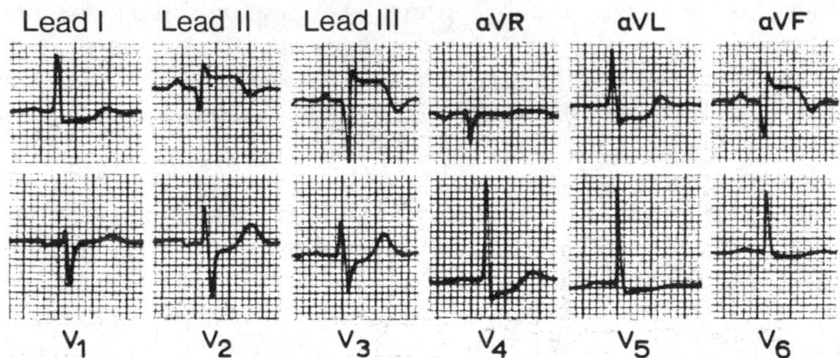


Fig. 6.24 Recent inferior myocardial infarction. In leads II, III and aVF there is ST elevation, inverted T and deep Q waves. In leads I, aVL and V2–V4 there is reciprocal ST depression.

The myocardial infarct, whether recent or replaced by a scar, transmits the changes of potential from within the ventricular cavity and hence produces what is sometimes called an 'electrical window'. The size of the Q and inverted T which results will depend in part on the size of this window. In established anterior infarction Q and inverted T waves are found in the anterior chest leads and in established anterolateral infarctions a prominent Q and inverted T is usually seen also in leads aVL and I (Fig. 6.25). In established inferior infarction a Q and inverted T in leads aVF, II and III is the usual pattern. With established posterior infarction Q waves are not detected in the standard leads and a tall R in VI, due to unopposed anterior depolarisation, may be the only evidence of the posterior scar (Fig. 6.26). Unipolar leads recorded from the back of the left chest may, however, also show evidence of the posterior infarction.

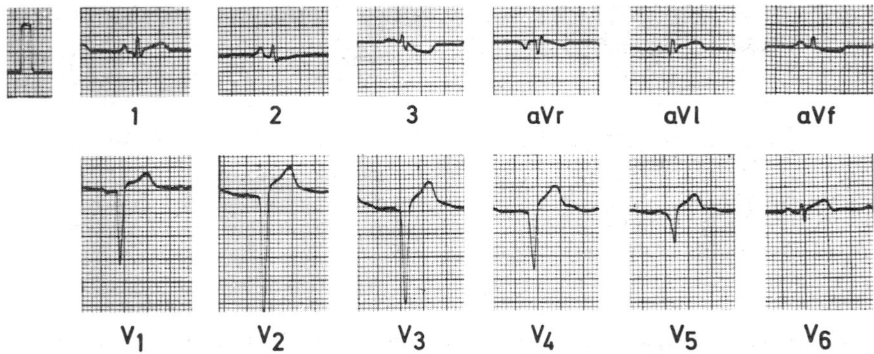


Fig. 6.25 Established anteroseptal myocardial infarction. There is a deep Q and absent R in leads V1–V5.

Often the ECG is normal in the early stages of the attack and it is a mistake to assume that this excludes myocardial infarction especially in a patient with a history strongly suggestive of the diagnosis. Although the ECG becomes abnormal in a high proportion of patients there are a few in whom no detectable change may be found although the history, enzyme changes or other evidence may support the diagnosis. The residual changes of an established infarct may obscure the effects of a fresh lesion.

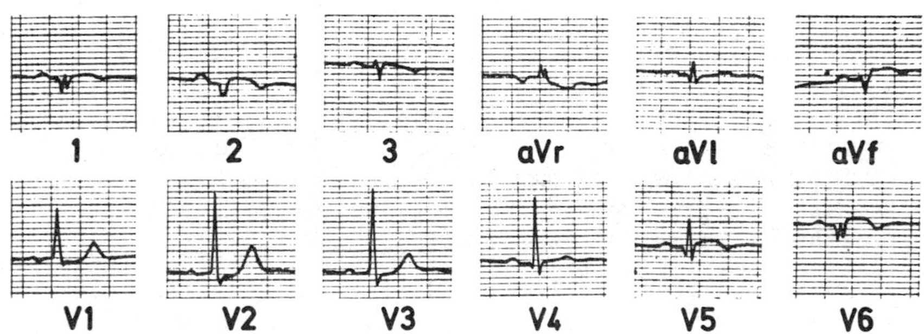


Fig. 6.26 Established posterior myocardial infarction. The depolarisation of the right ventricle is no longer opposed by the depolarisation of the back of the left ventricle and hence there is a prominent R in the right anterior leads. (Q1, II and V6 indicate antero-lateral infarction also).

SERUM ENZYMES. Experimental work in dogs shows that infarction of as little as 5% of the myocardium leads to a detectable rise, in the blood, of enzymes normally confined within cardiac cells and liberated as a result of myocardial necrosis. The enzymes most widely used in the detection of myocardial infarction are creatine kinase (CK), aspartate aminotransferase (AST), formerly known as glutamic oxalo-acetic transaminase (GOT), and lactic dehydrogenase (LD). CK which is also found in skeletal muscle, starts to rise at 4–6 hours, peaks about 12 hours and falls to normal in 48–72 hours. AST starts to rise about 12 hours after infarction and reaches a peak on the first or second day. LD is also liberated from haemolysed red cells and is therefore less specific. It starts to rise after 12 hours, reaches a peak after 2 or 3 days and may be elevated for about a week; it is useful when the diagnosis is in doubt several days after a possible infarct. Serial estimations are necessary, in doubtful cases, for it is the change in enzyme levels which is of diagnostic value (p. 906).

**Complications.** ARRHYTHMIAS. Nearly all patients with myocardial infarction have some form of arrhythmia, the minor varieties of which would be expected even in normal subjects subjected to similar monitoring.

*Sinus tachycardia* is the commonest; anxiety may contribute to it. *Sinus bradycardia* is a special feature of inferior myocardial infarction and may lead to ventricular escape and the development of more dangerous rhythms; occasionally it causes syncope. *Atrial tachycardia* or *fibrillation* occur in about 15% of patients; these arrhythmias may exacerbate cardiac failure or hypotension and require urgent treatment. *Ventricular ectopic beats* are almost invariable and are frequently numerous. They are usually of little consequence but may indicate an increased liability to ventricular fibrillation if they fall on the T wave of the preceding beat ('R on T'; Fig. 6.11).

*Ventricular tachycardia* is also common. If it persists at a fast rate for more than a few seconds it may have serious haemodynamic effects.

*Ventricular fibrillation* appears in about 10% of patients most of whom never reach hospital. The potential reversibility in those patients who do not have cardiogenic shock is one of the main foundations upon which the policy of acute coronary care and rapid hospital admission were built. Various degrees of *atrioventricular block* are also common and of these the most sinister is the development of complete heart block in a patient with anterior myocardial infarction, for it indicates that both bundles have been involved in the infarction of the interventricular septum. Because of the extensive damage such patients usually also have cardiogenic shock.

CARDIOGENIC SHOCK (p. 166). If there is a reversible arrhythmia as an important contributory factor its correction may bring about considerable improvement. If this is not the case and shock is persistent, all the other complications of myocardial infarction tend to be more likely, such as dangerous arrhythmias, extension of the infarct, pulmonary oedema and renal failure.

OTHER COMPLICATIONS. *Cardiac failure* may occur and *pulmonary oedema* is its commonest form. Regular examination for post-tussive crepitations, oliguria or radiographic evidence should lead to its early detection.

Rarer complications include *infarction of a mitral papillary muscle* which may lead to the development of *mitral regurgitation*; occasionally this precipitates or exacerbates pulmonary oedema. *Rupture of the interventricular septum* is diagnosed by the development of the characteristic murmur of a ventricular septal defect (p. 207) and may be followed by severe hypotension and venous hypertension. *Rupture of the myocardium* may lead to cardiac tamponade (p. 203). *Venous thrombosis* is less common than in the days when patients with myocardial infarction were kept in bed for about 6 weeks. It often first announces its presence by *pulmonary embolism*; even a careful watch on the legs for evidence of the primary lesion will reveal only about 50%. When a thrombus forms on the endocardium of the left ventricle *systemic embolism* can occur and occlude an artery.

The *postmyocardial infarction syndrome* (Dressler's syndrome) which is probably an autoimmune reaction to necrotic myocardium, is characterised by persistent fever, pericarditis and pleurisy. It occurs a few weeks or even months after the infarct and often subsides after a few days but may require aspirin, phenylbutazone or even steroid therapy for its control if it is prolonged.

**Treatment.** The main needs are for the relief of pain, the prevention and treatment of arrhythmias and other complications, and the rehabilitation of the patient.

In the acute stage when the risk of fatal arrhythmia is highest, it is desirable for most patients to be admitted, if possible, to a coronary care unit. Patients who are diagnosed after the first few hours may be cared for at home if they are free of cardiac failure or shock and are adequately supported domestically.

*Relief of Pain.* The patient with a severe attack is in pain and is frightened. The most effective remedies are morphine (10–20 mg s.c. or i.v.) or diamorphine (5–10 mg s.c. or i.v.) supplemented by cyclizine (50 mg i.v.) to reduce the likelihood of vomiting. The anxiety must be recognised even if it is not overt; it is essential to reassure the patient that recovery is the most likely outcome and that initially it is best to be where complications can most readily be treated should these arise.

*Arrhythmias.* During the acute phase of the illness, if there are multiple ectopic beats or particularly if there are the potentially dangerous 'R on T' extrasystoles or a ventricular tachycardia, the drug of choice is lignocaine (p. 166). If lignocaine proves to be ineffective alternatives are practolol (5 mg i.v. given slowly to a maximum of 25 mg) or mexiletine (p. 165). If ventricular fibrillation develops, DC shock should be used immediately without cardiac massage or artificial ventilation. Failing this the cardiac resuscitation procedure (p. 161) should be used until the defibrillator is available. Asystole is generally not amenable to treatment, but in some cases success has been achieved when resuscitation is followed by transvenous insertion of a pacemaker. Patients in shock prior to the development of asystole or ventricular fibrillation are very unlikely to prove amenable to resuscitation. Atrial tachycardia, flutter or fibrillation are best treated with digoxin if the ventricular rate is high. Sinus bradycardia usually does not require treatment, but if there is hypotension or ventricular escape, atropine (p. 166) should be used. In advanced heart block it is sometimes necessary to introduce a pacing catheter into the right ventricle in order to maintain a satisfactory rhythm.

*Cardiogenic shock* (p. 166) and *cardiac failure* (p. 170) are treated along the usual lines; digoxin may be prescribed unless precluded by the cardiac rhythm. Oxygen is indicated in pulmonary oedema or shock.

*Anticoagulants* (p. 600) are indicated in the treatment of venous thrombosis and pulmonary embolism and may be used prophylactically if the patient is at risk because of the need for prolonged immobilisation. There is no convincing evidence that anticoagulants are of value in the prevention of further coronary thrombosis.

*Rehabilitation.* There is pathological evidence that an infarct takes 4–6 weeks to undergo repair; it is then replaced by fibrous tissue. Accordingly it is generally thought reasonable to restrict physical activities during this period. When there are no complications the patient with a minor attack can sit in a chair within a few days, be ambulant within a week, return home in 10 days and gradually increase activity with the prospect of return to work after 6 weeks. When there are complications the regime has to be adjusted accordingly; a few patients are permanently disabled by heart failure or severe angina. Reassurance is essential at every stage for many patients are severely and even permanently incapacitated as a result of psychological rather than physical effects of a myocardial infarction. The success of restoring a patient to normal life depends very much on the attitudes of the physician. The naturally vigorous person may require restraint in the early stages but more often the anxious will need encouragement. The spouse has often to learn to stop reminding the patient of former disability. Such efforts, however well intended, often perpetuate worry and restrict rehabilitation.

Ventricular aneurysm, mitral regurgitation due to papillary muscle damage, and rupture of the interventricular septum are all amenable to surgical repair but preferably not earlier than 6 weeks after the infarct.

**Prognosis.** In about a quarter of all cases of myocardial infarction death occurs within the first few minutes without medical care. Half the deaths from myocardial infarction occur within 2 hours of the onset of symptoms and three quarters within 24 hours. About 40% of all affected patients die within the first month. Unfavourable features are old age, cardiogenic shock, cardiac failure, heart block, and ventricular arrhythmias. Bundle branch block and high enzyme readings both indicate extensive damage. In the absence of unfavourable features, the outlook is as good for those who survive ventricular fibrillation as for the others. Of those who survive an acute attack more than 80% live for a further year, about 75% 5 years, 50% 10 years and 25% 20 years. It is therefore appropriate to be reassuring to patients about their prospects. Most should be able to return to work in 2 or 3 months. Late dangerous complications include recurrence of myocardial infarction, cardiac aneurysm, cardiac rupture and pulmonary embolism.

There have been claims that the long term prognosis after myocardial infarction may be improved by the antiarrhythmic effect of a $\beta$-blocking drug or by the antiplatelet effect of aspirin, sulphinpyrazone or dipyridamole. The evidence is still inconclusive.

### Sudden Death

Many patients die suddenly and unexpectedly of ischaemic heart disease. Death may appear to be instantaneous, or nearly so; necropsy finding in such cases usually shows extensive coronary atherosclerosis but frequently there is no evidence of recent coronary occlusion or myocardial infarction. It is believed that most instances are the result of ventricular fibrillation; resuscitation, if promptly applied, may restore effective cardiac action.

## Systemic Arterial Hypertension

The maintenance of normal blood pressure even in health is now recognised to be a process of somewhat daunting complexity. The mean arterial pressure depends principally upon the cardiac output and the arteriolar tone. The blood pressure is constantly monitored by baroreceptors and a complicated autoregulation system immediately makes adjustments to maintain blood pressure despite changes in posture, a sudden fall in venous return — as with the Valsalva manoeuvre — or to counteract the effects of exercise, heat, changes in the salt and water intake, fluid loss and other variables.

In Western civilisation the normal blood pressure gradually rises with age. Hypertension is defined arbitrarily at levels above generally accepted normals, for example, 140/90 at the age of 20 rising gradually to 170/105 at the age of 75. Hypertension is present in about 15% of the population. The disorder is symptomless until complications arise so that diagnosis depends on whether there is special screening, as when patients attend their doctors for other reasons. It must be emphasised that to wait for symptoms attributable to hypertension is a very inefficient method of case finding. The blood pressure depends also on the circumstances of the measurement and is higher in anxious subjects. It is insufficiently appreciated that normal individuals may develop very high blood pressure levels under stress; continuous arterial readings have shown blood pressures of 230/130 in 20-year-olds in oral examinations; very high levels also occur at orgasm or immediately after straining at stool. Conversely, during sleep the blood pressures may fall to less than 90/50. Many patients find medical examination very stressful. Senior physicians record significantly higher blood pressure levels than appropriately trained nurses, who to the patient appear less formidable.

Vasomotor tone is dependent on sympathetic nervous, metabolic and hormonal factors. Vasodilation can be produced by the kallikrein system and the prostaglandins. Vasoconstriction may result from increased sympathetic activity, and adrenal catecholamines, but the most powerful vasoconstrictor is angiotensin II. It acts directly by causing contraction of arterioles, but also indirectly via the central nervous system and by increasing catecholamine release from sympathetic nerves. It also has a positive inotropic effect and leads to retention of sodium and water by the kidneys. Increased levels of renin and angiotensin II are a feature of severe essential — i.e. unexplained — hypertension, in the malignant and accelerated phases and in renovascular hypertension.

An excess of circulating aldosterone from an adrenal adenoma or from adrenocortical hyperplasia may cause hypertension. It is to be suspected from low serum potassium levels and is associated with low plasma renin activity.

In about 80 to 90% of patients with hypertension even the use of refined diagnostic methods will not establish a cause, and this is known as *essential hypertension*. This type of hypertension is a graded characteristic with a continuous unimodal frequency distribution with a multifactorial inheritance (p. 16); in 70% of patients another member of the family is affected. Essential hypertension is especially frequent in some races, particularly American Negroes and Japanese. It is commoner where salt intake is excessive.

*Secondary Hypertension*. In approximately 10–20% of cases of hypertension a cause can be found but only by a methodical approach. Its discovery is important because cure is often possible; the search is most likely to be rewarded in children and young adults.

The main causes of secondary hypertension are: 1. Coarctation of the aorta.

2. Renal disease: (*a*) Parenchymatous e.g. acute and chronic glomerulonephritis; pyelonephritis; systemic lupus erythematosus and polyarteritis nodosa. (*b*) Polycystic kidneys. (*c*) Renal artery stenosis.
3. Endocrine disorders and hormone therapy: (*a*) Phaeochromocytoma. (*b*) Cushing's syndrome, spontaneous and drug induced. (*c*) Primary aldosteronism (Conn's syndrome). (*d*) Oral contraception and oestrogen therapy.
4. Pregnancy.

In hypertensive children and young adults coarctation of the aorta should be particularly suspected; it is usually easy to detect from a weak femoral pulse delayed after the radial pulse. Renal parenchymal disease, identifiable usually by urine examination, is another important cause of hypertension in this age group. Renal arterial disease and phaeochromocytomas may also be found. In early middle-age, arterial and renal parenchymal disease and hypertension resulting from the use of oral contraceptives should all be considered, but phaeochromocytoma and primary aldosteronism also occur. By late middle age, essential hypertension accounts for the great majority of cases but renal artery stenosis and primary aldosteronism are also found. Over the age of 50 renal artery stenosis from atheroma, and oestrogen therapy, have also to be considered as possible causes.

*Systolic hypertension* is a feature of the non-compliant arteries of old age. Though diastolic hypertension is usually regarded as of more sinister prognosis than systolic, it is now established that systolic hypertension found at routine examination — so-called *casual hypertension* — is of comparable prognostic importance in middle age.

**Clinical Features.** Hypertension is frequently discovered on routine examination of apparently healthy subjects. Symptoms are rare and when present are generally attributable to the complications of the disease, whether from a cerebrovascular accident, from haemorrhages in the retina or visual pathways or from left ventricular failure. Coexisting arterial disease, causing for example angina or intermittent claudication, also occurs. Minor symptoms such as headache, dizziness, irritability, fatigue and insomnia are widespread in the population and tend to be inappropriately attributed to the hypertension when it is found. Such symptoms are commoner in patients who know that they have hypertension. The occasional patient with malignant hypertension has severe headache which is relieved by adequate treatment. Polyuria and nocturia may be due to renal failure.

Physical signs also tend to be few. Long-standing hypertension leads to left ventricular hypertrophy and may be indicated by a forceful apical impulse displaced to the left. The hypertrophied ventricle is less compliant than a normal ventricle so that left atrial hypertrophy follows and may be inferred from a palpable and/or audible fourth heart sound. The aortic second sound is often increased. There may be an ejection sound. In the elderly there may be an aortic diastolic murmur due to dilatation of the aortic ring. There may be evidence of left ventricular failure from basal crepitations. However, the symptom of sudden breathlessness awakening the patient from sleep is a more reliable indication of left ventricular failure.

In the child or young adult an arterial pulsation in the neck should arouse the suspicion of coarctation of the aorta and emphasise the need to look for the other physical signs of it. In renal artery stenosis a systolic bruit may be heard in the abdomen or lumbar region over the kidney. It should be sought in young patients with severe hypertension in whom it may be due to remediable fibromuscular dysplasia of a renal artery. In older persons coexisting atheromatous disease in other arteries may be suggested by absent peripheral pulses, by a systolic bruit over a major vessel or by a 'kinked carotid' (p. 148). In polycystic disease the large kidneys are often palpable. Protein and casts in the urine are to be expected in renal parenchymal disease and in the malignant phase of essential hypertension.

Examination of the ocular fundus is crucial. In the early stages of hypertension some decrease in tortuosity and a variation in calibre of the retinal arterioles becomes apparent, and at the arteriovenous crossings the thickened arteriolar wall is liable to compress the vein so that the vein appears empty at each side of it ('nipping'). Haemorrhages may occur, the most common being flame-shaped; these fade within a few weeks. Soft ('cotton wool') exudates are areas of retinal infarction resulting from occlusion of small arterioles. (Plate 1, p. 530). These indicate the onset of the malignant or accelerated phase. They also fade in a few weeks and leave no trace. Hard exudates are small, dense, whitish deposits containing lipid which may remain unaltered for months or years. Papilloedema indicates the most advanced stage of malignant hypertension and the coexistence of fibrinoid arteriolar necrosis. Early death from renal failure is likely unless prompt action is taken to maintain a lower arterial pressure.

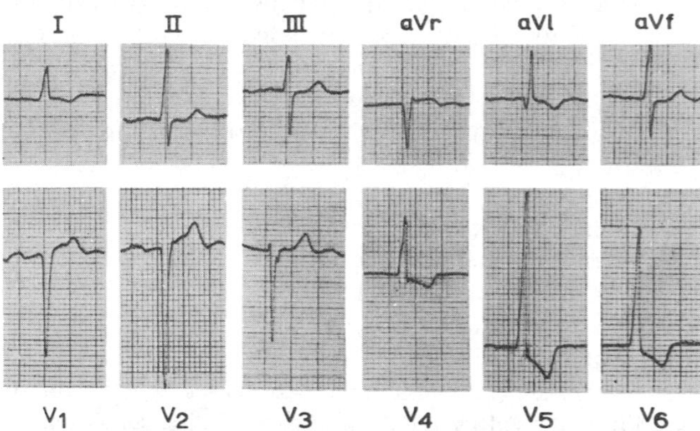


Fig. 6.27 Left ventricular hypertrophy. Note: (1) tall R waves over left ventricle (V5–6); (2) deep S waves over right ventricle (V1–2); (3) ST depression and asymmetrical inversion of T wave in leads I, aVL and V4–V6.

**Investigation.** Evidence of left ventricular and left atrial hypertrophy may be obtained from the electrocardiogram (Fig. 6.27) and help to indicate that the hypertension is not just temporary. The chest radiograph may show left ventricular enlargement but less reliably than the physical examination and the electrocardiogram. With coarctation of the aorta there may be characteristic 'notching' of the ribs. The plasma urea or creatinine are required as a measure of renal excretory function. Estimation of plasma electrolytes is essential as hypokalaemia is an indicator of primary or secondary aldosteronism if it is not due to diuretic therapy. Measurement of plasma urate is advisable because hyperuricaemia is associated with hypertension and gout is liable to be produced by diuretic therapy; examination of the urine for sugar is important because hypertension and its complications are commoner in diabetics. An elevated serum cholesterol is indirectly associated with atheroma.

Radioisotope studies or excretion urography is indicated in younger patients to detect potentially remediable unilateral lesions resulting from reduced blood flow. An excretion urogram is the less reliable method but may show a delay in appearance and/or increased concentration of dye on the affected side.

Further investigation is also required for patients with manifestations suggestive of a phaeochromocytoma (p. 496) or primary aldosteronism (p. 487). In older patients routine investigation so rarely leads to radical cure that it has been proved to be uneconomical unless there is some clinical indication or unusual difficulty in treatment.

**Complications.** CARDIAC. Hypertrophy of the left ventricle at first maintains a normal blood flow. Later the left ventricular output can no longer be maintained and cardiac failure may become manifest. Breathlessness on exercise may occur and paroxysmal noctural dyspnoea may be the presenting symptom in hitherto unsuspected hypertension. A fourth heart sound and pulsus alternans are serious signs. Atrial fibrillation sometimes occurs. Coronary artery disease is more frequent in patients with hypertension.

CEREBRAL. Ischaemia (p. 689) and cerebral haemorrhage (p. 694) are common complications. Visual disturbances occur if the optic pathways are involved in vascular lesions (Fig. 14.4).

*Hypertensive encephalopathy* is an infrequent condition due to acute focal cerebral ischaemia to which cerebrovascular spasm, oedema or minor degrees of cerebral thrombosis contribute. Transient disturbances of vision or speech, paresis, paraesthesiae, disorientation, fits or loss of consciousness may occur. The blood pressure is usually very high; complete recovery can be expected if it is rapidly and effectively lowered.

RENAL. The term *malignant hypertension* should be reserved for the syndrome of severe diastolic hypertension, papilloedema, retinal exudates and haemorrhages, and renal failure; its importance lies in the renal arteriolar necrosis which accompanies it. Malignant hypertension occurs mainly in males in the third and fourth decades and pursues a rapidly downhill course to death from uraemia within a year unless appropriate treatment is established and maintained. Most cases of malignant hypertension before the age of 30 are caused by renal parenchymal disease. When papilloedema and renal failure suddenly develop in a person known to have essential hypertension this is described as '*accelerated hypertension*'. Papilloedema may be present temporarily during an attack of hypertensive encephalopathy or may occur in cases of transient hypertension such as with acute nephritis or pregnancy.

**Treatment.** ESSENTIAL HYPERTENSION. When significant hypertension is discovered and found to be persistently present, it should be explained to the patient that unless the blood pressure is modified to more normal levels there is a risk of developing one of the complications of hypertension. The patient must realise that once treatment is embarked upon it will need to be continued for life — at least in the present state of knowledge. The establishment of a good relationship between the doctor and the patient is very important. The previously asymptomatic patient who develops side-effects of treatment needs particular help; appropriate readjustment of the dose or a change of drug may restore confidence. As with the diabetic the treatment has to be reviewed regularly; whether the supervision should be by a general practitioner or by hospital doctors with a special interest in hypertension, depends on many factors and should be decided for the individual patient so that responsibilities are recognised.

The discovery of hypertension and the planning of management provide an opportunity to search for other factors which may add to the cardiovascular risks. Among these are heavy cigarette smoking and obesity. If the patient can stop smoking, reduce weight, and, except in severe hypertension, increase physical exercise, well-being is likely to be greater. Those who pour salt over their food in large quantities should be advised against this practice. A low salt diet, i.e. a diet containing less than 1·0 g per day, reduces blood pressure but it is too irksome to be of practical use. With effective drug treatment the special risks of surges of hypertension should be significantly reduced. It is customary to advise patients to 'avoid stress', but this is usually a pious hope. Spouses should be dissuaded from perpetually reminding patients of their hypertension which, with adequate treatment, should be non-existent.

More relaxation may be appropriate for the patient whose life is unreasonably hectic. Rest in bed is required, and then temporarily, only for the patient with severe malignant hypertension or with heart failure or when a serious complication, such as a cerebrovascular accident, occurs.

*Antihypertensive Drug Therapy*. The present is a time of transition, partly as a result of still incomplete knowledge of the roles of renin and angiotensin, partly as a result of new antihypertensive agents becoming available and partly because of disagreement as to whether mild hypertension (e.g. 150/95 at the age of 30) requires treatment. There is no doubt that in greater degrees of hypertension the outlook for hypertensive patients has been transformed, particularly in the reduction in the incidence of stroke, by the advent of effective antihypertensive therapy. *Pari passu* there has been a steady reduction in unwelcome side effects of treatment.

Many agents are now available but there is a growing consensus as to policy. The most logical plan is to use the smallest possible number of drugs and in the smallest possible quantities to achieve effective blood pressure control, which is usually accepted as a lying diastolic pressure of 90 or less at rest. By combining drugs when necessary it is possible to avoid the undesirable side-effects which may result from an excess of any one of them. The drug regime has to be tailored to the individual, for there is considerable variation in the side-effects with any one drug from one patient to another. The physician should not be content until the patient's blood pressure is under good control with minimal or absent side effects. Elderly patients often tolerate hypertension better than ill-judged treatment for it. Currently the drugs most commonly used first are either a diuretic or a $\beta$ blocker. If either is inadequate alone, the two may be used in combination. If control of the blood pressure is still not satisfactory then it is usually a vasodilator which is chosen to be added.

*Oral diuretics*, combined with moderate salt restriction, are effective in lowering blood pressure, initially by reducing blood volume, and over a longer period by reducing peripheral arteriolar resistance, probably in part by removing salt from the arterial media. They are particularly useful for minor degress of hypertension, and more specifically when total body sodium and water are increased, as with aldosteronism and renal parenchymal disease. A cheap, long-acting thiazide diuretic with potassium supplements if necessary, or triamterine, which conserves potassium, are both appropriate. Rapidly acting diuretics such as frusemide are less useful, unless there is accompanying cardiac or renal failure. Diuretics are also a useful adjunct to other forms of treatment.

*$\beta$-adrenoceptor blocking drugs* are now the most widely used of the sympatholytic agents. In addition to an antihypertensive effect they may also relieve anxiety, palpitation and angina pectoris. The many $\beta$ blockers include some whose use has been too brief to ensure that they are safe; the occasional dangers of practolol, which now preclude its oral use, took 8 years to be revealed.

Propranolol is effective, reliable and relatively free from side effects. Its dose has to be adjusted to the individual's needs because a large but variable proportion of the drug is destroyed in its first passage through the liver; even with equivalent blood concentrations there is also a great variation in response. Often twice daily dosage will suffice, but in others high doses may be required, so that treatment initiated in a dose of 40 mg b.d. may have to be increased to as much as 160 mg q.i.d. or even more in some patients if adequate blood pressure control is to be achieved. The slow release form has the advantage that the patient has to remember only a single daily dose. Many patients have no side-effects, but minor gastric disturbance, undue bradycardia, cardiac failure, bronchospasm, tiredness, bad dreams, hallucinations, cold hands and, occasionally, muscle weakness are all recognised complications. The combination of propranolol and a diuretic usually with a potassium supplement achieves the therapeutic goal without significant side-effects in a high proportion of patients with essential hypertension.

Some physicians prefer to use oxprenolol or other beta blockers. Metoprolol and atenolol are appropriate if a more cardio-selective drug is indicated as in patients who may have problems with airways obstruction, peripheral vascular disease or insulin dependent diabetes. Cardio-selective drugs have a greater effect on the cardiac ($\beta_1$) receptors than on the $\beta_2$ receptors which subserve bronchodilatation and vasodilatation. They also delay less the return of the blood sugar to normal after hypoglycaemia.

*Other sympatholytic agents* may be effective. Methyldopa, starting with 250 mg t.i.d. and rising to 3 g in total per day, has both a central and peripheral action. It may cause excessive sedation or a haemolytic anaemia (p. 36). The *adrenergic blocking drugs* are useful in severe hypertension but have the considerable disadvantage of causing hypotension on rising from bed and on exercise and are therefore particularly unsuitable for the elderly. Debrisoquine, starting with 10 mg t.i.d., is increased by 10 mg increments until the standing blood pressure is controlled. Bethanidine is an alternative drug which is used similarly. The adrenergic blocking drugs may cause nasal stuffiness, diarrhoea and impotence.

*Vasodilators*, e.g. hydrallazine and prazosin, are becoming more popular antihypertensive drugs. Although there is still doubt about their precise mode of action it is believed that they are mainly arteriolar vasodilators. Hydrallazine is used in a dose of 50–200 mg per day in divided dosage. In a small proportion of patients an SLE-like syndrome may develop (p. 627). Prazosin in a few cases causes dramatic hypotension when first given and therefore has to be instituted in a small dose (0·5 mg t.i.d. for about 3 days) with due warning to the patient. The maintenance dose is 5–20 mg per day in divided doses.

MALIGNANT OF ACCELERATED HYPERTENSION. The patient has a high sustained pressure (e.g. 300/160) with retinal exudates, haemorrhages and papilloedema. This requires urgent treatment over a period of several hours avoiding too great a fall in blood pressure which may precipitate neurological damage. Diazoxide (300 mg in 20 ml ampoules by rapid i.v. injection), reserpine (1–5 mg intramuscularly), or sodium nitroprusside initially as 0·5–1·5 μg/kg/min are all useful. The dose of each has to be adjusted to individual requirements once a safe level of blood pressure has been established.

SECONDARY HYPERTENSION. In a very small proportion of younger patients an operation to relieve stenosis of a renal artery or the removal of an ischaemic kidney may be dramatically successful in reducing blood pressure. Primary aldosteronism (p. 487) is the cause of hypertension in about 1% of cases. Phaeochromocytoma (p. 496) is even rarer. The treatment of these conditions and of other primary causes of hypertension, for example coarctation of the aorta (p. 206), is described in the appropriate section. Oral contraceptives and oestrogen therapy should be discontinued in the presence of hypertension.

**Prognosis.** There is a progressive reduction in expectation of life from those who have low normal blood pressures up to those who have levels which are clearly abnormal. However, it does not follow that all who have high blood pressure necessarily have a bad prognosis. The condition is mild if the heart is not enlarged, the fundi show no abnormalities and there is no proteinuria or evidence of impaired renal function. Many such patients live a life of normal span, free from related illness. Individuals with high casual readings and normal ones after a period of rest used to be regarded as having a benign condition. However, more recent evidence from prospective studies indicates that it is from such patients that an older population with serious hypertension is disproportionately drawn. On the whole, women appear to withstand hypertension better than men. Many elderly women in whom pressures are persistently of the order of 220/110 but who have no abnormalities in the optic fundi or the heart remain in good health for many years. Young men, in particular, who when first seen have high diastolic pressures together with secondary manifestations in the fundi or heart require optimal control of the blood pressure without delay. Patients with untreated malignant hypertension rarely live for more than a year. When properly administered, modern treatment is effective in preventing or postponing complications and in prolonging life.

Treatment of hypertension continues to be difficult and necessitates much attention to detail and considerable patience on the part of both patient and doctor. Until the cause of essential hypertension is found it is too much to hope that any single drug used in its management can be entirely satisfactory; those currently available produce in some patients tolerance, undesirable side-effects or occasional unpredictable hypotension. In addition it must be remembered that once begun, treatment will almost certainly have to be continued for life. It is therefore evident that most careful consideration should be given to the issues discussed above before making the decision to administer antihypertensive drugs.

## Pulmonary Arterial Hypertension

Pulmonary hypertension results from an increase in pulmonary capillary pressure, pulmonary blood flow, or pulmonary vascular resistance.

Increased pulmonary capillary pressure occurs with left ventricular failure and with mitral valve disease. Pulmonary blood flow is increased with left to right shunts as in atrial and ventricular septal defects and in persistent ductus arteriosus. In both these groups the pulmonary hypertension is potentially reversible if the cause can be successfully treated. In some cases increased pulmonary vascular resistance may develop and be irreversible; it can also be irreversible when it results from repetitive pulmonary thromboembolism or when it arises from an unknown cause, i.e. primary pulmonary hypertension. Hypoxaemia and hypercapnia cause a reflex increase in pulmonary arterial resistance and this contributes to right ventricular failure in lung disease.

**Primary pulmonary hypertension** is a rare disease of unknown aetiology which mainly affects young women. There may be a family history of the disease. Symptoms include syncope on exertion, breathlessnes and sometimes angina pectoris.

There may be a left parasternal impulse either from right ventricular hypertrophy, or from an enlarged pulmonary artery, or both. If there is accompanying right atrial hypertrophy a large *a* wave is to be expected in the jugular venous pulse. There may be an ejection sound and a loud second sound over the pulmonary valve. The ECG usually shows evidence of right atrial and right ventricular hypertrophy. The radiograph may show enlargement of the pulmonary artery and its main branches. In treatment the use of vasodilators is under trial but death usually occurs within a few years of diagnosis.

## Pulmonary Embolism and Infarction

Pulmonary embolism occurs when a portion of thrombus in a systemic vein, or, less commonly, in the right side of the heart is discharged into the circulation. It may lodge in the main pulmonary artery and cause sudden death, or in a smaller pulmonary artery and result in pulmonary infarction.

**Aetiology.** Thrombosis in the deep veins of the legs (p. 216) is the most frequent source. As this is usually the result of stasis, pulmonary embolism most often affects people who have been confined to bed. It is particularly liable to occur within ten days after a surgical operation or after childbirth. The presence of phlebothrombosis is frequently not recognised until after the embolism.

In less than 10% of cases, thrombi responsible for pulmonary embolism form in the right atrium in patients with atrial fibrillation, especially if cardiac failure is present.

**Clinical Features.** PULMONARY EMBOLISM. The patient may suddenly be seized with a sensation of great oppression in the chest and intense dyspnoea followed by cyanosis and shock. Death may occur within a few minutes. Recovery is usual if the patient survives the first few hours, but there is at least a 25% risk of recurrence. Pain indistinguishable from that of myocardial infarction may occur due to a combination of decreased coronary blood flow and hypoxaemia. The blood pressure falls, the jugular venous pressure rises and cardiac failure may follow in severe cases. The pulmonary second sound may be accentuated and either a third or a fourth heart sound may develop. These signs are due to a combination of pulmonary arterial hypertension, right ventricular failure and a low cardiac output.

In cases of lesser severity, symptoms and signs may be absent or there may be transient dyspnoea, tachycardia or syncope. Recurrent embolism may result in pulmonary hypertension which may be followed by right ventricular failure.

PULMONARY INFARCTION. The usual symptoms are pleural pain which may be severe and haemoptysis which may be profuse and repetitive. There may be dyspnoea, tachycardia, central cyanosis, pyrexia and polymorphonuclear leucocytosis. Secondary infection may occur. Often pulmonary infarction produces no symptoms.

**Investigation.** *Radiological Examination.* In massive pulmonary embolism the lung fields often appear normal but sometimes there is a hilar opacity from the blocked vessel and ischaemia distal to the embolus causes a reduction in the normal vascular markings of a lung or lobe. Pulmonary angiography is the most reliable method of diagnosis and should be carried out prior to urgent treatment such as embolectomy or thrombolytic therapy.

In pulmonary infarction there may be a pulmonary opacity due to a recent infarct or a linear scar from an earlier one. A small pleural effusion is common. The ipsilateral hemidiaphragm may be elevated. These radiological abnormalities are usually most marked at the base of one lung but are often bilateral.

Venous thrombosis is demonstrated by bilateral ascending or femoral phlebography.

*Radio-isotope Studies.* The intravenous injection of isotope-labelled macroaggregated albumin can be used to delineate underperfused areas of lung not detected on a plain radiograph. This technique is of value in the diagnosis of pulmonary embolism especially if combined with ventilation scanning following the inhalation of an isotope-labelled gas, particularly when the radiograph is normal.

*Electrocardiography* in cases of massive embolism may show a suggestive pattern, namely right axis deviation and inversion of T waves in the right ventricular leads, displacement of the interventricular septum to the left, or the pattern of incomplete right bundle branch block. The ECG is usually normal in cases of lesser severity.

**Course and Prognosis.** Massive pulmonary embolism is frequently fatal. Minor and medium-sized emboli are much less dangerous unless they are followed by further embolisation which may itself be fatal. In retrospect it is often apparent that small 'herald' emboli have, been missed or misinterpreted. Recurrent emboli may cause chronic pulmonary hypertension and right ventricular failure. The vast majority of pulmonary infarcts resolve completely. Occasionally an infarct may become secondarily infected and result in a lung abscess.

**Treatment and Prevention.** Heparin should be administered immediately and thereafter oral anticoagulants should be given in order to prevent further venous thrombosis in the legs (p. 600). Depending on the circumstances such treatment should be continued for six weeks to six months. Thrombolytic drugs such as urokinase are under trial.

Pain and apprehension should be allayed but morphine must be avoided if there is severe hypotension. Oxygen should be administered if central cyanosis is present.

Management of massive pulmonary embolism is best conducted in an area where intensive care can be provided. Occasionally a large embolus may be successfully removed from the main pulmonary artery. The chances of survival are greatest if embolectomy is carried out with the aid of cardiopulmonary bypass. In cases of recurrent pulmonary embolism, despite anticoagulation, venous interruption may be necessary either by inserting a filter into or plicating the inferior vena cava.

The prevention of pulmonary embolism and infarction consists of those measures directed at prophylaxis against venous thrombosis in the legs (p. 217).

## Diseases of the Myocardium

The myocardium is involved in most types of heart disease, but the terms myocarditis and cardiomyopathy are usually applied to those relatively uncommon forms of myocardial disease which are not the result of rheumatic fever, coronary artery disease, hypertension or thyroid disease.

### Acute Myocarditis

Acute myocarditis usually occurs as a complication of infections such as diphtheria, pneumonia, typhoid fever, scrub typhus fever and meningitis. Chagas' disease (American trypanosomiasis, p. 820) is the commonest cause in South America. Myocarditis may also be due to viral infection as in influenza, poliomyelitis, infectious mononucleosis and particularly Coxsackie-B infections. Rheumatic myocarditis is described on page 172.

Often the only evidence of myocarditis is a sinus tachycardia which is out of proportion to the severity of the infection. In more severe cases there may be a third heart sound, arrhythmias, conduction defects or acute cardiac failure. Prognosis in most types of acute myocarditis is usually good, but it may cause death in diphtheria. In Chagas' disease, the patient usually recovers from the acute phase and after a latent period of 10 or 20 years, a chronic cardiomyopathy develops which is eventually fatal.

There is no specific therapy for acute myocarditis; the usual forms of treatment for cardiac failure and arrhythmias should be undertaken. Prolonged rest is sometimes necessary.

### Chronic Cardiomyopathies

**Aetiology.** In a considerable number of cases, the myocardial disease is part of a generalised disorder and the cardiac involvement may be of major or minor degree.

Such disorders include haemochromatosis, sarcoidosis, amyloidosis, uraemia, the muscular dystrophies, and connective tissue disorders such as systemic lupus erythematosus, systemic sclerosis and polyarteritis nodosa. Cardiomyopathy may be associated with alcoholism and rarely with the late stages of pregnancy and puerperium.

In the remainder there is no generalised disorder and frequently no aetiological agent can be found, although in a proportion of such cases there is a family history. Sometimes there is a definite or suspected history of acute myocarditis.

**Clinical Features.** The cardiomyopathies most often present in one or other of two clinical patterns: (1) The most common is '*congestive*' with cardiomegaly and valvular regurgitation, and progressive left-sided and, later, right-sided cardiac failure. (2) '*Hypertrophic*' *cardiomyopathy* is frequently associated with such severe thickening of the interventricular septum that obstruction to outflow from the left ventricle occurs. This produces a clinical picture simulating aortic stenosis (hypertrophic obstructive cardiomyopathy). There is usually no identifiable cause although a family history is common.

Two rarer types of presentation are (3) a '*restrictive*' type simulating constrictive pericarditis and (4) an '*obliterative*' type as in endomyocardial fibrosis which is a disorder confined to the tropics (p. 795) though eosinophilic myocarditis which occurs outside the tropics is very similar. Fibrotic tissue and thrombus obliterate the cavities of the left and right ventricles and may lead to mitral and tricuspid regurgitation. The cause of the disorder is unknown but nutritional or infective factors may contribute.

Arrhythmias occur in all types and are a common cause of death.

Cardiomyopathy should be considered whenever there is unexplained cardiomegaly or cardiac failure. The diagnosis is usually made only when the major causes of heart disease—rheumatic, hypertensive, ischaemic, thyrotoxic or congenital—have been excluded or when there is a generalised disorder of a type known to involve the heart.

**Treatment** remains unsatisfactory for the majority of cases for which the cause is not known and for which no specific therapy is available. A well-balanced diet is indicated in those cases in which a nutritional deficiency may be of aetiological importance and the avoidance of alcohol is essential if alcoholism is thought to be a provoking factor. Corticosteroid therapy is sometimes of value for cardiomyopathy due to sarcoidosis or associated with connective tissue disorders.

Cardiac failure must be treated and prolonged rest is necessary in resistant cases. $\beta$–receptor blockade or surgical resection of some of the hypertrophied septum is sometimes effective in relieving angina in the hypertrophic obstructive type but does not improve prognosis.

## Diseases of the Pericardium

### Pericarditis

There are numerous causes of acute pericarditis, the commonest being myocardial infarction and Coxsackie B viral infection. Rheumatic fever and tuberculosis are also important causes but both are now rare in Britain. Pericarditis may occur as a complication of bacterial infection and of malignant disease. Other causes include uraemia, trauma and connective tissue disorders such as systemic lupus erythematosus.

**Pathology.** Pericarditis may be fibrinous, serous, haemorrhagic or purulent. In the first there is a fibrinous exudate on the surface which leads to varying degrees of adhesion formation and hence to obliteration of the pericardial cavity. In serous pericarditis there is in addition a serous exudate of anything from a few ml to 2 litres. The effusion is straw-coloured and often slightly turbid with a high protein content. A haemorrhagic effusion suggests a malignant origin. Purulent pericarditis is due to a pyogenic infection and the effusion is rarely large.

**Clinical Features.** The characteristic pain of pericarditis is substernal and often radiates to the shoulders and neck. It may be present on, or be made worse by, a deep breath, movement, change of position, exercise or swallowing.

Friction is the diagnostic sign of pericarditis. It consists of a superficial scratching sound, best heard to the left of the lower sternum; it is usually systolic but may be audible also in diastole, sometimes with a pre-systolic accentuation. Friction is often better heard when the stethoscope diaphragm is pressed firmly upon the chest, the patient's breath being held for a time in expiration and for a time in inspiration.

If a pericardial effusion develops there is sometimes a sensation of substernal oppression. An effusion may be difficult to detect clinically but the heart sounds may become quieter; an effusion need not, as might be expected, abolish pericardial friction.

*Tamponade* refers to compression of the heart by a large or rapidly developing effusion which interferes with diastolic filling. The amount of fluid required to produce tamponade depends in part also on the compliance of the pericardium. Cardiac output and hence urinary flow may be reduced, the jugular venous pressure is usually increased and the blood pressure tends to fall; pulsus paradoxus (p. 147) may be found. The clinical picture of shock may develop.

Serial radiographs may show a rapid increase in the size of the cardiac shadow over days, or even hours and with a large effusion the heart may have a pear-shaped appearance. Echocardiography is particularly helpful in detecting a pericardial effusion. The ECG in acute pericarditis shows ST elevation with upward concavity over the affected area which may be widespread. Later there is inversion of T waves; with effusion the voltage is often reduced.

**Treatment, Course and Prognosis.** The pain can usually be relieved by aspirin but a more potent anti-inflammatory agent such as indomethacin may be required. Paracentesis of a pericardial effusion is rarely required but may have to be carried out for diagnostic purposes or to relieve severe symptoms from tamponade. The procedure is not without danger from puncture of a coronary vessel and should be carried out only when strictly necessary. The needle is best inserted to the left of the xiphoid process and insinuated deep to the left costal margin and then directed towards the left shoulder. Surgical drainage will usually be necessary on the rare occasions when pus is found.

Treatment, course and prognosis vary with the underlying disease.

*Viral pericarditis* often follows an upper respiratory infection and in about 10% of cases a Coxsackie viral infection can be established. Recovery usually occurs within a few weeks without after-effects but recurrences may follow and an occasional death has been reported. There is no specific treatment but corticosteroids may be helpful in accelerating recovery.

*Tuberculous pericarditis* may be secondary to manifest pulmonary or mediastinal tuberculosis, but the primary source may not be detectable. The disease sometimes begins with an acute febrile illness but is more commonly insidious in onset with vague malaise and low-grade fever. The subsequent course is chronic. An effusion usually develops and the pericardium may become thick and unyielding so that the heart is compressed. Pleural effusions are often associated.

The diagnosis may be confirmed by aspiration of the fluid and direct examination or culture for tubercle bacilli. Antituberculous chemotherapy is prescribed (p. 259). Aspiration may be carried out as required to relieve symptoms. Corticosteroids may prevent the development of constrictive pericarditis. In the inactive stage surgical relief may be necessary (p. 204).

*Purulent pericarditis* occurs rarely from direct spread from an intrathoracic infection, from septicaemia, or from a penetrating injury. It is now rare in Britain. Treatment is by surgical drainage and chemotherapy.

### Chronic Constrictive Pericarditis

Tuberculosis was formerly a frequent cause in Britain; some cases accompany rheumatoid disease (p. 608) and others follow a haemopericardium or, rarely, acute pericarditis. In many the cause is obscure. A slowly progressive fibrosis of the pericardium develops and constricts the movement of the heart, so that it cannot expand in diastole. The fibrous tissue is thick, dense and inelastic; calcification is common. The inflow of blood to the heart is impeded so that the cardiac output is diminished and the systemic venous pressure is increased with hepatic congestion, ascites and sometimes oedema. The heart is otherwise normal, though secondary atrophy of cardiac muscle occurs.

**Clinical Features.** Breathlessness is not a prominent symptom as the lungs are seldom congested. Raised jugular venous pressure is a notable feature. Enlargement of the liver and ascites occur relatively early compared with peripheral oedema.

The apical impulse may be difficult to feel and a third heart sound may be heard. The pulse is rapid and of small volume; there may be pulsus paradoxus (p. 147). There is usually a high plateau of venous pressure with a rapid and transitory *y* descent (Fig. 6.1). An important feature in most cases is the absence of much enlargement of the heart. This contrasts with almost all forms of cardiac failure. Atrial fibrillation occurs in about 30% of cases.

Calcification of the pericardium is frequently seen, particularly in lateral radiographs. Radioscopy may show a small 'quiet' heart with diminished pulsation.

**Treatment.** The problem is primarily a mechanical one and rapid improvement is usual if surgical resection of the pericardium is performed. However, it may take several months for maximum benefit to be obtained.

## Congenital Heart Disease

The incidence of congenital cardiac abnormalities is about 2% of live births. In most cases the cause of the abnormality is unknown, but some fetal defects are due to maternal infections in the early weeks of pregnancy, e.g. rubella. All degrees of severity occur. Many defects are not compatible with extrauterine life, or only for a short time. Early diagnosis is important because most types are amenable to surgical treatment. Infective endocarditis is a potential complication against which precautions must be taken.

Symptoms may be absent or consist principally of breathlessness and failure of development. Local signs vary with the anatomical lesion. Central cyanosis occurs when desaturated blood enters the systemic circulation. In the neonate the commonest cause of this is transposition of the great arteries in which the aorta derives from the right ventricle and the pulmonary artery from the left. In older children cyanosis is usually the consequence of a ventricular septal defect combined with severe pulmonary stenosis (tetralogy of Fallot) or with pulmonary vascular disease.

## Persistent Ductus Arteriosus

During fetal life, before the lungs begin to function, most of the blood from the pulmonary artery passes through the ductus arteriosus into the aorta just below the origin of the left subclavian artery. Normally the ductus closes soon after birth but sometimes it fails to do so. Since the pressure in the aorta is higher than that in the pulmonary artery there will be a continuous arteriovenous shunt, the volume of which depends on the size of the ductus (Fig. 6.28). As much as 50% of the left ventricular output may be recirculated through the lungs with a consequent increase in the work of the heart. The condition, which may be associated with other anomalies, is much commoner in females.

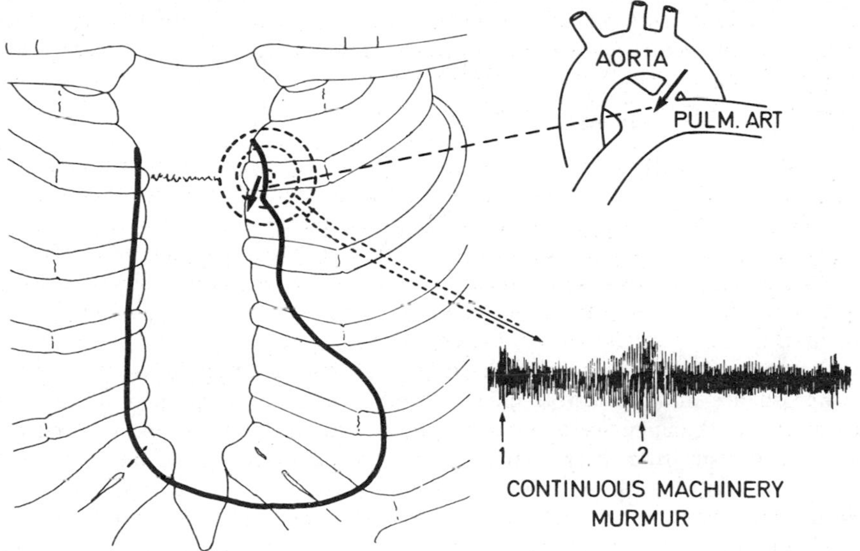


Fig. 6.28 Persistent ductus arteriosus.

With small shunts there may be no symptoms for many years but if the ductus is large, growth and development are retarded. There is usually no disability but cardiac failure may eventually ensue, dyspnoea being the first symptom. A continuous 'machinery' murmur is heard with late systolic accentuation, maximal at the second left rib near the sternum. It is frequently accompanied by a thrill. Enlargement of the pulmonary artery, but little enlargement of the heart, may be detected radiologically. The ECG is usually normal.

In uncomplicated cases, the ductus can be divided with little risk, especially in children, and there is general agreement that this should be carried out in all cases, preferably before the child goes to school. Few untreated patients live beyond the age of 40, death usually resulting from infective endocarditis or heart failure.

## Coarctation of the Aorta

Narrowing of the aorta occurs in the region where the ductus arteriosus joins the aorta, i.e. just below the origin of the left subclavian artery (Fig. 6.29). The condition is more common in males.

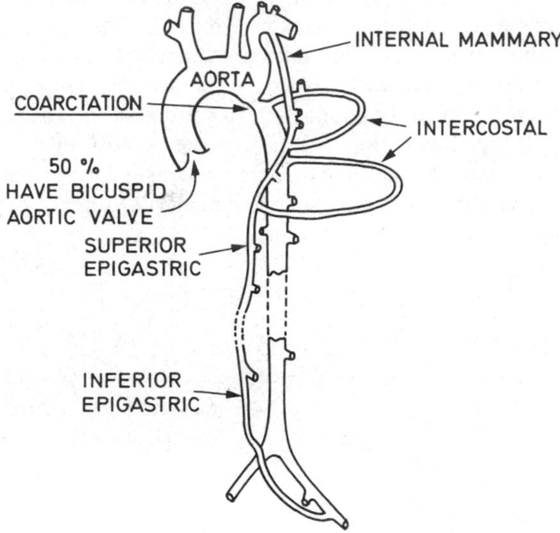


Fig. 6.29 Coarctation of the aorta.

Symptoms are often absent. Headaches and cardiac symptoms may occur from hypertension in the upper part of the body and occasionally weakness or cramps in the legs may result from decreased circulation in the lower part of the body. The blood pressure is raised in the arms but is normal or low in the legs. Unduly large arterial pulsations may be visible in the neck. The femoral pulses are weak and delayed after the radial. A systolic murmur is often present at the upper sternum but is usually loudest over the coarctation posteriorly. Evidence of collateral circulation is present in the older child and adult. Dilated, tortuous arteries may be visible or palpable around the scapulae and below the ribs posteriorly, especially if the patient bends forward.

Radiological examination in early childhood is often normal but at a later age may show changes in the contour of the aorta and notching of the under surface of the ribs from tortuous loops of enlarged intercostal arteries. The ECG may show left ventricular hypertrophy.

The constricted portion of the aorta can be resected and the divided ends of the aorta anastomosed. In untreated severe cases, death may occur from left ventricular failure, dissection of the aorta, cerebral haemorrhage or infection of the bicuspid aortic valve which is present in about half the patients.

## Atrial Septal Defect

Atrial septal defect is more common in females. Since the normal right ventricle is much more compliant than the left, a large volume of blood shunts through this defect from left to right atrium and thence to the right ventricle and pulmonary arteries (Fig. 6.30). As a result there is gradual enlargement of the right side of the heart and of the pulmonary artery and its main branches. In a few cases there may be a striking increase in the pulmonary vascular resistance causing pulmonary and right ventricular hypertension and sometimes reversal of the shunt.

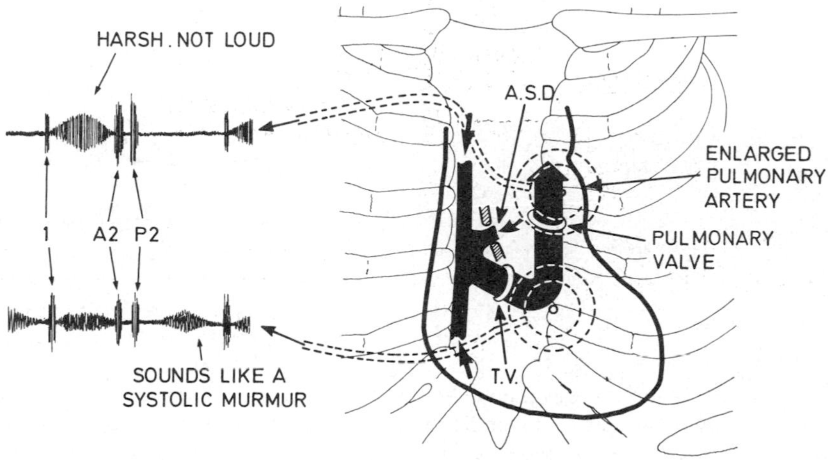


Fig. 6.30 Atrial septal defect.

There may be no symptoms for many years. Dyspnoea, cyanosis and cardiac failure develop in early adult life in most patients. The characteristic physical signs are (1) wide splitting of the second heart sound due to the increased right ventricular stroke volume and (2) pulmonary systolic and tricuspid diastolic murmurs due to increased flow. Enlargement of the pulmonary artery and its main branches is seen radiologically and a dynamic pulsation observed on the screen ('hilar dance') on radioscopy. The right ventricular enlargement can also be seen. The ECG shows incomplete right bundle branch block because depolarisation is prolonged as a result of dilatation of the right ventricle.

Surgical closure of a large defect should be carried out, preferably before the age of 10 years, following which the expectation of life is probably normal. Most patients used to die from cardiac failure.

## Ventricular Septal Defect

Since the pressure in the left ventricle is higher than that in the right ventricle, the shunt is normally from left to right (Fig. 6.31).

Usually there are no relevant symptoms. The characteristic signs are a harsh systolic murmur and thrill maximal in the fourth intercostal space to the left of the sternum. When the defect is small a murmur is the only abnormality; such defects often close

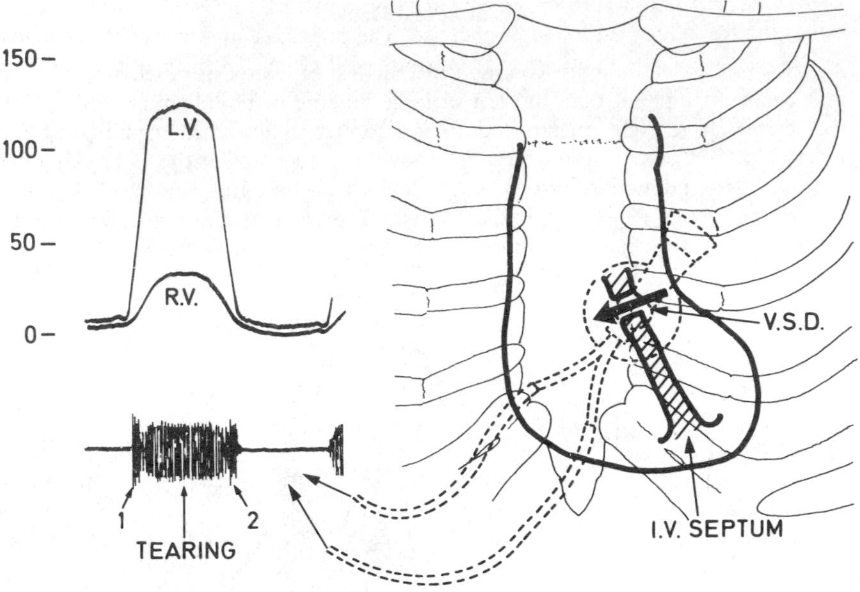


Fig. 6.31 Ventricular septal defect.

spontaneously. When there is a large shunt left ventricular failure may occur. Occasionally the pulmonary arteriolar resistance may increase to such an extent that the shunt reverses. Radiological and electrocardiographic examinations are normal except in the more severe cases when the heart is enlarged.

The defect can be repaired by open heart surgery. This is not necessary for small defects and is dangerous if there is a severe pulmonary hypertension. Surgical treatment is curative and should be used when the left to right shunt is large.

## Pulmonary Stenosis

Pulmonary stenosis may occur as an isolated anomaly in which case there is no cyanosis, or in association with an atrial or ventricular septal defect in which case there may or may not be cyanosis depending on the relative pressures on the two sides of the defect. Stenosis may occur at the level of the pulmonary valve or in the infundibular region of the right ventricle.

**Pulmonary Stenosis with Closed Interventricular Septum.** In many cases the stenosis is mild. In severe cases there may be dyspnoea, fatigue or, occasionally, syncope on exertion. The characteristic signs of pulmonary stenosis are present (p. 180). With slight stenosis, no treatment is necessary. When the stenosis is severe, pulmonary valvotomy should be carried out as sudden death or progressive cardiac failure may otherwise occur.

**Pulmonary Stenosis with Ventricular Septal Defect (Fallot's Tetralogy).** This is the most common form of cyanotic congenital heart disease in children or adults. The tetralogy comprises pulmonary stenosis, ventricular septal defect, dextroposition of the aorta which overrides this defect, and right ventricular hypertrophy (Fig. 6.32).

Dyspnoea and fatigue are the principal symptoms and the child characteristically assumes the squatting position after exercise. The principal signs are: central cyanosis; clubbing of the fingers; a loud systolic murmur, and often a thrill, maximal to the left of the upper sternum; soft pulmonary component of the second sound; enlargement of the right side of the heart; absence of the normal pulmonary artery curve on radiological examination.

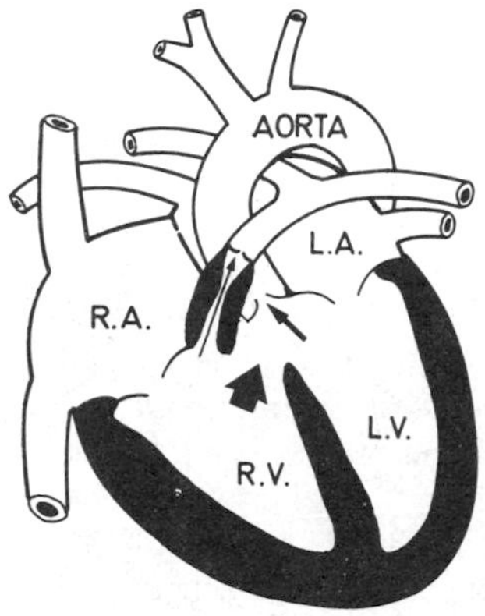


Fig. 6.32 Fallot's tetralogy. The stenosis is in the infundibulum of the right ventricle.

In infancy a palliative operation in the form of an anastomosis can be made either between the left or right pulmonary artery and the corresponding subclavian artery (Blalock's operation) or between the pulmonary artery and the aorta thereby increasing the blood supply to the lungs. Increasingly, total correction is carried out in infancy. This abolishes symptoms and restores life expectancy in most cases. Without surgical treatment few patients reach adult life.

## Surgery and Heart Disease

**The Surgical Treatment of Heart Disease.** Surgery is playing an increasingly important part in the management of heart disease; it is now possible, for example, to correct, to varying degrees, most types of congenital heart disease and to alleviate many cases of rheumatic and ischaemic heart disease.

Some operations, such as mitral valvotomy and the correction of coarctation, can be performed under normal circulatory conditions with blood continuing to flow through the heart. Most procedures, however, require an open heart so that the circulation must be temporarily occluded (open-heart surgery). In such cases, adequate time for intracardiac surgery can be obtained by the use of an extracorporeal circulation (bypass surgery). With this technique, venous blood is drained from the great veins into a reservoir and is then passed through an oxygenator before being pumped back into the aorta. The heart can then be stopped for several hours whilst an adequate circulation is maintained to the other vital organs. The mortality of bypass surgery should be less than 1% but patients subjected to this procedure are at risk from several hazards, including cerebral air embolism, trauma to the blood from the pump oxygenator and electrolyte and acid-base disturbances. The lungs may become abnormally rigid in the postoperative phase and pulmonary infection is common.

In certain types of disorder, such as persistent ductus arteriosus and atrial septal defect, complete correction can be achieved. In other cases, for example some instances of ventricular septal defect and coarctation of the aorta, prosthetic materials may be needed to effect the repair. In some cases of mitral stenosis a satisfactory result may be obtained by valvotomy. In most forms of mitral disease the valve must be replaced either by a prosthesis or a graft. Although results on the whole are satisfactory with prosthetic valves, they are liable to lead to complications which include thromboembolism and haemolysis. Because of the risk of thrombosis, patients with prosthetic valves are usually kept on long-term anticoagulant therapy. Grafts are usually of animal origin (heterograft); the risks of haemolysis and thrombosis are slight but the long-term results remain uncertain.

**Surgery in Patients with Heart Disease.** Patients with heart disease undergoing surgery are at risk from the anaesthetic and from the surgery itself. Skilled anaesthesia is particularly important and an appropriate anaesthetic should be chosen to take account of the nature of the cardiac abnormality and operation being undertaken. Thus, induction may be dangerous particularly when intravenous barbiturates are used; a fall in blood pressure is particularly undesirable.

On the whole, patients with heart disease tolerate surgery remarkably well. Exceptions to this rule are patients with recent myocardial infarction and those who have cardiac or respiratory failure. Only in exceptional circumstances should patients be operated on within 3 months of myocardial infarction; cardiac and respiratory failure should be brought under control before operation if possible. If heart block is present, a pacemaker should be inserted prior to surgery.

Hypertension is usually not a contraindication to surgery, but it is necessary for the anaesthetist to be aware of what antihypertensive therapy is being used as excessive hypotension may result from such drugs as adrenergic blocking agents.

In some patients it is better to defer surgery until the heart disease has been corrected or ameliorated. Thus, elective general surgery should be deferred until after mitral valvotomy, if this is indicated. On the other hand, if the cardiac surgery necessitates long-term anticoagulants it may be preferable to undertake general surgery first.

## Heart Disease in Pregnancy

Pregnancy leads to increases of blood volume and cardiac output of up to 50%. In the early weeks of pregnancy, this is probably mainly a consequence of endocrine activity. Subsequently, the increasing demands of the fetus and the arteriovenous shunt in the uterus are the main contributory factors. These changes produce characteristic physical signs. The extremities feel warm and the pulse is of large volume. Tachycardia is present and there may be a rise in venous pressure. The arterial diastolic pressure is lower than in the non-pregnant state because of vasodilation. The heart may be slightly enlarged and may be displaced outwards because of the high diaphragm. A pulmonary systolic murmur due to high flow is usual and there may also be a physiological third heart sound.

The increased load on the heart often provokes or worsens symptoms in patients with heart disease. These do not usually occur before about the 12th week and tend to become maximal from the 24th week onwards. The main symptom of heart disease in pregnancy is breathlessness but oedema may also occur. Angina is very unusual. Symptoms are a poor guide to the severity of the heart disease as some patients are totally asymptomatic until they develop acute pulmonary oedema in late pregnancy or shortly after delivery.

The commonest major form of heart disease encountered in pregnancy is mitral stenosis; other valvular lesions are not uncommon but seldom give rise to problems. Pregnancy should be deferred in patients with severe mitral stenosis, but it is usually safe after valvotomy has been performed. If a patient with advanced mitral stenosis does become pregnant, either valvotomy or termination should be carried out before the 16th week. With less serious degrees of mitral stenosis and with other forms of heart disease, pregnancy can be allowed to continue and in most cases is uncomplicated. However, if objective evidence of deterioration is taking place, bed rest must be enforced, combined if necessary with digitalis and diuretics. With careful management, even those with advanced heart disease can be carried successfully through pregnancy and delivery.

Patients with congenital heart disease are being seen with increasing frequency during pregnancy, but usually the lesion has been corrected beforehand. In most cases, no problems arise but pregnancy is a formidable hazard in those who have pulmonary vascular disease in association with congenital heart disease and it is usually wise to terminate the pregnancy early.

# DISEASES OF ARTERIES AND VEINS

For clinical purposes it is convenient to classify arterial disease under the general headings of degenerative, inflammatory and vasospastic causes.

## Degenerative Arterial Disease

**Arteriosclerosis** is a term which in the past has been applied rather indiscriminately to various unrelated forms of arterial disease. Its retention is justified only if it is confined to the degenerative changes which are part of the usual ageing process and which affect the whole arterial tree.

*Medial or Mönckeberg's sclerosis* is the name given to degenerative changes which occur in old age in the muscular coats of medium sized arteries such as the radial. Calcification of the media is the characteristic change and accounts for the 'pipe stem' arteries so commonly palpable in the elderly and of little clinical significance. Since the medium and large vessels are mainly affected and their lumina are not greatly reduced in size, clinical features are usually absent.

**Atherosclerosis** is a condition which principally affects the aorta, large and medium-sized vessels, particularly the coronary and cerebral arteries. It becomes increasingly common as age advances, but it is not an inevitable concomitant of ageing, and there is a great variation in its extent and severity. Although often associated with and accelerated by hypertension, atherosclerosis may be advanced even in the presence of a normal blood pressure. It may also occur in response to a persistent elevation of pressure in the pulmonary arteries.

The basic atheromatous lesion is the plaque, the most important constituents of which are cholesterol and other lipids which may be free in the intimal tissues or intracellular. At a later stage the plaque becomes sclerosed and calcified. Thrombosis is liable to occur on the surface of the plaque, particularly if it ulcerates. Embolism is frequent.

### Atherosclerosis Obliterans

This condition affects males more commonly than females and usually after the age of 50. It is particularly common in diabetics and is rare in non-smokers.

**Clinical Features.** These are usually confined to the lower limbs. The principal symptoms which follow impairment of blood supply to the extremities are (1) pain, which occurs on exercise (intermittent claudication) and (2) cold extremities. Although the pathological changes are usually present in both lower limbs, symptoms commonly present first on one side.

Intermittent claudication appears on walking and is rapidly relieved by rest. It most commonly occurs in the calf and causes the patient to limp or stop. Pain occurs at rest with severe ischaemia. Pain which is relieved by elevation of the part suggests venous obstruction, and pain which is relieved by dependency suggests gross arterial obstruction.

Ischaemia may lead to dryness, scaling and inelasticity of the skin, loss of hair, brittle nails, ulceration or gangrene. There may be a change of colour of the skin and delay in the return of colour after blanching with light finger pressure. Ulceration or gangrene may occur. Where gross lesions are present in one limb, the lower temperature is appreciable to the touch. If the ischaemic limb is first raised 75 degrees above the horizontal, it will blanch more quickly than normal. If then placed in the dependent position, there will be delay in flushing and in venous filling.

Loss of pulsation of one or more peripheral arteries is a common and important feature of arterial disease; bruits may be heard over the larger arteries if they are partially obstructed.

Patients seldom die from peripheral vascular disease but frequently succumb to myocardial infarction.

**Investigation.** A radiograph may show calcification. This is especially common in Mönckeberg's sclerosis but does not necessarily indicate that the arterial lumen is significantly narrowed. Intra-arterial injection of a radio-opaque dye will show the site of vascular occlusion and the extent of any collateral circulation. Where there are good facilities for arteriography, reactive hyperaemia and oscillometry are now little used. Research techniques include the use of ultrasonic blood flow detectors, clearance measurements using isotopes, and electromagnetic metering.

**Treatment.** Until the pathogenesis of atherosclerosis has been clearly established and until specific therapy is discovered the treatment of peripheral vascular disease must continue to be unsatisfactory. Diabetes or obesity may require attention. The patient may need help in getting rid of the tobacco habit.

Cold should be avoided and suitable woollen clothing worn, especially on the limbs. The application of heat to the affected limb is harmful because it increases local metabolism in the ischaemic area without improving blood flow. Pain at rest may be reduced by raising the head of the bed or by lowering the limb below the horizontal and keeping it cool.

Protection against trauma and the early treatment of sepsis are most important. Fungal infection between the toes should be treated. Detailed instructions on the care of the feet and nails must be given. The feet should be kept scrupulously clean, carefully dried after washing, especially between the toes, and dusting powder containing zinc oxide and salicylic acid applied. Nails should be cut carefully and corns pared with caution. It is wise to employ the services of a chiropodist. Socks and shoes should be well fitting. Even the slightest abrasion should be taken seriously and medical advice sought. Dressings to keep the part dry are required for any breach of the surface.

Regular exercise encourages the development of collateral vessels. Patients should not be alarmed by the development of pain and they should be encouraged to believe that with exercise and the stopping of smoking improvement is expected and that the occurrence of gangrene is improbable. Vasodilators are not recommended as they act by dilating normal vessels elsewhere and may divert blood from the affected site.

Areas of gangrene should be kept clean and dry until a clear line of demarcation appears. Thereafter surgical treatment may be required. Sympathectomy may be of value when the limb is cold or rest pain is present but it seldom helps claudication. Direct arterial surgery is indicated for disabling claudication, rest pain or gangrene provided the vessels are shown by arteriography to be suitable.

### Sudden Occlusion of a Major Artery

This is usually due to embolism from the heart as a result of rheumatic heart disease, myocardial infarction or, rarely, an atrial myxoma. Emboli lodge commonly at the aortic, iliac or popliteal bifurcations. The limb becomes painful, cold, numb and pale, and pulses distal to the block are absent. The outcome depends on the collateral circulation and on subsequent treatment. Pain should be relieved and the limb kept at rest and exposed to room temperature. The other limbs and the body should be kept warm and reflex vasodilation encouraged by an electric blanket or hot-water bottles applied to the trunk. Embolectomy is usually necessary when a major limb artery is occluded.

### Atherosclerosis and Aneurysm Formation

Atherosclerosis is frequently present in the aorta but seldom affects its function. It may, however, be responsible for aneurysms of any part of this vessel. An aneurysm in the ascending portion is usually due to tertiary syphilis and may cause pain because of erosion of the ribs or sternum; a pulsating mass may occasionally be visible. An aneurysm of the arch of the aorta may produce hoarseness from pressure on the left recurrent laryngeal nerve. Aneurysms of the abdominal aorta are generally due to atherosclerosis; their rupture leads usually to sudden death. The results of resection and replacement with a graft are improving and operation is therefore more frequently performed.

**Dissecting Aneurysm of the Aorta.** In this condition a tear occurs through the intima secondary to degeneration of the media. As a result blood makes its way in a split in the media to form a new channel. Death usually occurs from rupture through the adventitia into the pericardium, pleural cavity or elsewhere. Most patients have been hypertensive. There is an increased risk of aortic dissection in pregnancy and in patients with *Marfan's syndrome*, a connective tissue disorder characterised by long, thin extremities, a high arched palate and subluxation of the lens.

The onset of dissection is sudden with severe, tearing, chest pain which often radiates into the neck, abdomen, legs or back of the chest. It may be precipitated by exertion and may simulate or include myocardial infarction. Neurological features may result from occlusion of branches of the aorta supplying the spinal cord. One or more of the peripheral pulses may be obliterated.

Diagnosis is suggested by the sudden onset of the characteristic pain and the absence of the ECG and enzyme abnormalities of myocardial infarction unless the dissection includes a coronary artery. The chest radiograph may be helpful in showing a broadened mediastinum due to widening of the aorta. Aortography is required for precise assessment.

In the initial stages the blood pressure, if high, should be lowered by antihypertensive drugs to normal levels. Surgical treatment is usually necessary later.

## Inflammatory Arterial Disease

The principal types of inflammatory arterial disease are syphilitic aortitis, polyarteritis nodosa, thromboangiitis, obliterans cranial (giant cell) arteritis and Takayasu's syndrome (pulseless disease).

**Syphilitic aortitis** is now very rare in Britain. There is often a latent period of 15 to 20 years following an infection before clinical manifestations are evident in the cardiovascular system. Neurosyphilis sometimes coexists.

The disease begins just above the aortic valve cusps. In the adventitia there is infiltration of lymphocytes and plasma cells round the vasa vasorum, which are obliterated by intimal proliferation. Elastic tissue is gradually replaced by fibrous tissue and this leads to dilatation of the aorta. Proliferation of the intima occurs and may involve the mouths of the coronary arteries leading to myocardial ischaemia, or spread along the valve cusps which become thickened, everted and incompetent.

The diagnosis is difficult in the early uncomplicated stages. Suspicion may be aroused by an aortic systolic murmur, together with accentuation of the second sound. Later there are the characteristic signs of aortic regurgitation but the diastolic murmur is more commonly best heard to the right of the sternum. Dilatation and calcification of the ascending aorta may be demonstrated by radiological examination. The diagnosis is confirmed by serological tests (p. 66).

If adequate antisyphilitic therapy is given in the early stages of the infection cardiovascular manifestations in later life are prevented. Treatment of syphilitic aortitis consists of a course of procaine penicillin (p. 66). If cardiac failure is present this should first be controlled. Surgical treatment may be indicated for aortic regurgitation or aneurysm.

**Thromboangiitis obliterans** (*Buerger's disease*) is an uncommon condition of obscure origin. It usually begins before the age of 40 and is almost confined to males who smoke heavily. The lower limbs are principally affected. The wall of the artery is infiltrated with polymorphs and the lumen may be obstructed by thrombus. The adjacent vein is often involved.

The symptoms and signs are essentially those of diminished blood supply to the limb; persistent pain in a cold, cyanosed toe is often the presenting complaint. This is followed by intermittent claudication and rest pain. In the leg, atrophic changes and finally gangrene may develop. Involvement of the veins may cause recurrent thrombophlebitis.

There is no specific treatment but it is essential that cigarette smoking is stopped.

**Polyarteritis nodosa** is an uncommon condition most often seen in men between the ages of 20 and 50 and thought to have an immunological basis. The characteristic lesions consist of multiple nodules on the smaller arteries. The vessel wall is infiltrated by polymorphs and necrosis follows with resultant aneurysmal dilatation. Thrombosis may occur.

Clinical features such as fever, tachycardia, wasting, sweating and generalised pain are accompanied by local manifestations of ischaemia in various parts of the body. The vessels of the kidney, gastrointestinal tract, heart, peripheral nerves and skin are particularly affected giving rise to such varied manifestations as haematuria, abdominal pain, angina, myocardial infarction, pericarditis, peripheral neuropathy, subcutaneous nodules or localised oedema. Involvement of the lungs may cause asthma. There may be leucocytosis or eosinophilia. Hypertension is common.

The course is usually progressive although mild cases may recover. There is no curative treatment, but corticosteroids, administered before vascular damage is extensive, may produce a remission.

**Cranial or giant cell arteritis** is a panarteritis of medium-sized vessels affecting elderly persons. The cause of the disease is unknown; it is related to polymyalgia rheumatica (p. 634).

The vessel wall is infiltrated by mononuclear cells, plasma cells and giant cells. Thrombosis may occur. The temporal arteries are usually affected and may be thickened and tender. Other arteries may also be involved, notably the ophthalmic and cerebral.

Intense headache is usual and blindness may occur. Other manifestations include fever, pain and stiffness of hips and shoulders, weakness and loss of weight. Spontaneous recovery usually occurs after several months but cranial arteritis responds promptly to prednisolone; at least 50 mg daily should be given initially because of the risk of blindness; the dose is then reduced to the minimum for control of symptoms.

**Takayasu's syndrome** known also as *pulseless disease* and the *aortic arch syndrome*, is rare except in some communities, e.g. Japan. It predominantly affects young females. An arteritis of unknown origin involves the aortic arch with narrowing of its major branches. The pulses are diminished or absent in the upper extremities, neck and head. Headache, syncope, visual disturbance and muscular wasting may occur. The prognosis is poor but corticosteroids are sometimes of value.

## Vasospastic Disorders

**Raynaud's disease** is the name given to a peripheral vascular disturbance consisting of spasmodic contraction of the digital arteries, which is precipitated by cold, emotion and by other causative factors mentioned below. Primary Raynaud's disease is commonest in young women and is an exaggerated physiological response to cold. Secondary Raynaud's disease or phenomenon occurs in (1) disorders of connective tissue, especially systemic sclerosis, (2)obliterative arterial disease, (3) occupations in which the hands are exposed to vibration e.g. from pneumatic drills, or (4) occasionally from cold agglutinins and cryoglobulins. In the early, uncomplicated stages there are no pathological changes. Later, obliterative endarteritis may occur and result in thrombosis, ischaemic changes in the skin of the digits and nails, superficial necrosis and finally gangrene.

The disorder is usually bilateral and fingers are more affected than toes. Numbness, tingling and burning are more prominent than pain. Sensitivity to cold may be extreme and disabling. Colour changes usually consist of three phases; pallor, cyanosis and redness. If the limb is bloodless it will be pale. If blood flow is sluggish, excessive deoxygenation results in cyanosis. Redness is in some cases due to reactive hyperaemia which may follow the vasospasm.

Any primary disease should be treated and protection from cold is obviously indicated. Cigarette smoking should be stopped. In severe cases, sympathectomy, to remove vasomotor tone, should be considered; the long-term results are poor in the arms but fairly good in the legs.

## Venous Thrombosis

A distinction may be made between *thrombophlebitis* when the endothelium is injured by inflammation, and *phlebothrombosis* when thrombosis is the primary disturbance. The latter is the more common condition and carries a much greater risk of pulmonary embolism.

**Aetiology.** The following factors are of importance:

1. *Slowing or Obstruction of the Blood Stream.* This may result from rest in bed, particularly if a pillow is placed under the knees, especially in the elderly or from unduly prolonged sitting, e.g. in journeys by air. Cardiac failure also leads to slowing of the circulation.
2. *Injury to the Vein.* This may be due to trauma and may follow accidents, operations, childbirth, intravenous infusions or injections.
3. *Increased Coagulability of the Blood.* Many factors may disturb the dynamic equilibrium which normally exists between coagulation and fibrinolysis, notably an increase in platelet adhesiveness. This may occur for example in malignant disease or with the use of oral contraceptives. An increased liability to thrombosis also occurs in dehydration and polycythaemia due to an increase in the blood viscosity.

**Pathology.** At first the thrombus consists mainly of dense layers of platelets and fibrin; later it is a loose, friable, jelly-like mass of fibrin and red cells which readily becomes detached to form an embolus. After a few days inflammatory changes occur in the wall of the vein. The thrombus may undergo lysis or organisation.

Venous thrombosis is most common in the lower limbs, particularly in the venous sinuses of the soleus muscle in the calf and in the femoral and iliac veins. It is much less frequent in the upper limb but the axillary vein may be involved as a complication of trauma, neoplasm or radiotherapy. Superficial thrombophlebitis most commonly occurs in the saphenous vein, particularly if there are associated varicosities.

Suppurative thrombophlebitis is a rare but very serious condition usually involving the veins of the pelvis following sepsis.

Tropical phlebitis is described on page 796.

**Clinical Features.** The patient may complain of pain in the calf but the process is often silent and undiagnosed. An unexplained slight pyrexia may be the only warning. If the lumen of a main vein is occluded, there is dilatation of the superficial veins, the skin may be warm and pink and there may be oedema at the ankle. In extensive occlusive iliofemoral thrombosis the whole lower limb is swollen and white if the collateral channels remain patent. If the collaterals are also occluded, the leg is blue—a pregangrenous condition. In contrast there may be no sign in the presence of an extensive non-occlusive, potentially lethal thrombus. Pulmonary embolism is frequently the first clinical manifestation of venous thrombosis.

The most certain way of establishing the diagnosis is by phlebography. The veins from the ankle to the inguinal ligament can be demonstrated by ascending lower limb phlebography. Percutaneous iliofemoral phlebography may also be required. Ultrasound is used to assess the patency of deep veins in patients who present with a swollen leg or with pulmonary embolism. The uptake of $^{123}$ I labelled fibrinogen is used for the early detection of thrombosis, for example post-operatively; it has the advantage of being non-invasive but is less reliable than phlebography, particularly for the detection of thrombosis in the pelvic and common femoral veins.

**Prevention.** Efforts must chiefly be directed to the avoidance of venous stasis. This is easiest in surgical patients when the period of risk can be defined. Almost all post-operative thromboses begin during or within 72 hours of operation. Early ambulation should be encouraged after surgery and medical illnesses. This means more than simply transferring the patient from lying in bed to sitting in a chair. Active exercises should be prescribed and at other times the leg should be elevated. A graduated elastic support should be worn if the patient is at particular risk. If confinement to bed is unavoidable, the patient should be encouraged to move the lower limbs frequently. In hospital, exercises can be organised under the supervision of a physiotherapist. Faulty posture in bed must be corrected, constricting bandages avoided and cardiac failure and dehydration should receive attention.

For patients at particular risk other prophylactic measures include low dose subcutaneous heparin or intravenous dextran 70.

**Treatment** aims at preventing the propagation of thrombus and pulmonary embolism, damage to the valves of the vein and chronic venous insufficiency. Unless there is an obvious contraindication, such as active peptic ulceration or a bleeding surface as after prostatectomy, treatment is initiated with heparin and continued with warfarin (p. 600). Thrombolytic therapy with streptokinase is expensive but can be considered for iliofemoral thrombosis. Thrombectomy may occasionally be required for a recent non-occlusive thrombosis at this site.

The legs should be elevated to 15 degrees and physiotherapy commenced after 48 hours. Straining at stool often causes separation of venous thrombi and should be avoided. The venous flow is accelerated by the support of graduated elastic hose but care must be taken to avoid a constricting effect by the hose rolling up. The ambulant woman should wear elastic support tights and for men knee-length elastic hose is best. Support of this kind will probably be necessary permanently after a severe thrombosis to control chronic venous insufficiency. Superficial thrombophlebitis usually responds to an elastic support and phenylbutazone (200 mg t.i.d. for 6 days).

## Prospects in Cardiology

Some fetal abnormalities, such as Down's syndrome, which carry an increased risk of congenital heart disease can now be recognised antenatally (p. 21). Under these circumstances therapeutic abortion can for the first time result in a reduced incidence of congenital heart disease.

In regard to investigative procedures, cardiac biopsy is acceptably safe and provides tissue for microscopic and ultramicroscopic examination which is of occasional use in the diagnosis of myocardial diseases. Twenty-four to forty-eight hour portable ECG recordings, particularly where computer analysis is available, will continue to refine the management of arrhythmias.

Studies in cardiac metabolism and pharmacokinetics will further improve the understanding of myocardial function. The uses of calcium blocking agents for angina and vasodilators for resistant cardiac failure and other purposes are being investigated, notably captropril, an oral inhibitor of angiotensin converting enzyme.

Coronary bypass surgery offers improved vascularisation of the heart and usually good symptomatic benefit. Enthusiasm for it is such that in 1979 an estimated 80 000 operations for aorta-coronary saphenous vein bypass graft were performed in the United States. Doubt remains about the effect of such procedures on the prognosis but it seems likely that further studies will confirm that, for stenosis of the left main coronary artery at least, the outlook is definitely improved. The European controlled trial of coronary bypass surgery supports this view but such trials inevitably suffer from the problem of variation in surgical skills at different centres. Cardiac transplantation will no doubt continue to be in the news but offers expensive and unreliable help to only a miniscule proportion of patients with heart disease untreatable by other methods.

Already in the United States health measures such as reduction in smoking appear to be having an effect in reducing the impact of coronary artery disease though there is not yet much sign of this in Britain.

In the management of hypertension, poor case discovery, inadequate explanation of the aims of blood pressure control and unreliable patient compliance particularly when the disease is asymptomatic, all provide major challenges urgently requiring solutions.

D. G. JULIAN
M. B. MATTHEWS

*Further reading*:

Julian, D. G. (1979) *Cardiology*, 3rd edn. London: Baillière Tindall — An introduction to cardiology for the non-specialist.

Matthews, M. B. (1979) Examination of the cardiovascular system. In *Clinical Examination*, 5th edn, ed., Macleod. J. Edinburgh: Churchill Livingstone.

Report of a Joint Working Party of the Royal College of Physicians of London and the British Cardiac Society (1976) Prevention of coronary heart disease. *Journal of the Royal College of Physicians,* **10**, 213.— An expert committee considers all the risk factors.

Resnekov, L. & Julian D.G. (eds) (1981) *Friedberg: Diseases of the Heart*. Edinburgh: Churchill Livingstone.— A comprehensive reference book.

# 7. Diseases of the Respiratory System

## Anatomy

The *upper respiratory tract*, which includes the nose, nasopharynx and larynx, is lined by vascular mucous membrane. The rich blood supply ensures that the inspired air enters the lungs at body temperature and fully saturated with water vapour. The whole respiratory epithelium down to the terminal bronchioles is equipped with cilia, which, aided by the layer of sticky mucus covering them, have the important function of trapping foreign particles and bacteria, and propelling them towards the pharynx. They contribute to the prevention of respiratory infection, as do the alveolar macrophages by means of their secretory, phagocytic and bactericidal activity.

The maxillary, frontal, ethmoidal and sphenoidal *nasal sinuses* communicate with the nasopharynx by narrow openings and are frequently involved in upper respiratory infections. Adequate drainage of infected sinuses is often prevented by inflammatory oedema of the mucosa lining their narrow openings: as a result, resolution of sinus infection is often slow and sometimes incomplete.

The *larynx*, in addition to being the organ of voice production, has the function of preventing particles larger than can be dealt with by the cilia from reaching the lower respiratory tract. Together with the bronchi, the larynx is supplied with vagal receptors, which form the sensory side of the cough reflex and perhaps also of reflexes concerned with bronchoconstriction. The larynx is often involved in disease, particularly infection. It is sometimes obstructed by oedema or exudate, or by an impacted foreign body. Laryngeal paralysis is usually due to a lesion of the recurrent laryngeal branch of the vagus nerve. As the left recurrent laryngeal nerve runs part of its course within the thoracic cavity, in close proximity to the aortic arch and the left pulmonary hilum, a bronchial carcinoma in the left hilar region and, less frequently, an aortic aneurysm may cause paralysis of the left vocal cord. Paralysis of the right vocal cord is rare, most cases being due to an aneurysm of the right subclavian artery.

The *trachea* begins at the cricoid cartilage and ends at the level of the sternal angle by bifurcation into the two *main bronchi*. The trachea is usually palpable in the suprasternal notch, where in normal subjects it is exactly in the midline. Deviation of the trachea to either side, in the absence of a local lesion in the neck, is a valuable indication of displacement of the upper mediastinum.

The *right main bronchus* is more vertical than the left, with the result that a foreign body entering the trachea is more likely to lodge in that bronchus or one of its divisions than the left. The right main bronchus first gives off from its lateral wall the upper lobe bronchus and then from its anterior wall the middle lobe bronchus, after which it continues as the lower lobe bronchus. The left main bronchus gives off the upper lobe bronchus from its lateral wall and continues as the lower lobe bronchus.

The three lobar bronchi on the right side and the two on the left divide and subdivide like the branches of a tree (the term 'bronchial tree' is in common use) until the terminal bronchioles are reached. The portion of lung supplied by a terminal bronchiole is called an acinus, which is the basic functional unit of lung tissue. Each acinus contains branching respiratory bronchioles communicating with clusters of alveoli. The alveoli are lined by a single layer of flattened epithelial cells which are in direct contact with the pulmonary capillaries. Exchange of the respiratory gases, oxygen and carbon dioxide, takes place between the air in the alveoli and the blood in the pulmonary capillaries.

The *left lung* differs from the right in having two lobes instead of three. The left lung is divided into upper and lower lobes by the oblique fissure which extends from the junction of the fourth or fifth rib with the vertebral column behind to the sixth costochondral junction in front, crossing the midaxillary line at the level of the fifth rib. As the posterior end of the fissure is at a much higher level than its anterior end, the upper lobe, as well as being above the lower lobe, is also largely in front of it. It therefore follows that upper lobe lesions produce physical signs mainly on the front of the chest and lower lobe lesions on the back.

On the *right* side the oblique fissure corresponds in position to that on the left, but the lung above it is divided into *upper* and *middle lobes* by the *transverse fissure*, which runs laterally in a horizontal direction from the junction of the fourth costal cartilage with the sternum to join the oblique fissure at the level of the fifth rib in the midaxillary line. The middle lobe is thus situated behind the lower part of the anterior chest wall. Each lobe is composed of two or more *bronchopulmonary segments*, which represent the portions of lung tissue supplied by the main branches of each lobar bronchus. The situation of the various lobes and segments is shown in Figure 7.1.

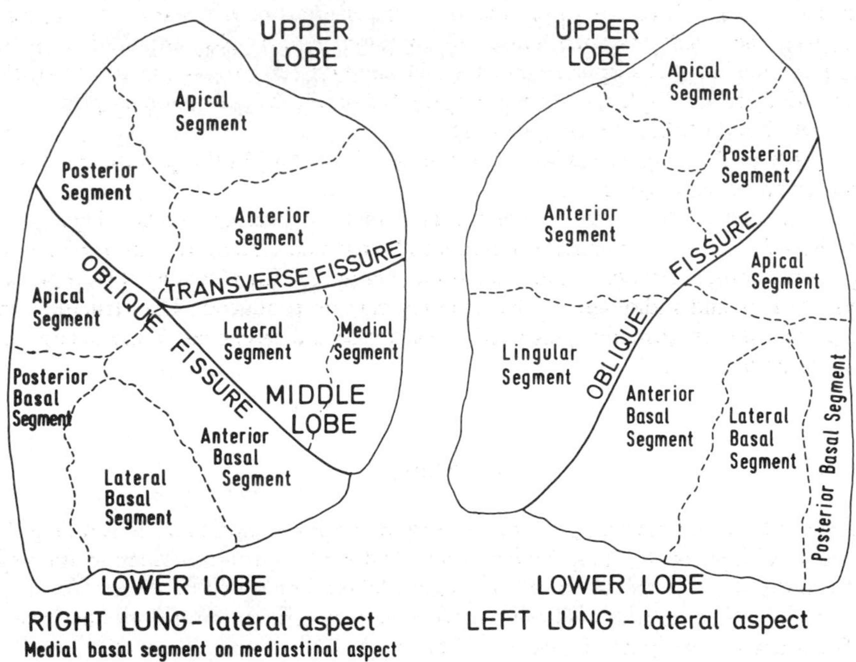


Fig. 7.1 The lobes and segments of the lungs.

In many diseases, e.g. pneumococcal pneumonia, collapse and lung abscess, the lesion is typically confined to a single lobe or segment. A knowledge of pulmonary anatomy, when applied to the interpretation of radiographs, is thus of value in determining the nature of the lesion as well as its situation.

Each lung is closely invested with *visceral pleura*. *Parietal pleura* lines the chest wall, mediastinum and diaphragm, and is continuous with the visceral pleura at the pulmonary hilum. In health the two pleural layers are separated only by a thin film of lymph, but between them there is a negative (subatmospheric) pressure. This results from the natural tendency of the lung to recoil towards the hilum, a property related to the rich supply of elastic fibres in the bronchi, blood vessels and lung parenchyma.

If a communication develops with the atmosphere as, for example, with a penetrating wound of the chest wall or from the rupture of an emphysematous bulla, the negative intrapleural pressure draws air between the pleural layers and the potential intrapleural space becomes a real one. There is then said to be a pneumothorax. When the space is created by the presence of serous fluid there is said to be a pleural effusion or a hydrothorax; by pus, an empyema; by blood, a haemothorax; by both serous fluid and air, a hydropneumothorax; by both pus and air, a pyopneumothorax; and by both blood and air, a haemopneumothorax.

When the pleural space contains air or fluid the elastic recoil of the underlying lung is to some extent released and the lung shrinks towards the hilum, this shrinkage being referred to as *pulmonary collapse*. The larger the amount of air or fluid between the pleural layers the more marked is the degree of pulmonary collapse and the greater the impairment of function of the collapsed lung. If the quantity of air or fluid is very large it causes displacement of the mediastinum towards the opposite side, with the result that function of the opposite lung is also impaired. A gross degree of mediastinal displacement may, in addition, embarrass the action of the heart. Mediastinal displacement is recognised clinically by alteration in position of the trachea and of the cardiac apex beat.

Collapse of the lung may also occur without air or fluid in the pleural space as a result of bronchial obstruction.

The anatomy of the *mediastinum* has an important bearing on the diagnosis of intrathoracic disease, particularly tumours and aneurysms. These lesions are liable to involve mediastinal structures and, as a result, certain readily recognisable symptoms, physical signs and radiological abnormalities may be produced. The structures involved and the abnormality produced in each case are discussed in the section on mediastinal tumours.

## Physiology

Knowledge of the normal processes of respiration is of value in understanding the effects of disease on the lungs and airways, and is of great importance in therapy. Oxygen therapy, the treatment of ventilatory failure and much of the treatment of chronic bronchitis and asthma have a rational basis in applied respiratory physiology.

The aspects of the physiology of respiration which merit special attention are:

1. *Ventilation*, which includes (*a*) the mechanical processes of inspiration and expiration and (*b*) the control of ventilation at a level appropriate to metabolic needs.
2. *Perfusion* of the lungs by the output of the right ventricle.
3. *Distribution* of ventilation and perfusion within the lungs.
4. *Diffusion* of oxygen and carbon dioxide between the terminal airways, the alveoli and the pulmonary capillary blood.

In a typical normal adult at rest the normal pulmonary blood flow of 5 *l*/min carries 11 mmol/min (250 ml/min) of oxygen from the lungs to the tissues and normal ventilation of about 6 *l*/min carries 9 mmol/min (200 ml/min) of carbon dioxide out of the body. The pressures of oxygen and carbon dioxide in the arterial blood are closely controlled. The normal range of $Po_2$ is 11–13 kPa (83–98 mmHg) and of $Pco_2$ 4·8–6 kPa (36–45 mmHg). Observation of changes in these pressures in disease is of importance in assessing the nature and severity of any disturbance of lung function (p. 227).

## Ventilation

The respiratory muscles, in ventilating the lungs, do mechanical work of two kinds, elastic and non-elastic. The first is performed against elastic forces in the lungs and chest wall which together tend to bring the chest to the position it occupies at the end of a normal expiration. Movement of the chest from this position of equilibrium involves the performance of elastic work and the storage of kinetic energy which is later available for non-elastic work during the return to the resting position. This second kind of work is largely expended in overcoming the resistance of the airways to the inspiratory and expiratory flow of air and to a smaller extent in displacing soft and inelastic tissues. Most of the resistance in normal subjects lies in the large central airways. The peripheral airways, although smaller in calibre, contribute less to total resistance because of their large number.

During quiet breathing inspiration is 'active' and expiration 'passive'. Inspiration against abnormal resistance (whether elastic or non-elastic) may bring accessory muscles such as the sternomastoids and scaleni into play; expiration, if forced or performed against abnormal resistance, is accomplished with the aid of the accessory muscles of expiration, chiefly those of the abdominal wall.

Elastic work is increased when the lungs are made more rigid (less compliant) by pulmonary oedema or fibrosis or when the chest wall is made more unyielding by ankylosing spondylitis or severe kyphoscoliosis. Rapid shallow breathing is often observed in these conditions. Non-elastic work is increased by rapid breathing and by conditions causing airflow obstruction such as asthma, chronic bronchitis, emphysema and tumours of major bronchi. The metabolic cost of breathing is normally low: an increase in ventilation of 1 *l*/min raises oxygen uptake by about 45 μmol/min (1 ml/min) at most. In disease, this figure may rise to as much as 450 μmol (10 ml) oxygen per min per *l*/min increase in ventilation. Under such circumstances breathing accounts for an important fraction of metabolic oxygen uptake.

Not all of the inspired air takes part in gas exchange in the lungs. Some of each breath ventilates the conducting airways down to the respiratory bronchioles, which constitute the 'anatomical' dead space; because of maldistribution (see below) some of each breath is wasted in ventilating underperfused parts of the lungs. The proportion of wasted ventilation in each breath (physiological dead space: tidal volume ratio, Vd/Vt) is normally one-fifth to one-third, but may be much increased, sometimes to as much as two-thirds, in disease. The volume which remains takes part in gas exchange and provides *alveolar ventilation*, which is normally about 5 *l*/min at rest. It follows that if the proportion of wasted ventilation is greater than normal a greater total ventilation is needed to achieve normal alveolar ventilation.

Normally, alveolar ventilation is closely matched to the excretion of carbon dioxide and this matching is reflected in a normal level of arterial $Pco_2$. If alveolar ventilation is reduced in proportion to carbon dioxide excretion, the arterial $Pco_2$ must rise (hypercapnia), and if alveolar ventilation becomes excessive, the arterial $P_{CO_2}$ will fall (hypocapnia). Indeed, the arterial $P_{CO_2}$ reflects alveolar ventilation and the production of carbon dioxide just as the blood urea concentration reflects renal urea clearance and the metabolic production of urea.

Generalised alveolar underventilation is most commonly found as a late result of chronic bronchitis and emphysema. It also occurs if respiration is depressed by narcotics, anaesthetics or intracranial disease. It may ensue when the respiratory muscles are paralysed or when gross deformity of the chest wall limits thoracic or diaphragmatic movement, as in kyphoscoliosis. Lowering of the arterial $P_{O_2}$ (hypoxaemia) is an inevitable result of alveolar underventilation when air is breathed. Giving oxygen will correct this, but the hypercapnia is corrected only when alveolar ventilation is improved.

Alveolar overventilation occurs in asthma of mild or moderate severity, in interstitial lung disease, in pulmonary vascular disease (e.g. pulmonary embolism), in salicylate overdosage, as a result of pontine lesions, or from anxiety or hysteria. It is often a prominent manifestation of metabolic acidosis (p. 140).

## Control of Breathing

Rhythmical discharges originating in the reticular substance of the brain stem provide the basis for co-ordinated respiratory movements; it is convenient to use the term 'respiratory centre' for the neurones involved in breathing, but the distribution and organisation of these neurones is highly complex. From the respiratory centre impulses reach the spinal motor neurones by the reticulo-spinal tracts, in contrast to impulses mediating conscious changes in breathing, which travel via the pyramidal tracts. Normal breathing is modified by afferent impulses from many sources, which are best considered in two groups:

1. Those arising within the central nervous system and from receptors other than chemoreceptors ('neural stimuli').
2. Those arising from chemoreceptors sensitive to the composition of blood or cerebrospinal fluid ('chemical stimuli').

Afferent impulses of the first group mediate (*a*) the changes in rate and depth of breathing which may be consciously induced for short periods, (*b*) the central neurogenic overventilation which occurs in certain lesions of the pons and mid-brain, (*c*) the respiratory depression associated with medullary compression and (*d*) the respiratory stimulation which originates in limb receptors, as in exercise. These impulses may also arise from receptors in muscles and joints in the chest wall, and from pulmonary receptors sensitive to stretch, bronchial irritation and pulmonary capillary distension. Pulmonary inflation and deflation (Hering-Breuer) reflexes are present in the newborn, but are weak in adults except under general anaesthesia.

The second group of afferent impulses arises in chemosensitive cells located in the carotid and aortic bodies (peripheral chemoreceptors) and intracranially (central chemoreceptors). In animals central chemosensitive areas are located on the ventrolateral surface of the medulla, but in man their situation is uncertain.

Ventilation is increased when the peripheral chemoreceptors are stimulated by arterial hypoxia; at rest, the stimulus is not strong unless arterial $P_{O_2}$ is below 8 kPa (60 mmHg), and becomes powerful at about 4 kPa (30 mmHg). The peripheral chemoreceptors are also stimulated by an increase in the hydrogen ion activity of arterial blood. Central chemoreceptors are stimulated by an increase in the hydrogen ion activity of cerebrospinal fluid (CSF). A rise in $P_{CO_2}$ of the arterial blood is accompanied by increasing acidity of both blood and CSF and therefore stimulates both central and peripheral chemoreceptors. For this reason, inhalation of carbon dioxide is one of the strongest known respiratory stimulants. In the presence of mild or moderate hypoxia its effect is increased, but severe hypoxia acts as a central depressant, as in asphyxia. Pyrexia increases the sensitivity of the respiratory centre; all sedatives, particularly opiates, depress it. Aspirin in large doses stimulates it.

In some patients with chronic bronchitis the normal sensitivity to increased arterial $P_{CO_2}$ is greatly reduced. In such patients chronic alveolar underventilation occurs and relief of the concurrent hypoxaemia may, by removing one of the remaining stimuli to breathing, be followed by worsening of the hypercapnia.

### Distribution of Gas and Blood in the Lungs

Gas exchange in the lungs is inefficient unless alveolar ventilation is distributed uniformly to different parts of the lungs and is matched by uniform distribution of blood flow. The composition of blood leaving an individual alveolus depends on the composition of the mixed venous blood entering the pulmonary capillaries and the ratio between the ventilation of and blood flow around the alveolus. The possible values of this ventilation:perfusion ratio ($\dot{V}_A/\dot{Q}$) lie between infinity (ventilation but no perfusion) and zero (perfusion but no ventilation). Thus areas of lung with $\dot{V}_A/\dot{Q}=\infty$ behave as dead space, giving rise to wasted ventilation, while areas with $\dot{V}_A/\dot{Q}=0$ behave as a physiological right-to-left shunt or venous admixture effect, giving rise to wasted perfusion.

The possible range of ventilation:perfusion ratios in lung units is so large that it has become conventional to treat the lungs *as if* they were made up of three compartments:

(*a*) a compartment normally ventilated and perfused,
(*b*) physiological dead space, contributed to by all alveoli whose $\dot{V}_A/\dot{Q}$ exceeds unity, and including the anatomical dead space,
(*c*) physiological shunt, contributed to by all alveoli with $\dot{V}_A/\dot{Q}$ less than unity, and including the small anatomical or 'true' right-to-left shunts through such pathways as bronchial-pulmonary venous anastomoses.

It follows that if the range of ventilation:perfusion ratios found in the lungs is wider than normal the physiological dead space and physiological shunt will be larger than normal and gas exchange will become less efficient.

Even in the normal lung, distribution of ventilation and perfusion is imperfect. In the erect posture, gravity affects distribution of both ventilation and blood flow, causing regional $\dot{V}_A/\dot{Q}$ to be increased at the apices and reduced at the bases of the lungs. In most forms of lung disease, distribution of ventilation and perfusion is further impaired, and it is easy to visualise how pathological mechanisms may have this effect. For example, distribution of ventilation may be impaired by

(*a*) bronchial or bronchiolar obstruction (tumour, secretions, mucosal oedema, bronchoconstriction),
(*b*) destruction of elastic tissue (as in emphysema),
(*c*) pulmonary collapse, consolidation, fibrosis or oedema,
(*d*) chest wall deformities.

Blood flow is reduced or abolished by pulmonary embolism or thrombosis or by obliteration of areas of the pulmonary capillary bed by necrosis or fibrosis.

The consequences of maldistribution are twofold. First, as has been shown above, an increase in physiological dead space means that a greater total ventilation is needed to achieve a given alveolar ventilation. Secondly, any increase in physiological shunt causes arterial hypoxaemia. Any tendency to hypercapnia due to perfusion of alveoli with low $\dot{V}_A/\dot{Q}$ ratios can be compensated for by overventilation of alveoli with high $\dot{V}_A/\dot{Q}$ ratios. This preserves a normal or low arterial $P_{CO_2}$, but the arterial hypoxaemia is little affected. Maldistribution, with areas of low $\dot{V}_A/\dot{Q}$ ratio, is therefore the most important single cause of hypoxaemia in disease, and is found in a wide variety of conditions. Fortunately, administration of oxygen raises the alveolar $P_{O_2}$, even in poorly ventilated alveoli, and corrects the hypoxaemia.

### Diffusion of Gases in the Lungs

Oxygen and carbon dioxide move by molecular diffusion in the gas phase along the terminal airways and alveoli, and are also exchanged across the alveolar membrane by diffusion in the liquid phase from a site of higher to one of lower partial pressure. It might be expected that if the alveolar wall became thickened, as in so-called interstitial lung disease, diffusion of gases, particularly of oxygen, would be impaired. However, most conditions which might be expected to have this effect can also give rise to maldistribution of ventilation and blood flow, and analysis suggests that the effect on distribution is usually the chief cause of hypoxaemia in these conditions.

If the area available for gas exchange is reduced (e.g. in emphysema) or if, because of maldistribution, the effective area is reduced, the ability of the lung to transfer gases will also diminish. Such a reduction may not be significant at rest, but may limit the amount of oxygen which can be taken up during exercise and may become a cause of hypoxaemia under these circumstances. It can be corrected by administration of oxygen.

The overall ability of the lung to transfer gases can be readily measured by relating the uptake of carbon monoxide to the alveolar CO pressure when a very weak mixture of the gas is breathed. By this method, values for *gas transfer factor* or *diffusing capacity* of the lung are obtained. The former name is preferable, since 'diffusing capacity' carries the implication that diffusion itself is being measured, whereas in fact the measurement is affected by other factors, such as maldistribution.

## Common Manifestations of Respiratory Disease

**Cough.** This is the most frequent of all respiratory symptoms. It may be short, painful and half-suppressed, as when dry pleurisy accompanies pneumonia. It may be loose and readily productive of sputum, as in bronchiectasis, or paroxysmal, ineffectual and exhausting, as in some cases of chronic bronchitis and asthma. It is usually an early symptom in bronchial carcinoma but may be a relatively late development in pulmonary tuberculosis. Generally it is worse at night or on waking. Often it is aggravated by changes in temperature or humidity. The explosive character of a normal cough is lost when laryngeal paralysis is present ('bovine cough'). It is accompanied by stridor (p. 227) in whooping cough and in the presence of laryngeal or tracheal obstruction.

**Sputum.** Purulent sputum is due to bacterial infection in the respiratory tract and is typically seen in acute bronchitis, infective exacerbations of chronic bronchitis, bacterial pneumonia, bronchiectasis and lung abscess. In the last two conditions the sputum may be copious and is sometimes foetid. Mucoid sputum is due to oversecretion of bronchial mucus. It is frequently present in chronic bronchitis and bronchial asthma. In early cases of pulmonary tuberculosis the sputum is mucoid but in advanced cases it is usually purulent.

**Haemoptysis.** Haemoptysis of all grades of severity may occur, from slight streaking of the sputum with blood, which is a common symptom in acute and chronic bronchitis, to a massive haemorrhage. Frank haemoptysis, however small, must always be regarded as of potentially serious significance and demands full investigation. Bronchial carcinoma, pulmonary infarction, bronchiectasis, pulmonary tuberculosis and mitral stenosis are its most common causes.

**Chest Pain.** There are three types of chest pain associated with respiratory disease:

(1) Central retrosternal pain of a sore, 'scratchy' character made worse by coughing, usually caused by tracheitis.

(2) Unilateral chest pain, usually in the pectoral or axillary regions but sometimes in the back, of a sharp stabbing character, made worse by deep breathing and coughing, and caused by inflammation of the pleura.

(3) Constant pain, unrelated to breathing, caused by invasion of the chest wall by a malignant tumour of the lung.

*Pleural pain* is thought to be due to stretching of the inflamed parietal pleura (the visceral pleura is insensitive to painful stimuli) and is maximal towards the end of inspiration. Patients with pleural pain try to minimise it by taking shallow breaths and by suppressing cough as much as possible. The pain is referred to the area of skin supplied by the same spinal nerves as those supplying the inflamed area of pleura. Usually it is referred to the chest wall, but when the pleura lining the diaphragm is inflamed it may be referred to the cutaneous distribution of the supraclavicular nerves which have the same spinal roots (third and fourth cervical) as the phrenic nerve. Pain in the front and top of the shoulder is thus characteristic of diaphragmatic pleurisy. Pleural pain may also be referred to the anterior abdominal wall, where it may be difficult to distinguish from the pain of an acute abdominal emergency.

A *pleural rub*, which is a common physical sign in dry pleurisy, is due to the rubbing together of pleural surfaces roughed by fibrinous exudate. The effusion of fluid between the layers of the pleura diminishes pain by reducing the movement of the chest wall and abolishes the pleural rub by separating the pleural surfaces.

**Dyspnoea.** It has been said that breathing is the only involuntary act which is carried out by voluntary muscle, and this is normally so. Dyspnoea is a subjective sensation in which the effort of breathing reaches consciousness, usually under circumstances in which a normal person would not be aware of breathing at all. It should be distinguished from *hyperpnoea*, where the volume of ventilation is increased, but no abnormal sensation is felt, and *tachypnoea*, an excessive respiratory rate.

Dyspnoea occurs as a symptom in a wide variety of diseases, and no single theory can adequately explain why it occurs. In conditions where resistance to airflow is high, such as asthma or chronic bronchitis, the increased mechanical work needed to achieve a given volume of ventilation may account for it. A similar explanation may be given for dyspnoea in diseases causing lung stiffness, such as fibrosing alveolitis, with the added factor that the hypoxaemia which occurs readily during exercise in such diseases may still further increase the drive to breathe. This explanation is less satisfactory for the dyspnoea of heart disease, and still less so for the dyspnoea found in anaemia, where both the lungs and the arterial oxygen pressure are normal. It has been suggested that the sensation arises from 'inappropriateness' between the amount of breathing which the patient feels is needed for a given task and the amount he has in fact to produce — a feeling comparable to that experienced when picking up what seems to be an ordinary rubber ball and finding it is filled with lead. This throws some light on the nature of the sensation, but still leaves its cause obscure.

In mild heart or lung disease, dyspnoea is noticeable only on effort, and the presence of dyspnoea at rest is an indication that the disease is severe or advanced. In conditions such as chronic bronchitis, much of the respiratory reserve may have been lost before a sedentary patient complains of dyspnoea, and measurements of ventilatory capacity show that irreversible airway obstruction is already established. Complaints of dyspnoea should therefore be taken seriously, for although the symptom is commonly found in anxiety states, it also may occur early in diseases such as pulmonary thrombo-embolism or allergic alveolitis at a stage when abnormalities may not be apparent clinically or radiologically. Tests of pulmonary function and objective assessment of exercise capacity are then of value.

**Wheeze.** In all diseases causing airflow obstruction, particularly bronchial asthma, wheeze is usually a conspicuous symptom. It is a musical sound heard best during expiration, and is associated with numerous rhonchi on auscultation. *Stridor*, on the other hand, occurs when one of the major airways (larynx, trachea or main bronchus) is obstructed. It is a crowing sound heard best during inspiration, and is associated with a persistent low-pitched rhonchus audible all over the chest.

**Hypoxaemia** is present if either the pressure or content of oxygen in arterial blood is reduced, and if severe enough may result in visible central cyanosis. The normal arterial $Po_2$ is over 12 kPa (90 mmHg) at the age of 20, and falls to around 11 kPa (82 mmHg) at 60. Above this age a further fall in $Po_2$ of up to 1·3 kPa (10 mmHg) occurs on recumbency because of closure of airways in the dependent regions of the lungs. The most frequent and important cause of hypoxaemia in respiratory disease is the presence in the lungs of areas where the distribution of ventilation and perfusion is disturbed and where ventilation is low in relation to perfusion. Hypoxaemia also inevitably results from alveolar underventilation (which increases alveolar and arterial $Pco_2$) or if an atmosphere poor in oxygen is breathed, as at high altitudes. Impairment of diffusion across the alveolar wall may cause hypoxaemia during exercise, but is hardly ever an important factor at rest. The hypoxaemia due to all these causes is reversed by giving oxygen. Hypoxaemia due to congenital heart disease or vascular anomalies, with shunting of blood from the right to the left of the circulation past the lungs, is never entirely reversed by oxygen. Hypoxaemia also occurs if the oxygen capacity of the blood is reduced, as in anaemia or carbon monoxide poisoning.

**Hypercapnia** is present if the pressure of carbon dioxide in the arterial blood ($Paco_2$) is above the upper limit of normal of 6·0 kPa or 45 mmHg at rest. Clinically significant hypercapnia occurs when the $Paco_2$ exceeds 7 kPa (52 mmHg). As has been seen, the finding of a raised $Paco_2$ implies that alveolar ventilation is inadequate in relation to the carbon dioxide production of the body; the causes of hypercapnia are therefore those of alveolar underventilation. Alveoli in which the ventilation: perfusion ratio is low also contribute to hypercapnia.

The finding of hypercapnia also implies either that the normal sensitivity of the respiratory centre to carbon dioxide has been reduced, or that mechanical limitation, or failure of neuromuscular transmission prevents a normally responsive centre from maintaining adequate alveolar ventilation.

Clinical features suggestive of hypercapnia include peripheral vasodilatation, with warm extremities and bounding pulses, sweating, muscle twitching, headache, drowsiness, coma, retinal venous distension and, rarely, papilloedema. Unfortunately, none of these signs is specific and the diagnosis must be made by measurement of the pressure of carbon dioxide in arterial blood.

Hypercapnia has three consequences of clinical importance: (a) it aggravates hypoxaemia by lowering the pressure of oxygen in the alveolar gas, (b) when acute, it increases the arterial hydrogen ion concentration (respiratory acidosis), although renal retention of bicarbonate tends to compensate for this over a period of hours or days (p. 144), and (c) when of a severe degree ($Paco_2 > 11$ kPa or 82 mmHg), it induces drowsiness, which may proceed to coma.

**Respiratory failure** is said to occur when the normal pressures of oxygen and carbon dioxide in the arterial blood are no longer maintained. For practical purposes, this means the finding of either a $Pao_2$ of less than 8 kPa (60 mmHg) or a $Paco_2$ of more than 7 kPa (52 mmHg).

It follows that two varieties of respiratory failure can be recognised. In so-called Type 1 respiratory failure the $Paco_2$ is normal or low, but $Pao_2$ is reduced. Type 2 respiratory failure, in which the $Paco_2$ is elevated and the $Pao_2$ is reduced, is often termed '*ventilatory failure*'. The mechanisms responsible for the hypoxaemia in each type have already been discussed (p. 227), but it must be stressed once more that the finding of hypercapnia means that the normal mechanisms controlling breathing have been disturbed.

The causes of Type 1 respiratory failure are many, and include any of the pathological causes of maldistribution of ventilation and perfusion in the lungs (p. 223). Among the most important are bronchial asthma, pneumonia, pulmonary collapse, pulmonary oedema, allergic and fibrosing alveolitis, myocardial infarction and shock.

The most common pulmonary cause of ventilatory failure is chronic bronchitis, particularly when complicated by acute respiratory infection. Other causes include respiratory paralysis (p. 710), deformities of the chest such as severe kyphoscoliosis, and depression of the respiratory centre, particularly by narcotic or sedative drugs.

The treatment of Type 1 respiratory failure, in which hypoxaemia is not accompanied by hypercapnia, must always include oxygen, which can be given without strict control of the inspired concentration. In addition, treatment appropriate to the particular cause of the failure must be given. Treatment of ventilatory failure is discussed on page 236.

**Clubbing of the Fingers and Toes.** The cause of clubbing, which is most readily recognised in the fingers, is not known but it is frequently found in patients with certain types of respiratory disease, notably bronchial carcinoma, chronic intrathoracic suppuration and fibrosing alveolitis. It does not occur in chronic bronchitis or emphysema unless there is accompanying pulmonary suppuration or if the patient has developed a tumour, nor in pulmonary tuberculosis except in advanced cases.

Clubbing also occurs in certain other conditions. It is usually present in infective endocarditis and cyanotic congenital heart disease, occasionally in Crohn's disease, malabsorption syndrome and cirrhosis of the liver, and rarely in healthy subjects as a familial trait. The earliest indication of finger clubbing is an abnormal degree of fluctuation at the bases of the nails. With more advanced clubbing there is, in addition, an increase in the curvature of the nails and bulbous swelling of the fingertips.

## The Investigation of Respiratory Disease

In most respiratory diseases a reasonably accurate diagnosis can be made from the history and physical examination alone, but in several important conditions, notably pulmonary tuberculosis and bronchial carcinoma, these methods are inadequate and the diagnosis can be confirmed or excluded only by more specialised procedures such as radiological, bacteriological or endoscopic examination. In taking the history, particular enquiry must always be made about symptoms such as cough, sputum, haemoptysis, pain, breathlessness, wheeze and nasal discharge. The patient must also be asked about any previous respiratory illness, about any family history of tuberculosis and about any occupational exposure to dust.

### Physical Examination

Before the chest itself is examined the temperature should be taken, and a note made of the rate and character of breathing, the type and severity of any cough and the amount and character of the sputum. In addition, particular care must be taken to determine whether or not there is cyanosis, clubbing of the fingers or enlargement of the supraclavicular lymph nodes, these features being of special significance in respiratory disease.

The upper respiratory tract should be examined next, with particular regard to nasal discharge or obstruction, oral sepsis, and infection or enlargement of the tonsils. The presence of hoarseness or a 'bovine' cough would draw attention to the need for laryngoscopic examination (p. 231). The chest wall should then be carefully inspected for soft tissue abnormalities such as cutaneous lesions, subcutaneous swellings (including lumps in the breast) and bulging or indrawing of intercostal spaces, and for skeletal abnormalities such as an increase in the anteroposterior diameter of the chest relative to its lateral diameter. The position of the trachea and of the apex beat should be noted and the chest expansion measured. Chest wall movement, vocal fremitus and the percussion note should be compared in equivalent positions on the two sides. The terms used to describe the various types of percussion note are: hyper-resonant, normal, impaired, dull and stony dull. At auscultation, attention should be directed in turn to the breath sounds, added sounds and vocal resonance.

BREATH SOUNDS. The following terms are used: vesicular, vesicular with prolonged expiration, diminished vesicular, absent breath sounds and high-pitched, low-pitched and amphoric bronchial breath sounds.

ADDED SOUNDS. *Rhonchi* seem to be related to narrowing of the lumen of the bronchi caused by spasm of bronchial muscle, swelling of bronchial mucosa or tenacious mucus adherent to bronchial walls. Rhonchi may be high-pitched, medium-pitched or low-pitched, according to the size of the bronchi in which they originate.

*Crepitations* usually indicate the presence of secretions within alveoli, bronchi or pulmonary cavities. They may be fine, medium or coarse in quality, and may either disappear or become more numerous after coughing. Crackling crepitations, unaltered by coughing, are a feature of interstitial lung disease (p. 292).

*Pleural rub* is a diagnostic sign of pleural inflammation. It is a grating or creaking sound, unaltered by coughing, audible during both inspiration and expiration.

VOCAL RESONANCE. The following terms are used: normal, increased, diminished or absent vocal resonance, aegophony, whispering pectoriloquy.

**The Interpretation of Physical Signs.** Certain groups of physical signs are typically associated with certain pathological changes in the lungs and pleura. Such changes are not necessarily specific for one particular disease. For example, consolidation may occur in pneumonia or tuberculosis, and fluid may be present in the pleural space in tuberculous pleurisy, empyema or congestive cardiac failure. Each group of physical signs should therefore be correlated with the gross pathological lesion by which the signs are produced rather than with any specific disease, the diagnosis of which depends on an analysis of all the clinical and other evidence.

The physical signs of the more common lesions are shown on Table 7.1.

Table 7.1 Summary of typical physical signs in the more common respiratory diseases

| Pathological Process | Movement of Chest Wall | Mediastinal Displacement | Percussion Note | Breath Sounds | Vocal Resonance | Accompaniments |
|---|---|---|---|---|---|---|
| Consolidation as in lobar pneumonia | Reduced on affected side | None | Dull | High-pitched bronchial | Increased (with aegophony) Whispering pectoriloquy | Fine crepitations early Coarse crepitations later |
| Collapse due to obstruction of major bronchus | Reduced on side affected | Towards lesion | Dull | Diminished or absent | Reduced or absent | None |
| Collapse due to peripheral bronchial obstruction | Reduced on side affected | Towards lesion | Dull | High-pitched bronchial | Increased (with aegophony) Whispering pectoriloquy | None early—coarse crepitations later |
| Localised fibrosis and/or bronchiectasis | Slightly reduced on side affected | Towards lesion | Impaired | Low-pitched bronchial | Increased | Coarse crepitations |
| Cavitation (typical signs only when cavity is large and linked with bronchus) | Slightly reduced on side affected | None, or towards lesion | Impaired | 'Amphoric' bronchial | Increased Whispering pectoriloquy | Coarse crepitations |
| Pleural effusion Empyema | Reduced or absent (depending on size) on side affected | Towards opposite side | Stony dull | Diminished or absent (occasionally high-pitched bronchial) | Reduced or absent (occasionally increased with aegophony) | Pleural rub in some cases (above effusion) |
| Pneumothorax | Reduced or absent (depending on size) on side affected | Towards opposite side | Normal or hyper-resonant | Diminished or absent (occasionally faint high-pitched bronchial) | Reduced or absent | Tinkling crepitations when fluid present |
| Bronchitis: Acute Chronic | Normal or symmetrically diminished | None | Normal | Vesicular with prolonged expiration | Normal | Rhonchi, usually with some coarse crepitations |
| Bronchial asthma | Symmetrically diminished | None | Normal | Vesicular with prolonged expiration | Normal or diminished | Rhonchi, mainly expiratory and high-pitched |
| Broncho-pneumonia | Symmetrically diminished | None | May be impaired | Usually harsh vesicular with prolonged expiration | Normal | Rhonchi and coarse crepitations |
| Diffuse pulmonary emphysema | Symmetrically diminished | None | Normal | Diminished vesicular with prolonged expiration | Normal or reduced | Rhonchi and coarse crepitations from associated bronchitis |
| Interstitial lung disease | Symmetrically diminished | None | Normal | Harsh vesicular with prolonged expiration | Usually increased | Crackling crepitations uninfluenced by coughing |

(From Macleod, J. (1979) *Clinical Examination*, 5th edn. Edinburgh: Churchill Livingstone.)

## Special Methods of Investigation

**Radiological Examination of the Chest.** Many pulmonary diseases, including bronchial carcinoma and pulmonary tuberculosis, cannot be detected at an early stage without radiological examination of the chest. Facilities for this investigation are now readily available to most doctors, and it should always be undertaken whenever any serious form of intrathoracic disease is suspected. A lateral film may provide additional information about the nature and situation of a pulmonary, pleural or mediastinal abnormality. Specialised techniques, such as bronchography, radioscopy, conventional tomography, computed tomography and radio-isotope ventilation and perfusion scanning may be of considerable diagnostic value in selected cases.

It may be very useful to obtain chest radiographs taken previously for comparison with a current film, since this may show whether a radiographic opacity is 'new' or progressive, and thus potentially serious, or 'old' and probably of no importance.

Some respiratory diseases, such as bronchial asthma and chronic bronchitis, and occasionally bronchial carcinoma, may not be associated with any radiographic abnormality, and a normal chest radiograph in these circumstances does not necessarily exclude serious intrathoracic disease.

**Bacteriological and Cytological Examination.** *Sputum.* Bacteriological examination of the sputum seldom provides conclusive diagnostic information except when *Mycobacterium tuberculosis* is isolated. The findings in other circumstances must be interpreted in conjunction with the results of clinical and, if necessary, radiological examination. Cytological examination, by demonstrating malignant cells in the sputum, may enable a diagnosis of bronchial carcinoma to be made.

*Pleural Fluid.* This should always be examined cytologically and bacteriologically. A special search should be made for *Myco. tuberculosis* if the fluid is serous and also for pyogenic organisms if it is purulent. When malignant disease is suspected, especially if the fluid is blood-stained, it should also be examined histologically for malignant cells.

**Blood Examination.** Serological examination may be of value in the diagnosis of viral infections and allergic disorders.

Estimation of the total and differential leucocyte count may help to distinguish pyogenic infection from tuberculous or viral infection.

**Skin Tests.** The tuberculin test (p. 254) and Kveim test (p. 294) may be of value in the diagnosis of tuberculosis and sarcoidosis respectively. Skin sensitivity tests (p. 268) are useful in the investigation of allergic diseases.

**Laryngoscopy and Bronchoscopy.** The larynx is inspected either by means of a mirror placed in front of the uvula (indirect laryngoscopy) or through an illuminated telescopic tube (direct laryngoscopy).

The trachea and larger bronchi are inspected by a bronchoscope of either the rigid or the fibreoptic type. Abnormal tissue can be removed for histological examination (bronchial biopsy). The range of vision with the rigid instrument extends to the origins of all segmental bronchi but the fibreoptic bronchoscope is more useful for the inspection and biopsy of lesions situated more peripherally, particularly in the upper lobes.

**Biopsy.** Histological examination of an enlarged lymph node removed from the neck or axilla, or from the mediastinum by the technique of *mediastinoscopy*, may provide a firm diagnosis in conditions such as bronchial carcinoma, tuberculosis, lymphoma and sarcoidosis.

In patients with pleural effusion it is possible to obtain a specimen of parietal pleura suitable for histological examination by means of Abrams' pleural biopsy 'punch'. This procedure is simple and safe and may be of considerable value in determining the cause of a pleural effusion. If it is unsuccessful, the pleural surfaces can be inspected with a thoracoscope inserted through an intercostal space, and if a pleural lesion is seen, a biopsy can be performed under telescopic vision.

When a diagnosis cannot be made in any other way it may be necessary to obtain a specimen of lung tissue for histological examination either by formal thoracotomy, by needle biopsy through the chest wall or by transbronchial lung biopsy via a fibreoptic bronchoscope.

**Tests of Pulmonary Function.** Many of the procedures mentioned above are of great assistance in arriving at a pathological diagnosis, but investigations of a different type are necessary to determine the effects of disease on pulmonary function and to assess the response to therapy (p. 270). Disturbances of the mechanical properties of the lungs, of ventilation, of control of breathing, of the distribution of ventilation and perfusion within the lungs and of diffusing capacity can all be measured (Fig. 7.2). Some of the tests require a high degree of skill and elaborate apparatus, but others are simple routine procedures which can be undertaken by any doctor without special training.

(a) ESTIMATION OF VENTILATORY CAPACITY. The patient is asked to take in as deep a breath as possible and then expel it as hard and as fast as possible. If the forced expiration is made into a recording spirometer of low resistance and low inertia, the *forced expiratory volume* in the standard time of 1 second ($FEV_1$) can be measured; if the forced expiration is continued till no more gas can be expelled, the *forced vital capacity* (FVC) is measured. The ratio of these two volumes may be expressed as a percentage (FEV/FVC %); normal people can expel between 80 and 65% of the FVC in 1 second, depending on age and sex.

In diseases which cause narrowing of the airways during expiration, such as asthma and chronic bronchitis, the FEV/FVC % is reduced, sometimes to 40% or less. This is due to a greater reduction in FEV than in FVC, and this type of ventilatory defect is called '*obstructive*'. In diseases such as interstitial lung disease or ankylosing spondylitis, which make the lungs or chest wall more rigid, FEV and FVC are reduced in the same proportion and FEV/FVC % is normal, as the airflow is relatively unaffected. This is called a '*restrictive*' ventilatory defect. Discovery of airflow obstruction is an indication to repeat the spirometric measurements after a bronchodilator drug has been given; reversibility of airflow obstruction is found in asthma and in some patients with chronic bronchitis.

During forced expiration, the *peak expiratory flow rate* (PEFR) can be measured by a device which is simpler and cheaper than the average spirometer. PEFR is reduced in conditions causing airways obstruction, and is a good indicator of the severity of the obstruction. The measurement has therefore become popular in clinical practice because of its speed and simplicity. PEFR is less affected by conditions causing a restrictive type of ventilatory defect, and is therefore of little value in diagnosing or assessing them.

Even if no apparatus other than a watch and stethoscope is available, forced expiration can still be used to assess ventilatory capacity. Normal people can empty

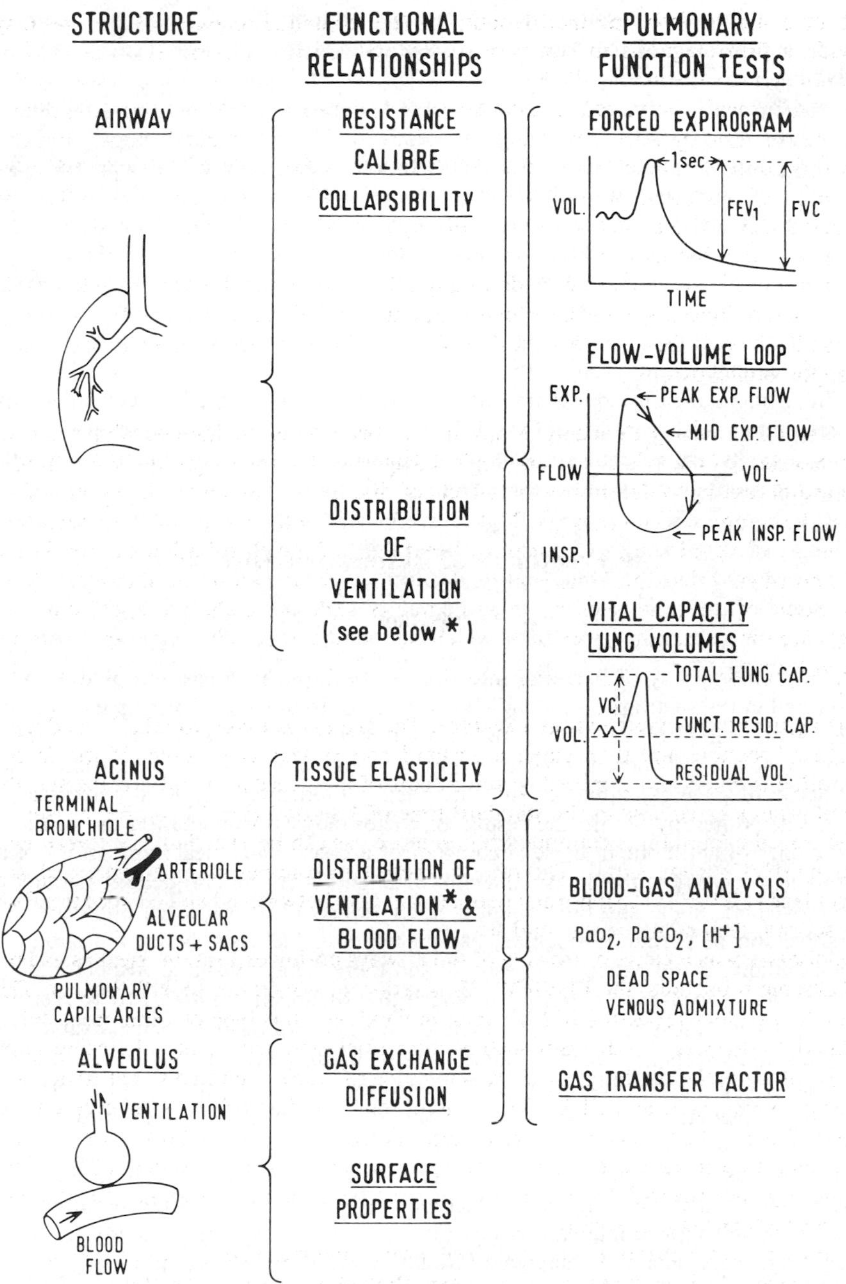


Fig. 7.2 Relationships between structure and function of lungs and pulmonary function tests. The forced expirogram gives information about airway resistance and calibre and the maximal flow-volume loop supplements this with information about inspiratory resistance, airway collapsibility and behaviour of small peripheral airways. Vital capacity and lung volume measurements are influenced by tissue elasticity and airway resistance. Distribution of ventilation and blood gases may be assessed by blood gas analysis and by measurement of dead space and venous admixture. Overall gas exchange is assessed by arterial $P_{O_2}$ and $P_{CO_2}$ and by gas transfer factor.

their chest from full inspiration in 4 seconds or less. Prolongation of the *forced expiratory time* (FET) to more than 6 seconds indicates airways obstruction and a reduction in FEV/FVC % to less than 50%. The end-point of FET is detected by placing the chest-piece of a stethoscope over the trachea in the suprasternal notch.

(b) ANALYSIS OF ARTERIAL BLOOD. Apparatus for arterial blood-gas analysis is now available in most hospitals. Knowledge of the $Paco_2$ provides the answer to the question, 'Is the patient breathing enough?', and is of particular value in the management of ventilatory failure (p. 236). If the arterial hydrogen ion concentration (activity) or pH and the $Paco_2$ are both known, it is often possible to deduce the type of any disturbance of acid:base balance (p. 144) which may be present. Knowledge of the $Pao_2$ or arterial oxygen saturation allows accurate assessment of hypoxaemia and of the effects of oxygen therapy.

These simple measurements are thus of value in distinguishing between some types of respiratory disorder, as well as in providing an index of their severity. Serial measurements are valuable in following changes in pulmonary function, whether occurring spontaneously or in response to treatment.

## The Treatment of Respiratory Disease

### Infection

The chemotherapy of bacterial infection of the bronchi, lungs and pleura will be described in the sections on individual diseases. Certain general principles are, however, applicable to all cases. Before any treatment is started a specimen of sputum, a laryngeal swab (if there is no sputum) or a specimen of pleural fluid should be sent for bacteriological examination. In acute bacterial infection it is usually necessary to begin chemotherapy before the results of bacteriological examination are available. The choice of antibiotic in these circumstances is based on clinical impressions of the nature and severity of the illness. If a clinical diagnosis of acute bronchitis, pneumonia or empyema is made and the patient is not seriously ill or if the acute infection is a complication of chronic bronchitis, asthma or bronchiectasis, ampicillin should be given initially. If the patient is gravely ill and there is any reason to suspect infection with *Staph. pyogenes*, an antibiotic to which that organism is unlikely to be resistant, e.g. cloxacillin, must be added. As soon as the results of bacteriological examination and sensitivity tests are received, modifications in antibiotic therapy can be made, if necessary. Factors which interfere with the response to antibiotics must be corrected, e.g. an empyema must be aspirated or drained, and bronchiectatic cavities and lung abscesses must be kept empty by postural drainage.

The viruses which infect the respiratory tract are uninfluenced by chemotherapy, but secondary bacterial infection, which occurs in many cases, often requires treatment with an appropriate antibiotic. Infection caused by small bacteria, such as coxiella, mycoplasma and chlamydia, usually responds to tetracycline.

The treatment of respiratory diseases caused by fungi is described on page 265.

### Oxygen Therapy

Oxygen is present in the air at a concentration of 21% and at sea level the pressure of oxygen in inspired tracheal air is almost 20 kPa (150 mmHg). Arterial blood of normal haemoglobin concentration contains about 9 mmol oxygen per litre (20 ml/

100 ml); at a $Pa_{O_2}$ of 13·5 kPa (100 mmHg) 135 μmol oxygen per litre (0·3 ml/100 ml) are dissolved in the plasma (i.e. a solubility of 10 μmol/*l*/kPa) and the rest is bound to haemoglobin.

**Therapeutic Indications.** The objectives of oxygen therapy are (1) to overcome the reduced pressure and quantity of oxygen in the blood found in hypoxaemia, and (2) to increase the quantity of oxygen carried in solution in the plasma even when the haemoglobin is fully saturated. The causes of hypoxaemia have already been discussed (p. 227). Raising the alveolar $P_{O_2}$ by administration of oxygen overcomes the hypoxaemia consequent upon a high alveolar $P_{CO_2}$; when the oxygen pressure is raised in alveoli which are poorly ventilated but perfused, the blood perfusing them becomes fully saturated and the hypoxaemia due to maldistribution of ventilation and perfusion is overcome. A raised alveolar $P_{O_2}$ will also correct hypoxaemia caused by limitation of diffusing capacity.

The cause of hypoxaemia least susceptible to oxygen therapy is right-to-left shunting, either through circulatory channels by-passing the lungs, or through parts of the lungs in which the alveoli are inaccessible to inspired oxygen. The increased amounts of dissolved oxygen carried by blood which has perfused alveoli with a high $P_{O_2}$ can saturate the haemoglobin in small quantities of shunted blood; persistence of cyanosis when pure oxygen is breathed indicates that the shunt is larger than 20% of the cardiac output. This accounts for the observation that the cyanosis of congenital heart disease is not relieved by oxygen.

In anaemia or in heart failure the arterial blood may be normally saturated with oxygen when air is breathed, but the delivery of oxygen to the tissues is reduced. In these conditions oxygen therapy may benefit seriously ill patients by increasing the amount of dissolved oxygen in the blood.

**Adverse Effects.** Pure oxygen is both irritant and toxic if it is inhaled for more than a few hours. Premature infants develop retrolental fibroplasia if exposed to excessive concentrations of oxygen. Normal subjects notice cough and bronchial irritation, and in patients ventilated with high concentrations of oxygen for several days pulmonary oedema and consolidation may occur. If such patients require oxygen it is important to give, whenever possible, an inspired concentration which corrects hypoxaemia but does not exceed 60 to 70%.

**Technique of Oxygen Administration.** Hypoxaemia is such a common consequence of respiratory diseases that oxygen may well be the most frequently prescribed 'drug' used in their treatment. It is important that prescriptions for oxygen should be in writing, and that flow rates or concentrations should be clearly specified. Administration of oxygen should be continuous though this may prove difficult in confused or restless patients. The risk of fire should never be forgotten when any patient is treated with oxygen.

*Oxygen masks* are of two types: 1. Those which are designed to produce a high concentration of $O_2$ in the inspired air. Examples of this type of mask are the Polymask (British Oxygen Co. Ltd) and the MC mask (Medical and Industrial Equipment Ltd), both of which deliver about 60% $O_2$ when the flow rate is 4–6 *l* per min.

2. Those which are designed to produce slight $O_2$ enrichment of the inspired air and do not permit the rebreathing of expired $CO_2$. Examples of this type of mask are the Edinburgh mask (British Oxygen Co. Ltd) and the Ventimask (Vickers Limited Medical Group). With the Edinburgh mask adjustments of the $O_2$ flow rate can provide inspired $O_2$ concentrations at any level between 23 and 35%. The Ventimask

is available in three models, which deliver 24, 28 and 35% $O_2$ respectively.

*Nasal Cannulae.* Double nasal cannulae fit comfortably into the nostrils. Their main advantages are that they do not permit rebreathing of $CO_2$ and do not interfere with eating, drinking and the wearing of spectacles. The inspired $O_2$ concentration they provide is somewhat unpredictable, but an $O_2$ flow rate of 2 *l*/min. will usually raise it to about 30%. They are of particular value if oxygen is administered for long periods.

*Humidification.* When Polymasks or MC masks are used, the oxygen must be humidified, either by passing it over the surface of warm water in an electrically heated canister (East-Radcliffe humidifier) or through a nebuliser. This is not necessary with Edinburgh masks, Ventimasks or nasal cannulae, as a high proportion of atmospheric air is mixed with the oxygen in these devices.

## Treatment of Ventilatory Failure

**Acute Ventilatory Failure.** A clear airway is essential. In conscious patients this can often be secured and maintained by determined efforts to encourage expectoration, every 15 minutes or so at first, under the strict supervision of a doctor, nurse or physiotherapist. If this policy fails, and particularly if the patient has become confused or unconscious, a cuffed endotracheal tube should be inserted through the mouth or nose under general anaesthesia, and connected to a mechanical ventilator. At frequent intervals the trachea and bronchi should be cleared of secretions by aspiration through a soft catheter. Most patients are intolerant of artificial ventilation in the early stages and require heavy sedation with opiates. Some patients recover adequate spontaneous ventilation within a few days but others require tracheostomy to allow tracheobronchial aspiration and mechanical ventilation to be continued for a longer period. These intensive methods of resuscitation are contraindicated in patients who have had severe respiratory disability for several months before the onset of ventilatory failure. Bronchoscopic aspiration may be of value as an initial measure to clear the airways of secretion, and, if the patient can thereafter cough effectively, tracheal intubation may not be required.

During mechanical ventilation through an endotracheal tube the depressant effect of a high $Pa_{O_2}$ on respiration can be ignored, and there is no objection to ventilating the patient with a high concentration (up to 60%) of $O_2$. When artificial ventilation is stopped, however, or in cases where it has not been employed, increasing hypercapnia is a potential hazard of $O_2$ administration, and the concentration of $O_2$ in the inspired air should initially be kept below 30% by using a Ventimask, an Edinburgh mask or a double nasal cannula. It is seldom necessary or desirable to increase the inspired $O_2$ concentration above this level. When $O_2$, even in a concentration of 30% or less, is being administered to patients with acute ventilatory failure, the $Pa_{O_2}$, $Pa_{CO_2}$ and hydrogen-ion concentration or pH should be measured at regular intervals. An indwelling cannula in the brachial or radial artery can conveniently and safely be used for obtaining blood samples. If a steady increase in $Pa_{CO_2}$ is accompanied by clinical deterioration and/or by a rise in hydrogen-ion concentration above 60 nmol/litre (fall in pH below 7·25 units), this is another indication for artificial ventilation, either short-term via an endotracheal tube or long-term via a tracheostomy tube. The disturbances in $Pa_{O_2}$, $Pa_{CO_2}$, and pH can usually be corrected within 24 hours, but it may be several days before the patient is capable of maintaining a sufficiently high level of alveolar ventilation to allow discontinuation of mechanical assistance.

In all cases respiratory infection should be treated. Water and electrolyte balance should be maintained, by intravenous infusion if necessary, as dehydration increases the viscosity of bronchial mucus and makes it difficult to dislodge.

Analeptic drugs have a limited but useful place in treatment. Nikethamide (2–4 ml of a 25% solution 1 to 2 hourly) or doxapram (infusions of up to 3 mg/min.) given intravenously for 24 hours, may successfully tide the patient over a period of under-ventilation and obviate the need for tracheal intubation or tracheostomy, particularly if bronchial secretions are not present in large amounts. Although analeptic drugs seldom produce sustained stimulation of respiration, they may improve the level of consciousness and thus restore effective expectoration. Should sedation be necessary, diazepam is probably the drug least liable to depress respiration.

**Chronic Ventilatory Failure.** Many patients with progressive respiratory disease eventually enter a state in which $Pa_{O_2}$ and $Pa_{CO_2}$ never return to normal. In such patients, treatment should be directed to the prevention of acute respiratory infections, the relief of airflow obstruction and the management of right ventricular failure. In chronic ventilatory failure a worthwhile increase in exercise tolerance has been shown to result from the use of light, portable oxygen equipment, but this benefit may be nullified by carboxyhaemoglobin in concentrations produced by cigarette smoking. The provision of such equipment for all patients who could derive benefit from it presents a formidable problem. However, patients confined to their homes may be helped by the intermittent use of low concentrations of oxygen obtained from a static supply; it must be admitted that such benefit may often be psychological rather than physical. The potential benefits of continuous low-concentration oxygen therapy in the home are still under investigation.

## Symptomatic Treatment in Respiratory Disease

*Cough*, when productive of sputum, should be encouraged and not suppressed. Those who are physically weak should be exhorted at regular intervals to clear their bronchi of secretion. Those with bronchiectasis or lung abscess should practise postural drainage, and those with tenacious sputum should be given hot drinks and inhalations of either steam or nebulised water to help them to bring it up more easily.

Unproductive, distressing cough should be suppressed, especially if sleep is disturbed. The two most effective preparations, suitable for use in bronchitis, pneumonia, bronchial carcinoma and pulmonary tuberculosis, are pholcodine and methadone.

*Airflow obstruction* in bronchitis and asthma is treated by bronchodilators (p. 270) and in some cases by corticosteroids given by mouth or by inhalation (p. 271).

*Chest Pain.* Pleural pain can usually be relieved by the application of a rubber hot-water bottle or by an electric heating pad to the chest wall, supplemented by an analgesic and, if necessary, by an antitussive drug. Mild analgesics, such as acetyl-salicylic acid, or codeine, are adequate in most cases but a few patients may require pethidine, 50–100 mg by mouth or intramuscular injection, or even morphine, 10–15 mg subcutaneously. Opiates must, however, be avoided in patients with poor respiratory function and in those who have difficulty in coughing up sputum.

The pain of acute tracheitis usually responds to the application of heat to the front of the chest, combined with inhalations of steam medicated with benzoin (p. 241). Pain due to invasion of the chest wall by a malignant tumour, if not relieved by radiotherapy, usually demands a powerful analgesic such as pethidine or morphine, given by injection. In advanced cases these drugs may become ineffective and neurosurgical measures may be required for the relief of intractable pain.

# INFECTIONS OF THE RESPIRATORY SYSTEM

Infections of the respiratory tract may be caused by large and small bacteria, by viruses and by fungi. 'Small' bacteria include coxiella, causing Q-fever, mycoplasma and *Legionella pneumophila*, causing pneumonia, and chlamydia, causing psittacosis and ornithosis. Infections of the respiratory tract are very common and the average person can expect to have three or four such infections every year. By far the commonest are those affecting the upper respiratory tract and of these about 80% are viral in origin. The types of viral infection and the upper respiratory tract illnesses they cause are shown in Table 7.2. Immunity is short-lived and is specific for each virus. Pulmonary tuberculosis and diseases caused by fungi are described in separate sections.

Table 7.2 Upper respiratory tract infections caused by viruses

| Aetiological Agent | Clinical Syndrome | Incubation Period (days) |
|---|---|---|
| *Adenoviruses | Acute coryza<br>Pharyngoconjunctival fever<br>Acute laryngitis | 6–9 |
| Coxsackie virus | Pharyngoconjunctival fever<br>Herpangina | 7–14 |
| Echo viruses | Acute coryza<br>Pharyngoconjunctival fever | 2–4 |
| *Influenza virus A, B, (C) | Epidemic influenza<br>Acute laryngotracheobronchitis (croup) | 1–3 |
| *Parainfluenza virus 1–4 | Acute coryza<br>Acute laryngotracheobronchitis (croup) | 4–7 |
| *Respiratory syncytial (RS) virus | Acute coryza<br>Acute laryngotracheobronchitis (croup) | 4–7 |
| Rhinoviruses | Acute coryza | 2–4 |

*May also cause pneumonia

## Upper Respiratory Tract Infections

The main diseases caused by viruses are acute coryza (common cold), pharyngo-conjunctival fever, acute laryngitis and acute laryngotracheobronchitis; those caused by bacteria are acute tonsillitis and otitis media.

**Acute Coryza.** The onset is usually sudden with a tickling sensation in the nose accompanied by sneezing. The throat often feels dry and sore, the head feels 'stuffed' and there is a profuse watery nasal discharge. These symptoms last for 1 to 2 days, after which, with secondary infection, the secretion becomes thick and purulent, and impedes nasal breathing.

Coryza may be complicated by sinusitis when there is usually more systemic upset. Sinus infection is liable to become chronic, particularly in the maxillary sinuses, causing persistent purulent discharge from the front and back of the nose, often accompanied by nasal obstruction and headaches.

Other complications are infections of the lower respiratory tract, catarrh of the auditory tubes causing deafness, and otitis media causing fever and aural pain.

Frequent attacks of sneezing and watery rhinorrhoea, without systemic upset, suggest nasal allergy rather than viral infection.

**Pharyngoconjunctival Fever.** The pharyngeal syndrome, which is sometimes accompanied by conjunctivitis, occurs particularly amongst school children in spring and summer and in holiday camps. It may be caused by several viruses (Table 7.2), especially adenoviruses. Herpangina may occur in infections with Coxsackie A viruses.

Conjunctivitis may be the first symptom, but sore throat is the dominant feature and may be slight or severe. The pharynx, tonsils and adenoids become inflamed, and yellow exudate may be present. Cervical lymph nodes are enlarged and tender. The degree of constitutional symptoms — shivering, malaise, anorexia, headache and fever — is variable. In herpangina, typical vesicles, which may become punched-out ulcers, are present on the fauces. Acute streptococcal sore throat may be clinically indistinguishable from pharyngoconjunctival fever, but *Strep. pyogenes* will be isolated from such cases. Infectious mononucleosis (p. 570) may also be difficult to differentiate from the pharyngeal syndrome in the early stages. The possibility of diphtheria and of gonococcal infection should not be overlooked.

**Acute Laryngitis.** This usually occurs either as a complication of coryza or as a manifestation of one of the infectious fevers, for example, measles. The laryngeal mucous membrane is swollen, congested and coated with mucus.

The throat is dry and sore. The voice is at first hoarse and then reduced to a whisper. Speaking may be painful. There is an irritating non-productive cough, but the general upset is usually mild. In children the small laryngeal opening may be obstructed by viscid secretion and spasm, giving rise to stridor (croup).

Acute laryngitis usually clears up in a few days, but frequently recurring episodes may predispose to chronic laryngitis. Downward spread of the infection may cause tracheitis, bronchitis or even pneumonia.

**Acute Laryngotracheobronchitis.** This illness, which is particularly serious in very young children because of the small calibre of their airways, may be caused by several viruses (Table 7.2). Superinfection with bacteria, especially *Strep. pyogenes* and *Staph. pyogenes*, may occur. The mucosa is intensely inflamed, the secretions are extremely tenacious and fibrinous casts of the bronchi may form.

The initial symptoms may be those of the common cold. These are followed by severe and sometimes violent cough which may be paroxysmal, accompanied by dyspnoea and stridor, contraction of accessory muscles and indrawing of intercostal spaces. The child may be cyanosed, and asphyxia may occur if appropriate treatment is not given.

### Investigation and Treatment of Upper Respiratory Tract Infections

Most patients with these infections recover rapidly and specific investigation is indicated only in the more severe cases. Viral infections may be identified by serological tests. Throat swabs may be helpful if streptococcal sore throat is suspected, and examination of the blood will identify infectious mononucleosis. Radiographic examination may be required to confirm the presence of chronic sinus infection.

The spread of infection can be reduced by voluntary isolation of patients for 2 to 3 days during the early, highly infectious stage. Excessive nasal secretions can be reduced by the periodic use of 1% ephedrine in normal saline either sprayed or dropped into the nose. Lozenges containing local anaesthetic, for example, benzocaine, are helpful when the throat is painful. A mild analgesic, such as codeine compound tablets, relieves systemic symptoms. Antibiotics are unnecessary except in the treatment of secondary bacterial infection, for example, sinusitis or otitis media, or of acute streptococcal sore throat.

Inhalations of medicated steam given 3 or 4 times a day are helpful in laryngitis. In acute laryngotracheobronchitis clearing of secretions is of the utmost importance, and bronchoscopy or tracheostomy may be required as a life-saving measure. Attention to adequate hydration is also important and oxygen therapy is necessary.

## Influenza

Influenza is a specific acute illness caused by a group of myxoviruses. It occurs in epidemics, and occasionally pandemics, often explosive in nature.

**Aetiology.** Three types of virus are described, A, B and C. At least four strains of influenza A, which is responsible for the pandemics, have been identified. The so-called 'Asian' strain has been implicated in most recent epidemics. Influenza B is usually associated with smaller and less virulent outbreaks. The C virus is found only rarely. The immunity which follows is type-specific and of short duration. This causes problems in providing effective immunisation.

**Clinical Features.** The incubation period is 24 to 48 hours. The illness starts suddenly with malaise, headache, pain in the back and limbs, anorexia and sometimes nausea and vomiting. Pyrexia to 39°C remits for 2 to 3 days, with chills and shivering but seldom rigors. The face is flushed, conjunctivae suffused and fauces hyperaemic with prominent lymphoid follicles. The pulse is rapid. There is often leucopenia. There may be a harsh unproductive cough, without physical signs over the lungs. At this stage the illness is indistinguishable clinically from a severe upper respiratory infection due to other respiratory viruses. The disease may spread rapidly throughout a household or institution.

During epidemics, the diagnosis is usually easy. Most sporadic cases are identifiable only as respiratory virus infections unless the virus is isolated or serological tests for specific antibodies are positive.

**Course and Complication.** In many cases, no further symptoms develop and recovery ensues within 3 to 5 days. The disease may, however, be complicated by tracheitis, bronchitis, bronchiolitis and bronchopneumonia. Secondary bacterial invasion by *Strep. pneumoniae*, *H. influenzae* and occasionally *Staph. pyogenes* causes these complications.

Toxic cardiomyopathy may cause sudden death, especially when there is pre-existing cardiac disease. Encephalitis and post-influenzal demyelinating encephalopathy are rare complications. Post-influenzal asthenia and depression are common, often marked, and may last for a week or two.

**Treatment and Prevention.** The patient should be kept in bed until the fever has subsided. A mild analgesic usually relieves the headache and backache. A linctus containing pholcodine or methadone may be used to suppress unproductive cough. The treatment of complications such as bronchitis and pneumonia is dealt with later.

Immunity is type-specific and if the antigenic constitution of a new strain can be detected early, a specific vaccine may give about 70% protection. Annual winter vaccination is recommended for patients suffering from chronic pulmonary, cardiac or renal disease.

## Acute Bronchitis

**Aetiology.** This condition is an acute inflammation of the trachea and bronchi caused by pyogenic organisms such as *Strep. pneumoniae, H. influenzae* and, rarely, *Staph. pyogenes*. Infection by these organisms is a common sequel to coryza, influenza, measles and whooping-cough, and is particularly prone to develop in patients with chronic bronchitis.

Other factors predisposing to bacterial infection include cold, damp, foggy and dusty atmospheres and cigarette smoking.

**Clinical Features.** The first symptom is an irritating, unproductive cough accompanied by upper retrosternal discomfort or pain caused by tracheitis. When the bronchi become involved there is also a sensation of tightness in the chest, and dyspnoea with wheezing respiration may be present. Respiratory distress may be particularly severe when acute bronchitis complicates chronic bronchitis and emphysema. The sputum is at first scanty, mucoid, viscid and difficult to bring up, and occasionally may be streaked with blood. A day or two later it becomes mucopurulent and more copious. As the infection extends down the bronchial tree there is a general febrile disturbance, with a temperature of 38–39°C and a neutrophil leucocytosis. In the vast majority of cases recovery takes place gradually over the next 4 to 8 days without the patient ever becoming seriously ill. Occasionally the dyspnoea and general symptoms increase in severity, cyanosis appears, and if the infection reaches the smaller bronchi and bronchioles ('bronchiolitis') the condition becomes indistinguishable from bronchopneumonia.

Tracheitis without bronchitis produces no abnormal physical signs. In bronchitis there is no impairment of chest wall movement or percussion note. The breath sounds are vesicular, or vesicular with prolonged expiration, and are accompanied by bilateral rhonchi and, occasionally, coarse crepitations.

The disease is usually mild and of short duration, the patient recovering within a few days if a suitable antibiotic is given. In severe cases it lasts longer, especially if bronchiolitis and bronchopneumonia develop.

**Treatment.** The patient should be confined to bed and tetracycline or ampicillin, 250–500 mg 4 times daily, given by mouth. Co-trimoxazole is equally effective in a dose of 2 tablets twice daily. In the early stages, when cough is painful and unproductive, the tough viscid secretion should be loosened by the inhalation 3 or 4 times a day of steam medicated with benzoin or menthol. A steam kettle or steam tent is more suitable for children. The cough should be controlled at night by the use of pholcodine or methadone. If symptoms or signs of airways obstruction are present a bronchodilator drug may be of some value. Oxygen is seldom required in uncomplicated acute bronchitis.

## The Pneumonias

Pneumonia is the term used to describe inflammation of the lung. There are many different kinds of pneumonia, some common, others rare. Aetiologically, they can be divided into the *specific pneumonias*, in which the disease is caused by a specific pathogenic organism, and the *aspiration pneumonias*, in which some abnormality of the respiratory system predisposes to the invasion of the lung by organisms of relatively low virulence, and infection generally reaches the alveoli by aspiration from other parts of the respiratory tract. In the aspiration pneumonias, *H. influenzae*, some types of *Strep. pneumoniae* and certain of the bacteria forming the flora of the upper respiratory tract and mouth are the organisms most frequently cultured from the sputum.

In some types of specific and aspiration pneumonia, prominent features are destruction of lung tissue by the inflammatory process, a high incidence of abscess formation and the subsequent development of pulmonary fibrosis and bronchiectasis. The term '*suppurative pneumonia*' has been applied to this group of cases and this condition merits separate description (p. 246).

## The Specific Pneumonias

This group may be further subdivided into pneumonias caused by 'large' bacteria, and by 'small' bacteria or viruses.

Pneumonia due to the pneumococcus still constitutes the largest proportion of all specific pneumonias. Other large bacteria causing such pneumonias are *Strep. pneumoniae*, *Staph. pyogenes*, *Klebsiella pneumoniae*, *H. influenzae*, *Myco. tuberculosis*, *Yersinia pestis* and *Y. tularensis*.

### Pneumococcal Pneumonia (Acute Lobar Pneumonia)

Pneumococcal pneumonia is characterised by homogeneous consolidation of one or more lobes or segments. The disease occurs at all ages but most frequently in early and middle adult life. The highest incidence is in winter. It is usually a sporadic disease, the mode of spread being by droplet infection.

**Clinical Features.** The onset is sudden, with rigor, or with vomiting or a convulsion in children. The temperature rises in a few hours to 39–40°C. Malaise, loss of appetite, headache, and aching pains in the body and limbs accompany the pyrexia. Localised pain of pleural type develops at an early stage in the illness. It is generally referred to the chest wall but may on occasion be referred to the shoulder or to the abdominal wall. There is a short, painful cough, dry at first but later productive of tenacious sputum which is often rust-coloured and occasionally frankly blood-stained. Respiration is rapid (30–40 per minute in adults, 50–60 in children), shallow and painful. The pulse is rapid, the skin is hot and dry, the face is flushed, and central cyanosis may be observed in severe cases. Herpes labialis is often present. A marked neutrophil leucocytosis is characteristic. *Strep. pneumoniae* can usually be isolated from the sputum, and a positive blood culture may be obtained in severe cases.

*Physical Signs in the Chest*. In the first 24 to 48 hours of the illness, there is diminution of respiratory movement, slight impairment of the percussion note and often a pleural rub on the affected side. At a variable time after the onset, generally within 2 days, signs of consolidation appear (p. 230), the breath sounds being of the high-pitched bronchial type. When resolution begins, numerous coarse crepitations are heard, indicating liquefaction of the exudate. If a serous or purulent effusion develops, the physical signs of fluid in the pleural space are usually found, but often bronchial breath sounds persist and the presence of an effusion may be suspected only from stony dullness on percussion.

**Radiological examination** shows a homogeneous opacity localised to the affected lobe or segment, appearing within 12 to 18 hours of the onset of the illness. Radiological examination is particularly helpful when the diagnosis is in doubt or if a complication such as empyema is suspected.

**Course.** Most cases respond promptly to chemotherapy and within a week the patient is well again. Delayed recovery suggests either that some complication such as empyema has developed or that the diagnosis is incorrect.

## Other Types of Specific Pneumonia

**Staphylococcal Pneumonia.** Pneumonia due to *Staph. pyogenes* may occur either as a primary respiratory infection or as a blood-borne infection from a staphylococcal lesion elsewhere in the body, for example, osteomyelitis. The second condition is essentially one of pyaemic abscess formation in the lungs. Unless an empyema is produced by rupture of an abscess into the pleura, the pulmonary lesions may pass unnoticed, overshadowed by the severe general illness.

Primary staphylococcal pneumonia, although it occurs much less frequently than pneumococcal pneumonia, is a relatively common illness, especially as a complication of influenza. It may present as a lobar or segmental pneumonia, which may be difficult to distinguish clinically from a severe pneumococcal infection, or as a suppurative pneumonia (p. 246) with multiple lung abscesses which may persist as thin-walled cysts after the acute infection has subsided. Culture of the sputum yields a growth of coagulase-positive staphylococci which are frequently resistant to penicillin, streptomycin, tetracycline and co-trimoxazole. At the present time, few strains of staphylococci causing pneumonia are resistant to erythromycin, cloxacillin, cephaloridine or sodium fusidate, but this relatively favourable situation may alter.

**Klebsiella Pneumonia (Friedländer's Pneumonia).** Pneumonia due to *Kl. pneumoniae* is a rare disease. There is usually massive consolidation and excavation of one or more lobes, the upper lobes being most often involved, with profound systemic disturbance, the expectoration of large amounts of purulent, sometimes chocolate-coloured, sputum and a high mortality. The diagnosis is made by the radiological appearances and the isolation of the causative organism from the sputum. Streptomycin plus chloramphenicol is the first choice in antibiotic therapy, modified according to the results of sensitivity tests.

**Actinomycosis.** Formerly included amongst the fungal diseases, this is now regarded as a bacterial infection. It is caused by *A. israeli*, an anaerobic organism, which exists as a commensal in the mouth. Actinomycosis may produce a widespread suppurative bronchopneumonia (p. 246). Empyema, often bilateral and associated with persistent chest wall sinuses, may develop later, or occasionally *de novo*.

**Pneumonia caused by Viruses and Small Bacteria.** A distinctive form of pneumonia may be produced by certain viruses, (Table 7.2) and by small bacteria which exhibit a similar pathogenicity to lung tissue. The clinical picture differs from that of the bacterial pneumonias in that fever and toxaemia usually precede the respiratory symptoms by several days. Severe headache, malaise and anorexia are characteristic features in the early stages. The physical signs in the chest, if there are any, appear later and are seldom gross. The existence of a pulmonary lesion may not be recognised without a radiograph. The spleen may be palpable in the first week. The white blood count is generally normal and the pyrexia does not respond to penicillin. The diagnosis can often be confirmed by isolation of the causal organism or by serological tests.

The disease is usually self-limiting. The pyrexia subsides by lysis after 5 to 10 days, and complete recovery and radiographic resolution follow, the latter sometimes being slow. Very rarely, death takes place from widespread extension of the pneumonia or from viral encephalitis.

The *influenza*, *parainfluenza* and *measles* viruses rarely produce a specific pneumonia. The pneumonia caused by *chickenpox* virus, however, is usually characteristic. The radiograph shows numerous miliary nodular shadows which may eventually calcify. It occurs almost exclusively in adults. The *adenoviruses* cause occasional mild epidemics of specific pneumonia.

*Respiratory syncytial virus* is the most important respiratory pathogen of early childhood, especially in the first 2 months of life. This is because it causes bronchiolitis and pneumonia, and carries an important risk of mortality in this age group. The infant is fevered, and cough, wheezy respiration and occasionally an erythematous rash are prominent features. The virus is not susceptible to any known antibiotic, and immunisation is ineffective.

*Psittacosis* (parrot-fever) and *ornithosis* are caused by *Chlamydia*. These used to be regarded as viruses but have in fact the structural and biochemical properties of bacteria and rickettsiae. The diseases are primarily infections of birds, and are transmitted to humans by inhalation of dust containing faeces from infected birds. The pneumonia caused by these organisms, which are susceptible to tetracyclines, is occasionally extensive and associated with severe toxaemia. Headache is prominent.

*Mycoplasma pneumonia* is a pleomorphic bacterium capable of passing through a filter. It is susceptible to tetracyclines though a few strains are sensitive only to erythromycin. Cold agglutinins (p. 563) can be demonstrated in a high proportion of cases. Antibodies can be detected, and haemagglutination and complement-fixation tests are available for diagnosis. Outbreaks of pneumonia caused by this organism are common in barracks and institutions. Most cases occur in children and young adults. Maculopapular rashes, haemolysis and meningoencephalitis occur rarely.

*Coxiella (Rickettsia) burneti* is the organism responsible for *Q-fever*. Endocarditis may occur, as well as pneumonia, in this disease (p. 181).

*Legionella pneumophila*, a coccobacillus, often causes severe respiratory illness (sometimes in epidemics) characterised by gastrointestinal symptoms, confusion, hyponatraemia and proteinuria, as well as pneumonia (Legionnaires' disease).

**Pneumonia due to Opportunistic Infections.** Patients whose immunological defences have been compromised by disease, or by immunosuppressive, corticosteroid or prolonged antibiotic therapy, may develop pneumonia due to opportunist infections. The commonest causes are gram-negative bacilli (coliforms and *Ps. aeruginosa*), fungi (*Cryptococcus neoformans*, *Candida albicans* and *Aspergillus fumigatus*), viruses (cytomegaloviruses, herpes viruses) and protozoa (*Pneumocystis carinii*).

**Tuberculous Pneumonia** (p. 256), **Plague** (p. 833) and **Tularaemia** (p. 835).

## The Aspiration Pneumonias

This group, sometimes described as the 'non-specific' pneumonias, comprises a large number of different conditions, their common features being the absence of any specific pathogenic organism in the sputum and the existence of some abnormality of the respiratory system which predisposes to the invasion of the lung by organisms of relatively low virulence derived from the upper respiratory tract or from the mouth, for example, streptococci, certain types of pneumococci, *H. influenzae*, Vincent's spirochaetes and fusiform bacilli.

Infection may reach the lungs in various ways. Pus may be aspirated from an infected nasal sinus, or septic matter may be inhaled during tonsillectomy or dental extraction under general anaesthesia. Vomitus or the contents of a dilated oesophagus may enter the larynx during general anaesthesia, coma or even sleep. Infected secretion in the bronchi and pus from acute bronchitis, dilated bronchi or a lung abscess may also be carried into the alveoli by the air stream or by gravity.

Ineffective coughing caused by post-operative or post-traumatic thoracic or abdominal pain, by debility or immobility, or by laryngeal paralysis may also predispose to the development of aspiration pneumonia.

Bronchial obstruction, partial or complete, as for example by a carcinoma, is another potential cause of aspiration pneumonia, as it allows infection derived from the upper air passages to become established in the inadequately ventilated portion of lung beyond the obstruction.

### Acute Bronchopneumonia

This type of aspiration pneumonia is invariably preceded by bronchial infection, which accounts for the widespread patchy distribution of the lesions. It occurs most frequently at the extremes of life, and may be described as 'hypostatic pneumonia' when it occurs in elderly or debilitated patients. In children, it is often a complication of measles or of whooping cough, and in adults of acute bronchitis or influenza. It is particularly common in patients with chronic bronchitis.

**Pathology.** There is acute inflammation of the bronchi, especially the terminal bronchioles, which are filled with pus. Collapse and consolidation of the associated groups of alveoli follow. The lesions are distributed bilaterally in small patches which tend to become larger by confluence and are often more extensive in the lower lobes. The alveolar exudate consists of neutrophil leucocytes with a small amount of fibrin. There is interstitial oedema and cellular proliferation in the alveolar walls, and compensatory emphysema around the collapsed alveoli. Resolution of bronchopneumonia may be incomplete, and in such cases pulmonary fibrosis and bronchiectasis are common sequelae.

**Clinical Features.** After 2 or 3 days of acute bronchitis, as bronchopneumonia develops, the temperature rises to a higher level, the pulse and respiration rates increase, and dyspnoea and central cyanosis appear. There is generally a severe cough with purulent sputum. Pleural pain is relatively uncommon, in contrast to pneumococcal pneumonia.

During the early stages the physical signs are those of acute bronchitis but crepitations later become more numerous. In many cases, no signs of consolidation can be detected, but these may develop when the lesions coalesce, and radiological examination shows mottled opacities in both lung fields, chiefly in the lower zones. A neutrophil leucocytosis is present.

**Course and Complications.** The disease is of more insidious onset and tends to run a more protracted course (up to 10 days) than pneumococcal pneumonia. Incomplete resolution may lead to bronchiectasis, but the number of patients developing this complication has fallen dramatically since antibiotics became available. The mortality is higher at the extremes of life, especially if the disease supervenes on chronic bronchitis and emphysema, chronic nephritis or heart disease.

**Prevention.** The incidence of bronchopneumonia can be reduced by careful attention to apparently benign upper respiratory infections such as coryza and acute bronchitis, especially when they occur in children or elderly subjects and in patients with chronic bronchitis. Measures to prevent whooping cough and measles, and adequate treatment of those diseases, are also important in prophylaxis.

### Benign Aspiration Pneumonia

This type of pneumonia is due to the aspiration of infected secretion into the lungs during the course of an upper respiratory infection such as coryza or sinusitis. It is thus often associated with segmental pulmonary collapse. The organisms causing the pneumonia, being derived from the upper respiratory tract, are generally of low virulence and the degree of systemic disturbance is usually slight. In fact, the symptoms are often no more severe than would be expected with an uncomplicated upper respiratory infection and the existence of a pneumonia may be discovered only by radiological examination. As a rule, however, the condition manifests itself by cough, purulent sputum, low-grade pyrexia and sometimes pleural pain, in association with a frank upper respiratory infection. Localised coarse crepitations are often the only abnormal physical finding. A neutrophil leucocytosis is usually present. The radiological lesions are typically unilateral, the characteristic appearance being a mottled opacity involving a single lobe or segment, which in some cases may be collapsed.

The condition is liable to be confused with viral pneumonia, but the coexistent upper respiratory infection and the minimal systemic upset are useful distinguishing features. Pulmonary tuberculosis may be erroneously diagnosed on the basis of a single radiograph. Re-examination 10 to 14 days later, following treatment with an antibiotic, will clarify the diagnosis as resolution is generally rapid in aspiration pneumonia.

## Suppurative Pneumonia
*(Including Pulmonary Abscess)*

Suppurative pneumonia is the term used to describe a form of pneumonic consolidation in which there is destruction of lung parenchyma by the inflammatory process. Although microabscess formation is a characteristic histological feature of suppurative pneumonia, it is usual to restrict the term 'pulmonary abscess' to lesions in which there is a fairly large localised collection of pus, or a cavity lined by chronic inflammatory tissue, from which pus has ruptured into a bronchus.

Suppurative pneumonia and pulmonary abscess may be produced by infection of previously healthy lung tissue with *Staph. pyogenes* or *Kl. pneumoniae*. These are, in effect, specific bacterial pneumonias associated with pulmonary suppuration. More frequently, suppurative pneumonia and pulmonary abscess are forms of aspiration pneumonia. They may develop after the inhalation of septic material during operations on the nose, mouth or throat under general anaesthesia, or of vomitus during anaesthesia or coma. In such circumstances gross oral sepsis may be an important predisposing factor. Bacterial infection of a pulmonary infarct or of a collapsed lobe, may also produce a suppurative pneumonia or a pulmonary abscess. The organisms isolated from the sputum may include *Strep. pneumoniae*, *Staph. pyogenes*, *Strep. pyogenes*, *H. influenzae*, and in a few cases, anaerobic streptococci and other anaerobes such as Vincent's spirochaetes and fusiform bacilli. In some cases, however, no pathogens can be isolated, particularly when antibiotics have been given.

**Clinical Features.** These depend to a large extent on the pathogenesis of the lesion. The onset of the illness may be either insidious or acute, but cough with purulent sputum, usually large in amount, sometimes foetid and occasionally blood-stained, is present from an early stage. There is high, remittent pyrexia with shivering and sweating, and a neutrophil leucocytosis. Pleural pain is common and clubbing of the fingers may develop as early as 10 to 14 days after the onset of the illness. Progressive deterioration in general health with marked loss of weight ensues if the patient remains untreated. The rupture of a large abscess into a bronchus can be assumed when a large quantity of pus is suddenly expectorated. Such an incident is often preceded by blood-staining of the sputum and followed by remission of the pyrexia.

Physical signs in the chest also depend on the nature of the primary pathological process. Signs of consolidation (p. 230) are the most frequent; signs of cavitation are rarely found. A pleural rub is often present.

**Radiological Examination.** There is a homogeneous lobar or segmental opacity consistent with consolidation or collapse. A large, dense opacity, which may later cavitate and show a fluid level within it, is the characteristic finding when a frank pulmonary abscess is present.

**Course and Prognosis.** In most cases, there is a good response to antibacterial therapy (p. 249), and although residual fibrosis and bronchiectasis are common sequelae, these seldom give rise to serious morbidity. Empyema (p. 301) may complicate the acute phase of the disease.

**Prevention.** Every precaution should be taken during operations on the mouth, nose and throat to prevent the inhalation of blood, tonsillar fragments, etc. Oral sepsis should be eradicated, especially if a general anaesthetic is contemplated.

### Investigation of Pneumonia

An attempt should always be made to establish a positive microbiological diagnosis, though this is not always possible, particularly if antibiotics have been given before specimens are submitted for examination. Direct smear examination of *sputum* by Gram and Ziehl-Neelsen stains may give an immediate indication of possible pathogens, and indicate what treatment should be prescribed. Culture (including anaerobic culture where indicated) and sensitivity testing should be carried out. Where a microbiological diagnosis is essential, as in severely ill immunosuppressed patients, and a specimen of sputum cannot be obtained, an attempt should be made to aspirate secretions from the trachea or bronchi either by bronchoscopy or by inserting a needle through the cricothyroid membrane. Transthoracic lung puncture has been advocated if the other techniques are unsuccessful, but carries the risk of producing a pneumothorax, which may have lethal consequences in dangerously ill patients.

*Blood culture* should be performed in patients with severe pneumonia, and may yield a positive result when sputum examination is negative, particularly in pneumococcal pneumonia. Pneumococcal antigen may also be detected in serum.

*Serological tests* may be helpful, specimens being examined at 10-day intervals for viral titres. A four-fold rise suggests recent infection. Nose and throat swabs, and post-nasal and bronchial aspirates, can be cultured for viruses or examined by immunofluorescence or electron microscopy.

The *total and differential white blood count* is often below $5{\cdot}0 \times 10^9/l$ in patients with viral infection, and a high neutrophil polymorph leucocytosis favours bacterial infection. The ESR is usually elevated, but is of no help in diagnosis.

*Arterial blood gas studies* are of vital importance in all patients who are seriously ill and in those with a previous history of chronic respiratory disease. It is impossible to make any rational decisions on oxygen therapy unless the $PaO_2$ and $PaCO_2$ and the hydrogen ion concentration or pH of arterial blood are known.

*Radiological examination* is essential for confirmation of the diagnosis and for the early detection of complications such as pleural effusion and empyema. Follow-up radiological examination is important, because if a pneumonia fails to resolve, it may be secondary to bronchial obstruction by a carcinoma.

## Complications of Pneumonia

*Pulmonary*: in most cases, the abnormal physical signs disappear within 2 weeks and the radiographic opacity within 4 weeks. Although resolution is occasionally delayed for longer periods, and may be incomplete, particularly in patients with suppurative pneumonia, this is always an indication for further investigation, including bronchoscopic examination. Bronchiectasis is a common complication of suppurative pneumonia.

*Pleural*: spread of the infection to the pleura may occur, with the development of a sterile pleural effusion or empyema. Staphylococcal lung abscess may be complicated by pyopneumothorax.

*Cardiovascular*: these are peripheral circulatory failure due to bacteraemia, acute pericarditis and endocarditis (rare).

*Neurological*: meningism is not uncommon in children and lumbar puncture may be required to distinguish it from meningitis. Pneumococcal meningitis is rare.

## Differential Diagnosis of Pneumonia

The following conditions may be difficult to distinguish from pneumonia:

*Pulmonary infarction*, in which pyrexia is less marked and is uninfluenced by antibiotics, frank haemoptysis is common, cough is inconspicuous and the source of an embolus can often be identified.

*Tuberculous pleurisy with effusion*, in which the correct diagnosis can usually be suspected from the insidious onset, the virtual absence of cough and sputum, the physical signs of pleural effusion, the absence of leucocytosis, the failure of the pyrexia to respond to antibiotics, the radiological findings and the aspiration of serous fluid, in which lymphocytes predominate, from the pleural space.

*Pulmonary tuberculosis*, acute cases of which may simulate pneumonia. The patient is, however, seldom as acutely ill as in other specific pneumonias, it is uncommon for the respiratory rate to be markedly increased and the white blood count is seldom above $12{\cdot}0 \times 10^9/l$. The diagnosis can usually be made by radiological examination, and the isolation of tubercle bacilli puts it beyond doubt.

*Pulmonary oedema*, particularly in the elderly, may be difficult to distinguish from pneumonia. If fever is present, pneumonia is the more likely diagnosis, but where there is any doubt, both an antibiotic and a diuretic should be given.

*Inflammatory conditions below the diaphragm*, such as cholecystitis, perforated duodenal ulcer, acute appendicitis, subphrenic abscess, generalised peritonitis, acute pancreatitis and hepatic amoebiasis, may occasionally be mistaken for pneumonia. A carefully taken history is one of the most valuable means of determining the site and nature of the primary disease. A high temperature and a rapid respiration rate favour a diagnosis of pneumonia, whereas tenderness of the abdominal wall suggests that the primary lesion is below the diaphragm. Sometimes radiological examination of the chest is necessary before the presence of pneumonia can be confirmed or excluded.

## Treatment of Pneumonia

**Chemotherapy.** The principles governing the specific treatment of bacterial infections of the respiratory tract have already been stated (p. 234). The appropriate antibiotic in relation to the various aetiological agents is shown in Table 7.3.

Table 7.3 Treatment of pneumonia with antibacterial drugs

| Organism | Choice of drug |
|---|---|
| *Streptococcus pneumoniae* | penicillin, ampicillin |
| *Haemophilus influenzae* | ampicillin, co-trimoxazole |
| *Staphylococcus pyogenes* | benzylpenicillin *plus* flucloxacillin; clindamycin and/or sodium fusidate. |
| *Klebsiella pneumoniae* | chloramphenicol, streptomycin |
| *Proteus mirabilis* | ampicillin, co-trimoxazole |
| *Pseudomonas pyocyanea* | ticarcillin |
| *Mycoplasma pneumoniae* | oxytetracycline, erythromycin |
| *Coxiella burneti* | oxytetracycline, erythromycin |
| *Chlamydia psittaci* | oxytetracycline, erythromycin |
| *Legionella pneumophila* | erythromycin, rifampicin or a tetracycline |
| *Anaerobes* | benzylpenicillin, metronidazole |

When a clinical diagnosis of pneumonia is made, provided the patient is not gravely ill, the initial treatment should consist of ampicillin, 500 mg four times daily, or co-trimoxazole, 2 tablets twice daily. Patients who are gravely ill and in whom a staphylococcal or a Gram-negative infection is suspected, should receive, in addition to ampicillin by intravenous injection, antibiotics to which the causative organism is unlikely to be resistant, for example, flucloxacillin, 250 mg 6-hourly by intravenous injection, and gentamicin, 80 mg 8-hourly by intramuscular injection.

1. If *Strep. pneumoniae*, *Strep. pyogenes* or an anaerobic streptococcus is isolated, or no pathogenic organisms are reported on culture, and the patient appears to be

making satisfactory clinical progress, treatment with ampicillin or co-trimoxazole should be continued, but the dose of ampicillin can be reduced to 250 mg 6-hourly.

2. If *Staph. pyogenes* is isolated, treatment must be modified in accordance with the results of sensitivity tests. Resistance to penicillin may be due to the production of penicillinase, and such infections can usually be controlled by a combination of benzylpenicillin (600 mg b.d./i.m.) and oral or intramuscular flucloxacillin (250–500 mg 6-hourly). In other cases lincomycin (500 mg t.i.d.), sodium fusidate (500 mg t.i.d.) or cephalexin (500 mg 6-hourly) by mouth, or gentamicin (80 mg t.i.d.) by intramuscular injection, may be indicated. There may be an advantage in combining two of these drugs.

3. If *Actinomyces israeli* is isolated, benzylpenicillin is given by intramuscular injection in a dose of 5 g daily for up to 6 weeks.

4. If bacteriological examination is uninformative and there is no neutrophil leucocytosis in the blood, the pneumonia may be due to *Coxiella burneti*, *Mycoplasma pneumoniae* or *Chlamydia*. In these circumstances, tetracycline, 500 mg four times daily is recommended. Erythromycin is to be preferred if infection with *Legionella pneumophila* is suspected. Pneumonia caused by viruses does not respond to antibiotic therapy.

5. If recovery is progressing satisfactorily, the isolation of an organism showing *in vitro* resistance to the antibiotic in use is not necessarily an indication for a change in treatment. If, however, the patient is not improving and is still febrile when such an organism is isolated, an appropriate change in antibiotic is imperative.

The impulse to substitute another antibiotic, where there is no bacteriological indication for doing so, should be resisted. The failure of patients to respond to treatment may be due to a complicating factor such as pleural infection, tuberculosis or bronchial obstruction by a tumour, and these conditions must be carefully excluded before the antibiotic is changed.

6. No definite rule can be laid down for the duration of chemotherapy. In most cases of uncomplicated pneumococcal pneumonia, a 7-day course of treatment is usually adequate but this may have to be extended if the response to treatment is slow. In staphylococcal and klebsiella pneumonia, and in other forms of suppurative pneumonia, chemotherapy should be continued for a minimum of 2 weeks and should not be stopped until the causative organism has been eliminated from the sputum.

**General Measures.** The usual regimen of treatment for an acute infection should be instituted. If respiratory distress is marked the patient should be propped up comfortably with pillows or a backrest.

*Cough*, when distressing and unproductive, should be controlled by the measures described on page 237. When secretions are present in the bronchi the patient should be firmly encouraged to cough up sputum, even if the effort to do so causes pleural pain. In these circumstances a mild analgesic and the support of a nurse's hand on the painful side of the chest may relieve the distress of coughing. Postural drainage is of value if the sputum is difficult to bring up, particularly if it is copious, as in suppurative pneumonia, or when pneumonia complicates bronchiectasis. Skilled physiotherapy may be invaluable.

*Pleural pain* should be treated with local heat and analgesics (p. 237). It is, however, dangerous to prescribe morphine if even a mild degree of ventilatory insufficiency is present, and the safest policy is not to use this drug at all in the treatment of pneumonia.

*Hypoxia* demands oxygen therapy (p. 234).

*Delirium*, which in the early stages is caused mainly by the high temperature, and later by cerebral hypoxia, may have to be controlled by sedation. The safest drug to use is diazepam (5–10 mg i.m.).

*Bacteraemic shock* (p. 80) carries a high mortality and admission to an intensive therapy unit affords the best prospect of survival. The three most important therapeutic measures are (1) the administration of appropriate antibiotics in high dosage, (2) the maintenance of oxygenation, if necessary by tracheal intubation and intermittent positive-pressure ventilation, and (3) restoration of the depleted circulating blood volume by intravenous infusion of a 5% glucose solution, dextran or plasma, monitored by measurements of central venous pressure. Massive doses of intravenous hydrocortisone (3 g per day or more) have been advocated, but this treatment is of doubtful value.

*Abscess Formation*. Suppurative pneumonia is not in itself a reason for any departure from standard antibiotic policy. When an abscess cavity is present, however, it must be kept empty by regular postural drainage. Medical treatment is almost invariably successful and surgical measures nowadays are seldom required. In occasional instances, however, a large abscess may have to be drained externally or residual bronchiectasis resected.

## Tuberculosis

Although tuberculosis is a problem of rapidly diminishing proportions in Western Europe and North America, it remains, in the words of a WHO report: 'the most important specific communicable disease in the world'. As the disease decreases in frequency there is a tendency for tuberculosis to be overlooked.

**Aetiology.** Three types of mycobacteria are responsible for the disease in man: (1) *Myco. tuberculosis* (human type) — now the cause of almost all infections in man; (2) *Myco. bovis* — endemic in cattle, but now rarely responsible for disease in man, and (3) the *atypical* or *opportunistic* mycobacteria. The clinical importance of the last group of organisms lies in their ability to cause infection in cervical lymph nodes in children and, rarely, pulmonary disease in adults, when treatment may be a problem because the mycobacteria are primarily resistant to many drugs.

Entry of the tubercle bacillus into the body by the alimentary or respiratory tract is not necessarily followed by a clinical illness, the development of which is dependent of several other factors. Those of most practical importance are:

*Age and Sex*. In Europe and America, tuberculosis used to affect predominantly the young people in the community, especially females, but there has been a radical change in the age and sex incidence. Twenty years ago, 80% of notifications were of patients under 45 years of age, but nowadays 60% of patients are over that age, males predominating. This change is important in case-finding.

*Natural Resistance*. Susceptibility to tuberculosis is not inherited in the strict sense of the word, but the fact that certain races, and even certain regional groups, such as the inhabitants of the Western Isles of Scotland and of Ireland, are more prone to develop tuberculosis suggests that natural resistance varies from race to race and even from region to region. The natural resistance of a community tends to rise as the period of exposure to tuberculosis increases. Immigrants to Britain from Asia are more prone to develop disease than the indigenous population, and tend to have the more florid types of disease.

*Standard of Living*. The prevalence of tuberculosis diminishes as social and economic conditions improve. Poor housing with associated overcrowding increases the risk of massive infection or reinfection if one of the occupants suffers from infectious tuberculosis.

*Conditions Affecting Individual Patients*. Diabetes mellitus, gastrectomy and silicosis all predispose to the development of tuberculosis, as does treatment with corticosteroids or immunosuppressive drugs.

**Pathology.** The initial *'primary' tuberculous infection* usually occurs in the lung but occasionally in the tonsil or in the alimentary tract, especially the ileocaecal region. The primary infection differs from later infections in that the primary focus in lung, tonsil or bowel is almost invariably accompanied by a caseous lesion in the regional lymph nodes, i.e. in the mediastinal, cervical or mesenteric groups respectively. In most people the primary infection and the associated lymph node lesion heal and calcify. In a few, healing, particularly in lymph nodes, is incomplete and surviving tubercle bacilli may under certain circumstances, such as a lowering of the general health or an alteration of the balance between allergy and immunity, be discharged into the blood stream. Such patients may in consequence develop tuberculous lesions elsewhere. The most common sites for *'haematogenous' lesions* of this kind are the lungs, bones, joints and kidneys. Such lesions may develop months or even years after the primary infection.

The primary infection may in some cases fail to heal. A primary pulmonary lesion, particularly when it occurs during adolescence or early adult life, may lead to progressive pulmonary tuberculosis. A tuberculous mediastinal lymph node, in children especially, may compress a lobar or segmental bronchus (rarely a main bronchus) and produce pulmonary collapse. Occasionally the node may ulcerate through the bronchial wall and discharge caseous material into the lumen, with the production of acute tuberculous lesions in the related lobe or segment. Infection may also be carried by lymphatics from tuberculous mediastinal lymph nodes to the pleura or pericardium with the production of tuberculous pleurisy or pericarditis. Comparable complications may occur when the primary lesion is in the tonsil or gut, e.g. 'cold abscess' of the neck or tuberculous peritonitis.

Rarely, a caseous tuberculous focus either at the site of the primary infection or, more commonly, in an associated lymph node ruptures into a vein and produces acute dissemination of the disease throughout the body, a condition known as *acute miliary tuberculosis*. Tuberculous meningitis often accompanies this condition.

Progressive pulmonary tuberculosis may develop directly from a primary lesion or it may occur later, following reactivation of an incompletely healed primary focus in the lung or as a result of haematogenous dissemination from an unhealed lymph node lesion. Alternatively it may be the result of reinfection from an outside source after the primary focus has healed completely. All these forms of pulmonary tuberculosis, although differing in pathogenesis, have similar pathological features and can be grouped together under the term *postprimary pulmonary tuberculosis*. The characteristic pathological feature of this condition is the tuberculous cavity, which forms when the caseated and liquefied centre of a tuberculous pulmonary lesion is discharged into a bronchus. Extension of the infection to the pleura either by direct or lymphatic spread causes tuberculous pleurisy, which is sometimes accompanied by effusion and is occasionally followed by the development of a tuberculous empyema. Blood-borne dissemination to other organs is uncommon in postprimary pulmonary tuberculosis.

**Clinical Features.** There are two groups of clinical features in tuberculosis:

1. Those due to the systemic effects of the disease, which include lassitude and malaise, impairment of appetite, loss of weight, anaemia, sweating especially during

sleep, tachycardia and pyrexia. The last is usually most marked in the late afternoon or evening and sometimes occurs only at these times. The absence of symptoms does not necessarily mean that the disease is inactive.

2. Those caused by the local effects of the tuberculous lesions, which are summarised below according to anatomical site:

*Lungs and bronchi*: cough, sputum, haemoptysis, dyspnoea.
*Pleura*: pleural pain, dyspnoea due to pleural effusion.
*Larynx:* hoarseness, with dysphagia at a later stage from involvement of pharynx.
*Tongue*: ulceration (rare).
*Intestine*: diarrhoea, malabsorption or intestinal obstruction.
*Peritoneum*: ascites, attacks of intestinal obstruction due to plastic peritonitis.
*Pericardium*: pericardial effusion, constrictive pericarditis later.
*Kidneys and bladder*: haematuria, increased frequency of micturition. These are relatively late developments, early renal lesions being symptomless.
*Epididymo-orchitis*: painless swelling, sinus formation later.
*Fallopian tubes*: salpingitis, tubal abscess, infertility.
*Brain*: tuberculoma with or without focal neurological signs.
*Meninges*: symptoms and signs of meningitis.
*Lymph nodes*: enlargement of nodes, often with 'cold' abscess and sinus formation later.
*Adrenal glands*: symptoms and signs of Addison's disease.
*Bones and joints*: arthritis, osteomyelitis, 'cold' abscesses.
*Skin*: lupus vulgaris, erythema nodosum.
*Eyes*: phlyctenular keratoconjunctivitis, iridocyclitis, choroiditis.

In the sections which follow an account is given of those manifestations of tuberculosis which involve the lungs, namely primary pulmonary tuberculosis, acute miliary tuberculosis and postprimary pulmonary tuberculosis. Tuberculous pleurisy is described on page 300. For information regarding other manifestations of tuberculosis the reader should refer to appropriate sections of the book. The treatment and prevention of tuberculosis are dealt with on pages 259–262.

## Primary Pulmonary Tuberculosis

The pathological features of this type of tuberculosis have been described on page 252. The primary infection usually occurs in childhood but is sometimes delayed until adult life. A history of contact with a case of active pulmonary tuberculosis is obtained in many instances.

**Clinical Features.** In the vast majority of patients the primary infection produces no symptoms or signs and passes unnoticed unless routine radiological examination of the chest happens to be carried out at the appropriate time or serial tuberculin tests show conversion from negative to positive.

In a few patients the primary infection produces a febrile illness. It is generally mild and lasts for no more than 7 to 14 days, but it may be accompanied by other systemic features of tuberculous infection. It is unusual for gross focal symptoms or signs to develop in an uncomplicated case, but a slight dry cough is occasionally present. The leucocyte count is usually normal but the ESR is invariably raised.

The primary infection may be accompanied by *erythema nodosum*. This condition is characterised by bluish-red, raised, tender cutaneous lesions on the shins and, less commonly, on the thighs, and is associated in some cases with pyrexia and polyarthralgia. Erythema nodosum may be the first clinical indication of a tuberculous infection. In such cases the tuberculin reaction (p. 254) is always strongly positive and evidence of primary tuberculosis can usually be detected on the chest radiograph. Erythema nodosum may, however, be seen in conditions other than primary tuberculosis, e.g. sarcoidosis, streptococcal infections and, rarely, following the administration of a sulphonamide drug. It may also occur as an isolated phenomenon without apparent cause.

Occasionally the primary pulmonary infection pursues a progressive course (p. 252). Symptoms and signs due to its complications may appear either during the course of the initial illness or after a latent interval of weeks or months. Such complications include dry pleurisy or pleural effusion (p. 298), lobar or segmental collapse (p. 284), acute miliary tuberculosis (p. 255), tuberculous meningitis (p. 255), and postprimary pulmonary tuberculosis (p. 256).

**Investigation.** The three most valuable diagnostic investigations in primary pulmonary tuberculosis are:

1. *Radiological Examination of the Chest.* In children this usually shows unilateral enlargement of the hilar lymph nodes and demonstrates the primary intrapulmonary lesion if it is large enough to be visible radiologically. In adolescents and young adults the lymph node component of the primary complex is usually less conspicuous than in children and the pulmonary lesion more prominent. Complications such as pleural effusion, collapse and acute pneumonic tuberculosis may be superimposed.

2. *Tuberculin test.* With the Mantoux technique a solution of Old Tuberculin or purified protein derivative (PPD) tuberculin is injected intradermally on the flexor aspect of the forearm. The test is regarded as positive if, 2 to 4 days after injection, there is a reaction consisting of a raised area of inflammatory oedema not less than 5 mm in diameter, with surrounding erythema. The test is regarded as negative if there is no reaction or if there is an immediate (non-specific) reaction which disappears completely within 48 hours. The test should first be carried out with 1 tuberculin unit (TU) in 0·1 ml of normal saline. If there is no reaction it should be repeated with 10 TU in the same volume of saline. In order to obtain accurate results it is essential to use freshly prepared dilutions of tuberculin. Differential tuberculin testing with antigens prepared from other mycobacteria, e.g. PPD-A (*Myco. avium*) or PPD-Y (*Myco. kansasii*) is often a satisfactory method of distinguishing atypical mycobacterial infection from tuberculosis.

The younger the patient the greater is the diagnostic significance of a positive tuberculin test. A repeatedly negative test over a period of 6 weeks from the onset of symptoms practically rules out a diagnosis of tuberculosis except in the elderly, after acute exanthemata, in the later stages of miliary tuberculosis and tuberculous meningitis and in patients taking immunosuppressive drugs.

Tuberculin testing is an essential part of the examination of the family contacts of cases of tuberculosis. Apart from its value as a diagnostic measure it indicates which of the contacts should be vaccinated with BCG. When large numbers are being tested, particularly children, the *Heaf multiple puncture tuberculin test* is preferable to the Mantoux technique as it is more rapidly performed and is less painful. For this test a solution containing 100 000 TU of PPD tuberculin per ml, to which adrenaline has been added, should be used. This test may be read from the third to the seventh day and four grades of positivity are recognised.

Grade I: At least four discrete papules
II: The papules coalesce to form a ring
III: The area encircled by the papules is completely indurated.
IV: Any reaction which is greater than III, including central necrosis.

Reaction in grades III and IV indicates infection with mammalian tubercle bacilli and a grade I reaction usually indicates infection with atypical mycobacteria. The significance of a grade II reaction is uncertain.

The *tuberculin tine test* is performed with a disposable unit thus avoiding any risk of transmitting hepatitis. The unit has four prongs or 'tines' 2 mm in length mounted on a disc, the tines having been coated with Old Tuberculin. The validity of the tine test is being questioned at present.

3. *Bacteriological Examination*. Sputum is seldom available in cases of primary pulmonary tuberculosis, but tubercle bacilli can sometimes be isolated by culture of fasting gastric washings or of secretion obtained by swabbing the larynx. At least three specimens should be examined. The isolation of tubercle bacilli is absolute proof of the diagnosis, but a negative result does not exclude it.

**Prognosis.** Since primary pulmonary tuberculosis and its complications respond satisfactorily to antituberculosis chemotherapy (p. 259), which should be given in every case, the prognosis is excellent.

## Miliary Tuberculosis

The pathogenesis of this condition has already been discussed. Hitherto it has occurred chiefly in children and young adults. With the changing age-structure of tuberculosis in many countries it is now affecting persons in older age groups in whom it takes the form of an insidious illness — the so-called 'cryptic' type — which is often difficult to diagnose. Before the introduction of chemotherapy the disease was invariably fatal but most patients now recover completely.

**Clinical Features.** The disease may start suddenly or may be preceded by a few weeks of vague ill-health. In children and young adults the systemic disturbance rapidly becomes profound. In particular there is high remittent or intermittent pyrexia with drenching sweats during sleep, marked tachycardia, loss of weight and usually progressive anaemia. Cough and dyspnoea are occasionally present. There may be no abnormal physical signs in the lungs, although widespread fine crepitations are not infrequently heard at later stages of the disease. The liver is often enlarged and the spleen often palpable and sometimes tender. Choroidal tubercles may be visible on ophthalmoscopy but are rarely present in acute miliary disease affecting the elderly. Leucocytosis is usually absent or slight and the ESR variable. If chemotherapy is not given the patient's condition deteriorates rapidly and death takes place from exhaustion or from tuberculous meningitis within 4 to 8 weeks.

*'Cryptic' miliary tuberculosis* occurs in older age groups, particularly females. Lassitude and eventual exhaustion, loss of weight, and anaemia are common presenting features. Respiratory symptoms are rare, and the characteristic miliary shadows are absent. Choroidal tubercles are never observed in this form of the disease. A variety of specific blood disorders — neutropenia, pancytopenia and leukaemoid reaction — may be found. The clinical features are often so non-specific that the diagnosis is frequently made only at autopsy.

**Investigation.** The diagnosis of acute miliary tuberculosis can be made with certainty only when radiological examination of the chest shows the characteristic fine 'miliary' mottling symmetrically distributed throughout both lung fields or when choroidal tubercles are seen. These changes take a few weeks to develop but the diagnosis can often be suspected at an earlier stage by the symptoms, progressive clinical deterioration, persistent pyrexia and splenomegaly. Bacteriological confirmation should be sought by culture of sputum, urine or bone-marrow. In difficult cases, liver biopsy may be diagnostic. Although the tuberculin reaction is usually positive, a negative result does not always exclude acute miliary tuberculosis, as tuberculin sensitivity is occasionally depressed in the later stages of the illness. In 'cryptic' cases, a therapeutic test of chemotherapy with ethambutol and isoniazid (p. 261) is essential as death is inevitable if treatment is not given.

**Prognosis.** Antituberculosis chemotherapy (p. 259) has reduced the mortality of miliary tuberculosis from 100% to less than 5%. The cause of death is often tuberculous meningitis, although many patients who develop this complication make a complete recovery, provided there has been no delay in starting treatment.

### Postprimary Pulmonary Tuberculosis

Most of the morbidity and mortality from tuberculosis is caused by this form of the disease. Although in developing countries it is most prevalent in adolescence and early adult life, the majority of cases in Western Europe and North America now occur in middle-aged and elderly subjects, particularly males.

The lesions are most frequently situated in the upper lobes. Another common site is the apex of a lower lobe. The disease is often bilateral; usually it starts in one lung and spreads via the bronchi to the other; less commonly it develops in both lungs at the same time. Occasionally, when the disease takes an acute form, the initial lesion is pneumonic or bronchopneumonic.

**Clinical Features.** The onset of postprimary pulmonary tuberculosis is usually insidious, with the gradual development of general symptoms or of cough and sputum. Sometimes a dramatic incident such as an haemoptysis, an attack of pleurisy or a spontaneous pneumothorax marks the onset of the disease, but the diagnosis is now frequently made by radiography before any symptoms have appeared.

The focal respiratory symptoms which may occur during the course of post-primary tuberculosis are the following. Cough may be one of the earliest symptoms or may not be troublesome until a late stage. Its absence does not exclude a diagnosis of pulmonary tuberculosis. Sputum, like cough, may not become a prominent feature until the disease has reached an advanced stage. It is usually mucoid at first but later becomes purulent. It is rarely foetid. Haemoptysis, in the early stages, is due to the erosion of a small vessel in a caseating lesion and the bleeding is usually slight. In the late stages it originates from a large vessel in the wall of a cavity and the haemorrhage may be large, occasionally fatal. Dyspnoea on exertion is usually a late symptom, but may develop acutely when due to a spontaneous pneumothorax or to a rapidly developing pleural effusion. Pleural pain is usually due to dry pleurisy but occasionally to spontaneous pneumothorax.

In the early stages no physical signs may be elicited, but despite this an extensive lesion may be visible radiologically. The earliest physical signs consist of a few medium or coarse crepitations, usually situated over one or other lung apex posteriorly. These crepitations may be present only after coughing.

As the disease advances the percussion note over the site of the lesion loses its normal resonance and there is a change in the character of the breath sounds, which may become either diminished in intensity or harsh vesicular with prolonged expiration. The crepitations become more numerous and more coarse. Ultimately the physical signs of consolidation, cavitation and fibrosis may appear (p. 230). Pleurisy, with or without effusion, and spontaneous pneumothorax may modify the pulmonary signs.

**Radiological Examination.** This is of paramount importance for diagnosis in the early stages before physical signs appear and for assessment of the extent and progress of the disease. The earliest radiological change is an ill-defined opacity or opacities, usually situated in one of the upper lobes. In more advanced cases opacities are larger and more widespread, and may be bilateral. Occasionally there is a dense, homogeneous shadow involving a whole lobe ('pneumonic tuberculosis'). An area or areas of translucency within the opacities indicates cavitation. Very large cavities may be visible in some cases. If there is progress towards healing the opacities shrink, become more clearly defined, and may later show calcification. When fibrosis is marked the trachea and heart shadow are displaced towards the side of the lesion.

In any case of tuberculosis it is common for lesions at different stages of development to coexist. Thus in one area there may be cavitation, in a second evidence of fibrosis and in a third an opacity due to recent disease.

The presence of cavitation in an untreated case usually indicates that the disease is active. When cavitation is absent, however, it may sometimes be difficult to assess the activity of a tuberculous lesion from a single radiograph. Observation of the lesion over a period of time will be necessary in doubtful cases.

The radiological appearances of pleural effusion and pneumothorax, which may accompany those of pulmonary tuberculosis, are described on pages 299 and 305.

**Diagnosis.** The symptoms and signs suggesting a diagnosis of tuberculosis have already been stated. The grounds on which pulmonary tuberculosis should be suspected are: (1) unexplained cough persisting for more than three weeks; (2) haemoptysis; (3) pleural pain not associated with an acute illness; (4) spontaneous pneumothorax (although most cases are *not* tuberculous); (5) unexplained tiredness or loss of weight, even in the absence of respiratory symptoms. The presence of any of these symptoms demands immediate radiological examination of the lungs and, if any abnormality is found, the examination of at least three specimens of sputum for tubercle bacilli. When bacilli are numerous, the diagnosis can readily be made by microscopical examination of sputum smears stained by the Ziehl-Neelsen method, but culture of sputum (or fasting gastric washings or laryngeal swabs, if no sputum can be obtained) is essential for the isolation of bacilli present in small numbers and for the detection of drug resistance (p. 261). Cultural methods are thus of great practical value and should be used in the examination of every specimen, if facilities permit.

In the vast majority of cases the diagnosis of pulmonary tuberculosis can be made with certainty by radiological examination of the chest, bacteriological examination of the sputum for tubercle bacilli, or a combination of the two. In some cases it is necessary to carry out further radiological examination after a course of treatment with an antibiotic in order to exclude an acute inflammatory cause for an abnormal shadow.

Pulmonary tuberculosis must be regarded as active and requiring treatment if one or more of the following features is present:

1. Local or general symptoms, particularly haemoptysis or pleural pain
2. A radiological opacity known or suspected to be of recent development, or one which has increased in extent during a period of observation
3. Radiological evidence of cavitation
4. Tubercle bacilli isolated from sputum, gastric washings or laryngeal swabs.

**Complications**

*Pleurisy with or without effusion* (p. 300).

*Spontaneous pneumothorax* may be due to rupture of a tuberculous lesion into the pleural space (p. 303).

*Tuberculous empyema or pyopneumothorax* (p. 301) may complicate spontaneous pneumothorax.

*Tuberculous laryngitis* usually occurs as a complication of advanced pulmonary disease.

*Tuberculous enteritis* is practically confined to advanced cases. It is due to the swallowing of heavily infected sputum.

*Ischiorectal abscess and fistula-in-ano.* The abscess forms as a result of tubercle bacilli passing through an abrasion in the rectal mucosa. Secondary pyogenic infection invariably occurs, and a fistula may form when the abscess is incised or if it ruptures spontaneously.

*Dissemination of tuberculosis via the blood stream* is very unusual in post-primary pulmonary tuberculosis, but may occur in advanced cases with the production of renal tuberculosis or tuberculous meningitis.

*Respiratory failure* (p. 228) and *right ventricular failure* (p. 168) are important late complications if extensive areas of lung tissue are destroyed by tuberculosis or were resected when surgery was the only effective treatment. Although the tuberculous infection itself can be controlled, the residual pulmonary damage and the fibrosis and emphysema with which it is invariably associated may leave the patient seriously disabled by exertional dyspnoea.

*Secondary infection* of a healed cavity with fungi such as *Aspergillus fumigatus* may lead to the development of a mycetoma (p. 264). Occasionally the rupture of a large blood vessel in the wall of a pulmonary cavity or a dilated bronchus may result in a massive or even fatal haemoptysis long after the tuberculous infection has been eradicated.

**Prognosis.** With the advent of effective chemotherapy there has been a remarkable decline in the mortality from pulmonary tuberculosis. Provided the tubercle bacilli are not initially drug-resistant and chemotherapy is used correctly, a fatal outcome is extremely uncommon, even if the disease has reached an advanced stage when it is first recognised. The advent of new effective antituberculosis drugs has also improved the outlook for those patients whose bacilli are resistant to two or three drugs. The late complications of respiratory failure and secondary infection with pyogenic bacteria or fungi can be prevented if pulmonary tuberculosis is diagnosed at a reasonably early stage and is efficiently treated.

## The Treatment of Tuberculosis

### General Principles

*Antituberculosis chemotherapy* is by far the most important measure in the treatment of all forms of tuberculosis and should be given to every patient with active disease.

*Rest* is unimportant except in a few specific circumstances. The current practice is to keep patients in bed only until acute symptoms have subsided. The majority of patients are ambulant throughout treatment, many of them remaining at work. Immobilisation is of course necessary in certain forms of skeletal tuberculosis.

*Isolation* of patients who are excreting tubercle bacilli and who are therefore potentially infectious has previously been an important principle. The observation made in Madras that the frequency of disease amongst contacts was no greater when the patient was treated at home than in a sanatorium has led to the adoption of a policy whereby the majority of patients, even those who are sputum-positive on smear examination, are treated wholly as out-patients. However, many authorities still prefer to isolate patients from contact with young children. Hospitalisation for an initial period of treatment, as distinct from isolation, may be recommended for patients who cannot be relied upon to take their drugs regularly and for those who present difficult therapeutic problems.

*Surgical treatment* such as pulmonary resection, nephrectomy or removal of superficial lymph nodes is now rarely required. However, an irreparably damaged kidney should be removed and drainage of an abscess from tuberculous lymph nodes or of an empyema may be necessary. Early surgical treatment of tuberculosis of the spine ensures stability and prevents deformity.

### Chemotherapy

Effective treatment of tuberculosis demands not only a detailed knowledge of the drugs available but also of the most appropriate regimen for the individual patient.

**Drugs.** In Britain, six drugs — rifampicin, isoniazid, ethambutol, streptomycin, pyrazinamide and sodium aminosalicylate (PAS) — are normally considered in the initial treatment of tuberculosis. Thiacetazone, which is cheap, is widely used in developing countries. Pyrazinamide is particularly useful in the treatment of tuberculous meningitis because it diffuses well into the cerebrospinal fluid. Apart from a few minor variations in dose and duration of treatment (pp. 260 and 261) the policy governing the use of antituberculosis drugs is the same for all manifestations of the disease.

With the exception of PAS (twice daily) the drugs should be used in the following once daily doses:

| | | |
|---|---|---|
| Rifampicin | Children | 10–20 mg/kg |
| | Adults weighing less than 50 kg and in the elderly | 450 mg |
| | Adults weighing more than 50 kg | 600mg |
| | Intermittent regimen | 600–900 mg |
| Isoniazid | Children | 3 mg/kg |
| | Adults | 200–300 mg |
| | Intermittent regimen | 15 mg/kg * |
| | Miliary/meningitis | 10–12 mg/kg * |

| | | |
|---|---|---|
| Ethambutol ** | Initial 8 weeks in short-course regimen | 25 mg/kg |
| | Other daily regimens | 15 mg/kg |
| | Intermittent regimen | 90 mg/kg |
| Streptomycin sulphate | Children | 30 mg/kg |
| | Adults under 40 years and weighing more than 45 kg | 1 g |
| | Adults 40–60 years or weighing less than 45 kg | 0·75 g |
| | Adults over 60 years or in patients with renal failure | According to serum levels |
| | Intermittent regimens | 0·75–1g |
| Sodium aminosalicylate (PAS) ** | Children | 300 mg/kg |
| | Adults | 10–12 g |
| | Intermittent regimen | 10–12 g |
| Pyrazinamide | Daily | 30 mg/kg (max 2.5 g) |
| | Intermittent regimen | 90 mg/kg |
| Thiacetazone | Children | 2 mg/kg |
| | Adults | 150 mg |

* Plus pyridoxine 10 mg to prevent peripheral neuropathy (p. 117)

** In patients with renal failure the doses of ethambutol and PAS may also need to be determined according to serum levels.

SIDE-EFFECTS. In choosing a suitable drug regimen for individual patients it is important to bear in mind those side-effects which are particularly liable to cause serious chronic disability, such as vestibular disturbance due to streptomycin and optic neuritis due to ethambutol. Streptomycin must be prescribed with caution in the middle aged and elderly, who find difficulty in compensating for vestibular disturbance. Even in the relatively low dose recommended for ethambutol, a few patients develop optic neuritis and some are left with a permanent visual defect. This potential hazard must be taken into consideration whenever ethambutol is prescribed. Patients should be instructed to test their own visual acuity daily.

Streptomycin and PAS, and occasionally isoniazid, ethambutol and rifampicin, may produce a hypersensitivity reaction, consisting of pyrexia and an erythematous skin eruption, which usually develops 2 to 4 weeks after treatment is started.

Rifampicin is a potent liver enzyme inducer (p. 380) and should be used with appropriate caution when the following drugs are prescribed: oestrogens (e.g. oral contraceptives), warfarin, corticosteroids and digoxin. It should, if possible, be avoided in patients with liver disease.

The principal side-effects are:

*Streptomycin:* vestibular disturbance (see above); hypersensitivity (see above); deafness (rare).

*PAS:* hypersensitivity (see above); anorexia, nausea, vomiting, diarrhoea (common); goitre and hypothyroidism (rare); hepatitis, usually associated with hypersensitivity (rare); intestinal malabsorption (rare); hypokalaemia (rare); haemolytic anaemia (rare).

*Isoniazid*: hypersensitivity (occasionally, see above); polyneuropathy (rare); lack of mental concentration (rare).

*Ethambutol*: optic neuritis (see above); hypersensitivity (rare, see above).

*Rifampicin*: drug interaction (see above); hypersensitivity (occasionally, see above); hepatitis (rare); purpura (rare); fever, respiratory, cutaneous and abdominal syndromes (intermittent regimens only). Rifampicin should not be given again if the respiratory syndrome or purpura has occurred.

*Pyrazinamide*: hepatitis; gout; hypersensitivity (rare).

*Thiacetazone*: nausea, vomiting, anaemia (rare); leucopenia (rare)

REGIMENS. The following regimens are now considered to be optimal in the treatment of tuberculosis, those containing rifampicin throughout having the advantage that the period of treatment can be shortened to nine months:

*Initial Phase* (2 months): ethambutol or streptomycin plus isoniazid plus rifampicin.

*Continuation Phase* (7 months): isoniazid plus rifampicin.

Rifampicin, which colours the urine pinkish-orange, should be administered about half an hour before breakfast, in combination with isoniazid. In young children, PAS is to be preferred to ethambutol because of difficulty in identifying ocular toxicity in this age group, and should be administered in combination with isoniazid.

A patient who may not take antituberculosis drugs regularly without supervision should be kept in hospital for the initial (two-month) phase of treatment. Thereafter, for 10 months, the following regimen should be given at home twice weekly (at 3 and 4 day intervals) in the following doses: streptomycin sulphate, (1 g i.m.) isoniazid, (15 mg/kg body weight by mouth) and pyridoxine, 10 mg to prevent peripheral neuropathy. This type of chemotherapy should be wholly supervised, the tablets being administered at the same time as the injections.

*Inexpensive Treatment Regimens.* In developing countries it will usually be impossible for economic reasons to adhere to the recommended chemotherapeutic regimen. The following inexpensive forms of treatment are reasonably effective if administered for 12 months: (1) Streptomycin (1 g) by intramuscular injection *plus* isoniazid (15 mg/kg) by mouth plus pyridoxine (10 mg) on 2 days per week. This is 90 to 95% effective: if one or preferably two months of daily treatment with streptomycin, PAS and isoniazid can be afforded as initial treatment, the effectiveness of this regimen is nearly 100%. (2) Isoniazid (300 mg) *plus* thiacetazone (150 mg) given in a single daily dose by mouth is extremely cheap, and is about 80 to 95% effective.

RESPONSE TO TREATMENT. If the bacilli at the start of treatment are fully sensitive to the drugs in use it is most unusual, even in advanced cases, for cultures of sputum, gastric washings, laryngeal swabs or urine to remain positive for longer than 6 months. Where facilities for sensitivity testing do not exist, reliance must be placed on smear examination. Persistence of a positive sputum culture after 6 months' treatment suggests that drug resistance has occurred. Alternatively, failure may have been due to irregular treatment. A simple urine test for isoniazid metabolites can be used to assess the patient's cooperation in treatment.

DRUG-RESISTANT TUBERCLE BACILLI. The treatment of patients infected with drug-resistant tubercle bacilli presents a problem requiring specialised knowledge for its solution. Additional drugs available for the treatment of such cases are:

Capreomycin (0·75–1 g i.m.), ethionamide (0·75–1 g), prothionamide (0·75–1 g), pryazinamide (30 mg/kg) and cycloserine (0·75–1 g). The last four are given in a single oral dose daily.

## Corticosteroid Drugs

These agents suppress the inflammatory reaction excited by the tubercle bacillus and by interfering with tissue defence mechanisms may promote a rapid dissemination of infection throughout the body. If, however, a corticosteroid drug is given in conjunction with effective antituberculosis chemotherapy, it may exert a favourable influence on the course of the disease by reducing the severity both of the local inflammatory reaction and of the associated systemic disturbance. In acute cases of pulmonary tuberculosis such treatment will rapidly relieve pyrexia and will often produce a dramatic improvement in the radiological appearances. The effect is temporary and ceases when the corticosteroid drug is withdrawn, but it may save the lives of patients with fulminating tuberculous infection by enabling them to survive until antituberculosis chemotherapy has had time to exert its influence. Prednisolone is given in a dose of 20 mg daily for about 3 months.

Corticosteroid drugs in combination with chemotherapy may also be of value in tuberculous pleural and pericardial effusion, tuberculous disease of intrathoracic or superficial lymph nodes, tuberculosis involving the eye and in tuberculous meningitis. Whenever there is evidence of ureteric obstruction in genitourinary tuberculosis, corticosteroids should be administered in addition to chemotherapy, for such treatment significantly reduces the need for surgery.

### Symptomatic Treatment

*Haemoptysis.* A sedative may be given to allay anxiety, e.g. diazepam. Morphine, which depresses the cough reflex, may have the effect of allowing blood clot to accumulate in the bronchi and should seldom be prescribed. Haemoptysis nearly always stops spontaneously and reassurance to this effect lessens the strain of what, to patient and relatives, is a most alarming experience.

If the haemorrhage is very severe a blood transfusion should be given and, if respiratory obstruction develops, the blood must be removed from the bronchi by aspiration through a bronchoscope. Control of the bleeding by surgical measures is occasionally required.

*Pleural pain* due to dry pleurisy or spontaneous pneumothorax and *cough* are treated as described on page 237. *Fever and sweating* usually subside soon after chemotherapy is started. When persistent and excessive they should be treated by repeated tepid sponging. *Hoarseness* is usually due to tuberculous laryngitis, which responds rapidly to specific chemotherapy provided the organism is not drug-resistant. Severe and continuous *diarrhoea* in a patient with pulmonary tuberculosis is usually due to tuberculous enteritis. In most cases it can be rapidly controlled by chemotherapy. Diarrhoea may also be caused by PAS.

## The Prevention of Tuberculosis

Mortality rates are no longer considered so important in the assessment of the success of control measures because of the very low rates now existing in some countries and the inaccuracy of certification in the many countries where tuberculosis remains a major problem. The frequency of tuberculous meningitis is, however, a crude yardstick of the progress being made towards eradication. Notification rates are of limited value because of the adoption of varying standards, but the annual recording of the number of smear-positive patients with pulmonary tuberculosis is a useful indication of the efficiency of preventive measures. Another useful parameter is the *tuberculin index*, i.e. the percentage of positive reactors to tuberculin at a standard age, e.g. 5 or 13 years. It is important to assess the possible influence of the prevalence of atypical bacteria in the community and of BCG vaccination policy on the tuberculin index. It is also useful to estimate periodically the percentage of patients who on initial diagnosis are found to excrete drug-resistant tubercle bacilli.

The following control measures are important in the achievement of the goal of eradication of the disease.

*Improvement in socio-economic conditions* mainly in respect of adequate housing, ventilation and nutrition may still be the most important control measure of all.

*Case-finding.* Mass radiography is an expensive method of case-finding and should now be used in a selective manner concentrating on certain specific groups. The highest yield by far is from patients referred by general practitioners because of symptoms. Open access to mass radiography for general practitioners and minimum waiting time for patients are essential for success. Other important groups are persons in prisons, borstals and mental hospitals, elderly men especially those in lodging houses, and immigrants (especially from Asia). Mobile units have only a very small role nowadays.

Sputum-smear examination is an important and inexpensive method of case-finding in developing countries. The provision of a microscope and the training of a health worker in the examination of smears can be readily organised.

Contact examination achieves a high yield in case-finding. Efforts should be concentrated on the immediate examination of household contacts of sputum-smear positive patients especially amongst contacts under 25 years of age. Asian immigrants should have a chest radiograph annually for two years but others may be discharged after one year.

*Chemotherapy.* The proper use of modern highly-effective chemotherapy, by rendering patients non-infectious rapidly, makes a very important contribution to the control of the disease.

*Isolation of patients* is rarely considered necessary nowadays even in smear-positive patients except where very young children are at risk, provided the source case is being properly treated by chemotherapy.

*BCG Vaccination.* This is carried out by the administration of freeze-dried vaccine, reconstituted at the time of use, by the intradermal route (0·1 ml) injected at the junction of the upper and middle thirds of the upper arm. The multiple puncture method (40 needles) is less commonly used. Complications such as local abscess formation and enlargement of regional lymph nodes are very rare. BCG vaccine should not be given in the presence of immunodeficiency. The duration of protection is from 3 to 7 years. Vaccination reduces the incidence of pulmonary tuberculosis in young adults by 80% and eliminates the risk of serious disseminated disease – miliary tuberculosis and tuberculous meningitis.

Policy in relation to BCG vaccination in a community depends upon the size of the problem locally. If the infection rate is very low (1% or less) vaccination is inappropriate on the grounds of cost and the fact that BCG interferes with the diagnostic value of the tuberculin test in such a situation. Where there are many positive tuberculin reactors, as occur in communities with low living standards, vaccination of the newborn is usually indicated. Where infection rates are falling to low levels, vaccination at puberty may be appropriate.

*Chemoprophylaxis.* The concept of administering chemotherapy to individuals in order to try to prevent the development of tuberculosis is adopted in different communities with varying degrees of enthusiasm. Chemoprophylaxis, using isoniazid (5 mg/kg by mouth) daily for 1 year, is indicated in: (a) tuberculin positive children under 3 years of age, as this is a vulnerable group in respect of miliary tuberculosis and tuberculous meningitis; (b) individuals who have recently become tuberculin-positive; (c) patients on immunosuppressive drugs.

Chemoprophylaxis may be considered in: (a) tuberculin-positive adolescents with a high level of tuberculin sensitivity; (b) infants of highly infectious parents, when isoniazid-resistant BCG vaccine may be administered, isoniazid chemoprophylaxis being given for 6 weeks thereafter to prevent infection until vaccination exerts its protective effects.

*Elimination of Bovine Infection.* Although such infection is now extremely rare in Western countries constant vigilance will be required to ensure that it remains so.

## Respiratory Diseases Caused by Fungi

Most fungi encountered by man are harmless saprophytes, but some species may in certain circumstances infect human tissue or promote damaging allergic reactions.

The term *mycosis* is applied to disease caused by fungal infection. Predisposing factors include metabolic disorders, such as diabetes mellitus, toxic states such as chronic alcoholism, diseases such as leukaemia and myelomatosis in which immunological responses are disturbed, treatment with corticosteroids and immunosuppressive drugs, and radiotherapy. Local factors, such as tissue damage by suppuration or necrosis and the elimination of the competitive influence of a normal bacterial flora by antibiotics, may also facilitate fungal infection.

Allergic reactions to fungi may cause bronchial asthma (*Aspergillus fumigatus* and *Cladosporium herbarum*), bronchopulmonary eosinophilia (*A. fumigatus*) or extrinsic allergic alveolitis (*Micropolyspora faeni*, *Thermoactinomyces vulgaris*, *Coniosporium corticale* and *A. clavatus*). These conditions are described in the following section on allergic diseases of the respiratory tract.

The diagnosis of fungal diseases is usually made by mycological examination of the sputum, supported by serological tests for precipitating antibodies, and in some instances by skin sensitivity tests.

**Aspergillosis.** This is the most common respiratory mycosis in Britain. Inhaled air-borne spores of *Aspergillus fumigatus* lodge and germinate in damaged pulmonary tissue. In some cases the fungal infection remains localised to the site of the original lesion, but, particularly in immunodeficient or immunosuppressed patients, it may extend widely throughout the lungs, with the production of pulmonary necrosis and grave systemic disturbance (*necrotising pulmonary aspergillosis*).

When a pre-existing pulmonary cavity or cyst is infected by *A. fumigatus*, a large spherical mass of fungal mycelium may form within the cavity, producing on radiological examination a tumour-like opacity to which the term *mycetoma* or *aspergilloma* is applied. This type of lesion can readily be distinguished from a peripheral bronchial carcinoma by the presence of a crescent of air between the mycelial mass and the cavity wall. An aspergilloma often produces no specific symptoms, but may be responsible for recurrent severe haemoptysis.

Whenever mycelium is present in large quantities in a pulmonary cavity, or in any other lesion, precipitating antibodies can be detected in the serum by means of a gel diffusion test, using an antigen derived from *A. fumigatus*. This test is of considerable diagnostic value.

**Candidiasis.** Occasionally, in debilitated subjects oral thrush extends into the respiratory tract, with the production of bronchial or pulmonary candidiasis.

**Other Pulmonary Mycoses.** These, all of which are rare, include nocardiosis, cryptococcosis (p. 885), mucormycosis, blastomycosis (p. 884) and sporotrichosis (p. 884). Only the first three of these conditions have been encountered in Britain. In a somewhat different category are histoplasmosis (p. 881) and coccidioidomycosis (p. 885), which are endemic in certain areas of North America and Africa, and produce local or systemic granulomatous lesions resembling tuberculosis.

**Treatment** of the pulmonary mycoses is difficult and unsatisfactory. The administration of antibacterial drugs should be stopped, and antifungal agents substituted. Nystatin and natamycin by inhalation may control the more superficial respiratory mycoses involving the trachea and bronchi. For grave pulmonary infections amphotericin, a potent but highly toxic antifungal agent may have to be given intravenously (p. 882). Surgical treatment for a mycetoma may have to be considered if severe haemoptysis occurs.

## ALLERGIC DISEASES

Many types of particle suspended in the atmosphere possess antigenic properties, and are capable of stimulating the production of specific antibody when inhaled. Further exposure to antigen of an individual 'sensitised' in this way may provoke an allergic reaction which causes pathological changes and disturbances of function in the tissue where the reaction occurs. Three types of allergic response are concerned in the production of respiratory disease. The Type I or anaphylactic response (p. 29), mediated by immunoglobulin IgE, is associated with an immediate hypersensitivity reaction, the clinical manifestations of which include allergic rhinitis and bronchial asthma. The Type III or immune complex response, mediated by immunoglobulin IgG, is associated with a late hypersensitivity reaction which may contribute to the production of allergic alveolitis. Both Type I and Type III responses may be concerned in the production of some forms of bronchopulmonary eosinophilia, such as allergic aspergillosis. Type IV or tuberculin-type allergic responses, which are cell-mediated and do not involve circulating antibody, are usually associated with delayed hypersensitivity reactions in conditions such as tuberculosis, but may be involved in predominantly Type III reactions, such as allergic alveolitis.

Ingested antigens, or drugs acting as haptens, such as aspirin and PAS, occasionally produce allergic respiratory disorders, such as bronchial asthma and bronchopulmonary eosinophilia, and auto-antigens may have a similar role in conditions such as polyarteritis nodosa and systemic lupus erythematosus.

In this chapter, allergic rhinitis, bronchial asthma, bronchopulmonary eosinophilia and allergic alveolitis will be described in some detail, but for a description of other forms of allergic disorder the reader should refer to Chapter 2.

### Allergic Rhinitis

This is a disorder in which there are episodes of nasal congestion, watery nasal discharge and sneezing. It may be *seasonal* or *perennial*.

**Aetiology.** Allergic rhinitis is due to an anaphylactic antigen-antibody reaction in the nasal mucosa (p. 29). The antigens concerned in the seasonal form of the disorder are pollens from grasses, flowers, weeds or trees. Grass pollen is responsible for *hay fever*, the most common type of seasonal allergic rhinitis in Britain, and this disorder is at its peak between May and July.

Perennial allergic rhinitis may be a specific reaction to antigens derived from house dust, fungal spores or animal dander, but similar symptoms can be caused by physical or chemical irritants, such as pungent odours or fumes, including strong perfumes, cold air and dry atmospheres. In this context the term 'allergic' is a misnomer.

**Clinical Features.** In the seasonal type there are frequent sudden attacks of sneezing, with profuse watery nasal discharge and nasal obstruction. These attacks last for a few hours, and are often accompanied by smarting and watering of the eyes and conjunctival injection. In the perennial type the symptoms are similar, but more continuous and generally less severe.

In seasonal allergic rhinitis skin sensitivity tests with the relevant antigen are usually positive, and are thus of diagnostic value, but these tests are less useful in perennial rhinitis, and may be completely negative.

**Treatment.** The following symptomatic measures, singly or in combination, are usually effective in both seasonal and perennial allergic rhinitis: (1) an antihistamine drug, such as chlorpheniramine maleate (4–8 mg t.i.d.), but in some cases this causes intolerable drowsiness. (2) a decongestant nasal spray, e.g. 1% ephedrine hydrochloride in saline. (3) sodium cromoglycate nasal spray, one metered dose of a 2% solution (10 mg), into each nostril 6 times daily. (4) beclomethasone dipropionate nasal spray, one metered dose of 50 μg into each nostril 4 times daily.

Patients failing to respond to these measures may obtain symptomatic relief from weekly intramuscular injections of 0·5–1 mg of tetracosactrin zinc, but this form of treatment should be reserved for those patients whose symptoms are very severe and interfere seriously with business and social activities.

**Prevention.** In the seasonal type an attempt should be made to reduce exposure to pollen, for example by avoiding country districts and keeping indoors as much as possible, with the windows closed, during the pollen season. Some patients with hay fever may benefit from preseasonal hyposensitisation with a grass pollen extract. The prevention of perennial rhinitis consists of avoiding, as far as possible, exposure to any identifiable aetiological factors. Specific hyposensitisation is probably of little value.

## Bronchial Asthma

Bronchial asthma is characterised by paroxysms of dyspnoea accompanied by wheezing, resulting from narrowing of the bronchial airways by muscle spasm, mucosal swelling or viscid secretion. The airflow obstruction causes mismatching of alveolar ventilation and perfusion and increases the work of breathing. Being more marked during expiration it also causes air to be 'trapped' in the lungs. The narrowed bronchi can no longer be effectively cleared of mucus by the act of coughing, and in patients with severe acute asthma many of the smaller bronchi become obstructed by inspissated and often very tenacious secretion. This is usually the most conspicuous finding at autopsy. The cause of death is progressive alveolar hypoventilation and severe arterial hypoxaemia, culminating in cardiac arrest.

**Aetiology.** Asthma in most cases starts either in childhood or in middle age. 'Early onset' asthma is slightly more common in males, and 'late onset' asthma in females. 'Early onset' asthma generally occurs in atopic individuals, i.e. those who readily form IgE antibodies to commonly encountered allergens (p. 29). Such individuals can be identified by skin sensitivity tests (p. 268), which produce positive reactions to a wide range of common allergens. They often suffer from other allergic disorders, such as allergic rhinitis and eczema, and a family history of these disorders and of 'early onset' asthma is common. It is unusual for a single allergen to be the sole cause of asthma, and clinical experience indicates that many different allergens are implicated in almost every case, although the importance of each of them may vary from time to time. 'Late onset' asthma generally occurs in non-atopic individuals, and it would appear that external allergens play no part in the production of this form of the disease, to which the term 'intrinsic asthma' is sometimes applied.

The allergens responsible for asthma in atopic individuals generally enter the bronchi with the inspired air, and are derived from organic material, such as pollen, mite-containing house dust, feathers, animal dander and fungal spores. Previous exposure to these agents will have stimulated the formation of reaginic antibody (the immunoglobulin IgE), and an anaphylactic antigen-antibody reaction in the bronchi may follow further exposure to specific allergen. This releases pharmacologically active substances, such as histamine, kinins and the slow-reacting substance of anaphylaxis from mast cells, which provoke bronchial construction and an inflammatory reaction of allergic type in the bronchial mucosa. Much less frequently, similar effects may be produced by ingested allergens derived from certain foods, such as fish, eggs, milk, yeasts and wheat, which presumably reach the bronchi via the blood stream.

An immune complex allergic reaction may also be implicated in the pathogenesis of bronchial asthma, particularly where antigens derived from fungi, such as *A. fumigatus*, are implicated. For reasons which are still obscure acute attacks of asthma may be caused by drugs such as aspirin and by occupational exposure to chemical substances such as di-isocyanates and epoxy resins.

Asthma is often aggravated by non-specific factors, such as bronchial irritation caused by tobacco smoke, dust and acrid fumes, bacterial infection in the respiratory tract, and emotional stress. In children and young adults, usually atopic subjects, an attack of asthma may follow strenuous exertion (*exercise-induced asthma*) or exposure to cold air.

**Clinical Features.** Bronchial asthma may be either *episodic* or *chronic*, and although there is a good deal of overlap between these two syndromes, the distinction is clinically useful, particularly in terms of prognosis and management. In general, atopic individuals tend to develop episodic asthma, and non-atopic individuals chronic asthma.

In typical cases of episodic asthma the paroxysms, which may occur at any hour of the day or night, are of sudden onset, but may be preceded by a feeling of tightness in the chest. The dyspnoea, which may be intense, is chiefly expiratory in character. Expiration becomes a conscious and exhausting effort, in contrast to inspiration which is short and gasping. The patient adopts an upright position, fixing the shoulder-girdle to assist the accessory muscles of expiration. Wheezing, chiefly expiratory, is heard, and there may be an unproductive cough which aggravates the dyspnoea. In severe attacks there is tachycardia, pulsus paradoxus, and central cyanosis.

The attack may end abruptly within an hour or two, sometimes with the coughing up of tough viscid sputum, or may persist for many hours or even for several days. The sputum, usually scanty, may contain numerous eosinophil leucocytes and, occasionally, gelatinous casts of small bronchi. In most cases there is an increase in the number of eosinophil leucocytes in the blood.

The term, *severe acute asthma*, has now replaced 'status asthmaticus' for the description of life-threatening attacks associated with extreme respiratory distress and arterial hypoxaemia.

In *chronic asthma* the paroxysmal character of the symptoms is usually less conspicuous, the chief clinical features being continuous wheeze and breathlessness on exertion. Cough and mucoid sputum, with recurrent episodes of frank respiratory infection, are common in this type of asthma, which may be difficult to distinguish from chronic bronchitis.

*Physical Signs in the Chest.* 1. During a paroxysm the chest is held near the position of full inspiration. The percussion note may be hyperresonant. The breath sounds, which are obscured by numerous high pitched rhonchi, are vesicular in character with prolonged expiration. In very severe asthma airflow may be insufficient to produce rhonchi, and a 'silent chest' in such patients is an ominous sign.

2. Between paroxysms there are usually no abnormal physical signs except in patients with chronic asthma, who are seldom without rhonchi. Severe asthma starting in childhood usually causes a 'pigeon chest' deformity.

**Investigation.** *Radiological Examination.* In an acute attack of asthma the lungs appear hyperinflated. In long-standing cases the features of emphysema may be present, and the lateral view may demonstrate a 'pigeon chest' deformity. Occasionally, when a bronchus is obstructed by tenacious mucus, there is an opacity caused by lobar or segmental collapse.

*Pulmonary Function Tests.* Measurements of the forced expiratory volume in 1 second ($FEV_1$) and forced vital capacity (FVC) or of the peak expiratory flow rate (PEFR) provide a fairly reliable indication of the degree of airflow obstruction (p. 232), and can also be used to determine whether and to what extent it can be relieved by bronchodilator drugs or corticosteroids, or to confirm that it is provoked by exercise. Such tests thus have an important place in the diagnosis and treatment of bronchial asthma. Frequent recordings of PEFR are useful in the assessment of those patients whose asthma shows marked diurnal variations in severity (the so-called 'morning dippers'). Measurements of arterial blood gas pressures ($Pa{O_2}$ and $Pa{CO_2}$) are indispensable to the management of patients with severe acute asthma.

*Skin Sensitivity Tests.* A prick is made in the skin with a fine needle through a drop of an aqueous extract of the substance to be tested, and a positive reaction is indicated by the development of a wheal and flare, which begins to appear within a few minutes. Tests are usually performed with solutions of common substances known to possess antigenic properties. It is seldom possible with these tests to identify one particular substance as the cause of asthma in an individual case, and their chief value is to distinguish atopic from non-atopic subjects.

**Course and Prognosis.** The prognosis of the individual attack is good, except in severe acute asthma where there is occasionally a fatal outcome, especially if treatment is inadequate or delayed. Spontaneous recovery is fairly common in episodic asthma, particularly in children, but rare in chronic asthma, which often causes permanent pulmonary damage. Seasonal fluctuations occur in both types of asthma. Atopic subjects with episodic asthma are usually worse in the summer, when they are more heavily exposed to antigens, while chronic asthmatics are usually worse in the winter months because of their increased liability to bacterial infection.

**Treatment.** The following measures may be of value in the management of patients with bronchial asthma: (1) Reduction of exposure to relevant allergens. (2) Hyposensitisation, which may prevent damaging antigen-antibody reactions. (3) Drugs, such as sodium cromoglycate, which prevent release from mast cells in the bronchial wall of pharmacological mediators of bronchoconstriction. (4) Drugs, such as bronchodilators or corticosteroids, which control or suppress clinical manifestations of asthma. (5) Measures to counter the effects of aggravating factors such as exercise, infection and emotional stress.

1. AVOIDANCE OF ALLERGENS. There are a few instances in which a single allergen can be identified as the cause of attacks of asthma. These include grass pollens, mites, animal dander, drugs such as aspirin, a few industrial chemicals such as di-isocyanates and certain articles of diet. The measures which can be taken to prevent or reduce exposure to these allergens, and the degree of success likely to be achieved, are summarised in Table 7.4. In the vast majority of cases, however, asthmatic patients are sensitive to a wide range of allergens and attempts to avoid them all are impracticable.

Table 7.4 Avoidance of allergens and other substances liable to provoke attacks of asthma

| Causative agent | Preventive measures | Efficacy |
|---|---|---|
| Pollens | Try to avoid exposure to seeding vegetation. Keep bedroom windows closed. | Low |
| Mites (e.g. *D. pteronyssinus*) | Vacuum-clean mattress daily. Shake out blankets daily. Dust bedroom thoroughly. | Doubtful |
| Animal dander | Avoid contact with dogs, cats, horses or other animals. | High |
| Feathers in pillows or quilts | Substitute latex foam pillows and terylene quilts. | High |
| Fungal spores | Try to avoid exposure to sources of fungal contamination. | Low |
| Drugs (e.g. aspirin) | Avoid all preparations of relevant drug. | High |
| Foods | Identify and eliminate from diet. | Low* |
| Industrial chemicals (e.g. di-isocyanates, epoxy resins) | Avoid exposure to chemical, or change occupation. | High |

*More effective in control of eczema

2. HYPOSENSITISATION. This is the only measure at present available for the prevention of damaging antigen-antibody reactions. It involves the subcutaneous injection of initially very small, but gradually increasing, doses of extracts of allergens believed to be responsible for the patient's asthma. It may be of some value when only a single allergen, such as grass pollen or animal dander, is implicated but it is not devoid of the risk of producing an acute anaphylactic reaction. Hyposensitisation with a mixture of allergens is irrational and cannot be recommended. Although allergy to the house dust mite is widely believed to be an important cause of nocturnal asthma, the results of hyposensitisation with a 'mite vaccine' have proved to be disappointing.

3. PREVENTION OF THE RELEASE OF PHARMACOLOGICAL MEDIATORS OF BRONCHOCONSTRICTION. The only drug which has so far been shown to exert this effect is sodium cromoglycate administered by inhalation. It seems to be of particular value in children with extrinsic (atopic) asthma, and should be given a trial of four weeks' duration in all such patients. If it is found to be effective, regular treatment with a dose of 20 mg four times daily may completely prevent recurrence of asthma in this group of patients and it may also be of value in a few cases of intrinsic (non-atopic) asthma. A similar mode of action has been claimed for ketotifen by mouth, but that drug appears to be less effective than sodium cromoglycate and has the serious disadvantage in some patients of causing drowsiness which may be a dangerous side-effect in patients driving cars or operating machinery.

4. DRUGS WHICH CONTROL OR SUPPRESS CLINICAL MANIFESTATIONS OF ASTHMA

(i) *General Principles.* It is important to distinguish between bronchodilators, which have a direct and immediate effect on airflow obstruction, and corticosteroids, which relieve or prevent airflow obstruction indirectly by their less rapid anti-inflammatory action. Thus a corticosteroid aerosol cannot be expected to relieve an acute episode of asthma. On the other hand, if a patient with severe acute asthma has ceased to respond to bronchodilator aerosols, systemic treatment with corticosteroids in high dosage by mouth or intravenously, is the only measure likely to be effective. In such a situation, there may be a delay of a few hours before a severe attack of asthma responds to corticosteroids and, during that period, intensive bronchodilator and oxygen therapy may be essential to the patient's survival.

There is considerable controversy about the relative efficacy of the various methods of administering bronchodilator drugs. In the case of selective $\beta_2$-adrenoceptor agonists, such as salbutamol, terbutaline or fenoterol, the inhalation of an aerosol has clear advantages over oral administration because it reduces airflow obstruction more rapidly. Since the effective dose is much lower, it is less liable to produce side-effects such as tremor and anxiety. When a patient fails to obtain the accustomed degree of relief from the inhalation of a bronchodilator aerosol, this means that the asthma is in a refractory phase, and that a more potent form of treatment, such as a course of prednisolone by mouth, is urgently required.

Methylxanthine derivatives, such as theophylline or aminophylline, can be given by intravenous injection, mouth or suppository. Intravenous aminophylline (375 mg) is often an effective form of treatment for severe acute asthma, although it is probably not superior to salbutamol (0·5 mg) administered by the same route. Although there has been a renewal of interest in oral methylxanthine preparations, mainly because it is now appreciated that they are effective only when they produce adequate serum levels, there is still considerable doubt as to whether they are of superior efficacy to the regular inhalation of $\beta_2$-adrenoceptor agonist aerosols, except possibly for the prevention of nocturnal wheeze.

(ii) *Episodic Asthma.* Where episodes of asthma are mild and infrequent, they can be controlled by inhalation of a bronchodilator aerosol, for example, 2 metered doses of salbutamol (200 μg) as required. When the episodes are more frequent, this should be supplemented by a regular prophylactic measure, such as sodium cromoglycate or a corticosteroid aerosol by inhalation. In general, sodium cromoglycate is more effective in atopic individuals, particularly children and corticosteroid aerosols in non-atopic individuals, particularly adults. Sodium cromoglycate has virtually no side-effects, but corticosteroid aerosols are apt to cause oropharyngeal candidiasis.

(iii) *Exercise-Induced Asthma.* This fairly common phenomenon, which occurs particularly in atopic children with episodic asthma, can often be prevented by regular treatment with sodium cromoglycate. If that fails, the inhalation of two metered doses of salbutamol (200 μg), a few minutes before the patient expects to undertake strenuous exertion, is usually effective.

(iv) *Chronic Asthma.* Some form of prophylaxis is necessary in all patients with chronic asthma. Sodium cromoglycate is always worth a trial in such cases, but there is usually a better response to the regular inhalation of a corticosteroid aerosol – three metered doses of beclomethasone dipropionate (150 μg) or of betamethasone valerate (300 μg) thrice daily. In severe cases, this may have to be supplemented by a small maintenance dose of prednisolone by mouth (5–7·5 mg/d) and/or by occasional short courses of prednisolone in higher dosage (20 mg/d or more for a week). Most patients with chronic asthma also require to inhale a bronchodilator aerosol either regularly or periodically to control recurrences of wheeze. When regular treatment is needed, it is best given a few minutes before the inhalation of sodium cromoglycate or a corticosteroid aerosol to ensure that the largest possible amounts of these drugs enter the bronchi. Oral bronchodilator drugs are seldom as effective as aerosols in the treatment of chronic asthma, but slow-release oral preparations of salbutamol and aminophylline taken at bedtime may prevent nocturnal wheeze, as may aminophylline suppositories.

(v) *Severe Acute Asthma.* When an acute attack of asthma becomes severe and life-threatening, the patient will have ceased to show any response to bronchodilator aerosols and it is futile, and perhaps dangerous in hypoxic asthmatics, to persist with this form of treatment. All such patients should be admitted to hospital as quickly as possible and emergency admission schemes, which eliminate the delays inherent in normal hospital admission procedures, can do much to reduce the number of unnecessary deaths from severe acute asthma. It is equally important that, before the ambulance arrives, the general practitioner should start effective treatment with an intravenous bronchodilator drug and large doses of corticosteroids by intravenous injection and by mouth (Table 7.5). Since all bronchodilator drugs may produce a significant increase in arterial hypoxaemia, which may have grave consequences in patients with severe acute asthma, it is strongly advisable for oxygen to be given from a portable cylinder for a few minutes before these drugs are administered. Oxygen therapy (35% by Ventimask) should be continued in the ambulance conveying the patient to hospital.

Table 7.5 Treatment of severe acute asthma in the home

1. Administer oxygen from portable cylinder (preferably by MC mask at 'high' setting).
2. Give bronchodilator intravenously: aminophylline (375 mg in 20 ml saline) *or* salbutamol (0·5 mg in 20 ml saline) *or* terbutaline (0·5 mg in 20 ml of saline)
3. Give hydrocortisone sodium succinate 200 mg intravenously.
4. Arrange for emergency admission to hospital in ambulance equipped for oxygen therapy.
5. Give prednisolone 60 mg by mouth.

N.B. The above doses are for adults — those for children should be proportionately smaller.

On arrival in hospital most patients respond to treatment with high doses of corticosteroid, supplemented by bronchodilator drugs administered by intravenous injection or infusion, or in the form of an aqueous aerosol delivered, if necessary, by intermittent positive-pressure breathing with a Bird or Bennett ventilator. Only occasionally is it necessary to employ major resuscitative measures, such as tracheal intubation, mechanical ventilation and bronchial lavage, because most patients nowadays are admitted before they have become desperately ill, and most of them have received adequate emergency treatment from their general practitioners.

5. GENERAL MANAGEMENT OF ASTHMATIC PATIENTS. Whether the patient suffers from episodic or chronic asthma, the following general principles are essential to successful management: (i) The nature of the disease and the action of the various drugs must be carefully explained to every patient. (ii) The patient should be taught how to recognise 'danger signs', such as failure to respond to bronchodilator aerosol, and how to deal with them. (iii) All patients must be shown exactly how to use the various types of inhaler. If they are unable to use one type efficiently, another type should be substituted. (iv) It is just as important to secure patient compliance in the dosage of aerosols as of tablets. Excessive use of a bronchodilator aerosol is as much the fault of the prescriber as it is of the patient. (v) A patient with potentially severe

asthma should be actively encouraged to call his or her general practitioner when things go wrong. Only a very small number of patients will do so unnecessarily. (vi) Antibiotics are of value only when there is evidence of bacterial infection, but they are no substitute for the effective treatment of airflow obstruction. (vii) Although asthma is basically not a psychological disorder, it can be aggravated by emotional and social problems; these must be carefully evaluated, and whenever possible resolved, in every patient suffering from the disease.

## Bronchopulmonary Eosinophilia

This term is applied to a group of allergic disorders of different aetiology in which lesions of the bronchi and/or the lungs are associated with an increase in the number of eosinophil leucocytes in the blood. In some of these diseases the bronchi appear to be primarily affected, although there may be secondary effects on lung tissue, while in others the pathological changes are confined to the lungs. It is therefore appropriate to subdivide the syndrome into bronchial and pulmonary eosinophilia (Table 7.6).

Table 7.6 Bronchopulmonary eosinophilia

| | |
|---|---|
| Bronchial eosinophilia: | Bronchial asthma |
| | Eosinophilic bronchitis with bronchial obstruction (including allergic bronchial aspergillosis) |
| Pulmonary eosinophilia: | Helminthic eosinophilic pneumonia |
| | localised |
| | diffuse |
| | Fungal eosinophilic pneumonia |
| | Drug-induced eosinophilic pneumonia |
| | Cryptogenic eosinophilic pneumonia |

### Bronchial Eosinophilia

Although bronchial asthma could logically be included in this category, it is not customary to do so, and the term is normally restricted to patients with a severe allergic reaction in the bronchi which gives rise to the production of inspissated mucus heavily coated with eosinophils ('eosinophilic bronchitis'). These casts frequently obstruct bronchi and produce lobar or segmental collapse. In some cases, the allergic reaction extends into the collapsed lung tissue, but because lung biopsy is seldom indicated in patients with bronchopulmonary eosinophilia, the frequency of this complication is uncertain. There is evidence that eosinophilic bronchitis is the result of dual anaphylactic and immune complex antigen-antibody reactions (p. 29) in the bronchial wall, and that an antigen derived from the fungus, *Aspergillus fumigatus*, is often the causal agent. In many cases that fungus can be isolated from the sputum or from a bronchial cast, skin tests (immediate and late) with an *A. fumigatus* antigen are positive and precipitating antibodies can be detected in the serum. The term, *allergic bronchial aspergillosis*, is commonly used to describe such cases. Occasionally all investigations are negative and the causal antigen cannot be identified.

**Clinical Features.** Chronic asthma is the dominant clinical manifestation of bronchial eosinophilia, but at irregular intervals bronchi, usually in the upper lobes, are obstructed by casts, with the production of lobar or segmental collapse, which may cause a mild febrile illness. When these episodes recur over a period of years, as they usually do, they result in permanent damage to the bronchi and lungs. Cast formation first produces dilatation of the larger bronchi ('proximal bronchiectasis'), and at a later stage bacterial and possibly fungal infection in lung tissue distal to the bronchial obstruction causes extensive pulmonary fibrosis and bronchiectasis. These changes, together with the associated chronic asthma, which seldom responds well to treatment, eventually cause respiratory failure, pulmonary hypertension and right ventricular failure.

**Diagnosis.** In early cases, the diagnosis is made by observing recurrent transient radiographic opacities, usually of lobar or segmental distribution, in young adults (seldom children) with chronic asthma and an increased eosinophil count in the blood. Often the investigations already described will identify *A. fumigatus* as the cause of the allergic reaction. In advanced cases, however, chronic respiratory failure overshadows the earlier and more specific features, and radiological examination shows extensive bilateral fibrosis and bronchiectasis predominantly affecting the upper lobes.

**Treatment.** Initially, a short course of prednisolone (5 mg by mouth 6 hourly for a week), presumably by relieving airflow obstruction, may be followed by the expectoration of bronchial casts and clearing of the pulmonary opacities. If not, it may be necessary to extract the cast or casts by bronchoscopy in an attempt to avert permanent bronchopulmonary damage. Further cast formation can in some cases be prevented by a small maintenance dose of prednisolone (5–10 mg per day), but in many cases this does not halt the development of progressive pulmonary fibrosis and bronchiectasis, particularly when bronchial eosinophilia is a manifestation of allergic aspergillosis.

## Pulmonary Eosinophilia

As the term implies, this condition predominantly involves lung tissues although in a few cases it may be associated with chronic bronchial asthma. There is a cellular infiltrate, chiefly consisting of eosinophil leucocytes, in the alveoli and alveolar walls, to which the term, *eosinophilic pneumonia*, can suitably be applied. This may be localised or diffuse, and appears to be an immunological reaction in the lung to a variety of antigens (Table 7.7). In some cases eosinophilic pneumonia, which may be severe and extensive, develops in the absence of any identifiable cause. The term, *cryptogenic pulmonary eosinophilia*, is applied to this form of the disease, for which an autoimmune mechanism may be responsible.

Table 7.7 Some causes of pulmonary eosinophilia

| | |
|---|---|
| Helminths | *Ascaris lumbricoides* (localised eosinophilic pneumonia).<br>Microfilaria (diffuse eosinophilic pneumonia). |
| Fungi | *Aspergillus fumigatus.* |
| Drugs | Nitrofurantoin, para-aminosalicyclic acid, sulphasalazine, imipramine, chlorpropamide, phenylbutazone, aspirin. |
| Chemicals | Toluene di-isocyanate. |

**Clinical Features.** These vary widely in severity, depending on the aetiology and on the extent of pulmonary involvement. Many patients have only a trivial febrile illness, the nature of which would have passed unrecognised in the absence of radiological and haematological investigation. Others, particularly those in whom the illness is an allergic reaction to microfilaria (*tropical pulmonary eosinophilia*) (p. 878) or to drugs, may become gravely ill with high fever and severe dyspnoea, and a similar clinical picture may be observed in cryptogenic pulmonary eosinophilia. In most patients with a severe clinical illness, the absolute eosinophil count in the blood is high, often exceeding $5{\cdot}0 \times 10^9/l$.

**Investigation.** Pulmonary eosinophilia should always be suspected in patients with unexplained radiographic opacities in the lungs, either localised or diffuse. It can readily be mistaken for pulmonary tuberculosis or bacterial pneumonia unless an eosinophil count is carried out. After the diagnosis is established, an attempt should always be made to discover the relevant aetiological factor, such as an intestinal helminth, filariasis or treatment with a drug or exposure to a chemical substance previously reported to have caused the disease. If all such causes are excluded, and tests for fungal allergy are negative, a diagnosis of *cryptogenic pulmonary eosinophilia* has to be accepted. It has been suggested that the last condition is an early manifestation of polyarteritis nodosa, in which transient pulmonary infiltrates and blood eosinophilia may occur, but this seems unlikely, since pulmonary vascular lesions are not a feature of cryptogenic pulmonary eosinophilia and there is no multisystem involvement.

**Treatment.** If a cause is found or suspected it must be treated or removed. Helminthic intestinal infections should be eradicated and any drug likely to be responsible for the pulmonary eosinophilia should be withdrawn. When the condition is due to microfilaria (p. 875) the patient should be given diethylcarbamazine and rapid clinical and radiographic improvement will follow. Cryptogenic pulmonary eosinophilia usually responds dramatically to prednisolone (5 mg 6 hourly by mouth) but because it is apt to recur after corticosteroid therapy is withdrawn, a small maintenance dose may have to be continued for some months, or even for a few years.

## Extrinsic Allergic Alveolitis

In this condition the inhalation of certain types of organic dust produces a diffuse allergic reaction in the walls of the alveoli and bronchioles. There is a cellular exudate consisting of polymorphs, lymphocytes and plasma cells, and small epithelioid granulomata may also be seen. These changes cause decreased pulmonary compliance and ventilation:perfusion maldistribution. They are presumably also responsible for the widespread coarse crepitations heard on auscultation, and for the diffuse micronodular shadowing seen on the chest radiograph. Precipitating antibodies in the serum against the relevant antigens would seem to indicate that allergic alveolitis is an immune complex reaction, but the finding of small pulmonary granulomata suggests that cell-mediated hypersensitivity may also be implicated (p. 33).

Some of the agents which produce extrinsic allergic alveolitis, the source of these agents, and the names applied to the resulting diseases are shown in Table 7.8. If patients with this disorder continue to expose themselves to the relevant antigen for long periods, they may eventually develop permanent pulmonary damage with severe respiratory disability.

Table 7.8 Types and causes of extrinsic allergic alveolitis

| Agent | Source | Disease |
|---|---|---|
| *Micropolyspora faeni* | Mouldy hay | Farmer's lung |
| Thermophilic actinomycetes | Compost | Mushroom worker's lung |
| | Mouldy sugar cane fibre | Bagassosis |
| *Aspergillus clavatus* | Malting barley | Maltworker's lung |
| *Coniosporium corticale* | Bark of maple trees | Maple bark disease |
| Avian protein in pigeon and budgerigar droppings | Pigeon loft or bird cage | Bird fancier's lung |
| Proteolytic enzyme derived from *Bacillus subtilis* | Air-borne dust in factory making 'biological' washing powder | Terminology undecided |

**Clinical Features.** Extrinsic allergic alveolitis should be suspected when a person regularly exposed to a heavy concentration of organic dust complains, a few hours after re-exposure to the same dust, of general malaise, dry cough and dyspnoea without wheeze. If the cause of these symptoms is not appreciated, and further exposure to the dust hazard permitted, they are likely to become continuous, and in some cases very severe. At this stage the patient may be febrile, cyanosed and dyspnoeic at rest, coarse crepitations (but no rhonchi) can be heard over both lungs and a chest radiograph may show diffuse micronodular shadowing. The $FEV_1$ and FVC are both reduced, but the $FEV_1$/FVC ratio is normal — indicating a restrictive ventilatory defect without airflow obstruction. The $Pa{O_2}$ is reduced, and the $Pa{CO_2}$ is slightly subnormal as a result of overventilation. Gas transfer (p. 225) is impaired.

The diagnosis of extrinsic allergic alveolitis is confirmed serologically by a positive precipitin test and, if necessary, by a positive provocation test, in which the inhalation of an aerosol containing the relevant antigen is followed after 3 to 6 hours by pyrexia and a reduction in FVC, often associated with a recurrence of symptoms.

**Treatment.** Mild forms of extrinsic allergic alveolitis rapidly subside when exposure to the dust ceases. In severe cases a corticosteroid preparation should be given for 3 to 4 weeks, starting with 40–60 mg of prednisolone per day. Severely hypoxic patients may require oxygen in high concentration (60%).

## DISEASES OF THE LARYNX, TRACHEA AND BRONCHI

Acute infections of the larynx have already been described (p. 239). Other common disorders of the larynx include chronic laryngitis, laryngeal tuberculosis (p. 253), laryngeal paralysis and laryngeal obstruction. Tumours of the larynx are relatively common, but for information on these conditions the reader should refer to a textbook of diseases of the ear, nose and throat.

### Chronic Laryngitis

Chronic laryngitis occurs as a result of repeated attacks of acute laryngitis, excessive use of the voice, especially in dusty atmospheres, e.g. in auctioneers, heavy tobacco smoking, mouth-breathing from nasal obstruction and chronic nasal and oral sepsis. The chief symptom is hoarseness and the voice may be lost. There is irritation of the throat and spasmodic cough with a little mucoid sputum. The disease pursues a chronic course frequently uninfluenced by treatment, and in long-standing cases the voice is often permanently impaired.

As chronic and progressive hoarseness may also be caused by tuberculosis and tumours of the larynx and by laryngeal paralysis, these conditions must be considered in the differential diagnosis if the hoarseness does not improve within a few weeks. In some cases a chest radiograph may bring to light unsuspected pulmonary tuberculosis or a bronchial carcinoma. If no such abnormality is found the patient should be referred to a specialist for laryngoscopic examination.

The voice must be rested completely. This is particularly important in the case of public speakers. Smoking should be prohibited. Some benefit may be obtained from frequent inhalations of medicated steam.

## Laryngeal Paralysis

**Aetiology.** Laryngeal paralysis may be organic or functional.

*Organic paralysis* is due to interference with the motor nerve supply of the larynx and may be caused by lesions of the brain stem, e.g. bulbar paralysis, or of the vagus nerve or its recurrent laryngeal branch.

Interruption of the recurrent laryngeal nerve, or of the vagus trunk above the origin of that nerve, by tumour, aneurysm or trauma is the most common way in which laryngeal paralysis is produced. The paralysis is nearly always unilateral and, by reason of the intrathoracic course of the left recurrent laryngeal nerve, usually left-sided. Accidental division of one or both recurrent laryngeal nerves is one of the hazards of thyroidectomy.

*Functional paralysis* of the larynx occurs as a manifestation of hysteria.

**Clinical Features.** *Hoarseness* always accompanies laryngeal paralysis whatever its cause. Paralysis of organic origin is seldom reversible, but when only one vocal cord is affected the hoarseness may improve or even disappear after a few weeks as a result of a compensatory adjustment whereby the unparalysed cord crosses the midline and approximates with the paralysed cord on phonation.

*'Bovine' cough*, which is a characteristic feature of organic laryngeal paralysis, results from the loss of the explosive phase of normal coughing consequent upon the failure of the cords to close the glottis. The difficulty in bringing up sputum which some of these patients experience can be explained on the same basis. 'Bovine' cough does not occur with hysterical paralysis.

*Dyspnoea* and *stridor* are occasionally present but are seldom severe except with bilateral laryngeal paralysis of organic origin.

*Laryngoscopy* is necessary to establish the diagnosis of laryngeal paralysis with certainty. The paralysed cord lies in the so-called 'cadaveric' position, midway between abduction and adduction. In hysterical paralysis only adduction of the cords, a voluntary movement, is affected.

**Treatment.** The cause of the laryngeal paralysis should be treated if that is possible. In unilateral paralysis the voice can be improved by the injection of teflon into the affected vocal cord. In bilateral organic paralysis, tracheal intubation, tracheostomy or a plastic operation on the larynx may be necessary. Psychiatric treatment is indicated for hysterical aphonia.

### Laryngeal Obstruction

**Aetiology.** The laryngeal opening (glottis) may be obstructed by (1) inflammatory or allergic oedema or exudate, (2) spasm of the laryngeal muscles, (3) inhaled foreign body, (4) inhaled vomitus in an unconscious patient, (5) tumours of the larynx, (6) bilateral vocal cord paralysis and (7) fixation of both cords in advanced rheumatoid arthritis. Laryngeal obstruction is more liable to occur in children than in adults because of the smaller size of the glottis.

**Clinical Features.** Sudden complete laryngeal obstruction by a foreign body produces the clinical picture of acute asphyxia — violent but ineffective inspiratory efforts with indrawing of the intercostal spaces and the unsupported lower ribs, accompanied by deep cyanosis. Unrelieved, the condition progresses rapidly to coma, and death ensues within 5 to 10 minutes. When, as in most cases, the obstruction is incomplete at first, the main clinical features are progressive dyspnoea and cyanosis, stridor and indrawing of the intercostal spaces and lower ribs on both sides. The great danger in these cases is that the obstruction may at any time become complete and result in sudden death.

**Treatment.** Transient attacks of laryngeal obstruction due to exudate and spasm, which may occur with acute laryngitis in children (p. 239) and with whooping cough, are potentially dangerous but can usually be relieved by the inhalation of steam.

Laryngeal obstruction from all other causes carries a high mortality and demands prompt treatment. The following measures may have to be employed:

1. *The relief of obstruction by mechanical means*. When a foreign body is known to be the cause of the obstruction it can often be dislodged by turning the patient's head downwards and thumping the back vigorously. In other circumstances the nature of the obstruction should be ascertained whenever possible by direct laryngoscopy, which may also permit the removal of a foreign body or the insertion of a tube past the obstruction into the trachea. Tracheostomy must be performed without delay if these procedures fail to relieve the obstruction, but except in dire emergencies the operation should be performed in the operating theatre by a surgeon.

2. *Treatment of the cause*. In cases of diphtheria, antitoxin should be administered and for other infections the appropriate antibiotic should be given. In angio-oedema the patient should receive adrenaline (0·5–1·0 ml of 1:1000 solution s.c.), chlorpheniramine maleate (10–20 mg i.v.) and hydrocortisone hemisuccinate (100 mg i.v.). These remedies take time to act and tracheostomy may be required in the intervening period.

## Diseases of the Trachea

**Acute tracheitis** is a common complication of viral and bacterial infection of the upper respiratory tract, and is usually associated with acute bronchitis. Other primary disorders of the trachea are rare.

**Tracheal Obstruction**. Intrinsic benign and malignant tumours may produce tracheal obstruction, but external compression by enlarged mediastinal lymph nodes containing metastatic deposits from a bronchial carcinoma is a much more common cause. Rarely, the trachea may be compressed by an aneurysm of the aortic arch, or in children by tuberculous mediastinal lymph nodes. Tracheal stricture is an occasional complication of tracheostomy.

Stridor (p. 227) can be detected in every patient with severe tracheal obstruction. Endoscopic examination of the trachea should be undertaken without delay in these patients to determine the degree of obstruction and its nature. Localised tumours of the trachea can be resected, but reconstruction of the resected segment may present complex technical problems. Radiotherapy or the administration of cytotoxic drugs may temporarily relieve compression by malignant lymph nodes. Tracheal strictures can sometimes be dilated, but may have to be resected.

**Tracheo-oesophageal Fistula.** This may be present in newborn infants as a congenital abnormality. In adults, it is usually due to malignant lesions in the mediastinum, such as carcinoma or malignant lymphoma, eroding both the trachea and oesophagus, to produce a communication between them. Swallowed liquids enter the trachea and bronchi through the fistula, and provoke a 'spluttering' cough. Surgical closure of a congenital fistula, if undertaken promptly, is usually successful, but malignant fistulae are incurable, and death from overwhelming pulmonary infection rapidly supervenes.

## Chronic Obstructive Airways Disease

Although chronic bronchitis and emphysema are pathologically distinct, they frequently co-exist, and it may then be difficult or impossible to determine the relative importance of each condition in the individual case. Generalised airflow obstruction is the dominant feature of both diseases. In chronic bronchitis it is chiefly due to swelling of the bronchial mucosa and the accumulation of tenacious mucus within the air passages. In emphysema, on the other hand, the main factor in the production of airflow obstruction is extramural bronchial compression and collapse caused by overdistended alveoli in which air has been 'trapped' during expiration. This phenomenon is aggravated by chronic bronchitis and bronchopulmonary infection.

Chronic bronchitis and emphysema are often grouped together under the heading of 'chronic obstructive airways disease', and can be regarded as forming a spectrum, with 'pure' chronic bronchitis at one end and 'pure' emphysema at the other. For descriptive purposes, however, it is convenient to deal with them separately, with emphasis on their similarities and differences, and on the relationships which frequently exist between them.

## Chronic Bronchitis

**Aetiology.** Chronic bronchitis is the name given to the clinical syndrome which many individuals develop in response to the long-continued action of various types of irritant on the bronchial mucosa. The most important of these is tobacco smoke, but they also include dust, smoke and fumes, occurring as specific occupational hazards or as part of a general atmospheric pollution in industrial cities and towns. Infection is sometimes a precipitating factor in the onset of chronic bronchitis, but its main role is in aggravating the established condition. Exposure to dampness, to sudden changes in temperature and to fog may also be responsible for exacerbations of chronic bronchitis.

The disorder occurs most commonly in middle and late adult life. More males are affected than females and there may be a familial predisposition. As might be expected, it is more common in smokers than in non-smokers, and in urban than in rural dwellers.

On culture of the sputum *Strep. pneumoniae* and *H. influenzae* are isolated in most cases. These organisms become more numerous during acute exacerbations.

**Pathology.** In all cases there is overactivity of the mucus-secreting glands and goblet cells in the bronchi and bronchioles. The vast excess of mucus so produced coats the bronchial walls and clogs the bronchioles. Mucosal oedema further reduces the calibre of the air passages and as the degree of obstruction is greater during expiration air is 'trapped' in the alveoli. With the passage of time the alveoli become permanently overdistended and there is extensive rupture of their walls. These changes, which constitute one form of 'emphysema', are also discussed on page 280.

**Clinical Features.** The disease usually starts with repeated attacks of 'winter cough', which show a steady increase in severity and duration with successive years, until cough is present all the year round. Wheeze, dyspnoea and tightness in the chest are common complaints, especially in the morning before the bronchial secretions are cleared, often with difficulty, by coughing. The sputum may be scanty, tenacious mucoid, and occasionally streaked with blood, or copious and watery. A frankly purulent sputum is indicative of bacterial infection, which supervenes from time to time in most cases of chronic bronchitis.

Dyspnoea in chronic bronchitis is caused by airflow obstruction, and is aggravated by infection or by an increase in mucosal oedema which may be produced by cigarette smoking and by adverse atmospheric conditions.

Variable numbers of inspiratory and expiratory rhonchi, mainly low and medium pitched, are present in most cases of chronic bronchitis and there may also be some coarse crepitations. Physical signs attributable to emphysema may coexist.

**Investigation.** *Radiological Examination.* Chronic bronchitis produces no characteristic abnormality in the radiograph, but bronchography shows various irregularities of bronchial calibre, outline and branching. The features of emphysema (p. 281) may be prominent in some cases.

*Pulmonary Function Tests.* 1. The forced expiratory volume in 1 second ($FEV_1$) is reduced, and the ratio of $FEV_1$ to forced vital capacity (FVC) is also subnormal. In advanced cases the $FEV_1$ may be less than 1 *l*, and the FEV/FVC ratio may be as low as 30%. Such changes are common to all forms of obstructive airway disease.

2. Because of 'air trapping' and alveolar distension the residual volume of the lungs is increased at the expense of vital capacity.

3. As the distribution of ventilation and perfusion within the lungs becomes disturbed (p. 224), the $Pa_{O_2}$ falls below normal.

4. In the later stages, when generalised alveolar underventilation supervenes, often following a bacterial or viral infection, there is a further fall in $Pa_{O_2}$ and a rise in $Pa_{CO_2}$ accompanied by respiratory acidosis (p. 144). Profound falls in arterial oxygenation may occur during sleep and may be a factor in the production of pulmonary hypertension (p. 199).

**Course and Prognosis.** Chronic bronchitis is usually a progressive disease, punctuated by acute exacerbations and remissions, and eventually causing ventilatory and cardiac failure. Some patients die within 5 years of the onset of symptoms, while others survive for 20 to 30 years, with gradually diminishing respiratory reserve.

**Treatment.** 1. *Bronchial irritation* must be reduced to a minimum. If a tobacco smoker, the patient should be urged to give up the habit completely and permanently. Dusty and smoke-laden atmospheres should be avoided, which may involve a change of occupation.

2. *Respiratory infection* must be promptly controlled, as it aggravates dyspnoea

and may precipitate ventilatory failure. The patient should be instructed to observe the colour of the sputum every morning, and, if it becomes purulent, should be given tetracycline or ampicillin in a dose of 250 mg four times daily or co-trimoxazole, 2 tablets twice daily, for 5 to 7 days. Intelligent patients can be provided with a stock of antibiotic tablets, and permitted to start a course of treatment on their own initiative when the need arises.

As the vast majority of bacterial infections in chronic bronchitis are caused by *Strep. pneumoniae* or *H. influenzae*, bacteriological examination of sputum is essential only when the response to standard treatment is unsatisfactory, and the sputum remains purulent. In that event a change of antibiotic, guided by the results of bacterial sensitivity tests, will be indicated. Continuous suppressive treatment with tetracycline or ampicillin given throughout the winter or even throughout the year, is not advised, since it is apt to promote the emergence of a drug-resistant respiratory tract flora, and may merely add to the therapeutic problems.

3. *Symptomatic measures* may be required to control unproductive cough during the night, to enable sputum to be coughed up more easily and to relieve breathlessness and wheeze. Nocturnal unproductive cough will often be less troublesome if the patient sleeps in a heated bedroom, but pholcodine or methadone may be required to control it. A hot drink or the inhalation of steam helps to liquefy sputum and make it easier to bring up. So-called expectorant cough mixtures are of little or no value. Measures for the relief of asthmatic symptoms are described on page 268.

4. *Ventilatory failure* must be promptly treated (p. 236).

**Prevention.** The abandonment of tobacco smoking and the prompt treatment of acute respiratory infections are the most important preventive measures. The control of atmospheric pollution in urban areas and the increased use of measures to prevent the inhalation of dust by industrial workers would also help to reduce the prevalence of chronic bronchitis.

## Emphysema

The word 'emphysema' means 'inflation' in the sense of unnatural distension with air, and this phenomenon, thus defined, can occur anywhere in the body. Air may, for example, enter the mediastinum (*mediastinal emphysema*) following the rupture of overdistended alveoli into the interstitial tissues of the lung in patients with severe bronchial asthma, or following rupture of the oesophagus. If a very large amount of air escapes rapidly into the mediastinum, it may produce cardiac tamponade (p. 203), but in most cases it tracks harmlessly upwards into the soft tissues of the neck, where it imparts a characteristic crackling sensation to the palpating fingers (*subcutaneous emphysema*). Penetrating wounds of the chest wall may also cause subcutaneous emphysema, and when a spontaneous pneumothorax is treated by pleural decompression with an intercostal tube (p. 305), widespread subcutaneous emphysema is an occasional complication, which is alarming but not serious.

### Pulmonary Emphysema

The term 'pulmonary emphysema' covers a wide variety of pathological processes, ranging from overdistension of otherwise normal alveoli in conditions such as bronchial asthma, obstructive emphysema and compensatory emphysema to the widespread disruption of the alveolar walls which occurs in the more serious forms of pulmonary emphysema. There is a close association between the latter and chronic bronchitis, but the physical signs and radiological changes attributable to 'emphysema' may be more conspicuous in some cases of chronic bronchitis than in others. Chronic bronchitis and emphysema can both cause severe pulmonary damage, but it is of a different type in the two conditions. In emphysema generalised destruction of the alveolar walls ('panacinar' emphysema) is the dominant lesion. Where emphysema occurs along with a major component of chronic bronchitis, it is usually 'centrilobular' or 'centriacinar', and principally affects these alveoli which are most closely related to the respiratory bronchioles. Although these two types of emphysema develop in different ways, factors such as bacterial infection, alveolar overdistension and distortion of the airways may eventually blur their distinctive features. The predominance of either chronic bronchitis or emphysema may, however, be sufficiently clear-cut to produce two separately identifiable syndromes. In the chronic bronchitis syndrome, ventilatory capacity is fairly well preserved, but severe hypoxia and hypercapnia, pulmonary hypertension and right ventricular failure occur at an early stage (the '*blue bloater*'). In the emphysema syndrome, on the other hand, grave impairment of ventilatory capacity and disabling exertional dyspnoea may antedate by many years the manifestations of respiratory and cardiac failure (the '*pink puffer*'). A mixed syndrome of chronic bronchitis and emphysema is, however, much more commonly seen than either of the two individual syndromes.

Emphysema in young adults may be associated with genetically determined $\alpha_1$-antitrypsin deficiency in the serum (p. 386). It is believed that connective tissue in the lung is digested by proteolytic enzymes normally inhibited by antitrypsin.

**Clinical Features.** Most patients with pulmonary emphysema complain of exertional dyspnoea, but since other causes of airflow obstruction, such as chronic bronchitis and bronchial asthma, often co-exist, it is seldom possible to assess the contribution of emphysema *per se* to the production of this symptom. In patients with chronic bronchitis and emphysema there is a progressive increase in respiratory disability, but the tempo of deterioration varies widely from one case to another. For example, in patients with a relatively minor component of chronic bronchitis, the exertional dyspnoea increases slowly over a period of several years, but the course of the disease tends to be more rapid where chronic bronchitis is a dominant feature.

The physical signs which may be observed in emphysema are summarised in Table 7.1. Other clinical abnormalities include (1) a reduction in the length of the trachea palpable above the sternal notch, (2) tracheal descent with inspiration, (3) contraction of the sternomastoid and scalene muscles on inspiration, (4) excavation of the suprasternal and supraclavicular fossae during inspiration, (5) jugular venous filling during expiration, (6) indrawing of the costal margins during inspiration, and (7) an increase in the anteroposterior diameter of the chest relative to the lateral diameter.

**Investigation.** *Radiological Examination.* A firm diagnosis of emphysema cannot be made by radiological examination alone, but the following abnormalities suggest that it may be present: 1. Unusually translucent lung fields, with loss of peripheral vascular markings. 2. Bullae (p. 282). 3. A low flat diaphragm, which moves poorly on radioscopy (2 cm or less). 4. Prominence of the pulmonary hilar arterial shadows.

Abnormalities caused by pulmonary infection ('inflammatory shadowing') may also be present. In the late stages, when pulmonary hypertension and right ventricular failure supervene, there is enlargement of the main pulmonary artery, the right ventricle and the right atrium.

*Pulmonary Function Tests*. See page 232.

**Complications.** 1. *Ventilatory failure* (p. 228); *secondary polycythaemia* (p. 566).

2. *Pulmonary hypertension* and *right ventricular failure* are the inevitable end-results of chronic bronchitis and emphysema. The increase in pulmonary arterial pressure is due to vasoconstriction mediated by the effect of hypoxia on pulmonary arterioles and ultimately to destruction of the pulmonary vascular bed. As hypoxia is aggravated by any increase in the degree of airflow obstruction, bacterial infection in the respiratory tract, oedema of the bronchial mucosa, oversecretion of bronchial mucus and spasm of the bronchial muscles (which can all cause hypoxia) are liable to increase the pulmonary arterial pressure and precipitate right ventricular failure. Conversely, effective treatment of these causes of hypoxia, combined with oxygen therapy and diuretics, may relieve pulmonary hypertension and cardiac failure, at least for a time.

3. *Pulmonary bullae*, single or multiple, large or small, may develop in emphysematous lung tissue, regardless of the primary pathology. Bullae are inflated thin-walled spaces created by rupture of the alveolar walls. They are usually situated subpleurally, and are commonly found along the anterior borders of the lungs. A small bulla may rupture, causing spontaneous pneumothorax. In other circumstances bullae may increase progressively in size, and eventually become so large that they interfere seriously with pulmonary ventilation.

**Treatment.** There is no specific remedy for emphysema, but the patient may benefit considerably from the treatment of associated chronic bronchitis (p. 279), and of respiratory failure (p. 236), which is a common complication. Obesity must be prevented or corrected, as excess weight is an intolerable burden on the reduced cardiorespiratory reserve. The purpose of physiotherapy should be to induce relaxation of the cervical muscles and to show the patient how to exhale slowly and steadily through pursed lips. It should also be used to encourage expectoration. Regular mild exercise has also been shown to increase mobility, even in severely disabled patients. The surgical ablation of giant bullae, where this is feasible, may allow relatively normal lung tissue compressed by the bullae to re-expand and may bring about a dramatic improvement in pulmonary function.

## Bronchiectasis

**Aetiology and Pathogenesis.** Bronchiectasis, which is the term used to describe abnormal dilatation of the bronchi, may be produced in different ways. In most cases bronchiectasis is secondary to severe bacterial infection, including tuberculosis, in the lungs. It is also a complication of bronchial eosinophilia (p. 272).

When pulmonary collapse follows obstruction of groups of small bronchi by secretion, the shrinkage of the affected portion of lung exerts outward traction on the walls of the medium-sized bronchi, which become dilated. Bronchiectasis arising in this way may be reversible if the obstructed bronchi can be cleared of secretion before the walls of the dilated bronchi are seriously damaged by infection. Bronchiectasis may be due to bronchial distension resulting from the accumulation of pus beyond a lesion obstructing a major bronchus, such as a bronchial carcinoma, a tuberculous hilar lymph node or an inhaled foreign body. In cystic fibrosis recurrent infection and chronic obstruction by viscid mucus are both factors in causing bronchiectasis. Rarely, it may be the result of congenital maldevelopment of the bronchi.

Because of the many different causes of bronchiectasis no precise age incidence can be stated. When it occurs following acute pulmonary infections or secondary to obstruction of a bronchus by tuberculous lymph nodes (the two most common causes), the disease usually starts in childhood but may not produce severe symptoms until some years later.

**Pathology.** Although bronchiectasis may involve any part of the lungs, depending on the site of the primary pathological process, the lower lobes are more frequently affected than the upper and middle, but the more efficient drainage by gravity of the upper lobes renders bronchiectasis there less liable to produce serious symptoms than when it involves the lower lobes. The bronchiectatic cavities may be lined by granulation tissue, squamous epithelium or normal ciliated epithelium, depending on the degree of infection present. There may also be inflammatory changes in the deeper layers of the bronchial walls and chronic inflammatory and fibrotic changes in the surrounding lung tissue.

**Clinical Features.** Three groups of clinical features occur in bronchiectasis:

1. *Those due to the accumulation of pus in the dilated bronchi* are chronic cough, usually worse in the mornings and often induced by changes in posture, and purulent sputum which in advanced cases is copious and sometimes foetid.
2. *Those due to inflammatory changes in the surrounding lung tissue and pleura.* Febrile episodes usually last for a few days but occasionally for weeks. Malaise, shivering and sleep sweating accompany the pyrexia; there is an increase in the amount of cough and sputum and a neutrophil leucocytosis is usually present. Dry pleurisy frequently accompanies the febrile episodes. Empyema is an occasional complication of bronchiectasis.

When chronic suppuration, either in the bronchi or in the lungs, is a marked feature it causes a decline in the patient's general health, with lassitude, anorexia, loss of weight, sleep sweating and clubbing of the fingers and toes. In many cases, however, symptoms are slight, consisting merely of recurrent episodes of cough and purulent sputum with no symptoms in the intervening periods and no deterioration in health.

3. *Haemoptysis* is caused by bleeding from thin-walled anastomotic vessels connecting the pulmonary and bronchial arteries, and situated in the walls of the dilated bronchi. It ranges in amount from blood-stained sputum to massive haemorrhage. It may be present in association with the first two groups of symptoms, but recurrent haemoptysis may also occur as an isolated symptom in the absence of cough and sputum ('dry' bronchiectasis).

Physical signs may be unilateral or bilateral and are usually basal. If the bronchiectatic cavities are dry and there is no collapse, there may be no abnormal physical signs. If a large amount of secretion is present, numerous coarse crepitations are heard over the affected areas. When collapse is present the character of the physical signs depends on whether or not the major bronchi in the collapsed lobe are patent.

In ordinary radiographs the dilated bronchi themselves may not be visible, but changes may be produced by associated pulmonary inflammation or collapse. A diagnosis of bronchiectasis can be made with certainty only by bronchography.

Bacteriological examination of the sputum is necessary in every case to exclude tuberculosis and to identify other pathogenic bacteria.

**Treatment.** *Postural Drainage.* The purpose of this measure is to keep the dilated bronchi emptied of secretion. Efficiently performed it is of great value both in reducing the amount of cough and sputum and in preventing the 'toxaemia' caused by associated bronchopulmonary infection. In its simplest form, postural drainage consists of adopting a position in which the lobe to be drained is uppermost, so as to allow secretions in the dilated bronchi to gravitate towards the trachea, from which they can readily be cleared by vigorous coughing. The optimum duration and frequency of postural drainage depends on the amount of sputum, but 5 to 10 minutes once or twice daily is adequate in most cases.

*Chemotherapy.* The policy governing the use of antibiotics in bronchiectasis is the same as that in chronic bronchitis.

*Surgical Treatment.* If surgical treatment is being considered, it is essential to obtain bronchograms demonstrating exactly the extent of the bronchiectasis. For this purpose the bronchi of all segments of both lungs must be outlined with a radio-opaque contrast medium. Pulmonary function should also be assessed.

The use of antibiotics has greatly reduced the need for surgical treatment. Unfortunately many of the cases in which medical treatment has been unsuccessful are also unsuitable for surgical treatment either because the bronchiectasis is too extensive or because most of the symptoms are due to coexisting chronic bronchitis. Emphysema of even moderate severity is a contraindication to surgical treatment, as the increase in exertional dyspnoea which inevitably results is more distressing to the patient than the symptoms of bronchiectasis. The most favourable cases for surgery are children and young adults in whom the bronchiectasis is confined to a single lobe or part of a lobe. Lobar or segmental resection in these patients is a highly satisfactory operation, carrying little risk.

*Prevention.* As bronchiectasis commonly starts in childhood following measles, whooping cough or a primary tuberculous infection, it is essential that these conditions receive adequate treatment. The early recognition and treatment of bronchial obstruction is particularly important in this respect.

**Prognosis.** With antibiotic therapy the prognosis, even in advanced cases, has greatly improved and the incidence of complications such as pneumonia, empyema, cerebral abscess and amyloidosis has fallen considerably.

## Bronchial Obstruction

**Aetiology.** The lesions most likely to obstruct a large bronchus are: (1) tumours, e.g. bronchial carcinoma or adenoma; (2) enlarged tracheobronchial lymph nodes, malignant or tuberculous; (3) inhaled foreign bodies; (4) bronchial casts or plugs, consisting of inspissated mucus or blood clot; (5) collections of mucus or mucopus retained in the bronchi as a result of ineffective expectoration.

Rare causes of bronchial obstruction include congenital bronchial atresia, fibrous bronchial stricture (often post-tuberculous), aortic aneurysm, giant left atrium and pericardial effusion.

**Clinical Features.** The manifestations of obstruction of a large bronchus depend on whether the obstruction is complete or partial, on secondary infection and on the effect on pulmonary function. The clinical features also vary with the cause of the obstruction.

1. COMPLETE OBSTRUCTION. When a large bronchus is completely obstructed, the air in the lung, lobe or segment it supplies is absorbed, the alveolar spaces close, and the

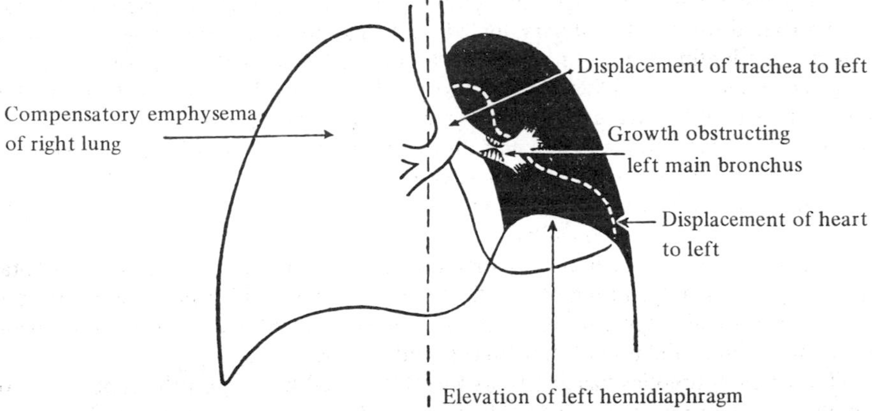


Fig. 7.3 The effects on neighbouring structures of collapse of the left lung.

affected portion of lung tissue becomes collapsed and solid. The percussion note over the collapsed lung or lobe is dull, the breath sounds are diminished or absent, and radiological examination shows displacement of the trachea and/or heart shadow towards the side of the lesion, elevation of the diaphragm on the same side and a dense pulmonary opacity of characteristic size, shape and position. If the collapse involves a smaller portion of lung (e.g. the right middle lobe or a bronchopulmonary segment), displacement of the mediastinum may not occur, and abnormal physical signs may be difficult to detect, but a characteristic radiographic opacity will be present. The radiological features of pulmonary and lobar collapse are shown in Figs 7.3 and 7.4. Semisolid material, such as mucus, mucopus or blood clot, obstructing a large bronchus is apt to fragment, and portions of it may then be aspirated into the peripheral bronchi, leaving the larger bronchus clear. The diminished or absent breath sounds are then replaced by bronchial breath sounds, but the other clinical and radiological abnormalities do not change.

2. PARTIAL OBSTRUCTION. If a large bronchus is partially obstructed, a situation occasionally arises in which there is less resistance to air flow through the narrowed bronchus during inspiration than during expiration, when the obstruction may become temporarily complete. This differential between inspiratory and expiratory airflow resistance, which is increased by coughing, results in over-distension of the lung, lobe or segment supplied by the partially obstructed bronchus (*obstructive emphysema*). The percussion note over such a lesion is resonant or hyper-resonant, and the breath sounds are diminished. A chest radiograph shows hypertranslucency of the affected part of lung, and on radioscopic examination the mediastinum can be seen to move towards the opposite side of the chest during expiration, because the pressure within the affected lung then exceeds that within the contralateral lung.

3. SECONDARY INFECTION. Whenever a bronchus is narrowed, bacterial infection of the lung tissue it supplies is virtually inevitable, and this may occur even when the degree of obstruction is insufficient to cause pulmonary collapse. This explains why pneumonia may be the first clinical manifestation of bronchial carcinoma. The infection is usually of low virulence, but in some cases severe pulmonary suppuration may occur, with empyema as a further complication.

4. PULMONARY FUNCTION. Bronchial obstruction impairs pulmonary function, but this is unlikely to produce symptoms unless a main or lobar bronchus is involved, or

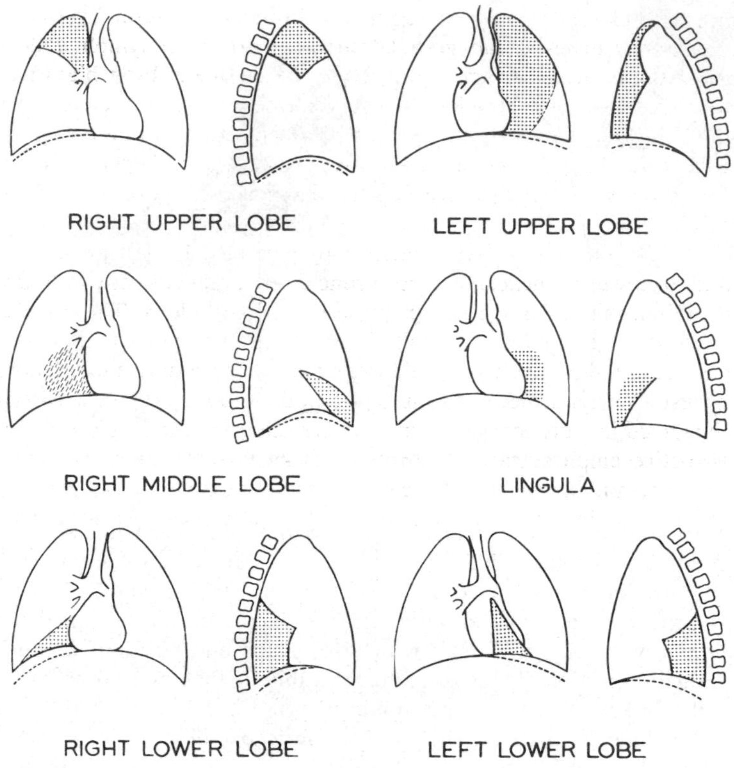


Fig. 7.4 Radiological features of lobar collapse caused by bronchial obstruction. The dotted line represents the normal position of the diaphragm.

if the patient's overall pulmonary function is so poor that obstruction of a smaller bronchus critically diminishes the respiratory reserve. Sudden occlusion of a main or lobar bronchus by mucus or mucopus occurring as a postoperative complication may cause severe dyspnoea and hypoxaemia.

5. CLINICAL FEATURES RELATED TO THE CAUSE OF THE OBSTRUCTION.

(i) *Tumours.* Bronchial obstruction by a carcinoma usually produces pulmonary collapse at an early stage and seldom causes obstructive emphysema. Pulmonary infection is common, and this may be complicated by empyema. The degree of exertional dyspnoea produced by a bronchial carcinoma is directly related to the size of the obstructed bronchus. The rate of growth of a bronchial adenoma is much less rapid than that of a carcinoma. Complete bronchial obstruction and pulmonary collapse are therefore later developments in the presence of an adenoma, and obstructive emphysema, caused by partial bronchial obstruction, may be observed during the intervening period.

(ii) *Enlarged Tracheobronchial Lymph Nodes.* By compressing or invading the bronchial wall, enlarged lymph nodes may produce the same clinical manifestations of bronchial obstruction as a tumour within the lumen, and in bronchial carcinoma both types of lesion may co-exist. Bronchial obstruction by enlarged lymph nodes in Hodgkin's disease and other forms of lymphoma is less common than in bronchial carcinoma, presumably because these are less invasive types of tumour. In children with severe primary tuberculous infection large caseous tracheobronchial lymph nodes may compress and erode lobar or segmental bronchi, occasionally even a main bronchus. Caseous material and granulation tissue from the lymph node may be extruded into the bronchial lumen and increase the degree of bronchial obstruction. Tuberculous infection may develop in the collapsed lobe or segment, and later complications include bronchial stricture and bronchiectasis. In all these conditions the supraclavicular lymph nodes may also be involved, and biopsy of one of these nodes may provide a positive histological diagnosis of tumour, lymphoma or tuberculosis.

(iii) *Foreign Bodies.* An inhaled foreign body generally lodges in the right main, intermediate or lower bronchus, as these bronchi are almost directly in line with the trachea. Children inhale foreign bodies more often than adults. These include nuts (usually peanuts), peas, beans and small pieces of metallic or plastic toys. Adults, on the other hand, are more likely to inhale fragments of tooth during extractions under general anaesthesia, and pieces of mutton or rabbit bone. When a foreign body becomes impacted in a bronchus, it first produces, after an initial episode of choking, either obstructive emphysema or absorption collapse, and a persistent low-pitched rhonchus may be audible all over the chest. Within a few days pathogenic bacteria, carried into the respiratory tract with the foreign body, give rise to a suppurative pneumonia in the collapsed lobe. The patient at this stage often has a high temperature, cough productive of purulent sputum, and pleural pain. On clinical examination there may be a pleural rub and physical signs of either pulmonary collapse or consolidation. Radiological examination shows either obstructive emphysema or collapse and/or pneumonic consolidation of the lobe or lobes supplied by the obstructed bronchus. A radio-opaque foreign body may be visible on the film.

(iv) *Bronchial Casts or Plugs.* These may consist of either inspissated mucus or blood clot. Plugs of mucus may cause bronchial obstruction in patients with asthma or bronchial eosinophilia (p. 272). Secondary bacterial infection of the collapsed lung may occur, but is seldom severe. Bronchial obstruction by blood clot frequently follows severe haemoptysis, but as this complication is usually recognised and treated at an early stage, secondary bacterial infection of collapsed lung tissue seldom occurs.

(v) *Retained Secretions.* A main, lobar or segmental bronchus may be obstructed by retained mucus or mucopus when a patient is unable to cough effectively because of chest pain, muscular weakness or general debility. Pulmonary collapse following an upper abdominal or thoracic operation, or an injury to the chest wall, is due to this type of bronchial obstruction. Secondary bacterial infection of the collapsed lung tissue supervenes at an early stage.

**Investigation and Treatment of Bronchial Obstruction.** The cause of the bronchial obstruction can be discovered by bronchoscopic examination, and in the case of tumour and tuberculosis histological confirmation of the diagnosis can usually be obtained by bronchial biopsy. Foreign bodies can be extracted by bronchoscopy or bronchotomy. If bronchial casts, plugs or secretions cannot be dislodged by postural coughing, they should be removed through a bronchoscope. In other forms of bronchial obstruction the treatment is that of the primary condition.

Postoperative pulmonary collapse can be prevented by forbidding patients to smoke for 3 weeks prior to operation, by vigorous pre- and postoperative breathing exercises, and by regularly supervised coughing during the immediate postoperative period.

# INTRATHORACIC TUMOURS

## Tumours of Bronchus and Lung

Bronchial carcinoma is by far the most common malignant pulmonary tumour. Benign tumours are rare. A primary carcinoma in any organ, but particularly in breast, kidney, uterus, ovary, testis, thyroid or in lung itself, may give rise to pulmonary metastatic deposits, as may an osteogenic or melanotic sarcoma.

### Bronchial Carcinoma

Bronchial carcinoma accounts for more than 50% of all male deaths from malignant disease. It is four times more common in men than in women, and occurs most frequently between the ages of 50 and 75. Cigarette smoking is responsible for most cases of bronchial carcinoma, and the increased risk is directly proportional to the amount smoked and to the tar content of the cigarettes. For example, the death rate from the disease in heavy cigarette smokers is 40 times that in non-smokers. It is slightly higher in urban than in rural dwellers, presumably because of atmospheric pollution. There is also a higher incidence in asbestosis.

**Pathology.** The tumour, which may be a squamous or small cell (oat cell) carcinoma or, occasionally, an adenocarcinoma, arises from bronchial epithelium or mucous glands and at an early stage may occlude the bronchial lumen. It also invades the deeper layers of the bronchial wall and the surrounding lung tissue. When the tumour obstructs a major bronchus it causes pulmonary collapse and infection (p. 284). A tumour arising from a peripheral bronchus may attain a very large size without producing a significant degree of collapse. A tumour of this type may undergo central necrosis and cavitation.

The tumour may involve the pleura either directly or by lymphatic spread, causing a pleural effusion which is often blood-stained. It may also extend into the chest wall and cause severe pain by invading intercostal nerves or the brachial plexus. The tumour or its lymph node metastases may extend into the mediastinum, involving the phrenic and recurrent laryngeal nerves, the sympathetic trunk, the superior vena cava, the pericardium and myocardium, the trachea and the oesophagus.

Lymphatic spread may occur to the supraclavicular ('scalene') lymph nodes as well as to the mediastinal lymph nodes and pleura. Blood-borne metastases occur most commonly in liver, bone, brain, suprarenals, skin and kidneys. Even a small primary tumour may cause widespread metastatic deposits. A carcinoma of the small cell type has often spread beyond the lung by the time it is diagnosed.

**Clinical Features.** Cough is the most common early symptom. The sputum is purulent if there is secondary bacterial infection. Repeated slight haemoptysis is a common and characteristic feature. Dyspnoea may occur early when a lobe or lung is collapsed, but in other circumstances is a late symptom unless the patient is coincidentally suffering from chronic bronchitis and emphysema. Pleural pain is a frequent symptom and may be due either to infective pleurisy or to malignant invasion of the pleura. Pain in the chest wall or in an upper limb with a nerve root distribution may be present if the tumour involves intercostal nerves or the brachial plexus. An apical bronchial carcinoma may cause Horner's syndrome. The symptoms and signs which may occur if the tumour invades the mediastinum are described in the section on mediastinal tumours (p. 290).

Occasionally the presenting symptom is due to metastases, e.g. headache, fits or personality change, jaundice, pathological fracture, haematuria or skin nodules which are usually tender. Clubbing of the fingers is often seen and a few patients present with the features of hypertrophic pulmonary osteoarthropathy, peripheral neuropathy or cerebellar degeneration; none of these manifestations is necessarily related to the presence of metastatic tumour. Rarely a small cell carcinoma may act as an ectopic source of adrenocorticotrophic, antidiuretic or other hormone, and the patient may present with symptoms and signs of endocrine dysfunction. Lassitude, anorexia and loss of weight are late symptoms except when pulmonary suppuration is an early complication.

Physical signs in the chest depend on the size of the tumour, but even more on the nature and extent of its secondary effects on lung and pleura. In the early stages a tumour may cause no abnormal physical signs. A tumour obstructing a large bronchus produces the physical signs of collapse or obstructive emphysema. Pulmonary infection beyond an obstructing tumour gives rise to pneumonia which is unusually slow to respond to treatment. A massive tumour may give rise to signs resembling those of a pleural effusion. Involvement of the pleura either by infection or by tumour may produce signs of dry pleurisy or of a pleural effusion.

**Investigation.** *Radiological Examination.* A bronchial carcinoma may produce (i) a dense, irregular, hilar opacity, (ii) a dense, fairly well circumscribed, peripheral pulmonary opacity, usually large when first discovered, sometimes irregularly cavitated or (iii) an opacity consistent with collapse of a whole lung, a lobe or a segment which may be associated with a hilar opacity due to the tumour itself.

In some cases radiological examination may also show a pleural effusion (indicating either infection or secondary tumour in the pleura), broadening of the mediastinal shadow (due to lymph node metastases), osteolytic lesions of the ribs (indicating either direct invasion by tumour or blood-borne metastases) or unilateral diaphragmatic paralysis (indicating involvement of the phrenic nerve). A paralysed hemidiaphragm is usually raised and on radioscopic examination moves 'paradoxically' when the patient sniffs, i.e. it moves upwards instead of downwards.

*Bronchoscopy* (p. 231). Inspection of the intrabronchial portion of the tumour and removal of tissue for histological examination is possible in over 70% of cases.

*Other investigations,* such as transbronchial or percutaneous lung biopsy, scalene node biopsy or mediastinoscopy may be required to confirm the diagnosis.

*Cytological* examination of sputum or bronchial brushings for malignant cells is a valuble diagnostic measure when practised by a pathologist with special expertise in this technique. Percutaneous needle biopsy is a useful method of obtaining a positive histological diagnosis in peripheral tumours.

**Treatment and Prognosis.** Unless surgical treatment is practicable the average period of survival after the diagnosis is made is less than a year. Resection of the lung (pneumonectomy) or, in some cases, of the lobe containing the tumour (lobectomy) offers the best prospect of survival. The operation can be performed only on the small number of cases (about 20%) in which the tumour is discovered at an early and relatively localised stage and pulmonary function is adequate. The tumour is liable to recur even after an apparently satisfactory operation, and only 30% of such patients survive for more than 5 years. Early diagnosis provides slightly better results, but the prognosis depends to an even greater extent on the histological type of tumour and on the presence or absence of metastatic deposits in the hilar lymph nodes. The outlook is particularly unfavourable when the tumour is a small cell carcinoma.

Small tumours can occasionally be eradicated by radiotherapy, but this form of treatment is more often used to relieve distressing complications such as superior vena caval obstruction, recurrent haemoptysis and pain caused by chest wall invasion or by skeletal metastatic deposits. Obstruction of the trachea and main bronchi can also be relieved temporarily by irradiation, but as the latter may initially produce tumour swelling and a dangerous increase in the degree of obstruction, a cytotoxic drug, e.g. cyclophosphamide intravenously or prednisolone by mouth, should be given first. The treatment of small cell carcinoma with combinations of cytotoxic drugs can increase the median survival of patients with this highly malignant type of bronchial carcinoma from 3 months to over a year. This form of treatment is, however, still in the experimental stage and because of problems arising from the toxicity of the drugs it should for the present be undertaken only in specialised centres. It is of little or no value in the treatment of other histological types of bronchial carcinoma.

### Bronchial Adenoma

This is an uncommon tumour occurring in a younger age group than carcinoma, and affecting females as often as males. Although classified as a benign tumour it possesses some of the properties of a malignant growth and may eventually give rise to metastases. There are two histological types of bronchial adenoma, the relatively more common carcinoid tumour and the rare cylindroma, or 'adenoid cystic carcinoma', which often arises at the tracheal bifurcation. A carcinoid tumour may secrete 5–hydroxytryptamine or a related substance, and give rise to the carcinoid syndrome (p. 359). The usual primary pathological lesion is a small, vascular tumour within the bronchial lumen with a large encapsulated extrabronchial extension.

The local clinical features, which may have a duration of several years, are recurrent haemoptysis, due to the vascularity of the tumour, recurrent pulmonary infection resulting from bronchial obstruction and, in rare cases, the carcinoid syndrome. The physical signs most frequently found are those of collapse. The diagnosis from bronchial carcinoma can be made only by bronchoscopy and histological examination of a portion of the tumour.

Treatment consists of resection of the pulmonary lobe or segment containing the tumour along with the bronchus from which it arises.

### Secondary Tumours of the Lung

Blood-borne metastatic deposits in the lungs may be derived from malignant disease almost anywhere in the body. The usual sites of the primary tumour have already been stated (p. 288). The secondary deposits are usually multiple and bilateral. Haemoptysis occurs in some cases but often there are no respiratory symptoms and the diagnosis is made by radiological examination.

Extensive infiltration of the pulmonary lymphatics by tumour may develop in patients with carcinoma of breast, stomach, pancreas or bronchus. This condition, *pulmonary lymphatic carcinomatosis*, causes severe and rapidly progressive dyspnoea.

## Tumours of the Mediastinum

**Classification.** *Tumours of the lymph nodes*, e.g. secondary carcinoma, usually from bronchus or breast; lymphomas, including Hodgkin's disease; leukaemia.

*Thymic tumours,* e.g. benign or malignant thymoma.

*Connective tissue tumours*, e.g. fibroma, lipoma (benign); sarcoma (malignant).

*Neural tumours*, e.g. neurofibroma.

*Developmental tumours and cysts*, e.g. teratoma; dermoid, bronchogenic and pleuro-pericardial cysts.

*Other lesions presenting as mediastinal tumours*, e.g. aortic aneurysm, aneurysmal dilatation of left atrium, intrathoracic goitre, sarcoidosis involving lymph nodes.

**Pathology and Clinical Features.** BENIGN TUMOURS AND CYSTS. The conditions in this category, which are all rare, include neural tumours, teratoma, developmental cysts and intrathoracic goitre. They may compress, but do not invade, vital structures. The diagnosis of benign tumour or cyst is usually made by chance, when radiological examination of the chest is undertaken for some other reason. Many of the cases are found by mass radiography. If a tumour becomes very large it may cause dyspnoea by compression of lung tissue, or occasionally by narrowing the trachea. A benign tumour in the upper part of the thorax occasionally compresses the superior vena cava (see below). A dermoid cyst occasionally ruptures into a bronchus.

MALIGNANT TUMOURS. Included in this category are mediastinal lymph node metastases, malignant lymphomas, leukaemia, malignant thymic tumours and mediastinal sarcoma. Aortic and innominate aneurysms have invasive features resembling those of malignant mediastinal tumours. All these conditions, except lymph node metastases, are uncommon.

The distinguishing feature of this group of tumours is their power to invade as well as to compress mediastinal structures, bronchi and lungs. As a result of this property even a small malignant tumour can produce symptoms, although as a rule the tumour has attained a considerable size before this happens. The structures which may be invaded or compressed and the symptoms and signs produced in each case are:

*Trachea:* dyspnoea, stridor, brassy cough.

*Main bronchus:* pulmonary collapse, dyspnoea.

*Oesophagus:* dysphagia.

*Phrenic nerve:* diaphragmatic paralysis.

*Left recurrent laryngeal nerve:* paralysis of left vocal cord, hoarseness.

*Sympathetic trunk:* Horner's syndrome.

*Pericardium*: pericarditis, either dry with pericardial rub, or with effusion.

*Superior vena cava:* oedema and cyanosis of head and neck, and sometimes of upper limbs also, with distension of external jugular veins and dilated anastomotic veins on anterior chest wall and in axillary regions.

**Investigation.** *Radiological examination.* A benign mediastinal tumour generally appears as a large, round, sharply circumscribed opacity, situated mainly in the mediastinum but often encroaching on one or both lung fields. A malignant mediastinal tumour seldom has a clearly defined margin and often presents as a general broadening of the mediastinal shadow.

As bronchial carcinoma is such a common primary cause of mediastinal tumour, *bronchoscopy* should be carried out in all cases. If enlarged mediastinal lymph nodes are suspected one of these can be removed for histological examination by the technique of *mediastinoscopy* (p. 232). In some cases, however, an exact diagnosis cannot be made without *surgical exploration* of the chest and removal of the tumour or a portion of it for histological examination.

**Treatment.** Benign mediastinal tumours should be removed surgically as soon as they are discovered because (a) they tend to produce symptoms sooner or later and (b) some of them, particularly cysts, may become infected while others, especially neural tumours, may become malignant. The operative mortality is low.

The treatment of lymphoma and leukaemia is described on pages 582 and 572 respectively. A malignant thymoma usually responds dramatically to radiotherapy. Lymph node metastases from bronchial carcinoma may respond well to radiotherapy or to cytotoxic chemotherapy, especially if the tumour is of the small cell type; complications such as superior vena caval and tracheal obstruction can often be relieved in this way.

## INTERSTITIAL LUNG DISEASE

This term is applied to a group of pulmonary diseases which have the following features in common: (1) thickening of the alveolar walls by oedema, cellular exudate or fibrosis; (2) increased stiffness of the lungs (reduced compliance), associated with exertional dyspnoea; (3) maldistribution of pulmonary ventilation and perfusion and a gas diffusion defect leading to hypoxaemia, hyperventilation and hypocapnia.

**Aetiology.** Interstitial lung disease is caused by several different pathological processes, but these all give rise to similar symptoms, physical signs, radiological changes and disturbances of pulmonary function. They are thus worthy of collective consideration. The most frequently recognised causes of interstitial lung disease are:

1. Chronic pulmonary oedema e.g. secondary to mitral valve disease (p. 176).
2. Extrinsic allergic alveolitis (p. 274).
3. Fibrosing alveolotis associated with the connective tissue disorders or of unknown aetiology (cryptogenic fibrosing alveolitis).
4. Pulmonary damage following radiotherapy to the thorax
5. Sarcoidosis (p. 293), asbestosis (p. 297), and idiopathic pulmonary haemosiderosis (p. 293).

### Fibrosing Alveolitis

This condition exemplifies many of the typical features of interstitial lung disease. It may be a manifestation of one of the connective tissue disorders, such as rheumatoid disease, systemic lupus erythematosus or systemic sclerosis, or it may occur as an isolated pulmonary abnormality. Progressive exertional dyspnoea is usually the presenting symptom, often accompanied by a persistent dry cough. In most cases there is gross clubbing of the fingers and toes. Chest expansion is poor, but hyperventilation is always a striking feature. Numerous bilateral coarse crackling crepitations are audible on auscultation. Radiologically, there are diffuse pulmonary opacities, the diaphragm is high and the lungs appear small. The $FEV_1$ and FVC are reduced proportionately, the carbon monoxide transfer factor is low, and there is arterial hypoxaemia and hypocapnia. The diagnosis can usually be made with confidence from these findings, but should in doubtful cases be confirmed by lung biopsy. Serological tests for antinuclear and rheumatoid factors may be positive, even in cases without evidence of connective tissue disorder. The rate of progression of the pulmonary changes varies considerably, from death within a few months to survival with minimal symptoms for many years. Treatment with corticosteroids is effective in perhaps 30% of the acute cases, but not in the others. It may have to be maintained for several years, or even for life.

**Honeycomb Lung.** The radiological phenomenon of 'honeycomb lung', in which diffuse pulmonary shadowing is interspersed with small cystic translucencies, may be observed in some cases of interstitial lung disease, but it may also be a characteristic feature of certain rare diseases, such as histiocytosis X and tuberous sclerosis. Honeycomb lung, whatever its cause, is associated with an increased incidence of spontaneous pneumothorax, and eventually produces respiratory failure, pulmonary hypertension and right ventricular failure.

### Idiopathic Pulmonary Haemosiderosis

This is a rare disease of unknown cause, in which spontaneous haemorrhage into the lungs causes recurrent episodes of pyrexia, haemoptysis and iron-deficiency anaemia. With every incident, red blood cells in large numbers are extravasated into the interstitial tissues of the lungs, where haemosiderin released from macrophages stimulates fibroblastic activity. If the patient survives the acute haemorrhagic episodes, the interstitial fibrosis may eventually cause respiratory failure and pulmonary hypertension. Pulmonary haemosiderosis may also be associated with acute glomerulonephritis (Goodpasture's syndrome, p. 431).

During the acute episodes, widespread coarse crepitations are present, and diffuse stippled shadowing, chiefly involving the mid-zones of both lung fields, is seen on the chest radiograph. In the later stages the clinical and radiographic abnormalities may be indistinguishable from those of fibrosing alveolitis.

## Sarcoidosis

Sarcoidosis is a systemic granulomatous disease of unknown cause. Apart from the absence of caseation and tubercle bacilli, the lesions are histologically similar to tuberculous follicles, but there is no convincing evidence to support the view that the disease is caused by any of the mycobacteria. Chronic beryllium poisoning produces a disease which mimics sarcoidosis both pathologically and clinically, but exposure to beryllium is extremely uncommon and few cases of sarcoidosis can be caused in this way. Histological changes resembling those of sarcoidosis are occasionally seen in individual organs, such as lymph nodes, in conditions such as carcinoma, reticulosis and fungal infections, but these localised 'sarcoid reactions' are not associated with systemic sarcoidosis.

**Pathology.** The mediastinal and superficial lymph nodes, lungs, liver, spleen, skin, eyes, parotid glands and phalangeal bones are most frequently involved. The characteristic histological feature consists of non-caseating epithelioid follicles. These lesions usually resolve spontaneously but in some cases they stimulate the production of fibrous tissue, which may have grave effects on local structure and function. The disease is seldom fatal, and then only when it affects vital organs such as the lungs, the heart or the central nervous system. Calcium metabolism may be disturbed causing hypercalcaemia and, rarely, nephrocalcinosis and renal failure.

**Clinical Features.** Sarcoidosis may present in a subacute or a chronic form. *Subacute sarcoidosis* is usually a benign and self-limiting disorder, spontaneous resolution occurring within a year in most cases. One of its most common manifestations is bilateral and often symmetrical enlargement of the hilar lymph nodes. The paratracheal lymph nodes may also be involved. Erythema nodosum, pyrexia and polyarthritis (p. 627) may be present at the outset. Later, transient pulmonary changes may be seen on radiological examination in addition to the lymph node enlargement. Other cases of subacute sarcoidosis may present with bilateral parotid swelling or iritis, which often persist for several weeks. Neurological manifestations, which are uncommon, include arachnoiditis, cranial nerve lesions and polyneuropathy.

*Chronic sarcoidosis* is a more serious condition, which is less likely to resolve spontaneously and is more liable to cause permanent damage to the structures it involves. Chronic pulmonary sarcoidosis may lead to the development of interstitial fibrosis, pulmonary hypertension and cor pulmonale. The vital capacity and carbon monoxide transfer factor (p. 225) are the most useful indices of impairment of lung function in this form of the disease. Myocardial sarcoidosis may produce arrhythmias and cardiomyopathy. The commonest ocular lesion is bilateral chronic iritis which, if untreated, may cause blindness. Various types of skin lesion may be seen, such as cutaneous 'sarcoids' (reddish-brown papules) or lupus pernio (raised purple plaques, usually on the face, resembling chilblains). Cystic lesions may develop in the phalangeal bones of the hands or feet.

**Investigation.** In most cases skin sensitivity to tuberculin is depressed or absent, and the Mantoux reaction (p. 254) is therefore a useful 'screening' test, a strongly positive reaction to 1 TU virtually excluding sarcoidosis. Although the diagnosis can often be made with a fair measure of confidence from the clinical and radiological features and the tuberculin test, it should, if possible, be confirmed histologically by biopsy of a superficial lymph node or of a skin lesion, when these are present. The Kveim test is also a useful diagnostic procedure, provided a potent antigen can be obtained from human sarcoid tissue. The antigen (0·1 ml) is injected intradermally and when the test is positive a small nodule develops about 4 weeks later, biopsy of which reveals typical sarcoid follicles.

**Treatment.** As subacute sarcoidosis usually resolves spontaneously treatment is seldom required, but occasionally patients with persistent erythema nodosum, pyrexia, parotid swelling or iridocyclitis may have to be given oral corticosteroid therapy for a short period. Patients with chronic sarcoidosis, particularly if it involves the lungs, eyes or other vital organs, are much more likely to require treatment with corticosteroids, which may have to be continued for several years. The dose should be kept to the minimum required to suppress the manifestations of the disease.

## OCCUPATIONAL LUNG DISEASES

In certain occupations the inhalation of dusts, fumes or other noxious substances may give rise to specific pathological changes in the lungs. The nature of each substance, the occupation in which the hazard occurs, the description of each disease and the pathological changes produced in the lungs are summarised in Table 7.9.

Since a diagnosis of occupational lung disease can easily be overlooked and the victims of it may be eligible for compensation, it is most important to take a detailed occupational history, past as well as present. It must also be emphasised that in many types of pneumoconiosis a long period of exposure to dust is required before radiological changes appear and these may precede symptoms by several years. Notes on

Table 7.9 Causes and effects of occupational lung disease

| Cause | Occupation | Description of Disease | Pathological Changes in Lungs |
|---|---|---|---|
| Mineral dusts: | | | |
| Coal dust | Coal mining | Coal-worker's pneumoconiosis | Focal and interstitial fibrosis<br>Centrilobular emphysema<br>Progressive massive fibrosis |
| Silica | Gold mining<br>Iron and steel industries (metal casting)<br>Metal grinding<br>Stone dressing<br>Pottery | Silicosis | |
| Asbestos | Manufacture of fireproof and insulating materials | Asbestosis | Asbestos bodies<br>Interstitial fibrosis<br>Bronchial carcinoma<br>Pleural mesothelioma |
| Iron oxide | Arc welding | Siderosis | Mineral deposition only |
| Tin dioxide | Tin ore mining | Stannosis | |
| Beryllium | Aircraft and atomic energy industries | Berylliosis | Granulomata<br>Interstitial fibrosis |
| Organic dusts: | | | |
| Cotton, flax or hemp dust | Textile industries | Byssinosis | Acute bronchiolitis<br>Bronchoconstriction |
| Fungal spores from mouldy hay, straw or grain, mushroom compost, bagasse, etc. | Agriculture and related industries | Farmer's lung<br>Maltworker's lung<br>Mushroom worker's lung<br>Bagassosis | Extrinsic allergic alveolitis |
| Gases and fumes: | | | |
| Irritant gases (ammonia, chlorine, phosgene, sulphur dioxide and trioxide) | Various industries (accidental exposure) | | Acute pulmonary oedema |
| Toluene di-isocyanate | Plastic and rubber industries | | Bronchial asthma |
| Cadmium | Welding and electroplating | | Chronic bronchitis and emphysema |

diagnosis and claims for benefits in pneumoconiosis and related occupational diseases in Britain are contained in a government pamphlet (p. 307). New industrial processes are constantly being introduced and it is necessary to remain alert to the possibility that they may be associated with new occupational lung diseases.

## Diseases Caused by Mineral Dusts (Pneumoconiosis)

The dust particles, after inhalation, are conveyed by macrophages from the bronchial mucosa to minute foci of lymphoid tissue throughout the lungs. There the irritation produced by solution of the particles in tissue fluid may initiate widespread pulmonary fibrosis. The fibrogenic capacities of mineral dusts vary, silica being markedly fibrogenic whereas iron is almost inert. The most important types of pneumoconiosis are coal-worker's pneumoconiosis, silicosis and asbestosis.

### Coal-worker's Pneumoconiosis

The disease results from prolonged inhalation of coal dust. For clinical purposes — and for certification — the condition is subdivided into simple pneumoconiosis and progressive massive fibrosis. It must be emphasised that for certification purposes in Britain the diagnosis rests at present on radiological, and not clinical, features.

*Simple Coal-worker's Pneumoconiosis*. This is categorised radiologically into 3 grades, depending on the size and extent of the nodulation present. It does not progress if the miner leaves the industry.

*Progressive Massive Fibrosis*. In this form of the disease, large dense masses, single or multiple, occur mainly in the upper lobes. These may be irregular in shape and may cavitate. This type of disease may be complicated very rarely by tuberculosis. It may be disabling, may shorten life expectancy and may progress even after the miner leaves the industry.

Cough and sputum due to associated chronic bronchitis are frequently present. The sputum may be black. Progressive breathlessness on exertion occurs in the later stages, and ventilatory and right ventricular failure supervene as terminal events. There may be no abnormal physical signs in the chest, but where present, they are those of chronic obstructive airways disease.

Antinuclear factor is present in the serum of about 15% of patients with coal-worker's pneumoconiosis. Rheumatoid factor is present in some patients — so-called *Caplan's syndrome* — in which rheumatoid arthritis coexists with rounded fibrotic nodules 0·5 to 5 cm in diameter, mainly in the periphery of the lung fields. This syndrome may also occur in other types of pneumoconiosis.

### Silicosis

This disease is becoming much more rare as the standards of industrial hygiene improve. It is caused by the inhalation of fine free crystalline silicon dioxide (silica) dust or quartz particles. It occurs in the following occupations: mining of coal, tin, gold and other minerals; quarrying, mining and dressing of sandstone and granite; the pottery and ceramics industry; the manufacture of silica bricks and abrasive soaps; iron and steel foundrymen; sand blasting, metal grinding and boiler scaling.

Silica is a very fibrogenic dust and causes the development of hard nodules which coalesce as the disease progresses. Tuberculosis may modify the silicotic process, and caseation and calcification may occur. The radiological features are similar to those seen in coal-worker's pneumoconiosis though the changes tend to be more marked in the upper zones. The hilar shadows may be enlarged and 'egg-shell' calcification in the hilar lymph nodes is a distinctive feature. The disease progresses even when exposure to dust ceases. The sufferer should be removed from the offending environment immediately.

Clinical features are similar to those described in coal-worker's pneumoconiosis.

### Asbestos-related Diseases of the Lungs and Pleura

The main types of asbestos are chrysotile, which accounts for 90% of the world's production, and crocidolite (blue asbestos). Exposure occurs in the following occupations: mining and milling of the material; manufacturing processes involving asbestos; pipe lagging and spraying of limpet asbestos; demolition workers, including those who may work alongside them, e.g. joiners, painters and electricians.

Three forms of disease related to inhalation of asbestos are recognised — calcified pleural plaques, progressive pulmonary fibrosis (pulmonary asbestosis) and malignant disease of pleura and peritoneum.

*Pleural plaques* are best seen in the early stages on oblique films. They are most commonly found on the diaphragm and anterolaterally.

*Progressive pulmonary fibrosis* is characterised by increasing shortness of breath on exertion and cough, by the presence of clubbing of the fingers and dry crepitations at the bases and anterolaterally, and by typical radiological and physiological abnormalities. The radiological abnormalities are usually confined to the lower two-thirds of the lung fields and consist of mottled shadows with some streaky opacities and sometimes 'honeycombing'. The cardiac silhouette becomes shaggy. The most important physiological abnormalities are a reduced carbon monoxide transfer factor (p. 225) and a restrictive ventilatory defect (p. 232). Respiratory and right ventricular failure eventually supervene. The incidence of bronchial carcinoma is much increased, about ten-fold, in persons suffering from asbestosis.

*Mesothelioma of the pleura* is usually linked with exposure, often relatively trivial, to blue asbestos. The patient frequently presents with an ache in the chest. A pleural effusion develops and this causes breathlessness. The effusion may be blood-stained. The diagnosis is often difficult to confirm on pleural biopsy and even at thoracotomy.

The *diagnosis of pulmonary asbestosis* is based on evidence of exposure, clubbing of fingers, characteristic crepitations, typical radiological features, and the physiological abnormalities of restrictive lung disease. Lung biopsy may be required to confirm the diagnosis, but is not without risk and should not be carried out solely for the purpose of allowing patients to claim benefits.

### Treatment and Prevention of Pneumoconiosis

No specific treatment is available. In the later stages treatment is required for associated conditions such as chronic bronchitis and ventilatory failure, pulmonary tuberculosis or malignant pleural effusion.

Improvement of standards of industrial hygiene are now enforced by law in many countries; such measures as wearing respirators, damping dust and efficient ventilation systems are already proving effective in a number of industries.

## Diseases Caused by Organic Dusts

In *byssinosis* the initial lesion is an acute bronchiolitis, associated with symptoms and signs of generalised airflow obstruction which tend to be worse after week-end breaks, but eventually become continuous. There is no radiological abnormality. Recovery usually follows removal from exposure to the dust hazard.

All the other diseases caused by organic dusts are forms of *extrinsic allergic alveolitis*, which have already been described (p. 274).

### Pulmonary Fibrosis

There are three main types of pulmonary fibrosis:

1. *Replacement fibrosis*, in which the fibrous tissue replaces lung parenchyma damaged by infection or by some other destructive process (e.g. infarction). Fibrosis of this type is a common feature of pulmonary tuberculosis and of all types of pulmonary suppuration (p. 246), and is often associated with bronchiectasis.
2. *Focal fibrosis*, which is a common manifestation of pneumoconiosis.
3. *Interstitial fibrosis*, which is the end-result of interstitial lung disease (p. 292).

If pulmonary fibrosis is extensive, it will cause exertional dyspnoea and hypoxaemia, and this is more likely to be the case in focal and interstitial fibrosis than in replacement fibrosis. On the other hand, the physical signs and radiological changes will usually be more conspicuous in replacement fibrosis, which generally produces gross localised abnormalities.

Pulmonary fibrosis cannot usefully be discussed as a single entity, and the reader is therefore referred to its various causes.

## DISEASES OF THE PLEURA AND CHEST WALL

### Fibrinous ('Dry') Pleurisy

This term is used to describe cases of pleurisy at the stage of fibrinous exudation when there is no significant degree of effusion. It is usually secondary to bacterial infection in the underlying lung, but may also occur in association with a viral infection (Coxsackie B), which primarily involves the intercostal muscles and is known as '*Bornholm disease*'. Dry pleurisy is a common feature of pulmonary infarction, and may be an early manifestation of pleural invasion by a pulmonary tumour or of pulmonary tuberculosis.

**Clinical Features.** The characteristic symptom of dry pleurisy is pleural pain. On examination, rib movement is restricted and the breath sounds, though vesicular, may be diminished on the affected side. A pleural rub is heard in a high proportion of cases. In all cases the rub is increased by deep breathing and is never heard when the patient is holding breath, except near the pericardium where a so-called pleuro-pericardial rub may be present. In the acute stage of dry pleurisy, respiration may be so painful that the limited range of movement of the chest wall may be insufficient to produce an audible rub.

The other clinical features depend on the nature of the lesion causing the pleurisy. Depending on the cause, complete clinical recovery may ensue or an effusion may develop, either serous or purulent.

Radiological examination must be performed in every case but a negative radiograph does not necessarily exclude a pulmonary cause for the pleurisy. A preceding history of a few days' cough, purulent sputum and pyrexia is presumptive evidence of a pulmonary infection which may not have been severe enough to produce a radiographic abnormality or which may have resolved before the film was taken.

**Treatment.** The primary cause of the pleurisy must be treated. The symptomatic treatment of pleural pain is described on page 237.

## Pleural Effusion

This term, by general consent, is applied only to serous effusions. The condition of purulent effusion or empyema is described on page 301. The passive transudation of fluid into the pleural cavity (*hydrothorax*) occurs in cardiac failure, nephrotic syndrome, advanced cirrhosis of the liver and severe malnutrition.

The most common causes of pleural effusion are pneumonia, tuberculosis, malignant disease and pulmonary infarction. Pleural effusion, often bilateral, may also be a manifestation of rheumatoid disease, systemic lupus erythematosus and lymphoma. Inflammatory lesions below the diaphragm, such as subphrenic abscess, amoebic liver abscess and pancreatitis, occasionally produce a pleural effusion. The cause of the majority of pleural effusions can be identified if a careful history is taken and comprehensive clinical examination performed.

Where the cause is obscure a lead may be given by enquiry regarding travel abroad, occupation (for example exposure to asbestos), contact with tuberculosis or sources of emboli (oral contraception; recent operation). Detailed investigations as described below may, however, be necessary.

**Clinical Features.** The symptoms and signs of dry pleurisy often precede the development of effusion, but the onset in other cases may be insidious with little or no pleural pain. Pyrexia occurs in most cases, whatever the primary cause, but is more severe in the presence of infection and more protracted when the infection is tuberculous. Dyspnoea is the principal symptom related to the effusion itself. Its severity depends on the size of the effusion and on the rate at which it accumulates. The physical signs in the chest are those of fluid in the pleural space (p. 230).

**Investigation.** *Radiological examination* shows a dense uniform opacity in the lower and lateral parts of the hemithorax shading off above and medially into translucent lung. Occasionally the fluid is localised below the lower lobe, the appearances simulating an elevated hemidiaphragm. When the effusion is loculated, for example, in an interlobar fissure, a localised opacity is seen.

*Ultrasonography* may be of value in detecting an effusion.

*Pleural aspiration.* Absolute proof that an effusion is present can be obtained only by the aspiration of fluid. A needle should be inserted through an intercostal space over the area of maximum dullness on percussion or, ideally, at the site of maximum radiological opacity as shown by postero-anterior and lateral films or by radioscopy. At least 50 ml of fluid should be withdrawn, 20 ml or more being placed in a sterile container for bacteriological examination, 20 ml in a citrated container for cytological examination and 10 ml in a chemically clean container for biochemical examination. Pleural biopsy (p. 232) is always indicated whenever a diagnostic aspiration of pleural fluid is performed.

The appearance of the fluid should be noted — straw coloured, blood stained, purulent or chylous. The protein content will give an indication as to whether the effusion is an exudate (> 30 g/*l*) or a transudate (< 30 g/*l*). The predominant cell type (polymorph, lymphocyte, red blood cell) gives useful information, and the fluid should be examined for malignant cells.

The glucose content is now considered to be unhelpful, but there is a high amylase level in effusions secondary to acute pancreatitis and a high concentration of cholesterol in most chronic rheumatoid effusions. Microbiological investigation, including culture for *Myco. tuberculosis* should be performed where appropriate.

*Other investigations* may be required to determine the primary cause of a pleural effusion. Estimation of the total and differential leucocyte count in the peripheral blood, a tuberculin test, and examination of the sputum for tubercle bacilli should never be omitted. Radiological examination of the chest may disclose underlying pulmonary disease and indicate its nature. If the lung is obscured by a massive effusion, this examination should be repeated after a large volume of fluid has been aspirated. Other investigations which may help to determine the cause of a pleural effusion include bronchoscopy, biopsy of a scalene lymph node, thoracoscopy and serological tests for antinuclear and rheumatoid factors.

The main features of the more important causes of pleural effusion are shown in Table 7.10.

Table 7.10 Important features of various causes of pleural effusion

| | Appearance of Fluid | Type of Fluid | Predominant Cells in Fluid | Other Diagnostic Features |
|---|---|---|---|---|
| Tuberculous | Serous, usually amber coloured | Exudate | Lymphocytes | Positive tuberculin test. Isolation of *M. tuberculosis*. Positive pleural biopsy (80%). |
| Malignant disease | Serous, often blood-stained | Exudate | Serosal cells and lymphocytes Often clumps of malignant cells | Positive pleural biopsy (40%). Evidence of malignant disease elsewhere. |
| *Cardiac failure | Serous, straw-coloured | Transudate | Few serosal cells | Other evidence of left heart failure. Response to diuretics. |
| *Pulmonary infarction | Serous or blood-stained | Exudate | Red blood cells Eosinophils | Contralateral evidence of infarction. Source of embolism. Factors predisposing to venous thrombosis. |
| *Rheumatoid disease | Serous Turbid if chronic | Exudate | Few lymphocytes and serosal cells | Rheumatoid arthritis. Rheumatoid factor in serum. Cholesterol in chronic effusions. |
| *Systemic lupus erythematosus | Serous | Exudate | Few lymphocytes and serosal cells Occasionally LE cells | Other manifestations of SLE. ANF or anti-DNA in serum. |

* Effusion often bilateral

**Treatment.** Aspiration of pleural fluid may be necessary to relieve breathlessness caused by a large effusion. It is inadvisable to remove more than one litre on the first occasion, since pulmonary oedema occasionally follows the aspiration of larger amounts. Even a careful operator may accidentally produce a pneumothorax and a radiograph of the chest should be taken after the procedure.

Treatment of the underlying cause, for example, heart failure, liver or subphrenic abscess, pulmonary embolism and systemic lupus erythematosus will often be followed by resolution of the effusion, but certain conditions require special measures.

In *postpneumonic pleural effusion*, aspiration may need to be repeated several times to make sure that an empyema has not formed and to prevent pleural thickening.

*Tuberculous pleural effusion* should always be treated with antituberculosis chemotherapy (p. 259). Aspiration is required initially if the effusion is large and causing dyspnoea, but the addition of prednisolone by mouth (20 mg/d for six weeks) will promote rapid absorption of the fluid and obviate the need for further aspiration. No restrictions need be placed on the activities of such patients.

*Malignant effusions* reaccumulate and to avoid the distress of repeated aspirations, an attempt should be made to obliterate the pleural space. The method most frequently used is to inject 20 mg of mustine hydrochloride in 60 ml of normal saline into the effusion, which is then drained by aspiration, or preferably through an intercostal tube, 24 hours later. By this time, the visceral and parietal surfaces are acutely inflamed and tend to adhere when the lung re-expands. Although mustine, a cytotoxic drug, may produce some necrosis of tumour cells on the pleural surfaces it is of value in the treatment of malignant pleural effusion chiefly or entirely because it is a chemical irritant, and other substances with similar properties (p. 306) may be equally effective. Some malignant effusions can be controlled at least temporarily by the use of cytotoxic drugs or hormonal therapy.

## Empyema Thoracis

This is the term used to describe the presence of pus in the pleural space. The pus may be as thin as serous fluid, or so thick that it is difficult to aspirate through even a wide-bore needle. Microscopically, neutrophil leucocytes are present in large numbers. The causative organism may or may not be isolated from the pus. An empyema may involve the whole pleural space ('total' empyema) or only part of it ('loculated' or 'encysted' empyema). It is almost invariably unilateral.

**Aetiology.** Empyema is always secondary to infection in a neighbouring structure, usually the lung. The principal infections liable to produce empyema are the bacterial pneumonias and tuberculosis. Other causes of empyema are infection of a haemothorax and rupture of a subphrenic abscess through the diaphragm. Empyema has become a relatively rare disease because pulmonary infection can now be so readily controlled by antibacterial therapy.

**Pathology.** Both layers of pleura are covered with a thick, shaggy, inflammatory exudate. In the course of time the exudate becomes converted into fibrous tissue which may encase the collapsed lung so rigidly that it cannot re-expand when the pus is removed by aspiration or by an external drainage operation. The pus in the pleural space is often under considerable pressure and if the condition is not adequately treated it may rupture into a bronchus, from which it is expectorated, or through an intercostal space with the formation of a subcutaneous abscess or sinus. When an empyema ruptures into a bronchus, a bronchopleural fistula is produced. This allows air to enter the pleural space, and a pyopneumothorax is formed.

The only way in which an empyema can heal is by apposition of the visceral and parietal layers of the pleura with obliteration of the empyema space by organisation of the intervening exudate. This cannot occur unless re-expansion of the collapsed lung is secured at an early stage by removal of all the pus from the pleural space. Re-expansion of the lung cannot take place if, through delay in treatment or inadequate drainage, the visceral pleura becomes grossly thickened and rigid, if the pleural layers are kept apart by air entering the pleura through a bronchopleural fistula, or if disease in the lung itself, such as bronchiectasis, bronchial carcinoma or pulmonary tuberculosis, renders it incapable of re-expansion. In all these circumstances an empyema tends to become chronic and healing may not take place without recourse to major thoracic surgery.

**Clinical Features.** Empyema should be suspected in patients with pulmonary infection if there is a recurrence of pyrexia which fails to respond or responds only partially to the continued administration of a suitable antibiotic. In other cases the illness produced by the primary infective lesion may be so slight that it passes unrecognised and the first definite clinical features are due to the empyema itself.

In the fully developed case two separate groups of clinical features are found:

*Systemic features*: (*a*) Pyrexia, usually high and remittent but sometimes slight. (*b*) Rigors, sweating, malaise, anorexia and loss of weight. (*c*) Neutrophil leucocytosis.

*Local features*: (*a*) Dyspnoea, when the empyema is large. (*b*) Pleural pain, usually confined to the initial stage of the illness. (*c*) Cough and purulent sputum usually related to the primary lung disease, but occasionally caused by the rupture of an empyema into a bronchus. An empyema usually produces the typical signs of fluid in the pleural space (p. 230), but a small localised empyema, particularly when situated in an interlobar fissure, may produce no abnormal physical signs.

**Investigation.** *Radiological Examination.* The appearances are indistinguishable from those of serous pleural effusion (p. 299). When air is present in addition to pus (pyopneumothorax), a horizontal 'fluid level' marks the interface of fluid and air if the film is taken in the erect position.

Confirmation of the presence of an empyema depends on the *aspiration of pus*. A wide-bore needle should be inserted through an intercostal space over the area of maximal dullness on percussion. Whenever possible the position of the empyema should have previously been confirmed by posteroanterior and lateral radiographs. Bacteriological examination of the pus may help to determine the cause of the empyema. In postpneumonic cases where intensive treatment with antibiotics has been given the pus is frequently sterile. The distinction between tuberculous and non-tuberculous cases can usually be made from the radiological changes in the lungs or by the isolation of tubercle bacilli from pus or sputum.

**Treatment.** NON-TUBERCULOUS EMPYEMA

1. *Acute*. When the patient is acutely ill, and the pus is thin in consistence:

(*a*) An intercostal tube should be inserted into the most dependent part of the pleural space and connected to a water seal drainage system (p. 305).

(*b*) An antibiotic to which the organism causing the empyema is sensitive should be given by intramuscular injection or by mouth.

If treatment is started early enough, and the organisms are drug-sensitive, an empyema can often be aborted by these measures. If, however, the intercostal tube is not providing adequate drainage, which is apt to happen when the pus thickens and clots, a short segment of rib should be resected, the empyema cavity cleared of pus and clot, and a wide-bore tube inserted.

2. *Chronic*. If the diagnosis is made before any drainage procedure is carried out, it may be feasible to resect the empyema sac *in toto*, provided the patient is fairly fit and the underlying lung is healthy. If open drainage has been performed, and re-expansion of the lung is prevented by gross thickening of the visceral pleura, 'decor-

tication' may be required. This procedure will allow the lung to re-expand and obliterate the pleural space. Few patients nowadays need to be left with a permanent pleural drain, but this may be unavoidable when respiratory function is poor, or if the underlying lung is badly damaged and the patient is unfit for a major pulmonary resection.

TUBERCULOUS EMPYEMA. Antituberculosis chemotherapy (p. 259) should be started immediately, and the pus in the pleural space should be aspirated through a wide-bore needle until it ceases to reaccumulate. In many cases no other treatment is necessary, but surgery is occasionally required to ablate the residual space.

**Prognosis.** With early drainage and antibiotic therapy most patients with acute empyema quickly recover. Chronic empyema, on the other hand, causes general ill-health, recurrent episodes of pyrexia, clubbing of the fingers and, in severe cases, amyloid disease, and always requires surgical treatment. With specific chemotherapy tuberculous empyema is no longer a serious condition, but complete recovery may take some months.

## Spontaneous Pneumothorax

**Aetiology.** The two chief causes of spontaneous pneumothorax are: (1) rupture of a subpleural emphysematous bulla or of the pulmonary end of a pleural adhesion; (2) rupture of a subpleural tuberculous focus into the pleural space.

In Britain the first cause is very much more common. Active pulmonary tuberculosis is, in fact, responsible for very few cases of spontaneous pneumothorax, a finding which is in sharp contrast with the experience of 50 years ago. Other conditions such as staphylococcal lung abscess, pulmonary infarction and bronchial carcinoma may, in rare instances, give rise to spontaneous pneumothorax.

**Pathology.** There are three types of spontaneous pneumothorax (Fig. 7.5):

1. *Closed.* The communication between pleura and lung seals off as the lung collapses, and does not reopen. In this type of case the air is gradually absorbed and the lung re-expands.

2. *Open.* The communication is generally with a bronchus (bronchopleural fistula) and does not seal off when the lung collapses. The air pressure in the pleural space thus approximates to atmospheric pressure on both inspiration and expiration and the lung cannot re-expand. Moreover, the large bronchial communication facilitates the transmission of infection from the air passages into the pleural space and empyema is a common complication.

3. *Valvular.* The communication between pleura and lung persists but is small and acts as a one-way valve which allows air to enter the pleura during inspiration but prevents it from escaping during expiration. Very large amounts of air may be 'trapped' in the pleural space during bouts of coughing and the intrapleural pressure may rise to well above atmospheric level. This results not only in complete collapse of the underlying lung but also in mediastinal displacement towards the opposite side with compression of the opposite lung. This type of pneumothorax is usually referred to as 'tension pneumothorax'.

**Clinical Features.** The onset is usually sudden, with pain or a feeling of 'tightness' on the affected side of the chest, which may be aggravated by deep inspiration. The

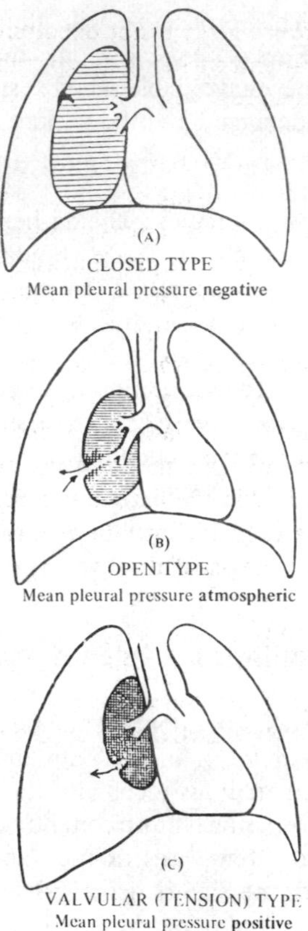


Fig. 7.5 The mechanisms of spontaneous pneumothorax.

patient then becomes increasingly breathless and in severe cases central cyanosis may be present. The physical signs in the chest are those of air in the pleural space (p. 230). When the pneumothorax is small and localised there may be no abnormal signs, and the condition may be revealed only by radiological examination.

*Closed spontaneous pneumothorax*. Dyspnoea, which is seldom severe, gradually abates over the course of a few days. Progressive spontaneous absorption of the air takes place and re-expansion of the lung is complete between 2 and 6 weeks later, depending on the initial size of the pneumothorax. Pleural infection is uncommon in this type of pneumothorax.

*Open spontaneous pneumothorax* is usually of tuberculous origin. The onset is similar to that of the closed type, but the dyspnoea, although it is not rapidly progressive, does not improve and within a few days the appearance of pyrexia and systemic disturbance, accompanied by physical and radiological signs of air and fluid in the pleural space, indicate the development of a pyopneumothorax. In tuberculous cases acid-fast bacilli can be isolated from the pleural fluid.

*Valvular pneumothorax* ('tension pneumothorax') produces the most dramatic clinical picture of all. The dyspnoea is rapidly progressive from the start and is accompanied by central cyanosis. The patient may die from asphyxia within a few minutes, but usually the course of events is less rapid and medical attention can be obtained in time to avert a fatal outcome.

*Recurrent spontaneous pneumothorax* is not uncommon, especially in patients with emphysematous bullae. Subsequent incidents are usually on the same side as the first but may also occur on the opposite side.

**Radiological examination** shows the sharp edge of the collapsed lung, and between this and the chest wall there is complete translucency with no lung markings. The degree of pulmonary collapse varies from case to case. Radiographs also show the degree of mediastinal displacement, and give information regarding the presence or absence of pleural fluid and underlying pulmonary disease.

**Treatment.** 1. *Closed Spontaneous Pneumothorax*. When the pneumothorax is small and the patient is only slightly dyspnoeic no treatment is required but observation should be continued until re-expansion of the lung is complete. If, however, the pneumothorax is large and causing moderate or severe dyspnoea, it is essential to employ more active measures. Immediate and complete re-expansion of the lung can be obtained by inserting a catheter into the pleural cavity through an intercostal space and connecting it to a water-seal drainage system (Fig. 7.6) or a non-return (Heimlich) valve. The catheter is left in place for 5 or 6 days. This form of treatment considerably shortens the period of incapacity.

If a tuberculous aetiology is suspected, specific chemotherapy (p. 259) should be started immediately. If a pleural effusion develops, the fluid may be drained through the catheter by suitable posturing or aspirated with a needle and syringe.

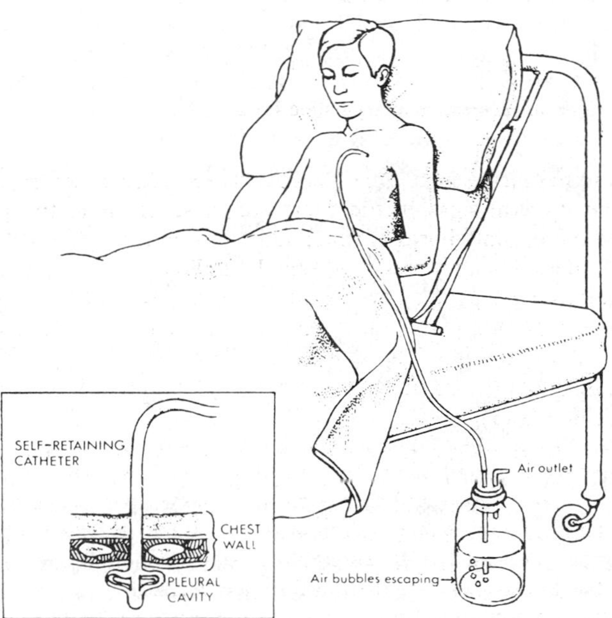


Fig. 7.6 Treatment of spontaneous pneumothorax by pleural intubation and 'water-seal' decompression. The water-seal allows air to leave the pleural space but prevents it from re-entering. This reduces the intrapleural pressure and promotes re-expansion of the lung. The insert shows the position of the self-retaining (Malecot) catheter in the pleural space.

2. *Open Spontaneous Pneumothorax*. There is a frank bronchopleural fistula, and pleural infection rapidly supervenes. Such cases are seldom amenable to medical treatment and, whether tuberculous or non-tuberculous, should be referred to a thoracic surgeon for treatment of the resulting pyopneumothorax.

3. *Tension Pneumothorax*. This constitutes an acute medical emergency. An intercostal catheter should be inserted at once and connected to a water-seal drainage system, as shown in Figure 7.6. Symptomatic relief is immediate and dramatic. If suitable equipment for this procedure is not at hand a wide-bore plastic cannula should be used instead. This should be attached to a length of tubing, the end of which should be placed under water in a bottle or basin. Surgical treatment may be required for a persistent tension pneumothorax.

4. *Recurrent spontaneous pneumothorax*, unilateral or bilateral, is first treated by the introduction of an irritant substance, such as an emulsion of kaolin, into the pleural space. This procedure (artificial pleurodesis) produces an aseptic pleurisy, which results in the formation of extensive adhesions between the parietal and visceral surfaces, and usually prevents further episodes of spontaneous pneumothorax. In a few cases thoracotomy and abrasion of the parietal pleura may be required to obliterate the pleural space.

## Deformities of the Chest Wall

An increase in the anteroposterior diameter of the chest relative to the lateral diameter is a common feature of emphysema, but only the most severe forms of this abnormality merit the description of 'barrel chest'. *Pectus carinatum* ('pigeon chest') is seen in patients who have suffered from severe obstructive airways disease (chronic bronchitis or asthma) since early childhood. *Pectus excavatum* ('funnel chest') is a condition in which the body of the sternum, often only its lower end, is curved backwards. The heart is displaced to the left, and may be compressed between the sternum and vertebral column, but only very rarely is this associated with disturbance of cardiac function. It may, however, restrict chest expansion and reduce the vital capacity. The impairment of cardiac or pulmonary function is seldom sufficiently severe to warrant surgical correction, but this may be indicated for cosmetic reasons.

Severe *thoracic kyphoscoliosis* causes ventilation:perfusion maldistribution in the lungs and pulmonary underventilation. Patients with this type of chest deformity later develop respiratory failure, pulmonary hypertension and right ventricular failure, and many die before the age of 50. The tempo of deterioration is often accelerated by bacterial infection in the bronchi and lungs. The prognosis in these cases can be improved only by early surgical correction of the spinal deformity. Respiratory failure may also occur in ankylosing spondylitis, particularly if there is any interference with the function of the diaphragm.

## Prospects in Respiratory Medicine

Advances in immunology, immunopathology and immunopharmacology have already opened the way to a clearer understanding of the nature of certain respiratory diseases, notably bronchial asthma, bronchopulmonary eosinophilia and extrinsic allergic alveolitis, and may in time help to elucidate the pathogenesis of conditions such as cryptogenic fibrosing alveolitis, some types of occupational lung disease and even bronchial carcinoma. Cytological and biochemical examination of material obtained from the bronchi and lungs by bronchoscopic lavage may also prove to be a useful diagnostic and research technique in many obscure forms of diffuse pulmonary disease. Immunology has a further contribution to make in the field of respiratory infection. Until recently research effort was concentrated mainly on the pathogenic properties of microorganisms, but with increasing awareness of the importance of the host reaction there is now a growing interest in methods of investigating the integrity of the various mechanisms, local and systemic, which protect the lungs against both acute and chronic infection by bacteria, viruses and fungi.

New non-invasive techniques are becoming available for the diagnosis of localised pulmonary lesions and of diseases which cause abnormalities of ventilation and perfusion, such as emphysema and pulmonary thromboembolism. These techniques, which include computed tomographic scanning and new methods of radioisotope scanning, are still in an early stage of development, but when fully exploited are certain to revolutionise the investigation of respiratory disease. On a more mundane level further improvement can be expected in the technique of bronchoscopy and of bronchial and pulmonary biopsy.

The empirical treatment of respiratory disease has recently seen many important advances, particularly in regard to antibiotics, bronchodilator drugs and corticosteroids. Efforts to discover drugs or other forms of treatment which can influence the basic causes of allergic and malignant disease and of chronic bronchopulmonary infection have so far met with only limited success, but this situation is bound to change when we have more precise knowledge of the pathogenesis of these diseases.

I. W. B. GRANT
N. W. HORNE
G. J. R. MCHARDY

*Further reading:*

Cotes, J. E. (1980) *Lung Function: Assessment and Application in Medicine*, 4th edn. Oxford: Blackwell.

Crofton, J. & Douglas, A. C. (1975) *Respiratory Diseases*, 2nd edn. Oxford: Blackwell.

Grant, I. W. B. (1979) Examination of the respiratory system. In *Clinical Examination*, 5th edn. ed. Macleod, J. Edinburgh: Churchill Livingstone.

Ross, J. D. & Horne, N. W. (1981) *Modern Drug Treatment in Tuberculosis*, 7th edn. London: Chest, Heart and Stroke Association.

Department of Health and Social Security (1979) Pneumoconiosis and related occupational diseases: Notes on diagnosis and claims for industrial injuries scheme benefits. London: DHSS.

# 8. Diseases of the Alimentary Tract and Pancreas

## Physiology of the Alimentary Tract

The alimentary tract is a coordinated structure with the function of ingesting and absorbing nutrients and excreting unabsorbed and waste products. It should not be regarded as a series of separate organs, since the role of each component is closely related to that of other parts of the tract. Its operation may be considered under the following headings:

(1) *Controlling and Coordinating Mechanisms.* The autonomic nervous system and hormones, including gastrin, secretin and cholecystokinin-pancreozymin, control and coordinate motility and secretion.

(2) *Motility*. The carefully controlled motility of the tract is responsible for the orderly progression of nutrients through the system so that the stage of digestion and absorption is appropriate to a given region of the tract.

(3) *Secretion.* The secretion of enzymes and detergents enables protein, carbohydrate and fat to be digested prior to absorption. The secretion of electrolytes provides the correct pH for each stage of digestion.

(4) *Absorption.* The absorptive system consists of specialised cells, together with the portal venous system and lymphatics.

(5) *Defence Mechanisms.* These are necessary to protect the mucosa from its own digestive enzymes and from the bacterial population to which it is exposed. These mechanisms include a rapid turnover of the epithelial cells, the production of mucus and a specialised immunological system.

### 1. The Controlling and Coordinating Mechanisms

The cells of the gastrointestinal tract are controlled by the autonomic nervous system and by chemical messages which are amino acids or their derivatives, amines or peptides. Their transmission is called endocrine when it is via the blood, neurocrine when it is across a synapse and paracrine when it is through an intercellular space.

### 2. Motility

Apart from the striated muscle in the upper oesophagus, smooth muscle is responsible for the motility of the gastrointestinal tract. The smooth muscle produces 'slow waves' which are conducted over long distances. These do not result in contraction but they enable contractions in different areas to be coordinated.

*Oesophagus.* The upper oesophageal sphincter is formed by the striated cricopharyngeus muscle which exerts constant tone to keep the sphincter closed except during swallowing. Once the upper oesophageal sphincter relaxes, peristalsis sweeps along the length of the body of the oesophagus, but occasionally, even in the normal oesophagus, the contractions are not coordinated. In the disorder of diffuse spasm these uncoordinated contractions predominate. The lowest few centimetres of the oesophagus form the lower oesophageal sphincter. This has a high resting tension which prevents reflux of gastric contents into the oesophagus. Normally the sphincter relaxes when the peristaltic wave arrives but the characteristic feature in achalasia is that it fails to do so. The sphincter is controlled by nervous and hormonal mechanisms.

*Stomach.* The normal tonic contraction of the stomach is inhibited by the arrival of food probably by means of a centrally mediated vagal reflex. This is termed receptive relaxation so that a large increase in volume is accompanied by only a small rise in pressure within the lumen. The gastric slow wave controls the frequency and direction of antral peristalsis which is responsible for the thorough mixing of the gastric contents and their progressive emptying into the duodenum. Several mechanisms exist to prevent the duodenum receiving more nutrient than it can deal with. Chemoreceptors for fat and acid and osmoreceptors in the duodenal mucosa control gastric emptying by means of local reflexes and the release of secretin, pancreozymin and other enteric hormones. Approximately half of a semisolid meal has left the stomach in about 30 minutes.

*Small Intestine.* Here also coordination is due to the slow wave in the longitudinal muscle fibres. It is the pacemaker which dictates the times at which any given segment of the gut can contract. The frequency of the slow wave in the duodenum is greater than in the ileum, thus enabling the proximal bowel to override more distal areas. By this means contractions are coordinated both to mix and propel the small bowel content so that all nutrients can be exposed to the absorptive cells. It is thought that the myenteric plexus and the enteric hormones determine the local response to the slow wave so that contraction may or may not occur depending on the state of affairs in the lumen at any one time.

*Colon.* Motility here is poorly understood. There is probably a slow wave but it is not known how it coordinates contractions. Observation of the colon suggests two main types of contraction occur which may be associated with two different functions. Firstly, there is segmentation which consists of contraction rings forming and disappearing over long periods of time: these produce a slow mixing of faeces but no propulsion, thus facilitating the absorption of water and electrolytes. Secondly, propulsion occurs through 'mass movement,' a peristaltic wave which occurs several times a day. This action carries out the second function of the colon, namely the elimination of faeces. All activity in the colon is increased after eating, and defaecation is more likely to occur post-prandially. The enteric hormones may be responsible for this activity. The main activity in the colon, segmentation, causes mixing only and is responsible for the resistance to flow along the lumen. In constipation, segmentation is increased and there is resistance to flow along the lumen whereas in diarrhoea there is a reduction in segmentation so that the semi-formed contents of the right colon have an unimpeded transit through the colon.

### 3. Secretion

The production of secretions for the digestion of nutrients is under nervous and hormonal control.

*Gastric Secretion.* In response to the sight or smell of food, the vagus stimulates acid and pepsin secretion by a direct effect on the parietal and peptic cells. It also initiates the release of gastrin from the antrum. More sustained output of this hormone is produced by a rise in pH and by ingested protein. Gastrin then enters the bloodstream and acts on the body of the stomach to produce acid and pepsin to digest the protein. It stimulates acid secretion through the release of histamine. Mechanisms are also required to turn off gastric secretion once digestion within the stomach is complete. These are largely the same as those which slow gastric emptying, i.e. the release of the enteric hormones, secretin and cholecystokinin-pancreozymin, and also the presence of a low pH in the gastric antrum which inhibits the further release of gastrin.

*Pancreatic Secretion, Bile and Intestinal Secretions.* Acid, fat and hypertonic solutions in the duodenum release the hormones secretin and cholecystokinin from the duodenal mucosa into the bloodstream. Secretin stimulates the acinar cells of the pancreas to produce bicarbonate which neutralises the gastric acid and provides a neutral pH for the activity of the pancreatic enzymes, lipase, amylase and trypsin. These are produced in response to cholecystokinin-pancreozymin, which also causes contraction of the gall bladder so that an adequate supply of bile acids reaches the intestine at a time when fat has to be digested. The enteric hormones are also responsible for the secretion, by the mucosa of the small intestine, of succus entericus which contains bicarbonate and additional enzymes.

### 4. The Absorptive System

The area for absorption in the small intestine is increased several hundredfold by the presence of villi and microvilli. The surface of the individual cell is formed of microvilli which possess a multitude of enzyme systems for the final stages of digestion of nutrients followed by their absorption. In coeliac disease and tropical sprue the surface area of the small intestine is reduced because of the decrease in villi, and malabsorption results.

Under normal circumstances nutrients are transported from the absorptive cell by the lymphatic system (e.g. fat and fat soluble vitamins) or by the portal venous system (e.g. amino acids and hexoses).

The absorptive system is discussed in more detail on page 346.

### 5. Defence Mechanisms

*Cell Turnover.* The epithelial cells of the gastrointestinal tract are constantly renewed so that, for example, the epithelial surface of the small intestine is replaced every 48 hours. The desquamated cells are digested and their products reabsorbed. In the intestine, cellular turnover has been shown to be slower than normal in germ-free animals and it can be argued that this turnover is to some extent a protective mechanism.

*Production of Mucus.* Mucus producing cells are present throughout the gastrointestinal tract and mucus has a protective function.

*Immunological System.* The lamina propria of the stomach and intestines contains many lymphocytes and plasma cells. Some of these cells synthesise secretory IgA (p. 28) which is resistant to digestion by intestinal enzymes and has a role in protecting mucosal surfaces from bacterial invasion. It is thus of particular importance in the small intestine where bacterial colonisation is deleterious.

## The Symptoms of Alimentary Disease

*Pain* is often the most important symptom of gastrointestinal disease. It must be analysed in relation to its main site, radiation, character, severity, duration, frequency, times of occurrence, aggravating and relieving factors and any associated phenomena. The characteristics of abdominal pain are often diagnostic, for example in peptic ulceration and acute appendicitis. *Loss of appetite* (anorexia) may have a local cause such as carcinoma of the stomach but may also be a feature of any debilitating disease or of a psychological disturbance. *Vomiting* may occur in diseases of the stomach or small intestine, peritonitis, appendicitis, or cholecystitis. Numerous other conditions may also be responsible, for example meningitis, uraemia, migraine, drugs such as digoxin or morphine and, in the child, infection. The type, timing and related features of the vomiting are important diagnostically. Sudden vomiting without preceding nausea may be due to direct stimulation of the vomiting centre in the medulla and thus be an indication of intracranial disease. Vomiting in the morning may be due to pregnancy or alcoholism. Vomiting of large quantities of food and secretions late in the day or night indicates gastric outlet obstruction. Vomiting which relieves pain is often due to a peptic ulcer. The complaint of persistent vomiting without loss of weight is nearly always indicative of a psychological disturbance. *Heartburn* is a burning retrosternal sensation due to reflux oesophagitis as in a sliding hiatus hernia. *Regurgitation* is the appearance of previously swallowed food in the mouth without warning. It usually has an acid or bitter taste because of the presence of gastric juice or bile but not in patients with obstruction in the oesophagus. *Dysphagia*, i.e. difficulty in swallowing, is discussed on page 319. *Flatulence* is often due to excessive swallowing of air (aerophagy) which in turn may be due to anxiety. Under normal circumstances a small amount of air is swallowed with food, drink and saliva. Some of this gas may be expelled as a belch. The remainder passes into the intestine. Some will be absorbed but most, particularly the nitrogen, will be expelled per rectum. A plain radiograph of the abdomen shows that gas is normally present in the stomach and colon but that very little is seen in the small intestine.

*Constipation and diarrhoea* are sometimes difficult to define. In Britain fewer than 10% of people have less than one bowel motion per day and only 1% have a bowel movement less frequently than 3 times a week. These latter should be regarded as constipated. In addition, if the stool is hard and difficult to pass the patient should be regarded as constipated whatever the frequency of bowel movement. In contrast, less than 1% of the population have more than three bowel movements daily and this should be regarded as abnormal, particularly if the stool is not formed. When the stool is liquid or semi-formed it must be regarded as abnormal whatever the frequency of bowel movement. The diet in Western countries is low in roughage; where a high residue diet is usual, more than three bowel movements daily may be normal. An explanation must be found for any change in bowel habits.

*Loss of weight* may be due to a reduced intake of food because of anorexia, nausea or vomiting, to malabsorption of nutrients or to the loss of protein from a diseased bowel as in ulcerative colitis. Carcinoma is the most important alimentary cause of loss of weight.

## Investigation of the Gastrointestinal Tract

In addition to systematic examination of the abdomen by inspection, palpation, percussion and auscultation and of the rectum by digital examination along the lines described in *Clinical Examination* (p. 375), further investigation is frequently required, notably radiological and endoscopic examinations.

## Radiological Examination

**Plain radiographs** show the normal soft tissue shadows due to the liver, spleen and kidneys and also abnormal shadows. Gas in the intestine acts as a contrast medium so that the distribution of the bowel within the abdomen can be assessed. In obstruction there may be an excessive amount of gas and fluid in the bowel above the obstruction and films with the patient erect will demonstrate fluid levels. Finally, areas of opacification due to stones or to calcification in the liver, pancreas, cysts or blood vessels may provide important diagnostic information. A chest radiograph is helpful in delineating the diaphragmatic areas and any subphrenic collections of gas with or without a fluid level. Pulmonary lesions, from which pain may be referred to the abdomen, can also be identified.

**Barium Studies.** These will demonstrate a break in the continuity of the outline of the organ, abnormalities in the appearance of the mucosa and disorders of motility. Preparation of the patient for each examination should always be undertaken so that mucosal detail will not be obscured by contents. For studies of the upper gastro-intestinal tract, the patient is fasted and for barium enema examination the colon should be cleared of faeces by means of laxatives and in some cases by washout.

*The Barium Swallow and Meal Examination.* The oesophagus is studied whilst barium is being swallowed. This may demonstrate a disorder of motility, filling defects caused by tumours or varices, a stricture, a diverticulum or a hiatus hernia.

The mucosa of the stomach can be examined by using a small amount of barium together with the introduction of gas — a double contrast study. An ulcer is usually seen face on as a small collection of barium with radiating folds of mucosa. An ulcer may also appear as a projection beyond the normal outline while tumours cause filling defects (Fig. 8.2). Small cancers can be detected by irregularity in the mucosal pattern. Observation of the motility of the stomach may indicate an inert area caused by infiltrating carcinoma. The duodenal cap is examined by studying its contours when it is completely filled with barium and its mucosal pattern when only a small amount of barium remains.

*The Follow-through Examination.* When disease of the small intestine is suspected, barium is observed during its passage through the small intestine and radiographs are taken at intervals. The outline of the barium may indicate structural abnormalities such as diverticula or strictures. When there is malabsorption, excess secretions may cause the barium to clump and flocculate.

*Barium Enema.* This procedure is uncomfortable and sometimes exhausting, particularly in the elderly or in those with cardiac disease in whom arrhythmia may be induced. Barium enema must always have been preceded by digital examination of the rectum and preferably also by sigmoidoscopy a few days earlier. Barium alone or, for double contrast examination, barium and air, is run into the bowel through a self-retaining catheter. Radiographs are taken with the whole colon filled with barium in order to see any filling defect or diverticula. In some patients there will be a reflux of barium into the terminal ileum which can be outlined. Then the patient empties the bowel and further radiographs are taken which show the texture of the mucosa coated by the small amount of remaining barium.

*Cautionary Note.* Exposure to X-rays in the early months of pregnancy may upset normal development of the fetus and be responsible for deformity or still birth. These risks apply not only to radiographic examination of the abdomen such as barium enema but also to procedures such as excretion urography and radiographs of the lumbar spine and pelvis. Inadvertent irradiation in the first few weeks of pregnancy can be avoided by restricting radiological examination of the lower abdomen in women at risk to the 10 days immediately following the onset of the last menstrual period — 'the 10 day rule'.

**Computed tomography** is used to depict intra-abdominal organs and masses. It may be of particular value in the detection of pancreatic cancer since the pancreas is inaccessible to most other radiographic techniques.

## Imaging Studies

**Ultrasonography.** The principles of this technique are described on page 154. It has the advantage of being non-invasive and is of value in detecting cysts, particularly of the pancreas, and abscesses.

**Radioisotope scanning** is little used apart from examination of the liver and spleen (p. 387), and pancreatic scanning is very inaccurate.

## Endoscopy

With fibreoptic instruments it is not difficult to examine the whole of the oesophagus, stomach, duodenum and colon. Two bundles of many thousands of fine glass fibres are contained in the instrument's shaft. One bundle carries light to the tip of the instrument in order to illuminate the organ being examined whilst the other can transmit an image back to the observer. The fibre bundles are flexible so that the whole shaft can be bent and easily passed into the upper gastrointestinal tract or colon. The shaft of the instrument also carries controls so that the tip of the instrument can be moved, and channels through which air or forceps can be passed to insufflate the organ or to take a biopsy from the mucosa. Endoscopic instruments can also be used for therapeutic procedures which would otherwise require laparotomy; examples include polypectomy, removal of stones from the common bile duct and sphincterotomy of the ampulla of Vater.

Rigid instruments are used to examine the rectum and lower pelvic colon (sigmoidoscope) and occasionally the oesophagus (oesophagoscope).

**Upper Alimentary Tract.** It is usual to carry out the procedure with the patient under sedation, often as an out-patient. After a 12-hour fast the pharynx is anaesthetised with a spray. The instrument is passed with the assistance of the patient in swallowing and the procedure, whilst uncomfortable, should be no more so than any other intubation. Possible complications are perforation of the oesophagus or stomach whilst passing the instrument or during biopsy, and the inhalation of secretions; these are rare with flexible fibreoptic instruments.

Where possible, the oesophagus, stomach and duodenum are all inspected at the same examination (panendoscopy), because the presence of one lesion does not exclude another and double lesions are not uncommon, e.g. oesophagitis and duodenal ulcer. This is particularly important when endoscopy is carried out in patients with haematemesis or melaena, since there may be more than one source of bleeding.

*Oesophagoscopy* should be carried out when there is dysphagia or when barium examination suggests a tumour or stricture. Other indications include suspected oesophagitis, varices or a motility disorder. Therapeutic procedures that can be carried out include dilatation of a stricture and injection of sclerosing material into oesophageal varices to control bleeding.

*Gastroscopy* is indicated so that a biopsy can be taken when a gastric ulcer which may be malignant has been demonstrated on barium studies. Healing of ulcers may be assessed. Gastroscopy is nearly always necessary in the investigation of patients with symptoms after gastric surgery because the appearances are difficult to define radiologically. *Duodenoscopy* is indicated in duodenal ulceration.

*Endoscopic Retrograde Cholangio-Pancreatography* (ERCP) is a special application of fibreoptic endoscopy. At duodenoscopy the ampulla of Vater is cannulated with a fine bore catheter passed through the shaft of the instrument and radio-opaque dye is injected into the biliary and pancreatic ducts. The procedure is of great value in patients suspected of having pancreatic disease since distortion or obstruction of the ductal system may indicate a diagnosis of chronic pancreatitis or pancreatic carcinoma. Obstruction or distortion of the common bile duct by a stone or a tumour can also be demonstrated and stones can be removed.

**Lower Alimentary Tract.** *Proctoscopy and Sigmoidoscopy.* These are simple procedures which should always be carried out in patients with symptoms referable to the lower bowel or anus. Both terms are inaccurate since proctoscopy visualises the anal canal and only 2–3 cm of the rectum, and sigmoidoscopy examines the rectum and the lower few centimetres of the pelvic colon. It is usual to carry out the procedures without preparation but if the rectum contains faeces, then endoscopy is repeated after the bowel has been emptied. The examination is carried out with the patient in the knee-elbow position, or on the left side with the knees drawn up. Digital examination of the rectum should always precede endoscopy and the instruments should be warmed and well lubricated. Proctoscopy is used for the demonstration and injection of haemorrhoids. Sigmoidoscopy is necessary for the diagnosis of polyps, cancer of the rectum, ulcerative proctitis or colitis and Crohn's disease of the large bowel. Biopsy of the mucosa or lesion is also taken. Sigmoidoscopy is carried out under anaesthesia when there is a painful condition of the anus such as a fissure; it should be performed only with extreme care in fulminating ulcerative colitis because of the danger of perforation.

*Colonoscopy.* The flexible colonoscope allows examination of the whole colon but the procedure is time-consuming and occasionally difficult. The bowel must be carefully prepared over several days, first with laxatives and then by lavage so that no faecal material remains. During colonoscopy it is possible to take a biopsy of suspicious lesions and polyps can be removed using a diathermy snare.

### Other Investigations

**Biopsy** of lesions is an essential part of each endoscopic procedure but the small size of the specimen may make interpretation by the pathologist difficult.

Biopsy of the small intestine is indicated if malabsorbtion is suspected and is carried out by means of the Crosby capsule. After an overnight fast the capsule is passed into the jejunum attached to a stiff radio-opaque catheter and the biopsy is taken just distal to the duodeno-jejunal flexure. Suction via the catheter draws mucosa into a small port on the side of the instrument. The negative pressure which develops within the capsule also fires the knife which severs the mucosa. The intubation and biopsy are completed in about one hour. Bleeding occurs occasionally and for this reason biopsies should not be carried out unless the platelet count and prothrombin time are normal. Another rare complication is perforation of the intestine. The biopsy specimens are inspected under the dissecting microscope immediately after removal from the capsule prior to fixation and histological examination.

**Secretory Studies.** *The Pentagastrin Test.* The acid output is measured in response to pentagastrin, a synthetic pentapeptide which exerts the biological effects of gastrin. Preparation consists of an overnight fast and cimetidine must be stopped for at least 48 hours before the test. The fasting contents of the stomach are aspirated and their volume measured; then the secretions are collected continuously for one hour. This is termed the 'basal acid output'. Then pentagastrin is given subcutaneously and the secretions are collected for a further hour. The acid output in this hour is termed the 'maximum acid output'.

The pentagastrin test is helpful because: (a) a large volume of fasting juice indicates obstruction of the gastric outlet; (b) a very high basal acid output suggests that the patient has the Zollinger-Ellison syndrome (p. 334); (c) in patients with peptic ulcer it provides a preoperative base line; (d) achlorhydria can be demonstrated.

*The insulin test* is used after gastric surgery to indicate the completeness of vagotomy. The preparation and procedure are similar to those described above but the gastric stimulant is soluble insulin which is given intravenously. The resulting hypoglycaemia stimulates the vagal centres and gastric acid is secreted if the vagal innervation of the stomach has not been completely divided.

*Pancreatic function tests* are described on page 340.

**Bacteriological Studies.** The malabsorption syndrome may be due occasionally to bacterial colonisation of the small intestine. When this is suspected, secretion can be obtained for bacteriological studies by passing a fine sterile tube into the upper small intestine. A mercury bag attached to the tip of the tube ensures that the tube moves rapidly to the correct site. The patient should not be receiving antibiotics.

**Motility Studies.** Barium examination gives some indication of the motility of the oesophagus, stomach and small intestine. Cineradiography or videotape studies are useful in the analysis of dysphagia arising in the pharynx. Motility can be studied more accurately by measuring the pressure changes in the lumen of the organ but only in the case of the oesophagus is this of diagnostic value. Fine open ended tubes are passed into the stomach and pressures are transmitted to transducers and measured at intervals whilst the tube is gradually withdrawn with the patient swallowing. The procedure may be of value in establishing the relationship between chest pain and abnormal oeophageal contractions, for the diagnosis of motility disorders of the oesophagus and in determining the position of the lower oesophageal sphincter.

**Examination of the Stool.** In malabsorption the stool may be pale and frothy; in the irritable bowel syndrome it may be like pellets or ribbon with or without mucus. In mild ulcerative disease of the colon there may be flecks of blood in the mucus. Inspection of the stool is sufficient to diagnose fresh bleeding from the lower alimentary tract while the loss of over 60 ml of blood from a site proximal to the ascending colon will produce a black tarry stool.

Tests for occult blood (e.g. Hemoccult) detect small amounts of blood in the stool and are performed for several successive days because bleeding from the gastrointestinal tract is often intermittent. Specimens obtained on the finger-stall at rectal examination can be readily examined.

Microscopic examination is of value particularly in distinguishing amoebic dysentery and other parasitic diseases.

## Parenteral and Enteral Nutrition

When normal nutrition cannot be maintained, nutrients can be given intravenously (parenteral nutrition) or by nasogastric intubation (enteral nutrition). There are many possible indications for the use of parenteral nutrition including preparation for major surgery, postoperative care of patients who have undergone extensive intestinal resection and the management of prolonged ileus, enterocutaneous fistula, acute pancreatitis with complications, and severe inflammatory bowel disease. Some patients with these disorders can be managed by enteral feeding which has fewer complications and is more manageable and economical.

*Parenteral nutrition* provides calories, nitrogen, water, electrolytes and vitamins. Calories are provided in the form of 20–30% glucose and fat emulsions; protein hydrolysates or amino acid preparations provide the nitrogen. These are made up in a balanced solution containing the requirements of electrolytes, water and water soluble vitamins. Various commercial preparations are available for different requirements of protein and electrolytes. The solutions are hypertonic and hence they must be given via a central vein with the risks of pneumothorax, thrombosis and sepsis. Numerous metabolic complications and nutritional deficiencies of therapy have been described.

*Enteral Nutrition*. The diet may be polymeric, i.e. protein, fat and carbohydrate in high molecular weight form; this is used when the patient's digestive and absorptive capacity is normal but when there is difficulty in swallowing, e.g. after oesophageal surgery. Alternatively the diet may be monomeric, i.e. amino acids, oligo- and monosaccharides; these are used when digestion is impaired, e.g. after bowel resection, or when stimulation of digestive secretions is to be avoided. Enteral feeding is usually given as a constant infusion via a nasogastric or nasoenteric fine bore tube; gastrostomy or jejunostomy can also be used.

# DISEASES OF THE MOUTH

The mouth acts as a receptacle in which food can be broken down into small particles during mastication. Into the mouth flows the saliva which is secreted in response to the act of chewing and to the sight, taste and smell of food. Saliva has several functions. It facilitates speech, moistens the food and lubricates the process of swallowing. By its solvent action on the foodstuffs, it enables tasting to take place. It also contains an enzyme ptyalin which is concerned in the digestion of polysaccharides to disaccharides.

### Disorders of the Teeth

Mastication of food to a soft pulp is a prerequisite for good digestion. The teeth should be inspected to determine if they are healthy, present in adequate numbers and in correct apposition in the upper and lower jaws to allow efficient mastication. If dentures are worn it should be ascertained if they are comfortable and efficient. Bacteraemia may have its source in gingivitis or an apical abscess. It is particularly liable to occur after dental manipulation and may cause endocarditis in patients with valvular disease of the heart; for this reason such patients should always be given prophylactic antibiotics both before and after dental extraction (p. 182). All patients should be advised to consult a dentist regularly in order to conserve the teeth and to prevent or treat foci of infection in the mouth.

## Stomatitis

The mouth harbours a population of commensal micro-organisms which normally is controlled by a reasonable standard of oral hygiene; if this is neglected the bacterial population may proliferate and cause gingivitis or stomatitis. This may also occur when resistance to the commensal population is lowered by disease especially in the compromised host.

*Stomatitis due to deficiency of nutritional factors* may arise directly from an insufficient intake or indirectly as a result of impaired absorption of vitamins, especially niacin, riboflavin, folate, and cyanocobalamin. When the deficiency is acute and severe, the tongue is red, raw and painful. When the deficiency is chronic and less severe the tongue appears moist and unduly clean because of atrophy of the papillae. Angular stomatitis often accompanies glossitis, especially in the case of severe iron deficiency. In severe vitamin C deficiency the gums become swollen and spongy and bleed readily.

*Ulcerative stomatitis* (Vincent's infection) occurs mainly in adults in conditions associated with malnutrition and poor dental hygiene; it is not commonly seen nowadays in Britain. Ulcers with ragged necrotic margins occur especially on the gums, but may involve the palate, the lips, or the inner aspects of the cheeks; the ulcers are covered by a grey slough surrounded by an erythematous margin. A stained smear shows many spirochaetes and fusiform bacilli; these organisms are present in small numbers in the normal commensal population of the mouth and the condition may be regarded as an endogenous infection due to proliferation of the organisms because of some alteration in host resistance. The condition is infectious, so that the patient's food vessels and cutlery should be sterilised. The acute phase responds to local treatment with metronidazole (200 mg t.i.d. for 4 d), or to penicillin. Necrosis of the gums may occur, so that when the acute phase has been controlled it is most important that proper dental treatment is undertaken; surgical correction of the deformities resulting from tissue necrosis may be necessary.

*Candidiasis* (*Moniliasis*). The fungus *Candida albicans* is a normal commensal in the mouth but it may proliferate to cause *thrush* in babies, the aged and particularly in debilitated patients. Thrush is also common in those receiving corticosteroids, immunosuppressive therapy or prolonged treatment with antibiotics, especially tetracycline. White patches appear on the tongue and buccal mucosa and may enlarge and coalesce to form an easily detached membrane; there is little surrounding inflammation. In severe infection, the lower pharynx and oesophagus may be affected, causing dysphagia, or the fungus may spread to the lungs. Candidiasis may be treated by gentian violet mouth wash three times a day for 4 days or a suspension or lozenges, containing 500 000 units of nystatin, should be retained in the mouth for as long as possible, and should be given four times daily for at least 4 days.

*Aphthous ulceration* is a common recurrent condition characterised by painful superficial ulceration in the mouth. The lesion begins as an indurated erythematous area followed in a day or so by ulceration. The ulcers are often multiple and may recur over several weeks. The aetiology is unknown and the patient is usually healthy otherwise. Emotional stress may precipitate an attack, and in some women ulcers tend to recur in cyclical fashion during the premenstrual phase. Severe chronic aphthous ulceration may be found in association with Crohn's disease, ulcerative colitis, coeliac or Behçet's disease.

Treatment involves the avoidance of trauma from ill-fitting dentures and overbrushing. Hydrocortisone hemisuccinate lozenges (2·5 mg t.i.d.) may be effective in the early phase of lesions. Pain can be reduced with topical anaesthetics and secondary infection controlled with tetracycline mouth washes.

*Other Forms of Stomatitis*. An allergic reaction to chemicals in toothpaste, dentures, foodstuffs and many drugs, especially antibiotics, can cause stomatitis. A characteristic blue-black punctate line may be seen where the gum margins adjoin the teeth in lead poisoning. Skin diseases such as lichen planus, pemphigus and erythema multiforme involve the mouth and sometimes before being seen on the skin.

## Disorders of the Tongue

In health the tongue is moist with only a slight white fur on the dorsum. The papillae are readily seen. Mouth breathing causes a dry tongue, but otherwise dryness of the tongue is an indication of dehydration. The tongue may be coated with a whitish-yellow fur in persons who smoke excessively but in general, the presence of fur on the tongue has little clinical significance.

*Glossitis* may be a prominent feature of stomatitis resulting from nutritional deficiency (p. 116). *Geographical tongue* is the name given to a chronic migrating superficial glossitis; it looks odd but has no clinical significance. *Carcinoma* must be considered in all cases of chronic ulceration of the tongue; if any doubt exists biopsy should be carried out. *Syphilis* may occur as a primary chancre, in the secondary stage as 'mucous patches', or in the tertiary stage as painless gummatous ulcers.

*Leukoplakia* is a chronic affection characterised by the presence of white, firm, smooth patches beginning at the side of the tongue and later spreading over the dorsum. In the early stages the tongue is not painful but later the patches are split by fissures with resultant pain and tenderness. The importance of leukoplakia is that it may precede the development of carcinoma, and a biopsy of such lesions should always be undertaken.

When the patient complains of a persistently painful tongue (*glossodynia*) which appears normal on inspection and, unlike true glossitis, is not exacerbated by hot liquids or vinegar, then the symptom is usually psychogenic. A bad taste in the mouth may be caused by local disease in the oropharynx, by some of the materials used in dental conservation and by some drugs; when these causes can be excluded the symptom is usually neurotic in origin. The complaint of an offensive breath (*halitosis*), when it cannot be confirmed by the physician, is usually due to psychoneurosis. The breath has characteristic odours in conditions such as liver failure or diabetic ketoacidosis and after the ingestion of alcohol or garlic. In these circumstances, the subject is either unaware of the smell or has become accustomed to it and does not complain.

## Disorders of the Salivary Glands

Excessive salivary secretion may be a response to irritation or inflammation in the mouth, e.g. oral sepsis. Dryness of the mouth (*xerostomia*) may be due to dehydration or may be caused by anticholinergic or antidepressant drugs; commonly it is due to anxiety. Xerostomia is one of the features of Sjögren's syndrome (p. 607).

*Parotitis* may be due to the virus of mumps or to bacterial infection of the glands. The latter tends to develop during severe febrile illnesses and after major abdominal operations if adequate attention is not given to oral hygiene and to the prevention of dehydration and toxaemia. Its treatment consists of the parenteral administration of penicillin and surgical drainage if abscess formation has occurred.

Enlargement of the parotid glands may be found in sarcoidosis.

*Salivary calculi* occur occasionally in the submandibular gland or its duct. They cause pain and swelling brought on by eating. Infection of the gland is a complication. Stones in the duct can be felt in the floor of the mouth and can be removed by incision over the duct. Stones in the gland may require excision of the gland.

*A 'mixed' salivary tumour* is essentially of epithelial origin but may contain stromal elements. It presents as a slow, painless enlargement of one parotid gland. The tumour shows a variable degree of malignancy and is treated by excision.

# DISEASES OF THE OESOPHAGUS

## Dysphagia

Since the only function of the oesophagus is the transmission of food from mouth to stomach, most diseases of the oesophagus and its adjacent structures cause difficulty in swallowing (dysphagia).

**Causes of Dysphagia.** 1. PAINFUL DISEASES of the mouth and pharynx, e.g. stomatitis, tonsillitis, tuberculous laryngitis or retropharyngeal abscess, produce dysphagia, the cause of which is usually apparent.

2. NEUROMUSCULAR DISORDERS. Pharyngeal causes of dysphagia include bulbar and pseudobulbar paralysis and myasthenia gravis. Motility disorders of the oesophagus e.g. achalasia, diffuse spasm, Chagas' disease and systemic sclerosis also cause dysphagia.

3. EXTRINSIC COMPRESSION — goitre or a mediastinal mass, e.g. malignant lymph nodes.

4. INTRINSIC DISEASE OF THE OESOPHAGUS

(a) *Congenital Abnormalities*. Atresia, the upper oesophagus ending blindly at about the level of the tracheal bifurcation, occurs occasionally requiring urgent surgery in the newborn. A short oesophagus with hernia and stricture can occur as congenital abnormalities, though most examples are probably due to acquired disease.

(b) *Ulceration and Stricture*. Oesophagitis is most commonly due to reflux of gastric contents through a sphincter made incompetent by a sliding hiatus hernia. There is acid-pepsin digestion of the oesophageal mucosa immediately above the hernia, with ulceration, spasm and eventual stricture formation.

Oesophagitis and stricture are occasionally caused by the ingestion, accidental or otherwise, of corrosives such as bleach and caustic soda.

(c) *Sideropenic Dysphagia (Plummer–Vinson Syndrome)*. This form of dysphagia is mostly seen in middle-aged or elderly women and is associated with iron deficiency anaemia, glossitis, and perhaps koilonychia and splenic enlargement. There is degeneration and atrophy of the epithelium of tongue, pharynx, oesophagus and stomach. A fold of atrophic epithelial cells — the 'postcricoid web' — may be demonstrable radiographically or endoscopically. The dysphagia is to solids rather than to liquids, is intermittent, and may therefore mistakenly be thought to be hysterical. The dilatation associated with diagnostic endoscopy is often sufficient to relieve the dysphagia. Treatment is with iron.

(d) *Carcinoma* of the oesophagus or of the cardia of the stomach is the usual cause of dysphagia in elderly patients with no preceding history of indigestion or heartburn.

**Investigation.** The exclusion of malignant disease is essential in the investigation of any patient who complains of dysphagia. Barium swallow and oesophagoscopy are required. Where the disorder appears to be one of function rather than structure, as for example in achalasia or systemic sclerosis, then manometry can give additional information.

## Oesophageal Hiatus Hernia and Reflux Oesophagitis

Several mechanisms operate to prevent reflux of food and fluid from the stomach into the lower oesophagus. The most important are the lower oesophageal sphincter situated just above the oesophago-gastric junction, the position of this sphincter below the diaphragm so that it is reinforced by intra-abdominal pressure, and the angle of entry of the oesophagus into the stomach. The latter two mechanisms are lost when the oesophagogastric junction 'slides' through the oesophageal hiatus in the diaphragm. This proximal displacement is usually sufficient to allow reflux although the lower oesophageal sphincter may remain operative. If reflux continues over a lengthy period, the exposure of the lower oesophageal mucosa to the effects of gastric juice results in oesophagitis.

Hiatus hernia and reflux oesophagitis are most frequent in middle-aged and elderly women. An increase in intra-abdominal pressure, as a result of pregnancy or obesity, promotes their development in earlier years.

**Clinical Features.** Heartburn is the characteristic symptom of reflux oesophagitis. It is a deeply placed 'burning' pain, felt retro-sternally and brought on by bending, stooping or by the exertion of lifting or straining with consequent increase in intra-abdominal pressure. It may also occur on lying down at night and keep the patient awake; relief is obtained by sitting up, or by taking food or alkali. When severe, some patients find it more comfortable to spend the night in an easy chair. No other pain produced in the alimentary tract is so closely linked to change of posture as that of reflux oesophagitis. Many patients with hiatus hernia have no symptoms as these are related to the presence of oesophagitis. Occasionally the latter is itself symptomless. Some patients with oesophagitis present with severe iron deficiency anaemia due to blood loss.

Other complications are chronic ulcer of the oesophagus, stricture of the oesophagus and gastric ulcer in the herniated gastric mucosa.

The diagnosis of oesophagitis is made on the visual and biopsy findings at endoscopy. The presence of a hiatus hernia is shown by a barium meal (Fig. 8.1) and ulcer in the hiatus hernia can be revealed by endoscopy or barium studies.

**Treatment.** There are several practical dietary and postural measures which the patient can take to minimise reflux and these should be explained. Meals should be of small volume and fatty foods should be avoided as they tend to promote reflux and delay gastric emptying. Weight reduction is essential in obese subjects and may be all that is required to relieve symptoms. Stooping from the waist should be avoided as far as possible. To reduce reflux at night, the patient should sleep with the head of the bed elevated. Smoking reduces lower oesophageal sphincter pressure and should be stopped.

Heartburn can be effectively relieved by antacids which, when symptoms are severe, should be taken one and three hours after meals, before sleep, and whenever heartburn occurs. Metoclopramide (10 mg t.i.d.) tends to increase lower oesophageal sphincter pressure and may be helpful. Cimetidine (p. 328) relieves symptoms and a prolonged course may induce healing of oesophagitis. Patients with dysphagia will require a liquid or semi-liquid diet, pending dilatation. Anaemia will usually respond to oral iron, but transfusion may be required if blood loss has been severe.

Surgery is indicated if severe symptoms persist despite adequate medical therapy. The aim of surgery is to return the lower oesophageal sphincter to the abdomen and to construct an additional valve mechanism.

### Paraoesophageal Hernia

Here a knuckle of stomach 'rolls' alongside the oesophagus through the hiatus. The lower oesophageal sphincter remains below the diaphragm and competent even in the extreme cases when most of the stomach rotates to follow the herniated knuckle into the chest. Often there are no symptoms but a big hernia in the posterior mediastinum may lead to cardiac arrhythmias and breathlessness. Occasionally symptoms become acute because of obstruction, distension and even gangrene of the herniated portion of stomach and then surgery may be required urgently. In a few patients, and as a planned procedure, surgical repair of the hernia may be required if the disability is severe.

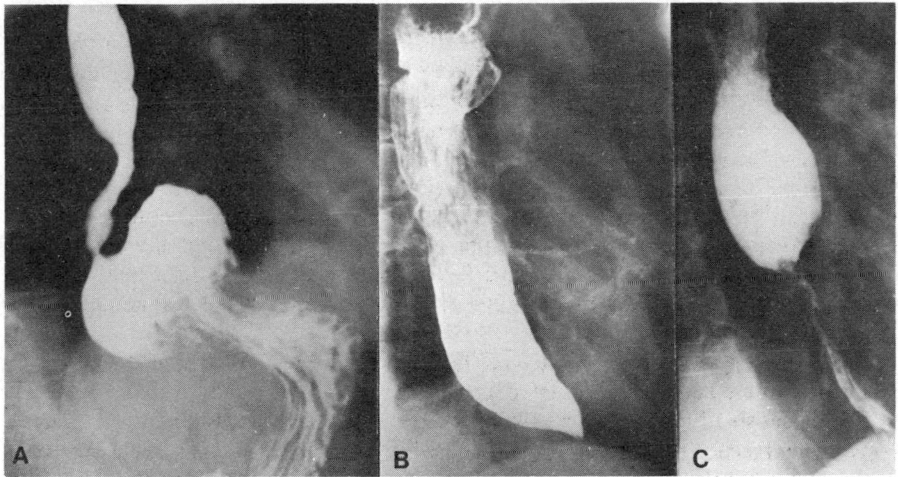


Fig. 8.1 A. Oesophageal hiatus hernia. B. Achalasia of cardia. C. Carcinoma of oesophagus.

### Diverticulum of Oesophagus

**A traction diverticulum** is most commonly situated in the anterior wall of the oesophagus just below the level of the tracheal bifurcation. It is due to chronic inflammation, usually tuberculous, in related lymph nodes. By the time the diverticulum is discovered, often accidentally during barium swallow, the disease in the lymph nodes has healed. It is seldom that the diverticulum itself causes symptoms and surgical treatment is rarely necessary.

**A pharyngeal pouch** develops at the site of the inferior constrictor of the pharynx. Its late onset and the fact that dysphagia precedes the formation of the pouch suggests that the condition is the result of muscle incoordination. It begins as a posterior bulge of mucosa which enlarges to form a sac that extends downwards and to the left between oesophagus and cervical spine. The fully-formed pouch causes dysphagia due to displacement forwards of the oesophagus. There is swelling and gurgling in the neck on swallowing. The patient may present with recurrent attacks of stridor, or inhalation of contents of the sac may lead to pneumonia.

The condition is seen almost exclusively in middle-aged subjects.

Treatment is surgical, a one-stage resection of the pouch with careful suture of its neck being carried out after preliminary cleansing and under antibiotic cover. The danger is leakage or contamination with consequent mediastinitis.

In Edinburgh, pharyngeal pouch is remembered as the affliction of Lord Jeffrey (1773–1850), a Scottish judge and wit who, in those days before surgery, emptied his pouch with a specially designed silver spoon.

## Achalasia of the Cardia

Although apparently confined to the lower end where there is failure of the sphincter to relax, this is in fact a motility disorder of the whole oesophagus which shows progressive atony and dilatation. The cause is probably a failure of nerve conduction due to diminution in the number of ganglion cells. Chagas' disease (American trypanosomiasis, p. 820) produces similar changes. Achalasia is also known, less appropriately, as *cardiospasm*.

**Clinical Features.** Dysphagia may at first be intermittent but later is always present. It is caused both by solids and liquids and can be localised behind the lower end of the sternum. In the initial stages, the patient continues to eat a normal diet but food accumulates in the capacious non-contractile oesophagus. Later the retained food cannot be expelled into the stomach and weight loss ensues. Inhalation of food and secretions may occur at night and cause recurrent pulmonary infection.

**Investigation.** A chest radiograph may be sufficient to show a dilated oesophageal outline, perhaps with a fluid level behind the heart shadow. A barium swallow shows the dilated atonic oesophagus coming to a smooth pointed termination (Fig. 8.1). There is absence of the usual gas shadow in the fundus of the stomach. While the appearances are typical, they are not diagnostic because they can be mimicked by a carcinoma at the lower end of the oesophagus or in the cardiac portion of the stomach. Treated or untreated, patients with achalasia have an increased liability to carcinoma of the oesophagus which makes initial endoscopy essential and periodic review after treatment desirable.

Oesophagoscopy should always be carried out. Usually cleansing of the oesophagus is required with mechanical removal of the larger retained food fragments, and this may involve repeated lavage, aspiration and oesophagoscopy. Once the oesophagus is clean it can be inspected and biopsies taken if necessary.

Motility studies are of value in establishing the diagnosis and in determining the extent and severity of the lesion.

**Treatment** may be by dilatation or cardiomyotomy. In the first a bag is guided through the narrow segment via an oesophagoscope and distended with water. A single dilatation may cure the patient. If not, it can be repeated.

Failure of hydrostatic dilatation or inability to introduce the dilator are indications for operation, which takes the form of cardiomyotomy (Heller's operation). Here the muscle at the lower end of the oesophagus, and for some distance above and below, is slit to expose but not to penetrate the mucosa. The operation is relatively effective and safe, even in the elderly, but either procedure may be complicated by reflux oesophagitis, or more occasionally by oesophageal perforation.

### Diffuse Spasm of the Oesophagus

Like achalasia, diffuse spasm is probably caused by a disorder of the oesophageal nerve cells. Often there is hypertrophy of the muscle wall of the oesophagus.

The main symptom is pain precipitated by eating or by emotional stress. The pain is retrosternal and there may be radiation to the back, neck or arms, thus making the differential diagnosis from coronary artery disease difficult. The pain may or may not be accompanied by dysphagia. The diagnosis is established by barium swallow which shows a hold-up of barium in the oesophagus due to multiple uncoordinated contractions. The appearance resembles a 'corkscrew'. Manometry shows strong uncoordinated contractions.

Treatment involves education in eating in a relaxed atmosphere with adequate mastication. Nitroglycerine may relieve pain. Since most patients are over the age of 60, the physician has to persist with medical management but in the occasional younger patient, an extended cardiomyotomy may be required.

## Carcinoma of the Oesophagus

There are wide geographical variations in the incidence of this tumour; it is very common around the Caspian Sea and some parts of Southern Africa. It is associated with smoking, alcohol and the consumption of spices.

In Western communities, the average age of patients with carcinoma of the oesophagus is between 60 and 70 years, and there is a slight male predominance. The most frequent site is the lower third of the oesophagus; it is less common in the middle third and least common in the upper third. The lesion is usually ulcerative and it extends circumferentially and longitudinally in the wall of the oesophagus, often producing stenosis. Direct invasion of surrounding structures and involvement of related lymph nodes is common by the time of diagnosis. Squamous carcinoma is most frequent. Of the 10–20% of adenocarcinomas, most have invaded the lower oesophagus from the stomach; the remainder arise from oesophageal glands.

**Clinical Features.** Progressive dysphagia is typical. It starts with the 'sticking' of solid food, at first intermittently and then regularly and proceeds to difficulty with semisolids and eventually with liquids. There is discomfort, not amounting to pain, at the site of the obstruction which is usually well localised by the patient. The development of symptoms occupies some months so that by the time the patient first attends, weight loss is already a feature and there may be metastases in lymph nodes, liver and related structures in the mediastinum.

**Investigation.** Obstruction and an irregular narrowing of the oesophagus, seen at barium swallow, are highly suggestive of the diagnosis (Fig. 8.1). At the lower end it may not be possible to distinguish between carcinoma of the oesophagus and achalasia of the cardia. Oesophagitis and a benign stricture may also simulate carcinoma.

Oesophagoscopy and biopsy should always be carried out. Repeated biopsy may be required to obtain positive confirmation of the diagnosis, and this is particularly so when stricture formation prevents further insertion of the oesophagoscope or the biopsy forceps. In these circumstances, the passage of a brush through the narrowed area and examination of dislodged cells is of value.

**Treatment.** The choice lies between palliation and radical treatment. The chances of cure seldom exceed 10%. In squamous carcinoma, particularly of the upper and middle thirds, high voltage radiotherapy is the treatment of choice in those centres possessing the necessary facilities. Otherwise, and with tumours of the lower third, oesophagogastrectomy offers the best hope. There is the possibility that a combined approach of surgery with preoperative radiotherapy may lead to enhanced survival.

Extensive tumours that are unsuitable for radical surgery or for intensive radiotherapy are treated palliatively, occasionally by bypass surgery, but more often by insertion of a permanent tube into the oesophagus. This allows liquids to be taken and is effective in relieving the patient of that most distressing problem — the inability to swallow saliva.

Gastrostomy as a palliative measure offers no relief to the patient, fails to prolong his survival and is therefore not advisable.

# DISEASES OF THE STOMACH AND DUODENUM

## Peptic Ulcer

The term 'peptic ulcer' refers to an ulcer in the lower oesophagus, stomach or duodenum, in the jejunum after surgical anastomosis to the stomach, or rarely in the ileum adjacent to a Meckel's diverticulum. Ulcers in the stomach or duodenum may be acute or chronic; both penetrate the muscularis mucosae but the acute ulcer shows no evidence of fibrosis. Erosions do not penetrate the muscularis mucosae.

Although the incidence of peptic ulcer is decreasing in many Western communities, it still affects, at some time, approximately 10% of all adult males. The male to female ratio for duodenal ulcer varies from 4:1 to 2:1 in different communities whilst that for gastric ulcer is 2:1 or less. Variations in the incidence of gastric and duodenal ulcer occur between different countries and between different parts of the same country; the incidence of peptic ulcer is higher in Scotland than in Southern England due to a preponderance of duodenal ulcers in Scotland. Peptic ulcer is becoming more common in many developing countries.

**Aetiology of Chronic Ulceration.** HEREDITY. Patients with peptic ulcer often have a family history of the disease; this is particularly the case with duodenal ulcers which develop below the age of 20 years. Gastric and duodenal ulcers are inherited as separate disorders; thus, the relatives of gastric ulcer patients have three times the expected number of gastric ulcers but duodenal ulcer occurs with the same frequency amongst them as in the general population.

ACID-PEPSIN VERSUS MUCOSAL RESISTANCE. The immediate cause of peptic ulceration is digestion of the mucosa by acid and pepsin of the gastric juice, but the sequence of events leading to this is unknown. Digestion by acid and pepsin cannot be the only factor involved, since the normal stomach is obviously capable of resisting digestion by its own secretions. The concept of ulcer aetiology may be written as 'acid plus pepsin vs mucosal resistance'. We will now identify some factors which affect this balance.

*Gastric Hypersecretion.* Ulcers occur only in the presence of acid and pepsin; they are never found in achlorhydric patients such as those with pernicious anaemia. On the other hand, severe intractable peptic ulceration nearly always occurs in patients with the Zollinger-Ellison syndrome which is characterised by very high acid secretion. Acid secretion is thought to be more important in the aetiology of duodenal than gastric ulcer, because patients with duodenal ulcer, as a group, secrete more acid than normal individuals and duodenal ulcer heals when gastric hypersecretion is reduced by drugs or by vagotomy.

*Mucosal Resistance.* Several mechanisms protect the gastric mucosa from hydrogen ions secreted into the lumen of the stomach. The surface epithelial cells secrete bicarbonate which creates an alkaline milieu at the surface of the mucosa; this bicarbonate secretion is under the influence of mucosal prostaglandins. The tight junction between the epithelial cells, and their surface lipoprotein layer provides a mechanical barrier. The normal turnover of epithelial cells and gastric mucus also has a protective function. Collectively, all these mechanisms can be described as the 'gastric mucosal barrier'. Its integrity is important in preventing gastric ulcer and some of the mechanisms may also operate in the duodenum.

*Factors Reducing Mucosal Resistance.* Several drugs, particularly those used in rheumatoid arthritis, will disrupt the gastric mucosal barrier. When aspirin is in solution at a pH below 3·5 it is undissociated and fat-soluble, so that it is absorbed through the lipoprotein membrane of the surface epithelial cells; during absorption it damages the membrane and the tight junctions. It also inhibits prostaglandin synthesis thus reducing bicarbonate secretion by the surface epithelial cells. Aspirin has been shown to be an important aetiological factor in gastric ulcer in Australia, and this may also be so in other countries where there is a high consumption of aspirin. There is also a relationship between aspirin ingestion and acute bleeding from the upper gastrointestinal tract.

Reflux of bile and intestinal secretions into the stomach occurs more frequently in patients with gastric ulcers than in normal individuals or patients with duodenal ulcer, due presumably to a poorly functioning pyloric sphincter. Bile damages the gastric mucosal barrier, predisposing the mucosa to ulceration. Chronic gastritis is more common in patients with gastric ulcer and it may be caused by damage from regurgitated bile and intestinal secretions.

**Aetiology of Acute and Stress Ulcers.** Many of the factors described above also contribute to the development of acute ulcers. Aspirin is particularly important. Acute peptic ulcers developing after head injury, burns, severe sepsis, surgery or trauma are termed stress ulcers. Gastric hyper-secretion is the usual cause of acute ulcer after head injury, while the reflux of duodenal contents and mucosal ischaemia may be responsible factors after burns or shock.

**Pathology.** Chronic gastric ulcer is nearly always single; 90% are situated on the lesser curve within the antrum or at the junction between body and antral mucosa. Chronic duodenal ulcer is usually situated in the first part of the duodenum just distal to the junction of pyloric and duodenal mucosa; 50% are on the anterior wall. More than one peptic ulcer is found in 10–15% of cases. Acute ulcers or erosions are frequently multiple, and are more widely distributed.

**Clinical Features.** A duodenal ulcer follows a chronic course for up to 20 years and whilst newer forms of treatment such as cimetidine may effect prompt healing, there is no evidence that the natural history of the ulcer is affected. The course of gastric ulcer is probably less chronic. While there are good grounds for believing that gastric and duodenal ulcers are different diseases it is convenient to describe the general features of 'peptic ulcer' as inclusive of both, noting differences where they occur.

Peptic ulcer may present in different ways. The commonest is chronic, episodic pain extending over months or years. However, the ulcer may come to attention as an acute episode with bleeding or perforation, with little or no previous history. Occasionally the patient presents with the symptoms of gastric outlet obstruction, having had negligible trouble previously.

Pain is the characteristic symptom of peptic ulcer, and it has three notable features — localisation to the epigastrium, relationship to food, and periodicity. Ulcer pain is typically referred to the epigastrium, in the midline or to the right; it is usually localised so that the patient can indicate the site with one finger, 'the pointing sign'. Occasionally ulcer pain is not clearly localised; it may be referred diffusely in the epigastrium, the lower chest or to the back in the interscapular region in the fifth to eighth thoracic segments. Pain referred to the interscapular area, especially if it is a new feature, suggests the possibility that the ulcer has penetrated posteriorly, involving structures such as the pancreas. The description of the pain is not especially helpful, although patients commonly describe it as gnawing or burning. Pain varies considerably in severity, and it is sometimes helpful to ask the patient to qualify the symptom as 'pain' or as 'discomfort' as a measure of its intensity.

Most patients recognise a relationship of the pain to food, although the relationship varies between patients, and in the same patient from time to time. Duodenal ulcer pain tends to occur between meal times, so that the patient may describe it as 'hunger' pain, which is characteristically relieved by food. A notable feature of duodenal ulcer is pain awakening the patient from sleep 2 to 3 hours after retiring. The pain of gastric ulcer occurs less regularly; it frequently occurs within an hour of eating, is less often relieved by food and it rarely occurs at night. Besides the characteristic relief obtained after eating, ulcer pain is almost invariably relieved by antacids or vomiting.

Ulcer pain is characteristically episodic occurring regularly each day for days or weeks at a time, then disappearing, to recur weeks or months later. Between attacks, the patient feels perfectly well, and may eat and drink with impunity. Bouts of pain may at first last only a day or so at a time, and occur only once or twice a year. As the natural history evolves, however, episodes begin to last longer and occur more frequently, so that in severe cases remissions of pain may be short lived and pain or discomfort becomes more or less persistent. The cause for these relapses is difficult to establish. Seasonal factors may be operative, sometimes psychological stress may be blamed, sometimes dietary indiscretion, and sometimes alcoholic excess. Most commonly, no reason can be found for the relapse.

Pain is sometimes absent or so slight as to be dismissed by the patient. Such individuals may complain of other symptoms such as a feeling of 'distension' in the epigastrium or a poorly defined sense of unease after eating. Other complaints include episodic nausea and sometimes anorexia, as well as heartburn or waterbrash. Vomiting in ulcer patients almost always relieves pain and when it is persistent may result in weight loss. This helps to distinguish it from vomiting of psychological origin, in which weight is usually maintained. Persistent vomiting in an ulcer subject usually indicates some degree of gastric outflow obstruction, whether due to spasm or organic narrowing. In such patients, vomiting is usually copious, so that the patient is 'surprised' at the volume; the patient often recognises food eaten twelve or more hours previously. Although there is no constant change in bowel rhythm during an ulcer relapse, some patients are aware of constipation or diarrhoea when dyspepsia reappears.

*Physical Signs.* The only physical sign that may be present is 'the pointing sign' which, when accompanied by localised tenderness, is practically diagnostic of an ulcer. However, tenderness may be completely absent. In patients with gastric outlet obstruction, the stomach may be visibly distended, a succussion splash may be present, and gastric peristalsis may be seen.

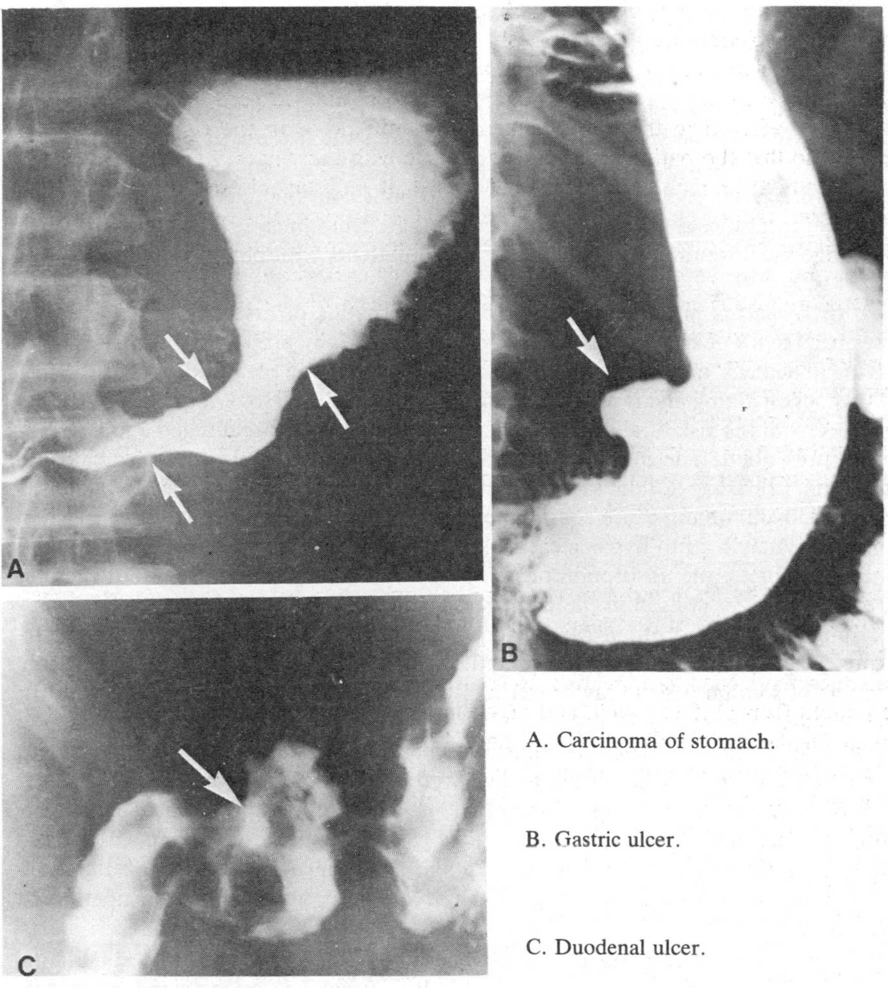


A. Carcinoma of stomach.

B. Gastric ulcer.

C. Duodenal ulcer.

Fig. 8.2

**Investigation.** A double contrast barium meal examination and endoscopy are equally effective in diagnosing peptic ulcers. The ulcer is seen as a niche or a collection of barium face-on (Fig. 8.2). Sometimes the crater is not detected but an ulcer is suspected because of a secondary sign such as deformity of the first part of the duodenum. Endoscopy is preferred by most physicians particularly when the ulcer is gastric, because a biopsy can be carried out to exclude carcinoma. Endoscopy will also locate some duodenal ulcers which are difficult to detect radiologically. In addition it will diagnose *duodenitis*, a generalised inflammation of the first part of the duodenum. This may be regarded as a variant of duodenal ulcer disease in which no ulcer crater is present.

**Treatment.** While various measures are available to alleviate symptoms and heal the ulcer, there is no evidence that the long term course of the disease is affected.

DIET, INJURIOUS DRUGS, TOBACCO AND ALCOHOL. There is no evidence that dietary manipulation affects symptoms or ulcer healing, and strict diets should be avoided. It is particularly important that aspirin and other anti-inflammatory drugs are not used in peptic ulceration. Their injurious action should be explained to the patient. There is evidence that stopping smoking accelerates the healing of gastric ulcers and it is likely that this also applies to duodenal ulcers. Patients should therefore be advised to give up cigarettes. Most patients cannot consume alcohol during exacerbations of ulcer disease because it aggravates their symptoms. It seems reasonable to encourage moderation in drinking habits in all patients with peptic ulceration.

DRUGS. *Antacids* provide symptomatic relief in peptic ulcers; if given in sufficient doses for 4 to 6 weeks they may also induce healing. Many preparations are available, varying in neutralising capacity, side effects, palatability and cost. Sodium bicarbonate is the quickest acting and is widely used for self-medication. However it is very readily absorbed with the risk of alkalosis, so that its use should be discouraged and it should not be prescribed. The majority of antacids are based on combinations of calcium, aluminium and magnesium salts, all of which may cause side-effects. Frequently calcium and aluminium cause constipation and magnesium causes diarrhoea. Calcium compounds may lead to hypercalcaemia if dosage is high and prolonged. Aluminium compounds block the absorption of phosphate and may cause phosphate depletion, an effect which is utilised in the management of renal failure; aluminium salts may also impair drug absorption. Magnesium compounds may cause toxic hypermagnesaemia when renal function is impaired. Almost all antacids contain appreciable amounts of sodium which may exacerbate fluid retention in patients with cardiac or liver disease.

For relief of minor discomfort, antacid preparations in tablet form are convenient; they may be carried in the pocket and chewed or sucked whenever pain occurs. For relief of more severe pain during exacerbations, 15–30 ml of liquid antacid are usually required. For duodenal ulcer, it is necessary to give 30 ml of liquid antacid one and three hours after food and at bedtime. Patient acceptance of this form of therapy is low because of poor palatability and the frequent occurrence of constipation or diarrhoea.

*Histamine $H_2$-receptor Antagonists*. It has long been known that the stimulating effect of histamine on gastric secretion could not be blocked by the standard antihistamines. This led to the idea that there might be a second type of histamine receptor situated on, or near, the parietal cells. The possibility of blocking this second type of receptor and so reducing gastric secretion led to the development of the group of drugs known as the histamine $H_2$-receptor antagonists. One of these drugs, cimetidine, is a powerful inhibitor of gastric secretion and is the treatment of choice for all forms of peptic ulcer. The drug is given in a dose of 200 mg three times a day with meals and 400 mg at bedtime for six weeks. The bedtime dose should be unaccompanied by food. It has been found that cimetidine, used in this way, will heal over 80% of duodenal ulcers and 70% of gastric ulcers. Furthermore, it has the advantage over other drugs of rendering nearly all patients asymptomatic within 48 hours of the commencement of therapy. For most patients it is sufficient to treat each exacerbation of the ulcer by means of a 6 week course of cimetidine. However, for those patients with frequent relapses and who have contraindications to elective surgery, such as age, respiratory or cardiac disease, further relapses can be prevented by giving cimetidine 400 mg nocte for 6 to 12 months at a time and occasionally on a permanent basis. Cimetidine appears to be a very safe drug; gynaccomastia or myopathy occur in a very small number of patients.

*Other Drugs used for Healing Ulcers.* It has been shown that carbenoxolone sodium accelerates the healing of both gastric and duodenal ulcers. However, because of its aldosterone-like effects, it may cause sodium retention with oedema, hypokalaemia and hypertension, so that it should not be prescribed in elderly patients or when there is a history of cardiac failure. The usual dose is 50 mg four times daily for six to eight weeks.

With the advent of cimetidine, there is little indication for the use of anticholinergic drugs.

SURGICAL TREATMENT. This has much to offer the patient with intractable peptic ulceration. It can relieve severe or persistent symptoms and prevent complications. While in many cases the assessment of the patient's disability is straightforward, in patients in whom anxiety or depression is present, the decision becomes difficult. Elective surgery should be considered in the following circumstances: 1. When an ulcer has failed to heal, and symptoms persist or recur so as to interfere with the enjoyment of life, or reduce the capacity to work. The indications for surgery are strengthened if the ulcer has developed in adolescence or young adult life, if there is a strong family history, or if there has been a previous complication such as haemorrhage or perforation.

2. When there is an ulcer which has produced gastric outlet obstruction, or an hour-glass stomach because of fibrosis.

3. When there is a gastric ulcer the nature of which is uncertain or which has failed to heal in three months.

4. In a recurrent ulcer following previous gastric surgery.

There is no single, ideal operation suitable for all ulcers and all patients. For a gastric ulcer, the operation of choice is partial gastrectomy preferably with a Billroth I anastomosis, in which the ulcer itself and the ulcer-bearing area of the stomach is resected (Fig. 8.3). For duodenal ulcer the acid secretory capacity of the stomach may be reduced by vagotomy which eliminates nervous stimulation (Fig. 8.3). At truncal vagotomy the main nerves are divided and thereafter gastric emptying may be retarded so that a drainage operation such as pyloroplasty or gastroenterostomy has to be added. One of these procedures is also required in selective vagotomy in which vagal innervation to the small intestine, pancreas and biliary tree is preserved. The aim of proximal (highly selective) vagotomy is to denervate only the acid-producing area of the stomach while leaving intact the vagal supply of the antrum and pylorus. Gastric emptying is thus not impaired and a drainage procedure is not required unless there is stenosis from ulcer scarring. The avoidance of a drainage procedure markedly reduces the incidence of post cibal syndromes and in particular dumping (p. 335). Vagotomy is preferred to partial gastrectomy because of the lesser mortality and lower incidence of long-term complications.

**Complications** of peptic ulcer are haemorrhage, perforation and gastric outlet obstruction. Ulcer-cancer is discussed on page 337.

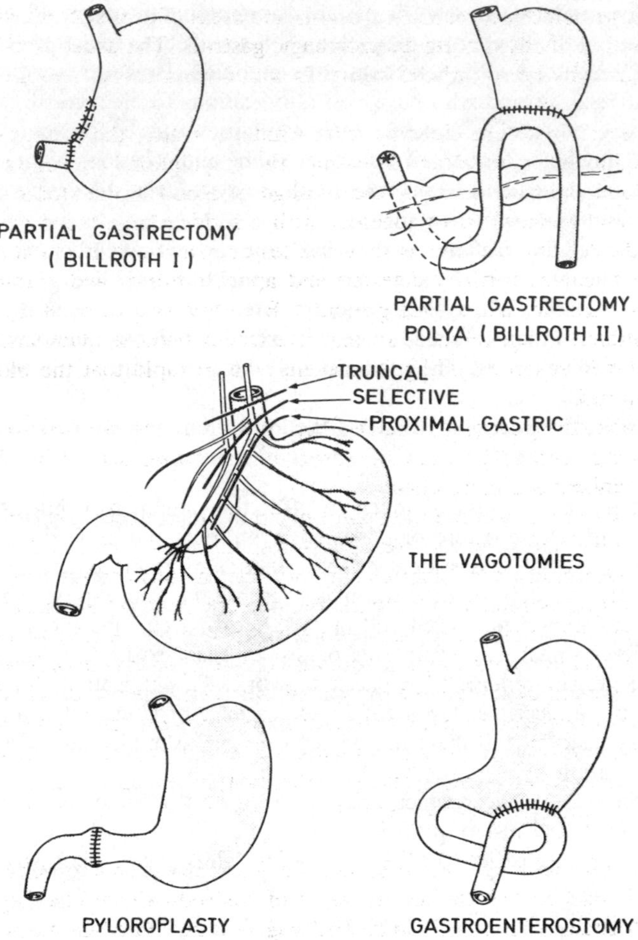


**Fig. 8.3 Operations for peptic ulceration**

## Gastroduodenal Haemorrhage

Bleeding as judged by a positive test for occult blood in the stools can often be detected in peptic ulcer. As a complication, gastro-duodenal haemorrhage is taken to mean bleeding sufficiently severe to cause symptoms. It carries a mortality that may reach 30% in elderly and shocked patients. A history of significant blood loss within the previous 48 hours should lead to immediate admission to hospital.

**Aetiology.** The common causes of bleeding are chronic gastric and duodenal ulcers (50%), erosions (15–30%), oesophageal varices (10%) and mucosal lacerations at the cardia due to vomiting (Mallory-Weiss syndrome — 7%). Less frequent causes are cancer of the stomach and other tumours such as leiomyoma, oesophagitis, stress ulcers and bleeding disorders.

Erosions are usually caused by the ingestion of aspirin either alone or in combination with alcohol or by drugs used to treat rheumatic disorders. In some patients the stomach shows petechiae, multiple erosions and areas of confluent mucosal bleeding; this appearance is called acute haemorrhagic gastritis. The usual presentation of stress ulcer, caused by burns or head injury, is with haematemesis and melaena.

**Clinical Features.** In severe bleeding from whatever cause, the patient complains of weakness, faintness, nausea, and sweating: these symptoms are followed by the vomiting of blood (*haematemesis*) or the passage of blood in the stools (*melaena*). Haematemesis and melaena occur together with a sudden large bleed whereas melaena alone indicates that bleeding is slow and lesser in amount. If blood remains in the stomach it becomes partially digested and appears brown and granular in the vomit or gastric aspirate, like 'coffee grounds'. Blood passing through the intestinal canal is also altered in appearance, so that the faeces become black and sticky, a 'tarry' stool. But in severe bleeding, transit may be so rapid that the blood in the rectum is bright red.

On examination, the patient may be shocked or restless and disorientated because of cerebral anoxia. These signs may be absent in the young patient in whom compensatory mechanisms are more effective.

The haemoglobin level will not alter until haemodilution occurs and this may not take place for some hours, nor be complete for some days. A reduced haematocrit on admission to hospital often indicates chronic bleeding prior to the acute episode. A raised urea with a normal serum creatinine indicates a blood loss of at least one litre. There is no simple laboratory procedure which will give a reliable estimate of the amount of blood loss until haemodilution is complete, so that in ordinary circumstances the assessment of the degree or rate of bleeding depends on clinical judgement. Serial recordings of the pulse rate and blood pressure give some indication, but for a more accurate assessment in patients who continue to bleed, measurement of central venous pressure is necessary. In patients with severe bleeding a record of urinary output by catheterisation is helpful.

**Investigation.** On admission there should be joint assessment by physician and surgeon and in large centres the management of gastroduodenal bleeding can with advantage be centralised in a single unit. The diagnosis and bleeding status should be established at the outset. Emergency endoscopy will show the source of the bleeding, whether it is continuing or whether it is likely to recur. Endoscopy is preferable to emergency barium studies in that it can demonstrate erosions and in the event of more than one lesion being present it can confirm which is bleeding.

The bleeding status is ascertained by passage of a nasogastric tube which should be aspirated at half hourly intervals and the quantity and type of aspirate recorded.

**Treatment.** Urgent treatment of shock requires rapid and adequate blood replacement. Whole blood should be given as soon as it is available; until then, a colloidal solution such as dextran can be used. A blood transfusion is also indicated if the pulse rate is faster than 100 per minute or the systolic pressure lower than 100 mmHg. Transfusion must keep pace with the estimated loss. This may be difficult in the elderly patient who is liable to develop cardiac or renal failure or cerebral anoxia and in whom coronary blood supply may also be impaired leading to angina or even myocardial infarction.

To control restlessness and anxiety, the injection of drugs such as diazepam is to be preferred to morphine which may itself cause vomiting.

Subsequent management depends on the initial response and on the site and cause of bleeding. In general, emergency surgery should be advised in patients over the age of 50 in whom there is continued or recurrent bleeding from a gastric or duodenal ulcer. Conversely operation is unlikely to be necessary in such patients under the age of 30 or in patients with erosions in whom conservative management, including cimetidine, will usually suffice. The greatest risks are in the shocked and elderly with continued severe bleeding and when operation is delayed too long.

The need for surgery does not disappear once the crisis is over. Early elective operation may still be indicated in patients with chronic ulcers which have bled, in those requiring continued treatment with salicylates or steroids, and in patients whose occupation or residence makes supervision difficult. In general, excision of the bleeding gastric ulcer, or exposure and suture of the duodenal ulcer coupled in either case with vagotomy is safer than partial gastrectomy which should be reserved for the complicated case in expert hands.

Bleeding from oesophageal varices secondary to portal hypertension can be extremely severe and demands special measures for its management (p. 409).

### Acute Perforation of a Peptic Ulcer

When free perforation occurs, the contents of the stomach escape into the peritoneal cavity. If perforation occurs without loss of contents, as in the accidental perforation of the empty stomach at gastroscopy, few symptoms are produced and the accident may even pass unnoticed. It follows that the symptoms of perforation are those of peritonitis, and they are in proportion to the extent of peritoneal soiling. Occasionally the symptoms of perforation appear and rapidly subside; presumably the perforation has then closed spontaneously, or more commonly the ulcer has perforated locally into an area confined by adhesions to adjacent structures. Perforation occurs more commonly in duodenal than in gastric ulcers, and usually in ulcers on the anterior wall. About one-quarter of all perforations occur in acute ulcers.

**Clinical Features.** Although perforation may be the first sign of ulcer, usually there is a history of recurrent epigastric pain. The most striking symptom is sudden, severe pain, the onset of which may be so incisive that the patient can time it to a minute. The pain is usually intense, and its distribution follows the spread of the gastric contents over the peritoneum. Thus, initially the pain may be referred to the upper abdomen, but very quickly it becomes generalised; shoulder tip pain may occur as a result of irritation of the diaphragm. The pain is accompanied by shallow respiration due to limitation of diaphragmatic movements and by shock. The abdomen is held immobile, and there is generalised board-like rigidity; intestinal sounds are absent, and liver dullness to percussion may decrease due to the presence of gas under the diaphragm. Vomiting is common. After some hours, the symptoms improve, though the abdominal rigidity remains. This period of improvement may deceive the clinician examining the patient for the first time; after this temporary improvement, manifestations of general peritonitis follow the initial peritoneal irritation and the patient's condition deteriorates.

A radiograph of the abdomen in the erect position may help to establish the diagnosis since free gas within the peritoneal cavity, if in sufficient amount, will show as a translucent crescent between the liver and diaphragm. Where doubt remains, an emergency Gastrografin meal may confirm that perforation has occurred.

**Treatment and Prognosis.** After initial treatment of the patient for shock, the acute perforation should be treated surgically either by simple closure, or occasionally in the case of perforation of a chronic ulcer by closure combined with vagotomy and drainage. More than half the patients who have a simple closure will eventually require a further elective operation for recurrence of ulcer symptoms, and for this reason some surgeons recommend a definitive procedure for the ulcer at the time of operation.

Acute perforation carries a mortality of about 5%, but the outlook depends on the degree of peritoneal soiling, and therefore on the size of the perforation and the amount of stomach contents released into the peritoneum. The time interval elapsing between the onset of perforation and the time of operation also determines the outcome — the longer the delay, the greater the risk of death from peritonitis.

## Gastric Outlet Obstruction

An ulcer in the region of the pylorus may result in gastric outlet obstruction. This may be due to fibrous stricture or to oedema or spasm produced by the ulcer; frequently it is a combination of all three. Long-standing obstruction may lead to severe 'retention' gastritis, or even to secondary gastric ulcer.

In addition to chronic duodenal ulcer, or benign gastric ulcer at or near the pylorus, gastric outlet obstruction may be caused by carcinoma of the antrum and by a rare condition known as *adult hypertrophic pyloric stenosis*. The syndrome of gastric outlet obstruction is loosely described as '*pyloric stenosis*', even when the cause is chronic duodenal ulcer, and the stenosis is distal to the pylorus; thus in 'pyloric' obstruction due to duodenal stenosis, the pylorus itself may be seen radiologically to be greatly dilated.

**Clinical Features.** Symptoms of obstruction are usually preceded by a long history of duodenal ulceration. Without such symptoms, a patient with gastric outlet obstruction is likely to have a pyloric carcinoma. When there has been an ulcer, the symptoms change, so that vomiting becomes a prominent feature, and nausea replaces normal appetite. Vomiting produces such striking relief that a patient may start to eat immediately after the stomach has been emptied. If the obstruction progresses, the stomach dilates so that, eventually, surprisingly large amounts of gastric content may be vomited. Articles of food which have been eaten 24 hours or more previously may be recognised in the vomit. An earlier symptom is a sense of repletion soon after eating a relatively small amount of food. The loss of gastric contents results in water and electrolyte depletion. The blood urea may be raised because of dehydration. Alkalosis develops if large amounts of hydrochloric acid are lost, as occurs particularly in obstruction due to duodenal ulcer.

Physical examination shows evidence of wasting and dehydration, and there may be signs of tetany (p. 482). A succussion splash may be elicited four hours or more after the last meal or drink. In normal persons splashing occurs for less than an hour after meals because gastric emptying is rapid. Visible gastric peristalsis is diagnostic of gastric outlet obstruction and the abdomen should be inspected for its presence. If the patient takes a fluid diet with large amounts of milk, the signs of obstruction may be masked and nutrition may be well maintained.

**Investigation.** *Aspiration of the stomach contents* will confirm the diagnosis if the volume is in excess of 100 ml after fasting overnight or if the aspirate contains food residue, or is foul. However, a fine bore nasogastric tube may become blocked by debris; if in doubt a wide bore stomach tube should be used. If obstruction is suspected the stomach should be emptied prior to radiological examination.

*The radiological signs* are (1) an increase in the fasting residue of the stomach, (2) dilatation of the stomach with or without excessive peristalsis, (3) a lesion at or near the pylorus, and (4) delayed gastric emptying.

*Endoscopy* may demonstrate the cause of the obstruction and its degree.

**Treatment.** The stomach is washed out to remove all food debris and then aspirated 2 to 4 hourly for 3 to 4 days at which point, if the volume of aspirate has decreased, it may be possible to allow fluids by mouth. Dehydration and electrolyte disturbance must be corrected by intravenous fluids. In the first 24 hours 4 litres of isotonic saline are given and thereafter the daily requirement is based on the volume of aspirate together with other body losses. Potassium, 80 mmol/day, is given in the infusion. When obstruction is not severe a homogenised diet may be prescribed. A multivitamin preparation should be given by injection to all but the mildest cases.

The majority of patients will be greatly improved by these methods; the volume of the gastric aspirate steadily declines, and the size of the stomach returns to near normal. It is then necessary to consider the timing of an operation; this should not be too long deferred. If obstruction persists, with no improvement after 5 to 7 days, nothing is gained by procrastination, and indeed the patient may deteriorate because of electrolyte imbalance. Relief of obstruction by conservative measures provides an opportunity to complete investigation and to render the patient as fit as possible for subsequent elective surgery.

## Zollinger-Ellison Syndrome

This is a rare disorder in which severe peptic ulceration occurs due usually to an adenoma or hyperplasia of the islets of the pancreas secreting large amounts of gastrin which stimulates the parietal cells of the stomach excessively. The acid output may be so great that the 'acid tide' may reach the upper small intestine, reducing the luminal pH to 2 or less; at this pH, pancreatic lipase is inactivated and bile acids may be precipitated, resulting in diarrhoea and steatorrhoea. Excessive gastric secretion results in large volumes on aspiration under 'basal' conditions. Pentagastrin does not increase the secretory rate much above 'basal' values, since the stomach is already continuously secreting at or near maximal rates.

The ulcers are often multiple and severe and may occur in unusual sites such as the jejunum or the oesophagus. The history is usually short and bleeding and perforation are common. The syndrome may present in the form of severe recurrent ulceration following a standard operation for peptic ulcer, the underlying cause not having been recognised.

The diagnosis should be suspected in all patients with unusual or severe peptic ulceration, especially if the barium meal examination shows abnormally coarse gastric mucosal folds. It may be confirmed by finding very high levels of gastrin in the circulation. Theoretically the condition should be cured by removing the pancreatic tumour, but this is not usually possible because of its diffuse nature. In these circumstances the only option is to eliminate, or very greatly reduce, acid secretion so that the ulcers may heal. In some patients, large doses of cimetidine may be effective. The alternative is total gastrectomy.

## Late Complications following Gastric Surgery

Although most operations carried out for the relief of peptic ulcer are successful, 10% of patients will develop complications months or years afterwards. Some of these, such as anaemia and nutritional impairment, develop insidiously, so that patients who have had an operation on the stomach should be reviewed at least once a year.

**Recurrent ulcer**, after surgery for duodenal ulcer, is usually due to insufficient reduction of the secretory capacity of the stomach because of incomplete vagotomy or inadequate gastrectomy. A jejunal ulcer develops just distal to the jejuno-gastric anastomosis, because the jejunal mucosa is more susceptible to acid-pepsin digestion than gastric or duodenal mucosa.

After months or years of freedom following the operation, ulcer pain recurs or the patient may present with melaena or severe anaemia without any dyspeptic symptoms. Occasionally perforation occurs. Rarely a jejunal ulcer penetrates the colon causing a gastro-jejunal-colic fistula; then there is bacterial contamination of the small bowel causing diarrhoea, malabsorption and wasting. The fistula can be demonstrated by barium enema.

Recurrent ulcer uncomplicated by perforation or fistula is best diagnosed by endoscopy which will also reveal the occasional ulcer due to an unabsorbed suture. This may be removed endoscopically. Cimetidine will heal some recurrent ulcers, but in those where secretion tests show the vagotomy or gastric resection to be grossly inadequate, further operative reduction of acid output is usually required.

**Biliary gastritis** is the result of reflux of bile into the stomach through a drainage stoma. It may be symptomless and observed only on routine postoperative endoscopy. There may be epigastric discomfort, nausea, heartburn or vomiting of bile. Reduction in fluid intake, the eating of meals dry, avoidance of alcohol and stopping smoking may bring relief. Drugs are of little value. Revisional surgery may be required if dietetic measures fail and especially when there is a mechanical cause for the reflux.

**Post-cibal syndromes** are mainly associated with gastrectomy and have become less frequent with the more general adoption of vagotomy.

1. *The small stomach syndrome.* Discomfort and distension with meals leads to diminished intake and weight loss or failure to regain weight. High calorie small meals, with food supplements and, in some cases, revisional surgery are indicated.

2. *Dumping syndrome.* After a meal and particularly after hot sweet foods, there is a feeling of intense drowsiness with weakness and nausea; there may also be flushing and palpitations. The syndrome usually disappears as the patient adapts and recognises the foods responsible. Occasionally further surgery may be necessary

3. *Hypoglycaemia.* Rarely, one to two hours after a meal, the patient experiences attacks of weakness, tremor and faintness. The hypoglycaemia responsible for these symptoms can be relieved by glucose or barley sugar.

**Diarrhoea** may occur after any operation on the stomach, but especially after vagotomy when most patients report some looseness of the stools. Moderate or severe diarrhoea occurs in about 10% and is characteristically episodic, several watery stools being passed daily for several days. A striking feature is the sense of urgency associated with the diarrhoea; defaecation may be precipitate, and the patient becomes worried because of the fear of soiling. Loperamide or codeine should be tried when diarrhoea occurs. If diarrhoea is severe and protracted it may be due to bacterial colonisation of the small intestine (p. 351) and respond to treatment with tetracycline. Mild steatorrhoea is common after all ulcer operations and does not require treatment, but if severe steatorrhoea occurs the cause (p. 347) should be identified so that appropriate treatment may be undertaken.

**Anaemia** is a common sequel to operations on the stomach, particularly partial gastrectomy, due to inadequate absorption of iron, or to recurrent minor blood loss from gastritis or oesophagitis. Its incidence increases in the first 10 years as the stores of iron are exhausted. The occurrence of anaemia is a measure of the adequacy of postoperative supervision, because it is preventable by and responds to the administration of iron. Megaloblastic anaemia may also occur (p. 551).

**Nutritional Impairment and Osteomalacia.** In a small proportion of patients there is some nutritional impairment following gastric surgery, and this increases with the extent of any resection. Severe weight loss is its most common manifestation. There may also be malabsorption with steatorrhoea and osteomalacia which may develop for the first time 15 to 20 years after partial gastrectomy, and may present as bone pain or as a pathological fracture. Treatment is described on page 105.

## Gastritis

Gastritis signifies an acute or chronic inflammation of the stomach. Knowledge of the changes that occur in the gastric mucosa has been obtained by direct studies of the gastric mucosa in patients with gastrostomies, by gastroscopic observation; and by histological examination of specimens removed at operation, biopsy or autopsy. There is poor agreement between these three approaches, so that the classification of gastritis is difficult. If histological specimens are examined, it is very rare to find a normal stomach completely free from any signs of inflammation. In this sense 'gastritis' is almost an invariable finding in adults. However, there are gross departures from this 'normal' state of affairs, even if they do not give rise to symptoms. For these reasons the condition is best defined in histological terms as acute or chronic gastritis.

### Acute Gastritis

This is most commonly caused by the ingestion of aspirin, anti-rheumatic drugs and probably alcohol. It is also caused by the regurgitation of bile into the stomach, especially after gastric surgery (p. 335). Macroscopically, there is engorgement of the mucosa with oedema and erosions or an acute haemorrhagic gastritis (p. 331). Microscopically there is loss of the surface epithelium, hyperaemia and some infiltration with inflammatory cells.

Acute gastritis may be asymptomatic. In some patients, there is anorexia, nausea, epigastric pain and heartburn. If gastritis persists, a slow loss of blood may lead to anaemia. The condition is diagnosed by the appearance of the mucosa at gastroscopy.

Drug consumption should be reviewed with a view to omitting or reducing drugs which are known to cause gastric mucosal damage. Alcohol should be avoided. The treatment of biliary gastritis is discussed on page 335.

### Chronic Gastritis

The classification is histological; there are three stages which are progressive over many years. In *chronic superficial gastritis*, the mucosa is normal in thickness and there is patchy infiltration of lymphocytes and plasma cells. In *atrophic gastritis* there is a reduction of the specialised cells in the glands of the body and of mucous cells in the pyloric glands. There is epithelial metaplasia and an infiltrate of lymphocytes and plasma cells. In *gastric atrophy* the thickness of the mucosa is reduced, metaplasia is common but round cell infiltration is slight.

In pernicious anaemia and other autoimmune disorders, the chronic gastritis is due to an immunological process, and circulating antibodies to parietal cells and intrinsic factor are frequently found. Chronic gastritis is common in gastric ulcer, gastric cancer and after gastric surgery. In these instances, the gastritis is thought not to be immunological and circulating antibodies are absent.

The condition is asymptomatic; its importance lies in its association with the disorders noted above. The diagnosis may be suspected from the absence of mucosal folds at barium meal examination or from the gastroscopic appearances. However, the diagnosis is confirmed only by gastric biopsy. No treatment is known for stimulating the mucosa to regenerate.

## Carcinoma of the Stomach

Carcinoma of the stomach is one of the commonest malignant tumours of the gastrointestinal tract, although its incidence varies considerably in different parts of the world — for example, the tumour is frequent in Japan and relatively uncommon in the USA. These variations have been attributed to environmental factors, such as trace elements in water, or differences in methods of food preparation: the incidence of gastric cancer in Japanese immigrants to America is much less than it is in Japan. Patients with pernicious anaemia have an increased risk of developing gastric cancer and this may extend to gastric atrophy from other causes.

**Pathology.** Almost 70% of all gastric cancers occur at the pylorus or in the antrum; the lesion does not spread to the duodenum. Such growths may produce symptoms of obstruction to the gastric outlet. Lesions of the body of the stomach often involve the greater curvature and produce a fungating ulcerating mass. Least common is a diffuse infiltrating lesion spreading throughout the body of the stomach and producing the so-called leather-bottle stomach. These are the descriptions of advanced cancer.

In the early stages, when the carcinoma is confined to the mucosa, the lesion may be represented only by a depressed area with obliteration or distortion of the mucosal folds, by irregular ulceration on an elevated base, or by a small polypoid lesion. Such changes can be seen and a biopsy taken during gastroscopy at a stage when the cancer is potentially curable by resection. The tumour is generally an adenocarcinoma and spreads by extension through the stomach wall, by lymphatic permeation and by embolism via the portal vein to the liver and thence to the systemic bloodstream.

Gastric carcinoma may present as a malignant ulcer, and whether it is then the result of malignant transformation of a benign ulcer is debatable. Most authorities believe that chronic peptic ulcer rarely becomes malignant, and that malignant ulcers, however long they have been present, have always been malignant. Whatever the truth of the matter the problem in the individual case is to decide whether a chronic gastric ulcer is benign or malignant.

**Clinical Features.** Loss of appetite, slight nausea and discomfort after meals occurring for the first time in middle age should always arouse suspicion. If the diagnosis is to be made early, then such patients require careful investigation. Unfortunately, the majority of patients have advanced gastric carcinoma before they seek advice. In some there have been no symptoms; in others symptoms have been present for 6 months or even a year. Dyspepsia, which is at first vague, becomes troublesome with increasing anorexia and nausea, discomfort or pain, vomiting and weight loss. There may be cachexia and pallor, a mass may be palpable or peristalsis visible. The abdomen may be distended by ascites from peritoneal metastases. Sometimes it is the presence of metastases in the liver, pelvis or scalene lymph nodes which first brings the patient to the physician.

Carcinoma of the stomach should always be considered as a cause of unexplained iron deficiency anaemia in the middle-aged person or as an uncommon cause of haematemesis or melaena. Tumours at the cardia may cause dysphagia, and tumours at the gastric outlet may cause vomiting. In the infiltrating type of tumour, diarrhoea may occur because of rapid emptying from the stomach.

**Investigation.** Early curable cancer is usually missed by a barium meal examination unless a double contrast study is carried out to show distortion of the mucosal pattern. The only method of establishing a positive diagnosis is by gastroscopy and biopsy of suspicious areas. These procedures are also necessary to distinguish malignant from benign gastric ulceration. The commonest appearance at barium meal is a filling defect in the antrum or body of the stomach (Fig. 8.2). In the rare diffuse infiltrating scirrhous carcinoma, the radiograph is that of a rigid tube through which the barium pours rapidly into the intestine. If dysphagia is the presenting symptom, a lesion in the cardia will probably be found, but symptomless lesions in this area can be very easily missed.

Exfoliative cytology can confirm the diagnosis of cancer of the stomach if the stomach washings contain obviously malignant cells.

**Treatment and Prognosis.** The only curative treatment is gastrectomy, but it is usually only at laparotomy that the possibility of resection can be decided. Only about one-third of patients coming to operation are found to have tumours capable of removal; in the remainder it is possible to perform only a palliative procedure. This is worthwhile if pyloric obstruction is present, even if there are secondary deposits; such an operation relieves the distressing vomiting and gives the patient some comfort. A total gastrectomy may be required for tumours involving the upper part of the stomach. Careful preoperative treatment is essential; this may require the restoration of fluid and electrolyte balance and the correction of anaemia. Every effort should be made to improve nutrition, if necessary by parenteral or enteral feeding (p. 316).

The prognosis in carcinoma of the stomach is very poor and has shown little improvement in the last 40 years. Among those who survive an apparently successful resection, the 5 year survival rate is in the region of 20%. Pending an entirely new approach to the problem, the only means currently available by which the prognosis can be improved is the detection of gastric cancer when it is at a curable stage; this requires a vigorous approach to the problem of dyspepsia in the middle-aged, including careful radiological and endoscopic examination and the critical follow-up of doubtful abnormalities.

### Malignant Ascites

Carcinoma of the stomach and other intra-abdominal tumours, including carcinoma of the colon and ovary, may be associated with the exudation of fluid into the peritoneal cavity. This follows the deposition of malignant cells on the peritoneal surface and is a sign of gross spread of the disease. The fluid is rich in protein and its sediment contains malignant cells which may be identifiable on microscopy.

Treatment is palliative. Relief of abdominal distension can be obtained by paracentesis, whilst instillation of an antimitotic agent such as methotrexate may slow the rate of reaccumulation.

## DISEASES OF THE PANCREAS

The pancreas is a gland producing exocrine secretions which play important roles in digestion and also endocrine secretions concerned with the regulation of carbohydrate metabolism. The exocrine tissue, composed of acinar cells grouped in lobules and drained by a duct system, forms almost the entire mass of the gland. The exocrine secretion is discharged into the intestine through the pancreatic duct, which usually enters the duodenum together with the common bile duct at the sphincter of Oddi; in about 10% of individuals, however, the main outflow of the pancreatic juice reaches the duodenum by a separate duct.

The endocrine tissue is composed of specialised cells collected together in the small islets of Langerhans scattered throughout the gland, and accounts for only 1% of the mass of the pancreas. The endocrine secretions include insulin, which is produced by the beta cells of the islets, and glucagon which is produced by the alpha cells; the functions of both are discussed in the chapter on diabetes mellitus.

Pancreatic juice is an alkaline secretion (pH 7·5–8·5) which is isotonic with plasma, the main cations being sodium and potassium while the main anion is bicarbonate which is produced by the cells lining the duct system. The juice also contains enzymes which digest carbohydrate, fat and protein, the main ones being amylase, lipase and trypsin. These enzymes are synthesised by the serous cells of the pancreatic acini, and they are secreted in parallel concentrations; they all require an alkaline medium for optimal efficiency, so that theoretically digestion may be impaired if the bicarbonate content of the pancreatic juice is reduced.

Exocrine pancreatic secretion is stimulated partly through nervous and partly through hormonal mechanisms (p. 310), and a maximum flow is reached between two and three hours after a meal; in all, about 1 litre is secreted daily.

### Investigation of the Pancreas

**Ultrasonography** will show the size and shape of the pancreas and the presence of tumours, cysts, oedema or dilated ducts. It is therefore particularly useful when carcinoma or pancreatitis is suspected.

**Radiological Examination.** A plain radiograph may show calcification in the pancreas, and in acute pancreatitis there is often evidence of ileus in the duodenum and jejunum. An intravenous cholangiogram may show narrowing or distortion of the common bile duct due to neoplastic or inflammatory changes in the head of the pancreas. A barium meal may show displacement of the stomach when the pancreas is enlarged by acute pancreatitis, cysts or tumours. The barium meal may also show abnormalities of the mucosal folds in the duodenum, particularly on the medial wall, but these features are seen better on hypotonic duodenography.

More specialised radiographic techniques include retrograde pancreatography of the duct system obtained by cannulating the ampulla of Vater during duodenoscopy (ERCP p. 314). Selective arteriography of the coeliac and superior mesenteric arteries can show distortion and compression of vessels from some tumours. CT scanning can also be used to detect tumours. Radioisotope studies are now little used.

**Tests of Exocrine Pancreatic Function.** Tubes are passed into the stomach and duodenum under radiological control. The gastric juice is aspirated throughout the test so that it does not mix with the pancreatic secretions. Secretin and pancreozymin are given by intravenous injection and the pancreatic secretions are collected for one hour. Measurements are made of the volume of secretion and of the concentration of bicarbonate and amylase or trypsin.

In pancreatic insufficiency low volumes of secretion may be obtained with reduction in the concentration and output of bicarbonate and enzymes. The test is also of use in excluding pancreatic disease as a cause of malabsorption. In patients with carcinoma of the pancreas, the duodenal aspirate may contain blood and cytological examination may reveal exfoliated malignant cells. Fibreoptic duodenoscopy may allow the direct collection of pancreatic secretion for cytological examination. The value of these tests is limited because of the technical difficulties involved and because early disease of the pancreas may not be detected.

**Tests of Endocrine Pancreatic Function.** A diabetic response to a glucose tolerance test in a patient with steatorrhoea suggests a pancreatic cause for the malabsorption of fat. When carcinoma of the pancreas is suspected, an abnormal glucose tolerance test is a frequent finding in a condition difficult to diagnose.

## Acute Pancreatitis

This is a serious disorder caused essentially by the digestion of the pancreas by its own enzymes. In mild cases the gland becomes swollen and oedematous; in more severe cases haemorrhagic necrosis occurs with the development of serious local and systemic complications. The disease is most common between the fourth and seventh decades, with an equal sex incidence.

**Aetiology.** In Britain about 50% of cases are associated with biliary disease and about 20% with alcoholism while in about 20% no cause can be identified. Alcoholism accounts for a much higher proportion in some countries, especially the USA and South Africa. Acute pancreatitis is a recognised complication of renal transplantation and may be caused also by drugs such as corticosteroids and oral contraceptives. It occurs occasionally after abdominal trauma or surgery and rarely in mumps, hyperparathyroidism, hyperlipidaemia or hypothermia.

The mechanisms which initiate the destruction of pancreatic tissue are not known. The frequent association with disease of the biliary tract led to the theory that obstruction of the sphincter of Oddi by a gallstone, oedema or spasm allows reflux of bile along the pancreatic duct, so activating the pancreatic enzymes and leading to autodigestion of the gland. This theory is no longer widely accepted because, while a common terminal channel for the bile and pancreatic duct is sometimes found, an impacted stone is rare. Alcohol may cause pancreatitis by increasing the protein concentration in the pancreatic secretions; precipitation of the protein may then result in obstruction of the smaller ducts leading to pancreatitis. Obstruction from other causes, such as a tumour or stone may produce pancreatitis in the same way.

**Clinical Features.** The onset is sudden with agonising pain in the epigastrium or right hypochondrium. It often occurs within 12 to 24 hours following the consumption of alcohol or a large meal. The pain is usually persistent and radiates most frequently through to the back, to either shoulder, or to one of the iliac fossae before spreading to involve the whole abdomen. Nausea and vomiting are frequent. In severe cases profound shock soon supervenes; occasionally the patient may present with shock and without pain. In milder cases moderate fever occurs, and slight jaundice may develop, especially in cases with gallstones.

Despite the severity of the pain, there may be little or no guarding of the abdominal muscles at first. Later the upper abdomen becomes tender and rigid as peritoneal irritation increases and the initial shock passes off. The condition may simulate acute cholecystitis (with which it may coexist), and myocardial infarction. About one-third of cases is recognised for the first time at laparotomy, having been diagnosed as perforated peptic ulcer or acute appendicitis.

**Investigation.** In the early stage of an acute case the serum amylase is elevated; this is short-lived because of rapid renal excretion. It follows that amylase measured in a 24-hour collection of urine may provide the diagnosis when serum levels are normal. A persistently raised serum amylase suggests the formation of a pseudocyst.

Biochemical findings may be helpful in the detection and monitoring of some complications. Hyperglycaemia is common in the first two days and hypocalcaemia may occur five to eight days after the attack because calcium is sequestered into the areas of fat necrosis which occur in severe pancreatitis.

A plain radiograph may show evidence of duodeno-jejunal ileus and absence of gas in the transverse colon. Ultrasonography may demonstrate an enlarged pancreas which at barium examination may displace the duodenum or stomach.

**Treatment.** When the diagnosis of acute pancreatitis can be established with certainty, the present tendency is to avoid operation in favour of conservative treatment. However, laparotomy is imperative if diagnostic uncertainty exists. Once the diagnosis is confirmed, the abdomen is drained and closed without any definitive procedure being performed unless there is associated disease in the biliary tract. Nasogastric suction is instituted as a treatment for ileus.

Medical management consists of measures to relieve pain, to combat shock, hypocalcaemia or hyperglycaemia and to prevent infection. For the relief of pain, repeated injections of methadone (10 mg) or pethidine (100 mg) should be given. If pain is very severe, hypodermic injections of morphine (10–20 mg) may be required, but this drug, and pethidine to a lesser degree, may have the undesirable effect of causing spasm of the sphincter of Oddi.

In the stage of shock, intravenous isotonic saline (1 to 2 *l*) is given initially followed by up to 4 *l* of plasma in the first 24 hours. In severe cases part of the requirement is given as blood. Total fluid needs are assessed by the measurement of central venous pressure, haematocrit and urine output. The initial treatment of shock is followed by continuous parenteral electrolyte therapy until the ileus has resolved.

Intravenous injections of calcium may be required if hypocalcaemia develops and blood sugar should be monitored regularly so that developing diabetes can be treated promptly.

Antibiotics may be administered with the object of preventing secondary bacterial infection of the damaged tissues. Corticosteroids have no specific place in the treatment of acute pancreatitis and indeed may be a cause of it.

**Complications.** Initial severe complications are shock, ileus and cardiorespiratory problems. The swollen pancreas may cause obstruction to the duodenum or common bile duct. Bleeding may occur from inflamed or eroded areas of the stomach or duodenum. A pancreatic abscess develops when the necrotic pancreatic tissue becomes infected; it must be drained surgically if the patient is to survive.

**Prognosis** depends upon the severity of the attack. Overall, the mortality is 10–20%. Patients with haemorrhagic pancreatitis have a mortality of over 50% whereas when there is only oedema of the pancreas, the mortality is less than 5%. Pancreatitis secondary to gallstones is unlikely to recur provided these are removed. Alcoholic pancreatitis will recur if alcohol consumption continues.

## Chronic Pancreatitis

In the Western world the majority of cases of chronic pancreatitis occurs as a result of high alcohol consumption. It is possible that a small number result from cholelithiasis, but a causative relationship is difficult to establish because coincidental gallstones would be expected in a significant proportion of patients. It is rare for acute attacks of pancreatitis to proceed to chronic pancreatitis. In a few patients chronic pancreatitis may be caused by stenosis or disease of the sphincter of Oddi. In some parts of the tropics, chronic pancreatitis is common and malnutrition may be an aetiological factor.

The microscopy of the pancreas shows fibrosis around the ducts and acinae which are gradually replaced. By contrast, there is preservation of the islets. The larger ducts are often irregular and dilated, and stones may be present in the lumen.

**Clinical Features.** The disease is most common in males between the ages of 35 and 45. Nearly all patients present with abdominal pain. Recurrent attacks occur at intervals of several weeks or months often within a few hours to two days of an alcoholic bout. In contrast to acute pancreatitis, the pain may begin gradually and persist for days or weeks. Pain is located in the epigastrium, right or left subcostal areas or around the umbilicus; characteristically it may radiate to the back between T10 and T12 and relief may be obtained by crouching forward or leaning forward over a chair.

Diabetes develops in about a fifth of patients and steatorrhoea in a third: occasionally one of these is the presenting feature. Both these complications are more likely when the pancreas is calcified. Jaundice may arise because of obstruction to the common bile duct and symptoms of duodenal obstruction due to the development of a pseudocyst. On examination there is often diffuse tenderness in the abdomen.

**Investigation.** In a small proportion of cases of chronic pancreatitis the plain radiograph of the abdomen shows calcification in the duct system or throughout the gland. The barium meal or hypotonic duodenography may show deformity of the duodenal cap as a result of oedema, and flattening and rigidity of the medial wall of the duodenum. Ultrasonography is usually performed first since it may show that the pancreas is abnormal. Evidence of pancreatic insufficiency is provided when pancreatic function tests show a normal volume of secretion and a reduced concentration of amylase and bicarbonate; with very advanced disease the volume of secretion is also reduced. The presence of steatorrhoea and a diabetic glucose tolerance curve provide further evidence of severe pancreatic insufficiency. Estimation of serum amylase activity is of value only in an acute exacerbation.

Endoscopic retrograde pancreatography often provides valuable evidence in favour of the diagnosis by showing stones and dilatation of the pancreatic ducts. This information is also important for planning surgical treatment.

**Treatment.** Pain is often severe and many patients require narcotics with the inevitable danger of addiction. When steatorrhoea is present, a diet containing over 2500 kcals per day is given, composed of carbohydrate and protein but only 40 g fat. Pancreatic extracts are given with and between meals to assist absorption; when they fail to bring about improvement, cimetidine given with meals will increase their effect by preventing their inactivation by gastric acid. In diabetic patients, oral hypoglycaemic agents should be tried initially, but if these fail, insulin is usually required. It is imperative that the patient abstains from drinking alcohol permanently.

Surgery should be contemplated for the relief of intractable pain. Drainage of the pancreatic duct into the small bowel, removal of part or most of the pancreas, or sphincterotomy are the most usual procedures. The ultimate result is so dependent on the alcoholic's ability to stop drinking that operation is not worth while in the patient who cannot do so. The indication for surgery is stronger when cysts and the possibility of cancer of the pancreas are present. The best results are obtained in those patients who are shown to have stones in the bile ducts or stenosis of the ampulla of Vater. Correction of these abnormalities may relieve pain and result in recovery of pancreatic function.

## Pancreatic Cysts

**A pancreatic pseudocyst** occurs as a complication of acute pancreatitis, chronic pancreatitis or trauma to the pancreas. A pseudocyst is a sac which contains fluid, pancreatic enzymes and blood. It usually occupies the lesser sac, displacing the stomach, and it may obstruct the duodenum. Most commonly the pseudocyst develops 3 to 4 weeks after the onset of acute pancreatitis. Epigastric pain, nausea and vomiting, weight loss, fever and jaundice are likely symptoms. On examination, a smooth, tender mass is felt in the upper abdomen in about half the cases.

There is a persistent leucocytosis and raised serum amylase activity. Ultrasonography will confirm the presence of a cyst in nearly all cases. An abdominal radiograph shows a mass in the epigastrium and a barium meal or hypotonic duodenogram confirms extrinsic pressure on the stomach, duodenum and small bowel.

Pseudocysts which fail to resolve spontaneously within six weeks are treated surgically by drainage into the stomach or small intestine.

**Intrapancreatic or retention cysts** are usually small and multiple and are found in chronic pancreatitis. These cysts may cause abdominal pain but the diagnosis is difficult to make except by retrograde pancreatography. Symptomatic cysts are treated surgically. Occasionally a cyst is secondary to carcinoma.

### Cystic Fibrosis

This autosomal recessive disease is the commonest serious genetic condition in Caucasian children. Cystic fibrosis is characterised by generalised dysfunction of all exocrine glands, including those which secrete mucus. Blockage by viscid secretion causes cystic changes in the pancreas and also bronchiectasis.

**Clinical Features.** Frequently cystic fibrosis presents in infancy with repeated attacks of respiratory infection. Defective pancreatic enzymes give rise to impaired digestion and malabsorption of fat. The stools are bulky, foamy and foul-smelling. The child is often poorly nourished. Complications include intussusception and obstruction due to faecal masses.

Increasing numbers of patients are surviving to adulthood because of better treatment of respiratory infection. The respiratory problems become progressively more important in the adolescent and adult and determine the fate of the individual; by contrast malabsorption is less troublesome. There may be bronchiectasis, recurrent spontaneous pneumothorax, recurrent haemoptysis, pulmonary fibrosis and right ventricular failure. Sometimes there is cirrhosis leading to portal hypertension. Females with cystic fibrosis may become pregnant but males are nearly always infertile.

In the child, the diagnosis is established by the finding of an increase in the concentration of sodium in the sweat to above 60 mmol/*l*. The test is difficult to interpret after adolescence; the diagnosis is then made on the presence of chronic pulmonary disease, pancreatic insufficiency and a family history of cystic fibrosis.

**Treatment.** In the child, surgery may be required for a variety of complications. The treatment of pancreatic insufficiency is very important to maintain adequate nutrition. The aims of treatment of respiratory disease are to control infection and to ensure adequate drainage of secretions by inhalation therapy, mucolytic agents, postural drainage and breathing exercises. In the adult these respiratory measures are of paramount importance.

Families with cystic fibrosis require long term support. Genetic advice should be made available to the parents (p. 19).

## Carcinoma of the Pancreas

The incidence of carcinoma of the pancreas is increasing in many Western countries. It is more common in males than in females and it occurs most frequently between the ages of 55 and 70 years. Most cancers are adenocarcinomas, commonly arising from the ducts but occasionally from the acinae; ductal carcinomas may be multicentric. Islet cell carcinoma (p. 345) and cystadenocarcinoma are rarer forms of cancer. Adenocarcinoma is of scirrhous nature and in two-thirds of cases it involves the head of the gland.

**Clinical Features.** Apart from carcinoma of the ampulla which may bleed into the duodenum, or cause jaundice at a relatively early stage, all cancers of the pancreas are advanced by the time they cause symptoms. Epigastric pain is common, but occasionally it may be absent throughout the course of the disease. The pain is variable in type but is characteristically dull and boring and radiates through to the back. It is often intensified by food and by lying supine, especially at night. It may be relieved by crouching forward. Vague dyspeptic symptoms are common and include anorexia, nausea, discomfort and sometimes vomiting. These symptoms may be the only manifestations until metastases occur.

Other clinical features depend largely on the site of the growth. In the majority of cases with involvement of the head of the pancreas, jaundice is the presenting feature and may be painless and progressive. A large firm liver eventually develops. An abdominal mass is present in one quarter of all patients and occasionally a distended gall bladder is palpable or ascites can be detected. Jaundice may not appear in cases where the lesion affects mainly the body and tail of the pancreas. The symptoms of diabetes mellitus or thrombophlebitis may occasionally be the presenting feature.

Carcinoma of the pancreas is a rapidly progressive emaciating disease especially in cases in which the head is involved, when death usually occurs within six months of the onset of obstructive jaundice.

**Investigation.** Pancreatic cancer is often suspected from the clinical features, a raised serum alkaline phosphatase and a diabetic glucose tolerance test. Ultrasonography is a useful initial investigation. Barium meal or hypotonic duodenography usually provides supportive evidence when cancer is in the head of the pancreas. This may show distortion or displacement of the stomach or duodenum with possible invasion by tumour. Duodenoscopy is important in detecting cancer of the ampulla; during this procedure, cannulation of the pancreatic duct may show stricture or obstruction of the duct and when jaundice is present, cannulation of the common bile duct may show the obstruction is within the pancreas. In some centres pancreatic function tests with the collection of juice for cytological examination are used to make the diagnosis. In some instances, ultrasonography, angiography and CT scanning show whether or not the tumour has spread to the portal vein and this determines operability.

**Treatment.** Carcinoma of the ampulla can be treated by excision of the duodenum and head of the pancreas; the prognosis in such cases is better than for cancers elsewhere in the pancreas. Radical surgery is rarely possible for pancreatic cancer. Usually the aim is to relieve obstructive jaundice by implanting the common bile duct or gall bladder into the jejunum or to forestall duodenal obstruction by gastrojejunostomy. Less than 10% of patients with cancer of the pancreas survive for one year after diagnosis and only 2% survive for two years.

### Islet-cell Tumours

A benign adenoma may arise rarely from the beta cells of the islets and produce hyperinsulinism with attacks of spontaneous hypoglycaemia (p. 518). Even more rare are tumours, usually malignant, from other islet cells which elaborate polypeptides, e.g. gastrin or allied substances, the secretion of which into the blood causes a variety of syndromes. The most common is the Zollinger-Ellison syndrome (p. 334).

# DISEASES OF THE SMALL INTESTINE

## Malabsorption

A number of disorders result in malabsorption of one or more of the essential nutrients, electrolytes, minerals or vitamins. Some or all of the following features may ensue: diarrhoea, abdominal pain and distension, loss of weight, anaemia, or other evidence of specific deficiency. However, some patients complain only of vague ill-health, and the diagnosis may not be made for many years.

The sequence followed in this section is first to review the basic processes of absorption and the means of testing them. Then the ways in which the processes of absorption can be deranged are discussed. Finally, the clinical presentation and treatment of malabsorption in general and then of specific disorders are described.

## Tests of Absorption

**Fat absorption** takes place predominantly in the duodenum and upper jejunum. Dietary fat occurs largely in the form of insoluble long-chain triglycerides. These are emulsified mechanically in the stomach and by detergents (mainly bile acids) in the small intestine. Then pancreatic lipase hydrolyses the triglycerides to monoglyceride and fatty acids. Pancreatic bicarbonate is required to maintain the optimum pH for this hydrolysis and for the next step in fat absorption, the solubilisation of the monoglycerides and fatty acids by bile acids. This consists of their incorporation into micelles which orientate the fatty acid and monoglyceride in such a way that they can be presented to the intestinal mucosal cell for absorption (Fig. 9.1). Once in the absorptive cell, the monoglycerides and fatty acids are reformed (re-esterified) into triglycerides which are then coated with phospholipid and protein to form chylomicrons. The chylomicron passes out of the cell to be transported by the lymphatic system into the blood (p. 377).

TEST OF FAT ABSORPTION. Fat excretion in the stool is measured over a 5-day period, whilst the patient is receiving a normal diet (which contains less than 100 g fat per day). The upper limit of normal for faecal fat excretion is 7 g per day.

The fat-soluble vitamins A, D and K are absorbed in the same way as dietary fat and measurement of their absorption can be used as an indirect assessment of fat absorption. For example, the plasma vitamin A level can be measured after oral administration of retinol for two or three days.

**Carbohydrate Absorption.** Carbohydrate in the diet is in the form of starch (60%), lactose (10%) and sucrose (30%). These are digested to glucose, galactose and fructose. Glucose and galactose are absorbed into the cell by active transport mechanisms, the process requiring sodium ions and energy. The fructose molecule is too large to move across the cell membrane by simple diffusion and it is thought that it must be facilitated by a carrier.

TESTS OF CARBOHYDRATE ABSORPTION. *The glucose tolerance test* (p. 507) is sometimes used and the absence of a rise in blood sugar can indicate malabsorption, but there are so many variables that the test is difficult to interpret in the context of malabsorption.

In the *xylose absorption test*, 25 g of d-xylose are given orally after an overnight fast. Only a small proportion is metabolised within the body and 5–8 g should be excreted in the urine over the next 5 hours.

In the *lactose tolerance test*, 50 g of lactose are given orally and blood glucose levels are measured as in the glucose tolerance test. Normally this disaccharide is broken down by intestinal lactase to glucose and galactose which are absorbed so that blood glucose levels rise. If the enzyme lactase is deficient in the intestinal mucosa, there may be no rise in blood glucose and the patient may complain of colic and diarrhoea because the unabsorbed lactose acts as an osmotic agent in the gut.

**Protein Absorption.** Initial hydrolysis of dietary protein molecules is performed by gastric pepsin and pancreatic enzymes. Further hydrolysis of peptides takes place at the brush border and a mixture of peptides and amino acids is absorbed into the cell. A large amount of protein, other than dietary, enters the lumen of the gastrointestinal tract each day, derived from various secretions, desquamated cells and the exudation of plasma proteins. These are absorbed by the same mechanisms as dietary protein.

TESTS OF PROTEIN ABSORPTION. Measurement of the amount of nitrogen in the stool provides a very crude estimate of the above processes. Stools are collected for 3 to 5 days and no more than 2·5 g of nitrogen per day should be excreted.

An excessive loss of nitrogen in the stool can result from the loss of albumin and other plasma proteins into the lumen of the tract. This is termed *protein losing enteropathy* and it can be detected by labelling serum proteins with radioactive chromium and measuring radioactivity in the stool.

A low serum albumin level in the absence of hepatic or renal disease may indicate protein malabsorption or protein losing enteropathy.

**Absorption of Other Substances.** The Schilling test (p. 549) is used in investigating the absorption of vitamin $B_{12}$. The serum levels of folate, iron and calcium provide an index of the absorption of these substances.

## Causes of Malabsorption

1. **Disorders of Intraluminal Digestion.** Here there is an insufficiency of a digestive enzyme or detergent within the lumen. The main feature is steatorrhoea with deficiency of fat soluble vitamins. Since the intestinal mucosal cells are normal, there is no impairment of absorption of other substances less dependent on intraluminal digestion, e.g. carbohydrate, protein, vitamin $B_{12}$, folate and iron.

(a) DISTURBANCES OF GASTRIC FUNCTION. After gastric surgery it is possible for the correct enzymes, detergents and electrolytes to be delivered into the intestinal lumen and yet malabsorption may occur. This is because gastric emptying is no longer co-ordinated with the correct stage of digestion. For example, after gastroenterostomy or a Polya partial gastrectomy, bile and pancreatic juice may be delivered after food from the stomach has already passed down the efferent loop.

(b) PANCREATIC INSUFFICIENCY. A deficiency of pancreatic lipase causes malabsorption of fat, for example, in chronic pancreatitis, cystic fibrosis and carcinoma of the pancreas.

(c) DEFICIENCY OF BILE ACIDS. This may occur in two circumstances:

(i) *Interruption of the Enterohepatic Circulation of Bile Acids*. When there is disease, e.g. Crohn's, or resection of the terminal ileum, bile acids cannot be reabsorbed (p. 379) and are lost in the faeces. In the colon they prevent water and electrolyte absorption and stimulate their secretion; diarrhoea results. Synthesis by the liver cannot compensate for the loss of bile acids. There is therefore an inadequate concentration of bile acid in the upper jejunum and micelles cannot be formed.

(ii) *Colonisation of the Small Bowel by Bacteria*. The upper part of the small intestine is practically sterile under normal conditions. If a large number of bacteria are present (p. 351) bile acids are deconjugated, micelle formation becomes inefficient and steatorrhea results. Bacteria in the small intestine can also utilise vitamin $B_{12}$ so that it is unavailable for absorption and anaemia ensues.

2. **Disorders of Transport in the Mucosal Cell.** In these disorders, the intraluminal digestive phase is normal, but the absorptive cells are not, because of:

(a) *Generalised mucosal damage* from coeliac disease, tropical sprue, giardiasis, Whipples disease (p. 623) or extensive Crohn's disease. In these conditions generilised malabsorption is usually demonstrated by tests of fat, xylose, folate, vitamin $B_{12}$, iron, calcium and amino acids in addition to steatorrhoea.

(b) *Disorders with histologically normal mucosa*. Here a specific substance is malabsorbed because of the absence of a particular enzyme. Thus there may be malabsorption of lactose because of an insufficiency of lactase in the mucosa. Another example is the malabsorption of vitamin $B_{12}$ because of a lack of intrinsic factor in pernicious anaemia.

3. **Disorders of Transport from the Mucosal Cell.** These are rare and result from the blockage of the lymphatic system which is responsible for the transfer of chylomicrons from the absorptive cell to the systemic circulation. This may occur in abdominal lymphoma or tuberculosis or in the rare condition of primary lymphangiectasia involving the mesenteric lymphatic system.

### Clinical Features and Investigation of Malabsorption

The patient can present in various ways. In severe forms there may be general malnutrition, with loss of weight and energy and a slow deterioration in health or, in a child, a failure to grow and thrive. Abdominal distension is often a striking feature. Steatorrhoea may be the presenting symptom. The patient complains of diarrhoea, with the passage of loose, pale, bulky and offensive stools which float on water. The patient may be anaemic due to a deficiency of iron, cyanocobalamin or of folate. Haemorrhagic phenomena due to a deficiency of vitamin K may be an occasional presenting feature. Hypocalcaemia may lead to tetany. The features of rickets or osteomalacia and various disorders due to deficiency of vitamins may be noted, such as sore tongue, angular stomatitis and dry, rough or cracked skin. Hypoalbuminaemic oedema may occur. In other patients, malabsorption may be suspected because of gastric surgery or intestinal resection. In patients with mild malabsorption, there may be no diarrhoea and the condition may be diagnosed only after investigation for non-specific abdominal complaints or anaemia.

The diagnosis may be suspected as a result of a barium follow-through examination in a patient with abdominal symptoms. The small intestine shows dilated loops with flocculation and segmentation of barium (Fig. 8.4).

Malabsorption is confirmed by the tests of absorption which may also provide a clue as to the cause of the disorder. For example, malabsorption of several substances is likely when there is a generalised disorder of the absorptive cells.

Biopsy of the small intestine (p. 314) may show the villous atrophy of coeliac disease. Partial villous atrophy can occur in a variety of disorders, such as tropical sprue, Crohn's disease and in mild cases of coeliac disease. If the intestinal biopsy is normal, other investigations may be necessary to provide the diagnosis — for example, pancreatic function tests (p. 340) or the culture of intestinal aspirates for bacteria.

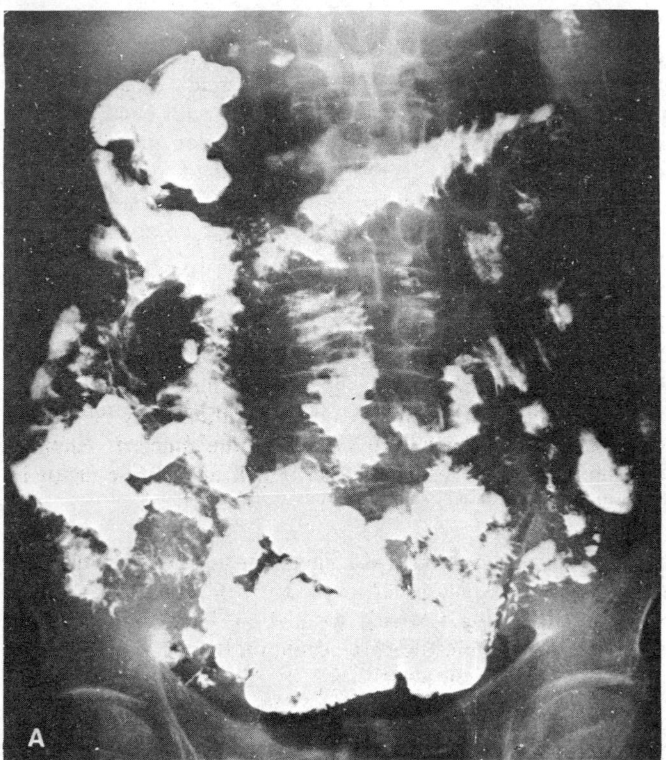


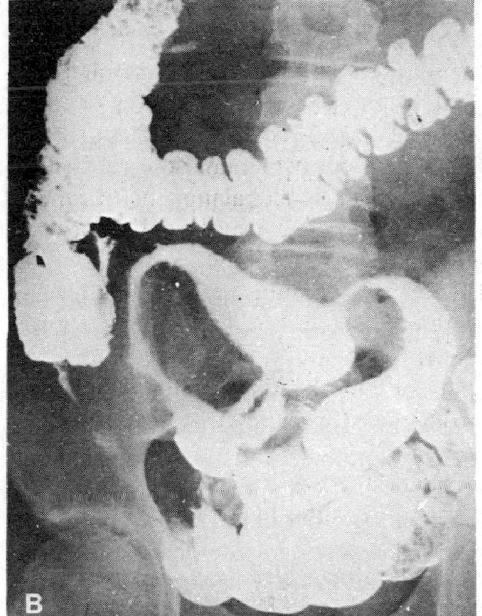


A. Malabsorption. Note dilated loops, segmentation and flocculation.

B. Crohn's disease. Note narrowed segments.

Fig. 8.4

### Treatment of Malabsorption

A gluten-free diet must be prescribed in coeliac disease. Pancreatic insufficiency is treated by pancreatic supplements (p. 343). Insufficiency of bile acids should not be treated with oral bile acids because these would pass into the colon, interfere with salt and water absorption, and so worsen the diarrhoea. The effect of the endogenous bile acids on the colon is counteracted by giving the binding agent cholestyramine in a dose of up to 12 g per day. In addition, a low fat diet should be given because cholestyramine will not improve the fat absorption.

In severe forms of malabsorptive disease, it may be necessary to treat dehydration and electrolyte deficiency by intravenous infusions.

Replacement therapy is necessary for those patients with anaemia, bone disease or coagulation defects. Folic acid and iron supplements are given orally and vitamin $B_{12}$ by a monthly injection. Vitamin D and calcium supplements may be required. Calcium is normally given as gluconate or lactate by mouth, but when there is tetany 10 ml of 10% calcium gluconate is given slowly intravenously. Glossitis and cheilosis are indications for the parenteral administration of vitamin B complex.

## The Principal Disorders Causing Malabsorption

### Coeliac Disease

Coeliac disease is characterised by an abnormal mucosa in the small intestine, induced by gliadin, a component of the gluten protein of wheat. Barley, rye and oats may also be injurious. It seems likely that local immunological responses to gluten are responsible.

**Pathology.** The mucosa of the normal small intestine has finger-like or leaf-like villi which can be seen with the dissecting microscope or on histological section. In coeliac disease the dissecting microscope appearance shows either (i) convolutions, like the surface of the cerebrum, which, when sectioned, appear as short wide villi, or (ii) a totally flat mucosa which is termed 'subtotal villous atrophy'. In addition, the height of the epithelial cells is reduced and there is an increase in the number of plasma cells in the lamina propria. All these histological features return towards normality during treatment with a gluten-free diet. In coeliac disease the mucosa at the duodeno-jejunal flexure is always abnormal and the abnormality extends distally for a variable distance.

**Clinical Features.** Coeliac disease usually begins in the first three years of life. The child ceases to thrive and becomes fractious and irritable, the stools become voluminous and pale and, as the disorder progresses, growth is retarded, anaemia develops, and the abdomen becomes distended. On the other hand, the disorder may manifest itself for the first time in adult life; the presenting symptoms range from those of a mild anaemia and listlessness of long duration, to a florid malabsorptive state developing rapidly over a period of weeks. The commonest features are diarrhoea, weight loss and anaemia, usually due to combined deficiency of folate and iron. There may be peripheral neuropathy and evidence of vitamin deficiency or hypoproteinaemia. Other features are finger clubbing, dermatitis herpetiformis, amenorrhoea and infertility.

Coeliac disease predisposes to the development of lymphoma of the small intestine;

colicky abdominal pain and unexpected weight loss in a previously well-controlled patient should arouse suspicion.

**Treatment.** A gluten-free diet must be taken indefinitely. This requires the exclusion of wheat, rye, oats and barley, and imposes severe restrictions which must be fully explained to the patient. A booklet produced by the Coeliac Society (PO Box 181, London) containing diet sheets and recipes for gluten-free flour is of great value in this respect. Mineral and vitamin supplements are also given when indicated. If the patient deteriorates on a strictly supervised diet, corticosteroids may be tried; a diagnosis of lymphoma must also be considered.

### **Tropical Sprue** (p. 841)

### Lactose Intolerance

This disorder is being seen more often in Britain because immigrant Asian and African races have insufficient lactase in the mucosa of the small intestine to digest the large amounts of lactose consumed in Britain.

The patient complains of abdominal discomfort, colic and diarrhoea after the ingestion of milk or milk products. The symptoms can be reproduced by the lactose tolerance test (p. 346) and respond to the reduction of lactose in the diet.

### Bacterial Colonisation of the Small Intestine

The effects of this proliferation have been discussed on page 348. The presentation is with steatorrhoea or anaemia due to vitamin $B_{12}$ deficiency. Radiological investigation shows a lesion causing stasis in the intestine such as jejunal diverticula, a long afferent ('blind') loop after gastrectomy or gastroenterostomy, Crohn's disease, stricture formation or a fistula between colon and small intestine. The Schilling test is abnormal (p. 549). The diagnosis is confirmed by the correction of steatorrhoea and vitamin $B_{12}$ malabsorption by the administration of tetracycline. Occasionally surgical correction of an abnormality may be required.

### Crohn's Disease

This disease is characterised by localised areas of non-specific, granulomatous inflammation of the bowel. It was formerly termed regional ileitis or enteritis. However, the eponymous designation 'Crohn's disease' is preferable since the alimentary tract can be affected anywhere from the mouth to the anus, the sites most commonly involved being, in order of frequency, terminal ileum alone, terminal ileum and right side of colon, colon alone, ileum and jejunum. The term 'inflammatory bowel disease' comprises Crohn's disease and ulcerative colitis (p. 359).

Crohn's disease may occur at any age, but most commonly between the ages of 20 and 40; it affects both sexes equally. In its chronic form, it is a debilitating disease which often interferes profoundly with a patient's life requiring repeated admission to hospital for treatment.

**Aetiology.** The cause is unknown. No specific organism has been identified from the bowel content, the bowel wall or the regional lymph nodes. One of the histological characteristics of the disease is the presence of granulomas composed of collections of epithelioid and giant cells. These granulomas closely resemble those found both in tuberculosis and sarcoidosis. However caseation does not occur in Crohn's disease which is now accepted as being unrelated to either. A current hypothesis is that Crohn's disease is the consequence of an abnormal immune response in the gut wall to an unidentified antigen. Crohn's disease, ankylosing spondylitis and ulcerative colitis all occur more commonly than might be expected amongst the families of patients with Crohn's disease, suggesting that all three diseases share a common but incomplete genetic basis.

**Pathology.** Although the disease may affect any part of the alimentary canal, the terminal ileum is most often involved. Macroscopically, the bowel is engorged and oedematous so that the lumen is markedly narrowed, sometimes enough to produce obstruction; the mucosa is oedematous, showing a 'cobble-stone' pattern with linear ulceration and fissuring. Characteristically, these changes are patchy; even when a relatively short segment of bowel is affected, it can be seen that the inflammatory process is interrupted by islands of normal mucosa occurring in the diseased area, the change from normal mucosa to the affected part being abrupt. The lesions may be discontinuous over a length of the bowel, a small lesion separated in this way from a major area of involvement being referred to as a 'skip' lesion. The affected lymph nodes are enlarged and the mesentery thickened.

Microscopically, inflammatory change involves all coats of the bowel wall. All grades of inflammation may be seen and characteristically there is oedema and hyperplasia of the lymphoid follicles. Granulomas are seen in about 50% of cases. Another feature is deep clefts or fissures opening on to the mucosal surface and sometimes passing through the entire thickness of the bowel wall. These clefts are responsible for the fistula formation which is such a characteristic feature of the disease. Fistulae may develop between adjacent loops of bowel or between affected segments of bowel and the bladder, uterus or vagina and may appear in the perineum.

**Clinical features** vary and depend in part on the site and extent of the bowel affected; many other diseases may be mimicked. Crohn's disease may present acutely with features indistinguishable from acute appendicitis. At laparotomy the terminal ileum is red and oedematous and provided the abdomen is closed without resection the prognosis is relatively good.

In the chronic form of the disease, pain is the commonest symptom and may be due either to peritoneal involvement, obstruction or both. Since the terminal ileum and right side of the colon are most commonly affected, this type of pain occurs most frequently in the right lower quadrant and it may be associated with local tenderness or guarding. A mass is palpable by abdominal and frequently by rectal examination. This consists of inflamed loops of bowel bound together, possibly including an abscess, and may be of any size. Colicky pain suggests obstruction, and may be associated with nausea and vomiting and excessive borborygmi. Indeed, recurrent episodes of colic due to attacks of subacute obstruction are a prominent feature in the life history of a patient with Crohn's disease; however, severe acute obstruction is uncommon.

Malabsorption occurs for a variety of reasons in Crohn's disease. The enterohepatic bile acid circulation may be interrupted by disease or resection of the ileum. Other areas of the small intestine may be involved, thus reducing the surface area for absorption. Strictures and fistula may lead to bacterial colonisation of the small intestine. The inflamed mucosa may cause a protein losing enteropathy.

Diarrhoea is frequent, but is rarely so marked as in ulcerative colitis. The stools may be formed or loose, and rarely contain frank blood, mucus or pus unless the colon is involved. In the latter case, the symptoms are indistinguishable from those of ulcerative colitis. A diagnostic feature, when present, is the occurrence of anal lesions such as oedematous skin tags or perianal abscesses and fistulas; they are more common when the colon is affected.

Weight loss is frequent and most patients have a low-grade fever and moderate anaemia. Clubbing of the fingers may be present. A number of other manifestations may occur, including enteropathic arthritis (p. 622), ankylosing spondylitis, iritis, aphthous stomatitis and erythema nodosum. Abnormal liver function tests are relatively common, while renal complications include hydronephrosis due to involvement of the right ureter in an inflammatory mass.

**Investigation.** Barium meal and follow-through examination may show alteration of the mucosal pattern, deep ulceration or the pathognomonic 'string sign' due to marked narrowing of a segment of affected bowel (Fig. 8.4). The lesions tend to be discontinuous along the length of the bowel. A barium enema should be carried out since the disease may affect the small bowel and the colon simultaneously. In some patients there will be involvement of the colon segmentally or in its entirety; in the latter case the radiological appearances may be indistinguishable from those of ulcerative colitis.

Pus cells and red blood corpuscles may be found on microscopic examination of the faeces, but culture of the stool yields no specific organism. Moderate anaemia is usually present because of blood loss, while protein loss from the inflamed, ulcerated mucosa may cause hypoproteinaemia. Vitamin $B_{12}$ absorption is likely to be impaired if there is extensive disease of the terminal ileum, and this can be shown by an abnormal Schilling test (p. 549). The diagnosis may be confirmed either by rectal biopsy or by excision of perianal skin tags; a rectal biopsy will sometimes show the characteristic granulomatous lesions although the mucosa appears normal to the naked eye.

Sometimes no conclusive proof of Crohn's disease is obtained, and the diagnosis can only be presumptive; such patients should be kept under observation until the natural history of the illness declares itself.

**Differential Diagnosis.** The symptoms, signs and radiological findings are usually sufficient to suggest a lesion in the lower part of the small bowel. The other common diseases in this part of the intestinal tract are appendicitis or an appendix abscess and carcinoma of the caecum. In the acute phase, it may be impossible to decide between these possibilities, so that a laparotomy may be necessary.

Ulcerative colitis is distinguished from Crohn's disease because it involves only the large bowel, whereas Crohn's disease may affect the alimentary tract from the mouth to the anus. The distinctive features of Crohn's disease are fistula and stricture formation, but when these are absent differentiation from ulcerative colitis may depend on demonstration of the extent and location of the disease and ultimately on biopsy.

Ileo-caecal tuberculosis usually occurs in association with an obvious pulmonary lesion so that the diagnosis is suggested by the chest radiograph. A 'negative' tuberculin test is common in patients with Crohn's disease and excludes an active tuberculous process.

Caecal amoebiasis may need to be excluded (p. 813).

**Treatment.** Crohn's disease is a chronic condition with remissions and relapses over many years. There is no known cure at present and treatment is largely a matter of managing particular problems as they arise and improving the general condition of the patient.

*General Measures.* A low residue diet will reduce the frequency of intestinal colic, while diarrhoea may be controlled with loperamide or codeine. When the terminal ileum is extensively diseased or has been resected, cholestyramine will reduce the diarrhoea due to the cathartic effect of the unabsorbed bile acids on the colon; hydroxocobalamin should be given to such patients for life since vitamin $B_{12}$ will not be absorbed.

Malabsorption with steatorrhoea may occur in patients with extensive involvement of the small intestine, contributing to weight loss and inanition. A low fat diet is then required and a course of oral antibiotics if bacterial colonisation of the upper intestine is suspected. Supplements of iron, folic acid, calcium, vitamins and electrolytes, especially potassium, may also be necessary. Hypoproteinaemia may require plasma or blood infusions in addition to a high protein diet.

An elemental diet is 'predigested' and absorbed high in the small intestine; it will relieve the symptoms of partial obstruction and restore nutrition. It is useful also in preoperative preparation, particularly for patients with external fistulas.

*Drugs.* Corticosteroids are beneficial when there is extensive active disease which is not improving with general medical measures. However they do not alter the long-term course of the disease. Prednisolone should be given in a dose of 40–60 mg daily in divided doses for 1 or 2 weeks depending on response, and the dose gradually reduced thereafter to 10–20 mg daily for 4 to 6 weeks and then withdrawn. Every effort should be made to stop the drug, but in the occasional case this may be difficult because of early relapse when the dose is reduced. In these circumstances, the effect of sulphasalazine (2–4 g daily) is worth a trial, much as it is used in ulcerative colitis (p. 364). Treatment with immunosuppressant drugs has been used with variable success in patients unresponsive to other forms of therapy.

*Surgical Treatment.* Although attacks of subacute obstruction can usually be managed conservatively by intestinal decompression and intravenous feeding (p. 316), operation may be necessary if attacks occur frequently. Surgery may also be required because of abscess or fistula formation. With localised disease, resection yields better results than bypass, but with extensive disease massive resection may result in malabsorption. Recurrence of the disease is always a danger, and therefore as much bowel as possible should be preserved. When the colon is extensively involved a total proctocolectomy as in ulcerative colitis may be the procedure of choice, though less extensive resection, for example a hemicolectomy, may suffice.

## Intestinal Obstruction

Intestinal obstruction may be complete or incomplete, acute or chronic, intermittent or continuous. The most important point to decide is whether the obstruction is *simple* or associated with *strangulation*. The latter occurs when there is interference with the blood supply to the intestine, as when the bowel is trapped or twisted. Urgent relief is required if the dangers of gangrene, perforation and peritonitis are to be avoided.

**Causes.** Obstruction may be mechanical, when the lumen of the bowel is blocked, or paralytic, when the propulsive power of the bowel is lost. In general the former type will require surgical relief, while the latter may respond to conservative measures, but the distinction is not always clear cut. Sometimes the mechanically obstructed bowel becomes exhausted and non-contractile, or it perforates at the site of the obstruction or proximally, the resultant peritonitis being responsible for paralysis of the adjacent bowel loops.

*Mechanical Obstruction.* At all ages adhesions and hernias are common causes of obstruction. In childhood, intussusception is frequent, while in the elderly, volvulus, tumours of the large bowel and diverticular disease account for a large proportion of cases. Impaction of faeces in the rectum presents with spurious diarrhoea but can also cause intestinal obstruction in the aged or bedridden. In children in unhygienic surroundings a mass of round worms may be responsible (p. 869).

*Paralytic obstruction or ileus* occurs temporarily after any abdominal operation and is a feature of shock, spinal injury and hypotension. Commonly it is due to peritonitis.

**Clinical Features.** *Pain.* In mechanical obstruction this is colicky and often originates at or about the site of the obstruction. Episodes of pain are accompanied by loud borborygmi. The advent of constant severe pain is indicative of strangulation. Paralytic obstruction is associated with a dull constant pain in an abdomen which is ominously silent.

*Vomiting.* This is copious in high obstruction and may be late or absent in obstructions of the lower small bowel or large bowel. The effortless trickle of foul-smelling fluid from the corner of the mouth of the lethargic patient is seen in untreated ileus, whereas in mechanical obstruction vomiting is projectile and intermittent.

*Distension.* This may be absent or confined to some loops of the bowel which can be seen in the thin patient as ridges across the abdomen forming the so-called ladder pattern. Diffuse distension is late and often indicative of a large bowel obstruction.

*Bowel Movements.* In complete obstruction neither faeces nor flatus is passed. In high obstructions, the bowels may move unaided or with enemas because of residual contents below the obstruction, while in large bowel obstruction, spurious diarrhoea may be due to a discharge of faecal-stained mucus.

*Physical Examination.* The diagnosis of obstruction and its cause can usually be made on physical examination alone. The hernial orifices should be palpated for the presence of a tender irreducible swelling. In fat patients particular care must be taken to check the femoral regions.

The presence of scars from previous abdominal operations is noted. Distension, particularly of individual loops, is significant. A distended caecum may be both seen and felt in thin patients and immediately points to a large bowel cause. Tenderness anywhere in the abdomen is suggestive of peritoneal irritation and bowel strangulation. A palpable mass is associated with large bowel tumours and diverticular disease. A transient mass, felt perhaps during bouts of colic, indicates intussusception. Classically bowel sounds are increased and tinkling in mechanical obstructions, but in advanced cases they are infrequent and auscultation must be prolonged to detect the occasional tinkle. In ileus, sounds are virtually absent.

Rectal examination usually reveals an empty ballooned rectum. In low obstructions there may be blood and mucus. Obstruction due to carcinoma of the rectum is rare.

In cases of doubt, and for confirmation of the diagnosis, serial measurements of abdominal girth will detect progressive abdominal distension. A diagnostic barium enema will confirm the presence of obstruction, particularly if repeated washouts yield neither flatus nor faeces.

*Fluid and Electrolyte Changes.* In obstruction of the upper small bowel, fluids and electrolytes are lost because of vomiting. When the obstruction is lower down, there is stagnation in the distended bowel loops, normal absorption from the gut is interrupted, and the body is deprived of fluid even in the absence of vomiting.

Biochemically, there is haemoconcentration with loss of water and electrolytes, particularly chloride, sodium and potassium. Elderly patients may develop secondary renal failure and this will add to the electrolyte imbalance. A vicious circle develops as increasing obstruction raises the tension in the bowel and further diminishes absorption; then increasing electrolyte imbalance interferes with intestinal peristalsis rendering the obstruction more complete. Recovery is heralded by diuresis, signifying return of peristalsis and re-absorption of fluid from the lumen of the bowel.

**Radiological Examination.** Plain radiographs, taken in the erect and supine positions, are most informative. The presence of fluid levels on the erect film, and of gas-distended loops on both films, indicate not only the diagnosis but also the site and probable cause of the obstruction. Where the completeness of the obstruction is in doubt, serial films can be compared for any change in the gas patterns. If further localisation is necessary, Gastrografin is preferable to barium which should be avoided lest it makes the obstruction worse.

**Treatment.** If intestinal obstruction is suspected, the opinion of a surgeon should be sought, even if non-operative measures are to be used.

The mainstays of treatment are decompression by gastrointestinal suction, the intravenous replacement of fluids and electrolytes, and operative relief of the obstruction. Urgent surgery is indicated for an irreducible hernia and where there is strangulation. In some countries, e.g. Uganda, volvulus of the sigmoid colon is a common cause of obstruction; it can be relieved by the passage of a rectal tube.

In cases of more gradual development where there is a possibility that the obstruction can be relieved even temporarily, and in ileus, conservative measures assume greatest importance. Passage of a nasogastric tube in an ill and nauseated patient requires skill and patience. Once in place, continuous suction with an electric pump, with periodic checks with a syringe to confirm that the tube is patent, will achieve upper intestinal decompression.

Intravenous infusion may require to be prolonged and biochemical estimations may be frequent, so that the veins should be treated with care. Where there has been blood loss, as in carcinoma of the bowel and diverticular disease, blood transfusion is required. Throughout conservative management, accurate fluid balance charts must be kept.

## Peritonitis

Peritonitis is the reaction of the peritoneum to an irritant. Usually this is infection, although sometimes the irritation is chemical, at least initially, as when bile or duodenal contents leak into the peritoneal cavity. Appendicitis is one of the commonest causes of peritonitis and *Esch. coli* is the organism usually responsible.

Infection or chemical irritation causes the peritoneum to become congested and oedematous. There is an exudation of fluid containing large quantities of leucocytes, protein and antibodies. Dilution and destruction of the irritant is accompanied by its localisation and by the formation of adhesions. Failure of these defence mechanisms is characterised by spread of the infection and by septicaemia and toxaemia. There is still a distressingly high mortality from generalised peritonitis.

**Acute Peritonitis.** In perforations, the onset is sudden, with severe abdominal pain, tenderness, rigidity and shock. The patient lies immobile, the respirations are short and grunting and the abdomen is retracted and motionless. These initial severe features then gradually decrease; the patient passes into a stage where he or she appears to have improved, and the diagnosis can be missed. Then, as ileus develops and fluid collects in the peritoneal cavity, there is increasing distension, the rigidity lessens, the tenderness remains and toxicity develops.

When peritonitis is secondary to inflammation of a viscus, such as appendicitis, the initial signs are those of the underlying disease, later to be replaced by the features of peritonitis. In advanced cases, only the history of onset remains to point to the probable cause.

Established peritonitis is treated by removal of the contaminating source when it is due to such conditions as appendicitis or perforation of the bowel or gall bladder. Anaerobic infection is controlled with metronidazole. Peritoneal toilet and lavage, intravenous replacement of fluids and electrolytes, and the treatment of the concomitant ileus by nasogastric suction are also required.

While the treatment of peritonitis is that of the cause, the ideal is its prevention. Thus acute appendicitis should be diagnosed before perforation and perforated peptic ulcer should be operated upon before the stage of chemical peritonitis is past.

General peritonitis may resolve completely, but often it localises to form an abscess at the primary site, in the subphrenic region or in the pelvis. Persistence of fever, or continued elevation of pulse rate, white blood count and ESR, should lead to efforts to locate such residual infections, for example by ultrasonography.

**Pelvic abscess** usually results from localisation of a general peritonitis and forms in the lowest part of the peritoneal cavity, in front of the rectum. The abscess may irritate the bladder causing frequency of micturition or involve the bowel causing diarrhoea with the passage of mucus and a feeling of incomplete emptying. It is evident on rectal or vaginal examination as a tender mass, which may discharge rectally or vaginally. Treatment with metronidazole is usually effective.

**Subphrenic Abscess.** Localisation of pus between diaphragm and liver on the right side, or between the diaphragm and the liver, spleen and stomach on the left, is a complication of peritonitis most commonly due to perforation of the stomach, duodenum or gall bladder or to operation on these organs.

There are signs of persistent infection; there may be dullness at the base of the lung and tenderness and slight oedema over the lower ribs posteriorly. Diagnosis is aided by ultrasonography or a radiograph of the diaphragmatic region which may show elevation of the diaphragm, a fluid level below it or an effusion above it. Treatment is by surgical drainage.

**Tuberculous peritonitis,** although now rare in Britain, is still relatively common elsewhere, notably in tropical countries. It is secondary to a tuberculous focus in the abdomen, usually in a mesenteric lymph node and it is characterised by wasting, malaise and abdominal distension. Masses caused by matted omentum and loops of bowel may be palpable. The abdomen contains fluid rich in protein from which tubercle bacilli may be cultured. Diagnosis may also be made by biopsy of granulomas seen at laparotomy or laparoscopy.

In the adult, the condition may be confused with advanced malignant disease and an unnecessarily hopeless prognosis given. The response to antituberculous chemotherapy (p. 259) is good and often dramatic.

## Acute Appendicitis

This condition occurs in both sexes and though it may develop at any age it is more common in young people. It is presumed that the rapid increase in the frequency of acute appendicitis since the turn of the century is connected with a change in dietetic habits to a highly processed, low residue diet and a general adoption of a more sedentary existence. Acute appendicitis is usually obstructive, the lumen of the appendix being narrowed by swelling of lymphoid tissue in its wall, or by stricture from previous inflammation. Obstruction is made complete by impaction of a retained faecolith. Infection and distension lead to gangrene, perforation and peritonitis.

**Clinical Features.** The classical history is of the sudden onset of vague central abdominal pain followed in a few hours by shift of the pain to the right iliac fossa, where it becomes localised to McBurney's point, situated one-third of the distance along a line from the anterior superior iliac spine to the umbilicus. There is nausea and general malaise. There may be vomiting, but this is seldom severe and is often absent. In the early stages there is little elevation of temperature, so that rigors and a high fever make the diagnosis of appendicitis unlikely. The pulse rate is increased and the breath foul.

Locally there is tenderness and guarding in the right iliac fossa, progressing to rigidity as peritonitis develops. Rectal examination should always be carried out; it may disclose tenderness to the right.

The 'classical' history and findings account for less than 50% of cases. The inflamed appendix may simulate many other diseases of the abdomen. In addition to pain, the patient may present with diarrhoea or with urinary or gynaecological symptoms. On occasion acute cholecystitis or perforated peptic ulcer may be mimicked.

**Differential Diagnosis.** In children and adolescents *non-specific mesenteric lymphadenitis* may resemble appendicitis. This condition is probably due to a virus. It is characterised by vague abdominal pain, slight fever and a doughy sensation on palpation. There is ill-defined tenderness in the right iliac fossa. The distinction from appendicitis may be difficult and if in doubt it is safer to operate; otherwise treatment is conservative, recovery taking place gradually over a few weeks.

Formerly a diagnosis of *chronic appendicitis* was made, often in young women, to cover a multitude of chronic or recurring abdominal pains. Removal of the appendix failed to give relief because these patients were suffering from conditions such as the irritable bowel syndrome or dysmenorrhoea.

**Treatment.** The diseased appendix should be removed as early in the acute stage as possible. Attempts to temporise in the belief that mild forms of appendicitis can be distinguished from severe are dangerous, because the condition is notoriously deceptive. When there is obvious peritonitis, vigorous treatment with an antibiotic such as ampicillin given intramuscularly is indicated from the time of the operation.

A conservative policy is allowable only when a clearly defined appendix mass is present, without generalised abdominal signs. Once the mass has subsided, probably within 2 to 3 weeks, the appendix should be removed. Not all patients presenting with an appendix mass require antibiotics. Some need no more than rest, restriction of diet and the avoidance of purgatives. Others in whom there is more marked local tenderness, with low grade fever and general malaise, benefit from ampicillin.

## Tumours of the Small Intestine

Tumours of the small intestine are rare, although there is some evidence that lymphoma is more likely to develop in patients who have coeliac disease. Simple tumours such as polyps and leiomyomas may cause chronic anaemia or intussusception or may be found unexpectedly in the course of radiological investigation or laparotomy.

**Carcinoid tumours** arise from argentaffin cells and are usually seen in the appendix or ileum, although they may occur anywhere in the alimentary tract and cause obstruction. The primary tumour may be elsewhere, for example in a bronchus. Spread to the liver is common where metastases produce 5–hydroxytryptamine causing flushing, borborygmi, diarrhoea and, occasionally, fibrosis of the tricuspid or pulmonary valve. The diagnosis is made on the clinical features and confirmed by finding an excessive amount of 5-hydroxyindoleacetic acid in the urine.

Although long-term survival is possible, even with the systemic manifestions, the primary tumour and associated lymphatic and visceral metastases should be removed whenever possible with the aim of reducing the total volume of secreting tumour. Hepatic lobectomy can be considered when spread appears localised to one lobe.

# DISEASES OF THE LARGE INTESTINE

The main functions of the large bowel are the removal of water from the intestinal contents, the storage of faeces and their evacuation at controlled intervals. Continence depends on training, on the function of a sphincter mechanism in the anal canal and on rectal sensation whereby the need to defaecate is appreciated.

The anal canal is sensitive to pain and touch, as is well demonstrated by the severe pain occasioned by fissures and inflamed piles. The rectum is insensitive to painful stimuli, so that the injection of a sclerosing agent for the treatment of haemorrhoids is painless. Rectal 'sensation' applies to an ability to appreciate distension and contraction.

In addition to clinical examination, including digital examination of the rectum, endoscopy (p. 314), stool examination (p. 315) and radiological investigation (p. 312) are all important aids to diagnosis.

## Ulcerative Colitis

Apart from the bacillary and amoebic dysenteries and tuberculous enterocolitis, there are certain non-specific chronic inflammatory bowel diseases which are associated with ulceration of the colon. One of these is Crohn's disease which may affect both the large and the small bowel; the other, commoner disease affecting the colon, is ulcerative colitis.

**Aetiology.** The aetiology of ulcerative colitis is not known. The disease may be due to an abnormal immune response, possibly to bacteria or to certain foods. In a few patients withdrawal of milk from the diet may improve the diarrhoea, but this could be due to the development of secondary alactasia (p. 351) rather than to specific allergy to milk protein.

A familial tendency is suggested by the increased incidence of the disease amongst relatives of patients and by the association between ulcerative colitis, ankylosing spondylitis and Crohn's disease (p. 351).

Some authorities believe that psychological disturbances are responsible and claim that patients with colitis have a particular personality structure characterised by traits such as undue dependence on others, extreme sensitivity to personal slight and obsessive tendencies. It seems probable, however, that these traits are largely due to the disease process itself, since they disappear or greatly improve during a remission; indeed, one of the most rewarding effects of successful treatment is the remarkable improvement that may occur in the psychological well-being of the patient. Moreover, similar psychological features occur in patients with severe long-standing diarrhoea due to specific causes such as dysentery; nevertheless the patient and the physician may relate the attack or exacerbation to a recent stressful event.

**Pathology.** The inflammatory process may be limited to the rectum, which is almost always involved (*proctitis*). The disease may also involve the distal colon (*distal colitis*) or the entire colon (*total colitis*). Whatever the extent of the disease, the inflammatory change is continuous throughout the affected part, in contrast to the patchy changes that occur in Crohn's disease of the colon. In the early stages the mucosa is swollen and reddened, and punctate bleeding points may be seen. Thereafter, ulceration develops; the ulcers may be superficial or penetrate deeply, spreading longitudinally beneath the mucosa. In severe disease the mucosa may slough in parts to expose granulation tissue; the mucosa that remains becomes oedematous, hyperplastic and raised, giving the appearance of pseudo-polyposis. In *acute fulminant disease* the bowel, especially the transverse colon, may be greatly dilated and the bowel wall becomes thin and may rupture. In long-standing disease, the colon is shortened and generally narrowed with a lack of haustrations.

Microscopically, in contrast to Crohn's disease, inflammation is confined to the mucosa. Initially there is congestion, oedema and intra-mucosal haemorrhage. The number of goblet cells is reduced and the lamina propria is infiltrated with lymphocytes and polymorphs; the latter also accumulate in the lumen of the crypts and are termed 'crypt abscesses'. These may progress to destruction of the mucosa which is replaced by granulation tissue. Finally, on healing, the mucosa has a reduced number of crypts.

**Clinical Features.** The disease occurs at all ages but most commonly between 20 and 40 years. The first attack is usually the most severe and thereafter the disease is characterised by exacerbations and remissions although a minority of patients develop chronic symptoms. The clinical features and the management are largely determined by the extent to which the colon is involved, the severity of the inflammation and the duration of the disease.

The principal symptom is diarrhoea with loose bloody stools containing mucus and pus; defaecation is often accompanied by lower abdominal discomfort, although severe pain is uncommon. Tenesmus may occur because of proctitis. Tenderness may be present on palpation of the colon, especially in the left iliac fossa; when peritoneal irritation is present, it signifies that the serosa is involved in the inflammatory process.

In severe ulcerative colitis, there is exhausting diarrhoea and dehydration. *Toxic dilatation* represents the most serious form with tachycardia, a high swinging temperature and abdominal distension. Untreated, the patient dies as a result of colonic perforation.

In chronic ulcerative colitis the bowel is permanently damaged as a result of fibrosis. The colon in such cases behaves as a rigid tube incapable of absorbing fluid properly or of acting as a faecal reservoir. There is no toxaemia, but the patient lives in chronic ill-health and with persistent diarrhoea.

When the disease is confined to the rectum, the symptoms may be trivial if the inflammation is mild and consist of loose motions and perhaps blood-streaking of the stool. However, a severe proctitis will cause tenesmus, and frequent small loose stools, together with bleeding per rectum, but systemic disturbance is absent. Paradoxically, in distal colitis, spasm may result in constipation, with hard faeces.

Occasionally relapse can be associated with emotional stress, intercurrent infection or the use of antibiotics. There is no special risk during pregnancy, when indeed it is usual for the disease to remit; in contrast there is a tendency for a severe relapse to occur early in the puerperium.

The patient is often anaemic and there may be leucocytosis and a raised ESR. In severe cases there are electrolyte disturbances and protein loss from the colon may lead to hypoalbuminaemia. Sometimes the liver function tests are abnormal. The stool should be cultured for pathogenic bacteria and a search of the mucus made for amoebae to exclude an infective cause for the colitis. Blood cultures are required if septicaemia is suspected.

**Investigation.** *Sigmoidoscopy* is essential in most cases; the mucosa appears engorged and hyperaemic and the normal vascular pattern is obliterated. In severe disease spontaneous bleeding will be seen; in less severe cases the mucosa appears intact, and bleeds only when it is gently rubbed, while in mild cases the only abnormality may be the absence of the normal vascular pattern. Rectal biopsy may be carried out to confirm the diagnosis and to exclude other causes of proctitis, such as Crohn's disease.

*Radiological Examination.* While sigmoidoscopy confirms the diagnosis of ulcerative colitis, a barium enema examination demonstrates its extent. If only the rectum is affected, no abnormalities may be seen. When the disease is more extensive, there is loss of haustration and shortening and narrowing of the colon with a ragged outline due to ulceration of the mucosa (Fig. 8.5). Occasionally the mucosa is undermined to produce a double contour, the final stages of this process being the formation of pseudopolypi.

Barium enema examination should not be attempted in patients with severe colitis because of the risk of perforation. In these cases, plain radiographs of the abdomen may allow a positive diagnosis to be made, since the colon will usually contain sufficient air to outline an abnormal mucosal pattern.

**Complications.** *Toxic dilatation* and *perforation* have already been mentioned. *Stricture* may occur at any level in the colon or rectum; on the barium enema it is usually smooth, but is sometimes difficult to distinguish from carcinoma. *Carcinoma of the colon* develops more often in patients with long-standing ulcerative colitis than it does in the normal population, the risk being related to the duration, extent and age at onset of the disease. The risk increases greatly after the disease has been present for 10 years or more. It is greatest in patients with total colitis who develop the disease under the age of 20 years; in this group the risk of cancer of the colon is about 40 times greater than it is in a comparable normal population.

*Extra-intestinal complications* include enteropathic arthritis (p. 622), aphthous stomatitis, cholangitis, iritis and skin lesions such as erythema nodosum and, rarely but characteristically, pyoderma gangrenosum. Cholangitis and septicaemia may also occur. These complications are most common in advanced cases.

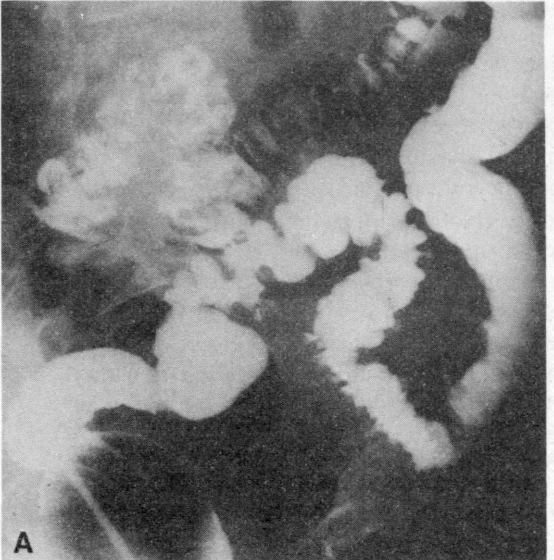


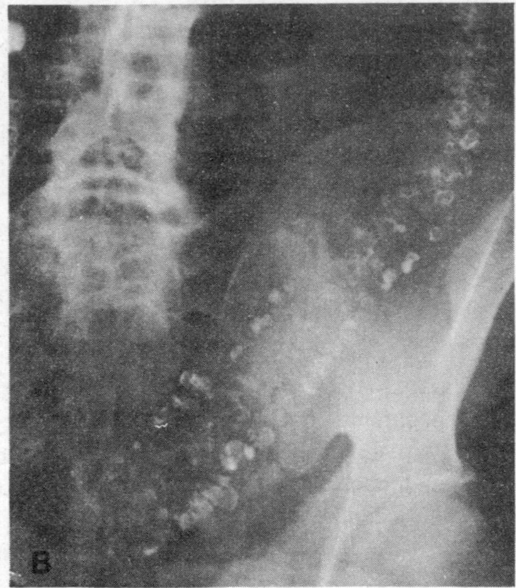


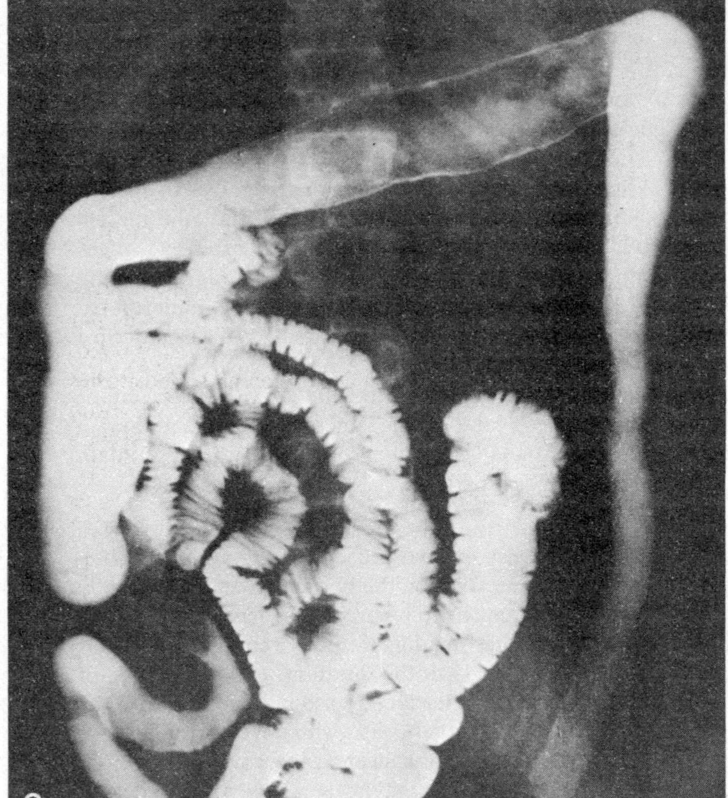


A. Diverticular disease. Spasm and diverticulae are seen in the pelvic colon.

B. Diverticular disease. After evacuation barium persists in the diverticula.

C. Advanced ulcerative colitis. The colon is shortened and its outline is smooth; haustrations are absent.

Fig. 8.5

**Differential Diagnosis.** Ulcerative colitis has to be distinguished from other causes of inflammation of the colonic mucosa namely Crohn's disease (p. 351), amoebic colitis (p. 812), bacillary dysentery (p. 59), campylobacter infections (p. 57), and pseudomembranous colitis (p. 76). Colitis can also occur as a result of ischaemia (p. 371) and radiation therapy. Gonorrhoea is frequently overlooked as a cause of proctitis.

**Treatment.** Admission to hospital is required for patients with severe bowel symptoms, especially when there are general disturbances such as weight loss, anaemia, fever or tachycardia. Such patients may require intense supportive treatment until the disease remits or as a preparation for surgery. Parenteral nutrition through a central venous line allows correction of these deficiencies in the severely wasted patient and will do much to hasten recovery after operation. The measures should include correction of dehydration and electrolyte deficiencies, especially hypokalaemia, blood and plasma infusions to correct anaemia and hypoproteinaemia, and a high protein, low residue diet. Blood cultures should always be taken initially and be repeated throughout the course of the illness if fever persists. Gram-negative bacteria are the commonest organisms involved; if septicaemia is suspected parenteral administration of broad spectrum antibiotics is necessary. However, antibiotics have no special place in the primary management of ulcerative colitis; indeed a broad spectrum antibiotic may precipitate a relapse. Moniliasis of the mouth and upper pharynx is common, especially in ill patients on corticosteroids and must be treated (p. 317).

There is no satisfactory drug for controlling diarrhoea. Codeine phosphate or loperamide may be helpful but these drugs should be avoided in severely ill patients since they may precipitate an attack of toxic dilatation of the colon.

ANTI-INFLAMMATORY DRUGS. 1. *Corticosteroids*. Although there is no specific treatment for ulcerative colitis, the introduction of corticosteroids and corticotrophin has greatly improved the outlook.

(*a*) Local Treatment. When the disease is confined to the distal colon or the rectum, symptoms may be limited to moderate diarrhoea (three or four stools per day) with the passage of blood from time to time, while general health is maintained. Such patients may be treated by administration of corticosteroids as suppositories when there is local rectal involvement, or as self-administered enemas if the distal colon is involved. The preparations commonly used are prednisolone-21-phosphate or betamethasone, and both are available in disposable enema form. The patient is taught to administer the enema, twice daily, retaining the material for as long as possible; suppositories may be inserted twice or three times daily for the treatment of proctitis. Either form of treatment may be continued for several weeks, the duration being judged by the sigmoidoscopic appearances.

(*b*) Systemic Treatment. Prednisolone is given in doses of between 40–60 mg daily by mouth for 3 to 6 weeks depending on response. The usual contraindications to the use of these drugs must be observed (p. 495) and supplements of potassium salts should be given (p. 132). Used in this way, the corticosteroids will induce remission in the majority of patients, the dose being reduced at weekly intervals as improvement takes place. Corticosteroids give rise to a sense of well-being and in addition improve appetite, so that the problem of persuading the patient to eat sufficient food is often solved; they are more effective in a first attack of ulcerative colitis, whereas corticotrophin may be more beneficial in the treatment of relapse. A long-acting form of corticotrophin (e.g. tetracosactrin zinc phosphate complex) should be used, and given in doses of the order of 1 mg daily by intramuscular or subcutaneous injection. This dosage is continued for a week after symptoms have remitted and it is then reduced at weekly intervals as in the case of corticosteroids. For convenience prednisolone may be substituted once the patient has responded adequately.

2. *Sulphasalazine* is split by bacteria in the colon into sulphapyridine and 5-aminosalicylic acid. The latter is probably the component responsible for reducing the chance of relapse of ulcerative colitis when corticosteroids have controlled the disease. It can also be used for mild or moderate attacks of colitis but is less effective than corticosteroids. The dose is 0·5–1 g q.i.d. with food for 1 to 2 years. Sulphasalazine can cause nausea, rashes and occasionally blood dyscrasias.

SURGICAL TREATMENT. If the appropriate medical measures are carried out assiduously, the majority of patients with proctitis or moderately severe colitis will pass into remission. In severe forms of ulcerative colitis, where there is toxic dilatation of the colon or perforation and in the occasional patient with severe haemorrhage, emergency surgical treatment is required. In these urgent circumstances surgery is usually restricted to colectomy with ileostomy, the rectum and distal colon being removed at a later stage when the crisis is over.

Acute ulcerative colitis which fails to respond to medical treatment, or which relapses in spite of adequate treatment, is an indication for proctocolectomy. This is also indicated in chronic forms, where the disease burns out but leaves a permanently damaged bowel, perhaps with stricture formation. Long-standing disease, particularly when the onset has been in childhood, carries a risk of carcinoma and accordingly total bowel involvement, with activity extending over more than 10 years, should lead to serious consideration of surgery.

At all stages of the disease, the timing of and preparation for surgery are important and require a joint medical and surgical approach. In emergency situations, intensive pre-operative replacement of blood, fluid and electrolytes is needed and operation is performed as soon as the patient is fit to withstand surgery. In less urgent situations, the timing of surgery depends on the degree of improvement in the patient's general condition to be expected from preoperative medical measures. Shrewd judgement is required to choose the optimum time before the patient's condition deteriorates again.

Whenever possible, in addition to a full explanation of ileostomy and its management, with a demonstration of the actual appliance to be used, the patient should have the opportunity before operation of meeting someone with an established ileostomy. Modern surgical techniques and the range of ileostomy appliances available make for easy management of the stoma and allow the patient to live an almost normal life with little restriction of physical activity. To be kept in touch with advances in techniques of ileostomy care, patients should join an ileostomy association or be enrolled in a stoma therapy clinic.

When the rectum is not grossly involved it may be preserved and ileo-rectal anastomosis performed. In selected cases ileo-anal anastomosis with formation of an ileal reservoir can be used. The risk of interference with sexual function is thus reduced and the need for a stoma avoided.

**Prognosis.** It is extremely difficult to give a prognosis in ulcerative colitis. The extent of involvement of the colon is an important consideration, the outlook being very much better, for example, if only the rectum is involved. The immediate death rate in patients with fulminating disease, however treated, is not less than 40%, and it is high also in patients developing an attack over the age of 60. In general, the overall mortality from ulcerative colitis is of the order of 10%, but this figure can be very greatly reduced when the patient is treated by those with special experience of the disease. Thus, the mortality from total proctocolectomy done during a remission by an experienced surgeon is about 2%, whereas mortality for proctocolectomy done as an emergency procedure is 10% in the best hands, and may be 20% or 30% in those with little experience of the disease. Attention has been drawn to the risk of carcinoma in long standing cases.

## Diverticular Disease

Though diverticula occur throughout the gastrointestinal tract, they are most common in the large bowel. The presence of diverticula is known as *diverticulosis*; when they are inflamed the condition is known as *diverticulitis*. Such inflammation occurs almost exclusively in colonic diverticula. Because it is often difficult to separate the two conditions on clinical or radiological evidence, they are grouped together under the term 'diverticular disease'.

**Aetiology.** In diverticulosis the muscular coat of the bowel is often greatly thickened, suggesting that the diverticula have formed as a result of increased intracolonic pressure. Manometric measurements support this view. It can be shown that pressure in the bowel is high and that there is an area of spasm or failure to relax at the pelvirectal junction. Epidemiological evidence suggests that dietary factors may be at least partly responsible. Diverticulosis is rare in areas of the world such as Africa and Asia where the usual diet is one of high residue; by contrast the incidence is increasing in Western countries where natural fibre is removed from the diet in the processes of food refining. Moreover there is evidence that intracolonic pressures vary with the bulk of the faecal residue, a high faecal residue being associated with a low intraluminal pressure and vice versa.

Diverticulosis occurs especially in middle-aged or elderly subjects and affects males and females equally.

**Pathology.** The pelvic colon is most commonly involved. Its muscle wall is thickened but the diverticula themselves are pouchings of the mucosa and have no muscle coat. It is not clear how they become inflamed. Radiological examination frequently shows the presence of a faecolith in a diverticulum, and it may be that faeces collect because of the inability of the diverticulum to contract. An area of inflammation may develop in the diverticulum and whilst this may resolve, it may become acute with perforation, local abscess formation, fistula and peritonitis. When there are repeated attacks of diverticulitis, the bowel wall becomes progressively thickened with narrowing of the lumen leading eventually to obstruction.

**Clinical Features.** Pain or discomfort felt in the left iliac fossa is a common complaint and there may be associated local tenderness. Acute diverticulitis can give rise to severe pain, guarding and rigidity on the left side, the signs of peritonitis and obstruction being combined. Change of bowel habit, either of increasing constipation or constipation alternating with diarrhoea, is frequent. This is the most important symptom of distal colonic disease and can occur with any lesion. Before middle age, bowel habits are firmly established and a definite alteration usually betokens organic disease in the colon such as carcinoma or diverticulitis and always calls for investigation. Another presenting feature may be severe rectal bleeding.

In the chronic forms, there may be symptoms of subacute obstruction with increasing abdominal distension, borborygmi and colicky pain. Urinary frequency and dysuria may be present. Occasionally a fistula to the bladder gives rise to pneumaturia and faecal contamination of the urine.

On examination, the thickened tender colon may be palpable in the left iliac fossa. A mass may be present in those patients who have developed diverticulitis, with or without abscess.

**Investigation.** *Sigmoidoscopy* is necessary to exclude cancer of the rectum or pelvi-rectal junction. Both diverticular disease and cancer may coexist or one may mimic the other to the extent that even at operation the true diagnosis is uncertain.

*Radiological Examination.* In diverticulosis, barium enema shows characteristic sacs along the contour of the gut (Fig. 8.5). After evacuation barium is frequently left behind in the diverticula which are clearly outlined. If diverticulitis is present, there will be narrowing, rigidity and lack of normal haustration of a segment of colon. Whether or not there are diverticula present, the main diagnostic difficulty is to distinguish the appearances from those of carcinoma and radiological differentiation may be impossible.

**Treatment.** Asymptomatic diverticulosis is common, is often found accidentally and requires no treatment. Patients who have mild or moderate symptoms will be relieved by regulation of the bowel. A high fibre diet with vegetables, fruit, or bran is usually sufficient. If not, a bulk laxative such as methylcellulose should be used in addition. Purgatives should be avoided.

During an attack of acute diverticulitis, bed rest, co-trimoxazole or ampicillin, fluids intravenously and orally, or even cessation of feeding and nasogastric suction may be required. Most severe attacks subside spontaneously but a few require emergency surgery which will probably be confined to a temporary defunctioning proximal colostomy, to be followed later by local resection. An emergency partial colectomy may be required for acute bleeding.

Elective surgery is indicated, after recovery from an acute attack, in patients who develop obstructive features, who have complications such as fistula and those in whom the possibility of carcinoma cannot be excluded. The treatment of choice is resection of the involved segment of pelvic colon with primary anastomosis.

A few patients fail to respond adequately to medical treatment and of these some will be considered suitable for treatment by primary surgical resection and anastomosis. In patients without advanced fibrotic changes the latter procedure gives good results but its long-term efficacy has still to be established.

## Haemorrhage from the Lower Gastrointestinal Tract

The commonest source is haemorrhoids. Bleeding per rectum may also originate in the rectum itself, in the colon or terminal ileum. With bleeding from the proximal colon or ileum, the blood may appear as melaena. The usual causes are diverticular disease or cancer of the rectum or distal half of the colon. Less common sources of bleeding are polyps, ulcerative colitis, ischaemic colitis and angiodysplasia in the mucosa of the bowel wall.

Rectal examination and sigmoidoscopy will detect most rectal causes of bleeding.

If bleeding is proximal to the rectum, the patient is treated conservatively, as for upper gastrointestinal haemorrhage, and in most cases bleeding will stop. Thereafter barium enema and colonoscopy will detect most lesions. If bleeding continues, angiography of the superior and inferior mesenteric arteries can be performed to detect the site of bleeding and possibly treat it by embolisation through the arterial catheter. If bleeding fails to stop, the appropriate segment of the colon can be resected.

## Carcinoma of the Colon and Rectum

In Britain, carcinoma of the large intestine is the most common malignant tumour of the alimentary tract. In contrast it is rare in Africa and Asia. The variation in incidence of the disease between different countries has led to speculation that dietary factors and differences in bacterial flora of the bowel may be of aetiological significance. Diseases known to be clearly associated with it are long-standing ulcerative colitis and familial multiple polyposis.

**Pathology.** In two-thirds of patients, cancer of the large bowel occurs in the left colon or rectum. Concomitant multiple tumours are present in 2% of cases. The risk of a second cancer may reach 10% in patients with adenomatous polyps. Macroscopically the tumour may be proliferative and fungating, ulcerative and infiltrating, polypoidal or encircling as a 'string' stricture. Perforation may occur at the site of the tumour, leading to peritonitis, localised abscess or a fistula.

Spread occurs directly in and through the bowel wall, by lymphatics and by the bloodstream through both portal and systemic circulations. Colonic carcinoma is capable of direct implantation on exposed surfaces, such as a suture line or area of trauma in the bowel. Metastases most commonly involve the liver.

**Clinical Features.** Symptoms vary depending on the site of the carcinoma. In tumours of the left colon, obstruction is early. Tumours of the right colon present with anaemia, cachexia and alteration of bowel habit, but obstruction is late because of the relatively fluid nature of the bowel contents. As a consequence left-sided tumours tend to be diagnosed earlier.

Change in bowel habit, anaemia, weight loss and sometimes excessive borborygmi, abdominal distension and colicky pains indicating subacute obstruction, all point to a large bowel tumour. Some, however, are relatively symptomless until the patient presents as an emergency with obstruction.

Carcinoma of the lower rectum will almost always cause early bleeding with mucus discharge; later there is tenesmus and a feeling of incomplete emptying of the bowel. Obstruction is a feature of tumours of the pelvirectal junction but not the rectum proper, which is capacious and distensible.

The findings on physical examination range from no obvious abnormality to the signs of advanced malignancy. The majority of rectal tumours can be palpated on digital examination. Fresh blood in the stool should always suggest the possibility of a tumour of the rectum or pelvic colon. Occult blood is found in the stool if an ulcerating lesion is present higher in the colon.

**Investigation.** *Endoscopy*. More than 50% of malignant tumours of the large bowel occur in a part accessible to direct inspection with the sigmoidoscope, i.e. the rectum and the lower pelvic colon and this procedure is mandatory. The whole or part of a growth may be seen and a biopsy carried out. Colonoscopic examination is valuable when a suspicious lesion is seen more proximally on the barium enema.

*Radiological Examination*. A barium enema will demonstrate advanced cancer as a filling defect or stricture (Fig. 8.6). For the demonstration of smaller, earlier tumours, careful preparation of the colon followed by a double contrast barium enema is necessary. A barium follow-through examination may be of value for tumours in the region of the caecum.

**Treatment** of choice is resection of the tumour as a one-stage procedure. If there is no colonic obstruction, or if it can be overcome by enemas, time should be spent in preparing the bowel by washouts and antibiotics. Anaemia should be corrected by preoperative transfusion.

Carcinoma of the rectum will almost always require total removal of the rectum with permanent colostomy and for this the patient requires pre-operative introduction to colostomy and its management (p. 364). However advances in suture techniques allow preservation of continuity in many more patients by means of a colo-rectal or colo-anal anastomosis. Success depends on early diagnosis and operation before spread has occurred and before obstruction renders the surgeon's task more complicated. The possibility of carcinoma must be considered when anyone of middle age presents with rectal bleeding, change of bowel habit or iron-deficiency anaemia.

Serial estimations of CEA levels (p. 40) may lead to the earlier detection of recurrence after operation.

## Benign Tumours of the Large Intestine

Only polyps are found with any frequency. These tumours may be single or multiple and are most commonly found in the left side of the colon. They are sessile or pedunculated; in the latter case the stalk may allow the polyp to move up and down the lumen of the bowel. These tumours may be found incidentally at operation or on barium enema, or they may cause bleeding, discharge of mucus, or intussusception. Occasionally, because of its mobility, a polyp may prolapse through the anus to appear as a red, cherry-like mass.

Although they are primarily benign, polyps of the colon may become carcinomatous. In general polyps of more than 1 cm in diameter are probably malignant. The malignant change may not extend into the stalk, so that removal of the polyp and stalk at colonoscopy may suffice. The stalk as well as the polyp itself should then be examined histologically.

## Multiple Polyposis

In this condition, transmitted by autosomal dominant inheritance, there may be thousands of small polyps diffusely scattered over the mucosal surface of the colon and rectum. They appear at adolescence and become malignant in about 15 years, the patient often dying from carcinomatosis before the age of 40. The disease can be recognised by radiological examination from adolescence onwards of members of affected families. Prevention of carcinoma means removal of the colon and rectum with permanent ileostomy, although symptomless members of the family may find ileorectal anastomosis with diathermy removal of rectal polyps and periodic surveillance more acceptable.

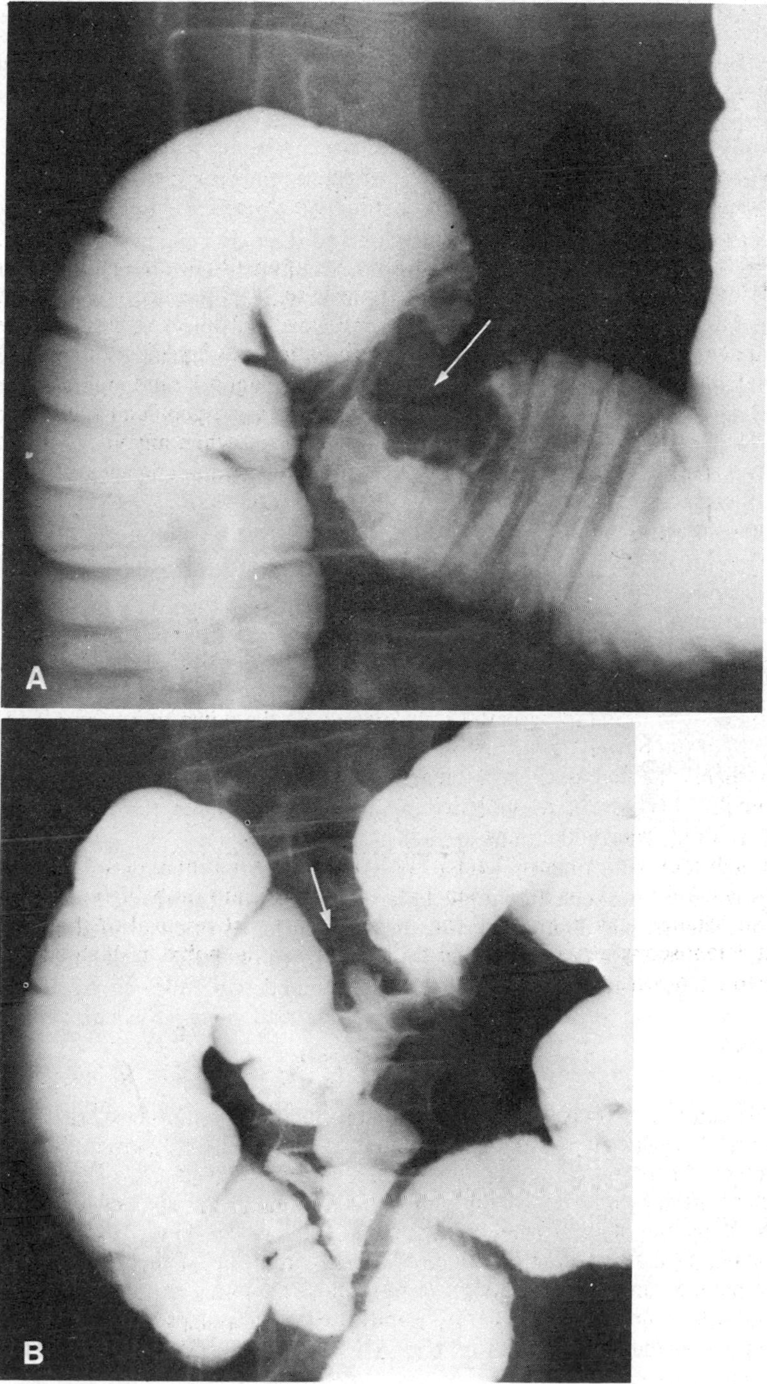


Fig. 8.6 Carcinoma of colon. A. Filling defect in transverse colon. B. Stricture in pelvic colon.

### Megacolon

Megacolon is a condition characterised by dilatation of the colon and obstinate constipation. The disease may be separated into two groups, congenital (Hirschsprung's disease) and acquired megacolon.

**Hirschsprung's Disease.** The cause is a congenital absence of the myenteric nerve plexus in the wall of the pelvic colon and upper rectum. Occasionally the defect extends proximally. Boys are often more affected than girls and symptoms of constipation, abdominal distension and vomiting date from birth. They may come in attacks, but even between attacks there is persistent pot-belly. The rectum is empty on digital examination.

Radiological examination with small amounts of barium shows a small rectum, a narrow segment above and then wide dilatation of the colon full of retained faeces. The diagnosis can be confirmed by rectal biopsy of sufficient thickness to include muscle of the bowel wall.

Treatment is by excision of the abnormal segment of colon and rectum.

**Acquired Megacolon.** In this group of cases, there is no defined aetiology and no defined age-group. Some are examples of a milder, short segment form of Hirschsprung's disease. Others are associated with cretinism. In Chagas' disease (p. 820) autonomic ganglia in the lower colon are destroyed by a trypanosome.

Radiologically, acquired megacolon usually shows no narrowed segment, the dilatation instead extending down to the anus. The rectum is full of faeces.

Most cases can be managed conservatively, by treatment of the cause where identifiable, by high residue diets, laxatives and perhaps saline enemas. In a few patients colonic resection has been used as a last resort in the relief of obstinate constipation.

### Incontinence of Faeces

Incontinence is most common in the elderly or debilitated in whom the appreciation of rectal distension is diminished and the sphincteric and pelvic floor muscles are weakened. It may also be due to faecal impaction with overflow incontinence of soft faeces and require manual or instrumental disimpaction followed by the use of laxatives to prevent recurrence. Senile dementia and psychiatric illness are often other factors.

Incontinence also occurs when the sphincters and the supporting muscles are injured, for example by obstetric tear; various operative procedures are available for their repair. The sphincter mechanisms can be damaged by cancer, Crohn's disease or third degree haemorrhoids or their neurological control may be impaired by spina bifida or trauma to the lumbar spine.

There can be incontinence of faeces even when anal function is normal as in behavioural disturbances in children or in the presence of severe diarrhoea. In both instances treatment must be directed at the primary cause.

## Infections of the Alimentary Tract

Infections of the mouth due to thrush and other organisms are discussed on page 317, and gastroenteritis caused by bacterial food poisoning on page 57. Epidemics of acute but transient gastroenteritis may be caused by Echo, Coxsackie, Rota and other viruses. Usually identification of the viral nature of the infection is not possible and diagnosis is presumptive on epidemiological grounds when no bacterial cause has been demonstrated.

The small intestine is involved in typhoid and paratyphoid fevers (p. 55), cholera (p. 830), staphylococcal enterocolitis (p. 52), tuberculosis (p. 253), giardiasis (p. 814), strongyloidiasis (p. 871) and ancylostomiasis (p. 869).

The principal infections involving the large intestine are bacillary dysentery (p. 59), amoebic dysentery (p. 812), antibiotic-associated pseudomembraneous colitis (p. 76) and schistosomiasis (p. 858).

**Treatment.** Bacterial resistance to antimicrobial agents is readily induced by their indiscriminate use in infections of the gut, many of which are not of bacterial origin. Specific therapy is usually not required in bacillary dysentery due to shigellae and in gastroenteritis due to *Esch. coli*. When it is indicated by the presence of systemic upset, local knowledge of sensitivity is important as resistance may have been acquired to one or more of the antibacterial agents commonly used in that area. Most forms of food poisoning due to salmonellosis similarly do not require specific chemotherapy but more severe attacks may be associated with bacteraemia and must be treated, usually with ampicillin.

Abdominal infection complicating surgical or gynaecological operations and diverticulitis are commonly caused by *Bacteroides fragilis* which respond to metronidazole or the lincomycins.

## Ischaemia of the Alimentary Tract

The intestines are supplied by the coeliac, superior mesenteric and inferior mesenteric arteries. Of these, the superior mesenteric, which supplies the mid-gut, has poor collateral support from the other two arteries. It follows that intestinal ischaemia is usually due to sudden or slow occlusion of the superior mesenteric artery. However, it may also arise from obstruction to the venous outflow from the intestine, or from a reduction in blood flow due to shock or cardiac failure, without evidence of obstruction to the arterial or venous supply. The usual causes of blockage of the superior mesenteric artery are atheroma, thrombosis due to blood diseases or oral contraceptives, and embolism. Most cases of intestinal ischaemia occur in the elderly and in those with cardiac failure or arrhythmias.

**Acute Intestinal Failure.** This term is used to describe the consequences of acute obstruction of the superior mesenteric artery. A variable length of the small intestine undergoes necrosis of the superficial epithelium and over several hours this progresses to gangrene. The patient has abdominal pain, vomiting, watery and later bloody diarrhoea. Signs of peritonitis and hypovolaemic shock develop. There is marked leucocytosis. Most patients will die unless the affected bowel is resected.

**Chronic Intestinal Ischaemia.** This occurs when there is a gradual reduction of blood flow in the superior mesenteric artery with resulting impairment of the normal postprandial increase in blood flow to the small bowel. There is abdominal pain some 30 minutes after each meal so that the patient is afraid to eat and loses weight. The condition is rare.

**Ischaemia of the Large Intestine.** Occlusion of the inferior mesenteric artery leads to ischaemia of the left colon, especially when blood flow in the superior mesenteric artery is also reduced. The disorder is termed *ischaemic colitis*. The patient presents with abdominal pain and bloody diarrhoea and the diagnosis is made by barium enema examination which shows oedema of the mucosa of the affected segment of colon. In contrast to ischaemia of the small intestine, the condition is usually transient, but in some patients it may proceed to gangrene or to stricture usually situated at the splenic flexure.

## Psychogenic Disorders

Gastric secretion, gastrointestinal motility and blood flow are influenced by emotion. Commonly psychological factors cause gastrointestinal disorders some of which mimic organic disease. Patients under stress, or with an anxiety neurosis, may develop a wide range of symptoms such as dry mouth, a lump in the throat, anorexia, nausea, vomiting, aerophagy with belching, abdominal discomfort and pain, diarrhoea or constipation. Patients with depressive illness may have anorexia, a bad taste in the mouth and constipation. It should not be forgotten that such patients may also have an organic lesion in the gastrointestinal tract.

A careful history will usually identify complaints of psychological origin; for example, pain of this type may have no discernible pattern with no clear time or food relationships and the patient often has difficulty in describing it. The more bizarre the description, the less likely is the symptom to be organic in origin. The history should also elicit features indicative of a psychological disturbance.

Occasionally the physical examination will reveal a manifestion of anxiety such as inappropriate sweating or tachycardia. If abdominal tenderness is elicited, this is often quite disproportionate both to the patient's physical well-being and to the complaint.

**Globus hystericus** describes the sensation of a lump in the throat which is independent of swallowing and indeed may be relieved by swallowing food or drink. The symptom occurs most frequently in tense, anxious individuals, but before accepting a psychogenic basis it is necessary to exclude organic disease by a barium swallow and if necessary by endoscopy.

**Psychogenic dyspepsia** is used to describe symptoms such as epigastric discomfort, feelings of undue satiety after eating, anorexia, nausea or vomiting and a complaint of excessive 'wind', associated with psychoneurosis. Sometimes pain is the main feature and may be difficult to distinguish from that of mild peptic ulcer disease. Pain which is diffuse, continuous, lacking in periodicity or present for months or even years is probably psychogenic. Quite often, the physician may suspect the diagnosis is 'nervous' dyspepsia, but is never quite sure; as a result barium meal or endoscopy is carried out. This is nearly always negative but occasionally an unexpected ulcer or cancer is found. When the diagnosis of psychogenic dyspepsia is suspected and the patient is young it is reasonable to proceed without prior investigation; this can be carried out later if the patient fails to respond. However, in the middle-aged, the onset of dyspepsia should never be attributed to neurosis without appropriate investigation.

The psychological origin of the symptoms should be explained. Frequently, such patients recognise that they have a 'weak stomach' which bears the brunt of recurrent stress, but they come to a doctor for reassurance from time to time. Some are helped by small doses of antacids or dicyclomine 10–20 mg with meals; this may be a placebo response.

**Psychogenic vomiting** is not an uncommon manifestation of anxiety neurosis. It occurs usually on wakening, or immediately after breakfast; only rarely does it occur later in the day. It is probably a reaction to awakening and facing up to the worries of everyday life; in the young it can be due to school phobia. There may be retching alone or the vomiting of gastric secretions or food. Although psychogenic vomiting may occur regularly over long periods, there is little or no weight loss and this is of value in distinguishing it from vomiting due to organic disease of the alimentary tract. Early morning vomiting also occurs in pregnancy, alcoholic abuse and depression.

It is essential in all cases to assess and, if possible, alleviate the underlying psychological disturbance. Tranquillisers and antiemetic drugs have only a secondary place.

## The Irritable Bowel Syndrome

One of the commonest disorders of the alimentary tract is that of long-standing colonic dysfunction associated with abdominal pain for which no organic cause can be found. Bowel habit is disturbed by diarrhoea or constipation occurring alone, or alternating. This irritable bowel syndrome is also known as *spastic colon* and *idiopathic* or *nervous diarrhoea*.

**Aetiology.** Manometric studies from the distal colon have shown various patterns. When constipation and pain are the predominant symptoms, intraluminal pressure is usually increased and there is an increased frequency of pressure waves, whereas motor activity is often reduced in patients with painless diarrhoea. These changes are not constant, and may not be detectable when the patient is symptom-free. Motility studies are not of value for diagnostic purposes.

Several factors may be involved in causation. Psychological disturbances, especially anxiety, are frequent; patients with the irritable bowel syndrome are often tense, conscientious individuals who worry excessively about family or financial affairs. Many relate the onset of their symptoms to an attack of infective diarrhoea. Some patients seem obsessed with bowel function and have taken purgatives constantly to ensure regular defecation.

**Clinical Features.** The syndrome occurs more commonly in women, usually between the ages of 20 and 40 years. The commonest symptom is abdominal pain, occurring in attacks and referred to the left or right iliac fossa or to the hypogastrium; it may be continuous or colicky, diffuse or localised and is rarely severe. It is generally relieved by defecation and is sometimes provoked by food. In some patients pain is associated solely with constipation, the stools being hard and pellet-like and accompanied by mucus. In other patients occasional bouts of diarrhoea are interspersed by periods of constipation when purgatives may be taken which precipitate another episode of diarrhoea, leading to a vicious cycle. Some patients complain of intermittent painless diarrhoea, passing several loose or watery stools daily during an attack. Diarrhoea occurs characteristically during the morning, either before or immediately after breakfast and it almost never occurs during the night. Defaecation is often precipitate after meals, presumably due to an exaggerated gastrocolic reflex.

Other symptoms include abdominal distension and an awareness of intestinal peristalsis or audible borborygmi. Nausea, anorexia and complaints of tiredness and weakness occur, especially during attacks of diarrhoea. Vomiting is uncommon.

The patient may appear anxious, but seems well otherwise. Tenderness is common over the pelvic colon which is often easily palpable because it is contracted. Rectal examination is normal and the rectum is usually empty.

**Investigation.** Although the diagnosis is usually suggested by the history alone, organic bowel disease has to be excluded, especially in patients developing symptoms for the first time over the age of 40 years. Sigmoidoscopy is essential to exclude an organic lesion of the distal colon. The mucosa appears normal in the irritable bowel syndrome but the colon may show marked motor activity, contracting and relaxing quite unlike the normal inert bowel. Barium enema examination is necessary principally to exclude organic disease; there are no diagnostic radiological features. There is no anaemia and ESR is normal. In patients whose principal complaint is painless diarrhoea, the possibility of lactose intolerance, mild hyperthyroidism or alcohol excess should not be overlooked.

**Treatment.** The patient must first be reassured on the basis of the normal findings on examination and investigation, as anxiety may precipitate or aggravate the condition and there is sometimes an underlying fear of cancer. In patients with persistent or troublesome symptoms, measures designed to modify the intestinal dysmotility are required. For constipation and pain, the patient should be encouraged to increase the roughage content of the diet and one of the hydrophilic colloids should be prescribed in a dose sufficient to ensure a normal bowel movement. It is important that the patient should stop laxatives. Pain and diarrhoea may be relieved by an anticholinergic drug such as dicyclomine or mebeverine hydrochloride thrice daily. The physiological basis of the symptoms should be explained without implying that the pain is not real. For patients with painless diarrhoea, improvement is commonly obtained with some dietary restriction, particularly the avoidance of fresh fruits and salads. Codeine phosphate and loperamide are useful drugs which act quickly and can be carried by the patient to use in emergency or they can be taken before any event which is known to precipitate diarrhoea.

## Prospects in Alimentary Disease

In the past decade a more accurate diagnosis of gastrointestinal disease has been made possible by the development of sophisticated endoscopic and radiological procedures. This precision is being still further improved by non-invasive methods, notably ultrasonography and computed scanning. In addition, radiographic techniques are being used increasingly for therapeutic purposes, especially for the control of gastrointestinal bleeding.

The ability to treat most cases of peptic ulceration with $H_2$-receptor antagonists and the success of highly selective vagotomy in those who require surgery, has led to more satisfactory management of the majority of patients. There remains the significant problem of those who develop ulcers or bleeding from erosions as a result of consuming aspirin or other drugs, particularly for the treatment of arthritis. It is likely that an increased understanding of the components of the gastric mucosal 'barrier' and the development of drugs to strengthen it, for example the prostaglandins, will avoid these complications.

Functional gastrointestinal disease remains a significant cause of illness. Our understanding of the mechanisms involved is rudimentary. The development of research into gastrointestinal motility and the increased awareness of the large number of interacting gastrointestinal hormones may eventually provide therapeutic benefits.

The surgical treatment of gastrointestinal disorders will continue to show technical improvement like the advent of new stapling techniques for safer anastomoses which is one factor in the development of sphincter sparing operations in the distal colon and rectum. Whilst these advances in technique offer more acceptable operations, the problem of gastrointestinal cancer remains; the utilisation of chemotherapy is in its infancy and the main hope still lies in the identification of carcinogens and their elimination from the diet and environment.

G. P. CREAN
D. J. C. SHEARMAN
W. P. SMALL

*Further reading*:

*Clinics in Gastroenterology*. London: Saunders.— A series of specialist volumes consisting of three numbers annually and each dealing with a specific disorder of the alimentary tract. Recommended for selective reading and as a reference library to current practice.

Cummack, D. H. (1969) *Gastrointestinal X-ray Diagnosis*. Edinburgh: Churchill Livingstone.— A comprehensive atlas of gastrointestinal lesions with informative legends and concise text.

French, E. B. (1979) Examination of the Alimentary System. In *Clinical Examination*. 5th edn, ed. Macleod, J. Edinburgh: Churchill Livingstone.— Complementary to this chapter and designed to be read in conjunction with it.

Shearman, D. J. C. & Finlayson, N. D. C. (1981) *Diseases of the Gastrointestinal Tract and Liver*. Edinburgh: Churchill Livingstone.— A new textbook primarily for clinicians.

Sleisenger, M. H. & Fordtran, J. S. (1978) *Gastrointestinal Disease*, 2nd edn. London: Saunders.— The most complete reference text presently available. Contains extensive bibliographies to each chapter.

# 9. Diseases of the Liver and Biliary Tract

## THE LIVER

### Anatomy

The liver is the largest organ in the body, weighing 1200–1500 g. It has right and left lobes separated by the falciform ligament anteriorly, the fissure of the ligamentum teres inferiorly and the fissure of the ligamentum venosum posteriorly. The right lobe is the larger; it contains the quadrate lobe on the anteromedial part of the inferior surface and the caudate lobe on the medial part of the posterior surface. The left lobe is relatively larger in infancy and contributes to the protuberant abdomen at that age.

Histologically, the liver is divided into lobules based on a central vein and peripheral portal tracts with regular radiating sinusoids and plates of liver cells between them. The central veins are tributaries of the hepatic veins which drain to the inferior vena cava; the portal tracts contain branches of the hepatic artery, the portal vein, lymphatics and the bile ducts; the sinusoids are channels, lined by endothelial and phagocytic (Kupffer) cells, which receive blood separately from the hepatic arterial and portal venous sytems and convey it to the central veins; the liver cells (hepatocytes) are arranged in single-cell plates which lie between and separate the sinusoids from one another. Between the liver cells and the sinusoidal cells is the space of Disse which contains fluid draining to the lymphatics in the portal tracts. Individual hepatocytes either line the space of Disse or abut on other liver cells; electron microscopically, the part of the membrane lining the space of Disse has irregular microvilli, while a part of the membrane adjacent to other liver cells helps to form the lining of the bile canaliculi, and here regular microvilli project into the canalicular lumen. These bile canaliculi form networks between the hepatocytes conveying bile towards the terminal bile ducts which link the intralobular bile canaliculi to the larger interlobular bile ducts in the portal tracts.

The liver has an arterial and a venous blood supply and total blood flow is normally about 1500 ml/min. The arterial supply is by the hepatic artery, a branch of the coeliac axis, which enters the liver in the porta hepatis and is distributed throughout the liver via the portal tracts. Its precise terminal distribution is uncertain, but most of its blood enters the sinusoids directly. In man, the hepatic artery supplies about 35% of the total liver blood flow and about 50% of its total oxygen supply. The portal vein drains its blood from the alimentary tract, spleen, pancreas and gall bladder. It also enters the liver in the porta hepatis, is distributed throughout the liver via the portal tracts and empties its blood into the sinusoids. The oxygen content of portal blood varies and is lowest during digestion.

**Clinical Aspects.** The upper border of the liver extends from the fifth rib medial to the right midclavicular line to the sixth rib in the left midclavicular line. Its lower margin crosses the epigastrium midway between the xiphisternum and the umbilicus.

As the liver descends 1–3 cm in inspiration, it can normally be palpated in adults below the right costal margin during deep inspiration. Heavy percussion from above and light percussion from below in the right midclavicular line helps to determine liver size; percussion is of greatest value in revealing a small liver. Auscultation over the liver may reveal a rub due to perihepatitis, a venous hum between the xiphisternum and umbilicus due to collateral vessels in portal hypertension, or, rarely, an arterial bruit due to hepatocellular carcinoma or acute alcoholic hepatitis.

## Physiology

Liver cells carry out a wide variety of metabolic functions facilitated by the rich blood supply derived from the gut as well as the systemic circulation, and by the intimate contact between hepatocytes and blood due to the highly permeable sinusoidal lining. All hepatocytes appear capable of performing the many functions of the liver.

**Carbohydrate Metabolism.** The liver is the most important organ for maintenance of normal blood glucose concentration. It can convert glucose, fructose, galactose, glycerol, certain amino acids and 2- and 3-carbon compounds such as lactate, pyruvate and oxaloacetate to glucose or to glycogen. When exogenous carbohydrate is not available, the blood glucose concentration is maintained by endogenous glucose production, 90% of which is derived from the liver by glycogenolysis or gluconeogenesis.

Glycogen stores become exhausted within about 24 hours of fasting, after which further glucose is provided directly by gluconeogenesis. Extrahepatic factors such as insulin, adrenaline, thyroxine, cortisol and glucagon profoundly affect carbohydrate metabolism in the liver.

**Protein Metabolism.** The synthesis of many proteins and their export into the blood is a major liver function. Indeed, all the plasma albumin and most of its globulins, other than the gammaglobulins, are made there. Globulins made in the liver, often exclusively, include coagulation factors I (fibrinogen), II (prothrombin), V, VII, IX and X, many of the components of the complement system, transport proteins such as transferrin and haptoglobin and proteins with no certain physiological function such as caeruloplasmin, $\alpha_2$-macroglobulin and $\alpha_1$-antitrypsin. Alpha-fetoprotein is made normally in substantial amounts only prior to and shortly after birth (p. 386). The result of this extensive synthetic activity is that the electrophoretic pattern of the plasma proteins is largely determined by liver function. The liver is also an important site of amino acid deamination prior to their interconversion and oxidation. Urea synthesis from the amino groups released by this process occurs solely in the liver.

**Lipid Metabolism.** Dietary fat is largely triglyceride, and it enters the body in chylomicrons (Fig. 9.1). Triglyceride is removed from the chylomicrons by lipoprotein lipase in the blood; the triglyceride is taken up by many tissues and the chylomicron remnants are removed by the liver. Triglyceride taken up by the liver is broken down to 2-carbon fragments which may be used in many metabolic processes. Free (non-esterified) fatty acids, liberated from the fat stores into the blood, are also taken up by the liver and used similarly. Among these processes is the synthesis of new lipid molecules — triglyceride, phospholipid and cholesterol — which are combined with specific apoproteins to form lipoproteins which are released into the blood. These include very low density (pre $\beta$) lipoproteins (VLDL) and high density ($\alpha$) lipoproteins (HDL). VLDL are converted by lipoprotein lipase in the blood to low density ($\beta$) lipoproteins (LDL) which transport triglyceride to muscles and other tissues as a source of energy or to the fat depots for storage. The functions of HDL are uncertain, but they may be important in cholesterol transport. The liver synthesises more cholesterol than any other organ and this can be incorporated into lipoproteins, converted into bile acids or excreted into the bile. In biliary obstruction of any severity the serum lipid concentration increases, largely due to the formation of an abnormal lipoprotein known as lipoprotein X.

**Bilirubin** is produced from the ferroporphyrin, haem, after removal of its iron component. Most (80%) is derived from haemoglobin breakdown by reticuloendoth-

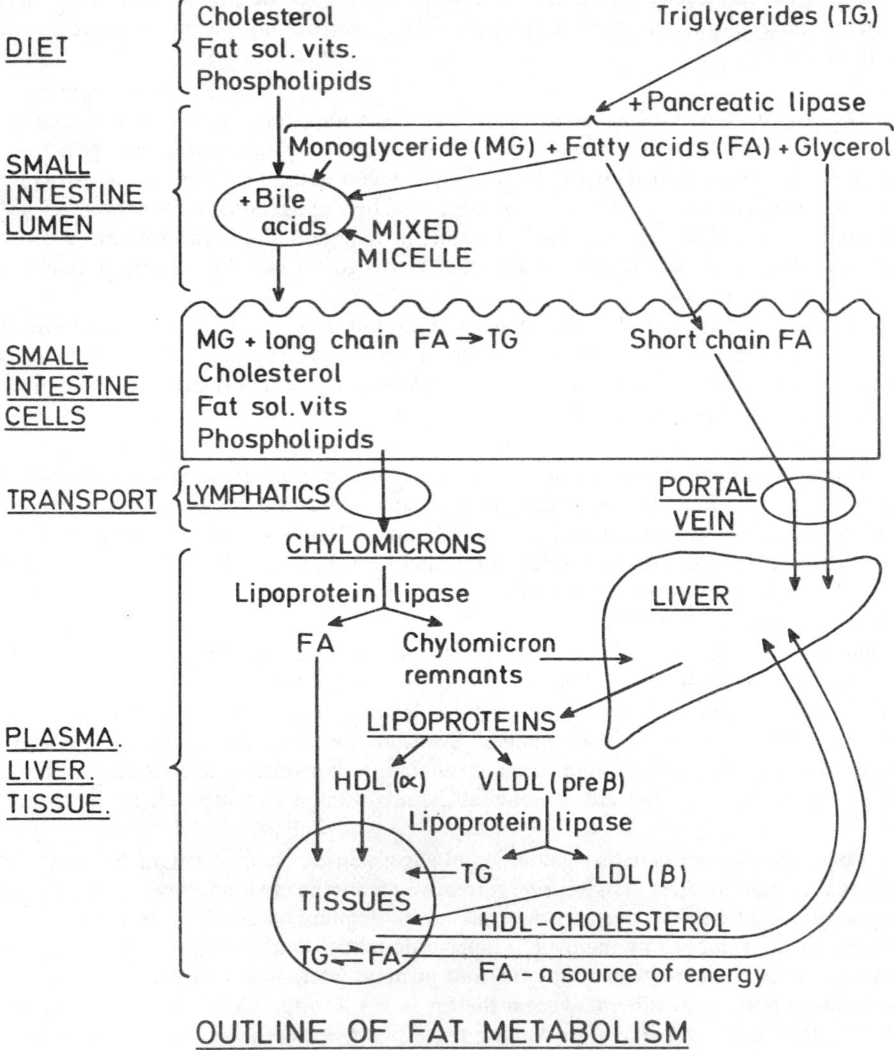


Fig. 9.1 See text pages 346 and 377.

elial cells in the liver, spleen and bone marrow, the rest being formed by catabolism of other haem-containing proteins, particularly enzymes (e.g. cytochromes, peroxidases, and catalase) and myoglobin. This bilirubin is unconjugated and is not water soluble; it is bound to albumin in the plasma and does not pass into the urine. It is taken up by the hepatocytes, conjugated with glucuronic acid and excreted into the bile. Bilirubin monoglucuronide is formed in the microsomes by the enzyme glucuronyl transferase and is then converted to bilirubin diglucuronide by an unknown mechanism either in the microsomes or at the biliary canalicular membrane. Bilirubin diglucuronide is water soluble and is the only form of bilirubin in bile. It is excreted into bile by active transport.

Conjugated bilirubin is not absorbed in the small intestine. Bacteria in the terminal ileum and colon, however, reduce it to a group of tetrapyrrolic substances. Most of these (stercobilinogen) are excreted in the stool (100–200 mg/day). Some are absorbed from the gut and pass to the liver where most are re-excreted in the bile; a small amount (4 mg/day) passes through the liver and is excreted in the urine where it is known as urobilinogen. Urobilinogen and its oxidation product urobilin in the urine are identical, respectively, with stercobilinogen and its oxidation product, stercobilin, in the faeces.

**Bile Acids.** Cholic and chenodeoxycholic acids, the primary bile acids, are produced in the liver from cholesterol. They are conjugated with glycine or taurine and secreted into the bile in which they reach the duodenum. Most (95%) of the bile acids are reabsorbed into the portal blood at specific sites in the terminal ileum; they pass to the liver and are almost completely re-excreted in the bile. Small amounts reach the colon and are metabolised by the colonic bacteria. Deconjugation and changes in the structure of the primary bile acids result in the production of secondary bile acids, deoxycholic acid from cholic acid, and lithocholic acid from chenodeoxycholic acid. Most of the secondary bile acids are excreted in the faeces. However, small amounts are absorbed, reach the liver where they are conjugated with glycine or taurine, and are excreted in the bile. Bile, therefore, contains two primary bile acids —cholic and chenodeoxycholic — and two secondary bile acids — deoxycholic and lithocholic. This *enterohepatic circulation* allows large amounts of bile acid to be delivered to the intestine daily from a relatively small total bile acid pool (6 mmols; 3 g) owing to frequent recycling (10 cycles/day) through the bowel. Synthesis of new bile acid compensates only for that lost in the faeces. The hepatic capacity for bile acid synthesis is limited, and large losses from the bowel cannot be replaced. Little bile acid reaches the systemic circulation normally, but the amount increases in liver disease.

Bile acids, as they enter bile, combine to form micelles (Fig 9.1). In the small intestine, provided the bile acid concentration remains sufficient to maintain the micellar state, this greatly increases the efficiency of fat absorption. Insufficiency of bile acids results in poor absorption of dietary fat and fat-soluble vitamins, notably D and K. Such deficiency may result from impaired synthesis in chronic liver disease, biliary obstruction, small intestinal overgrowth of bacteria capable of deconjugating and dehydroxylating bile acids, and loss of bile acids into the colon in disease of the terminal ileum or after its resection. In this last instance, the bile acids interfere with colonic water and electrolyte metabolism causing diarrhoea, while their absence from the small intestine results in steatorrhoea.

**Vitamin and Hormone Metabolism.** Some vitamins are stored in the liver. These include vitamins A, D, K, $B_{12}$ and folate. In addition, vitamin K is required by hepatocytes for production of coagulation factors II, VII, IX and X. Metabolic reactions in the liver involving vitamins include conversion of tryptophan to nicotinic acid (p. 113), phosphorylation of thiamin (p. 110), and 25-hydroxylation of vitamin D (p. 101).

Many hormones are metabolised and inactivated, including thyroxine, antidiuretic and steroid hormones such as cortisol and oestrogens. Some of the metabolic products, e.g. those of oestrogen, are excreted in the bile.

**Drug Metabolism.** The liver is quantitatively the most important organ for this function. Most drugs metabolised are fat-soluble and their conversion into water-soluble substances makes them suitable for excretion in bile or urine. These conversions are carried out by enzymes of low specificity located in the microsomes. Two types of reaction usually occur; first, oxidation, reduction, or hydroxylation reactions, and second, conjugation reactions in which glucuronides are usually produced. Methylation, acetylation, sulphation and amino-acid conjugation may also occur. The pharmacological results of drug metabolism vary. Barbiturates undergo oxidation with loss of activity; cyclophosphamide is metabolised from an inactive substance to an active alkylating agent; phenylbutazone is oxidised to another active agent, oxyphenbutazone; and codeine is converted in part to morphine. Conjugation, as occurs with salicylates, paracetamol and morphine, almost always causes loss of activity. Acetylation of sulphonamides makes them less soluble and therefore potentially more harmful. When two drugs are metabolised by the same microsomal enzymes, each retards the metabolism of the other, leading to prolongation of drug action and the danger of overdosage. This is an example of one mechanism causing an undesirable drug interaction in therapy.

The action of many drugs is determined largely by their speed of metabolism in the microsomal enzyme system, the activity of which may be altered by dietary and hormonal factors. In particular, microsomal enzyme activity may be greatly increased by certain drugs they themselves metabolise, an effect referred to as *enzyme induction*, due to an increase in enzyme protein which disappears when the drug is withdrawn. Drugs producing this effect — 'inducing agents' — are many and include barbiturates, phenylbutazone and phenytoin. Enzyme induction has important therapeutic consequences, for an enzyme inducer such as a barbiturate may increase the required dose of another drug, such as warfarin; if only the inducing drug is then stopped, bleeding from overdosage of the anticoagulant may occur.

The liver metabolises about 90% of alcohol (ethanol) ingested, the rest being excreted by the lungs and kidneys. It is oxidised via acetaldehyde to acetate with the eventual formation of carbon dioxide. These reactions are carried out mainly by alcohol dehydrogenase, a mitochondrial enzyme, and the microsomal ethanol oxidising system. The latter, like other microsomal enzyme systems such as $\gamma$GT (p. 383) may be induced by drugs, including alcohol itself, and this may in part account for increased alcohol tolerance in drinkers and for their resistance to the action of microsomally metabolised drugs. Conversely, the effects of alcohol may be enhanced when a microsomally metabolised drug such as chlormethiazole is taken concomitantly; this is a very important example of drug interaction.

In liver disease, drug metabolism may be impaired, and care is needed to avoid overdosage, particularly with sedative drugs. The extent to which individual drugs are affected is very variable and cannot be predicted. Special care should, therefore, be taken whenever hepatic damage is present, particularly where there is evidence of severe liver damage, such as ascites, encephalopathy, hypoalbuminaemia or a prolonged prothrombin time.

**Reticuloendothelial Function.** Approximately 20% of the hepatic cell mass is due to reticuloendothelial cells, including the Kupffer cells. Effete red cells are broken down by these cells. The Kupffer cells also have important but poorly understood immunological functions. Antigens from the gut normally gain repeated access to the body. They are carried in the portal blood to the liver where the Kupffer cells phagocytose them and prevent their eliciting immunological responses. Kupffer cells are also very efficient at removing immune complexes from the blood. The liver, therefore, is able to prevent undesirable immunological reactions.

## Liver Function Tests

The term 'liver function tests' refers to a group of biochemical investigations useful in confirming that the liver is diseased, in indicating whether hepatic cells (parenchymal liver disease) or the biliary tree (obstructive or cholestatic liver disease) is primarily involved, in giving an indication of the extent of liver damage and in assessing progress. The term is misleading in that many of the investigations do not measure liver functions and most liver functions are not tested in clinical practice; however, the term has become generally accepted. Liver function tests are variably abnormal in patients with liver disease and therefore a group of tests is usually done. It is important to realise that there are no patterns of abnormality indicative of specific diagnoses and that normality of all the commonly used tests does not prove that the liver is normal.

**Bilirubin.** The normal serum bilirubin is 5–17 $\mu$mol/*l* (0·3–1·0 mg/100 ml) and for practical purposes it is all unconjugated. Unconjugated hyperbilirubinaemia without any abnormality of other liver function tests may result from increased bilirubin production, as in haemolysis, or from inability to transport bilirubin across the liver, as in Gilbert's syndrome. Except in the newborn, the hyperbilirubinaemia rarely exceeds 100 $\mu$mol/*l*, and there is no bilirubin in the urine. Conjugated hyperbilirubinaemia without any abnormality of other liver function tests, as in the rare Dubin-Johnson syndrome, is accompanied by bilirubinuria but is uncommon. Estimates of unconjugated and conjugated bilirubin in the blood are hardly ever necessary, and cannot be done accurately when the total serum bilirubin is less than 70 $\mu$mol/*l* using generally available methods. Hyperbilirubinaemia in hepatobiliary disease is predominantly conjugated, bilirubinuria is present, and other tests of liver function are almost always abnormal. The serum bilirubin in parenchymal liver disease varies widely depending on the severity of the disease and its activity. It gives an accurate measure of the depth of jaundice and repeated estimations may be useful in following the progress of disease. Very high concentrations of bilirubin occur most frequently in biliary tract obstruction, with sustained high levels where this is due to malignant disease and more fluctuating levels where obstruction is caused by gallstones.

Simple, sensitive, inexpensive dipstick tests for bilirubin in the urine are available and useful. Unconjugated bilirubin is bound to albumin in the blood and does not pass into the urine and conjugated bilirubin is not detectable in the urine of normal persons. Consequently, bilirubinuria implies a conjugated hyperbilirubinaemia and points to hepatobiliary disease. Conversely, absence of bilirubinuria in a jaundiced patient suggests haemolysis or a congenital non-haemolytic hyperbilirubinaemia such as Gilbert's syndrome.

**Urobilinogen.** A simple dipstick test is available to detect excessive urobilinogenuria. There is normally a diurnal variation in the urinary output of urobilinogen, maximal excretion occurring in the afternoon when tests are best performed. Since it is readily oxidised to urobilin on exposure to air at room temperature, only fresh urine samples should be used. Excess urinary urobilinogen occurs in haemolytic diseases owing to increased bilirubin excretion leading to increased urobilinogen formation; in these patients bilirubinuria is not present. Any cause of hepatic parenchymal dysfunction — viral hepatitis, cirrhosis, malignancy, partial biliary obstruction, pyrexia or cardiac failure — will reduce the biliary re-excretion of urobilinogen and increase its excretion in the urine; bilirubinuria may or may not be present. In cholestatic jaundice, absence of urinary urobilinogen for over a week indicates complete biliary obstruction.

**Enzymes.** Liver cells contain many enzymes which may be released into the blood in various pathological processes. Measurement of the activity of these enzymes in the blood may give evidence of hepatocellular disease and of its general nature. In practice, maximum information may be obtained by measuring the activity of relatively few enzymes. It must be remembered in interpreting the results of these tests that none of the enzymes usually measured is specific to the liver and alternative sources should be considered, particularly where abnormalities have been found incidentally in patients with minimal or no clinical evidence of liver disease.

TRANSFERASES. The two important enzymes in this group are aspartate amino transferase, AST (glutamic oxaloacetic transaminase, GOT) and alanine aminotransferase, ALT (glutamic pyruvic transaminase, GPT); both are present in the cytosol of the hepatocytes, the former also being found in the mitochondria. Normal serum contains low enzyme activity (5–40 u/*l*) the source of which is unknown. Irrespective of the cause, whenever liver cells are damaged or killed the enzymes are liberated into the blood; this is therefore a test of the integrity of the liver cells. The highest activities are caused by any form of acute liver damage. In viral hepatitis there is generally increased activity even in the prodromal phase and maximal levels of 10 to 100 times the normal value are usually reached in the jaundiced phase after which activity falls rapidly. Equally high activity occurs in acute hepatitis due to drugs, in acute circulatory failure and in exacerbations of chronic active hepatitis. Most patients (80%) with infectious mononucleosis also have an acute hepatitis (few, 10%, become jaundiced) with serum transferase activity raised 2 to 10 times. Serum transferase activity rarely rises more than five-fold in acute alcoholic hepatitis. Patients with cirrhosis usually show only modest elevations of serum transferase. In obstructive jaundice, activity may rise up to four-fold but rarely more unless cholangitis is present.

Increased serum transferase activity is a very sensitive index of hepatic damage. Neither enzyme is specific to the liver, but as alanine aminotransferase is found there in much higher concentration than in other organs, increases in its activity indicate more specifically that hepatic damage is present. These enzymes are of principal value in the diagnosis of acute hepatitis and in differentiating hepatocellular from obstructive jaundice. They are of no prognostic value in either acute or chronic liver disease.

ALKALINE PHOSPHATASE. This enzyme occurs in almost all tissues; in liver cells it is situated principally in the canalicular and sinusoidal membranes. Normal serum contains alkaline phosphatase activity (40–100 u/*l*) derived mainly from bone and liver, and to a lesser extent intestine; in pregnancy additional activity of placental origin is found. When hepatocytes are damaged, relatively little alkaline phosphatase is liberated into the blood, most probably coming from cells which are killed. In hepatocellular disease, either acute or chronic, alkaline phosphatase does not usually exceed 250 u/*l*. When the biliary tract is obstructed at any level, new alkaline phosphatase is synthesised in the hepatocyte membrane much of which escapes into the blood. A greatly increased blood alkaline phosphatase activity is, therefore, the main indicator of biliary obstruction though it does not give any information regarding the site of that obstruction. The alkaline phosphatase activity has no prognostic significance in liver disease.

Sometimes a raised blood alkaline phosphatase activity may be found incidentally and may be the sole abnormality. Hepatobiliary disease may be present, but it is important to ensure that the alkaline phosphatase does not have an extrahepatic origin before investigating the liver further. This may be done by electrophoretic separation of the isoenzymes of alkaline phosphatase. Bone is the main alternative origin of a raised serum alkaline phosphatase: it results from increased osteoblastic activity, such as occurs in adolescents when it may reach 250 u/*l*, in Paget's disease, rickets, hyperparathyroidism, and in metastatic tumour in bone. Myelomatosis, though affecting bone extensively, is not associated with much bone repair and the blood alkaline phosphatase is not usually raised. During pregnancy, alkaline phosphatase of placental origin may increase the serum activity to 250 u/*l*.

OTHER ENZYMES. Measurement of the serum activity of numerous enzymes has been advocated in the investigation of liver disease. These include *5′ nucleotidase*, a membrane-bound enzyme the activity of which, like alkaline phosphatase, rises especially in biliary obstruction, and *γ-glutamyl transferase* (*γGT*), a microsomal enzyme, the activity of which rises in many liver diseases and in response to drugs, including alcohol, which induce microsomal enzymes. In practice, however, the transferases and alkaline phosphatases usually give all the information needed.

**Plasma Proteins.** *Albumin* is made solely in the liver and its production is impaired by severe parenchymal damage. In chronic liver disease, especially cirrhosis, the serum albumin concentration is frequently below normal, reflecting the clinical state and indicating impaired hepatic synthetic capacity; serial readings offer some guide to prognosis. Low serum albumin concentrations in patients with ascites may be partly dilutional, and other non-hepatic factors contributing to hypoalbuminaemia include malnutrition and fever. Serum albumin has a long half-life (20–26 days) and consequently changes in concentration occur slowly. Thus, even in severe acute hepatitis, the serum albumin remains normal unless the illness continues for many weeks.

*Globulins*. It is characteristic of chronic liver disease that hyperglobulinaemia occurs in addition to hypoalbuminaemia; it may be found irrespective of changes in the serum albumin concentration in prolonged viral hepatitis or chronic active hepatitis. Once established, hyperglobulinaemia tends to persist in most patients with cirrhosis. It represents a reaction of the reticuloendothelial system in general and does not directly reflect liver cell damage. The causes of hyperglobulinaemia are not fully understood; increases in gammaglobulins are prominent and probably reflect an increased activity of the immune system, to which many factors may contribute; in those with hypoalbuminaemia it may represent a response to a reduced colloid osmotic pressure in the plasma. Individual immunoglobulins are variably increased, IgG mainly in chronic active hepatitis and cryptogenic cirrhosis, IgA mainly in alcoholic liver disease and IgM in primary biliary cirrhosis. Variations, however, are so frequent that Ig measurements are not of much diagnostic value.

*Plasma Protein Electrophoresis*. Various changes occur in the electrophoretic pattern of the plasma proteins in cirrhosis. The commonest are a decreased albumin and an increased gammaglobulin peak. There is some relation between certain electrophoretic patterns and particular forms of liver disease, but this is not precise enough to be of great diagnostic value. Monoclonal gammopathy occurs rarely but does not have any clear diagnostic or prognostic implication.

**Coagulation Factors.** Severe liver damage impairs the production of several coagulation factors. This is most readily detected by the one stage prothrombin time which depends, among other things, on coagulation factors II, VII and X of liver origin. As the plasma concentration of any one of these factors has to fall to less than 30% of normal before the prothrombin time becomes abnormal, prolongation in chronic liver disease indicates severe liver dysfunction. Furthermore, as the normal plasma half-life of these factors is short (5–72 hours), prothrombin time changes occur relatively quickly after liver damage and abnormalities are found in severe acute hepatitis. Indeed, in acute hepatitis, such as viral heptatitis, the prothrombin time is a most valuable prognostic guide; an abnormal value indicates severe damage and an increasing prothrombin time indicates a progressively worse prognosis.

Vitamin K is required for coagulation factor production by the liver, and deficiency of this should be corrected by giving vitamin $K_1$ (10 mg) parenterally. This is particularly important in patients with biliary obstruction in whom vitamin K is poorly absorbed. A prothrombin time must be done in all such cases and any abnormality corrected prior to surgery.

**Bromsulphthalein (BSP) Excretion.** When injected intravenously, BSP is rapidly bound to albumin; little (2%) is excreted in the urine and the rest is taken up by the liver, partially conjugated with glutathione and excreted into the bile. Estimation of its clearance from the blood is a sensitive test of liver function. However, the effectiveness of the tests mentioned above, the misleading results with BSP in old, febrile, or hypoalbuminaemic patients, the fact that it is invalid in the presence of jaundice and the occasional hypersensitivity reaction which may even be fatal, make BSP excretion a test with limited applicability. It is of particular value in the diagnosis of the rare Dubin-Johnson syndrome (p. 390); blood concentrations of BSP are measured 45 minutes and 2 hours after injection, a higher value at 2 hours confirming the diagnosis.

## Other Investigations in Liver Disease

**Hepatitis A virus antigens and antibodies.** The hepatitis A antigen (HAAg) is located on a particle thought to be the hepatitis A virus (p. 396). It is excreted in the stools during the last two weeks of the incubation period, but disappears with the onset of the clinical illness. It is not found in the blood. Antibody to the hepatitis A virus (anti-HAV) appears at or soon after the onset of symptoms and is more important in diagnosis. The mere presence of the antibody is not enough for diagnosis as hepatitis A viral infection is common in all communities and antibody to it persists for years after infection. A rising antibody titre or antibody of the immunoglobulin M type which defines a primary immune response is diagnostic of recent infection. Anti-HAV measurements can be used in epidemiological studies of the prevalence of hepatitis A viral infection.

**Hepatitis B virus antigens and antibodies.** The hepatitis B virus (p. 395) contains several antigens to which infected persons can make immune responses. These anti-

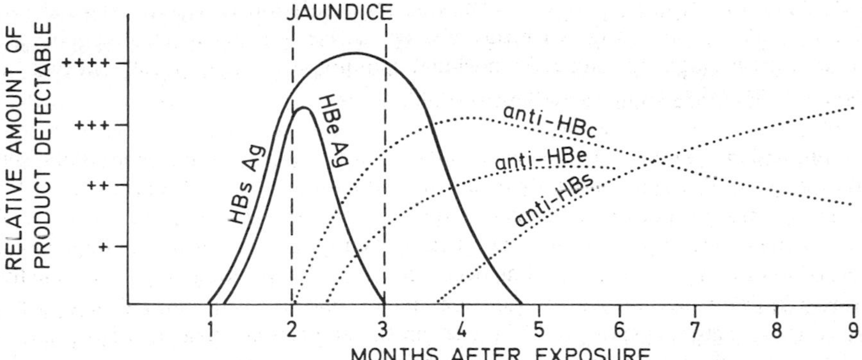


Fig. 9.2 Serological response to hepatitus B virus.

gens and their antibodies are important in identifying hepatitis B virus infection (Fig. 9.2). The hepatitis B surface antigen (HBsAg) is located in the capsular material of the virus; it can be identified by sensitive haemagglutination and radioimmunoassay methods and is a reliable marker of hepatitis B virus infection. It appears in the blood late in the incubation period or in the prodromal phase of acute type B hepatitis; it may be present for only a few days, disappearing even before jaundice has developed, but usually lasts for 3–4 weeks or may persist up to 3 months. It should therefore be sought as soon as possible in acute hepatitis. Antibody to HBsAg (anti-HBs) usually appears after about 3 months and persists for many years or perhaps permanently. The presence of anti-HBs implies only that infection has occurred at some time; seroconversion alone indicates recent infection. The hepatitis B core antigen (HBcAg) is located in the central part of the virus and is not found in the blood. However, antibody to the core antigen (anti-HBc) appears early in the illness, rapidly reaches a high titre, and then subsides gradually. This antibody is considered an index of infection and of viral replication. The central part of the virus contains another antigen, the e antigen (HBeAg), which appears only transiently at the outset of the illness and is followed by the production of antibody (anti-HBe).

About 5% of patients become chronic carriers of the hepatitis B virus after acute type B hepatitis, and they continue indefinitely with HBsAg and anti-HBc in the blood. In some cases the e antigen is also present (p. 396). Some healthy persons and a variable proportion of patients with chronic hepatitis (p. 403), cirrhosis (p. 406), or hepatocellular carcinoma (p. 412) are also chronic carriers of the virus. Any chronic virus carrier can transmit hepatitis, and the risk is greatest for those with chronic liver disease or with the e antigen in the blood. The risk of transmitting infection is low for healthy carriers who have anti-HBe and generally requires close bodily contact or direct inoculation of infected blood or other body fluids.

Hepatitis B antigens and their antibodies can be used to study the epidemiology of hepatitis B virus infection.

**Autoantibodies.** Three autoantibodies in the blood are important in liver disease; antinuclear antibody, smooth muscle antibody and antimitochondrial antibody. None is specific to liver disease; antinuclear and antimitochondrial antibodies occur in connective tissue diseases and in autoimmune diseases, including various thyroid disorders and pernicious anaemia, while smooth muscle antibody has been reported in infectious mononucleosis and in a variety of malignant diseases. In liver disease, smooth muscle antibody, and to a lesser extent antinuclear antibody, may occur transiently and at low titre in acute viral hepatitis. The autoantibodies are, however, more important in chronic liver disease where they are often present for long periods of time and at relatively high titres. They are found particularly in chronic active hepatitis, cryptogenic cirrhosis and primary biliary cirrhosis. In a patient with chronic liver disease, autoantibodies indicate the likelihood of one or other of these disorders, the differential diagnosis being made on other clinical and laboratory evidence. In a patient with cholestasis, the antimitochondrial antibody is of particular value in indicating that primary biliary cirrhosis is present. Antimitochondrial antibody occurs in primary biliary cirrhosis in 90% of cases and in less than 1% of patients with obstruction of the large biliary ducts. An antimicrosomal antibody has also been described which may become important in certain forms of chronic active hepatitis. None of the autoantibodies damages liver tissue, and they are therefore unlikely to have aetiological importance.

**Alpha-fetoprotein** is made mainly by the fetal liver, production falling to low levels after birth. The reappearance of substantial serum concentrations in adult life is almost always due to a hepatocellular carcinoma, though rarely it may be associated with embryonal tumours of the testes or ovary or with carcinomas derived from foregut epithelium, particularly the stomach. Such substantial serum concentrations can be detected by electrophoresis in a quarter to a third of patients with hepatocellular carcinoma in Europe and North America, and in up to three quarters of those in Africa and Asia. Lesser serum concentrations, detectable by radioimmunoassay, occur in 90% of all patients, but sometimes too in acute viral hepatitis and in chronic liver disease, particularly chronic active hepatitis. Increasing concentrations in chronic liver disease suggest hepatocellular carcinoma. Increased concentrations in the blood and amniotic fluid in pregnancy are associated with defects of the neural tube in the fetus.

**Caeruloplasmin** is a copper-containing globulin produced by the liver. It is important in the diagnosis of Wilson's disease (p. 410) in which serum concentrations are low or undetectable. Low levels may also occur in fulminant hepatic failure and in other advanced and severe chronic liver diseases, as well as in protein-losing enteropathy and malabsorption.

**Serum Iron and Ferritin.** The serum iron concentration (p. 907) and the saturation of the serum iron-binding capacity are usually high when the body iron stores are increased. A high serum iron and a highly saturated iron-binding capacity (>70%) in chronic liver disease suggests haemochromatosis but is not sufficient for a diagnosis as similar results occur in chronic alcoholic liver disease. The serum ferritin concentration reflects the total body iron more closely and is increased greatly in haemochromatosis. It is also the best single indication of iron overload in the asymptomatic relatives of patients. These tests can be used to follow the effects of venesection therapy. Haemochromatosis is excluded when they are all normal.

**Alpha$_1$-antitrypsin deficiency,** detectable by absence of the $\alpha_1$ peak on serum protein electrophoresis, is a well-established cause of liver disease in infancy and childhood. Rarely, it can cause cirrhosis or emphysema (p. 281) in adults, and occasionally both diseases occur together.

## Investigative Procedures in Liver Disease

**Liver biopsy** is a simple and safe procedure in the hands of an experienced clinician. It is carried out with a special needle, usually through an intercostal space, using local analgesia. It requires a co-operative patient who will stop breathing when the biopsy is actually taken. The haemostatic mechanisms must be intact as indicated by the prothrombin time and platelet count. After the procedure, the patient remains in bed for 24 hours, regular pulse and blood pressure measurements must be recorded and blood for transfusion (2 units) should be available. The main complications are abdominal and/or shoulder pain, bleeding and, rarely, biliary peritonitis which usually occurs when there is obstruction of a large bile duct.

Biopsy yields only a small sample of liver and consequently the best results are obtained in patients with diffuse liver disease. The procedure is essential in the diagnosis of chronic hepatitis and in separating its persistent and aggressive forms. It is also important in establishing a diagnosis of cirrhosis in which it may indicate a cause such as alcohol abuse or haemochromatosis. In cholestasis it may suggest obstruction of a large bile duct or give evidence of a disease of the smaller bile ducts or liver cells such as primary biliary cirrhosis. Other investigations are now preferred initially in obstructive jaundice (p. 389). It is not usually required in acute hepatitis in which the diagnosis can normally be made on other grounds; it may be needed, however, in atypical cases. Localised disease, particularly malignancy, is less accurately diagnosed unless the site of disease is first identified by some other method. Operative liver biopsy may sometimes be valuable, as in the staging of lymphoma.

**Laparoscopy** can be performed under local analgesia or general anaesthesia and involves the creation of a pneumoperitoneum. The laparoscope provides an excellent view of the anterior and superior surfaces of the liver as well as some of its inferior aspect and the gall bladder. The spleen, the prominent blood vessels of portal hypertension and evidence of peritoneal disease may also be seen. Biopsies can be taken directly from diseased areas which is valuable in focal disorders, especially malignant disease. The main contraindications are haemostatic abnormalities, marked ascites and previous surgery which may have caused adhesions.

**Imaging.** Radionuclides, ultrasound, or body computed tomography can be used for imaging of the liver and biliary tract. *Radionuclide imaging* is the simplest and is usually performed with technetium ($^{99M}$Tc) sulphur colloid which is taken up by the reticuloendothelial cells. Its greatest application is in the detection of focal hepatic disease, though lesions have to exceed 2–4cm in diameter to be seen. Patchy uptake of $^{99M}$Tc sulphur colloid by the liver and increased uptake by the spleen and bone marrow are most characteristic of cirrhosis with portal hypertension. Radionuclide imaging should be used primarily to localise liver disease prior to biopsy and should not be used on its own to make a definitive diagnosis.

*Ultrasonography* requires a skilled operator. It is most useful in identifying dilatation of the extrahepatic and intrahepatic bile ducts in jaundiced patients and in detecting gallstones which have not been revealed by cholecystography. It is similar to radionuclide imaging in detecting focal hepatic disease and can usually differentiate between tumours and abscesses or cysts. The portal vein can be identified. *Body computed tomography* requires expensive equipment. Its applications are similar to those of ultrasound.

**Radiology.** Specialised radiological techniques may be useful in investigating the liver. Angiography can define the site and nature of localised lesions and is valuable in planning hepatic surgery. Splenoportography, mesenteric angiography and transhepatic or perumbilical portography can all be used to investigate the portal venous system in portal hypertension prior to the surgical creation of portasystemic shunts. The portal venous pressure can be measured at splenoportography or direct portography and by catheterising the hepatic veins, as the wedged hepatic venous pressure closely reflects the portal venous pressure in cirrhosis. Hepatic venography can be used to identify hepatic venous obstruction.

**Paracentesis.** Analysis of ascites may give useful information. In cirrhosis, the fluid is clear, the protein content usually below 30 g/*l*, and in the absence of infection there are less than 500 cells/cu.mm. Ascitic protein concentrations above 30 g/*l* occur in peritoneal infection, especially tuberculosis, peritoneal tumour, hepatic venous obstruction and ascites associated with pancreatic disease. Amylase activity is high in ascites caused by pancreatitis. Infection, such as tuberculosis, can be determined by bacteriological examination of ascitic fluid.

## Jaundice

Jaundice is a clinical term referring to the yellow appearance of the skin and mucous membranes resulting from an increased bilirubin concentration in the body fluids. It is detectable when the serum bilirubin concentration exceeds 50 μmol/*l* (3 mg/100 ml); less marked hyperbilirubinaemia is called 'latent' jaundice. Internal tissues and body fluids are coloured yellow but not the brain as bilirubin does not cross the blood-brain barrier other than in the immediate neonatal period. Pathological mechanisms giving rise to jaundice fall into three groups: haemolytic, hepatocellular and cholestatic or obstructive.

### Haemolytic Jaundice

This results from an increased rate of destruction of red blood cells causing the production of more bilirubin. As a healthy liver can excrete a bilirubin load six times greater than normal before unconjugated bilirubin accumulates in the plasma, jaundice due to haemolysis is usually mild. Exceptions to this occur in the newborn when the hepatic bilirubin transport mechanism is immature and in patients with liver disease. Haemolysis may be due to intrinsic defects of the red blood cell or to various extracorpuscular factors (p. 554).

**Clinical Features.** Certain findings are common to all types of haemolytic jaundice. It is mild; the serum bilirubin is dominantly unconjugated and rarely exceeds 85 μmol (5 mg/100 ml). In some patients hyperbilirubinaemia is insufficient to cause jaundice. Bilirubin cannot be detected in the urine. Most patients have splenomegaly due to excessive activity of the reticuloendothelial system or congestion of the red pulp and also reticulocytosis and anaemia. The degree of anaemia depends on the severity of haemolysis and on the ability of the bone marrow to increase production of red blood cells. Increased bilirubin excretion leads to more stercobilinogen and stercobilin in the stools, which are therefore not pale, and to increased urobilinogen in the urine as more of this substance is absorbed from the gut. The urine rapidly becomes deep yellow on standing due to urobilin formation. Other tests of liver function are normal.

## Hepatocellular Jaundice

Hepatocellular jaundice results from inability of the liver to transport bilirubin into the bile as a result of liver cell damage. Bilirubin transport across the hepatocytes may be impaired at any point between uptake of unconjugated bilirubin into the cells and transport of conjugated bilirubin into the canaliculi. In addition, swelling of cells and oedema resulting from the disease itself may cause obstruction of the intrahepatic biliary tree. In hepatocellular jaundice the concentrations in the blood of both unconjugated and conjugated bilirubin increase, perhaps because of the variable way in which bilirubin transport is disturbed.

Acute parenchymal liver diseases, usually due to the hepatitis viruses (p. 393) or to toxins, usually drugs or alcohol (p. 392), are common causes. Immature bilirubin transport mechanisms in the newborn, especially in prematurity, and congenital defects in bilirubin transport (p. 390) are very specific metabolic defects in the liver cell causing jaundice. Chronic hepatitis and cirrhosis can also cause jaundice.

The clinical features vary depending on the underlying diseases. Jaundice ranges from mild to very severe.

## Cholestatic Jaundice

Cholestasis is a failure of bile flow, and its cause may lie anywhere between the hepatocyte and the duodenum. The concentrations of unconjugated bilirubin reaching the liver cells and of conjugated bilirubin unable to enter the canaliculi increase in the blood and cause jaundice if cholestasis is sufficiently severe.

CAUSES. The criterion for classifying cholestatic jaundice used to be whether or not it was amenable to surgical treatment. The terms 'surgical' and 'medical' jaundice fail to focus thought on particular disease sites, while the terms 'extrahepatic' (surgical) and 'intrahepatic' (medical) obscure the possibility that an obstruction to a large duct inside the liver is occasionally amenable to surgical treatment. Consequently, the terms used here are 'large (bile) duct obstruction' and 'small (bile) duct obstruction'.

*Large Duct Obstruction.* The most common causes are impaction of a gallstone in the common bile duct and carcinoma of the head of the pancreas. Other causes include carcinomas of the ampulla of Vater or bile duct, strictures of the bile duct usually the result of previous surgery, metastatic tumours impinging on the bile ducts, sclerosing cholangitis and, very rarely, involvement of the common bile duct by a duodenal ulcer.

*Small Duct Obstruction.* Widespread small duct obstruction is required to produce cholestatic jaundice. Drugs and alcohol are important causes which may exert their effects either on the liver cells or on the bile ducts. Other conditions causing obstruction are often primary diseases of the liver cells which also involve the small bile ducts, particularly the biliary canaliculi whose walls are formed by the hepatocytes, and such conditions include the cholestatic episodes which may occur in viral hepatitis, chronic active hepatitis, cirrhosis and the cholestasis of pregnancy. Cholestasis, sometimes with deep jaundice, may also occur for unknown reasons following surgery, in severe bacterial infections and in Hodgkin's disease. Diseases involving the smaller interlobular ducts and the ductules include primary biliary cirrhosis and the pericholangitis of ulcerative colitis. Widespread secondary carcinoma in the liver sometimes produces cholestatic jaundice.

**Clinical Features.** Apart from the manifestations of the causative disease, these include jaundice itself which, if prolonged and severe, may give the skin a greenish appearance, pale or clay-coloured stools due to deficiency of bilirubin and to steatorrhoea and dark urine due to the renal excretion of conjugated bilirubin. Some patients have generalised pruritus, anorexia, or a metallic taste in the mouth. Upper abdominal pain occurs particularly in large duct obstruction by a gallstone or pancreatic carcinoma. Fever, sometimes with rigors, suggests cholangitis, which occurs most often with gall-stone obstruction. A palpable gall bladder strongly suggests large-duct obstruction by a carcinoma, usually of the pancreas. The absence of this does not exclude a neoplasm. A very large and irregular liver indicates hepatic neoplasm. In prolonged obstructive jaundice, xanthomatous skin lesions, especially on the upper eyelids, occasionally appear as well as features due to secondary intestinal malabsorption; these latter include weight loss, a haemorrhagic tendency (vitamin K deficiency) and pain due to bone disease (calcium and vitamin D deficiency). In long-standing cases, clinical and biochemical evidence of hepatocellular dysfunction occurs.

## Congenital Non-haemolytic Hyperbilirubinaemia

With the exception of Gilbert's syndrome, the congenital abnormalities of bilirubin transport are very rare. In adults they all have an excellent prognosis, need no treatment and are clinically important only because they may be mistaken for more serious liver disease.

*Gilbert's Syndrome.* This common benign condition is usually first recognised in adolescents or young adults. It probably has varied aetiology, and in some cases may be inherited as an autosomal dominant. Gilbert's syndrome generally presents as mild jaundice, occasionally following viral hepatitis from which there has been an otherwise complete recovery, or is found incidentally. Many patients have no symptoms; others suffer episodes of malaise, anorexia and upper abdominal pain, the last occasionally severe, with increases in the jaundice. These episodes may be related to infection, fatigue or fasting. Apart from mild jaundice, examination is normal. Investigations show unconjugated hyperbilirubinaemia, generally below 100 $\mu$mol/*l* (6 mg/100 ml), with no abnormality of other liver function tests. No bilirubin is found in the urine. The peripheral blood count, reticulocyte count and the serum haptoglobin concentration are normal, giving no evidence of overt haemolysis. Liver biopsy is normal; in the absence of a history suggesting liver disease, a biopsy is not necessary.

The main cause of the unconjugated hyperbilirubinaemia is a deficiency of glucuronyl transferase; in some cases uptake of unconjugated bilirubin from the plasma may also be impaired. Glucuronyl transferase activity may be increased by phenobarbitone (60 mg thrice daily) which can be used to diminish jaundice and to ameliorate other symptoms.

*Crigler-Najjar Syndrome.* In the Crigler-Najjar syndrome (type I), there is complete absence of glucuronyl transferase from the liver. It causes severe unconjugated hyperbilirubinaemia and kernicterus in the newborn leading to early death, though a few patients have survived to adulthood. This autosomal-recessive condition is very rare. A less severe condition (type II), due to partial deficiency of the enzyme, does not cause kernicterus and patients usually survive to adult life.

*Dubin-Johnson Syndrome.* This very rare autosomal recessive condition is caused by a reduced ability to transport organic anions, such as bilirubin glucuronide, into the biliary canaliculi. It causes malaise and variable mild jaundice. The hyperbilirubinaemia is of the unconjugated type. Other organic anions which are poorly transported include BSP, which can be used to diagnose the condition, and the contrast agents for biliary radiology so that the gall bladder, though normal, is frequently visualised poorly or not at all on cholecystography. Liver biopsy shows a characteristic dark pigment. The prognosis is excellent.

*Rotor Syndrome*. This very rare conjugated hyperbilirubinaemia is caused by an inability of the liver to store bilirubin. The prognosis is excellent.

### Effect of Drugs on Bilirubin Metabolism

Numerous drugs and chemicals affect bilirubin metabolism. In normal adults, drugs interfering with bilirubin disposal produce only mild hyperbilirubinaemia, sometimes without jaundice, but more marked jaundice may occur where the ability to metabolise bilirubin is impaired. This occurs in the newborn, where hyperbilirubinaemia may become sufficient to cause kernicterus (p. 719), in those with congenital non-haemolytic hyperbilirubinaemia and in patients with chronic liver diseases such as cirrhosis. Hyperbilirubinaemia disappears readily when the drug is stopped.

The main sites at which drugs may interfere with bilirubin metabolism are shown in Table 9.1. Sulphonamides and salicylates displace unconjugated bilirubin from the binding sites on serum albumin; given to a newborn child with haemolytic disease or to the mother in late pregnancy, they may precipitate the development of kernicterus without increasing the serum bilirubin. Drugs which raise the serum bilirubin may increase either its unconjugated or conjugated forms depending on whether they act prior to or at the stage of conjugation or thereafter. Unconjugated hyperbilirubinaemia occurs when drugs produce haemolysis, impair transport from the plasma to the conjugating site or reduce conjugation itself. Conjugated hyperbilirubinaemia occurs when transport of conjugated bilirubin into the biliary canaliculus is impaired; drugs which do this also reduce BSP transport and increase BSP retention in the blood. Inducing agents, such as phenobarbitone can increase the capacity of the liver to conjugate bilirubin so that patients on long-term treatment with such agents, e.g. epileptics, tend to have low serum bilirubin concentrations.

*Oral Contraceptives*. These agents usually contain an oestrogen capable of causing cholestasis and a progestogen. Occasionally they cause jaundice, almost always within

Table 9.1 Sites of action of some drugs *reducing* the plasma protein binding of bilirubin or its uptake, transport, conjugation or excretion by hepatocytes

| Site of action | | | |
|---|---|---|---|
| Plasma | Hepatocyte | | |
| Protein binding | Uptake and transport | Conjugation* | Excretion into canaliculus |
| Sulphonamides<br>Salicylates | Rifampicin<br>Filix mas<br>Cholecystographic media | Novobiocin | Sulphadiazine<br>Oral contraceptives<br>Methyltestosterone<br><br>Anabolic steroids (C–17$\alpha$ alkyl substituted testosterones) |
| Unconjugated bilirubin | | Conjugated bilirubin | |

* Phenobarbitone *increases* conjugation of bilirubin.

the first three cycles. The serum bilirubin often exceeds 170 μmol/*l* (10 mg/100 ml) and the alkaline phosphatase activity is high indicating cholestasis. The reaction is a complex one, however, as the serum transferase activity is also moderately increased and liver biopsy shows some hepatocellular damage in addition to cholestasis. Those who develop jaundice due to oral contraceptives frequently also develop cholestasis of pregnancy and both conditions may reflect an unusual hepatic reaction to a steroid agent. This may have a genetic basis as both conditions show a similar geographic distribution.

## Acute Parenchymal Disease of the Liver

**Aetiology.** In acute parenchymal liver disease (acute hepatitis) there is a sudden episode of widespread damage in which variable numbers of hepatocytes undergo necrosis. These episodes are due largely to infective or toxic agents.

*Infections.* The most important infective causes are the hepatitis A and B viruses and the non A, non B virus. Cytomegalovirus, Epstein-Barr virus and yellow fever virus occasionally cause clinically apparent acute hepatitis. Other viruses, however, have been implicated only rarely. Less frequently non-viral agents such as *Leptospira icterohaemorrhagiae* (Weil's disease), *Toxoplasma gondii* (toxoplasmosis) and *Coxiella burneti* (Q fever) may cause acute hepatitis. Impaired hepatic function can also occur in severe extrahepatic infections, especially with septicaemia, but this is not due to infective agents reaching the liver.

*Toxic Substances.* Most substances causing acute hepatitis are drugs. How often an individual drug is responsible depends on the frequency with which it is used and in what proportion of cases hepatic damage occurs. Usually, liver damage caused by drugs is due to idiosyncratic reactions (i.e. not related to the dose of the drug and occurring in only a few individuals). Among the drugs more commonly responsible are: chlorpromazine and other phenothiazines, phenelzine and other monoamine oxidase inhibitors, imipramine, amitryptiline, erythromycin, isoniazid, rifampicin (and occasionally other antituberculous drugs), halothane, methyldopa, phenylbutazone, indomethacin, chlorpropamide and thiouracil. Liver damage due to drugs is reported increasingly, and any drug should be suspected. A few drugs cause liver damage in all people in a dose-related manner. These include tetracycline, especially in pregnancy or in those with renal dysfunction, and paracetamol which is often used in self-poisoning.

Potent liver poisons include carbon tetrachloride and yellow phosphorus. Where there are strict rules regarding their use, damage due to these agents is rare. Occasionally severe liver damage occurs from eating poisonous fungi (*Amanita phalloides*). Alcohol is by far the most important liver toxin; in addition to chronic liver damage it may produce acute alcoholic hepatitis.

*Circulatory Disturbances.* Acute hepatic damage, sometimes sufficient to cause jaundice, may be caused by any form of shock or by right ventricular failure.

*Other Conditions.* Rarely, severe fatty degeneration of the liver of unknown cause may be encountered, for example in pregnancy.

**Pathology.** Viral and most drug-induced hepatitis show similar lesions. Cell damage throughout the liver is the dominant abnormality, particularly in centrilobular areas, though individual lobules are variably affected. Damaged hepatocytes have a swollen granular appearance, while dead ones become shrunken and deeply stained, sometimes losing their nuclei to form eosinophilic Councilman bodies; these bodies, originally described in yellow fever, suggest acute hepatitis. The lobules may be infiltrated with mononuclear cells. Polymorphonuclear leucocytes and fatty change are not seen. The portal tracts are enlarged with a predominantly mononuclear cell infiltrate. More severe damage is accompanied by collapse of the reticulin framework, particularly between the central veins and portal tracts which become linked to one another; this is known as bridging or subacute hepatic necrosis. Very severe damage results in destruction of whole lobules (massive necrosis) and is the lesion underlying fulminant hepatic failure. Cholestasis is occasionally very prominent.

In some patients, the main histological abnormality is fatty change. This occurs in damage due to carbon tetrachloride, tetracycline and a number of other direct toxins as well as in the acute fatty liver of pregnancy. The changes are most marked in fatal cases. Circulatory disturbances cause centrilobular congestion and necrosis.

## Viral Hepatitis

Viral hepatitis is almost always caused by one or other of the hepatitis viruses. They give rise to illnesses which are similar in their clinical and pathological features and which are frequently asymptomatic.

### Acute Type A Hepatitis
*(Infectious, Epidemic, Short Incubation Hepatitis)*

**Aetiology and Pathology.** Type A hepatitis is due to a virus for which there is no generally available method of culture. It may belong to the picornavirus group of enteroviruses. It is highly infectious and is usually spread by human faeces entering the body via the oral route directly or indirectly. Infected persons may excrete viruses in the faeces for about 3 weeks before the onset of jaundice and for up to 2 weeks thereafter. Children are most commonly affected and conditions of overcrowding and poor sanitation facilitate spread. In occasional outbreaks, water, milk and shellfish have been the vehicles of transmission. Though faeces is the usual source, other body constituents may also spread disease; the hepatitis may, for example, be spread by blood transfusion. The sources in the community appear to be persons incubating or suffering from the disease; a carrier state, analogous to that for hepatitis B virus, has not been identified. The incubation period of type A hepatitis is about a month.

The disease is generalised with involvement of the gastrointestinal tract, heart, pancreas, spleen, etc., but the main lesion is in the liver (see above).

**Clinical Features.** In the case of average severity, prodromal symptoms precede the development of jaundice by a few days to 2 weeks. They are the usual manifestations of an acute infectious disease, and include chills, headache and malaise. Gastrointestinal symptoms may be prominent; anorexia and distaste for cigarettes are common and early complaints, and nausea, vomiting and diarrhoea may follow. A steady upper abdominal pain occurs as a result of stretching of the peritoneum over the liver as the organ enlarges; the pain is severe in some patients. Initially physical signs are scanty; the liver is usually tender, though not readily palpable, enlarged cervical lymph nodes may be found and splenomegaly may occur, particularly in children.

Dark urine and a yellow tint to the sclerae herald the onset of jaundice. As obstruction to the biliary canaliculi develops, the jaundice deepens, the stools become paler, the urine darker and the liver more easily palpable. At this time the appetite often improves and gastrointestinal symptoms diminish in intensity. Thereafter the jaundice usually recedes, the stools and urine regain their normal colour, the liver enlargement regresses and, in the course of 3 to 6 weeks, the great majority of cases gradually recover. Milder cases occur or the disease may run an anicteric course which is recognised by the association of vague gastrointestinal complaints or malaise with bilirubinuria and biochemical evidence of hepatic dysfunction.

**Investigation.** A serum transferase activity exceeding 400 units/*l*, even before jaundice develops, is the most striking abnormality. The serum bilirubin reflects the degree of jaundice, the alkaline phosphatase activity rarely exceeds 250 units/*l* (30 K.A. units/100 ml) unless marked cholestasis develops and the albumin concentration is normal. The prothrombin time is increased in severe cases and in these circumstances is a good guide to prognosis. Bilirubinuria is an early finding, occurring in the prodromal phase and usually continuing into the convalescent period. Urobilinogenuria appears just before jaundice, disappears at the height of the jaundice owing to intrahepatic cholestasis and reappears early in convalescence as a sign of recovery. Mild proteinuria may be present. The white cell count is normal or low in uncomplicated cases, sometimes with a relative lymphocytosis; this is of some value in differentiation from Weil's disease (p. 66). Measurement of anti-HAV allows a specific diagnosis to be made (p. 384)

Differential diagnosis is discussed on page 398.

**Course and Prognosis.** Almost all patients make a full recovery. During convalescence a small proportion relapse with a return of symptoms and signs; in these cases the relapse almost always subsides spontaneously. More frequently, the serum transferase activity increases without any return of clinical illness; these asymptomatic 'biochemical' relapses also subside spontaneously. Either from the onset or during the course of the illness, more severe jaundice of a clinically and biochemically obstructive type may develop and it may follow a prolonged course. Liver biopsy shows the features of hepatitis with prominent cholestasis and no evidence of chronic liver damage. This clinical syndrome is known as *cholestatic viral hepatitis* and, though it may continue for many months, the prognosis is good.

Following clinical and biochemical recovery, debility for 2 to 3 months is common. Sometimes, particularly in anxious patients, there may be prolonged malaise, anorexia, nausea and right hypochondrial discomfort without clinical, biochemical or histological evidence of liver disease. This syndrome, which may be exacerbated by too frequent clinical and biochemical assessment, is known as the *posthepatitis syndrome*; it is not due to liver disease and should be treated by reassurance.

Death from acute type A hepatitis is uncommon. In young adults, the mortality is around 0·2%. With increasing age, however, the frequency of severe episodes and death increases so that over the age of 60 years mortality reaches about 3%. Evidence regarding mortality during pregnancy is conflicting; most reports suggesting an increased mortality derive from countries in which the standard of living is low where factors such as poor nutrition may be important. In Europe and North America the mortality in pregnant women is probably not increased. Those who die of the acute illness do so after developing fulminant hepatic failure (p. 397). Rarely, aplastic anaemia may occur several months after recovery from viral hepatitis. Prolonged carriage of the virus and the development of chronic liver disease are not features of hepatitis A infection.

**Treatment and Prevention.** There is no specific therapy; general measures applicable to all forms of acute hepatitis are discussed on page 399. Although for many years patients have been treated in general medical wards without cross-infection occurring, indicating that isolation is not essential, precautions for preventing the spread of enteric infections are advisable.

The most effective prophylactic measures are to improve social conditions, particularly overcrowded and unhygienic situations. In sporadic cases, prevention of disease in contacts cannot be achieved as the patient is infectious during the incubation and prodromal stages. However, once the disease is recognised, contacts may be protected by gammaglobulin, especially those at particular risk such as close contacts, the elderly, those with other major disease and perhaps pregnant women. Persons travelling to endemic areas may be protected by gammaglobulin for about 3 months. A vaccine against type A hepatitis virus is not available.

## Acute Type B Hepatitis
### *(Serum Hepatitis, Long Incubation Hepatitis)*

**Aetiology and Pathology.** Type B hepatitis is due to a virus which cannot yet be grown but which can be transmitted to certain primates, such as the chimpanzee, in which it can replicate. The virus and an excess of its capsular material circulate in the blood where it can be identified (p. 384). The classification of the virus remains uncertain, but its core contains DNA and has DNA polymerase activity. Blood and certain blood products are the main sources of infection. Only those blood products subjected to pasteurisation (albumin solutions, $\gamma$–globulin fraction) can be regarded as largely free of risk. Spread may follow transfusion of infected blood or blood products or injections with contaminated needles, a mode of spread most common among parenteral ('mainline') drug abusers who share needles. Tattooing or acupuncture may also spread this disease as needles are reused frequently.

The ability to identify the hepatitis B virus has led to the realisation that it may cause sporadic infections which cannot be attributed to parenteral modes of spread. Infected serum can transmit disease orally and the discovery of the HBsAg in body fluids, such as saliva, urine, semen and vaginal secretions, suggests many alternative modes of spread. Close personal contact seems necessary for spread and sexual intercourse, especially in male homosexuals, seems an important route of transmission. Finally, the virus may be spread from mother to child; transmission at or soon after birth seems more likely than transplacental spread. Humans are the only source of the hepatitis B virus; in addition to those incubating or suffering from the disease, some asymptomatic individuals carry the virus in the blood over long periods, perhaps for life. The incubation period of type B hepatitis is about three months. A negative test for the HBsAg in the blood does not exclude type B hepatitis.

The pathology is as for type A hepatitis (p. 393).

**Clinical Features.** The clinical features are similar to, but usually more severe than those of type A hepatitis. Transient rashes, including urticaria, may occur and arthralgia or arthritis is common. Though these can occur in type A hepatitis, they are much more suggestive of type B hepatitis. Arthralgia and arthritis strongly suggest type B hepatitis.

Type B hepatitis tends to be a more severe disease than type A. The mortality depends on the virulence of the virus, the age of the patient and the underlying disease: In about 5% of cases chronic hepatitis B carriage follows the acute episode.

**Chronic Asymptomatic Carriers.** Some individuals with no history of acute hepatitis and lacking clinical evidence of liver disease are chronic carriers of the hepatitis B virus. They all have the HBsAg and anti-HBc in the blood, and some also have the e antigen (p. 385) and DNA polymerase activity (p. 395). The frequency of chronic carriers in northern Europe and in North America is about 0·1%, but higher frequencies (1–15%) are found in Mediterranean countries, in Africa, and in Asia. Most asymptomatic chronic carriers have normal liver function tests and need not undergo liver biopsy as significant histological abnormalities are uncommon. Persistent biochemical abnormalities are more common in those with the e antigen or DNA polymerase in the blood, and liver biopsy should be considered as aggressive hepatitis may benefit from treatment (p. 404).

The prognosis for chronic asymptomatic carriers is uncertain, but the virus can be carried for many years without severe chronic liver disease occurring. Close body contact and the body fluids of these individuals can transmit infection, particularly when the e antigen, DNA polymerase activity, or liver disease are present, and precautions are therefore needed when they undergo medical or dental treatment.

Patients with impaired immune responses are very liable to become chronic carriers; this occurs particularly in Hodgkin's disease and other lymphomas, in those on immunosuppressive drugs, in patients on long-term dialysis, and in institutionalised patients with Down's syndrome.

**Treatment and Prevention.** No specific treatment is available. Supportive therapy is described on page 399.

Post-transfusion type B hepatitis can be largely prevented by scrupulous blood transfusion technique, by using volunteer donors and excluding those with a history of jaundice and by screening all blood for the HBsAg, using highly sensitive methods. These precautions do not, however, eliminate post-transfusion hepatitis as the laboratory tests are not infallible and as the condition may be caused by other than the hepatitis B virus. Pooled dried plasma has proved a potent source of hepatitis which can be virtually eliminated by limiting the pool size to 10 donors. Sterile needles and syringes should always be used and if disposable equipment is not available these should be autoclaved for 20 minutes at 120°C. Washing in 2% carbolic acid and boiling in water for 20 minutes is an acceptable emergency procedure.

Type B hepatitis can be prevented or minimised by the intramuscular injection of gammaglobulin prepared from blood containing anti-HBs. Where available, it should be given to persons without HBsAg or anti-HBs in their blood within two days or at least a week of exposure to infected blood in circumstances likely to cause infection; these include accidental needle puncture, gross personal contamination with infected blood or exposure to infected blood in the presence of cuts and grazes.

## Non A, Non B Hepatitis

The existence of non A, non B hepatitis was recognised once infection with the hepatitis A and B viruses could be excluded by specific serological methods. The responsible agent or agents cannot yet be identified, but they can transmit infection in humans and confer specific immunity. Non A, non B hepatitis is diagnosed by excluding hepatitis A and B, cytomegaloviral, and Epstein-Barr viral infections. It may cause about a quarter of sporadic cases of acute viral hepatitis and it is known to cause 90% or more of post transfusion hepatitis in North America. It shares many features with type B hepatitis in that it has a long incubation period of two months or more, it causes a relatively prolonged illness and it may cause a chronic carrier state. Immune serum globulin, useful in type A hepatitis, may also prevent or ameliorate non A, non B hepatitis. Its contribution to the production of chronic liver disease is not yet known.

## Fulminant Hepatic Failure
*(Acute Massive Liver Necrosis)*

Fulminant hepatic failure is a rare syndrome in which hepatic encephalopathy, characterised by mental changes progressing from confusion to stupor and coma, results from sudden severe impairment of hepatic function. The syndrome is defined further as occurring within 8 weeks of onset of the precipitating illness, in the absence of evidence of pre-existing liver disease, to distinguish it from those instances in which hepatic encephalopathy represents a deterioration in chronic liver disease.

**Aetiology and Pathology.** Acute viral hepatitis is the commonest cause, drugs (p. 392) being the next most frequent. Rarely, it occurs in pregnancy, in Wilson's disease, following shock or from poisons such as carbon tetrachloride.

Extensive parenchymal necrosis is the most obvious lesion (p. 392). In fatal cases, less than 30% of the liver cells appear viable histologically and often few such cells are seen. Severe fatty degeneration is characteristic of such causes of this syndrome as tetracycline and pregnancy.

**Clinical Features.** Cerebral disturbance (encephalopathy) is the cardinal manifestation of fulminant hepatic failure. Its cause is unknown, but is thought to be due to toxic substances, including ammonia, fatty acids and nitrogenous compounds; these last may act as false neurotransmitters. The earliest features are reduced alertness and poor concentration progressing through behaviour abnormalities including restlessness, aggressive outbursts and mania, to drowsiness and coma. Confusion, disorientation, inversion of sleep rhythm, slurred speech, yawning, hiccoughing and, in the late stages, convulsions may occur. More general symptoms include weakness, nausea, and vomiting. Right hypochondrial pain is only an occasional feature.

Examination shows jaundice which develops rapidly and is usually deep in fatal cases though, rarely, death may occur before it develops. Fetor hepaticus, a sweet musty odour to the breath, may be present and is said to be due to methyl mercaptan. A flapping 'hepatic' tremor of the extended hands is characteristic. The liver may be enlarged initially, but later becomes impalpable. Hepatic dullness on percussion may disappear indicating much shrinkage and a bad prognosis. Splenomegaly is uncommon and never prominent. Ascites and oedema occur in a few patients surviving a week or more. Purpura and overt bleeding such as melaena reflect severe haemostatic disturbance. Neurological examination may show chorea, muscle spasticity and extensor plantar responses. Other features include fever, sweating, hypotension, tachycardia, hyperventilation and renal failure.

**Investigation.** The serum bilirubin reflects the degree of jaundice. Initially, serum transferase activity is very high, as in acute viral hepatitis, but with progression of damage activity falls; this investigation has diagnostic but not prognostic significance. Alkaline phosphatase activity is variable. Serum albumin concentration remains normal unless the course is prolonged. Increased serum and urine amino acids are characteristic but are not generally measured. The prothrombin time rapidly becomes prolonged as coagulation factor synthesis fails; this is the laboratory test of greatest prognostic value, a progressive and marked prolongation being a very bad prognostic sign. White blood cell counts vary, leucocytosis occurring even in the absence of infection. The urine contains protein, bilirubin and urobilinogen. Investigations required for the detection of complications are discussed on page 387.

**Course and Progress.** The progress of fulminant hepatic failure is closely related to the encephalopathy. When only minor signs are present and drowsiness is not prominent some two-thirds of patients survive. Once the patient is comatose only 10 to 20% survive. The prognosis is worse with increasing age and perhaps when due to certain agents such as halothane. In fatal cases, death usually occurs within a week. Life-threatening complications, some amenable to conservative therapy, may arise in the course of the illness. These include profound hypoglycaemia, cerebral oedema, respiratory failure, hypothermia, bacterial infections, bleeding due to coagulation disorders, pancreatitis and renal failure with severe oliguria. Electrolyte disturbances, particularly hyponatraemia, hypokalaemia and alkalosis, may also occur. The great majority of those who recover from fulminant hepatic failure regain normal hepatic structure and function.

**Treatment.** There is no specific therapy. Supportive measures are described on page 399.

## Differential Diagnosis of Acute Parenchymal Disease of the Liver

Most patients with acute parenchymal liver disease are suffering from viral hepatitis. This diagnosis depends on the clinical features described above, a history of contact with a jaundiced person or of transfusion, injection, or damage to the skin when handling blood within an appropriate incubation period, the results of liver function tests, and serological tests for the A and B hepatitis viruses. The possibility of drug-induced hepatitis should always be considered, the diagnosis depending on exposure to the drug within 2 weeks of the onset of symptoms with no other detectable cause for the illness. In the preicteric phase there may be confusion with other acute generalised infections, acute abdominal emergencies when pain is present, or gastroenteritis. Especially in young persons, there may be confusion with *infectious mononucleosis* in which sore throat, lymphadenopathy and splenomegaly are prominent, atypical blood lymphocytosis is present, and the Paul-Bunnell test generally positive; in this disease abnormal liver function tests are common and jaundice may occur. *Cytomegalovirus infection* should be considered in those with poor immune responses who have received blood transfusion; a specific antibody response occurs, virus may be isolated from the urine, and giant cells and intranuclear inclusions found on liver biopsy.

*Weil's disease* may cause severe jaundice and usually occurs in persons exposed to rats such as sewer workers, agricultural workers and miners. In contrast to viral hepatitis, there is a polymorphonuclear leucocytosis and protein, blood and casts are found in the urine. The diagnosis is made by demonstrating a rise in specific antibodies, and leptospires may be isolated from the blood or urine (p. 67).

A most difficult problem is to differentiate jaundice due to viral hepatitis from that due to *large-duct biliary obstruction* usually caused by a stone or a neoplasm. This is particularly so when an episode of viral hepatitis becomes prolonged and obstructive features develop. Clinically, a patient over 40 years old, previous attacks of abdominal pain, the gradual onset of fluctuant or progressive jaundice, marked pruritus, weight loss and right upper quadrant abdominal pain or a palpable gall-bladder indicate a large duct obstruction. Leucocytosis or a positive test for blood in the stool also suggest large-duct obstruction. Liver function tests are of greatest value at an early stage; in viral hepatitis serum alkaline phosphatase does not usually exceed 250 units/*l* (30 KA units/100 ml) and serum transferase activity almost always exceeds 400 units/*l*, while in biliary obstruction the reverse usually obtains. This laboratory differentiation becomes less clear as the disease progresses, however, and in biliary obstruction cholangitis may increase serum transferase activity. A plain radiograph of the abdomen may show gallstones, though only 10% of these are radio-opaque, and hypotonic duodenography may reveal an obstructing lesion arising from the head of the pancreas or ampulla of Vater. Oral cholecystography and intravenous cholangiography are of no value in these jaundiced patients; the biliary tract may be demonstrated by either transhepatic cholangiography or endoscopic retrograde cholangiopancreatography (p. 314). Liver biopsy may also be useful in revealing hepatitis or features of bile-duct obstruction. The HBsAg and the antimitochondrial antibody must always be sought. Where viral hepatitis is a possibility, laparotomy should be avoided as such patients withstand anaesthesia and surgery poorly.

### Treatment of Acute Parenchymal Disease of the Liver

*Aetiological Factors.* In most cases nothing can be done to eliminate the cause of the disease. It is important to detect drug-induced acute hepatitis so that the drug may be stopped and the patient warned to avoid its use in future. Penicillin, given early, is effective in Weil's disease (p. 67).

*Bed Rest.* When symptoms are marked, bed rest should be advised, the patient rising to the toilet if desired. Thereafter, the younger patient may be up and about taking care only to avoid exhaustion. For those in whom the risks of hepatitis may be greater, bed rest should be empirically prolonged until symptoms and signs have disappeared and liver function tests have returned substantially towards normal. These patients include those over 50 years, the pregnant, and those with other major disease.

*Diet.* A good general diet containing some 3000 kcal daily is desirable. Initially, owing to anorexia and nausea, this is usually not tolerated, in which case a light diet supplemented by fruit drinks and glucose is usually acceptable. The content of the diet should be dictated largely by the patient's wishes; however, a good protein intake should be encouraged. If vomiting is severe, intravenous fluid and glucose may be required for a few days.

*Drugs.* Corticosteroids have been advocated in viral hepatitis. Current evidence, however, is that they do not increase recovery and that they may cause serious side-effects. In general, therefore, they should not be used. On the other hand, in patients with marked malaise, anorexia or vomiting they may cause rapid regression of symptoms with return of appetite. In this small group of patients, prednisolone may be given provided the HBsAg test is negative as there is some evidence that corticosteroids may lead to chronic HBs antigenaemia. The dose is reduced rapidly from 20 mg daily as symptoms remit. Drugs metabolised in the liver should be avoided where possible, a principle applying especially to sedative and hypnotic agents. Alcohol must be avoided during the illness and should not be taken in the ensuing 6 months. Oral contraceptives may be resumed after clinical and biochemical recovery.

*Fulminant Hepatic Failure.* The development of hepatic encephalopathy greatly alters management. There is no specific treatment but certain measures should be instituted as soon as possible once cerebral changes occur. The patient's life is sustained in the hope that hepatic regeneration will occur spontaneously. There should be close observation so that steps may be taken quickly to correct complications as they occur. Encephalopathy is treated by withdrawing all nitrogen intake, by reducing the nitrogen-producing colonic flora with neomycin, 1 g orally 6 hourly and by increasing faecal output with lactulose 15 ml orally twice or thrice daily. If tests for stool blood are positive the colon should be washed out. Electroencephalography may be used to follow the course of the encephalopathy. Sedative drugs must be used with very great care, restlessness and excitement being best controlled, if necessary, with diazepam 5 mg intravenously.

Calories are provided as glucose 300 g daily either orally, if necessary by nasogastric tube, or into a large central vein as a 10–20% solution (0·6–1·2 mol/*l*). Fluid and electrolyte therapy depends on maintenance of accurate fluid balance records and on daily measures of serum urea, sodium, potassium and bicarbonate. Saline must be used cautiously to avoid sodium overload, and potassium deficiency, which occurs readily, should be corrected. The blood glucose should be measured 6 hourly in the severe phase as potentially fatal hypoglycaemia often occurs; its treatment may require large amounts of glucose.

As these patients have poor vasomotor control, early detection of bleeding and rapid correction of blood volume by transfusion are required. This is facilitated by regular recordings of pulse, blood pressure, hourly urine output and if possible central venous pressure. Impaired haemostasis leads to bleeding, particularly from the gastrointestinal tract. Intramuscular injections are best avoided. The development of a bleeding tendency is detected by regular haemoglobin, platelet count, prothrombin time and faecal occult blood measurements. Treatment is discussed on page 598. Cimetidine (30 mg i.v. hourly) may prevent gastrointestinal bleeding.

Infection is common and serious. As fever and leucocytosis may result solely from the liver disease itself, these are no guide and regular blood, urine, and throat cultures and chest X-ray should be carried out. Prophylactic antibiotics should not be used; if infection is strongly suspected they may be given once specimens have been taken for culture. A suitable regime is the use of parenteral gentamicin and clindamycin.

A close watch on the respiration is needed as initial hyperpnoea may rapidly become apnoea, requiring tracheostomy and assisted ventilation. Renal failure, revealed by a rising blood urea, may eventually require dialysis. The temperature must be measured 4 hourly as hypothermia can follow central loss of temperature control. Unexplained continuing coma may be due to cerebral oedema even in the absence of papilloedema; treatment with parenteral dexamethasone, 4 mg 6 hourly, can be given.

Fulminant hepatic failure requires intensive patient care, access to varied specialised help, and a hospital with great technical resources. Many special treatments have been tried. None is of proven value and some involve the risk of infecting staff; they include exchange transfusion, plasmaphoresis, haemodialysis, and extracorporeal circulation of the patient's blood through various animal livers, isolated or *in situ*, or through coated-charcoal columns. Corticosteroids, or gammaglobulin containing anti-HBs are of no value in HBsAg positive cases.

## Chronic Parenchymal Disease

There are two main forms of chronic parenchymal liver disease: (1) chronic hepatitis, which comprises (a) chronic persistent hepatitis and (b) chronic active hepatitis, and (2) cirrhosis.

**Aetiology.** There are many causes of chronic hepatitis and cirrhosis. In Britain, cirrhosis is usually associated with alcohol abuse, chronic active hepatitis or primary biliary cirrhosis. No cause can be found in 30% of cases. Haemochromatosis accounts for about 5% of patients and all other causes are rare.

*Alcohol.* The mechanism whereby alcohol damages the liver is unknown; it is now, however, accepted as a direct liver toxin in man and in other primates. The production of cirrhosis requires a prolonged intake of alcohol of about 100 g or more daily for 5 to 15 years. A daily alcohol intake may be more likely to cause cirrhosis than episodic drinking.

*Infection.* Rarely, patients can develop cirrhosis over a few months or years after viral hepatitis. In some patients with chronic hepatitis or cirrhosis, the proportion showing marked geographic variation (0–30%), the HBsAg is found persistently in the blood and in such cases the hepatitis B virus is presumably the causative agent. The non A, non B viruses can cause chronic infection and are likely causes of chronic liver disease. The hepatitis A virus does not cause chronic liver disease.

*Metabolic Disorders.* These include excess hepatic deposition of iron in haemochromatosis and of copper in Wilson's disease. Most metabolic conditions involving the liver occur in childhood, e.g. glycogen storage disease, fibrocystic disease and $\alpha_1$-antitrypsin deficiency.

*Drugs.* Chronic hepatitis and cirrhosis have been reported in patients on long-term treatment with methotrexate or methyldopa. Other drugs have been cited occasionally.

*Cholestasis.* Prolonged cholestasis anywhere in the biliary tree may cause cirrhosis. In primary biliary cirrhosis, obstruction results from damage to interlobular bile ducts. Cirrhosis from large-duct obstruction may occur with biliary strictures or in sclerosing cholangitis. Neoplastic lesions do not cause cirrhosis as survival is short.

*Congestion.* Prolonged hepatic congestion may eventually cause cirrhosis. This is rare, as death usually occurs before cirrhosis develops. Congestion may be due to hepatic venous outflow obstruction, as in the Budd-Chiari syndrome (p. 411) or chronic heart failure.

*Immunological Factors.* Some patients with chronic liver disease of unknown cause have abnormal serum antibodies (p. 384). Though the autoantibodies themselves are not cytotoxic, their presence has suggested that liver damage may be produced by abnormal immune mechanisms. Currently, the possibility that sensitised lymphocytes may do this is being actively investigated; lymphocytes from patients with chronic liver disease have been shown to react to antigens in liver and bile and to be capable of damaging liver cells *in vitro*. The importance of these reactions in chronic liver disease, however, remains to be established. Immune reactions could also be important in chronic liver disease caused by the hepatitis B virus.

*Malnutrition.* This may occur secondarily in patients with cirrhosis, but it is unlikely that it is primarily responsible for cirrhosis. Permanent liver damage does not follow marasmus or kwashiorkor.

*Cryptogenic Cirrhosis.* In this heterogeneous group, no cause can be found.

**Pathology**. 1. CHRONIC HEPATITIS. Two types of chronic hepatitis are recognised histologically. Their names — persistent hepatitis and aggressive hepatitis — are easily confused with the clinical syndromes they underlie — chronic persistent hepatitis and chronic active hepatitis; this should be avoided.

In *persistent hepatitis* the essential feature is an infiltration of chronic inflammatory cells confined to the portal tracts which may be expanded or show short fibrous septa extending into the parenchyma. Changes in the hepatocytes are absent or slight; there may be small foci of liver cell necrosis with inflammatory cell infiltration (spotty necrosis) and sometimes the residual changes of viral hepatitis. Lobular architecture is normal and cirrhosis occurs only rarely.

In *aggressive hepatitis*, the histological process underlying the clinical condition chronic active hepatitis, both the portal tracts and the parenchyma are involved, lobular architecture is distorted and cirrhosis often develops. The portal tract infiltration of mononuclear cells extends irregularly into the surrounding parenchyma so that swollen liver cells become isolated in the inflammatory cell infiltrate. This process of hepatocyte destruction is called 'piecemeal necrosis' and it leads to septum formation linking portal tracts and central veins. The ensuing disruption of lobular architecture is accompanied by the development of regenerative nodules and then by cirrhosis. Changes in the rest of the parenchyma are variable and resemble those of persistent hepatitis. These changes do not occur diffusely and may be more advanced in some areas than others, a point to be considered in interpreting biopsies.

2. CIRRHOSIS. In cirrhosis, widespread death of liver cells resulting from many causes is accompanied and followed by progressive fibrosis, regenerative (nodular) hyperplasia of surviving hepatocytes and distortion of liver architecture resulting in portal-systemic vascular shunts. The whole liver is involved, though not necessarily every lobule. Cirrhotic livers have an infinitely variable appearance limiting the usefulness of anatomical classifications. Currently, a simple classification into micronodular, macronodular and mixed cirrhosis is used. *Micronodular cirrhosis* is characterised by regular connective tissue septa, regenerative nodules approximating in size to the original lobules (1 mm in diameter) and involvement of every lobule. This form, also called portal, septal, nutritional, monolobular, or Laënnec's cirrhosis, is characteristic but not pathognomonic of the parenchymal damage induced by alcohol.

In *macronodular cirrhosis* the connective tissue septa vary in thickness and the nodules show marked differences in size, the larger ones containing histologically normal lobules. This form is also called posthepatitic or postnecrotic cirrhosis.

*Mixed cirrhosis* shows features of both micronodular and macronodular cirrhosis. None of these types of cirrhosis is static; micronodular cirrhosis may, for example, develop into a macronodular stage.

## 1. Chronic Hepatitis

It is important not to confuse gradually resolving acute hepatitis with chronic hepatitis. As there is no certain way to avoid this by clinical assessment or investigation, including biopsy, a diagnosis of chronic hepatitis should only be made firmly once liver disease has been present on clinical or other grounds for at least 6 months.

### (a) Chronic Persistent Hepatitis

Aetiology is discussed on page 401; pathology (persistent hepatitis) on page 402.

Symptoms are mild and comprise fatigue, poor appetite, fatty food intolerance and upper abdominal discomfort, especially over the liver. The condition may be asymptomatic and revealed by biochemical tests done for other reasons. There may or may not be a history of acute hepatitis. Examination may show slight hepatomegaly, but is often normal. There are no features of chronic liver disease.

Serum bilirubin is normal or slightly raised, serum transferase is raised up to five-fold and alkaline phosphatase is generally normal. Serum albumin and globulin are normal. The HBsAg may be present but autoantibodies are not found. Liver biopsy shows persistent hepatitis.

Differentiation should be made from the posthepatitis syndrome (p. 394) and Gilbert's syndrome (p. 390), as well as from the pericholangitis associated with Crohn's disease and ulcerative colitis (p. 361). The prognosis is usually excellent, the patient should be reassured and no treatment is required. Rarely, progression to chronic active hepatitis or cirrhosis may occur.

### (b) Chronic Active Hepatitis

*(Lupoid Hepatitis, Plasma-cell Hepatitis, Juvenile Cirrhosis)*

Aetiology is discussed on page 401; pathology (aggressive hepatitis) on page 402.

**Clinical Features.** This is a more severe disease than persistent hepatitis. It occurs predominantly but not exclusively in the second and third decades and more often in females. It shows a wide range of severity. The onset is usually insidious with fatigue, anorexia and jaundice. Other features include fever, arthralgia, epistaxis and ready bruising. Amenorrhoea is the rule. In about a quarter of cases the onset is acute, resembling viral hepatitis which, however, does not resolve normally. On examination, the general health appears good; jaundice is mild to moderate or occasionally absent. Signs of chronic liver disease, especially spider telangiectasia and hepatosplenomegaly, are almost always present. Sometimes a 'Cushingoid' face with acne, hirsutism and pink cutaneous striae, especially on the thighs and abdomen, are present. Bruises may be seen.

Though liver disease usually dominates the clinical syndrome, many associated conditions occur in chronic active hepatitis emphasising its essentially systemic nature. These include migrating polyarthritis of large joints, a variety of rashes, most non-specific but including inflammatory papules and urticaria, lymphadenopathy, thyroid disorders such as Hashimoto's thyroiditis, thyrotoxicosis and myxoedema, Coombs'-positive haemolytic anaemia, pleurisy, transient pulmonary infiltration, ulcerative colitis and glomerulonephritis. Some patients have Sjögren's syndrome (p. 607).

Some patients with chronic active hepatitis are chronic carriers of the hepatitis B virus. They are usually older males, clinical signs of chronic liver disease are less florid and associated conditions, except for arthralgia, are uncommon. Abnormalities of liver function tests are also less marked.

**Investigation.** Liver function tests are markedly abnormal; serum transferase activity is much increased, albumin concentration is often reduced, globulin concentration very high and the prothrombin time prolonged. The serum bilirubin reflects the degree of jaundice but usually does not exceed 170 $\mu$mol/*l* (10 mg/100 ml). Autoantibodies are often found; antinuclear antibody in half the cases, smooth muscle antibody in two-thirds and antimitochondrial antibody in a quarter. The HBsAg may be found, but almost always in patients without autoantibodies.

**Diagnosis and Prognosis.** Initially, differentiation from acute viral hepatitis may be impossible but the prolonged course and a biopsy at least 6 months after the onset will generally make the diagnosis clear. Wilson's disease must always be excluded (p. 410). Where ulcerative colitis coexists, cholestatic features suggest pericholangitis rather than chronic active hepatitis. Difficulty in differentiation from persistent hepatitis usually occurs where the liver biopsy does not confirm the clinical diagnosis and in these cases a further biopsy is needed.

The course is marked by exacerbations and remissions. Ultimately cirrhosis develops, about half the patients dying within 5 years of diagnosis, usually in the first 2 years. With the development of cirrhosis, ascites (p. 405), encephalopathy (p. 406), and portal hypertension (p. 404) occur. In patients with HBs antigenaemia, the progression of disease is slower so that survival is longer.

**Treatment.** Corticosteroids are life-saving in this disease, especially in the early stages, reducing activity and improving hepatocellular function. Initially, prednisolone 30 mg/day is given orally and the dose reduced gradually as the patient and liver function tests improve. Treatment for at least 6 months is needed, when gradual withdrawal of prednisolone may be tried. Relapse is frequent and prolonged maintenance therapy (10–15 mg/day) is often required. Where severe corticosteroid side-effects occur, azathioprine 50 mg/day orally may be given and the prednisolone reduced by half. Ascites, encephalopathy and portal hypertension are treated (p. 408).

## 2. Cirrhosis of the Liver

Aetiology is discussed on page 401 and pathology on page 402.

**Clinical Features.** These vary greatly and may include any combination of the manifestations described below. None are specifically related to particular causes of cirrhosis, though florid spider telangiectasia, gynaecomastia and parotid enlargement are more common in alcohol-associated cirrhosis. Autopsy experience shows that cirrhosis may be entirely asymptomatic, and in life it may be found incidentally or with minimal features such as isolated hepatomegaly. Enlargement of the liver tends to be more common in the early stages of the disease, disappearing as hepatocyte destruction and fibrosis reduce liver size. The patient may complain of weakness, fatigue or weight loss. Non-specific digestive symptoms such as anorexia, nausea, vomiting and upper abdominal discomfort may occur as does gaseous abdominal distension. Otherwise, clinical features are due mainly to portal hypertension and/or hepatic insufficiency.

*Portal Hypertension.* This results from destruction and distortion of the hepatic vasculature leading to obstruction of blood flow. In addition, there may be transmission of arterial pressure to the portal venous system. Cirrhosis is the commonest but not the only cause of portal hypertension; obstruction of the portal vein, e.g. from thrombosis, may have the same effect (p. 911).

*Splenomegaly* occurs as part of a general reticuloendothelial hyperplasia. It is, however, mainly caused by portal hypertension and is its cardinal sign. The splenomegaly is seldom marked in adults, the tip rarely reaching more than 5 cm below the costal margin. In children it may be much more marked. When the spleen is not enlarged clinically or radiographically, portal hypertension is unlikely.

*Haematological Changes.* Moderate leucopenia and thrombocytopenia frequently occur with splenomegaly and are attributed to hypersplenism (p. 589). Anaemia may occur and when hypochromic is usually due to blood loss from the gut. Macrocytes and target cells are common; though the marrow is usually normoblastic, megaloblastic anaemia sometimes occurs. Megaloblastic changes are usually due to nutritional folate deficiency; vitamin $B_{12}$ deficiency is rare.

*Collateral Circulation*. This occurs where there are portal-systemic communications. These are in the distal oesophagus and proximal stomach, in the anus and distal rectum, in the falciform ligament and between the colonic, omental, splenic and retroperitoneal veins. Collateral vessels may be seen on the anterior abdominal wall and rarely they radiate prominently from the umbilicus ('caput medusae'). The most important collateral vessels are in the oesophagus and stomach (oesophagogastric varices) as they can cause bleeding which may be severe and acute, or occult and chronic. Bleeding may occur from varices elsewhere in the gut but this is very rare. The presence of oesophagogastric varices establishes a diagnosis of portal hypertension. Special radiological procedures can demonstrate the patency of the splenic and portal veins, assess the extent of collateral circulation and allow the portal pressure to be measured (p. 388).

*Ascites*. In cirrhosis ascites is not due solely to portal hypertension. Several factors are responsible for general salt and water retention while portal hypertension and lymphatic obstruction in the cirrhotic liver predispose to the localisation of fluid in the abdomen. Liver failure leads to salt and water retention by decreasing renal blood flow which produces both a reduced glomerular filtration rate with excessive tubular resorption of water and sodium, and an increased renal release of renin leading to secondary aldosteronism. Failure of the liver to metabolise aldosterone intensifies the secondary aldosteronism and failure to metabolise vasopressin reduces renal water clearance. Hypoalbuminaemia lowers the colloid osmotic pressure of the plasma, encourages the formation of oedema and may contribute to a poor renal blood flow.

*Jaundice*. This is mainly due to failure of bilirubin metabolism. Intrahepatic cholestasis may also be a contributing factor. In cirrhosis jaundice is generally mild or absent. Increasing jaundice implies progressing liver failure.

*Circulatory Changes*. In cirrhosis the circulation tends to be hyperdynamic with increased peripheral blood flow and reduced visceral blood flow especially to the kidneys. The cause for this is unknown. Increased peripheral blood flow is indicated by palmar erythema. Arteriolar changes result in cutaneous spider telangiectases; these lesions comprise a central arteriole, which may raise the skin surface, from which small vessels radiate. They are usually confined to the area above the nipples and occur especially on the face, necklace area, forearms and dorsum of the hands. At an early stage they may appear as white spots on cooling the skin.

Reduced arterial oxygen saturation is frequent and central cyanosis may occur; this is probably due to the development of pulmonary venoarterial shunts and similar shunts may predispose to the development of clubbing of fingers.

*Endocrine Abnormalities*. Gynaecomastia, sometimes unilateral, may occur. It can result from the liver disease or may be induced by spironolactone therapy. Loss of libido occurs in both sexes; there is impotence and testicular atrophy in men and breast atrophy and irregular menses or amenorrhoea in premenopausal women.

*Haemorrhagic Tendency*. This is found in advanced liver failure and is due largely to underproduction of coagulation factors (p. 598). Thrombocytopenia may also occur particularly when splenomegaly is present. It is seldom sufficient to cause spontaneous bleeding but may aggravate bleeding from other causes such as varices. Serum fibrinogen concentration is not reduced until the terminal stages, though occasionally fibrinolysis may be significant. Bruising, purpura, epistaxis, menorrhagia or gastrointestinal bleeding can all occur.

*Skin Pigmentation*. Generalised hyperpigmentation due to increased melanin deposition occurs in a minority; haemochromatosis must then be excluded.

*Dupuytren's Contracture*. Various studies have suggested that there is an increased incidence of Dupuytren's contracture in patients with cirrhosis but the statistical evidence for this is poor.

*Fever*. About a third of cirrhotic patients have a low-grade fever not due to infection.

*Hepatic (Portal-systemic) Encephalopathy*. The mental and neurological features described in fulminant hepatic failure (p. 397) occur in cirrhosis in a more chronic and intermittent fashion. This complication sometimes overshadows the liver disease and leads to a diagnosis of primary mental disorder. Rarely, irreversible central nervous system changes occur with paraplegia, parkinsonism, epileptic fits and dementia. In addition to liver failure, the collateral venous circulation in cirrhosis bypasses the liver and allows nitrogenous substances from the gut to reach the systemic circulation thereby increasing the tendency to encephalopathy. Where anastomoses are extensive, encephalopathy may even occur despite relatively good liver function; this is rare in cirrhosis alone, but may be seen following a surgical portal-systemic shunt. A number of factors precipitate hepatic encephalopathy in the cirrhotic patient including sedatives, uraemia which itself is often precipitated by diuretics, a high protein diet, infection, trauma including surgery, gastrointestinal bleeding, hypokalaemia and constipation.

**Investigation.** The serum bilirubin may be normal; increases are usually slight. Bilirubinuria may or may not be present, but excessive urobilinogenuria is usual. Serum transferase activity is usually slightly increased by up to three-fold and serum alkaline phosphatase is raised similarly. All these tests may be normal and they are of no prognostic value. The serum albumin is reduced and the prothrombin time remains prolonged in spite of parenteral vitamin K in those with poor liver function; these tests, especially sequential results, are of considerable value as deteriorating levels indicate a poor outlook. The serum globulin is raised. BSP retention is almost always increased, though falsely normal values may occur in hypoalbuminaemia. Autoantibodies or the HBsAg may be found.

**Diagnosis.** Alternative diagnoses to be considered depend on how the patient presents, for example with haematemesis (p. 330) or ascites (p. 339). In those with hepatomegaly, secondary carcinoma should be especially considered where enlargement is gross, irregular and hard and where the spleen is not palpable. The site of the primary tumour may be found. A primary liver tumour is also possible (p. 412). Cardiac failure, tricuspid valve disease and constrictive pericarditis should be sought especially where the liver is large, smooth and tender. Rarer causes of hepatomegaly include lymphoma, leukaemia, amyloidosis, sarcoidosis, abscess and hydatid cyst. In the tropics, kala azar, malaria or schistosomiasis may be present. Finally, a cause for cirrhosis must be sought, especially one which is treatable, such as haemochromatosis or Wilson's disease.

**Prognosis.** Although cirrhosis is a progressive disease, the rate of progression varies and the outlook is related to many factors. The prognosis is better where the cause of cirrhosis can be corrected, as in alcohol abuse, haemochromatosis and Wilson's disease. Worsening liver function evidenced by jaundice or ascites indicates a poor prognosis unless a treatable cause such as bleeding or infection is present. Encephalopathy not associated with an extensive collateral circulation is a poor prognostic sign and, as with ascites, a poor response to therapy is ominous. Acute bleeding from oesophageal varices is fatal in about 50% of cases. Marked hypoalbuminaemia (below 25 g/*l*), hyponatraemia (below 120 mmol/*l*) not due to diuretic therapy and a prolonged prothrombin time are bad prognostic signs. The course of cirrhosis is uncertain as unforeseen complications such as severe infection or hepatocellular carcinoma may lead to death.

**Treatment** is discussed on page 408.

## Biliary Cirrhosis

Biliary cirrhosis is an uncommon condition resulting from prolonged obstruction anywhere between the small interlobular bile ducts and the ampulla of Vater.

**Primary Biliary Cirrhosis.** This disease affects predominantly women, usually in middle age. A chronic granulomatous inflammation of unknown cause destroys the interlobular bile ducts in the liver with the eventual development of cirrhosis. Immune complexes are found in the blood but their importance in producing liver damage is unknown. Pruritus is the commonest initial complaint and may precede jaundice by months or even years. When the patient is jaundiced, pruritus is almost always present. Although there may be upper abdominal discomfort, the abdominal pain, fever and rigors of large bile-duct obstruction do not occur. Diarrhoea resulting from malabsorption of fat and pain and tingling in the hands and feet due to lipid infiltration of peripheral nerves occasionally occur. Bone pain or fractures due to osteomalacia from malabsorption or osteoporosis are often prominent later.

Examination usually shows a well-nourished patient with or without scratch marks. Jaundice is only prominent late in the disease when the patient may become a bottle-green colour. Xanthomatous deposits occur in a minority especially around the eyes, in the hand creases and over the elbows, knees and buttocks. Hepatomegaly is virtually constant. Splenomegaly occurs later as portal hypertension develops. The disease generally lasts 5 to 10 years terminating in liver failure or alimentary bleeding.

The diagnosis is based on the clinical picture, on liver function tests showing cholestasis, especially a very high serum alkaline phosphatase activity greater than 250 units/*l* (30 KA units/100 ml), and on a positive antimitochondrial antibody test. It is confirmed by liver biopsy and the demonstration of normal large bile ducts on cholangiography. Laparotomy is rarely needed to determine the diagnosis.

No specific therapy is available. Azathioprine is of no value and corticosteroids are contraindicated as they exacerbate or precipitate bone disease. Penicillamine is under trial but cannot yet be recommended. Palliative measures, e.g. for pruritus, are described on page 409.

**Secondary Biliary Cirrhosis.** This develops after prolonged large duct biliary obstruction due to gallstones, bile duct strictures and, occasionally, sclerosing cholangitis (p. 418). There is chronic cholestasis with episodes of ascending cholangitis or even liver abscess manifested by upper abdominal pain, tender hepatomegaly, fever, rigors, leucocytosis and sometimes a positive blood culture or septicaemic shock. Finger clubbing is common and xanthomas and bone pain may develop. Cirrhosis, ascites and portal hypertension are late features.

## Treatment of Hepatic Cirrhosis

Although no treatment can reverse cirrhosis or even ensure that no further progression occurs, medical therapy can promote improved general health and alleviate symptoms. The main problems are to detect treatable causes, to correct malnutrition, to control fluid retention, encephalopathy and alimentary bleeding and to manage chronic cholestasis.

*Aetiological Factors*. Treatable conditions such as alcohol abuse, drug ingestion, haemochromatosis and Wilson's disease should always be sought. Relief of biliary obstruction will prevent biliary cirrhosis.

*Nutrition*. In the absence of encephalopathy or ascites, a high energy (3000 kcal/day), protein-rich (80–100 g/day) diet should be advised. Where cholestasis is not a feature, fat intake need not be restricted. Alcohol must be forbidden. When a good diet is taken, vitamins and other supplements are not required.

*Fluid Retention*. Treatment of ascites and oedema may relieve symptoms but does not improve the prognosis and, if overvigorous, may lead to fatal renal failure. In mild cases, therefore, only salt restriction need be advised; by using salt in cooking while avoiding salt at table, especially salty foods such as soups, ham and bacon, daily salt intake may be reduced to about 2 g of sodium chloride daily (40 mmol of sodium). More severe ascites requires diuretics. Initially, a potassium sparing drug such as spironolactone (100–200 mg/d) or triamterene (100–200 mg/d) should be used. Additional diuresis may be obtained from a medium potency diuretic such as bendrofluazide. Potassium supplements may not be necessary with this drug combination but hypokalaemia should be avoided as it may precipitate or worsen encephalopathy.

Patients with marked ascites should be admitted to hospital. They generally have more severe liver dysfunction and require more vigorous therapy to which they are apt to react adversely. Bed rest, restriction of water intake to 1 *l*/d, restriction of salt to 22 mmol of sodium daily (1 g salt) and potassium supplements may induce diuresis. If this does not occur within 4 days spironolactone or triamterene should be added and potassium intake reduced. Only when this has failed should high potency diuretics such as frusemide (80–160 mg) be used. Treatment should aim to produce a weight loss not above 0·5 kg/d, and regular checks should be made of the blood urea and electrolyte concentrations. Occasionally patients do not respond to treatment; many are continuing to take salt and this should be checked. The temptation to remove fluid by paracentesis must be resisted as patients tolerate this very badly. In special centres a Rhodiascit machine to ultrafilter ascites and return its colloid to the patient can be used. Salt-poor albumin (25 g) intravenously over 3 hours with frusemide (40 mg i.v.) may initiate diuresis in resistant cases.

*Hepatic Encephalopathy*. Episodes of encephalopathy develop in many patients with cirrhosis and are usually readily reversed until the terminal stages occur. The principles of treatment are as in fulminant hepatic failure (p. 399). All dietary protein is stopped or reduced below 20 g/d, and glucose (1500 kcal/d) is given orally or parenterally. The bowel flora is reduced with neomycin 2–4 g/d orally. Lactulose (10–30 ml t.i.d.) is given to produce two stools daily. Lactulose is a disaccharide which reaches the colon intact and is then split by colonic bacteria. It produces an osmotic laxative effect, reduces the pH of the colonic content thereby limiting colonic ammonia absorption and promotes the incorporation of nitrogen into bacteria. As encephalopathy improves, dietary protein is increased by 20 g/d on alternate days to an intake of 40–60 g/d which is usually the limit in these cirrhotic patients. Levodopa (0·5–2 g/d) and bromocriptine (15 mg/d) have been advocated for those who fail to improve adequately.

*Variceal Bleeding*. Acute bleeding from oesophagogastric varices is frequently severe and requires blood transfusion. Every effort should be made to avoid hypotension which may reduce liver blood flow and produce significant liver damage. Vasopressin, 20 units in 200 ml of 5% dextrose, should be given over 20 minutes to promote haemostasis by reducing portal venous pressure and blood flow to the variceal vessels. Abdominal colic, evacuation of the bowels and facial pallor from general arteriolar constriction indicate that vasopressin is active; absence of these suggests an inert vasopressin preparation. Cessation of bleeding is judged from nasogastric aspiration, pulse and blood pressure. This treatment can be repeated hourly if bleeding recurs. When initial bleeding has been controlled, its source should be determined by endoscopy as more than a third of patients with varices are bleeding from some other lesion, especially acute gastric erosions. Continued or recurrent bleeding from varices should then be controlled by a Sengstaken tube. This possesses two inflatable balloons which exert pressure in the lower oesophagus and gastric fundus. A useful modification, the Minnesota tube, allows secretions to be aspirated from the upper oesophagus when the balloons are inflated. Continued or recurrent bleeding can also be controlled by passing a catheter through the liver into the portal vein and obliterating the collateral vessels by injecting sclerosing material. If bleeding continues and liver failure has not occurred emergency surgery is necessary. Where oesophageal varices are bleeding, oesophageal transection or ligation of the varices may be done. Emergency portal-systemic shunt operations carry a high mortality and are reserved for those with good liver function. Emergency surgery is rarely applicable.

In patients with chronic variceal bleeding and in those who have recovered from an acute bleed, the surgical creation of a portal-systemic shunt is the only way to stop further bleeding. Portacaval, splenorenal and mesocaval shunts divert all portal blood flow from the liver. They virtually eliminate recurrent bleeding provided they remain patent, but there is a risk of postoperative hepatic encephalopathy which may be difficult to control. The distal splenorenal shunt, designed to decompress varices while preserving some portal blood flow to the liver, reduces encephalopathy at least during the five years after surgery. Portal-systemic shunts do not increase life expectancy, because they predispose to liver failure. Consequently they should be considered only for those under 60 years of age with good liver function evidenced by good general health, no ascites or evidence of encephalopathy, serum bilirubin less than 35 μmol/*l* (2·0 mg/100 ml), and serum albumin over 35 g/*l*. There is no place for the prophylactic use of these operations in patients with varices who have not bled.

*Chronic Cholestasis*. Where this is associated with irremediable biliary obstruction, episodes of cholangitis require antibiotics. Such treatment should be reserved for exacerbations and not given continuously.

Pruritus, believed to be due to bile acids, is the main symptom demanding relief. This is best achieved with the anion-binding resin cholestyramine, which reduces the bile acids in the body by binding them in the intestine and increasing their excretion in the stool. A dose of 4–16 g/day orally is used. The powder is mixed in orange juice and the main dose (8 g) is taken with breakfast when maximal duodenal bile acid concentrations occur. Cholestyramine may bind other drugs in the gut (e.g. anticoagulants); the latter should therefore be taken one hour before the binding agent.

Anion-binding resins are not helpful in complete biliary obstruction; then methyltestosterone (25 mg sublingually daily) or, for women, norethandrolone (10 mg orally thrice daily) is usually effective. These drugs, however, increase cholestasis at the canalicular membrane and jaundice invariably worsens. Anion-binding resins and the androgens usually relieve pruritus within a week.

Prolonged cholestasis is associated with steatorrhoea and malabsorption of fat-soluble vitamins and calcium. Steatorrhoea can be reduced by limiting fat intake to 40 g/day. Medium chain triglyceride supplements (Portagen) can be used to augment calorie intake. Monthly injections of vitamin $K_1$ (10 mg), vitamin D (calciferol 2·5 mg) and calcium supplements should also be given, the last as effervescent calcium gluconate (2–4 g/day). This preparation, however, contains much sodium and, where there is fluid retention, calcium gluconate alone should be used.

## Miscellaneous Diseases of the Liver

**Primary Haemochromatosis.** This is an uncommon disease in which excessive iron absorption over years leads to a gross increase in total body iron from the normal level of 4 g to 20–60 g. It is a genetic defect associated with the histocompatibility antigen HLA-A3. Iron is deposited widely: the important organs involved are the liver, pancreas, endocrine glands and heart. In the liver, iron deposition occurs first in the peripheral hepatocytes extending later to all hepatocytes. The gradual development of fibrous septa leads to the formation of irregular nodules and finally regeneration results in macronodular cirrhosis.

Clinical features generally occur in men aged over 45 years, menstruation and pregnancy providing protective mechanisms in women in whom the disease is ten times less common. There may be manifestations of hepatic cirrhosis, diabetes mellitus or heart failure. Leaden-grey skin pigmentation due to excess melanin and iron occurs especially in exposed parts, axillae, groins and genitalia, hence the term 'bronzed diabetes'. Impotence, loss of libido and testicular atrophy are also common.

The serum iron concentration is increased and the serum iron binding capacity is usually over 70% saturated. The serum ferritin is also high (p. 386). The diagnosis is confirmed by liver biopsy.

Haemochromatosis must be distinguished from other forms of cirrhosis, especially that due to alcohol in which there may be excess liver iron. Differentiation must also be made from other causes of excess body iron discussed below.

Treatment is by weekly venesection of 500 ml (250 mg iron) until the serum iron is normal; this may take 2 years or more. Thereafter, venesection is done to keep the serum iron normal. Other therapy includes that for cirrhosis and diabetes mellitus.

**Secondary Haemochromatosis.** Many conditions are associated with widespread secondary siderosis. Though they may cause features similar to haemochromatosis, these are rare and the history suggests the true diagnosis. Primary conditions include chronic haemolytic disorders, sideroblastic anaemia (p. 549), multiple blood transfusion (generally over 150 *l*) and Bantu siderosis (p. 96). Marked hepatic siderosis may also occur in alcoholic cirrhosis.

**Hepato-lenticular Degeneration (Wilson's Disease).** This rare condition is described on page 719. It is important to note that any of its hepatic features, including cirrhosis, may occur without neurological abnormality. Kayser-Fleischer rings occur in all patients with symptoms though their recognition may require slit-lamp examination. An episode of jaundice is often the first sign of disease; this may mimic acute viral hepatitis or be due to haemolysis consequent on red blood cell damage following sudden release of tissue copper. These episodes of jaundice may lead to fulminant hepatic failure. Later, the condition may proceed to active chronic hepatitis or a well-compensated cirrhosis. Slit-lamp examination of the cornea and measurement of the serum caeruloplasmin (p. 386) must be done in all patients under the age of 30 years with recurrent acute hepatitis or chronic liver disease of unknown cause irrespective of associated neurological abnormality.

**Non-cirrhotic Portal Hypertension.** Any obstruction to the portal blood flow results in portal hypertension; cirrhosis is much the commonest but not the sole cause. Portal or splenic vein obstruction is followed by the development of collateral vessels bypassing the obstruction as well as portal hypertension. Umbilical infection in the neonatal period is believed to be an important cause but other conditions leading to thrombosis include polycythaemia vera, malignant invasion from adjacent organs and pancreatitis. Portal tract lesions may also be responsible, including schistosomiasis, congenital hepatic fibrosis, myeloproliferative disease, exposure to arsenic or vinyl chloride and primary biliary cirrhosis. Other intrahepatic diseases causing portal hypertension include the Budd-Chiari syndrome and polycystic disease of the liver.

**Hepatic Venous Outflow Obstruction** *(Budd-Chiari Syndrome)* is an uncommon condition in which venous obstruction occurs anywhere between the efferent centrilobular veins and the right atrium. Obstruction may be due to thrombosis, especially in polycythaemia vera and in women taking oral contraceptives, to invasion by tumours of the liver, kidney, or adrenal, or to congenital venous webs. The syndrome may develop in constrictive pericarditis or right ventricular failure. It also follows damage to the central hepatic veins in *veno-occlusive disease*, occurring especially in children in Jamaica due to ingestion of toxic alkaloids in 'bush tea' infused from plants. In up to three-quarters of patients no cause can be found for the obstruction.

The condition generally develops fairly rapidly with abdominal pain, tender hepatomegaly and ascites. Liver biopsy shows severe centrilobular congestion. Hepatic venous obstruction is demonstrated angiographically. Mild cases recover completely; severer cases may die rapidly or go on to develop cirrhosis.

**Congenital hepatic fibrosis** is a rare condition in which broad fibrous bands are found in the liver. Most patients have associated polycystic renal disease. Many die in early childhood of renal failure. Those who survive often develop gastrointestinal bleeding due to portal hypertension, usually presenting between 5 and 30 years of age.

**The Liver in Protozoal and Helminthic Infections.** Protozoal infections associated with liver changes include malaria, trypanosomiasis, visceral leishmaniasis, toxoplasmosis and amoebiasis; the last is the most important as it causes liver abscesses which respond promptly to treatment (p. 814). In some cases of persistent malarial infection gross splenomegaly and portal hypertension develop (p. 809).

Schistosomiasis is the most significant helminthic infection as it may cause portal hypertension (p. 860). Echinococcosis, giving rise to hydatid liver cysts (p. 866), is the next most important. Rarely the roundworm, *Ascaris lumbricoides* (p. 868), may obstruct the common bile duct, and liver flukes (p. 864) may cause inflammation and adenocarcinoma of the bile ducts.

**Cysts.** Solitary cysts are rare, probably congenital, vary greatly in size and occur more frequently in the right lobe. Polycystic disease is characterised by many cysts of variable size; half the patients have associated polycystic disease of the kidneys (p. 453). Cysts may be found elsewhere as in the pancreas and lungs. Some patients have cerebrovascular aneurysms. Hepatic cysts are usually found incidentally. Occasionally a large cyst may cause upper abdominal pain, nausea, vomiting and a palpable mass. Complications are rare and include obstructive jaundice, torsion, bleeding and rupture. Portal hypertension may occur in the polycystic form. Liver function tests are usually normal. Cysts show as rounded filling defects on liver scan.

## Tumours of the Liver

**Primary Malignant Tumours.** *Hepatocellular carcinoma (hepatoma)* is the principal primary liver tumour. Its incidence shows great geographic variation — being common in Africa and S.E. Asia but rare in temperate climates. It occurs predominantly in males, and in 80% of cases cirrhosis is present. Cirrhosis may be of any type, but hepatocellular carcinoma appears most commonly in haemochromatosis and alcoholic cirrhosis, dominantly male diseases, and rarely in primary biliary cirrhosis, which mainly affects women. Other aetiological factors include chronic hepatitis B viral infection, ingestion of aflatoxin-contaminated foods in tropical countries (p. 799) and exposure to toxins such as thorotrast and arsenic. These last toxins usually produce angiosarcomas but they may also cause hepatocellular carcinomas. Oestrogens and androgens may cause adenomas or rarely hepatocellular carcinomas.

Macroscopically, the tumour may be a single mass or there may be multiple tumour nodules. Microscopically, the tumour is made up of trabeculae of well-differentiated cells resembling hepatocytes. Bile secretion by tumour cells may be seen.

Deterioration in a patient with cirrhosis should always lead to suspicion of hepatocellular carcinoma, the clinical features of which include weakness, anorexia, weight-loss, fever, abdominal pain, abdominal mass and ascites. Hepatocellular carcinomas are vascular so that a bruit may be heard over the liver or intra-abdominal bleeding may occur. Metabolic abnormalities are recognised increasingly and include polycythaemia, hypercalcaemia, hypoglycaemia and porphyria cutanea tarda.

The detection of high concentrations of $\alpha$–fetoprotein (p. 386) in the blood is virtually diagnostic. A liver scan almost always reveals a filling defect(s) and the diagnosis may be confirmed by liver biopsy. Surgical removal requires a tumour confined to one lobe in the absence of cirrhosis and is rarely feasible; the possibility should always, however, be considered. Doxorubicin (p. 579) can provide useful palliative therapy.

*Other primary tumours* are rare; they include haemangioendothelial sarcomas and adenomas. Cholangiocarcinoma is described on page 419.

**Secondary malignant tumours** are common and usually originate from carcinomas in the bronchus, breast, abdomen or pelvis. They may be single or multiple. Peritoneal dissemination frequently results in ascites.

Symptoms of the primary neoplasm are absent in about half the cases. Hepatomegaly may suggest cirrhosis, but splenomegaly is rare. There is usually rapid liver enlargement with fever, weight loss and jaundice. A raised alkaline phosphatase activity is the commonest abnormality but the liver function tests may be normal. Ascitic fluid has a high protein content, may be blood-stained and cytology may reveal malignant cells. Diagnosis can be made by needle biopsy in the area of a filling defect on liver scan or at laparoscopy.

**Benign Tumours.** Hepatic adenomas are rare vascular tumours which may present as an abdominal mass or with abdominal pain or intraperitoneal bleeding. They are more common in women and may be caused by oral contraceptives.

# THE GALL BLADDER AND BILE DUCTS

## Anatomy and Physiology

The junction of interlobular bile ducts leads to the formation of the right and left hepatic ducts which exit from the liver in the porta hepatis. These join immediately to form the common hepatic duct which, with the common hepatic artery and portal vein, lies in the free edge of the lesser omentum. The common hepatic and cystic ducts join to form the common bile duct which varies in length (2–9 cm) depending on where the junction occurs. The common bile duct, passing towards the duodenum, is usually divided into supraduodenal, retroduodenal, intrapancreatic and intraduodenal portions; it is, however, more useful to separate it into a thin-walled, wide-lumened proximal part up to 10 mm in diameter radiologically, and a thick-walled, narrow-lumened distal part 1–3 cm in length which may taper to a thread radiologically. The thick-walled part starts just outside the duodenal wall; it may be seen radiologically as a notch and is formed by the muscular choledochal sphincter (sphincter of Oddi). The common bile and pancreatic ducts fuse in the duodenal submucosa to enter the second part of the duodenum at the apex of the papilla of Vater.

The gall bladder is a pear-shaped sac of about 50 ml capacity situated under the right hepatic lobe. Its fundus lies close to the tip of the right ninth costal cartilage, its body and neck passing posterosuperiorly into the cystic duct which runs in a series of S-bends to join the common hepatic duct. Congenital abnormalities of the biliary system are rare; a folded gall bladder fundus ('phrygian cap') may be seen radiologically and biliary atresia or a choledochal cyst may occur.

The liver secretes bile continuously, producing 1–2 litres daily at a pressure of 15–25 cm of water. As the resting pressure in the common bile duct is somewhat higher than that in the gall bladder, bile enters the latter where it is concentrated about 10-fold by water and electrolyte absorption. The intraluminal pressure in the common bile duct is probably maintained by the choledochal sphincter. Bile duct pressures above 30 cm of water inhibit bile secretion. Reflux of bile into the pancreatic duct often occurs normally. The gall bladder receives an autonomic nerve supply, mainly from the vagus; acetylcholine causes contraction of gall-bladder muscle and it is likely that vagal innervation controls gall-bladder tone while the sympathetic nerve supply has little or no effect. Gall bladder contraction is due mainly to cholecystokinin secreted by the duodenal mucosa in response to food (p. 310). The choledochal sphincter normally opens and closes rhythmically; cholecystokinin and glyceryl trinitrate cause it to relax, while secretin and the analgesic drugs morphine, pethidine and pentazocine cause contraction. Of the analgesic drugs, pentazocine causes least sphincteric contraction. Acetylcholine has variable effects. Peristalsis does not occur in the common bile duct.

## Investigation

**Radiography.** *A plain radiograph* may show stones in the gall bladder or bile ducts, the soft tissue mass of an inflamed gall bladder, gas in the biliary tree due to a fistula into the intestine or pancreatic calcification. Only 10% of gallstones are radio-opaque.

*Cholecystography*. An iodine-containing compound is used which is absorbed from the gut, excreted into the bile and concentrated in the gall bladder so that it becomes radio-opaque; it is given the night before the investigation. The normal gall bladder shows as a homogeneous ovoid opacity. Non-opaque gallstones may show as 'filling defects' within the opaque area; much less commonly a tumour may do the same. Failure of the gall bladder to opacify is a frequent finding in gall bladder disease (non-functioning gall bladder). However, failure to take or vomiting of the tablets, pyloric stenosis, diarrhoea, occasionally intestinal malabsorption, poor liver function or a serum bilirubin above 35 $\mu$mol/*l* (2 mg/100 ml) can produce the same result. In addition, for unknown reasons, a normal gall bladder may fail to opacify in up to 20% of cases; for this reason the test should then be repeated, doses of the contrast medium being given on each of the 2 days prior to the test. If the gall bladder still fails to opacify, it is virtually certain to be diseased.

*Intravenous cholangiography.* Iodipamide methylglucamine (Biligrafin) given intravenously is excreted by the liver into bile. Provided liver function is good and the serum bilirubin not above 35 $\mu$mol/*l* the main biliary ducts and the gall bladder will be shown. This investigation may be used in those who have had a cholecystectomy. The extent of opacification of the biliary tree is much less than that achieved by cholecystography so that gallstones cannot be excluded confidently by this method. Furthermore side effects due to Biligrafin are fairly frequent; these can be reduced by infusing it slowly over an hour.

*Percutaneous transhepatic cholangiography* is of value in patients with obstructive jaundice and it may be done if the prothrombin time and platelet count are satisfactory. Under local analgesia, a narrow bore (Okuda) needle is passed into the liver and contrast material is injected under radiological control until a bile duct is entered. Where there is large-duct obstruction, the dilated biliary tree is usually entered readily allowing a demonstration of the site and often the nature of the obstruction. Less frequently the biliary tree is shown to be normal. Failure to enter the biliary tree cannot be taken to exclude fully a large duct obstruction. While narrow-bore needles have reduced the risk of surgery, facilities for operation should be available.

*Endoscopic Retrograde Cholangiopancreatography.* (ERCP, p. 314).

*Operative Cholangiography.* During operations on the biliary tract, the biliary tree should always be defined by injecting contrast material, either via the cystic duct or directly into the common bile duct.

**Ultrasonography** is the best method for the initial investigation of jaundice as it is capable of demonstrating dilatation of the biliary tree due to mechanical obstruction (p. 387). It can also detect gallstones and is particularly valuable for this in pregnancy.

## Gallstones

Gallstone formation is the commonest disorder of the biliary tract. Indeed, gall bladder disease in its absence is a rarity.

**Epidemiology and Pathology.** The prevalence of gallstones is not known as in most instances they are asymptomatic; however, they are exceptionally common among certain American Indians and in Sweden, common in North America, Europe, Australia and among South African whites, but less frequent in India and the Far East, and rare in African blacks. Gallstones are generally twice as common in females as in males and their frequency rises with age. In prosperous countries the incidence of symptomatic gallstones seems to be increasing and occurring at an earlier age.

In the past, gallstones have been classified by their macroscopic appearance into metabolic, inflammatory and mixed types. Biochemical analysis, however, has shown this to be misleading. In countries where gallstones are common, cholesterol is the most usual and frequently the major component irrespective of appearance. It is found in over three-quarters of gallstones accounting for 10–98% of their content. Some gallstones are composed almost wholly of calcium salts or bilirubin. The latter are commonest where there has been prolonged overproduction of bilirubin due to haemolysis; very little is known about the formation of calcium stones. Only the development of stones containing cholesterol will be considered here.

**Aetiology.** Current evidence suggests strongly that cholesterol gallstone formation is due mainly to physico-chemical changes in bile predisposing to cholesterol precipitation. Cholesterol, which is insoluble in water, is held in solution in bile by its association with bile acids and phospholipid in the form of mixed micelles (p. 346). In gallstone disease, the liver produces bile containing reduced amounts of bile acid and phospholipid relative to cholesterol with which the bile therefore becomes saturated or even supersaturated. Such bile is termed lithogenic. These changes precede gallstone formation and seem to be due mainly to a reduction in the size of the bile acid pool associated with reduced bile acid secretion into the bile. In a few patients there is also an increased secretion of cholesterol into bile. Although the liver produces the abnormal bile, the gall bladder is important in gallstone formation as it provides a site for cholesterol precipitation and a reservoir for gallstone growth. Infection and inflammation in the gall bladder may enhance the tendency to form stones.

Certain conditions predispose to gallstone formation. Disease or loss of the terminal ileum and long-term cholestyramine therapy lead to loss of bile acids in the faeces; cirrhosis reduces the secretion and pool of bile acids. Diets to lower serum cholesterol and long-term oral contraceptives also increase the frequency of gallstones.

**Clinical Features** are described in relation to the various illnesses which may be caused by gallstones.

**Treatment.** Currently, the only generally satisfactory treatment is cholecystectomy with the removal of any stones elsewhere in the biliary tree. Chenodeoxycholic acid (13–15 mg/kg/d) given orally dissolves stones with a high cholesterol content in patients with functioning gall bladders. Such stones are radiolucent on a cholecystogram. This treatment is recommended for those who are unfit for surgery or who refuse surgery. As dissolution takes six months to two years, symptoms may develop during treatment and stones can recur after treatment.

A frequent problem results from the incidental finding of asymptomatic gallstones. Follow-up of persons with these shows a high incidence of subsequent symptoms, sometimes with the development of serious complications, especially in older patients. Whether or not cholecystectomy should be carried out remains controversial, but it should be considered only in those with no contraindication to surgery.

## Acute Cholecystitis

**Aetiology and Pathology.** Acute cholecystitis is almost always associated with obstruction of the gall bladder neck or cystic duct by a gallstone. Occasionally, obstruction may be by mucus or rarely by a neoplasm. Initially, the inflammation is sterile being perhaps due to chemical irritation from an increasing concentration of the bile in the gall bladder. Later, enteric organisms, especially *Esch. coli* and *Strep. faecalis*, reach the gall bladder by unknown routes and secondary infection occurs. Culture of gall bladder contents within 24 hours of the onset of symptoms yields organisms in 30% of cases, whereas after 72 hours organisms are obtained in about 80%. Acute cholecystitis in the absence of stones is rare; it may develop in typhoid and paratyphoid fever or during bacteraemia.

All degrees of inflammation occur from mild congestion to gross swelling and tenseness of the gall bladder with ulceration of its wall. Occasionally, perforation takes place or the gall bladder may become distended with pus (empyema). Rarely, gas forms in the wall (emphysematous cholecystitis), a condition more frequent in males and in diabetes mellitus.

**Clinical Features.** The disease occurs at any age. Though more common in women, of the time-honoured factors — fair, fat, fertile, and 40 to 50 — only the fat remains true. The disease is seen increasingly in persons aged under 40 years. The cardinal feature is upper abdominal pain mainly in the epigastrium and right hypochondrium. It is commonly severe, causing restlessness, pallor, sweating and vomiting. Its onset is sudden and it increases quickly to its maximum intensity. The pain usually remains severe for up to an hour, though it may persist for many hours unless relief is obtained from powerful analgesics. Although called 'biliary colic' it rarely comes in waves like intestinal colic. There may be a history of previous similar pain.

Examination shows right hypochondrial tenderness and rigidity, worse on inspiration (Murphy's sign). Occasionally the gall bladder is palpable. Fever is present and rigors occasionally occur. Jaundice is seen in a minority and is usually slight; it suggests obstruction of the common duct.

Conservative therapy is followed by recovery in 80–90% of cases though recurrences are common. Sometimes there is deterioration due to the development of empyema, perforation and peritonitis or ascending cholangitis. In these cases increasing abdominal pain and rigidity, high fever, tachycardia and hypotension occur.

**Investigation.** A plain radiograph of the abdomen may show gallstones. Cholecystography fails to reveal the gall bladder and ultrasonography usually shows gallstones. Intravenous cholangiography may outline the common bile duct but not the gall bladder implying cystic duct obstruction. The serum amylase may be slightly raised and a moderate leucocytosis is common. Bilirubinuria may or may not be present.

Differential diagnosis has to be made from other causes of severe upper abdominal pain. These are mainly perforated peptic ulcer, acute pancreatitis, appendicitis (especially retrocaecal) and intestinal obstruction. Myocardial infarction should always be considered. Investigations useful in this differentiation are the raised serum amylase in acute pancreatitis, chest and abdominal radiographs, and an electrocardiogram. Occasionally there may be confusion with renal colic, herpes zoster, epidemic myalgia, pleurisy and acute intermittent porphyria.

**Treatment.** Initially, conservative therapy is usual. This consists of bed rest, relief of pain, maintenance of fluid balance and chemotherapy. Severe pain is relieved best by morphine 15–20 mg intramuscularly. Increased tone of the choledochal sphincter due to this drug may be minimised by atropine 0·6 mg intramuscularly. Less severe pain can be relieved by pethidine 100 mg or pentazocine 30 mg intramuscularly. Effective relief of pain may require repeated doses of analgesic every 2–3 hours. Provided persistent vomiting is not present, oral fluids can be given. Nasogastric aspiration is required only when there is persistent vomiting, in which case fluid must be given by the intravenous route. Co-trimoxazole or an antibiotic is usually prescribed. The development of complications, most common in the elderly, is an indication for surgery. However, over 90% of patients recover. The finding of stones or a non-functioning gall bladder should lead to cholecystectomy within 2–3 months.

Early operation has been advocated for acute cholecystitis. Therapy is begun as above, cholecystography or ultrasonography is carried out as soon as possible and operation done within a week of the onset of the illness. It is emphasised that this is not an emergency operation. The results of such therapy are similar to those of conservative treatment. It does, however, require only the one hospital admission, and it obviates the possibility of recurrent attacks.

## Chronic Cholecystitis

**Clinical Features.** Chronic cholecystitis is very common and almost always associated with gallstones. It usually manifests itself as recurrent episodes of biliary colic, unassociated with fever or leucocytosis. Severe pain lasts for about an hour and may be followed by upper abdominal soreness for a few days.

Sometimes a gallstone passes into the common bile duct and causes obstructive jaundice. Upper abdominal pain is present in three-quarters of these patients and there is frequently a history of biliary colic. Biliary infection causes fever in one third of cases; ascending cholangitis may then be severe, giving rise to liver abscesses or to septicaemia with shock. Obstruction is not usually complete so that the faeces remain pigmented and both bilirubin and excess urobilinogen are present in the urine. Occasionally, a gallstone may obstruct the common bile duct in the absence of abdominal pain or fever suggesting a pancreatic or biliary neoplasm. Alternatively, it may be associated with an attack of acute pancreatitis (p. 340). Rarely, a larger gallstone which has reached the intestinal tract, usually via a cholecystenteric fistula, may cause intestinal obstruction. This usually occurs in elderly patients. The clinical features are those of small intestinal obstruction with or without a history of biliary colic; the obstruction is usually in the terminal ileum. Abdominal radiographs show small intestinal obstruction, perhaps the gall-stone and possibly gas in the biliary tree.

Some patients with gallstones complain of non-specific symptoms such as eructations, nausea, vomiting and upper abdominal discomfort mainly in the epigastrium or right hypochondrium. These may be precipitated by fatty foods. This symptom complex has been termed 'gall bladder dyspepsia' and attributed to chronic cholecystitis. However, while such symptoms do occur in chronic cholecystitis and can be relieved by cholecystectomy, they also occur frequently in patients with other organic and functional bowel disease. Hence, when a patient complains only of dyspeptic symptoms, other bowel diseases must be excluded carefully before they are attributed to the gall bladder.

**Investigation.** The results of liver function tests and of urine tests for bilirubin and urobilinogen will depend on the degree of obstruction to the common bile duct. Abdominal radiographs occasionally show gallstones. Cholecystography will show either gallstones or a non-functioning gall bladder. Ultrasonography should be used when cholecystography fails to show gallstones in a patient with suggestive symptoms.

**Treatment.** Cholecystectomy and removal of gallstones from other parts of the biliary tree is the most satisfactory treatment. Stones may be removed from the common bile duct by perendoscopic sphincterotomy; this is a useful alternative to laparotomy in patients who are not suitable for surgery. Biliary colic is treated as in acute cholecystitis.

## Miscellaneous Diseases of the Gall Bladder and Biliary Tract

**Non-calculous cholecystitis** is rare. It may occur in typhoid fever, in polyarteritis nodosa, as emphysematous cholecystitis due to *Cl. welchii* in diabetes mellitus and in those on corticosteroid therapy. It may follow trauma and can complicate septicaemia.

**Cholesterolosis of the Gall Bladder.** In this condition lipid deposits in the submucosa and epithelium appear as multiple yellow spots on the pink mucosa. The changes are restricted to the gall bladder, symptoms are due to associated gallstones and the condition is recognised only at operation.

**Adenomyomatosis of the Gall Bladder.** In adenomyomatosis there is hyperplasia of all elements in the gall-bladder wall. This is usually localised to the fundus where it shows as a filling defect on cholecystography. It may also be generalised in which case cholecystography shows a distorted gall bladder possibly with intramural contrast medium in Rokitansky-Aschoff sinuses. Frequently there are associated gallstones. Although in most cases there are no symptoms, recurrent biliary colic sometimes occurs. In symptomatic cases, treatment is by cholecystectomy though where there are no gallstones operation should not be done before excluding other diseases, especially peptic ulcer and pancreatitis. Cholecystectomy should be carried out if it is thought that the filling defect might be a neoplasm.

**Postcholecystectomy Syndrome.** Where cholecystectomy is carried out for gallstones, 70% or more patients get complete relief of symptoms. When symptoms persist or biliary colic recurs, radiological examinations of the biliary tree for gallstones or unrecognised neoplasia should be carried out. Endoscopic retrograde cholangiopancreatography is specially valuable. In some patients, neither this nor investigation for other diseases such as peptic ulcer or pancreatitis shows any abnormality. The patients are then often considered to suffer from a functional abnormality of the biliary tree — 'biliary dyskinesia'. There is, however, no good evidence for such a condition and these patients should not be treated by procedures such as sphincterotomy or choledochoduodenostomy. Antacids, simple analgesics, sedatives, avoidance of foods clearly followed by symptoms and reassurance should be tried.

**Sclerosing Cholangitis.** In this condition there is fibrotic obliteration of the large bile duct system. It may be primary, associated with ulcerative colitis or retroperitoneal fibrosis, or secondary to cholelithiasis or biliary surgery. There is gradually progressive cholestasis and abdominal pain punctuated by episodes of cholangitis. Secondary biliary cirrhosis (p. 407) may occur. Diagnosis is usually made by biopsy of the bile ducts at laparotomy.

**Choledochal Cyst.** This cystic dilatation occurs in the common bile duct. It almost always presents by the age of 30 years with episodes of jaundice or abdominal pain. A mass is sometimes palpable in the right hypochondrium. Treatment is surgical, usually by drainage of the cyst or, rarely, excision.

### Tumours of the Gall Bladder and Bile Ducts

**Benign tumours of the gall bladder** are uncommon and usually found incidentally at operation or autopsy. Cholesterol polyps sometimes associated with cholesterolosis of the gall bladder, papillomas and adenomas are the main types.

**Carcinoma of the gall bladder** is an uncommon tumour occurring more often in women and hardly ever under the age of 50 years. It usually is in the fundus or neck of the gall-bladder and some 90% are adenocarcinomas. The remainder are anaplastic or, rarely, squamous tumours. Gallstones are usually also present and these are often held to be important in the aetiology of the tumour.

Clinically, there is frequently a history of repeated attacks of biliary colic and cholecystitis followed by general deterioration in health, weight loss and constant right upper quadrant abdominal pain. The gall bladder or a mass is palpable in the right hyponchondrium in half the patients. Jaundice is also present in half the patients and is occasionally an early feature in tumours of the gall bladder neck. Liver function tests most frequently show cholestasis. Gall bladder calcification (porcelain gall bladder), detectable on an abdominal radiograph, is strongly associated with cancer. Cholecystography may show a filling defect in the gall bladder but frequently jaundice prevents the procedure or a non-functioning gall bladder is found. Endoscopic retrograde or percutaneous transhepatic cholangiography may be helpful but frequently the diagnosis is made only at laparotomy.

In the majority of patients, the tumour is inoperable and survival is short.

**Benign tumours of the bile ducts** are extremely rare. Almost all are either papillomas or adenomas. They may cause biliary obstruction and generally are diagnosed only at operation.

**Cholangiocarcinoma** is an uncommon tumour arising anywhere in the biliary tree from the small intrahepatic bile ducts to the ampulla of Vater. It is not associated with cirrhosis. Virtually all the tumours are adenocarcinomas of varying degrees of differentiation and often with a marked connective tissue stroma.

Clinically, obstructive jaundice is the usual presenting feature though this may be delayed where the tumour involves only the right or left hepatic duct or an intrahepatic radical. Half the patients have upper abdominal pain and weight loss. Intrahepatic tumours are diagnosed as described for hepatocellular carcinoma (p. 412) with the exception that alphafetoprotein is hardly ever found. Transhepatic or retrograde cholangiography are the best methods for diagnosing large duct tumours preoperatively. Tumours above the junction of the hepatic ducts are often missed at operation despite operative cholangiography which may not show the intrahepatic ducts.

Treatment is surgical; it is rarely possible to remove the tumour but palliative surgery to bypass it is worthwhile as growth is slow and survival may be prolonged for a few years.

## Prospects in Liver Disease

The discovery of the HBsAg as a marker of the hepatitis B virus has been followed by the identification of several other antigens and antibodies associated with hepatitis B viral infection. These are likely to allow a better definition of the infectivity of patients and of the likelihood of their developing chronic liver disease. It has also led to the development of a vaccine, from formalin inactivated B viral particles, which has been proved effective. The ability to identify hepatitis A and B viral infection has revealed the existence of other (non A, non B) hepatitis virus(es) which can cause chronic carrier states. It is likely that these viruses will be identifiable by similar techniques, and this could reveal the cause of much chronic liver disease which is currently an enigma. Culture of the hepatitis viruses remain as elusive as ever.

In chronic liver disease, prevention must be the long term objective. Much will depend on how society faces the problem of alcohol abuse. Where disturbance of immunity seems to be an aetiological factor, recent observations indicate that the T lymphocyte has a significant role and advances in this area may lead to more rational therapy.

The development of a liver support system for the management of patients with liver failure has, as yet, met with only limited success. Difficulties include perfecting of materials such as polymer-coated charcoal capable of adsorbing substances toxic to the liver. Progress in this field is urgently required if we are to reduce the very high mortality in acute liver necrosis and also to facilitate liver transplantation. The latter is now technically feasible and there is steady progress in overcoming the immunity problems of organ transplantation and rejection.

Great advances have been made in understanding the pathogenesis of gallstones and perhaps these will lead to preventive measures in the future. Endoscopic retrograde cholangiography is an established diagnostic procedure, and the coming years are likely to see an increasing use of endoscopic techniques for removing stones from the biliary tree and for improving its drainage (e.g. papillotomy). The place of computed tomography in hepatobiliary disease needs to be defined.

N. D. C. Finlayson
John Richmond

*Further reading*:

Popper, H. & Schaffner, F. (eds.) *Progress in Liver Diseases*. Vol. IV (1972), Vol. V (1976) and Vol. VI (1979). New York: Grune and Stratton.

Schiff, L. (ed.) (1975) *Diseases of the Liver*, 4th edn. Philadelphia: Lippincott.— A very comprehensive reference book.

Shearman, D.J.C. & Finlayson, N.D.C. (1981) *Diseases of the Gastrointestinal Tract and Liver*. Edinburgh: Churchill Livingstone.— A new textbook primarily for clinicians.

Sherlock, S. (1975) *Diseases of the Liver and Biliary System*, 5th edn. London: Blackwell.— The standard textbook for reference purposes.

Sherlock, S. (1980) *Virus hepatitis. Clinics in Gastroenterology*. Vol 9, No. 1. Philadelphia: Saunders.

Wright, R., Alberti, K.G.M.M., Karran, S., Millward-Sadler, G.H. (eds) (1979) *Liver and Biliary Disease*. Philadelphia: Saunders.— A very comprehensive reference book.

# 10. Diseases of the Kidney and Urinary System

## Anatomy and Physiology

The kidneys are each composed of approximately one million nephrons, the basic structure of one of which is illustrated in Figure 10.1.

The blood supply of the kidneys is relatively large and amounts to about one-quarter of the cardiac output at rest, i.e. 1300 ml per minute. The afferent arterioles which give rise to the glomerular capillaries arise from branches of the renal artery. Emerging from the glomeruli the capillaries unite to form the efferent arterioles which then supply blood to the proximal and distal convoluted tubules surrounding the glomeruli. The medulla is supplied by arterioles which arise from those glomeruli situated in the deeper regions of the cortex.

For a short distance the afferent arterioles and distal convoluted tubules are in contact, and at this point the tubular cells become tall and columnar in character, forming the macula densa. The wall of the arteriole is thickened by cells which contain large secretory granules. These structures together constitute the juxtaglomerular apparatus which is intimately concerned in the regulation of the volume of the extracellular fluids and blood pressure.

The hydrostatic pressure within the glomerular capillaries of about 45 mmHg results in the filtration of fluid from the plasma into Bowman's capsule. This fluid is identical in its composition with plasma except that it normally contains no fat and very little protein. The filtrate thus formed then flows through the various parts of the tubule and is modified according to the needs of the body by tubular secretion and by the selective reabsorption of its constitutents.

### Functions of the Kidneys

In health the volume and composition of the body fluids vary within narrow limits. The kidneys are largely responsible for maintaining this constancy and the excretion of the waste products of metabolism represents merely one aspect of this task. The various renal functions are conveniently considered under the following headings and some are shown diagrammatically in Figure 10.1.

**Regulation of the Water Content of the Body.** About two-thirds of the water filtered by the glomerulus is reabsorbed iso-osmotically by the proximal tubules. The remaining water passes through the distal tubules and collecting ducts where its reabsorption is influenced chiefly by vasopressin, the antidiuretic hormone of the posterior pituitary. In the presence of vasopressin the collecting ducts become permeable to water which is then passively reabsorbed in response to the high concentration of sodium chloride and urea which exists in the medullary interstitium. The urine then becomes concentrated. In the absence of vasopressin the collecting ducts are impermeable to water. In these circumstances a dilute urine is formed by the tubular reabsorption of sodium without water. Disorders of the water-regulating mechanism which result in oliguria or polyuria are described on pages 425 and 426.

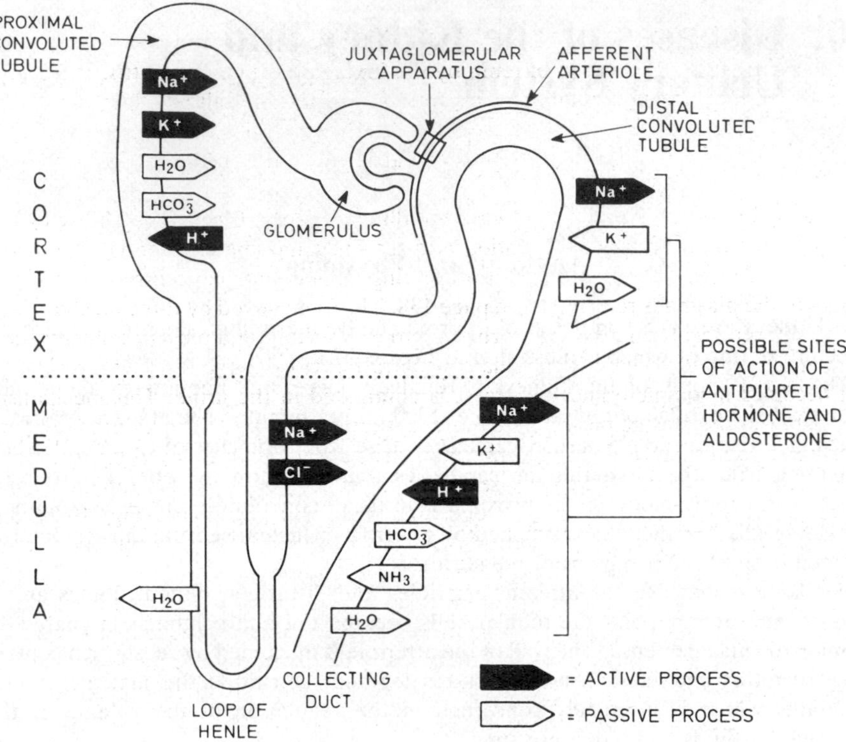


Fig. 10.1 Arrangements of some of the events concerned in urine formation. In the proximal convoluted tubule about two-thirds of the filtered sodium, potassium and water are reabsorbed. The greater part of the filtered bicarbonate is also reabsorbed here by a process which involves the secretion of hydrogen ions. The sodium and chloride reabsorbed in the ascending limb of the loop of Henle function as a counter-current multiplier and are largely responsible for the hyperosmolality of the medullary interstitium. In the distal convoluted tubule and collecting duct, potassium is transported into the cells and diffuses into the lumen in response to an electrochemical gradient. Hydrogen and ammonium ions are also secreted there and water is passively reabsorbed in the presence of antidiuretic hormone.

**Regulation of the Electrolyte Content of the Body.** The electrolyte content is kept remarkably constant as a result of selective reabsorption by the renal tubules. A large part of the sodium and probably all the potassium, which are freely filtered by the glomeruli, are actively reabsorbed in the proximal convoluted tubules and pars recta. The remainder of the sodium passes into the distal tubules and collecting ducts where its reabsorption appears to be under the influence of hormones of the adrenal cortex, especially aldosterone. With reduced secretion of these hormones, excessive quantities of sodium and chloride ions are lost in the urine, whereas with the administration of corticosteroids, sodium retention occurs. Urinary potassium is largely derived from potassium which diffuses into the tubular lumen from the distal tubular cells, in response to electrochemical gradients. The chemical gradient is created by the active transport of potassium into the cells and an intralumenal potential which is negative with respect to the peritubular fluid favours the diffusion of potassium into the lumen.

The dual actions of the adrenocortical hormones and of the antidiuretic hormone on the renal tubules play an important role in determining the total volume of water and the electrolyte content of the body. The rate of secretion of vasopressin is determined mainly by changes in osmolality of the blood; aldosterone secretion is influenced *inter alia* by changes in the pulse pressure within the renal arteries; this influences the rate of secretion of renin by the juxtaglomerular apparatus. It has also been shown that proximal tubular reabsorption of water and salt is influenced by the volume of the blood and the extracellular fluid. How this control is mediated is unknown but the activity of a third so-called natriuretic hormone has been postulated.

**Maintenance of the Normal Acid-base Equilibrium of the Blood.** The ability of the kidney to regulate urinary acidification and secrete ammonia is essential to normal acid-base balance. The importance of preserving an adequate concentration of bicarbonate in the plasma is referred to on page 138. This is achieved by three mechanisms. (1) All filtered bicarbonate is reabsorbed up to a threshold of a plasma concentration of about 25 mmol/*l*. When the plasma concentration rises above this level, reabsorption becomes incomplete and the excess is eliminated in the urine. This mechanism thus stabilises the plasma bicarbonate buffer system (p. 140). (2) The kidneys regulate bicarbonate and restore its concentration in the plasma when reduced by metabolic acids. This is achieved by actively secreting hydrogen ions into the tubular urine, where they are buffered by urinary disodium hydrogen phosphate (Fig. 10.2). (3) Ammonia formed within the distal tubular cells is secreted into the tubular lumen where it traps more of the hydrogen ions to form ammonium ions.

The degree to which these mechanisms operate is adjusted in accordance with the nature of the food ingested and the amount of endogenous acid production. In health, on a normal diet, 40–80 mmol of acid are excreted daily into the urine. When a diet consisting mainly of fruit and vegetables is taken, disodium hydrogen phosphate and bicarbonate are excreted in the urine and tubular secretion of hydrogen and ammonium ions is suppressed.

**Retention of other Substances vital to Body Economy, e.g. Glucose, Amino Acids, Phosphate, Bicarbonate, Proteins.** Glucose is normally reabsorbed so completely by the proximal tubules that none can be detected in the urine by clinical tests. Renal glycosuria is a genetically determined benign defect of tubular reabsorption in which glucose appears in the urine in the presence of normal blood glucose levels. More rarely other *congenital or acquired abnormalities of tubular transport* result in abnormal loss in the urine of amino acids, phosphate, sodium, potassium, calcium and water. These defects may occur singly or in combination. Examples are cystinuria, familial hypophosphataemia, nephrogenic diabetes insipidus and the Fanconi syndrome, a disease which usually does not present until the third decade of life.

In health the great bulk of the bicarbonate filtered by the glomeruli is removed from the urine by tubular reabsorption, and this becomes complete when the urine is acid. *Renal tubular acidosis* is a defect in the power either to reabsorb bicarbonate (proximal RTA) or to acidify the urine (distal RTA) which then usually contains significant amounts of bicarbonate in the face of metabolic acidosis. Such defects may be acquired as a result of renal disease such as pyelonephritis; they also occur as a consequence of myelomatosis, hyperparathyroidism, Wilson's disease and the use of degraded tetracycline. Idiopathic renal tubular acidosis is a rare, inherited form. All types are apt to lead to osteomalacia, nephrocalcinosis and hypokalaemia.

In health only a small amount of protein (0·2 g/*l*) reaches the fluid in Bowman's capsule. The volume of glomerular filtrate, however, is so great that if this small amount were not reabsorbed, more than 3 g of protein rather than the normal 50 mg would be excreted in the urine in 24 hours.

**Excretion of Waste Metabolic Products, Toxic Substances and Drugs.** The end-

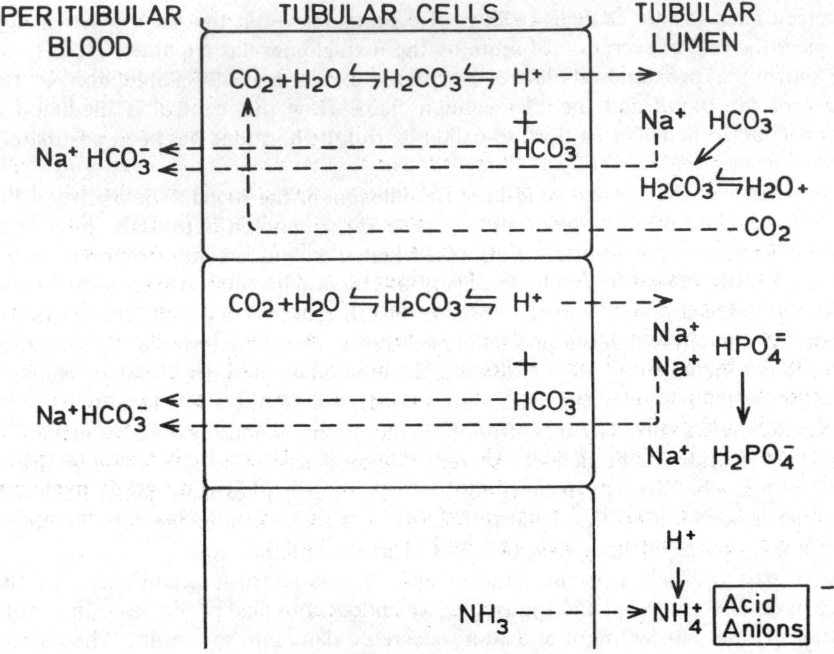


Fig. 10.2 Maintenance of the normal acid-base equilibrium of the blood. Carbonic acid is generated within the renal tubular cells from $CO_2$ and $H_2O$ released within the tubular lumen. The hydrogen ions of this acid are then actively secreted into the tubular lumen in exchange for filtered sodium which is then reabsorbed into the blood. The bicarbonate ions liberated from the carbonic acid are absorbed with the sodium into the blood; this restores the concentration of plasma bicarbonate to normal and also regenerates other buffers which have been titrated by the invading acids.

Some of the hydrogen ions are buffered in the urine by disodium hydrogen phosphate to form dihydrogen sodium phosphate and in the distal tubules by ammonia to form ammonium ions. Anions of the inorganic and organic acids are excreted in the urine largely as ammonium salts.

products of metabolism, especially those of protein, include urea, uric acid, creatinine, phosphates and sulphates, and are excreted in the urine.

**Hormonal and Metabolic Functions.** The juxtaglomerular apparatus within the kidneys is believed to secrete renin, which converts angiotensin I in the blood to angiotensin II. This substance increases the rate of aldosterone secretion by the adrenal cortex and also causes vasoconstriction. This may be the sequence of events by which renal ischaemia produces hypertension. The kidney is the main source of erythropoietin necessary for normal erythropoiesis (p. 535) and it is also responsible for the formation of 1,25 dihydroxycholecalciferol (p. 101). Two prostaglandins ($PGE_2$ and $PGI_2$) are also produced within the kidney. Both are powerful vasodilators and are natriuretic; $PGI_2$ is probably a mediator in renin release. Both may be concerned in the control of blood pressure.

## Investigation of Renal Disease

In the majority of patients suffering from renal disease, symptoms and signs are not usually referred to the anatomical site of the kidneys. This is due to the fact that clinical features of renal disease most frequently arise from abnormalities in the chemical composition of the body or from hypertension or anaemia. Their true origin therefore may be suspected only after the detection of urinary abnormalities and the importance of a routine examination of the urine in clinical practice cannot be overemphasised. The tests which may be of value include the determination of the volume of urine passed in 24 hours, the presence of abnormal urinary constituents and bacteriological examination. Under certain standardised conditions the determination of the specific gravity and pH of urine is of value. In addition it may be necessary to obtain further information by chemical analysis of the blood and by tests of glomerular and tubular function. The urethra and bladder can be inspected by urethroscopy and cystoscopy and catheterisation of the ureters can provide samples of urine from each kidney. Radiological examination includes a plain radiograph of the abdomen, excretion urography (intravenous pyelography), retrograde pyelography and renal angiography. Further information can be obtained by ultrasonic, radio-isotope and computed scanning, and by renal biopsy.

### Examination of the Urine

**Urinary Volume.** In health and in temperate climates the volume of urine excreted usually lies within the range of 800–2500 ml per 24 hours. There is a limit to the power of the kidneys to concentrate urine and on a normal diet a minimum volume of 800 ml is required to excrete the solid urinary constituents which consist mainly of urea and electrolytes. Less solute has to be excreted when a diet rich in carbohydrate and fat and low in protein and salt is eaten, and as little as 250 ml of urine per 24 hours is sufficient in these circumstances.

*Oliguria* is the production of insufficient urine to enable solute to be excreted in adequate amounts and the *milieu intérieur* of the body to be preserved. If the concentrating power of the kidneys is seriously reduced or if the solute to be excreted in the urine is increased above the normal, as occurs, for example, in severe infections or after traumatic injury, a daily output of as much as 2–3 litres of urine may even be insufficient. Oliguria develops in conditions associated with a reduction in renal blood flow and rate of glomerular filtration, e.g. diseases giving rise to water and salt depletion, hypotension, cardiac failure, acute glomerulonephritis, and other organic diseases of the kidneys. In these circumstances urine flow sometimes ceases completely and *anuria* develops. Anuria from this cause should be distinguished from urinary retention. In the latter case distension of the bladder will be found on examination of the abdomen, confirmed if necessary by catheterisation.

*Polyuria* denotes a persistent increase in urinary output. It must be distinguished from frequency of micturition, which may be defined as the frequent passage of small quantities of urine without an increase in the total volume.

There are two basic mechanisms which give rise to polyuria. It may be due either to the excretion of an abnormally large amount of solute so that elimination of an increased volume of water is required, or to a reduction in the ability of the kidney to concentrate urine so that an increased volume of water is needed to eliminate a given amount of solute. The latter defect may arise because of lack of circulating vasopressin or insensitivity of the concentrating mechanism within the kidney to its action. Polyuria occurs in the following clinical circumstances:

(1) Diabetes mellitus in which an osmotic diuresis occurs because of glycosuria due to hyperglycaemia.

(2) Renal disease with uraemia in which the elevated concentration of urea in the blood acts as the osmotic diuretic.

(3) Conditions in which there is decreased responsiveness of the collecting ducts to vasopressin, e.g. in some cases of chronic renal disease, during the recovery phase of acute renal failure, in hypercalcaemia such as may arise in hyperparathyroidism, in potassium depletion and in nephrogenic diabetes insipidus.

(4) Diabetes insipidus of neurohypophyseal origin in which there is diminished secretion of vasopressin.

(5) Inhibition of vasopressin secretion due to excessive drinking of fluid either from choice or from psychiatric causes, i.e. compulsive polydipsia.

(6) The elimination of oedema, e.g. in recovery from heart failure or the nephrotic syndrome.

**Specific gravity of urine** is a measure of the quantity of solids in solution and is an approximate measure of osmolality. In health, urea and sodium chloride are the main solutes contributing to the specific gravity of urine. In diabetes mellitus, on the other hand, the quantity of glucose in the urine may far outweigh the total of all the other solutes present; water containing 1% glucose has a specific gravity of 1·004, while, in the case of proteinuria, 4 g protein per litre, which gives a strong reaction with dipstix, raises the specific gravity by only 0·001. The specific gravity of urine varies with the nature and quantity of food eaten as well as with the amount of water or other fluid consumed.

The maximal capacity of the kidneys to concentrate urine may be determined after either depriving the patient of fluid or by the injection of vasopressin, but if a random or prebreakfast sample of urine is found to have a specific gravity of 1·020 or more there is clearly no need to carry out these tests.

**Reaction of the Urine and Acid Excretion.** In health urinary pH ranges from about 4·3 to 8·0. A very high pH (over 8·0) nearly always indicates urinary tract infection. In certain circumstances the ability of the renal tubules to excrete hydrogen ions is depressed and the demonstration of this is of clinical significance. Failure to acidify urine following the oral administration of ammonium chloride is characteristic of distal renal tubular acidosis occurring either as an inherited or acquired defect, and may also occur in potassium deficiency and in some patients with hypercalciuria and nephrocalcinosis.

**Abnormal Constituents of Urine Detectable by Routine Examination.** PROTEIN in the urine, detectable by dipstix or salicylsulphonic acid almost invariably indicates the presence of disease of the kidneys. Its magnitude bears little relation to any renal failure that may be present. Proteinuria does not occur in disease of the lower urinary tract, though a small amount can be detected in severe urinary tract infection or in obvious haematuria. Small amounts of protein are usually found in the urine in severe chronic renal disease, in the course of febrile illness and in heart failure. Larger amounts of protein (e.g. 3 g/day or more) are found in the nephrotic syndrome and invariably indicate glomerular disease. The great bulk of the urinary protein is albumin and larger molecular weight plasma proteins are present in only small amounts. The pattern of proteinuria can be determined and an index of selectivity assessed.

*A highly selective proteinuria* is one in which the larger molecular weight proteins are virtually absent, while a *non-selective proteinuria* is one in which the larger proteins are found in significant amounts. The degree of selectivity is an estimate of the amount of glomerular damage and is of help in predicting the response to be expected to the administration of corticosteroids (p. 436).

*Postural (Orthostatic) Proteinuria.* In a number of apparently healthy children and adolescents, and less commonly in adults, protein is excreted in the urine in variable but usually small amounts without associated disease of the kidneys. The urine formed while these individuals are recumbent is free from protein so that examination of the first specimen voided immediately on rising in the morning is normal. On the other hand urine formed while the individual is in the erect position or following vigorous exercise is found to contain protein. Tests of renal function show no abnormality. Postural proteinuria sometimes occurs in the presence of organic renal disease.

BLOOD is found in the urine in a wide variety of clinical conditions; haematuria commonly indicates serious disease of the urinary tract and the cause must always be sought without delay. The appearance of the urine varies with the amount of blood and is normal to the naked eye when only traces are present. When larger amounts of blood are present the urine may be smoky in appearance, bright red or reddish-brown. The brown discolouration is due to the formation of acid haematin from haemoglobin.

Red blood cells are found in varying number in the urine in acute glomerulonephritis, infective endocarditis, malignant hypertension, polyarteritis, systemic lupus erythematosus affecting the kidney, renal tuberculosis, congenital cystic disease, haemorrhagic diseases, renal infarction and trauma to the kidneys. Red cells occur in the urine also in inflammation and tumours of the kidney and of the urinary tract, in benign hyperplasia and carcinoma of the prostate, and in the presence of urinary calculi. Red cells are absent, or very scanty, in minimal lesion and membranous glomerulonephritis and in most cases of the nephrotic syndrome due to other causes.

Many of these conditions can be diagnosed by the presence of characteristic symptoms and signs in addition to haematuria. When haematuria is the sole or presenting symptom the cause is most likely to be renal carcinoma, papilloma of the bladder, benign prostatic hypertrophy or, in some localities, schistosomiasis (p. 860).

When blood appears only at the beginning of micturition, the rest of the urine voided being clear, the source of bleeding is distal to the bladder. When blood is uniformly mixed with the urine, it may have come from any part of the urinary tract other than the urethra. Renal colic accompanying haematuria indicates that the bleeding is renal or ureteric in origin.

Haematuria may be mimicked by other rarer causes of discolouration of the urine:

(1) *Haemoglobinuria*, which accompanies various intravascular haemolytic disorders (p. 554) and occasionally in normal people after strenuous exercise. The urine gives the chemical tests for haemoglobin, but no red cells are present on microscopic examination of the centrifuged deposit of a fresh sample of urine.

(2) *Acute intermittent porphyria* in which large amounts of porphobilinogen are excreted in the urine. Fresh urine from such cases may appear normal, but on standing for some hours a dark red colour may develop. The presence of porphobilinogen may be suspected from the red colour produced by the addition of Ehrlich's aldehyde reagent. In contrast to that produced by urobilinogen, this colour is not extracted by chloroform.

(3) *Beetroot, senna, dyes* used to colour sweets and *phenolphthalein* used in proprietary purgatives. These are rarer mimics of haematuria.

PUS CELLS AND BACTERIA. Pus cells may be found in the urine in inflammation of any part of the urinary tract. The urine should always be examined under the microscope and cultured when urinary tract infection is suspected. In obtaining the specimen for culture it is best to avoid catheterisation. A midstream specimen should be obtained from both male and female patients, and a culture should be made of this within 2 hours (p. 442).

CASTS are cylindrical structures of microscopic size which are found in the urinary deposit. They are formed in the renal tubules by the coagulation of protein. Red blood corpuscles or epithelial cells may be impressed upon this matrix, producing blood and epithelial casts respectively; such casts are found in the early stages of acute glomerulonephritis and other diseases in which there is glomerular inflammation. Granular casts are formed by degeneration of the impressed cells. Epithelial and granular casts are indicative of inflammation and degeneration of the renal tubules. Hyaline casts are formed by coagulated protein without the addition of cellular elements and are found in chronic glomerulonephritis and occasionally in small numbers in normal urine, especially after vigorous exercise.

OTHER ABNORMALITIES. Glycosuria is discussed on page 508; *biliuria* and *urobilinogenuria* on page 381.

## Chemical Analysis of the Blood

With progressive impairment of renal function the composition of the body fluids becomes abnormal. These abnormalities may be detected by blood analyses. The products of metabolism which in health are excreted in the urine are retained in the blood, and the concentration of urea, creatinine and the anions such as phosphate and sulphate increases. Determination of the concentration of blood urea gives a useful indication of the degree of renal failure, but it should be remembered that it does not rise above the accepted normal maximum until renal function is reduced by at least 50%. The diminishing capacity of the kidneys to secrete hydrogen ions results in their accumulation in the blood, and the severity of the consequent metabolic acidosis may be estimated by measurement of the concentration of bicarbonate. Estimation of plasma sodium, potassium, calcium and protein concentrations is of value in certain circumstances. A table of reference values for these and other biochemical factors, in SI and equivalent units, is given on page 906.

**Renal Clearance.** The ability of the glomeruli to perform their function is best studied by the measurement of renal clearance where clearance C = UVP, U and P being the urinary and plasma concentration of any given substance and V the minute volume of urine. If a substance in the plasma passes freely through the glomerular filter and is neither absorbed nor excreted by the tubules, the quantity excreted in the urine (UV) is identical with the amount filtered by the glomeruli; the clearance of such a substance therefore equals the rate of glomerular filtration (GFR) Endogenous creatinine and the polysaccharide, inulin, appear to be excreted in this way and their clearances are used to estimate GFR, which for the average adult is about 120 ml/min. In clinical practice the clearance of creatinine is usually carried out by collecting all the urine passed in a 24 hour period and withdrawing one sample of blood during the day of collection.

## Radiological and Imaging Investigation

A *plain radiograph* of the abdomen should always be taken before proceeding to excretion urography. Its main purpose is to reveal radio-opaque calculi or other areas of calcification such as nephrocalcinosis. Calculi are easily missed, especially if they are less than 1 cm in diameter as they are easily obscured by bowel shadows, or overlie bone. The plain film may also demonstrate the renal outline, though this is often better visualised during excretion urography.

*Excretion urography* is carried out by the intravenous injection of an organic iodine-containing compound, about one third of which is excreted largely by glomerular filtration within the first hour. Following the injection, films are taken at timed intervals. There is first an increase in the radiographic density of the renal substance (nephrogram), as the contrast medium enters the renal tubules. In the adult, healthy kidneys usually measure 11–14 cm and differ from each other by less than 2 cm; they are usually smooth in outline, but the nephrogram may reveal scars of pyelonephritis, often in association with a calyceal abnormality, or reveal localised masses of tumours; sometimes fetal lobulation, a normal variation, is seen. In diffuse renal disease with reduced function the nephrogram is faint and the kidneys may appear small. An increase in opacification occurs on the affected side in renal artery stenosis.

Normally within a few minutes the contrast medium begins to be excreted into the calyceal system, pelvis and ureters, which are best seen within the first 20 minutes, and may outline anatomical abnormalities there. Usually each kidney is seen to possess 2–4 major calyces, each of which possesses 3–4 minor calyces moulded around a renal papilla, and giving a concave or cup-like opacification. Clubbed calyces and slow excretion are commonly found in chronic urinary obstruction. When obstruction is severe there is often distension of the pelvis and thinning of the renal cortex and calyceal opacification is then often absent (negative pyelogram). Calyceal abnormalities may also suggest papillary necrosis, renal tuberculosis or atrophic pyelonephritis. In renal tuberculosis calcification and cavitation are common. Pools or streaks of contrast medium within the pyramids without calyceal deformity suggest medullary sponge kidney. Polycystic disease causes bilateral renal enlargement and the calyceal structure is stretched and spidery.

*Retrograde urography or pyelography* is mainly used to investigate lesions of the ureter and to define the cause of obstruction. Contrast medium is injected under screeening control into the ureteric orifice during cystoscopy; alternatively, a catheter can be introduced into the lower part of the ureters and the injection carried out later. Occasionally when retrograde pyelography is unsatisfactory or impossible, or a ureteric obstruction involves only the upper urinary tracts, percutaneous (antegrade) pyelography is carried out.

*A micturating cystogram* is of importance in the investigation of urinary infection in childhood, but because of risk to the gonads of radiation, it should be carried out only in those who show a urographic abnormality and are under the age of three years. It may also reveal abnormalities of the bladder outflow tract.

*Renal arteriography* is less often required than formerly, but may be helpful in identifying the nature of a renal mass detected by ultrasound examination and in revealing renal artery stenosis or intrarenal microaneurysms as occurs in polyarteritis.

*Ultrasonography* of the kidneys is complementary to other methods of investigation, but is most useful in distinguishing solid renal tumours and cystic lesions. Polycystic kidney disease is readily diagnosed by this means.

*Computed tomography* is particularly helpful in the diagnosis of masses in the kidneys and retroperitoneal tissues, and in defining the spread of bladder and prostatic tumours. Its use should be reserved for cases in which simpler methods fail to clarify the problem.

*Radioisotope studies* involve the injection of radioactive compounds which are concentrated and excreted by the kidney; the gamma radiation emitted is detected and the change in radioactivity with time is recorded by a gamma scintillation camera. The application of these techniques is of value in estimating the relative blood flow to the kidneys, in defining the size, shape, position and function, in the detection of tumours or abscesses and in estimating the effect of urinary tract obstruction on kidney function.

### Renal Biopsy

The technique of renal biopsy has greatly increased understanding of renal disease and in particular, knowledge of glomerulonephritis. Tissue obtained can be examined by light and electron microscopy; immunoglobulins, complement and fibrin can be identified by the use of immunofluorescence microscopy. Biopsy is especially useful in diagnosis in patients with proteinuria of unknown origin, in unexplained renal failure when the kidneys are of normal size, in suspected systemic disease associated with abnormal urinary constituents and in haematuria in which lesions of the lower urinary tract have been excluded. In experienced hands it is a safe procedure, but should be carried out only in patients possessing two kidneys and after the exclusion of any bleeding disorder by an appropriate coagulation screen. Hypertension, if present, should be under control.

## Glomerulonephritis

The term 'glomerulonephritis' is used to describe a bilateral disease of the kidneys which usually affects all the glomeruli. In practice, cases can usually be placed in one of three histologically defined categories which are described below under the headings of *proliferative*, *minimal lesion* and *membranous glomerulonephritis*. Within the proliferative group there are several variants, the most important of which are (1) *acute diffuse proliferative glomerulonephritis,* (2) *mesangiocapillary glomerulonephritis*, (3) *crescentic glomerulonephritis* and (4) *Goodpasture's syndrome*. These histological appearances reflect the different ways in which the glomerulus reacts to injury and to some extent they influence the presenting clinical features. In the early stages of these disorders the histological pictures are distinctive. In cases of proliferative glomerulonephritis which fail to recover completely, and in the later stages of membranous glomerulonephritis, the histological features become less clearly distinguishable. The fact that hypertension may accompany some stage of these diseases complicates the pathology still further by the changes due to arteriolosclerosis.

### Proliferative Glomerulonephritis

This condition is characterised by a diffuse inflammatory reaction of the glomeruli of both kidneys. When the disease appears abruptly, the terms *acute glomerulonephritis* or *acute nephritis* are often applied.

**Aetiology.** The great majority of cases of *acute diffuse proliferative glomerulonephritis* is due to the deposition of immune complexes in the capillary wall of the glomerulus. The classical disorder follows infection with $\beta$-haemolytic streptococci, and this may occur as acute tonsilitis, scarlet fever or upper respiratory infection. In developing countries streptococcal infection of wounds and skin infections are more often responsible but streptococcal infection anywhere may be the cause. Some viruses (e.g. varicella and E B) may also cause proliferative glomerulonephritis and a similar reaction can follow infection with organisms as different as staphylococci, pneumococci, *Myco. leprae*, *P. malariae* and schistosomiasis. It may also occur as a complication of infective endocarditis.

Glomerular disease caused by immune complexes also occurs in systemic lupus erythematosus (antibody to DNA) and polyarteritis, in the course of some tumours and lymphomas which induce circulating antibodies and as a consequence of an immunological reaction to drugs. However, in many patients and in the majority of cases that occur in Britain there is no clue to the nature of the antigen.

*Goodpasture's syndrome* is a rare form of acute proliferative glomerulonephritis associated with haemoptysis; it develops as a consequence of the formation of IgG antibodies to glomerular basement membrane.

**Pathology.** The commonest lesion is a diffuse reaction of the glomerular capillaries with variable swelling of the endothelial cells, proliferation of the mesangial cells and accumulation of polymorphonuclear leucocytes in the tuft and the glomerular space. Within the first few weeks of the illness EM examination shows characteristic deposits of antigen-antibody complexes on the subepithelial aspect of the basement membrane; these are associated with a granular appearance on immunofluorescence for IgG and C3. This is in contrast to Goodpasture's syndrome where antibodies are deposited in a linear fashion along the basement membrane. There may be proliferation of the outer layers of Bowman's capsule to form minor or segmental epithelial crescents. In many cases the changes resolve with clinical recovery and the kidney returns to normal.

In persistent and in rapidly progressive cases the epithelial crescents, which arise as a result of the presence of red blood cells, fibrin and inflammatory exudate in Bowman's space, increase in size and compress the glomeruli interfering with their function. This is the variant known as *crescentic glomerulonephritis*.

Progressive fibrosis of crescents and glomeruli occurs and the glomerular capillaries gradually become obstructed, resulting in secondary degeneration in the tubules. Ultimately many nephrons may be replaced by fibrous tissue, leading to small contracted kidneys. It appears likely that the immune complexes activate both the coagulation and the complement systems. The degree of intravascular glomerular thrombosis partly determines the rapidity of the deterioration and possibly also whether the condition resolves. This component of the disorder may be assessed by estimation of the breakdown products of fibrinogen and fibrin (FDP) in the urine. Another factor influencing the histological picture and the outcome is the way in which the mesangial cells react and fulfil their phagocyte role. In some cases proliferation of the mesangial cells is so marked that they project into the glomerular capillaries and seriously interfere with their function. They also send extensions of mesangial cell cytoplasm between the endothelial cells and the basement membrane giving a lobular appearance. This variant is called *mesangiocapillary glomerulonephritis*. The activation of complement in acute streptococcal glomerulonephritis is reflected in a transient fall in the C3 component of complement (p. 28) during the illness. In mesangiocapillary glomerulonephritis in many cases there is a persistent reduction of serum complement which probably antedates the disease. This abnormality, which is possibly genetically determined, may increase the susceptibility of the host to circulating immune complexes.

**Clinical Features.** Acute glomerulonephritis occurs most commonly in childhood and adolescence but may develop at any age. When it follows streptococcal infection a latent period is usual, the features of glomerulonephritis developing 1 to 3 weeks after the infection has subsided. The infection itself may be slight and may even pass unnoticed, and there is no relationship between its severity and the probability of the development of the disease.

In children the onset is usually abrupt, a striking feature being swelling of the face which is part of a generalised oedema caused by fluid retention. It is most marked around the eyes because the skin is more loosely attached to the subcutaneous tissues here and because the patient can usually lie flat. Oedema may be detected around the ankles if the patient is ambulant. Breathlessness due to pulmonary oedema may be present and in severe cases pleural effusions develop. Occasionally there is discomfort in the renal angles and epistaxis may occur. In acute cases there may be malaise, fever, anorexia, vomiting and headache. In most cases there is a moderate rise in blood pressure. In a few hypertensive encephalopathy occurs.

In adults, a history of acute streptococcal or other infection is less commonly obtained and the onset is insidious with progressive tiredness and slowly developing oedema of the lower limbs. Asymptomatic cases may be discovered after routine examination of the urine.

*Urine.* The daily output is usually reduced in volume due to a fall in the rate of glomerular filtration and increased tubular reabsorption of water and salt. Anuria may occur in very severe cases. The urine may appear red or smoky owing to the presence of blood and is usually concentrated. Proteinuria is of moderate degree, seldom exceeding 4 g/d, but the amount present is out of proportion to the haematuria. Microscopic examination of the urinary deposit reveals erythrocytes, some leucocytes, and red blood cell, epithelial and granular casts.

*Renal function tests.* In the early stages concentrating power is usually unimpaired, and the specific gravity of the urine is high. The rate of glomerular filtration is reduced and the concentration of urea in the blood is raised. A moderate degree of acidosis is usual. When recovery occurs the filtration rate rises and the blood urea concentration falls to normal.

**Course and Prognosis.** Complete recovery occurs in the great majority of children. The acute manifestations lessen in the course of 3 to 4 days, the temperature, pulse rate and blood pressure falling to normal. Diuresis occurs, and the oedema, haematuria and number of casts in the urine diminish. Small amounts of blood may be present in the urine for 10 to 14 days, while proteinuria may persist for several weeks or months. The prognosis is worse in adults and after middle age when complete recovery occurs in only about 50% of cases.

In about 10% of cases hypertension and haematuria subside and the patient apparently regains normal health. Proteinuria however persists, and after many years chronic glomerulonephritis, hypertension and renal failure develop.

While about one-third of patients with mesangiocapillary glomerulonephritis present an acute clinical picture, the remainder usually develop more slowly and go on to the nephrotic syndrome (p. 435).

In rapidly progressive crescentic glomerulonephritis, marked hypertension, extreme oliguria, recurrent convulsions and death may occur within a few days from acute cardiac failure and pulmonary oedema or in 2 or 3 weeks from uraemia. Treatment by dialysis has improved the mortality in this group but it still remains high.

**Differential Diagnosis.** Poststreptococcal nephritis may be diagnosed if haemolytic streptococci can be isolated or if there is evidence of streptococcal infection as shown by a rising titre of antistreptolysin antibody. In the absence of other infective causes (p. 431) acute glomerulonephritis should be distinguished from:

1. *Henoch-Schönlein purpura* (p. 624) in which focal or diffuse glomerulonephritis is associated with purpura and swollen joints and sometimes abdominal pain and melaena.
2. *Polyarteritis nodosa and systemic lupus erythematosus* in which red blood cell casts may also be found in the urine. Other organs are usually involved in the pathological process, and the diagnosis of these two diseases is suspected on this basis. Polyarteritis and systemic lupus erythematosus are occasionally confined to the kidney, when renal biopsy is necessary to establish the diagnosis.
3. *Infective endocarditis*, in which microscopic haematuria is a valuable diagnostic sign, and uraemia may develop.
4. *Acute recurrent focal nephritis*, a condition of unknown but probably multiple aetiology in which recurrent episodes of haematuria occur over a period of months or years. There are no other symptoms or signs of acute proliferative glomerulonephritis. The diagnosis is made by renal biopsy in which mesangial proliferation is found sometimes affecting only some glomeruli but commonly associated with the deposition of IgA. Repeated episodes may lead to progressive glomerular destruction with renal failure and hypertension in a few patients.

Other conditions which may need to be distinguished from acute glomerulonephritis are:

A. *Angio-oedema*, in which sudden swelling of the eyelids is a frequent feature. This condition is usually associated with swelling of the lips or tongue; urinary abnormalities are absent. In addition, the patient may be known to be an allergic subject, similar attacks may have occurred previously, and eosinophilia is often present.

B. *Acute pyelonephritis*, in which oedema is absent while pain and tenderness in the lumbar region and frequency of micturition may occur. The urine contains micro-organisms, more pus than red blood cells and red cell casts are absent.

C. *Haematuria due to tuberculosis or tumours* of the kidney or urinary tract in which oedema does not occur and there are no cellular casts in the urine.

**Treatment.** The patient should preferably remain in bed until haematuria, hypertension and oedema have disappeared and proteinuria has decreased. The intake of protein should be reduced to 40 g/d. While oedema is present fluid should be restricted to half a litre daily plus the volume of the previous day's output. Salt should not be added to food. If oedema is severe a low salt diet and diuretics may be necessary. When hypertension and haematuria have subsided and diuresis has occurred the protein content of the diet can be increased.

In the occasional rare case of severe nephritis with anuria or extreme oliguria the regime described on page 448 should be adopted.

Streptococcal infection should be treated with penicillin. Removal of infected tonsils or other septic foci should be delayed until convalescence is advanced, as operation may be followed by an exacerbation, especially if carried out during the acute stage. However, in a few cases with persistence or repeated recurrence of symptoms and signs, these features may disappear only after the removal of a focus of chronic infection, e.g. apical teeth abscesses. In the event of operative treatment being needed, benzylpenicillin should be given on the day of operation and for 3 days after it. When the condition is associated with other infections appropriate antimicrobial treatment should be given.

Hypertension does not require treatment in the majority of cases but hypertensive encephalopathy should be treated as described on page 198. Attempts to influence the course of the disease by the use of corticosteroids or immunosuppressive drugs have not been successful. Plasma exchange has been advocated to remove circulating immune complexes in a rapidly progressive glomerulonephritis and to remove anti-basement membrane antibodies in Goodpasture's syndrome. Its value has not yet been established.

### Minimal Lesion Glomerulonephritis and Membranous Glomerulonephritis

These conditions are associated with a marked increase in the permeability of the glomerular basement membrane. This leads to proteinuria which is often so severe that the nephrotic syndrome with hypoproteinaemia and oedema develop. The two conditions are described together because, although they tend to affect different age groups, their clinical presentation is similar.

**Aetiology and Pathology.** In membranous glomerulonephritis the histological appearances consist of a diffuse thickening of the glomerular basement membrane associated with sub-epithelial deposition of IgG. As the disease progresses the thickening becomes more severe and the glomerular tufts are converted into structureless hyaline tissue. Immunofluorescent studies show that while immunoglobulins are deposited in the basement membrane, there is little or no mesangial cell proliferation characteristic of proliferative glomerulonephritis. These findings taken together with experimental studies suggest that membranous glomerulonephritis is the result of antigen-antibody complexes sufficiently small to pass through most of the thickness of the glomerular basement membrane and become deposited on its external sub-epithelial aspect. While this could explain the lack of mesangial cell proliferation, the possibility of glomerular injury from other mechanisms cannot be excluded and the nature of the antigen or antigens is unknown in the vast majority of cases. Antibodies to type B hepatitis are occasionally associated with membranous glomerulonephritis.

In minimal lesion glomerulonephritis, the glomeruli show no lesion when examined by light microscopy. However, abnormalities of glomerular structure involving especially the epithelial cells are revealed by the electron microscope. The evidence suggests that this condition does not progress to glomerular destruction as is usually the case with membranous glomerulonephritis, and there is no evidence that the condition is due to the deposition of immune complexes. Minimal lesion glomerulonephritis may rarely follow exposure to pollen and this suggests an anaphylactic immune response (p. 29); however there is no immunofluorescent or other evidence to implicate IgE in the disease process.

**Clinical Features.** Minimal lesion glomerulonephritis occurs predominantly in children and young adults while membranous glomerulonephritis mainly affects those over 30 years of age. Both diseases are insidious in onset. If the proteinuria is slight they may persist without symptoms and remain undetected for months or years. When proteinuria increases in severity, oedema occurs and it is in this way that attention may be drawn to their existence. The patient may also notice the urine becomes frothy. The oedema is generalised, involving first the subcutaneous tissue and later the serous sacs and lungs. The face presents a pale and puffy appearance. The general health may remain good for some considerable time but eventually becomes progressively impaired, with increased liability to infection of the oedematous tissues or the serous cavities. Protein malnutrition with striae in the skin and osteoporosis may occur.

The urine contains protein in moderate amounts though as much as 30 g may be excreted per day in occasional patients. Granular and hyaline casts are seen on microscopic examination, red cells being scanty or absent.

At first chemical examination of the blood shows little or no increase in urea. Plasma cholesterol is slightly raised and the plasma and ascitic fluid may look milky due to an increase in fat and $\beta$-lipoproteins. Total plasma proteins are greatly reduced e.g. to 30–40 g/*l*. There are quantitative changes in the various globulin fractions, but the chief reduction affects albumin. Proteins of larger molecular weight, e.g. $\alpha_2$-macroglobulin, do not so readily pass the glomerular barrier and are retained in the blood and hence are increased relative to the other plasma proteins. The resulting fall of colloid osmotic pressure of the plasma is mainly responsible for the massive oedema which is the prominent clinical feature. The ensuing oligaemia stimulates the secretion of aldosterone which promotes further sodium and water retention and sometimes potassium loss.

In the early stage of the diseases renal function tests reveal no impairment of glomerular filtration rate or of the ability to concentrate urine.

**Course and Prognosis.** In the majority of cases the oedema persists for months or years, with occasional spontaneous but temporary remissions. Prior to the use of effective diuretics, antibiotics and corticosteroids, recovery rarely occurred. The majority of patients died either from intercurrent infection in the oedematous phase or from renal failure. There is now ample evidence that in patients with minimal lesion glomerulonephritis, corticosteroids and immunosuppressive treatment causes the proteinuria to subside and the condition to resolve in the great majority of cases. In membranous glomerulonephritis, however, the prognosis is less favourable. Arterial hypertension and hypertensive retinopathy develop and progressive renal destruction ultimately reduces the rate of glomerular filtration in most cases. Proteinuria diminishes, and consequently the plasma proteins rise and oedema becomes less. There is gradual impairment of renal function as the disease progresses to chronic glomerulonephritis with uraemia (p. 437). In a minority of cases, however, slow resolution of the glomerular lesion occurs and patients may recover completely.

**Differential Diagnosis of the Nephrotic Syndrome.** The term 'nephrotic syndrome' is used to describe the clinical state of hypoproteinaemic oedema associated with marked proteinuria irrespective of its aetiology. *Minimal lesion glomerulonephritis* is the most common cause of the nephrotic syndrome in children and is responsible for about 20% of cases in the adult. *Membranous glomerulonephritis* is more common in adults; both must be distinguished from other renal disorders which give rise to a similar clinical picture. Sometimes the aetiology of the nephrotic syndrome is obvious from the presence of other clinical features of the causative disease. In other patients it is necessary to carry out a renal biopsy in order to make the diagnosis.

*Proliferative glomerulonephritis* is occasionally associated with marked proteinuria and massive oedema. In many patients the clinical history and the course of the disease are sufficient to make this diagnosis clear, but in others the true nature of the syndrome is detected only after renal biopsy. Mesangiocapillary glomerulonephritis is often then found to be responsible (p. 431).

*Amyloid disease* is an uncommon cause of the nephrotic syndrome and is usually secondary to conditions such as rheumatoid arthritis, chronic suppuration or lepromatous leprosy. It gives rise to proteinuria as a result of the deposition of amyloid protein in the glomerular capillaries. The diagnosis can be made by renal biopsy. Primary amyloidosis is even rarer and affects other tissues, e.g. tongue, myocardium, peripheral nerves or joints (p. 627). It is also found in association with multiple myeloma.

*Renal vein thrombosis* is a rare cause of the nephrotic syndrome. It should be suspected when proteinuria occurs in a patient with evidence of deep venous thrombosis in the lower limbs or if an illness is complicated by pain in the loins and the subsequent development of the nephrotic syndrome.

*Other causes of the nephrotic syndrome* with individual distinguishing features are diabetic nephropathy (p. 523), drugs (e.g. penicillamine and gold), systemic lupus erythematosus (p. 627), polyarteritis nodosa, tumours and *P. malariae* infection in children in parts of Africa (p. 809).

The nephrotic syndrome must also be distinguished from:

*Cardiac failure* with severe oedema, in which dyspnoea is present, the venous pressure is increased, signs of underlying cardiac disease are present, oedema is usually absent from the face, and proteinuria is less severe.

*Hypoproteinaemic oedema*, due to causes other than loss of protein in the urine, namely impairment of intake, digestion, absorption or synthesis of protein and in protein-losing enteropathy.

**Treatment** is directed at relief of oedema and control of proteinuria. As long as the blood urea is not elevated, a liberal intake of protein is desirable in an attempt to make good the urinary loss of protein. At least 90–100 g protein should be given daily. This may be supplemented with proprietary salt-free protein concentrates.

Salt intake should be restricted by prohibiting extra table salt, avoiding salty foods and reducing the amount used in cooking. Although drastic salt restriction occasionally produces dramatic results, 'salt-free' diets are so unappetising that patients will not tolerate them for more than a few weeks.

Diuretics are of great value in controlling the oedema e.g. frusemide (p. 136). Because of the associated oligaemia these diuretics occasionally induce renal failure by causing further salt loss. In this event, or if the oedema is resistant, relief is obtained by giving plasma, salt-free albumin or dextran intravenously. Spironolactone is indicated in patients who show marked features of secondary aldosteronism, e.g. hypokalaemia.

*Corticosteroids* provide the main chance of cure in the treatment of minimal lesion glomerulonephritis in which the proteinuria is usually selective (p. 426). In the majority of cases this treatment abolishes proteinuria. Prednisolone should be given in doses of 1 mg/kg/d for about 3 weeks and then reduced to about one-third of this dose and continued for 2–3 months. In a minority of patients with minimal lesion glomerulonephritis the condition relapses after treatment when prednisolone is stopped. Such individuals are then best treated with cyclophosphamide in doses of 3 mg/kg body weight for 8 weeks. A weekly check of the white blood cell count should be made and the dose reduced if leucopenia develops. Temporary alopecia and chemical cystitis are other adverse effects.

Corticosteroids, cyclophosphamide and other immunosuppressive drugs are ineffective in membranous glomerulonephritis.

## Chronic Glomerulonephritis

**Aetiology**. Chronic glomerulonephritis develops when proliferative glomerulonephritis becomes progressive and in most cases of membranous glomerulonephritis. Frequently, no history of either disease is obtained and in these, post-mortem studies of the kidney suggests that the pathological change has been developing insidiously over many years. Chronic glomerulonephritis ends in chronic renal failure.

**Pathology.** The kidneys are small; the capsules strip with difficulty, leaving a granular surface; the peripelvic fat is increased and there is great reduction in renal cortical tissue. The normal distinction between cortex and medulla is obscured. On microscopical examination there is fibrosis or hyalinisation of most of the glomeruli with fibrous replacement of many tubules. Remaining nephrons may show hypertrophy and arteriolosclerosis is usually present.

**Clinical features** of chronic glomerulonephritis are attributable to the effects of chronic renal failure combined usually with arterial hypertension. As renal failure develops, the composition of the body fluid becomes abnormal, particularly with regard to its water and salt content, its acid-base equilibrium, and the concentration of nitrogenous compounds which are normally excreted by the kidney. These alterations ultimately combine to produce the clinical picture of severe uraemia which is the terminal stage of renal failure. A history of acute glomerulonephritis or of the nephrotic syndrome is obtained in some cases. The earlier stages of the disease may be unattended by symptoms but may come to light only by discovery of proteinuria or hypertension during the course of a routine examination. Later, because of the widespread consequences of renal failure, the symptoms and signs are referable to almost every system and patients suffering from the disease present with complaints which at first sight may not suggest their renal origin. Medical advice may be sought because of polyuria, thirst, itching, loss of energy, weakness, nausea, vomiting, or diarrhoea. Polyuria develops both because of diminished power for tubular reabsorption of water and because the elevated blood urea produces an osmotic diuresis. Anaemia is the main cause of the loss of energy and it is usually normocytic. The high blood pressure may have been detected in the course of a general examination or the patient consulted the doctor for headache, loss of vision or breathlessness or because of the occurrence of cerebrovascular insufficiency.

As the disease progresses, renal function deteriorates and uraemia increases. The blood concentration of urea and other nitrogenous compounds steadily rises. The patient looks more ill and the complexion is sallow, often accompanied by a yellow-brown discolouration attributed to the retention of urinary pigment. With the exception of those who develop cardiac failure from hypertension and those in whom the chronic stage of membranous glomerulonephritis has followed rapidly upon the initial oedematous stage, the patients are not only free from oedema but usually exhibit signs of water and salt depletion. The skin and tongue are dry and the blood pressure may fall from its previous high level. Acidosis contributes to the dyspnoea and the respirations are deep (Kussmaul's respiration). Hiccough, pruritus, muscular twitchings, fits, drowsiness and coma may occur. A tendency to bleed may develop in the terminal phase, as evidenced by epistaxis, bleeding gums, bruises, purpura, haematemesis and melaena. Hypertensive retinopathy of any degree may be present and visual impairment may result from numerous hard exudates arranged in star shapes around the macula (Plate I). Peripheral neuropathy due to uraemia also occurs.

Some patients complain of vague muscle or bone pain and in a few cases this becomes severe. These features are due to *renal osteodystrophy* which consists of osteomalacia, osteitis fibrosa and areas of osteosclerosis. Osteomalacia results from failure of the kidney to convert vitamin D to the active metabolite (p. 101). In young individuals this interferes with growth causing 'renal rickets'. Osteitis fibrosa arises as a result of secondary hyperparathyroidism, the parathyroid glands being stimulated by the low concentration of plasma calcium. The cause of osteosclerosis is unknown.

**Investigation.** During the early stages of the disease, and before nitrogen retention in the blood is detectable, the urine is found to contain protein, usually in small amounts; red blood cells and granular and hyaline casts are present in small numbers. Glomerular filtration may be reduced to less than 10% of normal and there is a gradual rise in the concentration of plasma urea, creatinine and phosphate. The ability of the kidneys to form concentrated or dilute urine is impaired. Ultimately this power is lost completely and the urine is of a fixed specific gravity. The plasma concentration of bicarbonate diminishes as acidosis occurs. The plasma concentration of calcium is frequently reduced due to defective vitamin D metabolism. Potassium occasionally accumulates in the blood and is one of the factors causing death by its effect on the heart.

A plain radiograph of the abdomen may show small, irregular kidneys and the changes of osteomalacia may be seen in the bones.

**Course and Prognosis**. The disease progresses steadily over months or years and, in the absence of treatment by haemodialysis or renal transplantation, leads to a fatal termination. The course may be punctuated by exacerbations of acute glomerulonephritis which hasten the progress of the disease. When nitrogen retention and acidosis are severe, the outlook is grave and most patients die in a few months or a year. Papilloedema is a bad prognostic sign and unless treatment with antihypertensive drugs is begun before uraemia becomes severe, most patients who show it die within a few months. The cause of death is generally uraemia, frequently complicated by infection to which such patients are susceptible; in other cases the patient dies from a cerebral haemorrhage, cardiac failure or myocardial infarction. A terminal non-bacterial pericarditis is common. Haemorrhage from any site or enterocolitis are also ominous features.

**Differential Diagnosis.** The distinction between chronic glomerulonephritis and other causes of chronic renal failure with hypertension is difficult and may be impossible. A similar clinical picture may arise in the following diseases.

1. Other conditions which primarily affect the glomeruli with their eventual destruction include systemic lupus erythematosus, amyloid disease and diabetes mellitus. Patients with these conditions may die ultimately of renal failure and uraemia.

2. Essential hypertension may occasionally lead to nephrosclerosis and uraemia. This should be suspected if there is a clear family history of high blood pressure; also in the malignant phase of hypertension from any cause, evidence of renal disease is invariably present and renal failure is rapidly progressive.

3. Congenital polycystic disease of the kidneys may be diagnosed by the family history, by palpation of the enlarged, irregular kidneys and by intravenous or retrograde urography. Medullary sponge kidney is also occasionally responsible (p. 454).

4. Chronic pyelonephritis is more common in women, and hypertension may be absent. There may be a history of acute pyelonephritis and organisms can sometimes be cultured from the urine. The diagnosis is often suggested by the radiological appearances seen after urography.

5. Analgesic nephropathy (p. 454) is suggested by a history of analgesic abuse.

6. Bilateral hydronephrosis may be confirmed by retrograde urography.

7. Congenital renal hypoplasia with bilateral small kidneys is occasionally the cause of death from uraemia in children.

8. Urinary schistosomiasis is a common cause in endemic areas in Africa and the Middle East (pp. 795 and 858).

**Treatment.** Although the natural history of the disease cannot be altered and there is progressive deterioration in renal function, the patient's feeling of well-being may be considerably improved with suitable treatment.

*Diet.* When there is nitrogen retention the onset of severe uraemia may be delayed by restricting protein intake to 40 g per day and by ensuring an adequate intake of carbohydrate (250 g) and fat (60 g), giving an energy value of 1700 kcal. In the later stages when the blood urea concentration rises above 35 mmol/*l* further protein restriction to 20 g/day is indicated.

*Fluid.* Restriction is contraindicated since, in view of the impaired concentrating power, a large volume of urine is needed to excrete end-products of metabolism. Except in the presence of cardiac failure the daily fluid intake should be sufficient to produce at least 2½ litres of urine.

*Salt.* In the absence of oedema, cardiac failure or arterial hypertension, salt restriction is contraindicated. In a few cases of chronic nephritis there is an excessive loss of salt in the urine due to a failure of tubular reabsorption, and this may be aggravated by an enforced high fluid intake. Water and salt depletion occur and this increases the uraemia. Clinical improvement results in such cases from the addition of 5–10 g salt per day. The limit to the additional salt is set by the occurrence of systemic or pulmonary oedema, or by an aggravation of the hypertension. Sodium bicarbonate should be substituted in part for sodium chloride when acidosis is severe and giving rise to symptoms.

When nausea, vomiting or coma make it impossible to control water and salt depletion and acidosis by oral administration, fluid and electrolytes should be given by intravenous infusion. The volume of fluid required depends upon the severity of the salt and water depletion and the degree of acidosis (p. 140). An average amount for a case of moderate severity is 5 litres given in 24 hours, one part of isotonic sodium bicarbonate, two parts of isotonic sodium chloride and two parts 5% glucose. The infusion should be continued until the bicarbonate concentration of the blood has been increased, if possible to within the normal range and until the patient is adequately hydrated.

*Infection.* Obvious foci of infection, e.g. tonsils, infected sinuses or root abscesses should be treated in order to reduce the likelihood of an exacerbation of acute glomerulonephritis. Antibiotics, as with other medication, must be used with special care in reduced dosage in the presence of chronic renal failure, notably benzylpenicillin, co-trimoxazole, streptomycin, gentamicin, kanamycin and cephaloridine. Tetracyclines should not be used because of their tendency to raise the blood urea.

*Anaemia.* This should be treated by slow blood transfusions though it is probably not desirable to increase the concentration of haemoglobin above 8·5 g/dl as a rapid rise in haematocrit causes a fall in renal plasma flow and a temporary aggravation of the uraemia. Iron therapy is ineffective unless there is evidence of iron deficiency.

*Nausea, hiccoughing or vomiting* may be relieved with chlorpromazine in reduced doses (e.g. 25 mg i.m.) because of the danger of accumulation.

*Bone Pain.* When the dominant radiological picture is that of osteomalacia, vitamin D should be given as 1–2 $\mu$g 1$\alpha$ OH vitamin $D_3$ orally daily for some weeks. The treatment should be controlled by chemical estimations of plasma calcium and alkaline phosphatase, for there is a significant risk of producing hypercalcaemia and calcification of the tissues. This tendency is also reduced by giving aluminium hydroxide gel by mouth to bind phosphate and lower its concentration.

*Cardiovascular Complications.* The presence of uraemia is no contraindication to the treatment of co-existing hypertension provided that care is taken to see that antihypertensive treatment does not cause a rise in the concentration of blood urea. The choice and use of drugs should be made according to the recommendations given on pages 196–198. Digoxin is normally excreted in the urine, and hence in renal failure the maintenance dose should not usually exceed 0·25 mg three times per week.

DIALYSIS AND RENAL TRANSPLANTATION. *Haemodialysis.* It is possible by repeated intermittent haemodialysis to preserve the lives of many patients with chronic renal failure who are devoid of all renal function. Haemodialysis is indicated when, in spite of adequate medical treatment, symptoms of uraemia become troublesome and preferably before the patient is obliged to give up employment. It should always be started before the serious features of uraemia, e.g. pericarditis, nausea, diarrhoea or vomiting and bleeding occur. Repeated access to blood vessels is achieved by establishing an arteriovenous anastomosis, usually in the arm. Haemodialysis using the cellophane membrane of the artificial kidney is best carried out for periods of 6–8 hours three times per week and in many instances patients can be trained to carry out their treatment at home, where survival of up to 10 years or more is common and where satisfactory mental and physical rehabilitation is best achieved.

*Renal Transplantation.* The practicability of transplantation of a normal kidney from a healthy donor or a cadaver to patients with chronic irreversible renal failure should also be considered and is especially suitable in young patients. If the patient has a healthy identical twin who is willing to act as a donor, the prospects of a successful renal transplantation are excellent. However, most kidney transplantations are carried out using either kidneys from living but less closely related siblings or from cadavers. It is customary to try to select donor kidneys on the basis of HLA-A and -B loci compatibility. When a living donor sibling kidney is used, the best results are obtained when the donor and recipient have 3–4 HLA antigens in common; there is less evidence that matching is important in cadaver transplants, but preliminary results of matching using HLA-D antigens are more promising. After three years the average survival rate in living related donor grafts is about 75%, and in the case of cadaver grafts, 60%. The postoperative course is complicated by the need to give immunosuppressive drugs such as prednisolone, azathioprine or antilymphocytic serum. Renal dialysis and transplantation are best used flexibly in an integrated fashion. It is wise and usually necessary to establish every patient on dialysis and carry out renal transplantation when a suitable kidney becomes available, especially in the patients under the age of 45 years. The commonest causes of death are myocardial ischaemia and infarction and infection.

*Continuous Ambulatory Peritoneal Dialysis.* This simple and less expensive form of long-term dialysis involves the introduction of a permanent intraperitoneal catheter, accessible from the skin surface on the anterior wall of the abdomen. Two litres of isotonic dialysate fluid are introduced into the peritoneal cavity from a plastic container bag worn around the waist and left for periods of 6 hours. It is then evacuated and fresh dialysate fluid reintroduced. This cycle is repeated 4 times in each period of 24 hours, during which time the patient carries on with normal daily tasks. This form of treatment remains at the exploratory stage; some patients respond well to it, but there is a risk of recurrent peritonitis.

# Infections of the Kidney and Urinary Tract

Infection of the urinary tract is an extremely common clinical problem. The infection may involve the urethra, the bladder, the ureters and the kidneys themselves. In any individual case it is difficult on clinical grounds to be certain of the extent of the invasion of the various parts of the urinary tract. Formerly it was assumed that the kidneys and the upper urinary tract are involved in every case, even when the symptoms of the infection are those solely of cystitis or urethritis. However, the great majority of patients develop recurrent symptoms of lower urinary tract infection without apparently suffering deterioration of renal function in later life, an important exception being children with vesico-ureteric reflux.

## Acute Pyelonephritis

This is characterised by an acute inflammation of the parenchyma and pelvis of the kidney. The disease may be unilateral or bilateral.

**Aetiology.** Acute pyelonephritis is commonly associated with some obstruction in the urinary tract. In men this is often due to prostatic enlargement, in pregnant women to obstruction by the uterus and atonia of the ureters due to the action of progesterone, and in infants and children to congenital malformation of the urinary tract or vesico-ureteric reflux. Calculi, cervical prolapse, cystocele, foreign bodies or tumours may also be responsible. Pyelonephritis may occur in infancy and in adult women, however, without evidence of an obstructive lesion. Diabetes also predisposes to infection. In most cases the infection ascends via the ureter but in some, and notably the newborn, it is blood borne. About 75% of the infections are due to *Esch. coli*, the remainder being mostly due to klebsiella, streptococci, staphylococci or the Proteus group of organisms.

The predominance of urinary infections in the adult female suggests that the anatomical relation of the short urethra to the rectum is a predisposing factor. Catheterisation of the bladder is particularly liable to introduce organisms into the urinary tract; when indicated it should be carried out with strict aseptic precautions.

**Pathology**. The renal pelvis is acutely inflamed and there is often a coincident inflammation of the bladder. In severe cases small abscesses may be seen on the surface of the kidney when the capsule has been stripped. On section, small cortical abscesses and linear streaks of pus in the medulla are often evident. On histological examination focal infiltration of the renal tissue by polymorphonuclear cells is evident.

**Clinical Features.** In many cases there is a sudden onset or pain in one or both loins, radiating to the iliac fossae and suprapubic area. There may by dysuria (difficult or painful micturition) and strangury (a painful desire to pass urine though the bladder is empty), with the frequent passage of small amounts of scalding, usually cloudy urine, due to an associated cystitis. The temperature rises rapidly to 38–40°C, with the general manifestations of fever. A rigor may occur, and there may be vomiting. Tenderness and muscular guarding may be present in the renal angle and the lumbar region. There is a leucocytosis. The urine in *Esch. coli* infections is nearly always acid; in other infections it may be acid or alkaline. On microscopic examination there are numerous pus cells and organisms, some red blood cells and epithelial cells. When the organisms are motile Gram-negative bacilli and the urine is acid, the infection may be assumed to be due to *Esch. coli.*

Acute pyelonephritis in infants and children, like infections of the throat and middle ear, often presents as fever without any localising symptoms. The initial feature may be a convulsion but apathy, abdominal distension and diarrhoea may occur. In the feverish child, particular attention should be paid to these sites and the urine should be examined for pus cells and organisms.

Routine culture of a midstream specimen of urine has revealed the presence of asymptomatic bacteriuria (>100 000 organisms/ml) in about 5% of all pregnancies during the early months. If no antibiotics are given, acute pyelonephritis occurs in about 40% of such cases whereas this is rare in those in whom the urine was sterile at the original examination. Investigation by intravenous urography after the termination of pregnancy shows a high incidence of abnormalities of the urinary tract in those women with bacteriuria. Suppressive chemotherapy at the asymptomatic stage has been found to prevent the development of acute symptoms.

**Course and Prognosis.** With adequate treatment the disease subsides rapidly in the great majority of cases. Fever, pain, frequency and dysuria disappear and the urine usually becomes sterile within a few days.

In some cases, although the acute symptoms subside, a low-grade infection may persist, and the disease may pass into the chronic stage. More rarely the disease may be severe and cause necrosis of the papillae (*acute necrotising papillitis*). Fragments of renal tissue are then excreted in the urine and can be identified histologically. This complication, which may lead to renal failure, is particularly liable to occur in diabetic patients and in those addicted to phenacetin (p. 454). In view of the frequency of acute pyelonephritis, the curable nature of the condition, and the fact that chronic pyelonephritis is a common cause of renal failure and hypertension, the importance of adequate treatment of the acute stage cannot be overstressed.

**Differential Diagnosis.** Acute pyelonephritis should be distinguished from: acute appendicitis, salpingitis, cholecystitis and diverticular disease, especially by the absence of pus and organisms in the urine in these conditions. Less commonly nowadays it may be mimicked by *perinephric abscess* due to infection by *Staph. aureus*. The characteristic clinical features are pain and tenderness in the renal region, fever and polymorphonuclear leucocytosis. Urinary symptoms are absent and there are no pus cells or organisms in the urine. Oedema may obliterate the normal hollow in the loin, and an abscess may eventually point in the loin or groin, or it may rupture into the peritoneal or pleural cavity.

**Treatment** depends upon the infecting organism and its sensitivity, and ideally a midstream specimen of urine should be sent to the laboratory before specific therapy is begun. This specimen should reach the laboratory within 2 hours of voiding or be refrigerated at 4°C for a period not exceeding 24 hours. Since infection is usually due to *Esch. coli* treatment with sulphadimidine or co-trimoxazole can be commenced and altered later if so indicated by the results of the culture or if the response is unsatisfactory. In the very severe case, and if septicaemia occurs, gentamicin is the drug of choice. Ampicillin is of value in proteus infections. Whatever drug is employed a second midstream specimen of urine should be sent to the laboratory from 4 to 6 weeks after the completion of the initial course of treatment to make sure that the infection has been eradicated. If this has not been accomplished further treatment with the appropriate antibiotic must be given, depending on the bacteriological findings.

In every case the possibility of calculus, an obstructive lesion of the urinary tract or renal tuberculosis must be considered and treated if found.

## Chronic Pyelonephritis

**Aetiology.** The disease in the adult may be caused by infection above an unrelieved obstruction to the urinary tract, e.g. calculus, stricture or prostatic disease. Other cases may follow cystitis due to stasis as a result of a cystocele or interference with the innervation of the bladder, e.g. in paraplegia or multiple sclerosis. In conditions in which the outflow tract of the bladder is deranged, reflux of urine into the ureters may occur during micturition and contribute to the persistence of infection. Vesico-ureteric reflux in the absence of such a lesion is an important determinant of infection and of progressive kidney damage in infancy and childhood. Chronic pyelonephritis also occurs in conditions leading to nephrocalcinosis (p. 451). *Esch. coli* is the organism responsible for most cases. Other infecting agents include proteus, *Ps. aeruginosa* and staphylococci.

Because of difficulty in culturing organisms from the urine of many patients with clinical and radiological features of pyelonephritis, the term *chronic interstitial nephritis* is often advocated as an alternative. Its use implies that the cause of the fibrosing destructive renal disease is unknown and that factors other than previous episodes of infection may be responsible. What these factors might be is unclear but they could possibly include reactions to analgesics and other drugs (p. 454).

**Pathology.** The changes may be unilateral or bilateral, and of any grade of severity. The fully developed case usually shows gross scarring of the kidneys, which may be much reduced in size with narrowing of the cortex and medulla. Microscopically there is patchy fibrosis with chronic inflammatory cell infiltration, tubular atrophy, periglomerular fibrosis and eventual disappearance of nephrons. The arteries and arterioles may show sclerosis and narrowing.

**Clinical Features.** In many cases no symptoms arise directly from the renal lesions, and the patient may consult the doctor because of lassitude, tiredness and vague ill-health or for symptoms of uraemia or arterial hypertension. The discovery of hypertension or proteinuria on routine examination may be the first indication of the presence of the disease. Symptoms arising from the urinary tract, however, may also be present and include frequency of micturition, dysuria and aching lumbar pain. Occasionally weakness and fainting may occur if the renal disorder is accompanied by excessive salt loss. The urine may contain pus cells, a small amount of protein and many epithelial cells, though in some cases it may be normal.

In all cases investigations such as rectal or vaginal examination, cystoscopy and urography must be carried out to discover the nature of any underlying mechanical factor causing obstruction to the flow of urine and to determine the extent of renal damage. Radiographs show affected kidneys to be reduced in size and localised contraction of the renal substance associated with clubbing of adjacent calyces.

**Course and Prognosis.** The course is usually a long one and is sometimes punctuated by acute exacerbations. The infection is difficult to eradicate, even when underlying mechanical obstructions are found and relieved. *Pyonephrosis* may occur, especially in the presence of renal calculi. It is characterised by persistent lumbar pain, intermittent pyrexia, often with rigors, emaciation, pyuria, and, if both kidneys are involved, uraemia; one or both kidneys may become palpable. Some cases progress to chronic uraemia, which may be alleviated for a year two by treatment. In elderly, diabetic or paraplegic patients a fulminating infection may be the immediate cause of death.

**Treatment** of chronic pyelonephritis is similar to that described for the acute disease. The chronic infection is usually more difficult to eradicate. Attempts should be made to remove obstructive lesions or renal calculi by appropriate surgical procedures. An antibiotic to which the organism is sensitive should be given for 14 days (p. 442). If the infection is not eradicated suppressive treatment may be required for many months, the antibiotic used being given in smaller doses and as indicated by the changing pattern and sensitivity of the organisms in the urine. Ampicillin, co-trimoxazole and nalidixic acid (1 g t.i.d.) are valuable for this purpose. A moderate degree of uraemia may be present which progresses little for months or years. This is especially so when hypertension is absent or minimal. When the renal infection is unilateral or if pyonephrosis has developed, nephrectomy may be indicated; rarely, high blood pressure may be cured by the removal of the diseased kidney.

## Cystitis, Urethritis and Prostatitis

Some infections of the urinary tract may be confined to the urethra or bladder. In these, the features of systemic illness are slight and the symptoms are those of frequency and dysuria. Scalding pain is felt in the urethra during micturition. Suprapubic pain of cystitis is felt before, during and for a few moments after voiding urine. Although the bladder is empty there may be an intense desire to pass more urine due to spasm of its inflamed wall. Tenderness is often present in the suprapubic region, and the urine may have an unpleasant odour and appear cloudy. Pus cells, red cells and organisms may be seen on microscopical examination. Sometimes the urine is grossly blood-stained. Cystitis is particularly common in women and girls, and the infection is usually due to *Esch. coli*.

In some patients with symptoms suggestive of urethritis and cystitis, no bacteria can be cultured from the urine. The term '*urethral syndrome*' has been applied to this category of patients who are predominantly female. The cause of the symptoms is unknown although a variety of explanations, which include allergy to deodorants, etc., congestion of the urethra possibly related to sexual activitiy and infection of the urethral glands, have been put forward. In some patients careful culture of urine reveals the presence of lactobacillus or a member of the *chlamydia* group.

In acute prostatitis there may be considerable systemic disturbance. On digital examination of the rectum the prostatic gland is usually very tender.

**Treatment** of infections is similar to that of acute pyelonephritis (p. 442). In the majority of instances this is effective and there is no recurrence of the symptoms. In some patients, however, the clinical features of infection persist or recur. In patients with a normal urinary tract, particularly women with recurrent urinary infection induced by sexual intercourse, the majority can be kept free of attacks by use of long-term low dose antibacterial drugs, taken after voiding urine before going to bed. Such a regimen should be commenced after a curative course of treatment, as evidenced by bacteriological culture. Some women with recurrent infection can remain free of attacks by practising pre- and postcoital micturition, or by applying an antiseptic cream such as 0·5% cetrimide to the periurethral area prior to sexual intercourse. It is preferable to attempt these simpler measures before embarking on a prophylactic course of treatment with an antibacterial agent.

The possible causes of failure to respond to treatment, or of relapse, are:

1. Infection with organisms e.g. trichomonas, resistant to the chemotherapeutic agent employed.
2. Tuberculosis, with or without secondary infection.
3. Continued infection from above, e.g. pyelonephritis associated with calculi.
4. Obstruction below the base of the bladder by (a) prostatic hyperplasia, carcinoma of the prostate, or urethral stricture in the male; (b) chronic urethritis or stricture in the female.
5. Atrophy of the urethra consequent upon oestrogen lack after the menopause.
6. Involvement of the bladder by: (a) malignant tumour arising in the bladder or in adjacent organs; (b) vesical calculus; foreign bodies may have been inserted into the bladder; (c) inflammation from adjacent structures, e.g. diverticular disease.
7. The presence of urethral caruncle, cystocele, urethrocele or cervicitis in the female or meatal fissure in the male. The latter may be noted as a tender induration on examination of the meatus.
8. Paraplegia, in which urinary infection is frequent, persistent and often the ultimate cause of death.

### Renal Tuberculosis

Tuberculosis of the kidney is invariably secondary to tuberculosis elsewhere and occurs as a result of blood-borne infection. The initial lesion develops in the renal cortex and if untreated may ulcerate into the pelvis with consequent involvement of the bladder, epididymes, seminal vesicles and prostate. The disease tends to occur in young people and may manifest itself with recurrent haematuria and dysuria due to secondary involvement of the bladder. In addition the general features of tuberculosis, i.e. malaise, fever, lassitude and weight loss, may be present. Culture of the urine by ordinary methods may be sterile in spite of pyuria. The extent of the infection should be ascertained by cystoscopic examination, by urography and by culture of the urine from both ureters. Chemotherapy should be given as for tuberculosis elsewhere (p. 259). Nephrectomy or epididymectomy may be necessary in those in whom the disease has advanced to the stage of producing serious destruction of tissue.

## Renal Failure

The term *uraemia* has been used for more than a century to describe the clinical state which arises from renal failure. The symptoms of chronic renal failure are attributable not so much to retention of abnormal amounts of urea in blood but to disturbances in hydrogen ion concentration, abnormalities in water and electrolyte balance and the accumulation of many other products of metabolism. In addition, renal failure is accompanied in the majority of cases by arterial hypertension, and this further complicates the clinical picture.

**Classification.** Renal function may be impaired by disease or drugs that affect the renal parenchyma (renal uraemia), by extrarenal disorders such as acute circulatory failure (prerenal uraemia) or as a result of conditions in which there is obstruction to the outflow of urine (postrenal uraemia). The deterioration of kidney function which ensues may be acute or chronic and of varying degrees of severity.

For descriptive purposes, renal failure is conveniently subdivided into four categories based mainly upon the site of the lesion responsible:

1. Renal failure due to disease of the kidneys (renal uraemia).
2. Acute renal failure due to prerenal disease (prerenal uraemia).
3. Acute renal failure due to acute tubular necrosis.
4. Renal failure as a result of conditions in which there is obstruction of the renal tract resulting in impairment of renal function (postrenal uraemia).

### 1. Renal Failure due to Disease of the Kidneys

The clinical features and treatment of renal failure occurring as a result of glomerulonephritis are described on pages 437 and 439. The manifestations of renal failure due to other kidney diseases are similar but there are also the features of the underlying process e.g. bilateral pyelonephritis, accelerated malignant hypertension and eclampsia, polyarteritis nodosa, systemic lupus erythematosus, polycystic disease, diabetic nephropathy, amyloidosis, conditions causing hypercalcaemia (p. 481) and disseminated intravascular coagulation (p. 601). Less common causes include lesions of major renal arteries and damage due to nephrotoxic drugs (p. 454). The haemolytic-uraemic syndrome which may follow viral or other infections, and in which glomerular coagulation is a prominent feature, is also an important cause of acute renal failure.

### 2. Acute Renal Failure due to Prerenal Disorder

Normal renal function is dependent upon the maintenance of an adequate renal circulation. The renal share of the cardiac output is normally about 25% at rest. If the cardiac output falls the blood flow to organs other than the heart or brain is reduced. In this event, the glomerular filtration rate is reduced and oliguria results. While systemic hypotension often precedes prerenal uraemia, renal ischaemia may occur in its absence. Regional vasoconstriction is a means by which the blood pressure may be maintained in the face of oligaemia, and the success of this mechanism may deprive the kidneys of a large part of their blood supply. The urine is usually small in volume and the concentration of urea in the blood gradually rises. The more important causes of prerenal failure include:

1. *Loss of blood* from any cause including complications of pregnancy, trauma or gastrointestinal bleeding and severe haemolysis as in blackwater fever (p. 809) or incompatible blood transfusion.
2. *Loss of plasma* as in burns and crushing injuries.
3. *Loss of fluid and salt.*
   (a) *from the gut* in severe vomiting, diarrhoea, acute intestinal obstruction, pancreatitis, paralytic ileus and fistulous drainage.
   (b) *in the urine* in diabetic ketoacidosis.
   (c) *from the skin* in excessive sweating.
4. *Hypotension* due to bacteraemic or cardiogenic shock or during the course of a surgical operation may reduce renal blood flow and precipitate renal failure particularly in those whose blood volume is precariously balanced.

These conditions should be treated by appropriate fluids given intravenously and by specific measures as indicated in the treatment of diabetic ketoacidosis, Addison's disease, infection, etc. Prompt and effective replacement of blood, water and salt is essential. In many cases vigorous treatment in the early stages prevents the occurrence of significant degrees of renal failure. If oliguria or anuria persists in spite of the return of the blood pressure to normal, the functional integrity of the nephrons has become disrupted due to 'acute tubular necrosis'.

### 3. Acute Renal Failure due to Acute Tubular Necrosis

This disease is due to acute ischaemia affecting both kidneys, and is characterised by oliguria or anuria with urine of low specific gravity and rapidly developing uraemia. 'Tubular necrosis' is a misleading term because it does not accurately reflect the histological abnormality but it is in wide general use except in the United States where the condition is known as 'vasospastic necrosis'.

**Aetiology.** Acute tubular necrosis occurs as a complication of various conditions which are associated with renal ischaemia, and which are listed above as causes of prerenal uraemia. Certain drugs are also capable of producing acute renal failure, e.g. paracetamol, sulphonamides and cephaloridine. Poisoning by substances, such as sodium chlorate, which produces renal parenchymal necrosis, may also be responsible.

**Pathogenesis.** Severe shock and water and salt depletion are accompanied by widespread vasconstriction. Blood flow is reduced by the fall in cardiac output and in the kidneys afferent arteriolar vasoconstriction further curtails glomerular filtration. The latter sometimes occurs even when the systemic blood pressure is maintained. If the ischaemia is severe and of sufficiently long duration the basement membrane of the renal tubules is ruptured and focal necrosis of the cells occurs. Stasis of the circulation within the kidney is associated with some degree of intraglomerular coagulation. In addition, casts of haemoglobin or of plasma proteins sometimes form within the tubular lumen and interfere with the passage of fluid; interstitial oedema around the tubules may also raise the intrarenal pressure and constrict nephrons externally so contributing to the renal failure.

In cases due to agents such as sulphonamides or sodium chlorate, direct damage to the renal tubular cells from toxic or allergic reactions is responsible.

Rarely, but notably in cases of retroplacental haemorrhage occurring as a complication of pregnancy, the whole or a large part of the renal cortex is involved, the glomeruli as well as the tubules becoming necrotic. This is called *renal cortical necrosis*.

**Clinical Features and Course.** The clinical features are those of the causal condition together with those of rapidly developing uraemia. Initially the urine volume is commonly but not invariably greatly reduced to between 200 and 500 ml/d and this stage of the illness is called the *oliguric phase*. Any urine that is formed contains protein, casts and red and white blood cells. The specific gravity is usually about 1·010 early in the course of the disease, and this persists for several days or weeks. The patient may feel well at first but after some days the features of uraemia appear. Initially these are anorexia, nausea and vomiting; apathy is followed by mental confusion and later muscular twitching, fits, drowsiness, coma, and bleeding episodes occur. At this stage the main dangers to life are (1) pulmonary oedema due to the injudicious administration of excessive amounts of fluid, (2) potassium intoxication due to the rise in the concentration of plasma potassium which is especially likely if there is haemolysis or massive soft tissue damage, (3) the occurrence of severe systemic infection to which such patients are susceptible, (4) uraemia and metabolic acidosis, and (5) renal cortical necrosis.

The oliguric phase of the disease usually lasts for 1 to 3 weeks. If the patient does not succumb the daily volume of urine increases and rapidly may reach several litres. This is called the *diuretic* phase and coincides with healing of the renal tubules, reduction in intrarenal tension and resolution of intratubular casts and intraglomerular coagulation. During this phase there is uncontrolled water and sodium loss, and sometimes flaccid paralysis due to loss of potassium occurs in the absence of treatment. The concentration of blood urea ceases to rise and then gradually falls. Virtually complete recovery of renal function then takes place slowly over a period fo 3 to 6 months.

**Treatment.** With a view to preventing or minimising the renal lesion, the underlying cause should be treated urgently. The blood volume should be quickly restored by appropriate transfusion and water and electrolyte deficits should be replenished. The adequacy of blood transfusion and fluid therapy is best monitored by the use of an in-dwelling atrial catheter (p. 167) and assessed by clinical response.

THE OLIGURIC PHASE. Clinical and pathological studies have shown that the ischaemic renal lesions are usually reversible provided the patient can be kept alive during the oliguric phase. Treatment is therefore designed to minimise the need for renal function until healing occurs and this can often be achieved by simple dietary restrictions.

*Water and Electrolyte Balance.* This is maintained by replacing the obligatory losses of water through the skin and lungs, estimated to be about 600 ml water/d, and by giving no electrolytes since none are being lost from the body. In febrile patients an extra allowance of water is required to replace the fluid lost through sweating and a further small supplement equal to the volume of urine passed each day should be added. Should abnormal losses of fluid occur, as in diarrhoea, additional fluid will be required in appropriate amounts.

*Protein and Energy.* Dietary protein is restricted to about 20 g/d and attempts are made to suppress endogenous protein catabolism to a minimum by giving as much energy as possible as fat and carbohydrate. For this purpose a diet restricted in its protein and electrolyte content may be supplemented by a liquid glucose preparation. In the event of vomiting, oral treatment should be avoided and carbohydrate should be given in the form of 20% glucose via an in-dwelling central venous catheter.

In many patients in whom the acute renal failure is mild in degree and relatively short in duration this treatment prevents the blood urea from rising more than 4 mmol/*l* (20 mg per 100 ml) per day, and the accumulation of potassium from protein catabolism is usually not sufficient to have serious consequences. If elevation of plasma potassium concentration should occur attempts should be made to reduce it by employing methods described on page 133; these include (1) the use of a sodium or calcium charged resin which removes potassium from the body, (2) giving 20 units of soluble insulin i.v. and an intravenous infusion of 50 g of glucose; and (3) controlling acidosis by intravenous administration of isotonic sodium bicarbonate.

*Haemodialysis.* In some patients, however, and especially in those suffering from severe infection or massive tissue damage, or in whom blood has become loculated in one of the tissue spaces, the rate of rise of blood urea and potassium is much more rapid and occurs in spite of the application of conservative methods; in these circumstances life may be threatened from acute renal failure within a few days. The patient should then be transferred to a centre equipped with the means for extracorporeal dialysis. Daily haemodialyses may then be required over a period of several weeks before renal function returns. When such a policy is adopted it is usually possible to be much more liberal regarding the intake of protein, fluid and energy. This is desirable from the point of view of encouraging repair of damaged or diseased tissues and is rendered possible by the daily correction of the composition of the blood and volume of body fluids achieved by the artificial kidney.

*Peritoneal dialysis* can sometimes be used as an alternative to haemodialysis. While this method has a place in the treatment of small children, it is a prolonged, uncomfortable, sometimes painful procedure and fraught with complications, notably peritonitis.

RECOVERY OR DIURETIC PHASE. When diuresis commences, the concentration of blood urea tends to remain constant for a few days and then begins to fall. When this occurs, a light diet, containing not more than 40–60 g protein per day and ample fruit, should be provided. Sufficient fluid must be given to replace the increased and uncontrolled loss of water in the urine. The fluid intake must be increased by the volume of the previous days urinary output. Salt supplements are usually needed during the diuretic phase to compensate for increased urinary loss. On average about 3 g of sodium chloride and 2 g of sodium bicarbonate are needed for each litre of urine passed. The fruit usually compensates for the potassium loss, though in many cases an oral supplement of potassium chloride may also be required. As renal function improves and blood urea falls, a normal diet may be taken.

Patients with severe acute renal failure are seriously ill and require skilled nursing, preferably in single rooms designed to prevent infection. Great care must be exercised in the use of drugs which are normally excreted by the kidneys.

**Prognosis.** The high mortality accompanying acute renal failure of ischaemic origin has been greatly reduced by the measures described above. Prognosis depends upon the speed and efficiency with which the therapeutic measures are put into operation, the prompt recognition and effective treatment of complicating infection, and the nature and the severity of the condition precipitating the syndrome. In cases of uncomplicated acute renal failure, such as those due to simple haemorrhage, the mortality should now be less than 10% even when haemodialysis is required. In severe renal failure complicated by serious infection or multiple injuries it is about 50%, the outcome being determined by the severity of the underlying disorders and their complications rather than by the renal failure itself.

### 4. Renal Failure due to Postrenal Causes

Renal failure may result from obstruction at any point in the urinary tract due to the causes given below. In the presence of two functioning kidneys ureteric obstruction causes uraemia only when it is bilateral.

The diagnosis may be suggested by a history of previous urinary symptoms such as pain in the loins, haematuria, renal colic, nocturia or difficulty in micturition. However, in many instances the onset is clinically silent and the cause of the obstruction discovered only after appropriate investigations. In contrast to acute renal failure associated with tubular necrosis, anuria is common and the complete absence of urine suggest the need for cytoscopy, ureteral catheterisation and retrograde pyelography.

Surgical treatment is required for all cases of renal failure due to postrenal obstruction. Uraemia may be severe, yet relief of the obstruction followed by a high fluid intake results in recovery of adequate renal function in many patients, provided that this treatment has not been delayed too long.

## Obstruction of the Urinary Tract

Obstruction to the flow of urine from the kidney through the pelvis, ureter, bladder and urethra is a common disorder; it causes stasis and a rise in pressure within the urinary tract which predisposes to infection, stone formation and renal failure. Obstruction may occur at any level but is most often found at the pelvi-ureteric junction, in the ureter, at the neck of the bladder or in the urethra. Obstruction at the pelvi-ureteric junction causes hydronephrosis; obstruction of the ureter results in hydroureter and later hydronephrosis; obstruction of the bladder neck or urethra distends the bladder, causes hypertrophy of its muscle seen on cystoscopic examination as trabeculation, and hydroureter and hydronephrosis. If obstruction is unrelieved, slow progressive destruction of renal tissue occurs superimposed infection may cause cystitis, ureteritis or pyonephrosis in which renal damage may become more rapid.

**Aetiology.** Obstruction may be due to an organic lesion in the lumen or in or around the wall of the urinary tract or it may arise because of a congenital neuromuscular defect at the pelvi-ureteric junction, ureter or bladder neck preventing the contraction wave and therefore the flow of urine. Organic causes include stone, blood clot, tumour or fibrosis following infection. An aberrant renal artery, retroperitoneal fibrosis, accidental ligation at operation, carcinoma of the cervix, prostatic enlargement or phimosis may compress the lumen from outside.

**Clinical features** vary with the cause and site of the lesion and in particular whether it is above or below the bladder. When the obstruction is supravesical, renal colic may occur, especially if the onset is sudden. More commonly the obstruction is gradual and an aching pain in the loins, sometimes aggravated by drinking, develops. Superimposed infection causes systemic manifestations with fever and dysuria. Haematuria is common. Transmission of the increased hydrostatic pressure to the kidney in partial obstruction interferes with the counter-current concentrating mechanism and may result paradoxically in polyuria.

When the obstruction is below the bladder, there is difficulty in micturition and the urinary stream is thin in calibre and poor in force. Complete urinary retention may occur with consequent distension of the bladder, which may be visible as a swelling of the lower abdomen and palpable; anuria or overflow incontinence may ensue. In the latter event catheterisation reveals the presence of residual urine in the bladder after the patient has voided.

**Treatment.** In all cases the ultimate objective is to remove the source of obstruction; this is often possible, as in the case of a stone, prostatic hypertrophy or urethral stricture. In the first instance it is necessary to relieve the obstruction in order to alleviate symptoms and preserve renal function. The action required varies with the nature of the underlying disease, but sometimes it may be dealt with initially and temporarily by draining the kidney, i.e. nephrostomy, the ureter, i.e. ureterostomy, or the bladder, i.e. suprapubic or urethral catheterisation. Antibiotics should be given if infection is severe but it is preferable to wait until the obstruction has been removed or relieved. When the hydronephrosis or pyonephrosis affects one kidney and this is severely damaged, nephrectomy is indicated. When obstruction affects both kidneys and is irremediable appropriate treatment for renal failure should be given.

## Renal and Vesical Calculi and Nephrocalcinosis

**Aetiology.** Urinary calculi have long presented fascinating aetiological problems which are still largely unsolved. Two or three centuries ago vesical calculus was so common in Britain that a respectable living could be made as lithotomist, but the incidence is much lower at the present time for reasons that are not clear. It is indeed surprising that renal and vesical calculi or nephrocalcinosis do not occur more frequently since some of the constituents of urine are present in a concentration in excess of their maximum solubility in water. It seems likely that urine contains certain substances, e.g. mucopolysaccharides, and citrate, which, by forming complexes, keep otherwise insoluble salts in solution in the urine. The concentration of urate is also important as it interferes with this function. Other authorities believe that the primary cause of urinary calculi is a pre-existing renal or vesical lesion which acts as a nidus on which urinary constituents precipitate.

The following conditions are frequently associated with stone formation:

(a) Climate or occupation which necessitates living or working under conditions where excessive loss of water from sweating occurs, thus causing constituents to be precipitated because of their high concentration in the diminished volume of urine excreted.

(b) Urinary infection, obstruction and stagnation.

(c) Conditions associated with hypercalciuria which increases the liability to the formation of stones consisting mainly of calcium phosphate and calcium oxalate. These include idiopathic hypercalciuria in which the main defect is increased intestinal absorption of calcium, excessive intake of milk or cheese, prolonged immobilisaton, hyperparathyroidism, Cushings syndrome, renal tubular acidosis, sarcoidosis, multiple myeloma and vitamin D intoxication.

(d) Certain rare inherited disorders, e.g. cystinuria and primary hyperoxaluria, which may lead to the production of cystine or oxalate stones respectively.

(e) Conditions causing increased excretion of uric acid, e.g. gout and myeloproliferative disease.

(f) The pH of the urine influences the extent to which some of these conditions lead to stone formation thus an alkaline urine tends to increase the precipitation of calcium phosphate stones and so may be responsible for their occurrence in renal tubular acidosis from any cause. Likewise an acid urine reduces the solubility of uric acid and cystine.

Today, however, in prosperous countries the great majority of renal calculi occur in well nourished, healthy young men in whom the most careful investigations reveal no cause for stone formation.

**Pathology.** Urinary concretions vary greatly in size. There may be particles like sand anywhere in the urinary tract or large round stones in the bladder. Staghorn calculi fill the whole renal pelvis and branch into the calyces; they are usually associated with hydronephrosis and chronic pyelonephritis. Over 90% of renal stones contain calcium but the nature of the salt varies with their origin. Deposits of calcium may also be present throughout the renal parenchyma, giving rise to nephrocalcinosis. This is especially liable to occur in cases of chronic pyelonephritis, renal tubular acidosis, hyperparathyroidism, renal tubular acidosis, vitamin D intoxication, and in healed renal tuberculosis.

**Clinical features** vary according to the size, shape and position of the stone, and the presence and nature of the underlying condition. Renal calculi or nephrocalcinosis may be present for many years and yet themselves give rise to no symptoms. While nephrocalcinosis never gives rise to pain, the most common complaint arising from renal calculi is an intermittent dull pain in the loin or back, increased by movement or a sudden jolt. Some abnormal constituents of the urine, e.g. red cells, protein or pus cells, can be found at one time or another.

*Renal Colic.* When a stone is small enough to enter the ureter and large enough to obstruct it, an attack of renal colic develops. The patient is suddenly aware of pain in the loin, which soon radiates round the flank to the groin and often into the testis or labia in the sensory distribution of the first lumbar nerve. The pain steadily increases in intensity to reach a maximum in a few minutes. The patient is restless, and generally tries, unsuccessfuly, to obtain relief by assuming various positions, both lying and sitting, and by pacing about the room. There is pallor, sweating, and often vomiting, and the patient may groan in agony. Frequency and haematuria may occur. Without treatment the intense pain usually subsides within two hours but may continue unabated for several hours or some days. In many cases the pain is constant during the attack, though slight fluctuations in severity may occur. Contrary to what is often believed, it is rare for attacks to consist of intermittent severe pains, coming and going every few minutes for some hours.

**Investigation.** When renal colic occurs the diagnosis is usually easily made as it can be established by the history and by the finding of red cells in the urine. All patients suspected of having renal calculus, including those with renal colic, should have a radiological examination of the urinary tract, including retrograde urogram in some instances. If there is doubt about the cause of the abdominal pain, an intravenous pyelogram during the attack may be helpful. When the pain is due to a stone in the ureter, the radiograph shows a dense renal shadow with delay in the appearance of the dye in the renal pelvis. Appropriate investigations should be undertaken to discover the presence of any underlying condition which might be responsible for the development of renal calcification or lithiasis.

**Treatment and Prevention.** The immediate treatment of renal pain or renal colic is rest in bed, the application of warmth to the seat of pain, and the administration of analgesic drugs, e.g. pethidine (100 mg) or morphine (15–30 mg), and antispasmodic drugs, e.g. atropine sulphate (0·8 or 1·2 mg). These should be given intramuscularly and may be repeated within 2 hours. Attempts to dissolve calculi in the kidneys have not been successful. Stones in the renal pelvis and urinary bladder must be removed surgically. Stones in the ureter usually pass naturally if left alone and surgical removal is apt to be followed by stricture and its complications. When, however, pain persists or frequent bouts of pain become intolerable, the insertion of a ureteric catheter is often followed by the passage of the stone. Urgent surgical intervention is necessary in the event of anuria. It is also required if the stone has not moved for some months and hydronephrosis is developing or there is continuing infection in the urinary tract. A stone larger than 1 cm in diameter generally requires surgical removal.

Suitable medical or surgical measures should be instituted for the correction of any primary cause of renal lithiasis that may have been discovered. In idiopathic hypercalciuria a diet low in calcium, by reducing the intake of milk and cheese, is advisable.

If this is not effective, bendrofluazide in a dose of 5 mg/d reduces urinary calcium excretion by about 30%, In recurrent oxalate stones the elimination from the diet of articles which have a very high content of oxalate, such as rhubarb or spinach, may be worthy of trial. Persons who have passed several uric acid or urate stones, as may occur in gout or in patients with leukaemia benefit from allopurinol (p. 638) which also has a place in treating calcium oxalate stone disease to which urates may contribute.

Since the distribution of phosphorus occurs so widely in foodstuffs, dietary restriction for the treatment of phosphate calculi is unlikely to be of any value. Phosphatic calculi are found only in alkaline urine, hence acidifying the urine by administering ammonium chloride daily may be effective. In contrast, cystine and urate stones may be prevented or sometimes dissolved by making the urine persistently alkaline, especially if combined with a high output of urine.

Lastly, the most important therapeutic and prophylactic measure for all forms of stones is the provision of an adequate fluid intake which assists in preventing deposition of crystalloids in the renal tissue. A daily output of urine of at least 3 *l* is advisable hence the intake of fluid should be approximately 4 *l* daily. If the climate or the patients occupation causes much sweating the fluid intake requires to be greatly increased.

## Congenital Abnormalities of the Kidneys

Congenital anomalies of the urinary tract affect more than 10% of infants and, unless they are immediately lethal, some are prone to lead to complications in later life. About 1 in 500 infants is born with only one kidney and, although usually compatible with a normal life, it is often associated with abnormalities in other organs.

**Polycystic Disease.** This genetically determined abnormality of renal structure may be associated with other congenital abnormalities, e.g. cystic liver (p. 411). There are two modes of inheritance. The infantile form is very rare and is inherited as an autosomal recessive; it is usually fatal within the first year of life. The commoner or adult type is inherited as an autosomal dominant trait. It may be found during infancy, but symptoms often do not develop until adult life. Both kidneys are affected, are several times the normal size and consist of masses of cysts, predominantly cortical, with a variable amount of renal parenchyma which often shows extensive fibrosis and arteriolosclerosis.

The clinical features include pain in the renal angles, haematuria, uraemia and usually a slowly developing arterial hypertension. Often one or both kidneys can be palpated and the surface may be nodular. In addition to polycystic disease, other diseases in which the kidneys may be palpable are hydro- or pyonephrosis, solitary cyst, renal carcinoma and other tumours. It should be remembered, however, that in some normal people all of the right kidney, and occasionally the lower pole of the left kidney may be felt on clinical examination. This is particularly true in slim women. On the other hand, pathologically enlarged kidneys are not always palpable. When a kidney can be felt, as in polycystic disease, it may be possible to appreciate departures from the normal size, smooth surface and firm consistency. Diagnosis can be confirmed by ultrasound or retrograde pyelography.

In course, prognosis and treatment, polycystic disease resembles chronic glomerulonephritis and death occurs in middle age from uraemia, cerebrovascular accident or cardiac failure.

**Medullary Cystic Disease.** Medullary cysts are found in two widely different conditions. In *medullary sponge kidney* the cysts are confined to the collecting ducts in the medulla. Affected patients are usually middle aged and present with pain, haematuria or urinary tract infection. The diagnosis is made on radiographic examination and the prognosis is generally good.

In *uraemic medullary sponge kidney* small cortical cysts are also present and these lead to progressive destruction of the nephrons; this condition occurs in younger patients and there is often a family history. Sometimes affected kidneys are salt-losing; this aggravates the degree of renal failure but, even when treated appropriately, serious renal failure is usual.

## Drug-induced Renal Disease

The susceptibility of the kidney to damage by drugs stems from the fact that it is the route of excretion for many water soluble compounds. Acute renal damage may arise in the course of treatment with a number of antimicrobial drugs. Sulphonamides may precipitate in the renal tubules, calyces or ureter and cause obstruction to urine flow, and occasionally lesions similar to polyarteritis nodosa may develop. Streptomycin, kanamycin, gentamicin and some cephalosporins may cause proximal tubular damage and proteinuria. Penicillins, cephalin and phenylbutazone may induce an allergic acute interstitial nephritis and acute renal failure. Tetracycline accentuates uraemia by its antianabolic effect on protein metabolism; tetracycline and amphotericin B, kept and used after the expiry date, can induce renal tubular acidosis and sometimes a Fanconi-like syndrome. Lithium may reduce renal concentrating power and induce polyuria.

**Analgesic Nephropathy.** The occurrence of chronic renal damage as a consequence of long-continued ingestion of analgesics is an important potential cause of renal failure. Although phenacetin is the major culprit it is possible that other analgesics, such as aspirin or codeine, may be partly responsible.

The pathological changes predominantly affect the corticomedullary junction with diffuse interstitial fibrosis and tubular atrophy. Ultimately there is a loss of tubules in cortex and medulla and acute papillary necrosis may develop. The changes are probably the result of ischaemia due to interference with the blood flow through the postglomerular vessels of juxtamedullary glomeruli. A recognised complication is the development of carcinoma of the renal pelvis.

The majority of affected patients are women who suffer from anxiety or headaches or have personal or marital problems. They are commonly divorced, anxious, apprehensive and smoke or drink alcohol to excess. Other patients have taken analgesics over many years for rheumatoid arthritis or osteoarthrosis. Symptoms include polyuria and thirst and the features of recurrent urinary tract infection. Renal colic may be caused by the passage of fragments of necrotic renal papillae which can be recognised by microscopic examination of the urine.

Apart from the history of drug ingestion, diagnosis is made by the characteristic radiological appearances of the papillae on retrograde pyelography. The contrast medium is seen as a small tract within the papillary substance; later the papillae may separate giving a ring shadow. Treatment consists of withdrawing the offending drug and substituting another analgesic, e.g. paracetamol, if such therapy is essential. Provided the analgesic is withdrawn sufficiently early there is a reasonable prospect of some recovery of renal function; otherwise severe renal failure develops and becomes irreversible.

## Tumours of Kidney and Genito-Urinary Tract

**Renal carcinoma** is the most common tumour of the kidney. It was formerly called a hypernephroma on the mistaken view that it arose from adrenal rest tissue within the kidney. Haematuria is the most frequent presenting feature and blood clots may give rise to renal colic. Sometimes the tumour causes vague abdominal pain and it may also be responsible for long continued fever. Occasionally patients present first with symptoms arising from metastases in the lungs, liver or bones. On rare occasions polycythaemia occurs, and this is believed to be due to excessive production of erythropoietin. The tumour may be palpable and is defined by radiological investigation and ultrasonography. Early surgical treatment affords the only prospect of cure.

**Nephroblastoma (Wilm's Tumour)** is the second most common malignant tumour of the kidney and presents in the first decade, and often the first year of life. The tumour is radiosensitive and the best hope of cure is early diagnosis and surgical removal followed by radiotherapy.

**Tumours of the renal pelvis, ureter and bladder** are histologically similar and are almost always transitional cell carcinomas. They tend to spread locally by direct invasion but also by implantation to other parts of the urinary tract. While some are benign, e.g. papillomas, all urinary tract tumours are liable to recur even after apparently adequate treatment. The bladder is by far the most common site and epidemiological studies have shown that it is particularly likely to develop in patients who work in industries where exposure to aniline is likely such as dyeing and printing and in areas of endemicity for urinary schistosomiasis (p. 859). Haematuria as a sole presenting symptom is almost universal. Features due to obstruction to the urinary tract also occur and symptoms of urinary tract infection may be superimposed. Diagnosis is made by cystoscopy, biopsy and radiography. Bladder tumours are treated by diathermy or radiotherapy. Cystectomy with transplantation of the ureters to colon or skin may be necessary.

**Prostatic carcinoma** usually presents with symptoms of urethral obstruction similar to those of benign prostatic hypertrophy. On digital examination of the rectum the prostrate is felt to be very hard and the median furrow may be obliterated. Spread through the capsule and metastases in bone occur and are often associated with a rise in the plasma acid phosphatase. Both the primary growth and metastases can be controlled with oestrogens, e.g. dienoestrol. Painful gynaecomastia is a troublesome side-effect. In some cases orchidectomy may also be necessary.

**Benign enlargement of the prostate gland** is of unknown cause but it may be associated with a fall in androgen secretion. It is most commonly found in men over 60 years. Histologically the inner zone of the gland undergoes hyperplasia and hypertrophy and there is an increase in the fibromuscular stroma. The enlarged prostate obstructs the outflow of urine from the bladder by compressing, displacing, distorting and elongating the prostatic urethra with the effects on bladder and renal function referred to on page 450.

The clinical features are those of progressive obstruction to urinary flow. Acute urinary retention may arise if the gland suddenly increases in size because of superimposed infection or congestion, or when cardiac failure develops in the elderly. Then the patient has a sudden desire to micturate but is unable to do so, the bladder becomes tense and is tender. More chronic retention may pass unnoticed for some time but there is a gradual increase in the volume of urine which remains in the bladder after micturition. Haematuria and bleeding from the urethra may also occur and may be the presenting symptom. On rectal examination the prostate may feel large, elastic and is uniform in consistency; however, when the median lobe alone is affected, the prostate feels normal and the condition can be recognised only by cystoscopy.

Prostatectomy is the only effective treatment and the important decision is when to operate. Acute retention should be relieved by catheterisation and drainage; sometimes this reduces congestion and the ability to pass urine spontaneously can be regained. If this does not occur, operation should be carried out in a few days.

**Testicular tumours** are uncommon but as they are usually malignant and sometimes spread to the abdomen and lungs at an early stage they are the main cause of death from neoplasia in young men. A seminoma presents as a painless and often uniform, rapid enlargement of the testis. A teratoma causes more nodular changes and may secrete gonadotrophic hormones producing gynaecomastia. A testicular tumour may be overlooked if it is obscured by a hydrocele or if the examination is inadequate. Seminomas can be treated successfully by orchidectomy and radiotherapy. Chemotherapy is also required for other tumours in which the prognosis is poorer.

## Prospects in Nephrology

The last 25 years have seen major advances in understanding the nature of renal disease and in its therapeutic control. Since 1950, renal transplantation and haemodialysis for acute and chronic renal failure have passed through a tentative and experimental phase and become established clinical procedures. Studies of renal biopsies by light, electron and immunofluorescence microscopy have transformed concepts of glomerular disease; knowledge of immunological mechanisms and their associated effects on complement, the mediators of inflammation and coagulation, are beginning to clarify the origin of glomerular damage, and awareness that the kidney acts as an endocrine organ has increased understanding of some forms of hypertension, of vitamin D resistance, and renal osteodystrophy and of renal anaemia.

Progress in the foreseeable future is likely to consist of a steady consolidation of these foundations rather than any dramatic discovery that might otherwise transform the picture. Knowledge of renal structure will be further advanced by the use of scanning electron microscopy and the application of immunofluorescent techniques to electron microscopic preparations. Improved methods of detecting and measuring immune complexes and the identification of further unknown specific antigens, including viruses, will add to the list of agents known to be responsible for glomerulonephritis. At present immunosuppressive therapy is disappointing in controlling both the naturally occurring immunological renal disorders and in the immunologically based rejection of transplanted kidneys. The non-specific nature of the action of immunosuppressive drugs gives rise to serious problems of toxicity and of opportunist infection. The ultimate goal in renal tranplantation is the induction of specific tolerance by which ideally the immune response against the transplantation antigens of a grafted kidney only is suppressed and all other immunological responses remain normal. Experimental work in rats gives rise to optimism that this might be ultimately achieved. A significant improvement in cadaver graft survival has resulted from the empirical use of blood transfusion given several weeks before the graft is carried out.

Its mechanism is unknown, but it may act by inducing some form of non-responsiveness to non-HLA and HLA antigens.

Estimates of plasma 1,OH and 1,25 OH cholecalciferol and of parathyroid hormone and calcitonin will increase the capacity to prevent renal osteodystrophy, but the isolation, precise measurement and therapeutic availability of erythropoetin appear to be more distant.

The prevention of chronic pyelonephritis and renal failure by the eradication of urinary tract infection at an early stage appears to be a goal which recedes with the passage of time. Even if it is accepted that a significant proportion of chronic pyelonephritis arises from recurrent infections in infancy, the cost and difficulties of screening large numbers of children sufficiently often to detect them present formidable obstacles.

Finally, steady miniaturisation of artificial kidneys using improved synthetic membranes and adsorbents with the ultimate aim of producing a portable, round-the-clock working artificial kidney is likely to continue.

J. S. Robson

*Further reading*:

Black, D. A. K. (1979), *Renal Disease,* 4th edn. Oxford: Blackwell.
Macleod, J. (1979) *Clinical Examination*, 5th edn. Edinburgh: Churchill Livingstone.— For further information about examination of the kidneys and the urine.
Passmore, R. & Robson, J. S. (1976) *Companion to Medical Studies.* Vol. 1, 2nd edn. p. 35.1. Oxford: Blackwell.
Passmore, R. & Robson, J. S. (1980) *Companion to Medical Studies.* Vol. 2, 2nd edn. p. 12.1 Oxford: Blackwell.
Passmore, R. & Robson, J. S. (1974) *Companion to Medical Studies.* Vol. 3, p. 22.1. Oxford: Blackwell.

# 11. Endocrine and Metabolic Diseases

The advances that have been achieved in the technology of hormone assay have resulted in a better understanding of clinical endocrinology in physiological terms. The isolation and synthesis of hormones or biologically active analogues have made many endocrine diseases eminently amenable to treatment. Formerly many hormone assays were confined to research laboratories but with improved techniques and understanding of their clinical application a wide range of assays is now available to the clinician. Among the methods in use are radioimmunoassay, competitive protein binding and fluorimetry. In addition, cytochemical techniques provide a new degree of sensitivity in the measurement of certain pituitary hormones. In order to take full advantage of such improvements in laboratory aspects of endocrinology the physician, while clearly having to maintain clinical acumen, must also be familiar with the investigative aspects of the subject.

The application of the science of immunology to endocrinology has been responsible for many of the advances, notably radioimmunoassay of all the hormones produced by the anterior pituitary gland and of many of the hormones produced by its target glands, thyroid, adrenal, testis and ovary. The study of immunology has thrown much light on the possible pathogenesis of many endocrine diseases in terms of autoimmunity, including certain of the thyroid diseases, insulin-dependent diabetes, a form of adrenal insufficiency and of parathyroid insufficiency and certain types of gonadal failure. The combined study of the patient's HLA type and TSH receptor-binding antibodies in the serum now enable us to predict the clinical course of Graves' disease with greater accuracy.

One of the most impressive clinical advances in endocrinology in the past decade has been the firm establishment of prolactin as a human pituitary hormone and the detection of hyperprolactinaemia in many patients with gonadal disorders. Dopamine is recognised to be the physiological hypothalamic prolactin-release inhibitory hormone. Pharmacological control of excessive prolactin secretion in these disorders and reduction in growth hormone secretion in acromegaly has become possible with the introduction of bromocriptine, a dopamine agonist.

While the metabolic aspects of the commonest of the endocrine diseases, diabetes mellitus and thyrotoxicosis, can be readily controlled, some of the complications of these conditions remain poorly understood, particularly angiopathy in diabetes mellitus and exophthalmos in thyrotoxicosis.

Endocrinology also permeates many other clinical disciplines, not only because disordered function of the endocrine glands may affect every organ in the body, but because corticosteroids are extensively used for the control of inflammation and adverse immune reactions in a variety of serious disorders. When used in pharmacological doses for these purposes there may be both beneficial and adverse effects because the anti-inflammatory action of the corticosteroids cannot be separated from their hormonal activity.

Among the benefits which will accrue if clinicians make full use of new knowledge in endocrinology is that disease will be more readily detected in its early stages and unnecessary morbidity avoided.

# THE HYPOTHALAMUS AND THE PITUITARY GLAND

**Anatomy and Physiology.** The pituitary gland is enclosed in the sella turcica, bridged over by the diaphragma sellae, with the sphenoidal air sinuses below, and the optic chiasma in the subarăchnoid space above. The gland is composed of two lobes, anterior and posterior, and is connected to the hypothalamus by the infundibular stalk carrying the portal vessels from the median eminence of the hypothalamus to the anterior lobe of the pituitary gland and nerve fibres to the posterior lobe.

The anterior lobe consists of three main histological types of cell using conventional staining: chromphobe, eosinophil and basophil. However, the correlation between these types of staining and hormone secretion is not close. Through the action of its seven hormones, four of which act on target endocrine glands while the remainder act primarily on target tissues it affects growth, thyroid activity, sexual function, lactation, the metabolism of water, carbohydrate protein and fat, as well as skin pigmentation. Melanocyte-stimulating 'hormone' is now believed to be a fragment from a large adenohypophysial polypeptide called $\beta$-lipotrophin, which is also associated with the polypeptide endorphins (endogenous substances with morphine–like actions) and their closely related pentapeptides the enkephalins. The only known function of melanocyte-stimulating hormone (MSH) in man is to increase pigmentation of the skin by increasing melanin synthesis in the melanocytes.

The posterior lobe (pars nervosa or neurohypophysis) contains neuroglial fibres which emanate from the supraoptic and paraventricular nuclei of the hypothalamus.

HORMONES OF THE ANTERIOR LOBE. Secretion of each of the hormones formed by the anterior lobe of the pituitary gland is influenced by a stimulus provided by the

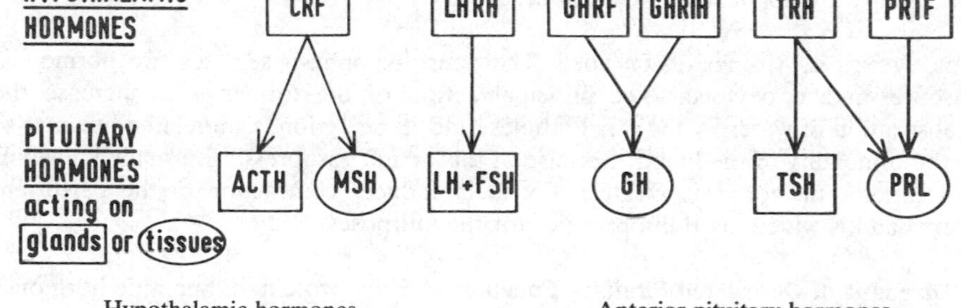


| Hypothalamic hormones | | Anterior pituitary hormones | |
|---|---|---|---|
| CRF: | Corticotrophin releasing factor | ACTH: | Adrenocorticotrophic hormone (corticotrophin) |
| LHRH: | Luteinising hormone (follicle stimulating hormone) releasing hormone | MSH: | Melanocyte stimulating 'hormone' |
| | | LH: | Luteinising hormone |
| | | FSH: | Follicle stimulating hormone |
| GHRF: | Growth hormone releasing factor | GH: | Growth hormone (somatotrophin) |
| GHRIH: | Growth hormone release inhibiting hormone (somatostatin) | TSH: | Thyrotrophin |
| | | PRL: | Prolactin |
| TRH: | Thyrotrophin releasing hormone | | |
| PRIF: | Prolactin release inhibiting factor | | |

Fig. 11.1 The principal direct relationships between the hypothalamus and the anterior lobe of the pituitary gland. Hypothalamic releasing (R) and inhibiting (I) activities are described as hormones (H) when they have been chemically identified and synthesised, and as factors (F) while their recognition still depends upon biological activity only, as determined in animal studies.

hypothalamus, either in the form of a releasing hormone or factor, or by an inhibitor which suppresses secretion or by both (Fig. 11.1).

The secretion of the hypothalamic factors in turn is dependent upon a wide variety of stimuli of nervous, metabolic, physical or hormonal origin, in particular from the appropriate target organs of the pituitary hormones, the thyroid gland, the adrenal cortex and the gonads. The secretion of corticotrophin and presumably of the hypothalamic corticotrophin releasing factor (CRF), is partly time-dependent, being most active in the morning, and least in the evening, except when this physiological diurnal (circadian) rhythm is overridden by other stimuli, particularly emotional or physical stresses.

The thyrotrophin releasing hormone (TRH) formed in the hypothalamus, like the other hypothalamic releasing or inhibiting factors, passes through the portal system of vessels connecting the hypothalamus to the pituitary gland, where it promotes the secretion of the thyroid stimulating hormone (TSH). The luteinising hormone and follicle stimulating hormone releasing hormone (designated LHRH for simplicity) acts on the pituitary to release both LH and FSH. Growth hormone (GH) however is controlled by a dual system, namely growth hormone releasing factor (GHRF) and an inhibitory hormone (GHRIH). The latter is known also as somatostatin and has many other functions, including reduction in plasma gastrin, glucagon, insulin and in platelet stickiness. It is also produced in sites other than the hypothalamus such as the delta cells of the pancreatic islets. Prolactin-release is under the control of an inhibitory factor (PRIF). The secretion of $\beta$-lipotrophin (MSH) is under the control of CRF. The actions of the hypothalamic hormones are not always as specific as their names suggest: in addition to the example of somatostatin cited above, TRH stimulates the secretion of prolactin (PRL).

To date there are no methods for measuring plasma levels of hypothalamic hormones that are applicable to clinical practice.

HORMONES OF THE POSTERIOR LOBE. The neurohypophysis secretes two hormones, vasopressin and oxytocin. The principal action of the former is to increase the reabsorption of water by the renal tubules, and its secretion is stimulated by any rise in the osmolality of the blood. Because of this action vasopressin is usually known as the antidiuretic hormone (ADH). Oxytocin induces contraction of the parturient uterus and is widely used in obstetrics for this purpose.

**Diagnosis of Disordered Pituitary Function.** All the protein and peptide hormones of the pituitary gland can be measured in body fluids by radioimmunoassay. In addition the hypothalamic hormones, TRH and LHRH have been synthesised and can be used clinically to stimulate the release of the appropriate pituitary hormones. Furthermore, assays for the hormones produced by the target glands of the pituitary are available. Thus it is possible to assess very fully and specifically the functional activity and the secretory capacity of the pituitary gland and its target organs. Several pituitary hormones, namely TSH, ACTH, GH, and gonadotrophins are available in suitable forms for the investigation and treatment of endocrine disorders, and are useful in distinguishing between primary insufficiency of the adrenal cortex, the thyroid gland and the gonads, and secondary failure due to reduced or absent secretion of one or more pituitary trophic hormones.

The application of assay procedures to the diagnosis of pituitary disease should be discussed in advance with the laboratory staff responsible for the hormone assays, so that standardisation is achieved. In assessing increased production of growth hormone in acromegaly; a standard glucose tolerance test is performed with radioimmunoassay of growth hormone at half-hourly intervals along with measurements of blood glucose. Under physiological conditions growth hormone secretion is promptly suppressed by a rise in the blood glucose level, while there is only partial or absent suppression in patients with pituitary tumours secreting growth hormone.

In assessing impaired secretion of growth hormone, insulin hypoglycaemia may be used (p. 492); this has the added advantage of stimulating the pituitary to secrete ACTH, which may be measured directly or can be monitored by estimating plasma 11-OH corticosteroids and also prolactin. In children insulin hypoglycaemia is also used unless there is an adequate increase in GH secretion 30 minutes after a standardised exercise test. If plasma is to be measured for ACTH it must be chilled promptly and stored frozen on account of its short half life and instability. However, $\beta$-lipotrophin, which is secreted with ACTH, is stable.

The ability of the pituitary to secrete TSH and PRL can be tested by TRH given intravenously and by measuring the serum TSH and PRL concentration after 20 minutes. LHRH can be given intravenously at the same time and the plasma LH and FSH measured also.

## Tumours of the Pituitary Gland

**Pathology.** Pituitary tumours may be macroadenomas (associated with enlargement of the pituitary fossa or involvement of the adjacent structures) or microadenomas (associated with a normal sized pituitary fossa or with minimal alteration such as a double floor). Such adenomas may be functional or non-functional. They may also produce hypofunction of the rest of the pituitary through pressure atrophy; such failure of function may be progressive and sequential with the secretion of gonadotrophins usually declining first, followed by GH, PRL, ACTH and finally TSH.

Excess production of a pituitary hormone may not necessarily be due to a tumour but to hyperplasia of the secreting cells on account of a disorder in hypothalamic control (excess production of a releasing hormone or insufficient production of an inhibiting hormone). In the case of PRL it has been claimed that the response in PRL secretion to TRH or to dopamine-receptor blockers (such as metoclopramide) is helpful in distinguishing between hyperplasia (associated with an augmented secretion) and tumour (associated with little or no response). In the case of GH, excess production is usually due to an acidophil (or mixed acidophil and chromophobe) macroadenoma of the pituitary. On the other hand, excess secretion of ACTH (and of $\beta$-lipotrophin) is usually associated with a microadenoma or hyperplasia of basophil (or mixed basophil and chromophobe) cells with little or no evidence of enlargement of the pituitary fossa, except in cases of longstanding or after bilateral adrenalectomy undertaken several years earlier (Nelson's syndrome, p. 485).

Craniopharyngiomas are tumours or cysts developing in cell rests of Rathke's pouch, and may be located within the sella turcica, or commonly in the suprasellar space, where they frequently calcify. In either situation their clinical presentation is likely to be due to pressure on one or both lobes of the pituitary gland, on the stalk, on the hypothalamus, or on the visual pathways. Primary carcinoma of the pituitary gland is particularly rare, but a metastatic tumour from a primary in the breast, lung, kidney or elsewhere may occur in the hypothalamus and thus reduce pituitary function. Other tumours, for example pinealoma, ependymoma or meningioma, may occasionally be associated with some disturbance of pituitary function. Granulomatous lesions of the pituitary or hypothalamus such as sarcoidosis or syphilis may mimic pituitary tumours.

**Clinical features** of pituitary tumours vary, depending on the type of lesion in the pituitary gland, whether both lobes are involved or only one and whether there is any hypothalamic involvement. Enlarging tumours of the gland may present with signs attributable to increased output of hormones or to failure of secretion. Some tumours secreting hormones compress the remaining pituitary tissue, so that there may be failure of some functions of the gland in the presence of an excess of others.

Clinical features also depend upon the site and size of the tumour. Headache is the most constant but least specific symptom. Involvement of an optic nerve, the optic chiasma, or an optic tract leads to impaired visual fields. The patient occasionally notices a visual field defect, but, more commonly, examination of the visual fields by confrontation or by perimetry will be required to identify the likely point of interference within the visual pathway (Fig. 14.4). A bitemporal field defect is the most characteristic finding associated with pressure upon the chiasma. Optic atrophy may be apparent on ophthalmoscopy. Diplopia and strabismus may follow pressure on the third, fourth or sixth cranial nerves. Some tumours expand sufficiently to interfere with ADH secretion and so cause diabetes insipidus. Tumours which expand upwards to impinge on the hypothalamus may cause disturbance of sleep and appetite and also obesity.

Enlargement of the sella turcica and erosion of the clinoid processes may be detected on radiological examination, or suprasellar calcification may be seen in a craniopharyngioma. A 'double floor' of the sella may be present if the tumour is expanding downwards. Computed tomography may be helpful, making the distressing investigation of air encephalography less necessary than previously.

**Treatment of Pituitary Tumours.** If there is evidence of pressure on the visual pathways, surgical treatment is required. If hyperfunction, as confirmed by suitable assays, is sufficiently severe to affect the patient's welfare and prognosis, then treatment aimed at destroying the tumour or its capacity to secrete should be considered. Hypophysectomy may be performed from below by a trans-sphenoidal approach or, if there is suprasellar extension, through a transfrontal craniotomy.

It is sometimes possible to remove microadenomas trans-sphenoidally by microdissection so as to leave sufficient normal pituitary tissue to maintain normal function.

Suppression of secretory capacity may be achieved without surgery using radiotherapy applied externally, but its effect is often slow and unpredictable in the individual patient. In the case of the excess production of GH and PRL, bromocriptine may be used as an adjunct until such times as external radiotherapy has become effective (perhaps 6 months or a year). Prolactinomas must be especially carefully supervised during pregnancy (fertility having been restored with bromocriptine) as they may undergo rapid expansion. The implantation of yttrium in the pituitary fossa is now seldom used on account of the complications it may cause.

## Syndromes due to Anterior Pituitary Hypersecretion

**Giantism and Acromegaly.** Hypersecretion of growth hormone by eosinophil cells may develop very rarely before the epiphyses have united and produce giantism. Much more frequently it occurs in adult life, after union of the epiphyses, to cause acromegaly (large extremities). If hypersecretion begins in adolescence and persists into adult life, giantism and acromegaly may be associated.

Acromegaly is characterised by an increase in the size of the bones and soft tissues of the hands, feet, supraorbital ridges, sinuses and the lower jaw. The skin becomes thick and coarse; the subcutaneous tissues increase in depth, while enlargement of the tongue, lips, nose and ears may be conspicuous. The viscera, for example the heart, thyroid and liver, enlarge. Sweating is common. Carbohydrate tolerance is reduced in about 30% of cases to the extent that diabetes mellitus develops. As the disease progresses, the patient often develops arthritis (p. 627), kyphosis and muscular weakness. Arterial hypertension is a common complication. The disease tends to progress slowly over several years, but patients are frequently seen with certain features of acromegaly in whom the progress of the condition has apparently been arrested, or a phase of hyperpituitarism may pass into hypopituitarism. Sensitive radioimmunological methods of assaying growth hormone in blood make it possible to assess with precision the activity of these tumours as well as the results of treatment. Bromocriptine is used to reduce GH levels as an adjunct to hypophysectomy or irradiation.

**Cushing's Disease.** Hypersecretion by basophil cells, or sometimes by chromophobe cells, leads to Cushing's disease (p. 485)

**Hyperprolactinaemia Syndrome.** Hyperprolactinaemia (due to adenoma or hyperplasia of the pituitary lactotrophs) will suppress gonadal function. In women amenorrhoea and infertility and sometimes galactorrhoea may occur. In man it is a cause of infertility associated with loss of libido or impotence. Serum prolactin levels may be raised by the stress of a bad venepuncture, by manipulation of the breasts, by certain drugs (e.g. oestrogens; some antidepressants and tranquillisers) and by primary hypothyroidism.

## Syndromes due to Anterior Pituitary Hyposecretion

### Pituitary Dwarfism and Infantilism

In children hyposecretion causes dwarfism and pituitary infantilism. The term 'dwarfism' means that growth is retarded; 'infantilism' implies that sexual development is subnormal for the individual's age. While pituitary tumours are an uncommon cause of dwarfism, delayed growth and development are characteristic of most pituitary tumours in children. In addition to assessment by assays of pituitary hormones, for example TSH, GH, ACTH and gonadotrophins, or if the techniques are not available, by the assay of target organ hormones, accurate records must be kept of the child's height, weight and bone age. Radiographs of the left hand and wrist taken at intervals of 1 year can be compared with a standard atlas to assess the progress of bone development. Children in whom growth hormone secretion has been shown to be absent may be treated by GH; this is obtainable only from appropriate national sources because of the need to extract GH from human pituitary glands. Intramuscular injections are given twice weekly for several years according to the response judged by serial readings recorded on standard height and weight charts.

DIFFERENTIAL DIAGNOSIS OF DWARFISM. Growth may be delayed or impaired for many reasons. Tallness and shortness of stature have genetic components. One form of dwarfism is Turner's syndrome (p. 11). Persistent stunting of growth is a recognised association with premature birth, anoxic forms of congenital heart disease, chronic liver or renal disease, many chronic infections, and persistent undernutrition (p. 94). Pituitary dwarfism must also be distinguished from:

1. *Cretinism and juvenile hypothyroidism.* If these conditions are not recognised and treated promptly, stunting of growth will occur (p. 476).

2. *Dwarfism due to coeliac disease* (p. 350). This disability is associated with steatorrhoea and defective absorption, especially of fat, minerals and vitamins. Dwarfs of this type are usually larger than the pituitary type; they may be further distinguished by a history of the passage of pale, bulky, offensive stools. Cystic fibrosis may simulate malabsorption due to coeliac disease.

3. *Achondroplasia.* This hereditary disorder of endochondral ossification is characterised by failure of the long bones of the arms and legs to grow properly, while the trunk and head develop normally. Dwarfs of this type are sexually and intellectually normal and frequently used to appear in circuses.

4. *Renal dwarfism.* Renal failure arising in early childhood may be caused by neuromuscular incoordination at the outlet of the bladder, which produces back-pressure and hydronephrosis, or it may be due to congenital cystic disease, congenital hypoplasia of the kidneys, or most commonly, chronic nephritis. In some cases hereditary defects of renal tubular function may be responsible (p. 423). Many of the characteristic features of renal failure may be found, for example hypertension, a raised blood urea and changes in the fundus of the eye.

## Hypopituitarism

**Aetiology.** At one time destruction of the anterior lobe of the hypophysis was commonly due to infarction and this was often a sequel to post-partum haemorrhage (*Sheehan's syndrome*). Improvements in obstetrical care have greatly reduced the incidence of this accident and the disorder is now most commonly due to a chomophobe adenoma. Other causes include nonsecretory tumours, trauma, granulomas (syphilis, sarcoidosis) and the presence of simple cysts. Idiopathic cases are probably the result of failure of the hypothalamus to secrete the appropriate releasing hormones or may conceivably be due to an autoimmune hypophysitis, although the evidence for this is poor. Surgical treatment or radiotherapy of tumours of the gland is often followed by a degree of hypopituitarism calling for replacement therapy, and hypophysectomy is sometimes performed in the treatment of malignant disease elsewhere, for example carcinoma of the breast.

**Clinical Features.** In Sheehan's syndrome, a history is usually obtained that, several years before the onset of the presenting illness, the patient had a difficult confinement with haemorrhage and a need for blood transfusion. Lactation failed or was never established, amenorrhoea persisted indefinitely and other changes attributable to the absence of the trophic hormones gradually made their appearance. Some of the features of hypothyroidism (p. 475) may be present, but myxoedema is seldom prominent. Absent or scanty axillary and pubic hair are characteristic findings. Symptoms of adrenal insufficiency (p. 489) may be noted, but the changes in serum electrolytes found in severe adrenal insufficiency do not occur in hypopituitarism and the blood pressure is usually not so low. This is because aldosterone continues to be secreted by the glomerulosa layer of the adrenal cortex, since this function is largely independent of corticotrophin. Cortisol production, however, falls to a minimum because the essential corticotrophic stimulus from the pituitary gland is absent or inadequate. In contrast to the pigmentation of the skin in Addison's disease, a striking degree of pallor is often one of the signs suggesting hypopituitarism. Although a mild degree of normochromic anaemia is usually present, this is insufficient to explain the pallor of the skin which is due to capillary vasoconstriction and the absence of melanin.

*Coma in Hypopituitarism.* Patients with hypopituitarism are peculiarly liable to go into coma if inadequately treated. While the onset of coma may occur for no apparent reason, it usually follows some mild infection or injury, in the same way that an Addisonian crisis may follow some relatively trivial stress. The coma may be due to one or more of the effects of hypopituitarism. These include increased sensitivity to insulin and spontaneous or reactive hypoglycaemia. Water intoxication is another important factor, due to a disturbance of water control in patients with adrenal insufficiency. Hypothyroidism is also an important component in the causation of coma; hypothermia with a rectal temperature as low as 32°C or less may develop. Failure of ventilation with anoxia and respiratory acidosis may be a lethal complication of hypopituitarism.

**Differential Diagnosis.** Hypopituitarism is sometimes confused with anorexia nervosa. The distinguishing features lie in the history and the presence of pubic, axillary and lanugo hair in anorexia nervosa. In addition, anorexia nervosa is characterised by an absent appetite and gross wasting, whereas in hypopituitarism neither is striking unless some other cause is present. Assays of pituitary trophic hormones of or the products of the target glands will help to distinguish these two disorders and others which might be confused with hypopituitarism. In anorexia nervosa the endocrine failure is restricted to the gonadotrophins and ovarian hormones. The excellent response of patients with hypopituitarism to treatment with corticosteroids will also help to distinguish between the two conditions.

**Treatment.** The aim should be to provide adequate substitution therapy, according to the deficiencies demonstrated, so that the patient can lead a normal life. Cortisol should be given by mouth in doses of 20 mg in the morning and 10 mg in the evening or according to the cortisol blood profile. Thyroid hormone will usually be required and should be given orally as thyroxine 0·15 mg daily. It is dangerous to give thyroid hormone to these patients until they have been protected by cortisol against the possibility of an Addisonian type of crisis. Excessive doses of corticosteroids may lead to hypertension. Oedema occasionally is troublesome, and may be corrected by substituting a corticosteroid with weaker electrolyte effects, for example prednisolone, in a dose of 5 mg in the morning and 2·5 mg in the evening. In some circumstances it may be helpful to add ethinyl oestradiol 50 $\mu$g daily, and for adolescent or adult men an androgen may be required. Fertility may be restored in young patients with appropriate gonadotrophin therapy.

## Diabetes Insipidus

This uncommon disease is characterised by the persistent excretion of excessive quantities of urine of low specific gravity, and by constant thirst.

**Aetiology.** The disease develops after damage to the neurohypophyseal mechanism for the production of ADH (antidiuretic hormone; arginine vasopressin, AVP). It may occur with tumours of the pituitary, with a craniopharyngioma, or after operations in this region, and as a sequel to encephalitis, basal meningitis, syphilis, and trauma. Metastatic disease involving the neurohypophysis may occasionally be responsible. In panhypopituitarism, the symptoms of diabetes insipidus may not be apparent until corticosteroid therapy has been provided; an adequate level of corticosteroids is required for the condition to be expressed. A rare genetic form exists due to unresponsiveness of the renal tubules to ADH (nephrogenic diabetes insipidus), but in some cases no cause can be identified.

**Clinical Features.** The most marked symptoms are polyuria and polydipsia. The patient may pass 5–20 or more litres of urine in 24 hours. The urine is clear and of low specific gravity and osmolality, i.e. less than the plasma osmolality, (p. 406)

A positive diagnosis of diabetes insipidus depends on demonstrating that a rise of plasma osmolality induced by withholding fluids is not accompanied by a rise in the osmolality or specific gravity of the urine, but that when vasopressin is given, such a rise does occur. The latter test is necessary in order to show that the kidney is capable of concentrating the urine which it cannot do in nephrogenic diabetes insipidus.

It may be difficult to differentiate the polyuria of diabetes insipidus from that found in *hysterical polydipsia*. In such cases, if fluids are not taken for 24 hours, the urine is found to concentrate to a normal specific gravity. Accurate weighing of the patient will show whether there has been surreptitious drinking; it should be repeated at regular intervals during such a test in order to avoid the risks inherent in excessive dehydration. If the weight falls by more than 3% the test should be terminated.

Other causes of polyuria are discussed on page 425.

**Treatment.** The minimum amount of vasopressin required to keep the patient in water balance must be determined by controlling the fluid output and then reducing the dose of hormone without permitting polyuria or excessive thirst to recur. A synthetic analogue of vasopressin, desmopressin is given intranasally; 20$\mu$g once or twice daily elicits a response as effectively as vasopressin given by injection.

### Inappropriate Secretion of ADH

Although there is no reported case of excess secretion of ADH (AVP or similar anti-diuretic peptides) by the pars nervosa, excessive secretion may occur in a wide variety of conditions giving rise to the syndrome of 'inappropriate' secretion of ADH as, for example, occasionally in bronchial carcinoma.

## THE THYROID GLAND

**Anatomy and Physiology.** The thyroid gland consists of an isthmus and two lateral lobes, and lies in front of and on either side of the upper part of the trachea and the laminae of the thyroid cartilage. Posteriorly it is closely related to the recurrent laryngeal nerves which lie between the trachea and the oesophagus; the gland is separated from these nerves by its fibrous sheath. The thyroid gland is provided with a rich blood supply through the superior and inferior thyroid arteries. The parathyroid glands are usually to be found lying on the posterior aspect of the thyroid, in its substance or in the sheath of the gland and in relation to the upper cornu of the thymus.

Thyroxine ($T_4$) and triiodothyronine ($T_3$), the hormones secreted by the gland, are dipeptides containing respectively 4 and 3 atoms of iodine in each molecule. Both are normally stored in the colloid vesicles as thyroglobulin. Because it is less strongly bound to serum proteins, $T_3$ acts more rapidly than $T_4$. It is also effective in smaller doses than $T_4$. Thus the effects of $T_3$ may be apparent in a number of hours while an equivalent dose of $T_4$ may take several days to be effective. Both hormones act directly on most of the tissues of the body to increase cellular metabolism.

Thyroid function is controlled by thyrotrophin, the thyroid stimulating hormone (TSH) secreted by the anterior pituitary gland which in turn is controlled by thyrotrophin releasing hormone (TRH) secreted by the hypothalamus. TRH is a tripeptide which has been synthesised and is available for clinical use. There is also a negative feed-back mechanism whereby the thyroid hormones act principally on the anterior pituitary to suppress the secretion of TSH. The synthesis and release of thyroid hormones from the colloid into the circulation are stimulated by TSH.

Calcitonin, secreted by the parafollicular C (calcitonin) cells of the thyroid gland, is discussed on page 479.

## Hyperthyroidism

The clinical condition consequent upon overproduction of $T_3$ or of both $T_3$ and $T_4$ is referred to as hyperthyroidism or thyrotoxicosis. In a significant minority of patients the excess production of thyroid hormone is confined to $T_3$ ($T_3$ thyrotoxicosis) but it is likely that a greater number of cases have an initial phase of excess $T_3$ production followed by an overproduction of both $T_3$ and $T_4$, and it is usually at the latter stage that the diagnosis is made.

**Aetiology and Pathology.** The serum TSH levels in patients with thyrotoxicosis are either reduced or undetectable using current radioimmunoassay techniques. Cases of thyrotoxicosis due to excess TSH production by pituitary tumours are exceptionally rare.

In many patients with hyperthyroidism the IgG autoantibody, human specific TSH receptor antibody, can be detected in the serum and it is possible that antibodies that can stimulate the TSH receptor may be the cause of hyperthyroidism in most instances of Graves' disease, as defined below. Other evidence of autoimmune activity directed against the thyroid gland in hyperthyroidism is the presence of lymphocytic infiltration in the gland which may be negligible, focal or extensive.

In the majority of patients with hyperthyroidism the thyroid gland is either diffusely hyperactive (*Graves' disease*) or the gland consists of multiple active nodules interspersed with inactive areas. This latter state is probably the outcome of alternate stimulation and degeneration or results from the development of thyrotoxicosis upon a multinodular goitre. Toxic nodular goitres tend to occur in older patients and diffuse goitres in younger subjects. Histologically, in Graves' disease, the increased activity of the gland is manifest by reduction in the size of the thyroid vesicles which are relatively empty of colloid; the epithelium is tall and columnar in contrast to the flat cuboidal epithelium of the normal gland. The vascularity is markedly increased. In a small percentage of patients, thyrotoxicosis is due to the presence of a hyperactive solitary nodule with suppression of the remainder of the gland through the normally functioning feed-back mechanism.

**Clinical Features.** Thyrotoxicosis is found much more frequently in women than in men (8:1), usually in the third to sixth decades, but it may occur at any age. There may or may not be clinically detectable enlargement of the thyroid gland (goitre). The increased blood supply to the thyroid often causes a bruit, and sometimes a thrill.

Most of the clinical features of thyrotoxicosis may be explained in terms of excess production of $T_3$ or of $T_3 + T_4$, although it is possible that $T_4$ is nothing more than a prohormone. The increased metabolism accounts for the loss in weight in spite of the increased appetite that is so often a striking feature in the clinical history. Occasionally, however, the patient overcompensates in terms of food intake and may gain weight.

Thyroid hormones potentiate the action of catecholamines, possibly by modulating amplification of the $\beta$-adrenergic signal at the level of the cell membrane. The increased cardiac output required to meet the metabolic demands, together with the effect of $T_3$ and $T_4$ on the sympathetic nervous system, tends to produce a tachycardia, or, particularly in elderly patients, arrhythmias such as atrial fibrillation or ectopic beats. The patient may complain of palpitations with or without the symptoms of cardiac failure. Sinus tachycardia, persisting during sleep, is one of the earliest and most constant signs. The pulse pressure is increased and capillary pulsation may be detectable. In the presence of coincident systolic hypertension a collapsing pulse may be noted. In the older patient cardiovascular manifestations may be the only clinical evidence of hyperthyroidism and it should be remembered that thyrotoxicosis is, along with coronary and rheumatic heart disease, one of the three commonest causes of atrial fibrillation.

There are other consequences of the effect of excess thyroid hormones on the $\beta$-adrenergic receptors. Patients commonly complain of increased frequency of bowel motions, usually with formed stools but there may be an element of malabsorption; a lag curve in a glucose tolerance test may be demonstrable partly as a result of intestinal hurry. Retraction of the upper eyelids and a fine tremor of the fingers may occur, while the hands are often hot and sweaty because of the increased metabolic rate and the need to lose excess heat. Intolerance of warm environments is characteristic. Thyrotoxic patients, although they are hyperdynamic, have a low efficiency in terms of what they achieve. They suffer from an inability to relax both mentally and physically; anxiety is frequent.

Less common clinical features that cannot be so readily explained in terms of disturbed physiology include exophthalmos (p. 474), pretibial myxoedema and finger clubbing, reduced fertility and menstrual irregularities. In addition there may be thyrotoxic myopathy (p. 740), which recovers when normal thyroid function is restored.

In some cases thyrotoxicosis undergoes spontaneous remission within a period of months or years, while in other cases it follows a prolonged or intermittent course.

*Thyrotoxic crises* are now uncommon, as cases of hyperthyroidism are recognised and treated earlier and more effectively. They may be seen shortly after thyroidectomy in patients who have not been adequately prepared for operation or in patients who have been operated on for some other disability without hyperthyroidism having been recognised. Alternatively a crisis may be precipitated by a severe infection. The patient in crisis suffers from severe mental and physical exhaustion with delirium, delusions or mania, dehydration, ketosis, tachycardia, cardiac failure and fever.

*Hyperthyroidism in the newborn and in children.* Thyrotoxicosis may occur rarely in the newborn when it is thought to be due to the transplacental transmission of thyroid stimulating antibody. This form of hyperthyroidism is self-limiting. If thyrotoxicosis occurs before puberty there is an increase in the growth rate so that affected children are unusually tall for their age.

**Investigation.** The diagnostic facilities available are so precise that it should not be necessary to treat patients in the absence of a high degree of certainty concerning the diagnosis.

*Total serum thyroxine* measured by competitive protein binding or radioimmunoassay is not influenced by exogenous iodine, but is altered by factors which affect the concentration of thyroid hormone-binding proteins (TBG). Thus, concentrations (p. 906) may be raised in people with normal thyroid function when levels of TBG are increased in pregnancy, oestrogen administration or as a congenital anomaly. Decreased levels of TBG may be due to the nephrotic syndrome, androgen therapy, liver failure or be inherited. TBG may appear to be low if binding sites are saturated with drugs such salicylates, phenylbutazone, sulphonylureas and phenytoin.

*Total serum tri-iodothyronine* is necessary for the diagnosis of $T_3$ thyrotoxicosis when $T_3$ is elevated in the presence of a normal total serum $T_4$ and other tests. It is subject to the same limitations as total serum $T_4$ in relation to the level of TBG, although to a lesser extent.

*$T_3$ resin uptake, free thyroxine index and effective thyroxine ratio* The $T_3$ resin uptake test is an indirect measure of circulating thyroid hormone levels. It measures the degree of saturation of the binding sites on the thyroid hormone-binding proteins. High values are found in thyrotoxicosis but low values are recorded in euthyroid patients either pregnant or on oestrogen medication. The role of such a test is in the calculation of the *free thyroxine index* derived from the product of the total serum thyroxine and the $T_3$ resin uptake. In euthyroid patients with abnormalities of the thyroid hormone-binding proteins and in whom the total serum thyroxine is elevated, the $T_3$ resin uptake will be depressed and the free thyroxine index is more likely to lie in the normal range. Measurements of total $T_4$ which have been corrected for the patient's TBG are available and the result is referred to as the *effective thyroxine ratio*.

*The uptake of radioactive iodine or technetium.* The overactive gland synthesising excess $T_4$ has an increased uptake of iodine which can be shown by measuring the proportion of an oral tracer dose of $^{131}$I taken up by the thyroid gland in a given time (e.g. 4 hours) by using an appropriate 'counter' over the neck. Alternatively, an isotope of technetium (Tc99m) may be used intravenously with the thyroid uptake measured at 20 minutes, giving an even smaller dose of radiation which can be regarded as insignificant. The major fallacies in such studies are caused by iodine deficiency or enzyme deficiency beyond the stage of iodide uptake (which can give an increased uptake measurement without the presence of thyrotoxicosis) and iodine excess (which can give a low uptake measurement in spite of the presence of thyrotoxicosis). It is necessary to know how avid is the uptake of the gland before treating a thyrotoxic patient with radioactive iodine.

Either $^{131}$I or Tc99m may also be used to obtain a scan of the gland, indicating the amount and the distribution of functioning tissue. Scans are useful in thyrotoxic patients for detecting a solitary 'hot' nodule or a retrosternal extension of the gland. *In vivo* isotope tests should not be done on subjects who may be pregnant.

*Serum TSH levels in response to TRH stimulation.* In thyrotoxicosis the secretion of TSH by the anterior pituitary is suppressed so that serum levels of TSH are either reduced or absent. Moreover, the TSH response of the pituitary 20 minutes after the injection of TRH is absent. This is a most useful test of thyroid function in otherwise equivocal cases of thyrotoxicosis.

*Choice of test* or combination of tests is made in the light of the foregoing and in relation to the individual problem and the local resources. It must be remembered that when thyrotoxicosis is due to excessive production of $T_3$ alone, the total serum $T_4$, the effective thyroxine ratio and the thyroid uptake of radioisotopes may give normal results. The measurement of the total serum $T_3$ concentration together with the TRH test are, therefore, the two most useful diagnostic aids in relation to thyrotoxicosis.

**Treatment.** Three effective methods of treating thyrotoxicosis are available: (1) Antithyroid drugs, such as carbimazole, initially supplemented as necessary by beta-adrenergic blocking agents, for example propranolol. (2) Surgery, after a euthyroid state has been achieved with antithyroid drugs or under propranolol and potassium iodide cover. (3) Radioactive iodine, with or without the use of propranolol or antithyroid drugs.

ANTITHYROID DRUGS. The site of action of the different antithyroid drugs is indicated in Figure 11.2. Most commonly used are those that act by blocking the organic binding of iodine to tyrosine, carbimazole in Europe and its active metabolite, methimazole, in North America. Other drugs which act in this way are propyl and methyl thiouracil, which may occasionally be useful in the event of hypersensitivity to the drug of first choice.

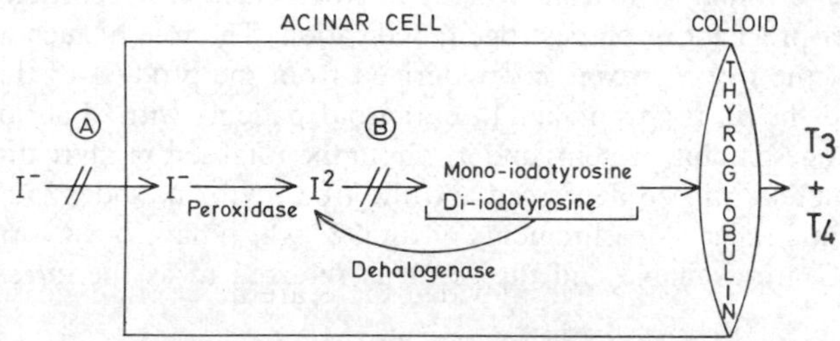


Fig. 11.2 Diagrammatic representation of the synthesis of thyroxine ($T_4$) and of triiodothyronine ($T_3$), illustrating the main sites of block induced by (A) potassium perchlorate and (B) by carbimazole, methimazole and the thiouracil group of drugs. The possible sites for enzyme deficiency in thyroid dyshormonogenesis (p. 478) are also shown.

Carbimazole is given initially in full suppressive doses of 15–20 mg at 8-hourly intervals for 3 to 4 weeks, according to the severity of the condition and the size of the goitre. Thereafter the dose can gradually be reduced, and, as the patient's clinical state responds, the aim should be to maintain a euthyroid state with as little of the antithyroid drug as necessary; this ranges between 5–30 mg daily. Overtreatment with antithyroid drugs will result in TSH production by the anterior pituitary with a risk of increase in size of the thyroid. In patients in whom the natural history of the underlying process is one of exacerbation and remission, stable control may be achieved with drugs only when an excessive dose of carbimazole (but not greater than 45–60 mg/day) is combined with continuous thyroxine administration in a dose of 0·15 mg/day. The patient's response should be monitored by measuring the plasma/serum levels of $T_4$, $T_3$ and TSH.

Carbimazole or methimazole may be selected as the definitive therapy or may be used to prepare the patient for surgery. If antithyroid drugs are being used as definitive therapy they should be continued for at least 1 year and restricted to patients who do not have a large goitre. By selecting cases in this way rather less than 50% of thyrotoxic patients will go into lasting remission and will not require further therapy. The probability of remission or relapse after 6–12 months treatment with antithyroid drugs can be assessed by determining whether the patient is HLA-DR3 or not and whether TSH receptor antibodies are present in the serum.

Carbimazole, methimazole and the thiouracil group of drugs as well as potassium perchlorate, may produce toxic effects, of which the commonest is a rash and the most serious are the blood dyscrasias, agranulocytosis being most frequent. Routine white cell counts are of little value in its early detection as it occurs with dramatic suddenness, usually, but not necessarily, in the first few weeks of treatment. Patients taking these drugs must be told to report a sore throat and to stop the drug immediately until it is clear whether agranulocytosis has occurred or not. By stopping the drug promptly and by using antibiotics prophylactically serious consequences will be avoided and the leucocyte count will return to normal within 1 to 2 weeks. Potassium perchlorate induces blood dyscrasias more commonly than other antithyroid drugs, including red cell aplasia which is usually lethal. For this reason, potassium perchlorate should be used only as a temporary expedient if hypersensitivity to other drugs has occurred and if radioactive iodine therapy or surgery under propranolol cover are not acceptable alternatives. It should never be used in a dose greater than 1 g/day.

There is no place for the use of potassium iodide as an antithyroid drug except in combination with propranolol or when the patient has already been made euthyroid with carbimazole or methimazole, or in the management of a thyrotoxic crisis.

BETA-ADRENERGIC BLOCKING DRUGS are very useful as they can produce much symptomatic improvement by countering the effect of $T_3$ and $T_4$ on catecholamine action. Thus anxiety, palpitations, increased bowel activity, lid retration and finger tremor may be alleviated with propranolol, 40 – 80 mg 6 hourly. It can therefore be useful during the interval of several weeks which is required for antithyroid drugs or radioactive iodine to be fully effective provided there are no contraindications to its use such as cardiac failure or asthma.

SURGICAL TREATMENT. This is the treatment of choice if the patient is considered too young for radioactive iodine therapy (i.e. during the reproductive years), if the antithyroid drug therapy has failed to produce a lasting remission, or there have been sensitivity reactions to antithyroid drugs. Thus a thyrotoxic patient younger than 40 years with a large goitre should be treated by surgery rather than by a prolonged course of antithyroid drugs in the somewhat vain hope that the condition will remit in the interval and not recur when antithyroid drugs are withdrawn.

For a girl a thin thyroidectomy scar may be more acceptable cosmetically than a goitre. Men are thought to relapse more frequently after prolonged antithyroid drug therapy than are women and some authorities advocate surgery as the treatment of choice in men under the age of 40, irrespective of the size of the goitre. The patient may state a preference once the possibilities have been explained.

Preparation for thyroidectomy is either by propranolol in increasing dosage until $\beta$-blockade has been achieved, or by carbimazole until euthyroid. In either event potassium iodide is given for 10–14 days before surgery in a dose of 60 mg twice daily. Potassium iodide should not be used as a means of achieving a euthyroid state except in thyrotoxic crisis. It makes the gland firmer and less vascular and the operation easier. The effects of potassium iodide are transitory so that it is important to reserve the drug for use in the circumstances described.

If propranolol is used substantially as preoperative preparation it is essential that tachycardia is controlled (by increasing the dose above 40 mg 4 times per day if necessary), that the dose on the morning of operation is not omitted and that propranolol is continued for 7 days after operation. Before surgery, evidence for adequate beta-blockade should be demonstrated on exercise tolerance. Some thyrotoxic patients are very resistant to beta-blockade by propranolol; the high doses of the drug in these subjects should be reduced immediately after surgery when the serum levels of $T_4$ and $T_3$ will drop rapidly. The advantages of propranolol preparation are greater flexibility in the timing of surgery, less blood loss and quicker permanent control of the thyrotoxicosis.

Some 80% of thyrotoxic patients treated by subtotal thyroidectomy should have no complications at least within 3 to 5 years. In some 15% there will be either recurrence of the thyrotoxicosis or post-operative hypothyroidism requiring continuous thyroxine replacement therapy. The relative proportion of each depends on the amount of thyroid tissue left at operation. Thyrotoxic patients with high titres of thyroid complement fixing antibody in the serum before operation tend to have an appreciable degree of lymphocytic infiltration in the gland and tend to develop hypothyroidism post-operatively. While the majority of patients who become hypothyroid after surgery do so within the first 6 months or a year, there is a low but steady further incidence with each year after surgery making annual review of the patient desirable. Transient hypothyroidism may occur in the first few months following surgery, presumably due to the supression of the hypothalamo-pituitary axis following a prolonged period of elevated serum $T_4$ and $T_3$ levels.

Damage to the recurrent laryngeal nerve occurs in a small percentage of patients and will produce temporary hoarseness with subsequent appreciable recovery as the other vocal cord compensates. The normal function of both vocal cords should be confirmed before surgery.

The parathyroid glands may be rendered temporarily ischaemic by interruption of their blood supply or they may be inadvertently removed, producing transient or permanent hypoparathyroidism respectively. The late onset of hypoparathyroidism is a complication of partial thyroidectomy which should be looked for in the follow up of surgical patients, as cataract and mental disturbance may develop insidiously in the presence of persistent mild hypocalcaemia. On account of the high incidence of recurrent laryngeal nerve damage and of hypoparathyroidism following second operations, thyrotoxic patients who relapse after surgery should be treated with radioactive iodine.

RADIOACTIVE IODINE is the treatment of choice for thyrotoxic patients over the age of 40 years and also for younger patients who for some other reason appear to have a short life expectancy or who have been sterilised. It has no established complications other than hypothyroidism in the years following therapy. The incidence of thyroid cancer or leukaemia following $^{131}I$ therapy has been shown not to be increased. Although an effect on the spontaneous mutation of the gametes in the ovary or testis has not been proved it is difficult to disprove and therefore the administration of radioactive iodine to persons of reproductive age who have not been sterilised should be discouraged unless there is no suitable alternative.

The assessment of the appropriate therapeutic dose of $^{131}I$ (half-life 8 days) presents some difficulties for the following reasons. The amount of functional thyroid tissue is not easy to assess with accuracy, the amount of radiation to the gland following a given dose can be assessed only by time-consuming dynamic studies, and even if a predicted amount of radiation per gram of thyroid tissue could be given, there remains the variation in radiosensitivity among thyroid glands of different patients. For these reasons the empirical assessment of dosage using clinical criteria gives results as good as those dependent on sophisticated physical methods, provided that an avid uptake of the isotope by the gland has been established.

Using a dose as small as 5 mCi $^{131}I$ with a diffuse uptake of the isotope as shown on a scan in a small thyroid or as high as 15–30 mCi for a large multinodular gland, the patient's thyrotoxicosis will be controlled in some 70% of cases following a single oral administration. It may take 2 months or longer for the dose to be effective. If the thyrotoxicosis is severe, more rapid relief may be obtained by the addition of propranolol. Carbimazole should preferably not be given prior to the administration of $^{131}I$ as there is some evidence that it reduces the effective radiation dose by virtue of the enzyme block which it induces. When given after $^{131}I$, carbimazole masks the effectiveness of the $^{131}I$ and makes the assessment of the need for a further dose of $^{131}I$ more difficult. The use of carbimazole in conjunction with $^{131}I$ should therefore be reserved for patients with cardiac failure or asthma, in whom propranolol is contraindicated. After 2 months a further dose of $^{131}I$ should be given in the 30% who have not responded adequately to the first dose, using a 50 to 100% higher dose in order to avoid the undesirable occurrence in a few patients of the need for repeated doses of the isotope. Large doses of $^{131}I$ should be given to thyrotoxic patients in cardiac failure or atrial fibrillation to ensure prompt control of thyroid function with a single dose, even though this will produce a high incidence of hypothyroidism. The patient's thyroid state can then be stabilised by replacement doses of thyroxine.

Thyrotoxicosis associated with a solitary 'hot' nodule should be treated with a large dose of $^{131}I$ (if the patient is over 40 y.) or by excision of the nodule.

The continuing incidence of new cases of hypothyroidism for many years following radioactive iodine therapy makes regular review essential until such time as the patient has become hypothyroid and is on a suitable life-long replacement dose of thyroxine. The overall incidence of hypothyroidism may be of the order of 50% at seven years depending on the dosage of $^{131}I$ given. Transient hypothyroidism with low plasma TSH levels may occur in the first six months after $^{131}I$ therapy due to the suppression of TRH and TSH secretion consequent upon sustained elevated $T_4$ and/or $T_3$ levels before therapy. Subsequent to that a rise in the plasma TSH level is an early warning that hypothyroidism may develop with low serum $T_4$ levels.

THYROTOXIC CRISIS. The treatment of thyrotoxic crisis consists of intravenous fluid and glucose replacement; parenteral hydrocortisone on account of possible adreno-cortical exhaustion; sedation and suppression of hyperpyrexia with chlorpromazine; digoxin for cardiac failure; propranolol if cardiac failure is not pronounced; intravenous potassium iodide 60 mg twice daily as the most rapidly acting antithyroid drug; and reduction of body temperature by tepid sponging. Antithyroid drugs such as carbimazole are administered as soon as the patient is capable of taking medicines orally. Precipitating causes must be dealt with, e.g. acute infection. Prevention and early recognition are essential if deaths are to be avoided.

HYPERTHYROIDISM IN CHILDREN AND IN PREGNANCY. As the results of thyroidectomy in children and young teenagers may be less satisfactory than in adults and as radioactive iodine therapy is contra-indicated in this age group, treatment should be with carbimazole or methimazole for as many years as is necessary.

In pregnancy hyperthyroidism may be treated with antithyroid drugs or by surgery provided the operation can be carried out in the middle trimester after appropriate preparation with antithyroid drugs and preoperative potassium iodide. If antithyroid drugs are used throughout it is important to give the smallest dose that will control the thyrotoxicosis and to use an index of thyroid function that is not altered by pregnancy (p. 469). Towards term, the dose of antithyroid drugs should be further reduced in the hope of withdrawing them for the last 3 weeks of pregnancy. In this way the uncommon complication of the fetus being born with a goitre may be avoided. If antithyroid drugs are to be continued after pregnancy the baby must not be breast fed. Radioactive iodine treatment should never be used for therapy in pregnancy. The baby should be checked for neo-natal thyrotoxicosis (p. 468).

### Exophthalmos

Autoimmune mechanisms involving the extraocular muscles, the retro-orbital fat and connective tissue are thought to be important in the pathogenesis of endocrine exophthalmos. Defined as the protrusion of one or both eyeballs, exophthalmos may be detected clinically in the majority of cases by observing the white sclera both above and below the iris. In other cases periorbital oedema which is frequently also present may obscure this sign. The degree of protrusion and especially any progression or regression of exophthalmos should be recorded by use of an exophthalmometer.

Exposure of the cornea as a consequence of the eyelids failing to close properly will result in keratitis producing a feeling of grit in the eye and excessive watering. The conjunctiva may become injected and oedematous (chemosis). Weakness of the extraocular muscles may give rise to an ophthalmoplegia with double vision, which is often first detected when the patient is asked to look upwards and outwards.

In a small minority of cases the exophthalmos takes a relentlessly progressive course so that the increased intra-orbital pressure causes a severe aching in the eyes and reduction in visual acuity. Pressure within the orbit must be relieved urgently if permanent deterioration in vision is to be avoided. Decompression of the orbital cavity by surgical means may be required, but large doses of oral corticosteroids may be used as an interim measure if surgery is not immediately possible. Fortunately, in most cases exophthalmos is less severe; its progression ceases and there is a prolonged phase of gradual improvement although the eyes seldom return to the normal state. In mild cases, chloromycetin eye drops and the wearing of slightly tinted spectacles with protective side pieces to the frames will prevent the irritation of glare, dust and wind. In more severe cases lateral tarsorrhaphy, stitching together the outer margins of the eyelids, may be all that is required, thereby improving their appearance and preventing exposure keratitis.

In relation to the treatment of thyrotoxicosis it is particularly important that hypothyroidism is avoided as this does seem to aggravate any associated exophthalmos.

In some patients exophthalmos may precede the development of frank thyrotoxicosis and present a problem in differential diagnosis, especially if the exophthalmos is unilateral when orbital or retro-orbital tumours and infections may require consideration. CT scanning is particularly helpful in this context. Support for an endocrine aetiology may be obtained by eliciting a family history of thyroid disease or by demonstrating an abnormal TRH stimulation test or thyroid or gastric antibodies in the serum.

## Hypothyroidism

Hypothyroidism may be due to causes within the thyroid gland itself (primary) or, less commonly, to failure of TSH production following pituitary or hypothalamic disease (secondary). Hypothyroidism, especially when it is due to primary thyroid failure, is often, but not necessarily, associated with myxoedema, a thickening of the skin or other tissues by deposition of mucopolysaccharide giving the patient a characteristic appearance.

**Incidence and Aetiology.** Hypothyroidism commonly occurs as a sequel to $^{131}I$ therapy for thyrotoxicosis. Spontaneous primary hypothyroidism is much less common than thyrotoxicosis and principally affects middle-aged females, although it can occur in either sex at any age.

Spontaneous primary hypothyroidism may be associated with a goitre or with thyroid atrophy. The commonest cause of spontaneous goitrous hypothyroidism in an adult female is Hashimoto's thyroiditis. It is believed that Graves' disease, Hashimoto's thyroiditis and primary atrophic hypothyroidism belong to a continuous spectrum of disease. This is characterised by a common familial trait towards organ-specific autoimmune disease and by the frequent occurrence in the serum of thyroid and gastric parietal cell antibodies. The natural history of Graves' disease in the absence of destructive forms of therapy is the incipient development of hypothyroidism over a period of one or several decades, a further indication that both belong to the same spectrum of autoimmune thyroid disease.

Less commonly hypothyroidism may be associated with other types of goitre; for example an enzyme deficiency in the synthesis of thyroid hormones (dyshormonogenesis, Fig. 11.2). This form is more likely to present in children or in young adults. When hypothyroidism is secondary to pituitary insufficiency, myxoedema is unusual.

**Clinical Features of Primary Hypothyroidism.** *Adults.* In contrast to thyrotoxicosis the symptoms are the result of decreased metabolism, with slowing of mental and physical activity. The onset is gradual and often mistaken for ageing alone. Often the patient is the last to complain and has to be persuaded by relatives or friends to seek medical help. Frequently, the general practitioner will recognise the condition on meeting the patient for some other reason, especially after a long interval. On questioning, the patient may admit to sensitivity to cold, dryness of the skin, coarse and dry hair, constipation, gain in weight, tiredness, vague generalised pains, deafness, forgetfulness and disordered menstrual function. The patient may also complain of tingling in the fingers from compression of the median nerve in the carpal tunnel, although it is to be remembered that patients with primary spontaneous hypothyroidism are also predisposed to Addisonian pernicious anaemia which may give rise to similar symptoms from polyneuropathy. Anaemia may also be a direct result of thyroxine deficiency.

In an advanced case the face appears swollen with puffy eyelids, thick lips and an enlarged tongue. There is often a malar flush but elsewhere the skin is pale as a consequence of thickening with myxoedema. Sweating is conspicuously absent and the skin is dry and readily flakes on rubbing. The hair tends to be more sparse than normal and lustreless. Speech is slow, monotonous and husky or, in advanced instances, deep and croaky.

Characteristically the pulse rate is slow, but if the condition has progressed to cardiac failure, tachycardia may be found. The blood pressure in uncomplicated hypothyroidism is usually normal. However, since degenerative vascular disease is frequent in hypothyroidism, the patient may have systolic hypertension. Commonly there is evidence of coronary artery disease with angina pectoris or ECG changes of myocardial ischaemia. On radiological examination the heart is frequently seen to be enlarged; in some cases there may be a pericardial effusion which is usually reversible with treatment.

Marked slowing of the recovery phase of the ankle jerk due to delayed relaxation of the calf muscles is a useful clinical sign. Patients with severe hypothyroidism may show frank psychosis with hallucinations and delusions ('myxoedema madness') or pass into a state of coma. In a severe case, failure to control body temperature is one of the most lethal complications; mortality rises markedly as the body temperature (measured by a low reading rectal thermometer) falls below 32°C.

*Children.* Hypothyroidism presents as a deterioration in performance at school, lack of interest in games and an arrest or slowing of growth. These features will precede the development of clinically obvious myxoedema. As in adults there may or may not be a goitre. While it is easy to detect the disease in its advanced state a high index of suspicion is required to avoid missing the early case and to prevent many years of unnecessary ill health.

*Infants.* Failure of thyroid development is responsible for the condition of *cretinism*. The defects leading to failure of thyroid development may be genetic and may be inherited as autosomal recessives: in the heterozygous state the child may be goitrous only, but in the homozygous state both goitrous and a cretin.

It is important to diagnose the state and initiate thyroxine replacement therapy as early as possible. The development of the brain is dependent on the thyroid hormones so that delay in starting treatment will inevitably lead to permanent mental impairment which will be the more severe the longer the delay. The diagnostic features are failure to achieve the normal milestones of development, constipation, poor feeding and a characteristic cry. Only in advanced cases will the child develop the obvious features of cretinism, which include a coarse facies with a broad flat nose, thick lips and a large tongue protruding from the mouth, and a pot belly with umbilical hernia.

**Investigation.** The measurement of total serum $T_4$ should be combined with a plasma TSH measurement. If abnormalities of thyroxine binding proteins are suspected, a form of free thyroxine index should be used. The measurement of serum $T_3$ is not helpful in suspected hypothyroidism.

All patients with primary hypothyroidism have an elevated plasma TSH level but not all patients with an elevated plasma TSH necessarily have a significant degree of hypothyroidism. While a normal or low TSH level may be associated with secondary hypothyroidism due to pituitary or hypothalamic disease, a normal serum TSH level would exclude primary hypothyroidism. No purpose is achieved by doing TRH tests when an elevated plasma TSH has already been demonstrated but a TRH test may be helpful in deciding whether secondary hypothyroidism is due to pituitary or hypothalamic disease. Screening of neonates for elevated serum TSH levels facilitates the early diagnosis of cretinism.

A single measurement of uptake of radioactive iodine by the gland is of very little value in the diagnosis of hypothyroidism, but the response in the uptake to adequate stimulation by parenteral TSH (10 i.u. bovine TSH on each of 3 consecutive days) is a good index of the capacity of the gland to function. Patients with primary hypothyroidism fail to respond. Radioimmunoassay of plasma TSH has largely superseded the need for TSH stimulation tests, but the latter are still useful in determining whether thyroxine medication empirically started in the past for suspected primary hypothyroidism is actually required.

Radiographs of the epiphyses in children, or of ossification centres in the wrist or heel in infants, will indicate whether the bone age is delayed relative to the chronological age. Hypothyroidism in young people is invariably associated with impaired bone development; fragmentation of the epiphysis at the head of the femur is a striking radiological sign.

**Treatment.** In uncomplicated adult cases treatment with thyroxine should start with 0·05 mg/day increasing to 0·1 mg/day after 3 weeks provided cardiac failure or angina have not arisen. After a further 3–6 weeks the dose may be increased to 0·15–0·2 mg/day. this is the normal full replacement dose, but a few patients may require up to 0·3 mg thyroxine/day. Patients must understand that their well-being depends on continued treatment and must not stop thyroxine when they feel better. There is no advantage in divided doses or taking tablets that consist of a mixture of $T_3$ and $T_4$.

In a patient known to have ischaemic heart disease it will usually be desirable to keep the dose of thyroxine between 0·05 and 0·1 mg/day and to use a beta-adrenergic blocking agent such as propranolol. In patients with secondary hypothyroidism it is essential to treat any adrenocortical insufficiency before starting thyroxine.

*Myxoedema Coma with Hypothermia.* Small doses (10 μg) of triiodothyronine may be given intravenously 8 hourly together with hydrocortisone and glucose. The body temperature should be restored very slowly to a level of 32°C; above this level active warming should be abandoned in favour of heat conservation.

## Goitre

This term is applied to any enlargement of the thyroid gland and on clinical examination its size, shape, consistency, symmetry, irregularity of surface, mobility and the presence of a bruit should be established. The level of thyroid activity should be determined in the manner already described. Goitre associated with thyrotoxicosis will not be discussed further. The common diagnosis of simple goitre is arrived at by the exclusion of other causes, such as Hashimoto's thyroiditis, subacute thyroiditis, dyshormonogenesis, or carcinoma of the thyroid gland.

**Hashimoto's thyroiditis** is characteristically a firm diffuse enlargement of the thyroid gland with or without hypothyroidism. It may give rise to an aching discomfort in the neck and to mild dysphagia. It occurs most commonly in middle-aged women. Almost all cases have antibodies in the serum to thyroglobulin or to the microsomal fraction of thyroid cytoplasm, frequently in high titre. The ESR is often elevated. Histologically the gland consists of rather small thyroid vesicles with columnar epithelium showing a varying degree of eosinophilic granularity, infiltration by lymphocytes and plasma cells, sometimes with germinal centre formation and an increase in the fibrous tissue stroma.

In most instances there will be a satisfactory regression in the size of the goitre in response to thyroxine 0·2 mg/day, which can be hastened by giving 20 mg prednisolone 8-hourly for 10 days only. Adults with Hashimoto's thyroiditis should remain on life-long thyroxine therapy irrespective of whether or not they were initially hypothyroid. In adolescence, Hashimoto's thyroiditis may be transitory. In cases of diagnostic doubt a needle biopsy of the gland under local anaesthesia may be helpful. Partial thyroidectomy in such patients rapidly produces hypothyroidisim if it did not already exist and is usually unnecessary.

**Subacute (de Quervain's) thyroiditis** is a painful condition generally associated with some thyroid enlargement. It is thought to be due to a viral infection of the thyroid (e.g. Coxsackie B) and viral antibody studies are sometimes helpful diagnostically. Thyroid function is suppressed as indicated by a very low uptake of radioactive iodine or technetium by the gland and histologically the characteristic feature is the presence of giant cells. The ESR may be markedly elevated and thyroid antibody tests are generally negative. The condition tends to regress spontaneously but may be persistent.

Thyroxine 0·2–0·3 mg/day should be given to suppress TSH secretion and, in some cases, it may be necessary to give a course of oral corticosteroids. Surgery is seldom indicated even in the protracted case.

**Dyshormonogenesis.** The patient who has a partial enzyme defect related to one of the steps in the synthesis of thyroid hormones (Fig. 11.2) is likely to develop a goitre in response to continued TSH secretion induced by the low serum thyroxine. While all these defects are rare, the commonest and the easiest to detect is a genetically determined defect in the binding of iodine to tyrosine which, when associated with nerve deafness, is known as *Pendred's syndrome*.

**Tumours of the Thyroid Gland.** CARCINOMA is uncommon, forming about 1% of all cases of cancer in Britain. The tumours may be well differentiated papillary or follicular carcinomas (or a mixture of the two) or be anaplastic. Advanced cancers are obvious by their hardness, irregularity, adhesion to surrounding tissues and associated lymphadenopathy. Early carcinoma of the thyroid gland presents as a single nodule which almost invariably has poorer function than the surrounding normal thyroid tissue. If the nodule is sufficiently large it will be detectable as a 'cold' area on radioisotope scanning. It is not possible to distinguish clinically between a single nodule that is malignant and one that is benign; all single (solitary) nodules should therefore be removed for histological examination.

Well differentiated thyroid tumours should be treated by total thyroidectomy followed by life-long oral thyroxine 0·2–0·3 mg/day according to the patient's age. Occasionally metastases from a well differentiated tumour may take up sufficient radioactive iodine, after all normally functioning thyroid tissue has been ablated by surgery and $^{131}I$, to allow effective therapy with a further large dose of $^{131}I$. Non-functioning secondaries can be treated by local radiotherapy. Anaplastic tumours may show a good initial response to external radiotherapy, but invariably recur.

*Medullary carcinoma* of the thyroid arises from the parafollicular C-cells; although rare, it is of particular interest as it is associated with high levels of plasma calcitonin, prostaglandins or 5-hydroxytryptamine, causing symptoms such as flushing, borborygmi and diarrhoea. Patients with this form of thyroid cancer may have neuromas on the tongue, lips or eyelids, Marfanoid skeletal proportions (p. 213), and, occasionally, phaeochromocytomas.

Total thyroidectomy and removal of affected lymph nodes are required. The tumour is not very radiosensitive. It does not take up $^{131}I$. Relapse can be detected by calcitonin assay.

BENIGN TUMOURS. Solitary 'cold' lesions in the thyroid may consist of adenomas or cysts; they can be differentiated by isotope scanning and ultrasonography. Calcification in cysts is common. Cysts without an admixture of solid constituents may be aspirated and the fluid sent for cytology. Haemorrhage occasionally occurs into adenomas and for this reason, in addition to the risk of malignancy, their removal is justified.

**Simple goitre** may occur sporadically, but in certain parts of the world it is found more frequently and is then referred to as endemic goitre.

The aetiology is not fully understood, but it is generally believed to be closely related to iodine deficiency, mainly in the diet. Less commonly factors in the diet or water such as excess calcium may interfere with iodine absorption; goitrogens in the diet may prevent concentration of iodine by the thyroid. Fish is a main source of iodine and thus simple goitre due to iodine deficiency is endemic in the mountains of New Guinea, in the Alps and in the Himalayas.

Apart from the antithyroid drugs, a number of other drugs are known to interfere with the synthesis of thyroid hormones; thus prolonged treatment with sulphonamides or PAS may produce a goitre. Iodides taken persistently in large doses in the form of cough mixtures or 'asthma cures' may likewise cause a goitre. In each of these examples the secretion or release of thyroid hormones is suppressed and presumably the goitre results from continuing increased secretion of TSH. An intermittent shortage in supply of iodine to the gland over prolonged periods is thought to result in the multinodular character of long-standing goitres.

A small, soft, diffuse, simple goitre may occur at puberty or during pregnancy and may regress spontaneously thereafter, but in other cases it persists. If already present, it may enlarge further at these times. A simple goitre of long standing may achieve considerable size, become grossly nodular and give rise to obstructive symptoms, particularly if there is a retrosternal extension. Deviation of the trachea may be noted clinically or radiologically and obstruction in the thoracic inlet may lead to venous engorgement of the head and neck. Bruits and thrills do not occur in simple goitres. Cretinism (p. 476) is associated with endemic goitre in areas where iodine deficiency is severe.

The treatment of sporadic simple diffuse goitre at puberty should be with thyroxine for 1 to 2 years and not potassium iodide. An adequate dietary intake of iodine should be ensured. Multinodular simple goitres are unlikely to respond to thyroxine and may require partial thyroidectomy for cosmetic reasons, or if obstructive symptoms are present or likely to occur. Postoperative life-long treatment with thyroxine may prevent a recurrence, although hypothyroidism after partial thyroidectomy for simple goitre is uncommon.

An adequate intake of iodine, particularly in the early years of life, is the only really satisfactory way of preventing sporadic simple goitre. The incidence of endemic goitre can be greatly reduced by correcting iodine deficiency, for example, by legislation that ensures that table salt contains traces of iodine (p. 96).

### Calcitonin

The parafollicular cells (C-cells) of the thyroid gland secrete a polypeptide hormone, calcitonin, apparently unrelated to the other functions of this gland. When administered by injection, the hormone lowers the serum calcium concentration. Its main effect on bone is to inhibit resorption, so that in these two important respects it could be regarded as a physiological antagonist of parathyroid hormone. It is secreted in very large quantities by medullary carcinomas of the thyroid gland, without however producing significant hypocalcaemia, and after complete removal of the source of the hormone, namely the thyroid gland, hypercalcaemia is not a feature.

Therapeutically, the hormone has been used to reduce hypercalcaemia, but corticosteroids may be more effective in doing so in sarcoidosis, vitamin D intoxication and in metastatic malignant disease in bone. In Paget's disease calcitonin relieves pain in the minority of patients in whom pain is a dominant feature (p. 644).

## THE PARATHYROID GLANDS

**Anatomy and Physiology.** These glands, usually four in number, each measure about 5 mm in diameter. Their relation to the thyroid gland is described on page 466. The parathyroid glands control the concentration of calcium and inorganic phosphorus in the blood, both by enhancing the removal of mineral from the skeleton, and by promoting the excretion of phosphorus by the kidney.

Calcium occurs in plasma in two forms, 'diffusible' and 'non-diffusible'. The former consists of ionised calcium, and a small amount of non-ionised calcium salts of organic acids. From the point of view of neuromuscular function and the occurrence of tetany, as well as the secretion of parathyroid hormone, it is the ionised plasma calcium concentration which is important. The non-diffusible fraction is that portion which is bound to the plasma albumin; if the latter is very low, the total plasma calcium might be 2·0 mmol/*l* (8 mg/100 ml) or less and yet the ionised calcium could be normal. When the plasma albumin concentration is high, the plasma calcium might be 3·0 mmol/*l* or even more, but this would not necessarily constitute evidence of hyperparathyroidism.

In addition to parathyroid hormone, calcitonin and vitamin D metabolites also affect the metabolism of calcium and phosphorus, so that these factors must be considered in disorders of these elements. Assays of parathyroid hormone (PTH) are becoming more widely available. Controversy continues regarding the reliability and relevance of calcitonin assays, except in the diagnosis of medullary carcinoma of the thyroid gland.

## Hyperparathyroidism

*Primary hyperparathyroidism* is usually due to a single parathyroid adenoma. Very occasionally it may be caused by simple hyperplasia or multiple adenomas: a functioning parathyroid carcinoma can also occur.

*Secondary hyperparathyroidism* is due to hypertrophy of the glands and is found in chronic renal failure which causes hypocalcaemia followed by an increase in parathyroid activity. Secondary hyperparathyroidism also occurs as a sequel to osteomalacia, malabsorption or rickets.

*Tertiary hyperparathyroidism* is used to describe the cases of the secondary variety of long standing in which a continuing stimulus is responsible for parathyroid hyperplasia being replaced by autonomous function in one or more parathyroid adenomas.

*Osteitis fibrosa* or *von Recklinghausen's disease of bone* occurs in the rare event of hyperparathyroidism involving the bones to such an extent that cyst formation occurs.

**Clinical Features.** Mild, asymptomatic hyperparathyroidism is not uncommon, particularly after middle age. Patients with more severe hypercalcaemia frequently complain of weakness, loss of appetite, nausea, vomiting, drowsiness or confusion. Some of these patients also have a peptic ulcer, the symptoms from which may obscure those of hyperparathyroidism. Acute pancreatitis is sometimes a presenting feature. When bone involvement is marked, backache is a common complaint. Pseudogout (p. 638) may occur.

Renal calculi frequently form in association with the increased excretion of calcium in the urine. While many patients with hyperparathyroidism develop symptoms due to renal calculi, relatively few presenting with renal calculi owe their disorder to increased parathyroid activity. In other cases of hyperparathyroidism deposits of calcium form in and around the renal tubular epithelium (nephrocalcinosis p. 451). Tubular reabsorption of water may be impaired as a consequence or from the direct effects of parathyroid hormone. Polyuria and thirst may be sufficiently severe to suggest diabetes insipidus. In cases of long standing, and in those with associated pyelonephritis, the renal disease may progress to uraemia in spite of the relief of the hyperparathyroidism.

Physical examination is usually unhelpful. Occasionally a parathyroid adenoma is sufficiently large and suitably placed to be palpable or even visible as a swelling in the region of the thyroid gland.

A parathyroid adenoma may occasionally coexist with secreting adenomas or hyperplasia in the pituitary, pancreas or adrenals. This association is known as *multiple endocrine adenomatosis* and may account for unusual manifestations.

**Investigation.** *Hypercalcaemia and related findings.* Hypercalcaemia is the most significant chemical finding. The fasting plasma calcium may be considerably increased above the upper limit of normal (2·62 mmol/*l*). It may be necessary to carry out estimations at intervals in doubtful cases, since hypercalcaemia may be episodic. A tourniquet should not be used in obtaining samples since this may be responsible for raising the plasma calcium. If the plasma albumin is low the value for the plasma calcium should be adjusted upwards.

Causes of hypercalcaemia other than hyperparathyroidism include metastatic malignant disease of bone, cancer (without bone secondaries) producing a PTH-like polypeptide, and chronic renal failure. Less common causes are sarcoidosis, myelomatosis, overdosage with vitamin D, hyperthyroidism, and immobilisation.

The plasma inorganic phosphate is usually lowered in hyperparathyroidism. The plasma alkaline phosphatase, an index of osteoblastic activity, may be raised (p. 906) depending on the degree of involvement of bone.

*Radiological Examination.* In the early stages there may be demineralisation or subperiosteal erosions may be noted in the phalanges. A 'pepper-pot' appearance seen in lateral radiographs of the skull is virtually diagnostic of hyperparathyroidism. Cystic changes are rare. In nephrocalcinosis scattered opacities may be visible within the renal outline. There may be soft tissue calcification elsewhere. Arteriography can be helpful in locating the site of an adenoma.

*Parathyroid Hormone Radioimmunoassay.* An inappropriately high plasma PTH, even within the normal range, in the presence of hypercalcaemia, is indicative of hyperparathyroidism. Such assays may also be helpful in localising small tumours by identifying high concentrations of parathyroid hormone in specific veins in the root of the neck or mediastinum.

**Treatment.** Removal of a solitary adenoma is usually sufficient to produce clinical cure, provided advanced renal disease is not already present. Patients with multiple adenomas or generalised hyperplasia of all the parathyroids may be difficult to manage, especially when the glands lie in unusual situations such as the superior mediastinum, but surgical treatment offers the only prospect of cure. Patients with bone involvement may, following removal of the tumour, show the 'hungry bone' syndrome characterised by tetany and magnesium depletion. It is not certain whether people, especially the elderly, with mild symptomless hypercalcaemia come to any harm from the continued presence of a parathyroid tumour.

## Hypoparathyroidism

This unusual condition may arise from a variety of causes, but with each the clinical feature in common is tetany. Biochemically, a depressed concentration of calcium and a raised concentration of phosphate in plasma are characteristic.

*Postoperative Hypoparathyroidism.* A transitory form of the disorder is common after a partial thyroidectomy, presumably due to interference with the blood supply of the parathyroid glands. After a complete thyroidectomy permanent hypoparathyroidism may occur. Hypoparathyroidism may be transient following removal of a hyperfunctioning parathyroid adenoma, the other three parathyroid glands having been suppressed by the high calcium levels.

*Infantile hypoparathyroidism* may be transient and associated with maternal hyperparathyroidism or calcium deficiency, or it may be associated with thymic aplasia (Di George syndrome, p. 41).

*Idiopathic hypoparathyroidism* may develop at any age, and is sometimes associated with autoimmune disease of the adrenal, thyroid or ovary especially in young people. In addition to tetany other features include psychoses, cataracts, aberrant calcification and moniliasis, particularly of the finger nails.

*Pseudohypoparathyroidism* is the term applied to a congenital variety, which may be familial. It presents with the biochemical features of hypoparathyroidism, and in addition aberrant calcification, cataracts, mental retardation and skeletal abnormalities, for example small, stocky stature and short 4th metacarpals. These patients are resistant to the action of administered parathyroid hormone; their own parathyroid glands appear to be normal histologically, plasma parathyroid hormone levels are raised, and high concentrations of calcitonin have been found in their circulation and in their thyroid glands.

**Treatment.** Commercial preparations of parathyroid hormone available for the treatment of parathyroid insufficiency are unsatisfactory because they have to be given by frequent injections, and soon become ineffective because of antibody formation. In the acute phase, calcium is given intravenously as for tetany; substitution therapy for persistent hypoparathyroidism and for pseudoparathyroidism is provided by calciferol, or an analogue of vitamin D, dihydrotachysterol (p. 483).

## Tetany

**Aetiology.** There is an increased excitability of peripheral nerves due either to a low plasma calcium concentration or to alkalosis in which the proportion of the plasma calcium in the ionised form is decreased, although the total calcium concentration remains unaltered. Magnesium depletion should also be considered as a possible contributing factor, particularly in the malabsorption syndrome.

CAUSES OF DEPLETION OF PLASMA CALCIUM. (1) *Inadequate intake or absorption of calcium.* This occurs in rickets, osteomalacia and the malabsorption syndrome. (2) *Hypoparathyroidism.* (3) *Chronic renal failure* where, although the plasma calcium is often low, coincident acidosis usually prevents tetany.

CAUSES OF ALKALOSIS. (1) *Repeated vomiting* of acid gastric juice, as in gastric outlet obstruction from peptic ulceration. (2) *Excessive quantities of absorbable alkalis* given by mouth especially when associated with repeated vomiting. (3) *Hyperventilation*, commonly due to hysteria, lowers the arterial $P_{CO_2}$. (4) *Primary aldosteronism* (p. 487)

**Clinical Features.** In *children* a characteristic triad of carpopedal spasm, stridor (laryngismus stridulus) and convulsions may occur, though one or more of these may be found independently of the others. The hands in carpal spasm adopt a characteristic position. The metacarpophalangeal joints are flexed, the interphalangeal joints of the fingers and thumb are extended and there is opposition of the thumb (*main d'accoucheur*). Pedal spasm is much less frequent. Stridor is caused by spasm of the glottis.

*Adults* complain of tingling in the hands, feet and around the mouth. Less often there is painful carpopedal spasm while stridor and fits are rare.

*Latent tetany* may be present when signs of overt tetany are lacking. It is best recognised by eliciting *Trousseau's sign*. Inflation of the sphygmomanometer cuff on the upper arm to more than the systolic blood pressure is followed by characteristic spasm in the forearm muscles within 4 minutes.

**Treatment.** *Control of Tetany*. Injection of 20 ml of a 10% solution of calcium gluconate slowly into a vein will raise the plasma calcium concentration immediately. An intramuscular injection of 10 ml may also be given to obtain a more prolonged effect. In severe cases of alkalotic tetany, intravenous calcium gluconate often relieves the spasm, while more radical treatment of the alkalosis, which will vary with the cause, is being applied. If tetany is not relieved by giving calcium the administration of magnesium may be required.

*Correction of Alkalosis*. 1. In persistent vomiting, intravenous isotonic saline is the most effective treatment.

2. When alkalis have been given to excess their withdrawal may suffice to stop the tetany, but if not, ammonium chloride 2 g should be given 4–hourly by mouth until relief has been obtained.

3. The inhalation of 5% carbon dioxide in oxygen may be prescribed for the correction of the alkalosis of hyperventilation, or more simply, the patient should be made to rebreathe expired air from a suitable bag. The hysterical patient should also be treated by appropriate psychotherapy (p. 767).

*Treatment of the Underlying Condition*. When tetany follows removal of a parathyroid gland and if there is any residual parathyroid tissue, this usually undergoes compensatory hypertrophy. In the interval intravenous calcium gluconate may be required to control the tetany. If all the parathyroid tissue has been removed, prolonged replacement therapy with calciferol is commonly used to maintain a normal plasma calcium concentration. One tablet (1·25 mg) daily is usually adequate, but less, or more, may be required. The maintenance dose is determined by careful monitoring of the plasma calcium at intervals, as persistent hypercalcaemia which might follow prolonged high doses of vitamin D would lead to widespread metastatic calcification and rapidly progressive renal failure.

Dihydrotachysterol, an analogue of vitamin D, is also a useful substitute in parathyroid insufficiency, but it is more expensive than calciferol.

In chronic renal failure temporary benefit is usually the most that can be expected unless haemodialysis or transplantation is being employed; symptoms should be treated with parenteral calcium as they arise.

Treatment may also be required for rickets (p. 103), osteomalacia (p. 105) or malabsorption (p. 350).

## THE ADRENAL GLANDS

**Anatomy and Physiology.** The adrenal glands lie in relation to the upper poles of the kidneys. Each consists of an inner medulla which secretes adrenaline and noradrenaline and an outer cortex formed of three layers. These, from without inwards, are the zona glomerulosa, fasciculata and reticularis. Although over 40 steroid compounds have been extracted from the adrenal cortex, the principal hormones are cortisol, corticosterone (glucocorticoids), aldosterone (mineralocorticoid) and androstenedione, androsterone and dehydroepiandrosterone (androgens).

Adrenocorticotrophic hormone (ACTH) is the only substance so far recognised that will alter the rate of biosynthesis and secretion of the glucocorticoid cortisol from the zona fasciculata and reticularis. ACTH also increases the secretion of the adrenal androgens. Aldosterone secretion by the zona glomerulosa is primarily controlled by the renin-angiotensin mechanism (p. 424) and is not markedly affected by physiological alterations in ACTH levels.

Three major mechanisms appear to control ACTH release and thus cortisol secretion, namely, negative feedback, diurnal rhythm and stress.

The negative feedback mechanism is thought to operate via the hypothalamus rather than directly on the pituitary but there is still uncertainty about this. The corticotrophin releasing factor (CRF) from the hypothalamus has not yet been isolated in man and cannot be measured in serum. Reduction in the level of plasma cortisol leads to an increased secretion of ACTH from the basophil cells of the anterior pituitary, probably effected by increased release of CRF from the hypothalamus. Conversely, a rise in plasma cortisol produces a rapid suppression of the secretion of ACTH. Cortisol secretion is thus presumably determined at the hypothalamic level, controlled by an inherent diurnal rhythmicity of CRF secretion and consequently of ACTH release. The normal range of plasma cortisol levels in an unstressed subject would be 220–720 nmol/*l* (8–26 $\mu$g/100 ml) at 0800 to 1000 h and less than 275 nmol/*l* (10 $\mu$g/100 ml) at 2200 to 2400 h.

Stress such as trauma, pain, apprehension, nausea, fever and hypoglycaemia can override the negative feedback mechanism and the diurnal rhythm.

It is from an understanding of the normal physiological mechanisms involved in adrenocortical hormone secretion that procedures have been developed to test various components of the hypothalamo-pituitary-adrenal axis and so determine the site of the lesion in cases of adrenocortical over- or underactivity.

The glucocorticoids have effects which are antagonistic to insulin, tending to raise the blood sugar by converting amino acids derived from protein breakdown into glucose (gluconeogenesis). Glucocorticoids such as cortisol have other important actions including the suppression of inflammatory reactions which may occur in response to injury, infection or immunological mechanisms. Glucocorticoids are also lipogenic and have some mineralocorticoid effects especially when used in pharmacological doses.

Aldosterone produces retention of sodium and increased excretion of potassium and if given in pharmacological doses over a prolonged period also causes hypertension. Weight for weight, aldosterone has far greater mineralocorticoid activity than the glucocorticoids.

In addition to androgens, the adrenal cortex also synthesises oestrogen and progesterone in small quantities in both sexes. The nitrogen-retaining (anabolic) activity of the androgenic hormones is antagonistic to the catabolic effect of the glucocorticoids.

## Hyperfunction of the Adrenal Gland

**Cushing's Syndrome.** This can be defined as the symptoms and signs associated with prolonged exposure to inappropriately elevated plasma corticosteroid levels. The patients may be divided into two main groups depending on whether or not the condition derives from exposure to excessive ACTH.

ACTH dependent causes of Cushing's syndrome:

1. Iatrogenic—administration of excessive quantities of ACTH or its synthetic analogues.
2. Pituitary-dependent bilateral adrenocortical hyperplasia, conventionally called *Cushing's disease*.

3. The ectopic ACTH syndrome—secretion of ACTH by malignant or benign tumours of non-endocrine origin.

Non-ACTH dependent causes of Cushing's syndrome:
1. Iatrogenic—administration of supraphysiological doses of corticosteroids.
2. Adenomas or carcinomas of the adrenal cortex.

Cushing's syndrome associated with pituitary-dependent adrenocortical hyperplasia and adrenal tumours is four times more common in women than in men with a peak age incidence between 35 and 50 years. This contrasts with the male predominance and later age incidence found in Cushing's syndrome secondary to the ectopic production of ACTH by non-endocrine tumours, commonly carcinoma of the bronchus.

**Clinical Features of Cushing's Disease.** These can be interpreted largely in terms of the action of the glucocorticoids. Thus the gluconeogenic effect is seen as an elevation of the blood glucose level and glycosuria; a proportion of patients develop diabetes. The effect on the blood sugar is however not invariable because of other mechanisms that counteract any disturbance in carbohydrate metabolism, such as insulin secretion. The breakdown of protein to form glucose is reflected in the reduction of muscle, bone and connective tissue, leading to weakness, proximal myopathy, osteoporosis, easy bruising and purple striae of the skin over the abdomen, buttocks and thighs. Osteoporosis may be sufficiently severe to produce backache; radiological changes in the vertebral bodies may progress to collapse, kyphosis and shortening of stature.

The most striking features of Cushing's disease are the rounded plethoric appearance (moon face), central obesity and 'buffalo hump' (accumulation of fat at the lower part of the back of the neck) due to redistribution of body fat. There is also arterial hypertension caused by sodium retention. The loss of potassium may contribute to muscular weakness. The overproduction of adrenal androgens may lead to the development of hirsutism and acne in some patients with perhaps temporal recession of hair in females. Amenorrhoea or other disorders of menstrual function are common. Mental symptoms, in particular depression, may be prominent.

The pituitary gland in Cushing's disease is seldom grossly enlarged either in the presence of hyperplasia or of an adenoma of the basophil or chomophobe cells. Although some enlargement may be detectable on a radiograph of the pituitary fossa, usually no abnormality can be seen. Expansion of the pituitary fossa and pressure on the optic chiasma may occur due to an adenoma some years after treatment by bilateral adrenalectomy and replacement doses of steroids. In such cases the secretion of MSH accompanying the very high levels of ACTH in the plasma, causes marked brown pigmentation of the skin (Nelson's syndrome).

*In the case of an adrenocortical tumour affecting the zona fasciculata/reticularis*, the clinical features will depend on the type of steroid that the tumour is synthesising. If the tumour is making glucocorticoids almost exclusively the clinical features will be indistinguishable from Cushing's disease, whereas if the tumour is making androgens predominantly the female patient will be virilised, with pronounced hirsutism, deepening of the voice, recession of the hair on the forehead, acne and clitoral enlargement, possibly with increased libido. In males an adrenal tumour may induce feminisation if the tumour is mainly making oestrogens. Although many adrenocortical adenomas are benign, functional carcinomas also occur with metastases to other organs.

*When Cushing's syndrome is due to the production of ectopic ACTH* the striking features are the rapid development of brown pigmentation due to the very high plasma levels of ACTH or MSH or biologically active analogues associated with the rise in ACTH. Frequently such patients show a marked alkalosis and potassium depletion. Characteristically they do not appear Cushingoid (moon face and central obesity) presumably because of the short survival time of the underlying malignant process.

**Differential Diagnosis.** The main differential diagnosis of Cushing's disease or syndrome is simple obesity and simple hirsutism, especially when either is associated with mild hypertension and menstrual irregularity or when both coexist. Functional ovarian tumours may give a similar clinical picture. It can sometimes be difficult to decide when to investigate and when to exclude the possibility of Cushing's disease or syndrome on clinical grounds alone. Overactivity of the adrenal cortex is comparatively rare while simple obesity, hirsutism, menstrual irregularities and hypertension are common.

**Investigation of Suspected Overactivity of the Zona Fasciculata/Reticularis.** Disordered function of the zona fasciculata/reticularis is almost invariably reflected in an alteration of the normal diurnal rhythm of cortisol secretion with high levels of plasma cortisol in the evening; the simple measurement of plasma fluorogenic corticosteroids can be taken as a close approximation to the level of plasma cortisol. The demonstration of such an abnormality does not establish the diagnosis since stress, obesity or hypertension may produce similar findings. In subjects with normal adrenocortical function the secretion of cortisol should be readily suppressible with biologically active analogues of cortisol such as dexamethasone. These substances do not contribute to the measurement of fluorogenic corticosteroids which therefore continue to reflect the endogenous level of cortisol in the plasma. Normal subjects and patients suffering from simple obesity or from hypertension due to causes other than Cushing's syndrome will show suppression of cortisol secretion following 0·5 mg oral dexamethasone 6-hourly for 48 hours. The majority of patients with Cushing's disease will show significant suppression following 2·0 mg dexamethasone 6-hourly for 48 hours, while most patients with adrenal tumours and the ectopic ACTH syndrome will fail to do so at this dosage. A further test of glucocorticoid production is the cortisol secretion rate (normal range 250–850 $\mu$mol/24 hours); this involves the administration of $^{14}$C-labelled cortisol and the measurement of one of its metabolites in a 24–hour collection of urine. The estimation of urinary free cortisol is useful in distinguishing between Cushing's syndrome and simple obesity.

An assessment of the secretion of adrenal androgens (of which dehydroepiandrosterone (DHEA) is the most important) may be made by measuring the 17-oxosteroid excretion in 24-hour urine samples. They are particularly likely to be elevated in adrenal carcinoma. In the rare feminising adrenal tumour in males the oestrogen output may also be estimated in urine.

Once a diagnosis of excess activity of the zona fasciculata/reticularis has been made, some indication of the cause may be obtained by radioimmunoassay of the plasma ACTH concentration. Moderately elevated levels are seen in Cushing's disease, low or undetectable levels occur in adrenal adenoma and strikingly high levels are found in the ectopic ACTH syndrome. Further information may be obtained by CT scan or adrenal arteriography. In the ectopic ACTH syndrome the tumour producing the ACTH is frequently highly malignant and is usually only too obvious.

About 70% of cases with overactivity of the zona fasciculata/reticularis are due to Cushing's disease, (i.e. pituitary dependent bilateral adrenal hyperplasia), 20% to an adrenal adenoma or carcinoma and 10% to the ectopic ACTH syndrome.

**Treatment of Overactivity of the Zona Fasciculata/Reticularis.** This clearly depends on establishing the cause. The adrenal which is the site of an adenoma or carcinoma should be excised. In the case of the ectopic ACTH syndrome the primary tumour should be removed but unfortunately this is rarely possible. Transitory improvement may be achieved by using metyrapone (which inhibits the enzyme 11-beta-hydoxylase that is involved in the final step in the synthesis of cortisol) or aminoglutethimide to block cortisol synthesis together with appropriate electrolyte replacement with particular reference to potassium.

In relation to the more common Cushing's disease opinions vary as to the best treatment. The most usual is bilateral adrenalectomy preceded by the control of adrenocortical function with metyrapone and followed by replacement steroid therapy (p. 493). Nelson's syndrome (p. 485) may be a later postoperative complication; this can be prevented either by giving external irradiation to the pituitary at the time of bilateral adrenalectomy or should there be evidence of rising plasma ACTH levels in excess of 1000 pg/ml after the operation; external irradiation as a sole form of treatment is another possibility. However, as in the case of excess GH and PRL secretion, its effect is slow and somewhat unpredictable in the individual patient. Hypophysectomy should be considered as a definitive form of therapy.

### Aldosteronism (Overactivity of the Zona Glomerulosa)

Hypersecretion of aldosterone may be primary in origin or secondary to some other pathological process.

In *primary aldosteronism*, usually associated with an adenoma and known as *Conn's syndrome*, the most consistent symptom is weakness, often episodic, and attributable to potassium deficiency. Polyuria and polydipsia, also due to the effects of potassium depletion and impaired renal tubular reabsorption of water, commonly occur. Tetany may be an occasional presenting symptom precipitated by the metabolic alkalosis associated with potassium depletion. The blood pressure is usually raised and the condition may be mistaken for essential hypertension, or for myasthenia gravis because of the weakness. Oedema is most unusual although its presence might be anticipated from the sodium retaining effect of aldosterone. Primary aldosteronism should be treated by removal of the affected gland or if this is not possible, spironolactone should be given.

*Secondary aldosteronism* occurs in cirrhosis of the liver with ascites, in the nephrotic syndrome and less consistently in severe cardiac failure.Potassium depletion may not be detected in the plasma and hypertension is less likely to occur; oedema is usual from hypoalbuminaemia or heart failure. The use of spironolactone in the management of these conditions is discussed on page 137. Secondary aldosteronism may also occur in patients with unilateral renal ischaemia due to renal artery stenosis, a form which can occasionally be cured by surgery.

Plasma renin and plasma and urinary aldosterone assays are used in assessing overactivity of the zona glomerulosa.

## Insufficiency of the Adrenal Cortex

Inadequate secretion of the adrenocortical hormones may be primary from acquired disease of the adrenals (Addison's disease) or because of congenital deficiency of the enzymes required for the synthesis of adrenocortical hormones (congenital adrenal hyperplasia). It may be secondary to failure of ACTH secretion due to pituitary or hypothalamic disorders (Fig. 11.3).

## Addison's Disease

Autoimmune adrenal failure and, much less commonly, tuberculous destruction of the adrenals are the main causes of Addison's disease in the developed countries, while other causes such as those listed in Figure 11.3 are rare.

Autoimmune adrenal failure (previously referred to as 'idiopathic' or 'simple' atrophy) affects females twice as frequently as males and may occur at any age. It is characterised by adrenocortical antibodies in the serum, by cell mediated hypersensitivity to adrenocortical antigens, the presence of HLA-B8 and HLA-DR3 and by a high incidence of other organ-specific autoimmune diseases such as thyrotoxicosis, Hashimoto's thyroiditis, primary atrophic hypothyroidism, pernicious anaemia, premature ovarian failure, idiopathic hypoparathyroidism and also insulin dependent diabetes. Histologically both adrenals show atrophy of the cortical cells in all three zones with lymphocytic infiltration and increase in fibrous tissue. The medulla is not

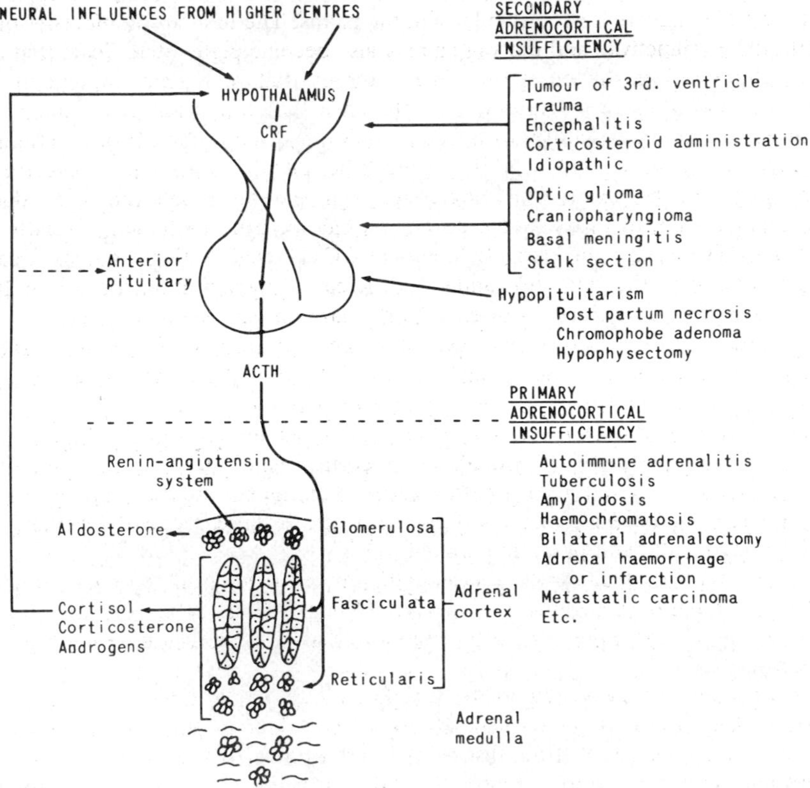


Fig. 11.3 Diagrammatic representation of the control of adrenocortical function and the sites of action of the various causes of disordered function. (Irvine & Barnes (1972) *Clinics in Endocrinology*, Vol. 1, No. 2.)

significantly affected. The adrenals are usually smaller than normal and appear atrophic.

In tuberculous destruction of the adrenal there is caseation with giant cells, and calcification which may be detected radiologically in long-standing cases.

**Clinical Features.** The onset of adrenal insufficiency may be acute or chronic, or more commonly acute following upon chronic. The main clinical features of chronic primary adrenal insufficiency are weakness, weight loss, hyperpigmentation or vitiligo, hypotension and gastrointestinal disorders. The invariable symptoms of tiredness and malaise, both physical and mental, gradually increase. Loss of weight does not occur until the adrenal failure is well advanced and then it is invariable. Anorexia, nausea and constipation alternating with diarrhoea occur with increased frequency as the disease progresses. Eventually in adrenal crisis the gastrointestinal complaints may be the oustanding feature and an erroneous diagnosis of severe gastroenteritis may be made; pain may simulate an acute abdomen. A wrong diagnosis may cost the patient his or her life.

Pigmentation of the skin is often the clinical sign that first raises the suspicion of primary hypoadrenalism. A history of its recent onset is more significant than pigmentation of long standing. This feature is due to increased melanin and is most obvious in regions normally pigmented and exposed to light or pressure, e.g. face, neck, back of hands, knuckles, elbows and knees, or in areas of the body subject to friction and in skin creases, particularly in the palms. The mucous membranes of the mouth, the conjunctivae and the vagina may also become pigmented. Scars that have been present before the onset of primary adrenal failure remain unpigmented in contrast to those that are acquired after the onset of adrenal failure. Pigmentation may precede the other features of hypoadrenalism by many years. It often manifests itself initially by the patient acquiring a much better suntan than usual and the tan taking longer to disappear. The progressive pigmentation is believed to be due to increased secretion of MSH by the pituitary which occurs simultaneously with augmented ACTH release and possibly in part to ACTH itself. Vitiligo, patchy areas of depigmentation of the skin surrounded by increased pigmentation, occurs in 10 to 20% of patients with Addison's disease, particularly in dark-skinned races.

The patient may give a history of very slow recovery from an illness or operation, having escaped an acute crisis at such a time. Likewise, there may be a history of extreme sensitivity to drugs such as morphine or pethidine.

Hypotension is almost invariable whether the patient is erect or supine. It is uncommon for a patient with primary adrenocortical failure to have a systolic blood pressure greater than 110 mmHg before appropriate replacement therapy is started. Normal reflex maintenance of the blood pressure is impaired and dizziness and syncope may result from postural hypotension.

Reactive hypoglycaemia after a carbohydrate meal may occur, cortisol being one of the physiological antagonists of insulin. Hypoglycaemia is usually manifest by tiredness and lethargy, the patient having more than usual difficulty in getting up in the morning.

Loss of body hair, especially in the female, is occasionally found but is generally not so marked as in hypopituitarism. Menstrual disorders, usually amenorrhoea, are common during the onset of the disease before treatment is instituted. A significant proportion of patients with autoimmune Addison's disease suffer from premature failure of ovarian function on account of an immunological reaction against antigens that are shared between the adrenal cortex and the steroid producing cells of the ovary.

### Secondary Adrenal Insufficiency

The secretion of ACTH and TSH is more resistant to pituitary damage than is the secretion of the gonadotrophins or growth hormone, so that patients with adrenal insufficiency secondary to organic pituitary disease generally show clinical features of impaired gonadotrophin secretion or of growth hormone secretion if the patient is of appropriate age for such manifestations. There is usually marked loss of axillary and pubic hair and the skin is fine provided hypothyroidism is not pronounced. A patient with secondary adrenal insufficiency will differ from one with Addison's disease by showing pallor instead of increased pigmentation of the skin. Because the secretion of aldosterone is largely independent of the pituitary, the blood pressure is better maintained than in primary adrenal insufficiency and the threat to life is less marked. Otherwise the symptoms are similar to those of primary adrenal insufficiency. In the absence of ACTH secretion the zona fasciculata/reticularis undergoes disuse atrophy.

Adrenal insufficiency induced by the prolonged use of therapeutic doses of corticosteroids is discussed on page 495.

### Congenital Adrenal Hyperplasia with Insufficiency

The synthesis of aldosterone and of the glucocorticoids involves a series of enzymatic steps involving hydroxylases. Congenital adrenal hyperplasia with insufficiency may present at birth, in infancy, or in childhood, depending on the precise type and severity of the hydroxylase deficiency. In the attempt to overcome the enzyme block, negative feedback control results in increased secretion of ACTH with overproduction of the compounds synthesised before the enzyme block is encountered. This usually means the production of large quantities of androgenic steroids. The metabolic consequences of deficiency of enzymes at the different stages of synthesis of cortisol and aldosterone are illustrated in Figure 11.4. Thus at birth, female infants may show signs of virilisation with clitoral hypertrophy and variable degrees of fusion of the labia. Male infants particularly may die from adrenocortical insufficiency, because the genital stigmata to be seen in female infants are not present to provide an appropriate warning of adrenal disease. If the enzyme defect is less severe the patient may survive infancy and present in childhood with evidence of precocious puberty. Growth may be abnormally advanced at first but is restricted later by early fusion of the epiphyses. Thus patients with mild examples of the enzyme defects usually come under supervision when excessive tallness, premature appearance of secondary sexual characteristics or libidinous tendencies arouse parental anxieties.

### Investigation of Adrenal Insufficiency

The symptoms and signs of adrenal insufficiency are so non-specific that confirmation of the diagnosis must be sought whenever suspicion arises. Tests of adrenocortical function are based on: (1) The metabolic effects of corticosteroids. (2) The measurement of cortisol levels in the resting state and following stimulation. (3) Measurement of ACTH levels in the plasma.

1. **Metabolic Effects.** Patients with Addison's disease, in contrast to those with secondary adrenal insufficiency, may show alteration in their serum electrolytes with depressed sodium and elevated potassium levels; this is by no means invariable even in advanced cases and must not be depended upon for diagnosis. Some degree of

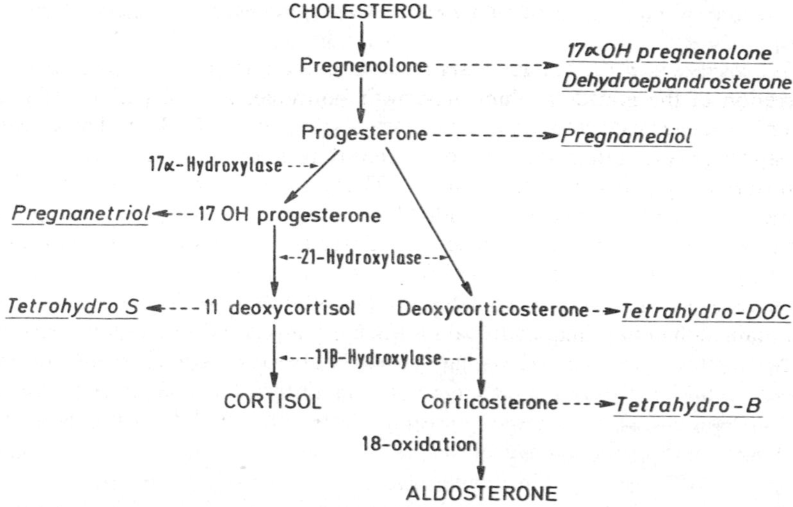


Fig. 11.4 The enzymatic steps involved in the synthesis of cortisol and aldosterone in the adrenal cortex and the urinary metabolites (underlined in italics) that are likely to be increased should there be an enzyme block (e.g. in congenital adrenal hyperplasia) at the next enzymatic step. The fall in the secretion of cortisol will activate the anterior pituitary to secrete ACTH with increased stimulation of the enzymatic steps preceding the block.

hypoglycaemia may occur but this also is of little diagnostic value. In past years the inability of patients with adrenal insufficiency to excrete a water load rapidly was used as a diagnostic test.

2. **Cortisol Levels.** Provided the patient is not in crisis or approaching crisis, time may be taken to determine the presence or absence of a diurnal rhythm in plasma cortisol levels by taking blood at 0900 hours and 2300 hours for 2 or 3 consecutive days for determination of fluorogenic corticosteroid levels before treatment is started. Low levels and the absence of a diurnal rhythm could be due to a lesion at any point in the hypothalamic-pituitary-adrenal axis. Normal levels and a normal rhythm would suggest that the whole axis is normal, but the possibility exists that, while overall function is maintained, there has been a significant reduction in reserve function which could be of paramount importance in times of stress. For this reason, if either primary or secondary adrenal insufficiency is suspected clinically, the diurnal rhythm studies should be supplemented by stimulation tests.

*ACTH Test.* The stimulation tests should be done in a logical sequence, starting with the administration of ACTH or a potent analogue. The preparation of choice is tetracosactrin which consists of the biologically active first 24 amino acids of human ACTH and has an action of about 30 minutes when given in a dosage of 250 μg intramuscularly. Oestrogen-containing oral contraceptives, spironolactone or glucocorticoids taken within the previous 12 hours may invalidate the test. In normal subjects the plasma corticosteroid level at 30 minutes reaches at least 550 nmol/*l* with an increment above basal which exceeds 200 nmol/*l*. A normal response excludes primary adrenocortical insufficiency, but an impaired or absent response requires further investigation using tetracosactrin depot, lmg. i.m. every 24 hrs for 3 days. Special care should be taken in patients with a history of allergic disease in view of occasional hypersensitivity reactions to tetracosactrin depot.

In secondary adrenal insufficiency there is a characteristic stepwise increase in plasma cortisol levels on each day of tetracosactrin depot administration, while in primary adrenal insufficiency (Addison's disease) there is little or no response. For practical purposes the criteria for primary adrenal insufficiency would be failure of the plasma fluorogenic corticosteroid levels to rise above 700 nmol/*l* by 5–12 hours after the third intramuscular injection of 1·0 mg tetracosactrin depot given on three consecutive mornings.

Since highly biologically active analogues of cortisol, such as betamethasone or prednisolone, do not cause fluorescence, tetracosactrin stimulation tests can be effectively carried out even though the patient may have recently started replacement therapy using these anlogues. As different steroid analogues may interfere with the assessment of plasma cortisol if the methods of radioimmunoassay or competitive protein binding are used, it is desirable to check with the laboratory beforehand.

*Insulin Induced Hypoglycaemia.* In a patient in whom secondary adrenocortical insufficiency is suspected, the next procedure should be insulin induced hypoglycaemia. Unless radioimmunoassay of ACTH is readily available, a normal adrenal response to ACTH stimulation should have been demonstrated before giving insulin because a cortisol rise in response to hypoglycaemia depends upon ACTH secretion and the patient is thus being used for bioassay. Insulin induced hypoglycaemia is a safe procedure provided certain precautions are taken. A history of epilepsy or myocardial ischaemia is a contraindication. Patients with hypopituitarism are very sensitive to small doses of insulin and the dose should not exceed 0·1 unit soluble insulin/kg body weight. This is given in the form of a single intravenous injection, an in-dwelling cannula with a slow infusion of saline having previously been established. The patient must be observed throughout the test with the physician at hand checking the condition of the patient repeatedly. A good index of adequate hypoglycaemia is the presence of sweating. Should hypoglycaemia become profound and the clinical features indicate that the test should be abandoned, the situation can be readily corrected by giving glucose and hydrocortisone if necessary via the intravenous cannula. In addition to the clinical criteria of sweating, the blood sugar should fall to less than 2·2 mmol/*l* or to less than 50% of the basal level at 30 minutes, whichever is the lower. Blood glucose and plasma fluorogenic corticosteroid levels should be estimated half-hourly for 120 min. Normal peak values of the latter show a mean of 785 mmol/*l* with a range of 560–1060 nmol/*l*, the increment being a mean of 420 with a range of 200–670 nmol/*l*.

Useful information of growth hormone secretion and prolactin can be obtained from the same samples. The corticosteroid response to insulin induced hypoglycaemia is probably the most sensitive of the tests currently available for assessing hypothalamic-pituitary-adrenal function.

3. **Measurement of ACTH Levels in Plasma.** In the presence of low levels of plasma fluorogenic steroids, if the plasma ACTH level is high, one would have strong evidence of primary adrenocortical insufficiency. The measurement of plasma ACTH levels greatly facilitates the study of hypopituitarism as it is no longer necessary to use the patient's potentially normal adrenals in an *in vivo* bioassay.

## Treatment of Adrenocortical Insufficiency

All patients with adrenocortical insufficiency will require replacement therapy with a glucocorticoid, while the majority of patients with Addison's disease will also need a mineralocorticoid. In congenital adrenal hyperplasia, full replacement doses of glucocorticoid will suppress ACTH secretion and prevent excessive formation of metabolites with consequent regression of the clinical features. If the nature of the enzymic block demands it, a mineralocorticoid should be added.

*Cortisol* (hydrocortisone) is the drug of choice for routine glucocorticoid replacement therapy. Cortisone acetate, although widely used, has the disadvantage that it has to be metabolised by the liver to cortisol before having any physiological action. Abnormal liver function results in reduced conversion of cortisone acetate to cortisol and the possibility of impaired liver function is particularly relevant in cases of secondary adrenal insufficiency taking oral androgens for concomitant hypogonadism. Other synthetic glucocorticoids, e.g. prednisone, prenisolone, dexamethasone and betamethasone are useful in keeping a patient in good health while adrenal function tests are being done, but have the disadvantage in terms of continual replacement therapy in that they do not react in the fluorogenic corticosteroid assay so their blood levels cannot be monitored. Cortisol, cortisone acetate and the synthetic glucocorticoids have a biological action of some 6 to 8 hours.

For maintenance treatment it is best to give the glucocorticoid medication in a regime which mimics the normal diurnal variation of cortisol output. For most patients this would be 20 mg cortisol at breakfast time and 10 mg at about 1800 hours. The equivalent doses of cortisone acetate would be 25 mg and 12·5 mg respectively. While it is not possible to be dogmatic about how much glucocorticoid any individual may require as absorption and metabolism may vary, the regime described will meet the needs of most patients. To assess the requirements of those whose response appears to be unsatisfactory a *corticosteroid profile* should be carried out. Plasma fluorogenic corticosteroids should be estimated before and half an hour, 1 hour and then at 2-hourly intervals after an oral dose of 20 mg of cortisol, or whatever dose seems to be clinically indicated. The plasma level usually reaches a peak after 30–60 minutes and the amount of cortisol should be adjusted to give a peak of 700–830 nmol/*l* and a level of about 165 nmol/*l* before the evening dose.

*Fludrocortisone* is the most useful mineralocorticoid for maintenance therapy, and the dose should be adjusted according to the serum electrolytes, the state of hydration of the patient and the blood pressure. Most patients require 0·05–0·15 mg in a single morning dose. The signs of overdosage of mineralocorticoid are those of sodium retention, i.e. hypertension, oedema, headaches and arthralgia, and also potassium depletion, hypokalaemic alkalosis and muscular weakness. The occasional patient is unable to tolerate fludrocortisone and in these cases a long-acting preparation may be given intravenously in a single dose of 50–100 mg every 2 to 4 weeks, e.g. deoxycortone pivalate.

The regime to be followed in secondary adrenocortical insufficiency is the same as in Addison's disease except that a mineralocorticoid is not required as aldosterone production is little affected. Any associated condition due to lack of other trophic hormones will require therapy along the usual lines.

*During periods of stress,* e.g. trauma, infection or operations, it is necessary for the dose of glucocorticoid to be increased to mimic what would happen in an individual with normal function of the hypothalamic-pituitary-adrenal axis. Thus if a patient develops a severe cold or influenza the dose of oral steroids should be increased to twice their normal maintenance level for 2 to 3 days. Should gastroenteritis with or without vomiting occur the oral glucocorticoid should be changed to intramuscular hydrocortisone at an increased dose level. Consequently, it is essential that patients with impaired adrenal function, either primary or secondary, should have available ampoules of hydrocortisone hemisuccinate for injection which are not outdated and which they know how to use.

Every patient on oral steroids of whatever form should have a steroid card or preferably a bracelet giving details of the diagnosis, steroid dosage and the medical attendant's address. Should the patient be involved in an accident and be taken unconscious to a casualty department a disastrous outcome may be avoided if information that the patient is taking steroids is available. Even the most minor operation is a potential hazard to a patient with adrenocortical insufficiency. On no account should such a patient be given morphine or pethidine. For dental extraction the patient should be admitted to hospital for the day. It is usually only necessary to give twice the normal dose of glucocorticoid on the day of the extraction and possibly the following morning. Normal replacement dosage may then be resumed provided there are no complications. Larger doses of steroids and more careful monitoring of cortisol levels are required before and after more major surgery.

ACUTE ADRENAL CRISIS. This is a medical emergency. If promptly treated with intravenous hydrocortisone (as sodium succinate or sodium phosphate) and intravenous fluids there is in most cases a dramatic improvement over 12 to 24 hours in a previously moribund patient. Occasional cases will need more protracted treatment depending upon how quickly the precipitating cause, e.g. infection, is brought under control. In incipient crises, intravenous fluids may not be necessary, but in frank crises with peripheral circulatory failure the patient may succumb in spite of massive doses of intravenous hydrocortisone. The intravenous fluids should consist of 5% of dextrose in isotonic saline to correct hypoglycaemia and sodium loss. Hydrocortisone is best given parenterally over the first 24–48 hours until gastrointestinal symptoms settle completely and one can be sure that oral medication will be retained. The initial dose should be 100 mg intravenously 6 hourly for the first 24 hours and then 50 mg 6 hourly for the next 24 hours. If progress is satisfactory, oral cortisol (hydrocortisone) can be given thereafter in a dose of 20 mg 8 hourly. The dose of oral cortisol can then be further reduced in a stepwise fashion by 10 mg daily until normal maintenance levels are reached. Below 40 mg of oral cortisol per day a mineralocorticoid is best added to the therapeutic regime, initially in a single morning dose of 0·1 mg fludrocortisone.

### Prognosis in Adrenal Insufficiency

With modern therapy the life expectancy of patients with adrenal insufficiency should be normal, within the limits imposed by any associated disease such as pituitary tumour, or other clinical disorders such as insulin dependent diabetes mellitus which may co-exist with autoimmune adrenal insufficiency. Otherwise the main risk to life is the avoidable occurrence of acute adrenal crisis and delay in its prompt management.

## Corticosteroids and ACTH in the Treatment of Disease

Extensive use is made of the anti-inflammatory actions of corticosteroids and their synthetic analogues. Alternatively, ACTH may be administered parenterally to augment the endogenous production of cortisol. The doses of steroid analogues therapeutically equivalent to 20 mg cortisol for an anti-inflammatory effect are cortisone (25 mg), prednisolone (5 mg), betamethasone (0·75 mg) and dexamethasone (0·75 mg). Of these prednisolone is the most commonly used for purposes other than replacement therapy. It is widely prescribed in the treatment of connective tissue diseases, of autoimmune disorders and conditions involving other forms of immune reaction. Corticosteroids may be used to suppress inflammation, for example in conjunction with chemotherapy in acute tuberculosis (p. 259). The use of corticosteroids in pharmacological doses is discussed under the heading of the various diseases for which they may be employed.

## The Dangers of Corticosteroid Therapy

The use of corticosteroids in doses exceeding those required for replacement therapy carries certain risks which must be balanced against the possible therapeutic advantages. These risks can be subdivided into two types: (1) the undesirable metabolic consequences that cannot be separated from the anti-inflammatory effect of the steroid and (2) the suppression of the hypothalamic-pituitary-adrenal (HPA) axis that may follow the use of pharmacological doses over a prolonged period. It should be realised that when large amounts of steroid are applied to the skin a significant proportion is absorbed.

1. *The metabolic consequences* are those that are encountered in Cushing's syndrome and are naturally more pronounced the higher the dose and the longer the treatment. Thus, although certain corticosteroid analogues may have slightly less mineralocorticoid activity than cortisol, fluid retention, moon face, hypertension, central obesity, striae, etc., may all be induced. The glucocorticoid action not infrequently precipitates diabetes mellitus and the catabolic effect is responsible for osteoporosis—an insidious but frequent complication of long term steroid therapy. Corticosteroids may modify the normal response to a major illness so that pain, tenderness, fever or a raised ESR may be abolished, while the response to inflammation and therefore the defences against infection may be poor and healing impaired. In this way treatment with these drugs may be responsible for masking the more typical and sometimes dangerous consequences of a variety of illnesses. For example, oral corticosteroids may induce peptic ulceration with perforation without pain, and the physical signs indicative of inflammation in the peritoneal cavity may not be present. As in Cushing's syndrome, mental symptoms may be troublesome, ranging from euphoria to depression which may be so severe as to lead to suicide.

2. *The suppression of the HPA axis* following prolonged corticosteroid therapy in doses greater than 7·5 mg prednisolone per day or its equivalent may be long standing, especially with regard to the hypothalamic-pituitary portion of the axis. This may make it difficult to withdraw steroid, the patient being as vulnerable as someone with secondary adrenocortical insufficiency due to organic pituitary disease. Stimulation of the adrenal cortex in such cases is usually possible with adequate ACTH dosage, but there is no known way of producing a comparably strong and prolonged stimulus to the hypothalamic-pituitary axis without risking adrenocortical failure. When trying to wean a patient off corticosteroid therapy, one should first ensure that the adrenal cortex is functional by giving tetracosactrin depot (1·0 mg i.m. on 3 consecutive mornings) and measuring the plasma cortisol response at 30 minutes, 1 hour and 5 hours (p. 491). Then, after gradually reducing the dosage of oral steroid, a maintenance dose of 20 mg cortisol should be given at 0800–0900 hours and no cortisol in the evenings; the hypothalamo-pituitary axis will then have no exogenous steroid to suppress the secretion of CRF or ACTH in the early hours of the morning. In this way a normal diurnal rhythm may be restored and the HPA axis should thereafter

respond normally to stress. This may take many months to achieve, while in other cases, normal function may be restored shortly after steroid therapy has been withdrawn.

Because it can be such a difficult task to withdraw corticosteroid therapy when it has been used in pharmacological dosage for a prolonged period, attempts have been made to use synthetic ACTH preparations such as tetracosactrin depot in place of oral corticosteroids. When used in appropriate doses, there is evidence that therapeutically useful elevation in the plasma cortisol level may be achieved in some patients without suppression of the HPA axis. However, this may be only a reflection of the amount of corticosteroid secreted in response to this stimulus. In children ACTH therapy has the distinct advantage over treatment with oral steroids in that it causes less inhibition of growth.

The incidence of mooning of the face and obesity is similar with oral corticosteroids and ACTH. Peptic ulceration and bruising are commoner with corticosteroids, and hypertension, pigmentation and acne with ACTH. In view of the serious risks involved very careful consideration must be given before either is employed and the practitioner must be convinced that the therapeutic benefits outweigh the disadvantages.

## Phaeochromocytoma

Phaeochromocytomas are tumours of chromaffin tissue which secrete catecholamines, predominantly noradrenaline but also adrenaline. The tumours, most of which are benign, may occur at any site along the sympathetic chain, but 90% are found in the adrenal glands. Rarely the lesions may be multiple. Phaeochromocytoma is an uncommon tumour but of considerable interest because of its pharmacological effects. The clinical presentation depends upon the relative amounts of noradrenaline and adrenaline secreted. The most common sign is hypertension which may be sustained or, characteristically, paroxysmal with associated episodes of extreme skin pallor, sweating, palpitations, headache, epigastric pain and chest discomfort. Apprehension is common during a paroxysm.

Confirmation of the diagnosis of phaeochromocytoma depends on the demonstration of increased levels of catecholamines or their metabolites in the urine, e.g. metanephrine and normetanephrine. The location of the tumour is best shown by adrenal venography or CT scanning.

The treatment of phaeochromocytoma is by excision of the tumour if it can be identified or, failing this, alpha and beta receptor blockade may be used. In order to avoid hypertension and arrhythmias during induction of anaesthesia and handling of the tumour at operation, the preoperative preparation of the patient with $\alpha$ and $\beta$ adrenergic blocking agents (phenoxybenzamine and propranolol) is essential. Emergencies associated with hypertensive crises should be dealt with by the intravenous administration of phentolamine in doses of 5 mg. Careful preparation before and during operation should prevent any severe fall in blood pressure resulting from hypovolaemia. If hypotension persists noradrenalin should be given intravenously in saline.

## Sexual Disorders in the Male

These may present in many forms. Some are due to faults arising in the mechanism of sex determination as early as conception, others to errors later in sexual differentiation of the embryo and fetus, and after birth, in sexual development. Abnormalities of the sex chromosomes may be associated with failure of sexual development so that the individual may show some of the characteristics of both sexes (intersex). The term hermaphroditism is reserved for patients in whom male and female gonadal tissue is found to coexist; it occurs much less commonly than the intersexes.

The anatomical characteristics of the male are influenced by essential hormonal factors, particularly androgen secretion. The personality and behaviour of the male are further attributes which must be considered in assessing the individual patient's needs. A few only of the more common sexual disorders occurring in the male will be discussed here.

## Hypogonadism

This term is used to include failure of one or both of the main functions of the testis, namely the production of spermatozoa and the secretion of androgens. The defect may involve only impaired spermatogenesis in the seminiferous tubules of the testis, or the interstitial (Leydig) cells of the testis may also be affected so that the secretion of testosterone by these cells is reduced or abolished. If the function of the interstitial cells is defective, then tubular dysfunction is inevitable.

**Aetiology.** Hypogonadism may be part of the syndrome of hypopituitarism. Hypogonadotrophic hypogonadism with an apparently normal pituitary gland appears to be due to failure of the hypothalamus to secrete the appropriate gonadotrophin releasing hormones. In addition there are patients in whom the anterior pituitary is intact but the testes have been destroyed or damaged (primary testicular failure). Trauma, tuberculosis, gonococcal infections, syphilis, malignant disease and orchitis as in mumps, are recognised causes of primary testicular failure. Maldescent or failure of descent will also lead to failure of the tubular epithelium to develop. Haemochromatosis, cirrhosis of the liver and oestrogen administration may all be associated with testicular insufficiency. The disorder may also be due to abnormalities of the sex chromosomes (p. 11). Many cases remain, however, for which an aetiological diagnosis is still not possible, and these form the majority of patients who present with infertility as their only complaint (idiopathic oligospermia).

**Clinical Features.** The results of failure of function of the interstitial cells depends upon the age of the patient at the time of the onset of the disease. When this occurs *before puberty* the external genitalia and the secondary sex characteristics fail to develop. In these circumstances the epiphyses of the long bones do not close at the usual age and in consequence the patient may grow to an excessive height. The typical pre-pubertal eunuch develops into a tall man with a hairless face, a high-pitched voice, small genitalia and an immature personality.

When the onset of the disease is *postpubertal* the changes are less striking. Growth is not affected and there is regression rather than disappearance of the secondary sex characteristics. The external genitalia undergo partial atrophy. Fatigue, loss of initiative and libido are the usual complaints. In some patients, particularly when the deprivation is sudden as after surgical castration, there may be 'menopausal symptoms' such as hot flushes and profuse sweating, unless replacement therapy is provided.

**Treatment.** Hypogonadism due to deficiency of androgens may be corrected by replacement therapy with testosterone. A satisfactory and the most economical form of therapy is the implantation of 200–600 mg of testosterone, in pellets, into the anterior abdominal wall. Renewal may be required after six to eight months. Alternatively fluoxymesterone, a synthetic analogue of testosterone, can be given sublingually in doses of 2·5–10 mg daily. In some cases of deficiency of the germinal epithelium, especially when this is due to lack of FSH, increased spermatogenesis may be achieved by treatment with human chorionic gonadotrophin and mentotrophin (FSH).

## Cryptorchidism

Cryptorchidism (undescended testis) usually occurs in otherwise normal boys but may be the presenting feature of hypogonadotrophic hypogonadism. Highly retractile testes, particularly in an obese boy, may be mistaken for cryptorchidism. If the glands remain in the inguinal canal they are more liable to trauma than if situated in the scrotum. The seminiferous tubules will fail to develop in an undescended gland, and if the condition is bilateral, sterility will follow. Even in testes which remain undescended into adult life the interstitial cells function normally, so that the secondary sex characters develop in the usual way. A course of chorionic gonadotrophin should be given at about 6 years of age. If this is unsuccessful the testis or testes should be placed in the scrotum surgically.

In maldescent the testis takes an abnormal route and is liable to develop malignancy.

## Impotence

Impotence, that is inability of the male to have an erection, is due to psychological causes in the majority of cases, and in these circumstances is not due to abnormality of the testes. Rarely it may be an important early symptom in organic disease such as diabetes mellitus, multiple sclerosis and tabes dorsalis. In hypogonadism due to anterior pituitary deficiency, a complaint of impotence is unusual; such patients usually have little interest in sexual function, and are unlikely to make this complaint spontaneously until they have received treatment for adrenal and thyroid insufficiency. They may then become aware of their impotence and require treatment with an androgen, e.g. testosterone. Gonadotrophins may be used to restore fertility if desired. Some impotent patients are found to have hyperprolactinaemia which may be treated successfully with bromocriptine.

## Infertility in the Male

Sterility in the husband is believed to be responsible for the infertility of approximately one-half of all childless marriages. The cause is usually defective development of the germinal epithelium in the seminiferous tubules, with oligospermia or azoospermia, but may follow hypogonadism due to any of the causes described earlier. Antibodies to sperm (p. 36) may explain a small number of cases.

Additional X chromosomes may be recognised by examination of a buccal smear for Barr bodies, but usually confirmation requires a full karyotype analysis (p. 6). Seminal analysis is a simple procedure and a low sperm count, or the presence of abnormal and immotile forms may be detected in this way. Testicular biopsy frequently provides valuable information on the development of the spermatic tubules and on the maturation of the germinal epithelium. This investigation should be undertaken before declaring a hopeless prognosis since the use of clomiphene for a period of 6 months or longer, as a means of promoting gonadotrophin secretion, may occasionally stimulate spermatogenesis.

Treatment of a varicocele has sometimes corrected infertility. Obstruction of the vas deferens may also be amenable to surgery.

## Sexual Disorders in the Female

Many conditions regarded as primarily gynaecological in nature may have much wider implications. *Primary amenorrhoea*, for example, may provide an important indication of systemic disorder; it may be due to a chromosomal anomaly such as Turner's syndrome or it may be due to an autoimmune reaction against antigens shared between the steroid producing cells in the ovary and in the adrenal cortex. Hermaphroditism may present with amenorrhoea. Congenital adrenal hyperplasia, if unrecognised and untreated in childhood, pituitary tumours and developmental disorders in the genital tract may all require full gynaecological and endocrine assessment for precise diagnosis. *Secondary amenorrhoea* also requires further investigation, but it is so common a feature of a wide range of conditions that by itself it has little diagnostic value. Hyperprolactinaemia (p. 463) must be considered.

**Risks of Oral Contraception.** A low level of mortality is associated with all major reversible methods of fertility control, including oral contraception (OC), compared with the risk of death from pregnancy and delivery in women using no method of fertility control, with the important exception of OC use in women over 40 years who also smoke. There is an increased risk of coronary artery disease, hypertension, cerebrovascular accident, deep vein thrombosis and pulmonary embolism in OC users. Immediate adverse effects which may influence the patients' acceptance of OC include breast discomfort, weight gain, jaundice (p. 391), bleeding occurring during courses of treatment (breakthrough bleeding) and failure to bleed between cycles. These complaints may subside after the first few courses of treatment. Other troublesome complaints include abdominal fullness, depression, fatigue, hirsutism, skin pigmentation and decreased libido.

### Disorders of the Menopause

The term menopause is used to describe the cessation of the menstrual cycle, which occurs in most women between the ages of 45 and 50; it is the direct result of the failure of the ovaries to produce oestrogens and progesterone. As a consequence the pituitary gland becomes more active and produces FSH and LH in greater quantity. Assays for these hormones may be of value in distinguishing amenorrhoea due primarily to failure of the ovaries from amenorrhoea due to failure of the pituitary to secrete gonadotrophins.

**Clinical Features.** The ease with which a woman adapts herself to the change of circumstances associated with the menopause varies widely. In some the loss of reproductive capacity is associated with psychological symptoms; in others adjustment is readily achieved and may be unattended by any emotional reaction. In the group of patients who are troubled by symptoms, anxiety, emotional instability, irritability, insomnia, and particularly hot flushes and cold sweats are common complaints. Depression is frequent and occasionally may be severe with suicidal tendencies.

Obesity may first appear, or, if previously present, may increase. Hirsutism, especially the appearance of hair on the upper lip and chin, is not uncommon. Osteoarthrosis may be responsible for considerable disability, particularly in the obese. Osteoporosis commonly presents for the first time in the early years after the menopause. Pruritus vulvae is a complication which is frequently associated with changes in the mucous membrances of the genital tract. Leukoplakia vulvae may develop, and if untreated may progress to carcinoma. Senile vaginitis may cause considerable distress from dyspareunia, dysuria and vaginal discharge, especially if complicated by secondary infection.

**Treatment.** The essential treatment is explanation of the nature of the condition, coupled with specific treatment for the complications. Features attributable to oestrogen deficiency call for replacement therapy with a synthetic oestrogen such as ethinyloestradiol. The daily dose required to suppress menopausal symptoms in different individuals varies from 10 to 50 μg daily, but 20 μg is often adequate; this should be given in courses lasting for 21 days, repeated if necessary after an interval of 7 days. The patient must be warned that this treatment may be followed by vaginal bleeding as in a normal menstrual period. Other appropriate measures, such as treatment of obesity and osteoarthrosis, may also be required. Depression complicating the menopause responds well to psychiatric treatment.

W. J. IRVINE

*Further reading:*

Hall, R., Anderson, J., Smart, G.A., & Besser, M. (1980) *Fundamentals of Clinical Endocrinology*, 3rd. edn. London: Pitman Medical.
Hall, R., Evered, D. & Greene, R. (1979) *A Colour Atlas of Endocrinology*. London: Wolfe Medical Publications.
Irvine, W.J. (1979) In *Medical Immunology*, Edinburgh: Teviot Scientific Publications: New York. MacGraw-Hill.
Lee, J. & Laycock, J. (1978) *Essential Endocrinology*. Oxford: Oxford Medical Publications.
Martini, L. (ed.) (1979) *Comprehensive Endocrinology*. New York: Raven Press.

## DIABETES MELLITUS

Diabetes mellitus is a clinical syndrome characterised by hyperglycaemia, due to deficiency or diminished effectiveness of insulin. The disease is chronic and affects the metabolism of carbohydrate, protein, fat, water and electrolytes, sometimes with grave consequences. The metabolic derangement is frequently associated with permanent and irreversible functional and structural changes in the cells of the body, those of the vascular system being particularly susceptible. The changes lead in turn to the development of well-defined clinical entities, the so-called 'complications' of diabetes, which most characteristically affect the eye, the kidney and the nervous system.

Diabetes mellitus is the most common of the endocrine disorders. The prevalence in Britain is over 1%, although about half of those affected remain undetected.

**Aetiology.** On the basis of aetiology two main categories of diabetes are recognised, namely primary (idiopathic) diabetes and secondary diabetes.

PRIMARY (IDIOPATHIC) DIABETES. The great majority of cases seen belong to this group, which consists of two main clinical types: *insulin-dependent diabetes* (IDD) most frequent in those less than 30 years old and *non insulin dependent diabetes* (NIDD) occurring mainly in the middle-aged and elderly. Although the precise aetiology is still uncertain, several contributing factors are known to be involved and in both types heredity and environment interact to determine which of those with a genetic predisposition actually develop the clinical syndrome and the timing of its onset. However, both the pattern of inheritance and the environmental factors differ in IDD and NIDD.

*Age.* The disease may appear at any time, but 80% of cases occur after the age of 50 years and the highest incidence of new patients is in the 60–70 age group. Diabetes is, therefore, principally a disease of the middle-aged and elderly.

*Sex.* There are rather more young male diabetics than female; in middle age women are more often affected. Repeated pregnancy adds to the likelihood of developing diabetes in middle age, particularly in obese women.

*Heredity.* In both types of diabetes a familial tendency exists and twins are more often both diabetic when they are identical than when they are not. Genetic factors seem to be stronger in NIDD and most pairs of identical twins are concordant. In contrast, concordance is between 50–60% in IDD pairs of identical twins. Susceptibility to IDD is associated with particular HLA phenotypes (p. 38), and affected diabetic siblings tend to have at least one and, in many cases, both HLA haplotypes in common. Both these findings are consistent with the presence of a diabetogenic gene or genes at a locus closely linked to the HLA chromosomal loci. Since genes closely linked in this way probably influence immune responses, a possible mode of action for the HLA-linked gene may be to permit destruction of the $\beta$ cells of the pancreas to occur, perhaps in response to a viral infection or because of a primary autoimmune disorder.

NIDD is not HLA–linked and the nature of the inherited abnormality is totally obscure.

*Autoimmunity.* Considerable evidence now exists in support of the hypothesis that, in some instances at least, IDD is an autoimmune disorder irrespective of the age of onset of the disease. Diabetes coexists with other autoimmune disease such as pernicious anaemia, hyperthyroidisim, Hashimoto's thyroiditis, primary hypothyroidism and Addison's disease more often than can be accounted for by chance. Thyroid, gastric, cytoplasmic, intrinsic factor and adrenal antibodies are all many times more common in diabetic than in non-diabetic populations. More direct evidence is provided by: (1) the lymphocytic and plasma cell infiltration found in the pancreas of young diabetic patients dying within 6 months of developing the disorder; (2) the demonstration of T lymphocytes sensitised against antigens derived from the pancreas in 20–30% of young IDD patients; and (3) the fact that antibodies reacting with human pancreatic islet cells have been found by immunofluorescence in the serum of over 50% of IDD patients soon after diagnosis, irrespective of age. In contrast, islet-cell antibodies are not found more commonly in the serum of diabetics requiring only dietary restriction than in control subjects. A number of diabetics requiring oral hypoglycaemic agents have islet-cell antibodies in the serum; such patients have an increased risk of becoming insulin-dependent eventually.

*Infection.* There is some evidence that viral infection may be involved in the aetiology of IDD. It is known that certain viruses can induce diabetes experimentally in some laboratory animals and a high incidence of diabetes has been known to occur after outbreaks of mumps. A seasonal variation in the incidence of diabetes in children has been demonstrated, with peaks occurring in October and June, and antibodies to Coxsackie B4 virus have been found significantly more often in the plasma of recently diagnosed young diabetics than in controls. NIDD does not show this excess of Coxsackie B4 infection, but infection of any kind may be important in unmasking latent diabetes in the middle aged and elderly. Staphylococcal infections, in particular, are frequently associated with the development of clinical diabetes.

*Obesity*. The association of obesity and NIDD has long been recognised but it is still uncertain whether obesity is the result or the cause of diabetes. The majority of middle-aged diabetic patients are obese, but only a minority of obese people develop clinical diabetes. Most of the evidence supports the view that obesity is diabetogenic in those genetically predisposed to the disorder and that the rising incidence of diabetes in older people is related to the increasing prevalence of obesity in the population as a whole.

*Diet*. Overeating, especially when combined with underactivity, is associated with a rise in the incidence of diabetes in the middle-aged and elderly. Studies of the incidence in war and peace and in immigrants whose material standards of living suddenly rise provide evidence of this. Studies of diabetic sibships also demonstrate that diabetic patients eat significantly more than their non-diabetic siblings.

SECONDARY DIABETES. A minority of cases of diabetes occur as a result of a recognisable pathological process or secondary to the treatment of some other condition.

1. *Pancreatic diabetes*. Diseases such as pancreatitis, haemochromatosis and carcinoma cause destruction of the pancreas and lead to impaired secretion and release of insulin. Diabetes will also follow pancreatectomy.

2. *Insulin antagonists*. Diabetes may occur in conditions where there are abnormal concentrations of hormones antagonistic to the action of insulin in the circulation.

(a) *Growth hormone* can produce permanent diabetes in experimental animals and about 30% of patients with acromegaly are diabetic.

(b) *Adrenocortical hormones*, such as cortisol, raise the concentration of glucose in the blood by increasing gluconeogenesis and by inhibiting utilisation of glucose by the peripheral tissues. Thus, many patients with Cushing's syndrome show impaired carbohydrate tolerance; diabetes may be precipitated by ACTH or corticosteroid therapy and the stress of physical injury may operate in this way. Conversely increased sensitiviy to insulin is an important feature of Addison's disease and of hypopituitarism, and this can be corrected by the administration of corticosteroids.

(c) *Adrenaline* raises the blood glucose concentration by increasing the breakdown of liver glycogen and by suppressing the secretion of insulin. Patients with phaeochromocytoma frequently show a diabetic blood glucose curve on glucose tolerance testing and the incidence of these uncommon tumours is relatively high among diabetic patients.

(d) *Thyroid hormone* in excess will aggravate the diabetic state and some patients with hyperthyroidism show impaired glucose tolerance.

(e) *Gestational diabetes* refers to the hyperglycaemia which can occur temporarily during pregnancy in individuals who have an inherited liability to develop the disorder. During normal pregnancy there is an increased production of hormonal antagonists to insulin, which in turn demands an increased rate of secretion and release of insulin. A failing pancreas may be unable to meet this demand.

3. *Iatrogenic diabetes*, in those genetically susceptible, may be precipitated by various forms of therapy, notably corticosteroids, and thiazide diuretics.

4. *Liver disease*, particularly cirrhosis and hepatitis, may be associated with impaired glucose tolerance.

**Chemical Pathology.** Whatever the aetiology, in all cases of diabetes hyperglycaemia results from deficiency of insulin. This is absolute in IDD and relative in NIDD. Increased gluconeogenesis and lipolysis follow as compensatory reactions under the influence of such hormones as growth hormone, glucagon and adrenocortical hormones, in what is basically a situation of glucose lack. Thus the hyperglycaemia characteristic of diabetes arises from two main sources, namely a reduced rate of removal of glucose from the blood by the peripheral tissues and an increased rate of release of glucose from the liver into the circulation.

CONSEQUENCES OF HYPERGLYCAEMIA AND GLYCOSURIA. When the glucose concentration in the blood exceeds the capacity of the renal tubules to reabsorb it from the glomerular filtrate, glycosuria occurs. In most people the level of blood glucose at which this happens is approximately 10 mmol/*l*(180 mg/100 ml). Glucose increases the osmolality of the glomerular filtrate and thus prevents the reabsorption of water as the filtrate passes down the renal tubular system. In this way the volume of urine is markedly increased in diabetes and polyuria and nocturia occur. This in turn leads to loss of water and minerals which results in thirst and polydipsia. Severe depletion of water and electrolytes may ensue.

CONSEQUENCES OF POOR GLUCOSE UTILISATION. Impaired utilisation of carbohydrate results in a sense of fatigue, and causes two main compensatory mechanisms to operate in an attempt to provide alternative metabolic substrate. Both of these lead to loss of body tissue, that is *wasting*, which may occur in spite of normal or even an increased intake of food, and which is additional to any loss of weight resulting from loss of body fluid. The compensatory mechanisms are:

1. *Increased Glycogenolysis and Gluconeogenesis.* As glycogen and protein are catabolised, glucose, nitrogen, water and electrolytes, particularly potassium, are released from cells into the extracellular space. An increased urinary excretion of potassium, magnesium and phosphorus therefore occurs.

2. *Increased Lipolysis.* This is seen as a raised fasting plasma concentration of non-esterified fatty acid (NEFA), and a diminished fall in plasma NEFA in response to a carbohydrate load. The extent to which increased lipolysis occurs is proportional to the degree of insulin deficiency. If the latter is marked, the normal response to feeding, namely suppression of lipolysis, may be lost and the plasma concentration of NEFA may remain consistently elevated to three or four times the normal level.

Fatty acids are taken up by the liver and degraded through eight steps within the mitochondria of the liver cells. Each stage yields one molecule of acetyl coenzyme A. Normally most of these molecules enter the citric acid cycle by condensing with oxaloacetic acid, but in severe diabetes more is formed than can enter the citric acid cycle. Instead acetyl coenzyme A is converted to acetoacetic acid. Most of this is then reduced to beta-hydroxybutyric acid, while some is decarboxylated to acetone. These ketone bodies, when formed in small amounts, are usually oxidised and utilised as metabolic fuel. However the rate of utilisation of ketone bodies is limited. When the rate of production by the liver exceeds that of removal by the peripheral tissues, then the blood level rises. Ketone bodies increase the osmolality of the plasma and so also lead to the withdrawal of water from the cell. They are strong acids which dissociate readily and release hydrogen ions into the body fluids. The fall in pH is reduced by the buffers of the blood, the most important being bicarbonate. The dissociation of carbonic acid is reduced, and the ratio of bicarbonate ions to carbonic acid falls, and measurement of plasma bicarbonate will show a lower value than normal. This state is called *ketoacidosis*. The rise in hydrogen ion concentration and increase in $P_{CO_2}$ in the arterial blood stimulate pulmonary ventilation so that clinically hyperpnoea or 'air hunger' is observed.

The extent to which the clinical features of dehydration and ketoacidosis are seen in the individual will depend on such factors as the speed at which the condition develops and the extent to which the patient increases the intake of fluid, as well as on the degree of insulin deficiency present.

**Pathology.** In IDD there is degeneration of pancreatic islet tissue, from which the beta cells have largely disappeared, leaving behind a variable number of alpha cells and a majority of small undifferentiated cells. The few remaining beta cells show evidence of excessive activity; the nuclei are commonly enlarged with degranulation of the cytoplasm. These appearances of the pancreas are consistent with the extremely low plasma insulin levels found in these patients.

In NIDD the moderate reduction in the total mass of islet tissue which is commonly seen does not appear to be sufficient in itself to account for the degree of impaired carbohydrate tolerance present. On the other hand, the observation that in many cases the beta cells, despite prolonged hyperglycaemia and their reduced number, fail to develop cytological signs of hyperactivity, suggests that in these diabetics the beta cells may be relatively insensitive to the stimulus of an elevated blood glucose. Failure to respond to hyperglycaemia could result from vascular lesions or from alterations in the islet stroma, interfering with the exchange between the blood and the islet cells. Fibrosis, hyalinisation, and fibrin deposits in the pericapillary space and changes in the islet epithelial basement membrane are often present in older diabetics.

Long-standing diabetes is commonly associated with an abnormal thickening of the basement membrane of the capillaries throughout the body. This *per se* is not pathognomonic of diabetes. It occurs for example as part of the normal ageing process; however the increased permeability of the thickened basement membrane in diabetes is a unique pathological feature. The main clinical and pathological impact of this micro-angiopathy is to be found in the retina, kidney and nervous system. (p. 523).

**Clinical Features.** Two main types of diabetes have long been recognised, and it is now clear that the level of plasma insulin correlates well with the clinical picture and the type of treatment subsequently required.

1. IDD usually develops during the first 40 years of life in patients of normal or less than normal weight. The majority develop severe symptoms of diabetes acutely, over a period of several weeks or months and if treatment with insulin is withheld they rapidly develop fatal ketoacidosis.

2. NIDD usually appears in middle-aged or elderly patients who are often obese and in whom hyperglycaemia can usually be controlled by dietary means alone or, if not, by an oral hypoglycaemic compound. Insulin is detectable in the plasma of nearly all patients in this category, and they are therefore less prone to develop ketosis. In this sense the disease is less severe than IDD; however, the complications associated with long-term diabetes occur in both types. Many patients with NIDD have a long history of mild symptoms which may come and go, and which may frequently be ignored or misdiagnosed for years before the true diagnosis is made.

Apart from patients with established clinical diabetes, two other categories are recognised.

1. *Potential diabetics* are persons with a normal glucose tolerance test who nevertheless have an increased liability to develop diabetes for genetic reasons, e.g. the children of two diabetic parents; the children of parents where one is diabetic and

the other has a first degree relative who is diabetic; the non-diabetic member of a pair of identical twins where the other is diabetic.

2. *Latent diabetics* are persons in whom the glucose tolerance test is normal, but who are known to have given an abnormal result under conditions imposing a burden on the pancreatic beta cells, e.g. during pregnancy, infection or other severe stress, mental or physical, during treatment with cortisone or other diabetogenic drugs, or when overweight.

PRESENTATION. Diabetes may be discovered in one of several ways:

1. Many patients are first noted to have glycosuria in the course of some routine examination. They may have had few or no symptoms, and no abnormal physical signs may be found.

2. Some patients present complaining of some or all of the classical symptoms of diabetes, including thirst, polydipsia, polyuria, nocturia, tiredness, loss of weight, white marks on clothing, pruritus vulvae or balanitis, impotence, a change in refraction usually in the direction of myopia and parasthesiae or pain in the limbs.

The severity of many of the classical symptoms of clinical diabetes are directly related to the severity of glycosuria. If relatively mild hyperglycaemia has developed slowly over many years the renal threshold for glucose will rise, glycosuria may be slight, and the symptoms of diabetes correspondingly trivial.

3. Diabetes may first present as a fulminating ketoacidosis associated with an acute infection or even without evidence of a precipitating cause, and in such cases epigastric pain and vomiting may be the presenting complaints. This is more likely to occur in IDD and such cases are acute medical emergencies.

4. Patients may present with symptoms due to the complications of diabetes.

PHYSICAL SIGNS depend very much on the mode of presentation. Cases without complications will usually show no abnormal physical signs attributable to diabetes. In some cases vulvitis or balanitis may be found, since the external genitalia are especially prone to infection by fungi (Candida) which flourish on the skin and mucous membranes contaminated by glucose. In the fulminating case the most striking features are those of dehydration.

The intraocular pressure may be obviously reduced. A rapid pulse and a low blood pressure may then be anticipated. Breathing may be deep and sighing in the acidotic patient; the breath is usually fetid and the sickly sweet smell of acetone may be noticeable. Apathy and confusion may be present or there may be stupor or even coma.

Evidence of complications of diabetes may be noted. Ophthalmoscopy may show the typical appearance of diabetic retinopathy (p. 524). The most constant early signs of diabetic neuropathy are depression or loss of the ankle jerks, and impaired vibration sense in the legs (p. 735).

The presence of diabetic nephropathy may be indicated by proteinuria in addition to glycosuria; rarely the other features of the nephrotic syndrome may be apparent.

Potential and latent diabetics usually complain of no symptoms and show no abnormality on examination. However certain features are recognised as being characteristic of potential diabetes without necessarily implying that such individuals will progress to clinical diabetes. For example genetically constituted potential diabetics are predisposed to coronary and peripheral arterial disease. They may show abnormal lipid patterns in response to oral contraceptives. They have a high incidence of stillborn or abnormally large and heavy babies and babies with congenital defects.

Potential and latent diabetics may be much overweight at a time when there is no detectable abnormality in terms of carbohydrate intolerance.

**Diagnosis.** By definition hyperglycaemia remains the *sine qua non* of the clinical diagnosis of diabetes mellitus. In the individual case when the classical symptoms are present, the diagnosis is often beyond reasonable doubt by the time the history taking and physical examination are complete, and it may then be confirmed by the finding of marked glycosuria, with or without ketonuria, and a random blood sugar greater than 14·0 mmol/*l* (250 mg/100 ml). However in many cases, particularly those with NIDD who have few if any symptoms, and where glycosuria is frequently discovered by chance, the diagnosis is less obvious and a glucose tolerance test will be required.

URINE TESTING. *Glycosuria.* For individual screening purposes sensitive and glucose-specific dip-stick methods are available. Clinistix consists of a paper stick impregnated with an enzyme preparation which turns purple when dipped in urine containing glucose. No other urinary constituent gives this reaction: it therefore provides a rapid and specific qualititative test for glucose. A positive response indicates that the urinary glucose concentration exceeds 0·55–1·11 mmol/*l* (10–20 mg/100 ml), but does not measure the amount accurately. Semiquantitative measurement of urinary reducing activity can be obtained using copper reduction methods, most conveniently with the Clinitest tablet.

If a sample collected during the 2 hours following a meal is examined, then more of the milder cases of diabetes will be recognised than if an overnight specimen is tested. The most serious disadvantage in the use of the urine test diagnostically arises from individual variations in renal threshold, so that on the one hand some undoubtedly diabetic people have a negative urine test for glucose due to a raised renal threshold, and on the other those with a low renal threshold give a false positive test. In order to distinguish cases of this type from patients with mild diabetes, suitable tests of carbohydrate tolerance are required.

*Detection of Ketone Bodies in Urine.* Clinically important amounts of ketone bodies can be recognised by the nitroprusside reaction which is conveniently carried out using Acetest tablets or Ketostix test papers. Ketonuria may be found in normal people who have been fasting for long periods, who have been vomiting repeatedly or who have been eating a diet very high in fats and low in carbohydrate. Ketonuria is therefore not pathognomonic of diabetes, but if both ketonuria and glycosuria are found, the diagnosis of diabetes is practically certain.

RANDOM BLOOD SUGAR. In many cases the clinical diagnosis of diabetes can be made with the help of a single blood sugar estimation, which may be used as the final confirmatory test when the symptoms strongly suggest the diagnosis. In these circumstances a random blood sugar exceeding 14·0 mmol/*l* (250 mg/100 ml) is almost certain to indicate diabetes. However, a random blood sugar below this level does not exclude diabetes, and in this case some degree of standardisation of the conditions under which the blood sugar is measured is necessary. In practice, the oral glucose tolerance test is the cornerstone of the diagnosis of diabetes unless a grossly elevated single blood sugar measurement, with or without clinical symptomatology, has already made this clear.

THE ORAL GLUCOSE TOLERANCE TEST (Fig. 11.5). The patient, who should have been on an unrestricted carbohydrate intake of at least 150 g for 3 days or more, fasts overnight. Out-patients should rest for at least half an hour before starting the test,

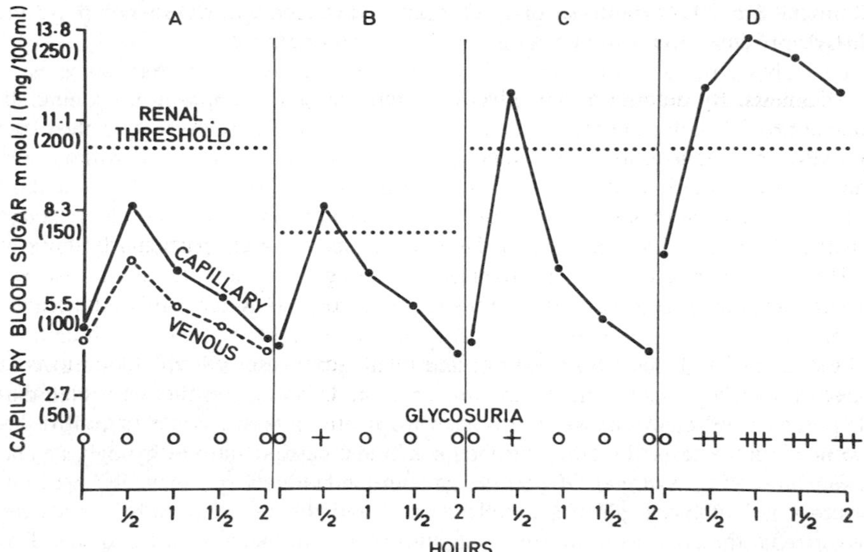


Fig. 11.5 The Glucose Tolerance Test: blood glucose curves after 75 g glucose by mouth, showing (A) normal curve, (B) renal glycosuria, (C) alimentary (lag storage) glycosuria and (D) diabetes mellitus of moderate severity.

and should remain seated and refrain from smoking during the test. A sample of blood is taken to measure the fasting blood glucose level and 50–100 g glucose dissolved in 250 – 350 ml of water is then given by mouth. Thereafter samples of blood are collected at half-hourly intervals for at least 2 hours, and their glucose content is estimated.

The WHO Expert Committee on Diabetes (1980) recommended that a 75g glucose load should be used and that the following concentrations of glucose in venous whole blood (estimated by a specific enzymatic assay) should be accepted as normal or diabetic respectively. Values for plasma glucose are about 15% higher than those for whole blood.

| | Glucose concentration mmol/*l* (mg/100 ml) | |
|---|---|---|
| | Normal | Diabetic |
| Fasting | <5·5 (100) | >7·0 (120) |
| 2 hours after glucose | <7·0 (120) | >10·0 (180) |

Intermediate readings indicate the need for further evaluation of the patient, including the history obtained. It may be necessary to keep the patient under observation and to repeat the test at a later date. In pregnancy those with intermediate readings should be treated as diabetic.

**Differential Diagnosis of Glycosuria.** *Renal Glycosuria.* Apart from diabetes, the commonest cause of glycosuria is a low renal threshold for glucose, or renal glycosuria (p. 423). This is a benign condition unrelated to diabetes. Renal glycosuria also commonly occurs temporarily in pregnancy, due probably in this case to an increase in the glomerular filtration rate. Renal glycosuria is unrelated to diabetes, and is not accompanied by the symptoms of glycosuria in diabetes, i.e. thirst and polyuria, although pruritus vulvae and even ketonuria may occur.

Renal glycosuria is a much more frequent cause of glycosuria than diabetes in young persons, particularly in the age group 20 to 30 years, when they are commonly examined prior to entering the armed services, professions and industry. In the older age groups the reverse holds, and significant hyperglycaemia can occur without any or minimal glycosuria. For this reason if urine tests for glucose are used as a method of screening for diabetes, some cases will be missed, so that a glucose tolerance test or at least a single blood glucose estimation 2 hours after an oral dose of 75 g of glucose should be used whenever possible.

It may be important to determine the renal threshold for glucose; this can be done reliably only by testing samples of urine for glucose taken at intervals of half an hour in the course of a glucose tolerance test and relating the results to the blood glucose concentration (Fig. 11.5). This information may be important in the occasional diabetic with a low renal glucose threshold who, if attempts are made to control his diabetes on urine tests alone, may to be kept in a persistent state of hypoglycaemia.

*Alimentary (Lag Storage) Glycosuria.* In some individuals an unusually rapid but transitory rise of blood glucose follows a meal and the concentration exceeds the normal renal threshold; during this time glucose will be present in the urine. This response to a meal or to a dose of glucose is traditionally known as 'lag storage', although alimentary glycosuria is a better term; it is not uncommon as a cause of symptomless glycosuria. It may occur in otherwise normal people or after a partial gastrectomy, when it is due to rapid absorption, or in patients with hyperthyroidism or hepatic disease. This type of blood glucose curve is usually regarded as benign and unrelated to diabetes; although the peak blood glucose is abnormally elevated, the value 2 hours after oral glucose is normal (Fig. 11.5).

*Other Metabolic Disorders.* Impaired carbohydrate tolerance with associated glycosuria may occur with any of the forms of secondary diabetes (p. 502).

*Carbohydrate deprivation* can lead to the development of a diabetic type of blood glucose curve with associated glycosuria in normal people. It would seem, however, that the daily carbohydrate intake has to be less than about 50 g before it has a notable effect. This effect of a low carbohydrate intake may be of importance clinically in relation to the diagnosis of diabetes in a person on a weight reducing diet or if acutely ill with a low daily intake of food.

## The Management of Diabetes Mellitus

**Aims of Treatment.** The ideal treatment for diabetes would allow the patient to lead a completely normal life, to remain not only symptom-free but in positive good health, to achieve a normal metabolic state, and to escape the complications associated with long-term diabetes. Nowadays diabetic patients rarely die in ketoacidosis in any number, but the major problem which has emerged is the chronic invalidism, due to disease of both large and small blood vessels (p. 523), of many of those whose duration of life has been extended.

Although the relationship between the degree of control and the development of serious diabetic complications is not a simple one, it would appear that the vascular abnormalities are secondary to the metabolic abnormalities occurring in diabetes, since they are found in both primary and secondary diabetes and can be produced experimentally in animals rendered diabetic by various methods. Moreover data from clinical studies strongly suggest that although genetic factors affect the susceptibility to develop complications, the incidence of serious retinopathy is related to the degree of diabetic control achieved. It is therefore incumbent on all those who are involved in looking after diabetic patients to strive in every way to achieve as good control as is practicable in terms of blood glucose concentration.

Bearing these general principles in mind the immediate aims of treatment are therefore, first, the abolition of symptoms of diabetes while avoiding hypoglycaemia, second, the correction of hyperglycaemia and glycosuria and, third, the attainment and maintenance of an appropriate body weight.

Patients should realise as early as possible that it is upon themselves that success or failure will depend. The doctor can only advise. As adherence to a diabetic regimen demands from the patient self-discipline and a sense of purpose, every effort should be made to ensure that the object of each aspect of management is understood. Accordingly, time must be spent on the education of the patient, and the doctor must be responsible for ensuring that all diabetic patients are educated to the limit of their abilities and that as far as possible they have adjusted adequately to their condition and have sufficient knowledge to undertake the day-to-day management of their diabetes competently.

As soon as the diagnosis is certain the patient should be told and instruction and treatment begun forthwith. The average patient suffers initially from an acute anxiety reaction for which explanation is the best remedy. Moreover understanding is likely to lead to better cooperation in treatment.

**Types of Treatment.** There are three methods of treatment, namely diet alone, diet and oral hypoglycaemic drugs and diet and insulin. Each obliges the patient to adhere to a lifelong dietary regimen. Approximately 60% of new cases of diabetes can be controlled adequately by diet alone, about 20% will need an oral hypoglycaemic drug and another 20%, mainly younger patients, will require insulin. The principles governing the choice of therapeutic regimen when a diabetic patient is seen for the first time are discussed on page 515. A patient may pass from one group to another temporarily or permanently.

**Diet.** GENERAL PRINCIPLES. The treatment of all diabetic patients, especially those who require insulin, involves some dietary restrictions if control is to be satisfactory. By regulating the amount and the time of food intake, particularly of carbohydrate, and by dove-tailing the dose of insulin, or of oral hypoglycaemic agent, an attempt is made to achieve a flat profile of glycaemia throughout the day and night. It is obvious that if the intake of food varies from day to day it is impossible to work out a steady insulin or other regime to cover it. Patients should understand that this is the main reason for dietary restriction and not the exclusion of certain 'bad' foods.

If one is to achieve a fixed daily intake and avoid the monotony of a static diet sheet, some kind of exchange system is necessary; this is the basis for the construction of nearly all diets in use today. Many doctors are intimidated by the number and variety of diet sheets published and feel that, since they are not trained dietitians, they cannot treat diabetes. A dietitian is certainly most helpful but is not indispensable; the basic principles of an exchange system of dietary treatment are simple, although the education of a patient in their use is time-consuming.

The first step in preparing any dietary regimen is to map out a time-table of the patient's day including a description of the usual meals. This is an essential step and one which is too often omitted. The total daily requirement of calories must next be decided. The diet must be nutritionally adequate for the patient's needs, and it must, therefore, be estimated for each individual patient after considering such factors as age, sex, actual weight in relation to desirable weight (Table 18.2 p. 905), activity, occupation and financial resources. An approximate range for the various groups might be (1) an obese, middle-aged or elderly patient with mild diabetes 1000–1600 kcal daily, (2) an elderly diabetic but not overweight, 1400–1800 kcal daily, (3) a young, active diabetic, 1800–3000 kcal daily. The body weight must be maintained at or slightly below the ideal for the patient's height. Thus the calorie range of group 2 may have to be extended if it is not sufficient to maintain weight, and young patients in group 3 who are overweight may have to reduce their daily intake to below 1800 kcal, perhaps temporarily.

Next the proportion of calories derived from carbohydrate, protein and fat must be allocated. The approximate ratio in the British national diet is, protein 12%, fat 42% and carbohydrate 46%. Although all sucrose should be eliminated from the diet the percentage of calories derived from carbohydrate should usually remain about the same or be increased slightly, those from protein increased if this is practicable, and those from fat reduced. In most diabetic diets, therefore, the percentage of calories derived from carbohydrate should be 45–50%, from protein 15–20% and about 30–35% from fat.

The daily intake of *carbohydrate* to be prescribed ranges from the minimum sufficient to prevent ketonuria, that is, 100 g daily, to a maximum of 240–260 g. The upper limit is imposed by the fact that it is difficult to achieve satisfactory blood glucose levels throughout 24 hours with a daily carbohydrate intake greater than this. If the daily intake of carbohydrate is 240 g, approximately 50 g carbohydrate will usually be provided by each of the three main meals, 20 g by each of three snacks and 30 g by one pint of milk (540 ml) taken in the course of the day. It is very difficult to prevent an excessive rise in the blood glucose concentration after each meal with amounts larger than this even when all the carbohydrate consumed is in the form of starch. A simple method of calculating the carbohydrate content of the diet is to allocate a figure equivalent to one-tenth of the total calories plus approximately 30–50 g to carbohydrate, that is, if a diet of 1800 kcal is prescribed it should contain about 210 – 230 g of carbohydrate, providing 840 – 920 kcal or approximately 50% of the total. All the carbohydrate eaten should be in the form of starch. Readily absorbed carbohydrates, such as glucose and sucrose, should generally be avoided because they produce a sudden rise in the blood glucose. A high intake of fibre will increase satiety and reduce constipation and may help to lower serum lipid and blood glucose.

The consumption of *protein* is largely determined by social and economic considerations and will frequently be lower than would be considered desirable. If this is the case, every effort should be made to increase the protein intake and to try to ensure that some protein is eaten at each main meal. An adequate consumption of protein is necessary in children and adolescents to ensure satisfactory growth, and since amino acids stimulate the beta cells of the pancreas to secrete insulin, in both normal subjects and those with NIDD, a smaller rise in blood glucose occurs when carbohydrate is consumed along with protein. In both categories of diabetic patients consumption of protein will also promote satiety and so help them to keep more strictly to their carbohydrate allowance. A minimum amount of protein should therefore be specified in all diabetic diets, but in the case of those who are not obese it should be emphasised that more may be taken if desired. The daily consumption of protein will usually lie in the range of 60–110 g.

The *fat* intake should be adjusted to bring the total calories to the level desired, and will usually amount to 50–150 g daily. Because diabetic patients have an increased risk of death from ischaemic heart disease which may be related to the amount of saturated fat in the diet, the total amount of fat should be restricted even in those who are not obese. Plasma lipids, particularly cholesterol, should be checked regularly and if significantly elevated the diabetic diet may be appropriately modified (p. 532).

When the patient's requirements have been assessed the figures must be translated into practical and comprehensible instructions for the patient with the help of a diet sheet (p. 902). Each patient should be given a list of exchanges with instructions regarding the meals at which they may be taken. The diet sheet and exchanges must be discussed with the patient repeatedly and with a relative if necessary until the system is fully understood.

TYPES OF DIET. Basically there are two types of diet: (1) measured, in which the amount of food to be eaten at each time of the day is specified, and (2) unmeasured, in which the patient is supplied with a list of foods grouped in three categories: foods with a high sucrose content which are to be avoided altogether; foods containing carbohydrate in the form of starch which are to be eaten in moderation only; and non-carbohydrate foods which may be eaten as desired.

*Measured Diets.* In these diets the portions of food may be measured either by weighing with scales or more simply by using household measures. Measured diets are required for two groups of patients, (a) those who require insulin or an oral hypoglycaemic agent, and (b) those who are overweight and require a strict reducing regimen.

Patients in group (a) should if at all possible weigh out the portions of food initially. They should be provided with simple dietetic scales for this purpose. After a few weeks most patients are capable of assessing the weight of portions with sufficient accuracy by eye, and regular weighing becomes less necessary. However it is often valuable to check visual assessments by weighing from time to time. A method of constructing a sample diet of 1800 kcal suitable for patients in group (a) is described on page 902. It is important to realise that the exchanges or portions employed as units are arbitrary and are decided mainly in the light of the food habits of the population as a whole. The British Diabetic and Dietetic Associations have recommended that the carbohydrate unit should contain 10 g carbohydrate. In Britain the staple carbohydrate food is bread, and the basic carbohydrate exchange for the purposes of calculation is therefore taken to be $^2/_3$ oz bread which contains 10 g carbohydrate, along with 2 g protein and $^2/_3$ g fat. This is the reason why a carbohydrate exchange contains some protein and fat in addition to carbohydrate. Note also that a protein exchange contains some fat.

Diabetics who are obese should be urged to accept a reducing regime (p. 122). The method of achieving reduction in weight is the same for obese diabetic patients as for those with simple obesity. The diet on page 900 will meet the needs of many. The portions in this diet can be weighed with scales but more usually are dispensed using household measures as described in this diet. It should be explained that such a strict diet is to be followed only temporarily until the standard weight is reached; thereafter the diet may be increased, and if the patient is sufficiently intelligent, advice can then be given on how to avoid monotony by using a list of exchanges for diabetic diets (*Human Nutrition and Dietetics* 1979).

*Unmeasured Diets.* If insulin or oral hypoglycaemic agents are not required and marked obesity is not present it may not be necessary for the patient to follow such an accurate diet. Sometimes it may be impracticable to do so because of the patient's mental, visual or other physical incapacity or unwillingness to cooperate. Many patients develop the disease when they are already middle-aged or elderly and have a mild type of diabetes often associated with moderate obesity. For such patients an unmeasured diet of the type described on page 903 may be adequate.

*Alcohol.* There is no medical objection to taking alcoholic drinks in moderation provided the patient realises that account must be taken of their calorie value and sometimes of their carbohydrate content. Beer may contain 10–30 g of carbohydrate per half litre (1 pint approx.) and with the alcohol this will provide 150–400 kcal, depending on the strength of the beer. Sweet wines and cider all have a high carbohydrate content, and spirits such as whisky and gin, while free of carbohydrates, contain about 70 kcal per 30 ml.

*Sweetening Agents.* Advice may also be asked about sweetening agents and so-called diabetic foods and drinks. Saccharin has been employed as a sweetening agent for many years. It has no calorie value. Sorbitol, a glucose derivative, and fructose are also added to 'diabetic' foods and drinks for sweetening purposes. In moderate quantities neither will interfere with the action or requirements of insulin. If a patient is having difficulty in reducing weight or in maintaining a normal weight, then the use of substitutes for sugar should be discouraged, since they may perpetuate the patient's desire to eat sweet foods and thus make it more difficult to tolerate dietary restrictions. Diabetic chocolate has a high fat content and this must be taken into account.

**Oral Hypoglycaemic Drugs.** A number of compounds are effective in reducing hyperglycaemia in patients who would otherwise require insulin. The sulphonylureas, tolbutamide and chlorpropamide, and to a lesser extent the biguanide, metformin, have a place in the management of about 20% of diabetic patients. Although their mechanism of action is different, the action of both groups depends upon a supply of endogenous insulin, and it is therefore futile and dangerous to attempt to control IDD with these compounds.

SULPHONYLUREAS. These drugs are valuable in the treatment of patients with NIDD who fail to respond to simple dietary restriction and who are not overweight.

*Tolbutamide* is the mildest, and probably also the safest, of the sulphonylureas. Since its effective action does not exceed 6 to 8 hours it should be administered two to three times a day. The dose varies between 1 and 2 g daily. It is very well tolerated and toxic reactions such as rashes occur only rarely. Tolbutamide is a useful drug in the elderly where the risk and the consequences of inducing hypoglycaemia are increased. Unfortunately, the relapse rate is relatively high.

*Chlorpropamide* has a biological half-life of about 36 hours, and an effective concentration can be maintained in the blood by a single dose at breakfast. The usual maintenance dose is between 100 and 375 mg daily; larger doses should not be used on a long-term basis, since above this level there is an increased risk of toxic effects, such as jaundice, rashes, and blood dyscrasia.

If alcohol is taken following chlorpropamide an unpleasant flushing of the face occurs in some patients. This is a dominantly-inherited trait associated with NIDD. The demonstration that this reaction can be blocked with naloxone suggests that these patients may have inherited an unusual sensitivity to endorphins.

Chlorpropamide may lead to severe hypoglycaemia, which can be very refractory to treatment. Great care must be taken to avoid this, particularly in elderly patients, and once glycosuria has been abolished and symptoms relieved, the daily dose of chlorpropamide must be reduced to the minimum required to maintain control. In fact many patients who require 375–500 mg daily initially can be maintained on a long-term basis on 100 mg or less per day.

*Other sulphonylureas* such as acetohexamide, tolazamide, glibenclamide, glipizide and glymidine usually offer little advantage over chlorpropamide but may be useful in individual patients.

BIGUANIDES. The biguanides, metformin and phenformin, are less widely used in Britain than the sulphonylureas, because of the higher incidence of side-effects, particularly gastrointestinal symptoms and because there have been a significant number of deaths from lactic acidosis in patients taking these drugs, particularly phenformin. However, metformin is useful in two clinical situations. Firstly, since its administration is not associated with an increase in weight it may be preferred when it is essential to treat a patient with NIDD who is overweight but in whom hyperglycaemia persists despite efforts to adhere to a diet and reduce weight. Secondly, as the hypoglycaemic effect of the biguanides appears to be synergistic with that of the sulphonylureas, there is a place for combining the two when the sulphonylureas alone have proved inadequate and when, as happens with 5 to 10% of patients, initial success is followed after several months, or even years, by loss of control.

Metformin is given with food in two or three daily doses of 0·5–1·0 g each. Its use is contraindicated in patients with impaired renal or hepatic function and in those who take alcohol in excess, as the risk of lactic acidosis occurring is significantly increased in such patients. Its administration should be discontinued, at least temporarily, if any other serious medical condition develops, and treatment with insulin substituted.

CLINICAL USE OF SULPHONYLUREAS AND BIGUANIDES. Patients may be started on an oral hypoglycaemic drug as soon as it is clear that dietary measures alone are inadequate. Evidence of some response is usually apparent within a week, though a full response may not occur for considerably longer. Diabetics treated successfully in this way for prolonged periods may ultimately need an alteration of dose or a change of regime temporarily or permanently; in particular they may require insulin to meet the need created by a severe infection, an operation or other stress.

There is some evidence that those taking an oral hypoglycaemic drug are at increased risk of dying from ischaemic heart disease. This may be due to a high incidence of ventricular fibrillation in diabetic patients on oral therapy who sustain a myocardial infarct. Efforts should therefore be made to control as many patients as possible by diet alone for this and other reasons (p. 515). Furthermore those taking oral hypoglycaemic drugs who develop a myocardial infarct should have these replaced by insulin during the acute illness and have a longer period of close supervision than non-diabetics, preferably in a coronary care unit.

**Insulin.** With one or more of the preparations of insulin available it is usually possible to keep the blood glucose within reasonable, although not physiological, limits throughout the day and night without undue risk of hypoglycaemia.

Two main therapeutic forms of insulin are available, namely (1) unmodified, rapid-onset, short-acting and (2) modified or depot, delayed-onset, long acting preparations. There are various varieties of each type some of which are shown in Table 11.1. The older insulins contain varying amounts of glucagon, pro-insulin, altered insulin and other peptides, which are largely responsible for the insulin-binding antibodies found in the plasma of all patients treated with these insulins. Highly purified, 'monocomponent' or 'single peak' insulins are now available which are much less antigenic and are gradually superseding the older preparations. Care must be taken to avoid hypoglycaemia when transferring patients from the older to the newer preparations, and the higher the dose of conventional insulin, the stricter the super-

Table 11.1 Main types of insulin and duration of effect

| Type | *Approximate* duration of effect in hours |
|---|---|
| *Rapid/Short* — unmodified | |
| Soluble (Regular) Insulin Injection<br>Neutral Insulin Injection | 6 |
| *Intermediate* — modified — depot | |
| Insulin Zinc Suspension Amorphous (Semilente) | 12 |
| Isophane Insulin Injection | 12+ |
| *Slow/Long* — modified — depot | |
| Insulin Zinc Suspension Crystalline (Ultralente)<br>Protamine Zinc Insulin Injection | 24 |

All these insulins are available in 'highly purified' form. This description covers several levels of purity since no precise specifications for purity are available at present.

vision required. Insulins are available in concentrations of 20, 40, 80 and 100 International Units per ml. If required they may also be supplied in a concentration of 320 and 500 IU/ml.

UNMODIFIED INSULINS. These are clear solutions in contrast to the depot insulins which are cloudy. When injected subcutaneously, unmodified insulin is effective in 20–30 mins but the action is relatively short-lived (Table 11.1). A patient stabilised on unmodified insulin alone would therefore need at least two injections in the day.

Unmodified insulin is essential in (1) new cases with severe dehydration or ketoacidosis (2) emergencies associated with ketosis, such as acute infection, gastroenteritis and some surgical operations and (3) the treatment of nearly all young patients.

MODIFIED (DEPOT) INSULINS. In some elderly patients with mild diabetes satisfactory control can be established by a single morning injection of depot insulin. Most insulin-requiring diabetics however need a depot insulin with one or two supporting doses of unmodified insulin to achieve good control throughout 24 hours. The choice of depot insulin in an individual case is determined by consideration of the patient's way of life, including the meal pattern, type of occupation, hours of work and recreation, in relation to the time of action of the various depot insulins. More insulin will be required to cover main meals and periods of inactivity, and vice versa.

*Protamine Zinc Insulin (PZI).* The addition of zinc and protamine to unmodified insulin delays its release from the site of injection, so that the effect of PZI is slow to start and is prolonged. Despite its prolonged action PZI alone does not usually keep the blood glucose within acceptable limits throughout the 24 hours. Glycosuria is most likely to occur before the morning injection has taken full effect, and an additional dose of unmodified insulin is generally required in the morning and sometimes in the evening, especially in young patients. Merely to increase the morning dose of PZI may result in severe hypoglycaemia later in the day or night. Indeed it is a good rule that the dose of PZI should not exceed 40 units at a single injection. When giving unmodified insulin and PZI together, the two should not be mixed in the syringe since the excess protamine in the PZI will convert some of the unmodified insulin into PZI.

*Insulin Zinc Suspensions (IZS).* The rate of release of these insulins from the tissues is related to the size of the insulin particles which are suspended in acetate buffer. Three preparations are available: (1) IZS amorphous (*semilente*) insulin has a duration of action which is intermediate between that of unmodified and protamine zinc insulin. (2) IZS crystalline (*ultralente*) insulin is slower in action than IZS amorphous insulin (Table 11.1). (3) IZS (*lente*) insulin is a mixture of three parts of amorphous with seven parts crystalline.

*Isophane insulin* is another depot insulin similar in action to PZI, though its effect is less prolonged. Since isophane insulin contains an excess of unmodified insulin it can be mixed in the same syringe as unmodified insulin. This is convenient particularly if an automatic injector is used. Many younger patients are best treated with highly purified isophane and soluble insulin taken twice daily.

In practice one must be prepared to try combinations of the various insulin preparations, and to vary the time at which they are administered in the light of the results of urine tests and blood glucose estimations at different times of the day until smooth control is achieved over 24 hours. It is impossible to forecast the response of a patient to insulin, and the daily dose required to establish control varies from 10 to 100 units or more.

**Choice of Therapeutic Regime.** It must be emphasised that the regime eventually adopted in each case of diabetes is chosen by a process of trial, and that changes may be needed as more is learned about the patient. The chief indications for the main types of therapeutic regimen are:

1. Practically all young patients who develop diabetes before the age of 40 require treatment with insulin. The majority will be best controlled by taking unmodified insulin along with one of the depot insulins in the morning, and a second dose of unmodified insulin, or of unmodified and depot insulin before the evening meal. Examples of suitable preparations are Velosinsulin and Insulatard (Nordisk Laboratories) or Actrapid MC and Semitard MC or Monotard MC (Novo Industries) taken twice daily.
2. The majority of patients developing the disease over the age of 40 can and should be controlled by diet alone. This applies particularly to obese patients, but others who are not overweight may also do well on dietary therapy alone.
3. Those over the age of 40 who fail to achieve satisfactory control by dietary measures alone will usually respond well to a sulphonylurea if they are not obese, or to a biguanide if they are obese. If adequate control is not achieved by one drug, a combination of sulphonylurea and biguanide may be tried. If this fails insulin will be required.
4. Elderly patients who require insulin will often do well with a relatively small dose (20 units) of a depot insulin alone. A few, particularly those who would otherwise require more than 40 units a day, should be given unmodified insulin in addition and some may require insulin twice daily.

It must be stressed again that obese patients should be treated by dietary restriction and weight reduction rather than by the administration of insulin or oral hypoglycaemic agent. The advent of the 'insulin era' has obscured the remarkable improvement in glucose tolerance which usually results from reduction in weight. Insulin and the sulphonylureas increase the appetite, and thus may increase weight and intensify the total disability.

**Initiation of Treatment.** It is desirable that the patient learns to manage all aspects of the disorder as quickly as possible, and this can best be done on an outpatient basis while leading a relatively normal existence at home and at work. However, patients being stabilised on insulin have to be seen daily at first and if this is not practicable, admission to hospital will be necessary. Hospital admission will also be necessary for patients with severe ketoacidosis. The therapeutic plan must include measures directed at any of the complications to which the diabetic is prone and which may already be present at diagnosis, namely coronary artery disease and hypertension, obliterative arterial disease, nephropathy, retinopathy, cataract, neuropathy, pulmonary tuberculosis and other infections, particularly of the skin and urinary tract (p. 525).

A practical point worth mentioning, since it may give rise to distress if not anticipated, is that blurring of vision, which may occur in a severe diabetic before treatment, may become noticeably worse after starting treatment with insulin or tablets. It is due to transitory osmotic abnormalities in the eye, especially the lens, and may persist for as long as several weeks after initiating treatment.

PATIENT'S EDUCATION. Every patient who is capable of learning must be taught how to test his urine with a Clinitest set (and sometimes with Acetest tablets also), to keep a record of the results and to understand their significance.

All patients requiring insulin must learn to measure their dose of insulin accurately with an insulin syringe, to give their own injections and to adjust the dose themselves on the basis of urine and/or blood tests and other factors such as illness, unusual exercise and insulin reactions. They should be made to experience an insulin reaction (p. 518).

All patients must have a working knowledge of diabetes, i.e. they must be able to recognise the symptoms associated with marked glycosuria and to understand their significance. They must be told that many drugs have undesirable effects on the diabetic state, as may also such other factors as illness of any kind or emotional upset. They should be advised to consult their doctor or clinic at once as soon as they are aware of any deterioration in health or urine tests which does not respond rapidly to the simple measures that they take themselves.

All patients must know how to take care of their feet, and learn to treat any infected lesion with respect. Regular chiropody is important especially for elderly patients.

Education of the patient is time-consuming and repeated practical demonstrations may also be required. It may be supplemented by reading appropriate booklets. It is only in this way that diabetic patients can safely undertake all normal activities while maintaining good control of their disease. If the patient is a child, or is blind, mentally defective or otherwise incapable, instructions must be given to a parent or other attendant.

It is a wise precaution for diabetic patients who are taking insulin or oral hypoglycaemic drugs to carry a card with them at all times stating their name and address, the fact that they are diabetic, the nature and dose of any insulin or other drugs they may be taking, and, in addition, giving the name, address and telephone number of their family doctor and any special diabetic clinic they may be attending. Suitable cards are provided by the British Diabetic Association for the use of members.

SUPERVISION OF PATIENT. Diabetics should be seen at regular intervals for the remainder of their lives. The object is to check the degree of control and if necessary to make appropriate alterations in treatment and to watch for any complications. Records should be kept so that the doctor is immediately on the alert if changes in health occur. The frequency of visits is determined by the severity of the disability and the reliability of the patient. For the general practitioner with diabetic patients scattered widely in his practice, this supervision may be difficult. For this reason and because of the need to develop and apply new and better techniques for the control of diabetes, many hospitals arrange diabetic clinics.

ASSESSMENT OF CONTROL. At the patient's regular visit to the diabetic clinic or general practitioner, the degree of control should be assessed by considering the patient's weight in relation to standard weight, the results of urine tests, the blood glucose concentration and the presence or absence of symptoms of either hyper- or hypoglycaemia.

*Urine Testing.* Proper assessment of control is impossible unless in the course of normal activity the patient tests samples of urine regularly. By selecting suitable times for the tests and tabulating the results, it is easy for the doctor or the experienced patient to decide whether the dose of insulin or hypoglycaemic drug should be changed, or whether the carbohydrate content of the diet or the time when it is taken should be altered.

Diabetics taking insulin should test samples of urine obtained before breakfast, before the mid-day and evening meals, and at bedtime (prior to a bedtime snack if this is taken). The patient must empty the bladder and discard the urine about 30 minutes before passing a specimen for testing. Patients treated by diet alone or with oral hypoglycaemic agents should test the first morning specimen and a sample passed about 2 hours after the main meals of the day. The majority of all the above specimens should be either free of glucose or contain ¼% or less.

While the patient is being stabilised, tests will have to be carried out three or four times daily; when control is established the frequency can be greatly reduced. One daily preprandial test taken serially at different times of the day is much more informative about the state of control than a single test carried out at the same time daily. Alternatively, three or four tests can be performed on a single day once or twice weekly.

*Blood Glucose Estimations.* It is advisable to measure the blood glucose concentration at different times of the day as an additional index of the degree of control. Some patients can be taught to take capillary blood samples and measure the blood glucose concentration in these by means of enzyme impregnated sticks (Dextrostix), if possible with a simple colorimetric meter, to improve accuracy. In assessing the result it is important to consider the interval between taking the sample and the last meal and also previous physical activity. The aim should be to keep the fasting blood glucose level less than 7·0 mmol/*l* (120 mg/100 ml) and the post-prandial peak under 10·0 mmol/*l* (180 mg/100 ml).

*Glycosylated Haemoglobin ($HbA_1$).* When haemoglobin from a normal adult is passed through a chromatographic column it separates into the major component HbA (94% of the total) and several minor, faster-moving components collectively known as $HbA_1$ (6% of the total). These are structurally identical to HbA except for the addition of a glucose group to the terminal aminoacid of the $\beta$ chain. This is a post-synthetic, non-enzymatic reaction and the rate of synthesis of $HbA_1$ is a function of the blood glucose concentration. Since the glucose linkage is relatively stable, $HbA_1$ accumulates throughout the life span of the erythrocyte and its concentration reflects the mean blood glucose concentration over the previous few months. Measurement of $HbA_1$ can therefore be used as a supplement to urine tests and blood glucose estimations to monitor the degree of diabetic control achieved.

**Insulin Reactions and Hypoglycaemia.** If unmodified insulin is administered to a normal person the blood glucose falls, producing symptoms that may begin to appear when the concentration is about 2·7 mmol/*l* (50 mg/100 ml) and are fully developed at about 2·2 mmol/*l*. In diabetics who are constantly hyperglycaemic, the same symptoms may develop at much higher levels, e.g. 6·6 mmol/*l* or more. The symptoms may include any one or more of the following: a feeling of being weak and empty, hunger, sweating, palpitation, tremor, faintness, dizziness, headache, diplopia and mental confusion. Abnormal behaviour, leading occasionally to arrest on a charge of being drunk and disorderly, may also occur. Alternatively, and particularly in children, there may be lassitude and somnolence or muscular twitchings. Eventually coma, sometimes with convulsions, may follow.

Hypoglycaemia induces secretion of adrenaline, and this in turn causes tachycardia and tremor. Adrenaline, by mobilising liver glycogen, combats the hypoglycaemia. This homeostatic reaction partly explains why patients rarely die of hypoglycaemic coma from too much unmodified insulin. By contrast, coma is dangerous when it arises from a large dose of depot insulin or from an overdose of a sulphonylurea, particularly chlorpropamide. The latter condition although relatively uncommon is resistant to treatment, since the drug reduces the hepatic release of glucose, and because the half-life of the drug is so long. The brain is dependent on the blood glucose for the energy necessary for its activity. Permanent brain damage may result from prolonged hypoglycaemia which should be prevented from recurring by prompt reduction of the dose of insulin or of sulphonylurea.

Hypoglycaemia due to overdosage with unmodified insulin comes on rapidly, at the time when the insulin is having its maximum effect that is, through the morning or in the early evening, and usually elicits classical symptoms and responds rapidly to treatment. Reactions from excessive depot insulin given before breakfast usually occur in the later afternoon, at night or early next morning. These reactions may begin gradually with little adrenaline response, become persistent and profound and respond more slowly to treatment. The predominant warning symptoms are very variable and include headache, malaise, night sweats, nausea leading sometimes to troublesome vomiting, mental confusion and drowsiness, especially in the morning.

TREATMENT OF HYPOGLYCAEMIC REACTIONS. Since hypoglycaemia can easily be corrected if recognised early, diabetic patients should experience the condition under supervision. In this way they learn to recognise the early symptoms. They must be made to realise that the most frequent causes of the condition are unpunctual meals and unaccustomed exercise, and seek to avoid both or to make adjustments to meet these circumstances. They should always carry some tablets of glucose or a few lumps of sugar for use in an emergency. Unless an attack of hypoglycaemia is adequately accounted for, the patient should reduce the next and subsequent doses of insulin by 20% and seek medical advice.

If the patient is so stuporous that swallowing is impossible an intravenous injection of 25 g of glucose (50 ml of a 50% solution) should be given. This may have to be repeated. Alternatively, the insulin-dependent patient may be given a subcutaneous or intramuscular injection of 1 mg of glucagon, repeated if necessary after 10 minutes. This raises the blood glucose by mobilising liver glycogen, and has the advantage of convenience in that it can be given by anybody capable of using a syringe, but it may not be effective in severe and prolonged hypoglycaemia due to depot insulins. In addition to increasing hepatic glycogenolysis, glucagon stimulates the secretion of insulin and therefore should not be used to treat hypoglycaemia induced by an oral hypoglycaemic agent.

As soon as the patient is able to swallow, glucose should be given orally. Full recovery may not occur immediately. Further, when hypoglycaemia has occurred in a diabetic using a depot preparation of insulin or a sulphonylurea, particularly chlorpropamide, the possibility of relapse within a day or more should be anticipated.

Repeated episodes of hypoglycaemia may lead to permanent intellectual deterioration; accordingly, adjustments to prevent recurrences are essential.

## The Complications of Diabetes Mellitus

### Diabetic Ketoacidosis

Prior to the discovery of insulin more than 50% of diabetic patients ultimately died of ketoacidosis. Today this complication is preventable and accounts for less than 2% of diabetic deaths. However, both the incidence and the mortality rate are still regrettably high. Failure of the patient to understand the disease, and failure to appreciate the significance of symptoms of poor control are the most common causes. Thus its prevention is largely a problem of education of patients and at times of their physicians. A clear understanding of the biochemical disorders involved (p. 503) is essential for its efficient treatment which should aim at having the patient out of danger within 24 hours.

*Water and Mineral Depletion.* The deficit of total body water in a severe case may be about 6 litres. About half of this is derived from the intracellular compartment and occurs comparatively early in the development of acidosis with relatively few clinical features; the remainder represents loss of extracellular fluid sustained largely in the later stages. It is at this time that marked contraction of the size of the extracellular space occurs, with haemoconcentration, a decrease in plasma volume, and finally a fall in blood pressure with associated renal ischaemia and oliguria.

The concentration of sodium and potassium in the serum gives very little indication of total body losses, and may even be raised due to disproportionate losses of water. Sodium loss, mainly from the extracellular space, may amount to as much as 500 mmol. Potassium loss from the cells may be 400 mmol or more. The concentration of potassium in the plasma in these circumstances is dependent on the balance between catabolism of protein and glycogen and haemoconcentration on the one hand, and urinary excretion on the other. Since the former generally exceeds the latter plasma potassium is likely to be high initially, in spite of a total body deficit. However, within a few hours of beginning treatment with insulin, there is likely to be a precipitous fall in the plasma potassium. At least three mechanisms are responsible for this; dilution of extracellular potassium by the administration of potassium-free fluids, the movement of potassium into the cells as the result of insulin therapy, and the continuing renal loss of potassium.

*Ketoacidosis.* The mechanism of the development of this state has been described (p. 504). Apart from the clinical findings, its severity can be rapidly assessed by measuring the plasma bicarbonate, less than 12 mmol/*l* indicating severe acidosis. The hydrogen ion concentration in the blood is an even more valuable guide but it may not be as readily available. There are no simple and accurate quantitative methods for the determination of plasma ketones.

**Clinical Features.** Any form of stress, particularly an acute infection, can precipitate severe ketoacidosis in even the mildest diabetic. The most common cause is neglect of treatment due to carelessness, misunderstanding or illness, and failure to adjust the therapeutic regimen in the event of an acute infection.

The symptoms of diabetic ketoacidosis invariably include intense thirst and polyuria. Constipation, cramps and altered vision are common. Sometimes, especially in children, there is abdominal pain, with or without vomiting. Hence diabetic ketoacidosis is important in the differential diagnosis of the acute abdomen. Weakness and drowsiness are commonly present, but it should be remembered that the state of consciousness is very variable and a patient with dangerous ketosis requiring urgent treatment may walk into hosptial. For this reason the term diabetic ketoacidosis is to be preferred to 'diabetic coma', which suggests that there is no urgency until unconsciousness occurs. In fact it is imperative that energetic treatment is started at the earliest possible stage.

The signs include a dry tongue and soft eyeballs due to dehydration; 'air hunger' indicated by long, deep, sighing respirations; a rapid, weak pulse, and low blood pressure; sometimes abdominal rigidity and tenderness; the smell of acetone in the breath; ultimately coma supervenes.

*Investigation* shows (1) ketonuria and severe glycosuria; (2) blood glucose usually between 22·2 and 44·4 mmol/*l* (400 and 800 mg/100 ml), but it may be much higher and in some cases lower; (3) low plasma bicarbonate and blood pH; (4) normal or raised serum sodium and potassium; (5) leucocytosis.

Hyperglycaemia and ketoacidosis do not always necessarily correlate well. Even at a level of blood glucose as low as 19·4 mmol/*l* (350 mg/100 ml), life-threatening acidosis may be present. In contrast diabetic coma can occur, usually in elderly patients, with extreme hyperglycaemia and dehydration but no ketoacidosis. This is known as *hyperosmolar diabetic coma*.

**Treatment.** Ketoacidosis should be treated with urgency in hospital. Intravenous therapy is required since even when the patient is able to swallow, fluids given by mouth may be poorly absorbed. Establishing an intravenous infusion can be technically difficult because of collapsed veins, but cutting down and tying in a cannula should be avoided if at all possible, because the veins may be needed again. Treatment must be checked against the blood concentration of glucose, potassium and bicarbonate estimated at intervals at first of not longer than 2 hours. Only in this way can the metabolic disorder be corrected accurately and rapidly. The aim should be to overcome with all speed: (1) ketosis, by means of insulin to permit glucose utilisation; (2) shock, acidosis, and water and electrolyte depletion, by means of appropriate intravenous fluids; (3) infection, if present, by means of antibiotics.

Only unmodified insulins should be used. Ketosis and dehydration render the comatose patient relatively resistant to insulin. The conventional treatment of diabetic ketoacidosis has, therefore, involved the use of large doses of unmodified insulin. It is now known that such large doses of insulin are unnecessary and that low-dose regimens are just as effective, are less complicated and may be safer. An infusion of saline is started and 20 units of unmodified insulin given by intramuscular injection immediately and 4–6 units hourly thereafter, either by intramuscular injection or intravenous infusion, preferably using a constant-rate pump. The blood glucose concentration should fall by 3–6 mmol/*l*/hour. If there is no fall in the blood glucose concentration by two hours after starting treatment, then the dose of insulin should be doubled until a satisfactory response is obtained. When the blood glucose concentration has fallen to 10·0mmol/*l* (180 mg/100 ml) 5% glucose should replace or be added to the saline infusion and the dose of insulin reduced to 1–3 units i.v. hourly, or 8–16 units four hourly by subcutaneous injection.

The deficit of extracellular fluid, which is usually about 3 litres, should be made good by infusion of saline isotonic with plasma (0·9% NaCl). A suitable regimen is 1 litre in half an hour, 1 litre in one hour, and then 1 litre in two hours until there is clinical improvement. Elderly patients or those with cardiovascular disease will require modification of this regimen and monitoring of central venous pressure may be necessary. If during treatment the serum sodium rises above 150 mmol/*l*, 0·45% saline should be given.

In cases which are also severely acidotic (pH <7.0), 500 ml of the isotonic saline may be replaced by isotonic sodium bicarbonate (1·4%) and this may be repeated if the pH remains < 7·1 mmol/*l*. Correction of the total deficit should not be attempted since there is some evidence that rapid correction of acidosis in diabetic ketoacidosis may aggravate tissue hypoxia and may also reduce the level of consciousness by causing a paradoxical acidosis of the cerebrospinal fluid. The combined administration of bicarbonate and insulin will also increase the risk of hypokalaemia and potassium should be given along with bicarbonate.

The intracellular deficit of water, usually about 2–3 litres, must be replaced by giving 5% glucose and not by more saline. It is best given when the blood glucose is approaching normal. It is important to continue the intravenous glucose together with appropriate doses of insulin until the ketonuria has disappeared and the water deficit has been made good.

Shock should be treated as described on page 167.

Every patient in diabetic ketoacidosis is potassium depleted and nearly all will require intravenous potassium (p. 132) to prevent the development of dangerous hypokalaemia during the course of treatment. As the serum potassium is often high at presentation, potassium therapy should be started cautiously and carefully monitored by frequent estimations of plasma potassium. ECG is sometimes helpful, a change in the T wave indicating a falling plasma potassium. Approximately 80 mmols of potassium may safely be given by vein in the first 16 hours, but much more than this may be required and sufficient must be given to maintain a normal plasma concentration. It is customary to add 1·5 g potassium chloride (20 mmol potassium) to each 500 ml of fluid given intravenously. Once oral feeding has started potassium chloride (p. 132) should be given four hourly for two to three days to restore the total body deficit.

In a stuporose or comatose patient, gastric aspiration should be undertaken to avoid the risk of inhaling vomitus. The stomach will often contain a large amount of brown fluid containing altered blood.

Infections must be carefully sought and vigorously treated since it may not be possible to abolish ketosis until they are controlled.

Once ketosis has been overcome and the salt and water deficit made good (usually in about 24 hours), feeding by mouth can be started with frequent small fluid feeds each containing 25 g carbohydrate. Two examples of such feeds are:

1. 100 ml (3½ oz) fruit juice plus 15 g (½ oz) of cane sugar or glucose.
2. 200 ml (7 ozs) milk plus 10 g (⅓ oz) cereal plus 7g (¼ oz) sugar.

Sufficient insulin should be given to prevent further ketonuria or glycosuria. Control of blood glucose can be lost very quickly and frequent blood glucose estimations are needed. Unmodified insulin should be given before each oral feed, even if the urine is free of sugar and only very small doses are required.

HYPEROSMOLAR, NON-KETOTIC DIABETIC COMA. Treatment differs from that of ketoacidotic coma in two main respects. These patients seem to be relatively sensitive to insulin and it is probably best to give approximately half the dose of insulin usually employed in diabetic ketoacidosis. Once it is known that plasma osmolality is high (calculated by the formula 2 × sodium mmol/*l* + glucose mmol/*l* = 285 mosmol/*l* normally) 0·45% saline should be given until the osmolality approaches normal, when 0·9% should be substituted.

COMA DUE TO LACTIC ACIDOSIS. Clinically the patient is likely to be a diabetic taking a biguanide, who is very ill and overbreathing, but not so profoundly dehydrated as is usual in coma due to ketoacidosis, and whose breath does not smell of acetone. Ketonuria is no more than mild, yet plasma bicarbonate and pH are markedly reduced. Diagnosis is confirmed by a high (usually >5·0 mmol/*l*) concentration of lactic acid in the blood. Treatment is with large amounts of intravenous bicarbonate; as much as 2500 mmols may be needed. Insulin is given by continuous intravenous infusion and glucose added when the blood level falls to about 10·0 mmol/*l*. Dialysis may be required in very severe cases (pH <7) if sodium overload results from the administration of large quantities of sodium bicarbonate. Despite such measures the mortality in this condition is greater than 50%.

**Differential Diagnosis of Coma in a Diabetic.** Confusion between coma due to hypoglycaemia and that associated with ketosis should seldom arise; the distinction is clear (Table 11.2). Diabetic coma may occasionally pass undetected into hypoglycaemic coma through too enthusiastic treatment; likewise, vomiting induced by hypoglycaemia from a depot insulin may continue until diabetic coma develops.

Table 11.2 Differential diagnosis of coma in a diabetic

| | *Hypoglycaemic Coma* | *Coma with Ketosis* |
|---|---|---|
| History: | no food; too much insulin; unaccustomed exercise | too little or no insulin; an infection; digestive disturbance |
| Onset: | in good previous health; related to last insulin injection | ill-health for several days |
| Symptoms: | of hypoglycaemia; occasional vomiting from depot insulins | of glycosuria and dehydration; abdominal pain and vomiting |
| Signs: | moist skin and tongue<br>full pulse<br>normal or raised BP<br>shallow or normal breathing<br>brisk reflexes | dry skin and tongue<br>weak pulse<br>low blood pressure<br>air hunger<br>diminished reflexes |
| Urine: | no ketonuria<br>no glycosuria, if bladder recently emptied | ketonuria<br>glycosuria |
| Blood: | hypoglycaemia<br>normal plasma bicarbonate | hyperglycaemia<br>reduced plasma bicarbonate |

## Vascular Disorders

Vascular disease, arterial, arteriolar and capillary, is the largest and most intractable problem in clinical diabetes. Arterial disease is easily the commonest cause of death in diabetics over the age of 50, while nephropathy accounts for more than half the deaths under 50. Strict control probably offers the best chance of delaying the onset and progress of the vascular complications of diabetes.

Atherosclerosis occurs commonly and extensively in diabetes. The pathological changes in diabetics are not specific in a qualitative sense but they occur earlier and are more widespread than in non-diabetics. Thus diabetics are more prone at an earlier age than other people to myocardial infarction and hypertension. The peripheral pulses in the legs are often diminished or impalpable, and particularly in elderly patients, intermittent claudication and ischaemic changes in the feet are frequently present. Defective circulation in the legs resulting in poorly nourished tissues predisposes to gangrene. If a painless peripheral neuropathy is present, this may also be of aetiological importance, since the patient will tend to ignore or neglect injuries and other damage to the tissues. Diabetic gangrene usually starts in one foot, following a trivial injury, such as the cutting of a corn, or a burn from a hot water bottle. Toxic absorption from necrotic tissue and secondary infection may kill the patient unless the limb is amputated. A great deal can be done to prevent these complications by instructing diabetics with a poor circulation to wear properly fitting shoes, to use bed-socks rather than hot water bottles, never to cut their own corns and 'to keep the feet as clean as the face'. The services of a skilled chiropodist are invaluable.

### Diabetic Nephropathy

*Diabetic Glomerulosclerosis.* A specific type of renal lesion may occur as a result of the changes in the basement membrane of the glomerular capillaries. There are two types, diffuse and nodular. The former is the more common and consists of a generalised thickening of the basement membrane. The nodular type is a development of this, in which rounded masses of hyaline material sometimes called Kimmelstiel-Wilson bodies are superimposed upon the diffuse lesion. Diabetic glomerulosclerosis can be seen by light microscopy in about 70% of diabetic patients at autopsy. Even with well-established diabetic glomerulosclerosis the patient may exhibit only slight to moderate proteinuria. In some cases, however, marked proteinuria and nephrosis develop with increasing renal failure and uraemia.

There is no way of preventing or modifying the progression of nephropathy once this is clinically apparent as proteinuria. In the later stages the management is the same as in other forms of chronic renal disease. Regular haemodialysis is technically possible although access to the circulation or maintenance of a shunt may be affected by diseased peripheral vessels. Results are less good than in non-diabetics and may not justify the burden placed on the patient. The place of continuous ambulatory peritoneal dialysis (p. 440) is still uncertain. Renal transplantation is more hopeful and in some centres results, in carefully selected cases, are almost as good as in non-diabetics. Unfortunately many will not qualify for active intervention because of other disabilities such as severe large blood vessel disease, neuropathy, and retinopathy.

### Diabetic Retinopathy

Retinopathy is the commonest long-term complication of diabetes. In most cases it produces no symptoms but it can cause blindness and in Britain diabetic retinopathy is now the single most common cause of blindness in the middle-aged.

**Clinical Features.** These are shown in Plate II (p. 531) and occur in varying combinations in different patients. Abnormalities of the capillary bed are the earliest lesions. They include capillary dilatation and closure which are not clinically visible.

In most cases *microaneurysms* are the earliest clinical abnormality detected. They appear as minute, discrete, circular, dark-red spots near to, but apparently separate from, the retinal vessels. They look like tiny haemorrhages but photography of injected preparations of retina show that they are in fact minute aneurysms arising mainly from the venous end of capillaries near areas of capillary closure. *Venous abnormalities* are among the commonest manifestations of diabetic retinopathy. Dilatation, irregularity and increased tortuosity of the retinal veins are all seen. *Haemorrhages*, most characteristically occurring in the deeper layers of the retina and hence round and regular in shape, are also a relatively early feature. The smaller ones may be difficult to differentiate from microaneurysms and the two are often grouped together as 'dots and blots'. *Soft exudates*, similar to those seen in hypertension, occur and represent areas of infarction. *Hard exudates* are more common and are specific to diabetic retinopathy. They are yellow, with irregular, sharply defined edges, varying in size from tiny specks to large confluent often circular patches. They probably result from leakage of plasma from abnormal retinal capillaries and lie over areas of neuronal degeneration. *New vessels* may arise from mature vessels on the optic disc or the retina. The earliest appearance is that of fine tufts of delicate vessels forming arcades on the surface of the retina. As they grow they may extend forwards towards the vitreous. They are fragile, readily leak and at first have no visible connective tissue covering. They are liable to rupture, causing haemorrhage which may be intraretinal, preretinal (subhyaloid) or intô the vitreous. Serous products leaking from these new vessel systems stimulate a connective tissue reaction *retinitis proliferans*. This first appears as a white cloudy haze among the network of new vessels. As it extends the new vessels are obliterated and the surrounding retina is covered by a dense white sheet. At this stage bleeding is less common but retinal detachment can occur due to contraction of adhesions between the vitreous and the retina.

CLASSIFICATION. Patients with only microaneurysms, retinal haemorrhages and exudates are classified as having *simple* or *background retinopathy*, while those with preretinal haemorrhage, new vessel formation, or fibrous proliferation are classified as having *proliferative* or *malignant retinopathy*. As with nephropathy, duration of diabetes is the most important factor influencing the occurrence of retinopathy and some abnormality, even if only a single microaneurysm, can be seen in the fundi of at least 60% of diabetics who have had the condition for 30 years.

INTERFERENCE WITH VISION. In general, prognosis for vision is good for patients with simple retinopathy and bad for those with proliferative retinopathy, of whom half are blind within 5 years. Microaneuryms, abnormalities of the veins, blot haemorrhages and exudates will not interfere seriously with vision unless they are associated with macular oedema or directly involve the macula. Unfortunately all these lesions occur most commonly in the perimacular area. New vessels may be completely symptomless until sudden visual loss occurs from a haemorrhage into the vitreous. Although these frequently clear, the risk of recurrence is high and the more frequent the haemorrhage the slower and less complete the recovery. New vessel formation is potentially reversible and therefore treatable. Fibrous tissue may obscure the retina and seriously damage sight, and retinal-vitreal adhesions may pull the retina forward and produce retinal detachment causing blindness. Retinitis proliferans is the irreversible end-stage of diabetic retinopathy which cannot be influenced by any form of treatment at present available. Early detection and treatment of new vessel formation is therefore of vital importance.

**Prevention.** As microangiopathy seems to be secondary to the metabolic abnormality and there is evidence to suggest that good control of the diabetes reduces the chance of its development and may delay the progression of severe diabetic retinopathy, every effort should be made to maintain a normal metabolic state in all diabetic patients. It is a common error to suppose that diabetes which is 'mild', i.e. controlled by diet alone, carries little risk of complications.

**Treatment.** There is no specific treatment for simple retinopathy without maculopathy which is usually not associated with significant impairment of vision. The administration of clofibrate will clear hard exudates from the retina but will not affect the underlying neuronal degeneration. It may be of value in preventing further exudation but the possible benefits must be weighed against the risks (p. 532). The diabetes and any hypertension must be well controlled.

In simple retinopathy visual loss results from macular exudates, haemorrhage or oedema. Photocoagulation can be used to destroy abnormally leaking vessels in the perimacular area and thus reduce oedema. Coagulation of the centre of rings of hard exudates may hasten absorption of the exudates. The smaller spot size and shorter duration of the argon laser enables lesions nearer the macula to be treated.

The primary aim in treating proliferative retinopathy is to destroy new vessels by photocoagulation before vitreous haemorrhage, macular damage or retinal detachment occur. If photocoagulation fails, pituitary ablation can be considered in a few, carefully selected patients. However, the morbidity and mortality associated with this procedure is particularly high in diabetics.

Light coagulation of new vessels on the retina can be done under local anaesthesia, and in skilled, experienced hands is a simple procedure which carries little risk and can be very effective. Because diabetic retinopathy is now a treatable condition if diagnosed early, when it is commonly symptomless, diabetic patients must have their eyes examined regularly, every 6 to 12 months, by a competent observer. To obtain adequate visualisation of the retina the pupils must be dilated with a mydriatic. Once there is evidence of progression of simple retinopathy, and particularly whenever new vessels are seen, the patient must be referred to an ophthalmologist for further supervision and treatment.

**Cataract.** Very rarely a specific type of opacity of the lens (cataract) occurs in diabetic children whose disease has not been adequately controlled. Cataract also occurs in elderly diabetics, but is said to be no more common than in other elderly people.

### Infections

Poor control of diabetes is associated with a lowered resistance to infection. Alternatively latent diabetes may be unmasked by a severe infection such as a carbuncle or pneumonia. Glucose tolerance may return to normal, at least temporarily, when the infection is controlled by appropriate chemotherapy. Cleanliness is a special virtue in the prevention of skin infection which is common in diabetes.

*Pulmonary Tuberculosis.* If a diabetic under treatment shows unexplained loss of weight, increase in insulin requirements or symptoms of pulmonary disease, clinical and radiological examination of the lungs should be undertaken. Pulmonary tuberculosis can be arrested in its early stages by prompt recognition and specific treatment.

*Urinary Tract Infections.* The presence of glucose in the urine provides a favourable medium for the growth of bacteria. Persistent infections of the urinary tract frequently occur, and for this reason catheterisation in particular should be avoided. Treatment consists of controlling the glycosuria and chemotherapy for the urinary tract infection.

*Pruritus vulvae* is very commonly associated with moniliasis in the diabetic woman. *Candida albicans* is nearly always present. In the majority, the treatment is abolition of glycosuria which brings rapid relief. In a few cases local treatment with nystatin cream and pessaries may be required.

### Diabetic Neuropathy

Mononeuropathy, generalised polyneuropathy and autonomic neuropathy are frequent complications of diabetes at any stage and may give rise to troublesome manifestations. Involvement of the autonomic nervous system may result in an impaired sympathetic response to hypoglycaemia so that the patient no longer experiences the classical warning symptoms. Motor, sensory and autonomic nerves may be involved in varying combinations (p. 735).

## Special Problems in the Management of Diabetes

**Diabetes in Children.** Fortunately diabetes is not common in childhood, but when it occurs it is relatively severe and always requires treatment with insulin. The therapeutic problem of matching the dose of insulin to the food intake raises practical difficulties but the principles of treating children with diabetes are the same as for adults who have insulin-dependent diabetes. It is important to achieve as good control of the diabetes as possible and diabetic children and their parents need to be educated in the management of their disorder to the limit of their ability.

*Diet.* The nutritional needs of diabetic children are essentially no different from those of other children but because of growth their caloric requirements are large in proportion to their size, by comparison with adult standards. It may be difficult to provide enough calories because children's preferences for foods are often unpredictable. On the other hand the child must not become too fat; hypoglycaemia due to too much insulin can lead to excessive appetite and hence to obesity. A dietitian can do much to help the child and the parents. Diabetic children must not have sugar or sweets, but otherwise the diet need differ little from that of their friends. It is important that everything possible should be done to avoid distinguishing them from their contemporaries. Once trained, they may take part in the same range of activities as their peers, provided that appropriate supervision is arranged. The British Diabetic Association runs special camps for diabetic children.

*Insulin.* Day-to-day requirements for insulin are often very variable. Children's emotions and activities fluctuate unexpectedly — sometimes wildly active and sometimes sulking. This may have an important effect on their daily needs for insulin; excessive activity may result in hypoglycaemia, whilst lethargy may lead to hyperglycaemia. The latter may also be caused by any one of the numerous infectious diseases to which all children are prone. A combination of unmodified insulin and one of the depot insulins before breakfast, repeated if necessary before the main evening meal is a suitable arrangement for most diabetic children, providing the necessary flexibility. Children and parents need to have sufficient knowledge to make daily alterations in the dose of insulin on the basis of the results of preprandial urine tests and other relevant factors such as exercise and illness.

**Diabetes in Pregnancy.** If a diabetic woman wishes to have a child there is no reason, apart from genetic aspects (p. 530) why she should avoid pregnancy, provided that she suffers from none of the more serious complications of diabetes and provided she remains constantly under expert medical care. Nevertheless pregnancy in a diabetic woman carries certain definite risks; in the later stages of pregnancy she may develop an excessive accumulation of amniotic fluid; in addition the fetus is sometimes unusually large leading to difficulty in labour. Moreover the chances that a diabetic mother may lose her baby, either from a stillbirth or in the early neonatal period, are greater than those of a non-diabetic mother, even with the most careful supervision. Congenital malformation is more common in diabetic pregnancy and now accounts for the majority of deaths.

The proper treatment of a pregnant diabetic patient requires the close and coordinated supervision of a team consisting of physician, obstetrician, anaesthetist, nurse and dietitian. The sooner the pregnancy is diagnosed the better. Some non-pregnant diabetic women often miss one or more menstrual periods, especially if their disease is poorly controlled. For this reason a laboratory test for pregnancy is often helpful. There are grounds for suggesting that oral hypoglycaemic agents might be teratogenic, and any diabetic patient who is taking these drugs and wishes to become pregnant should change to a preparation of insulin.

Good control of the diabetes is the key to a successful pregnancy. A normal blood glucose concentration before and at the time of conception and throughout the pregnancy should be the aim. Further education of the patient may be needed in the proper management of her diet and insulin while at home. The diet, at first at least, need differ in no important respect from the diabetic diet to which she has been accustomed, but may need adjustment later, particularly with additional milk. Practical problems may be created for the physician and dietitian by bouts of vomiting that may occur in the early stages of pregnancy, and by the peculiar food fads which some pregnant women develop. The administration of highly purified unmodified and depot insulins twice daily is the best regimen for most pregnant diabetic patients.

After the diagnosis of pregnancy has been made the patient should be seen at first at fortnightly and later at weekly intervals. Continued control of the diabetes may be complicated by other factors. First, the renal threshold for glucose often falls as pregnancy advances. This is a normal phenomenon, but in the diabetic it means that the tests for glycosuria may cease to be a reliable index of diabetic control. Further, in the later stages of pregnancy, lactosuria may occasionally occur and may lead to confusion. For these reasons and because good diabetic control is mandatory, some patients will benefit from being taught to estimate their own blood glucose concentration. If excessive amounts of glucose are lost in the urine because of the lowered renal threshold, it may be necessary to give additional carbohydrate feeds between meals and sometimes at night, covered by suitable amounts of unmodified insulin to avoid ketosis. Then, too, the requirements for insulin usually increase as pregnancy advances. Frequent estimations of blood glucose are needed to ensure that an increase in insulin dosage, based on misleading urine tests, is not producing hypoglycaemia; or alternatively, that hyperglycaemia is not insidiously building up through failure to give enough insulin to meet an increase in insulin requirements.

Because of the risk in late pregnancy of sudden intrauterine death, pregnancy in a diabetic woman is seldom, if ever, allowed to proceed to term and most are delivered between the 37th and 38th week by induction of labour or if necessary by Caesarean section. Estimation of the lecithin/sphingomyelin ratio in the amniotic fluid is helpful in choosing a date for delivery. If the ratio is above 2·0 the risk of respiratory distress in the infant is low. On the morning of delivery the usual breakfast and insulin should be replaced by an intravenous infusion of 10% dextrose with 10 units of unmodified insulin added to each 500 ml. This should be given at a rate of 100 ml hourly. The blood glucose should be monitored at intervals of 1 – 2 hours and the rate of infusion and the dose of insulin adjusted to keep the blood glucose concentration at about 6·0 mmol/*l*. An alternative method is to give the insulin separately from the glucose infusion, by means of a constant-rate infusion pump at a rate of 1–2 units hourly. Whatever method is used administration of insulin should be stopped immediately on delivery and subcutaneous insulin resumed according to need as determined by urine and blood tests. Little or no insulin may be required for 12 hours after delivery. Thereafter, the pre-pregnancy dose can be gradually resumed.

A final word of warning is necessary. It has already been indicated that sugar in the urine is not unusual during normal pregnancy, either because of a fall in the renal threshold for glucose or through lactose appearing in the urine. The finding, however, of reducing substances in the urine of a pregnant woman should never be lightly dismissed as a normal phenomenon. Full clinical investigation to exclude diabetes is essential; otherwise a preventable catastrophe may follow.

**Diabetes and Surgery.** Any surgical operation, however minor, and the accompanying anaesthetic cause metabolic stress which the diabetic is less well able to meet than the normal person. Operations under local anaesthesia do not usually require special treatment of the diabetes. For operations under general anaesthesia two points must be kept in mind: the need to provide an adequate supply of energy for the tissues, and the need to be constantly on the alert for acidosis.

In practice there are two separate problems related to elective and emergency surgery:

1. *Elective surgery in a stabilised diabetic.* All diabetics should be admitted to hospital about three days before even a minor operation. During this period the control of the diabetes can be checked thoroughly. Provided a diabetic goes to the theatre in good condition, there is unlikely to be any significant change in the blood glucose, plasma bicarbonate or ketone levels during the operation.

A diabetic who is not on insulin can usually be managed without special care other than careful postoperative observation of the clinical state, glycosuria, ketonuria and blood glucose concentration. However, care must be taken to avoid hypoglycaemia in those taking a sulphonylurea and conversely insulin may be required if significant loss of control occurs.

In the case of insulin treated patients it is desirable that the operation should take place as early as possible in the morning. The patient should receive no breakfast and nothing by mouth before operation and the normal dose of insulin should be omitted. Before being transferred to the theatre the fasting blood glucose level should be determined. If this lies between 7·0 and 10·0 mmol/*l* (120 to 180 mg/100ml) and surgery is minor, then no glucose or insulin need be given. If the level is below 5·0 mmol/*l*, then about 25 g of glucose should be given intravenously, preferably in hypertonic solution, in order to prevent possible hypoglycaemia (from the action of the previous day's depot insulin) during the operation. If the fasting blood sugar is over 10·0 mmol/*l* then some insulin will be required. About one-third of the usual total daily dose is indicated, in the form of unmodified insulin, but its administration can usually be postponed until after operation. If a major surgical procedure is to be performed, intravenous 5% dextrose or dextrose saline should be given at a rate of 500 ml over four hours, along with unmodified insulin i.v. Either 4 – 20 units can be added to each 500 ml dextrose or 1 – 3 units hourly can be given separately from the glucose infusion by a constant-rate infusion pump. The blood glucose concentration should be estimated frequently and the dose of insulin adjusted appropriately.

Recovery from the anaesthetic must be carefully supervised. The sooner the patient returns to the usual diet the better. This interval may be a few hours or several days, depending on the nature and severity of the operation. Within a few hours of recovery from the anaesthetic many patients are able to take fluid or semi-fluid feeds containing 25 g carbohydrate (p. 521) at three to four hourly intervals covered by suitable doses of unmodified insulin. After a major operation some insulin-dependent diabetics may need to have most of their energy requirements supplied as glucose, either intravenously or by mouth. If all has gone well, a single determination of the fasting blood glucose each morning will suffice. If recovery is stormy, measurements may be necessary at four hourly intervals or even more frequently. The determination of the plasma bicarbonate and electrolytes in the blood will also be helpful. The insulin dosage will depend on these findings, and until stability has been regained only unmodified insulin should be used.

Each specimen of urine must be tested for sugar and ketone bodies. If ketosis develops it is essential to take immediate steps to increase the metabolism of glucose by adjusting the dose of insulin.

2. *Diabetes and surgical emergencies.* Circumstances vary so much that it is impossible to consider them except in the most general way. The essentials are to maintain the oxidation of glucose by the tissues at a sufficient rate and to combat acidosis and electrolyte disturbances when they occur. This can be done effectively only if the state of the diabetic control is assessed continuously and accurately. A laboratory service that can provide rapid results is thus essential. As long as the surgical condition remains untreated and the 'metabolic stress' continues, the diabetic condition is likely to get worse. Once the patient's surgical condition is under control a prompt response may be expected to appropriate therapy for the diabetes.

## Prevention of Diabetes

NIDD is a disease of the prosperous, and in wealthy countries it is one of the major health problems. The hardships of the Second World War were associated with a marked decline in the incidence of NIDD in European countries; rationing of both food and petrol was probably responsible. The importance to health of sufficient exercise and of avoiding dietary excess has been stated repeatedly. Diabetes, like obesity and atherosclerosis, is likely to arise in genetically predisposed persons who eat too much and exercise too little. Excess of dietary carbohydrate may strain the limited capacity of the pancreas to produce insulin, especially if it is in the form of sugar or other refined carbohydrate; excess of dietary fat may accelerate the complications of diabetes; atherosclerosis is a common cause of death in diabetics. In any event the public should be warned primarily against an overall excess of calories.

Investigation of the HLA system has shown that certain individuals have an increased risk of developing IDD and that genetic factors may also play a part in individual susceptibility to develop complications. These genetic characteristics of susceptibility and the relevant environmental factors need to be defined more precisely before appropriate preventive measures can be taken.

*Screening.* It is much easier to control the disease and to maintain the health of the patient in a state which allows a normal life to be led, if the diagnosis is made early in the course of the disease. In many patients the biochemical changes can be detected before the symptoms are sufficiently severe to make them seek medical advice. Any screening technique is expensive and should be used only if it is likely that a significant number of new diabetics will be recognised. High-risk groups, for example the first degree relatives of known diabetics, the obese and the mothers of babies weighing more than 4·5 kg at birth, will give a particularly high yield. The prevalence of diabetes in different communities varies from 0·5 to 5%. These figures vary widely according to the social and economic state of the people and the educational and medical services available.

Urine testing has been widely used as a screening procedure. As up to 3% of people may have renal glycosuria and so will have to be recalled for blood tests, and as a number of undoubted diabetics will be missed owing to their raised renal threshold for glucose, this is an unsatisfactory procedure. Whenever practicable, estimation of the blood glucose 2 hours after 75 g glucose orally is recommended as the screening procedure. Auto-analysers enable many samples to be tested daily.

Quite apart from screening high-risk groups it is not difficult to make out a case for a routine test of the urine for glucose in every full clinical examination; and all those with glycosuria (albeit of minor degree) should be considered diabetic until proved otherwise.

*Genetic Counselling*. Diabetic patients will often consult their doctor about the advisability of having children. They can be told that the risks of pregnancy and delivery are little greater for a diabetic mother than for a normal woman, provided she submits to the strict discipline required. The chances that she will produce a healthy baby are also good, but not quite so good as for a normal mother. The chances that her child will subsequently develop diabetes are higher than normal (Table 1.5) but most diabetics have healthy children, and how strongly a doctor should word these necessary warnings is a matter for judgement in each case. The family history, the severity of the disease in the parents and their educational and economic background, must all be considered.

**Conclusion.** The management of a patient with diabetes mellitus offers a special opportunity for good medical practice, there being few other chronic diseases in which efficient management makes so much difference to the patient's life. The problems presented by the aetiology of diabetes and its long-term complications continue to offer some of the most demanding and fascinating challenges in medical research today.

## Other Metabolic Disorders

Metabolism is as fundamental as life itself; in medicine the term is usually restricted to disorders which can best be described in biochemical terms.

Many metabolic disorders are acquired. Others are congenital. The genetic aetiology of numerous inborn errors of metabolism has been identified with abnormalities of the structure or function of DNA and the pattern of their inheritance mapped by the study of a particular biochemical disorder. Metabolic disorders therefore may be classified in many ways, for example by the mode of inheritance or by the chemical factors involved. The specific enzyme deficiency responsible for the disorder, or the body system principally affected may be named. Disorders of carbohydrate, protein or amino acid, lipid or mineral metabolism may be predominant features, and a few examples of these are given below.

The vast majority of inborn errors of metabolism are rare and it would be inappropriate to describe them here. The reader will find much further information in specialised textbooks (p. 533).

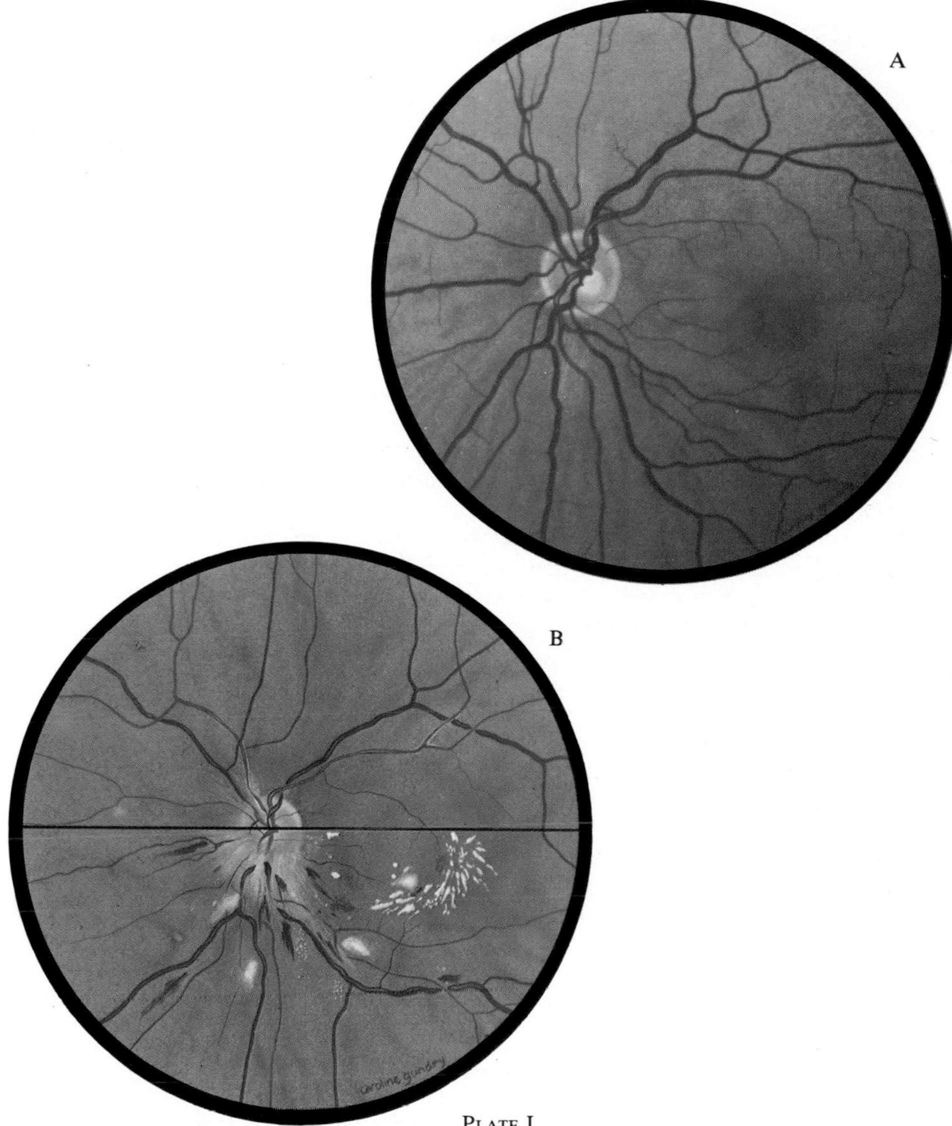


PLATE I

A. Painting of normal retinal vessels. B. Hypertensive retinopathy. The upper half of this painting shows the retinal blood vessels in hypertension of moderate severity. The arteriolar blood column is narrower than normal and a central white streak (light reflex) is visible or is more prominent than normal. Irregularity of breadth of the arteriolar blood column indicates an irregular lumen. Veins at arterial-venous crossings are narrowed ('nipping'), partly because of pressure by arterioles and also because opacity of the arterial wall obscures the venous blood column. The lower half of the painting shows severe hypertensive retinopathy. Haemorrhages and 'soft' exudates are added to the abnormalities seen in the upper half and these are also more marked.

*(By permission of Professor C. I. Phillips, Department of Ophthalmology, University of Edinburgh)*

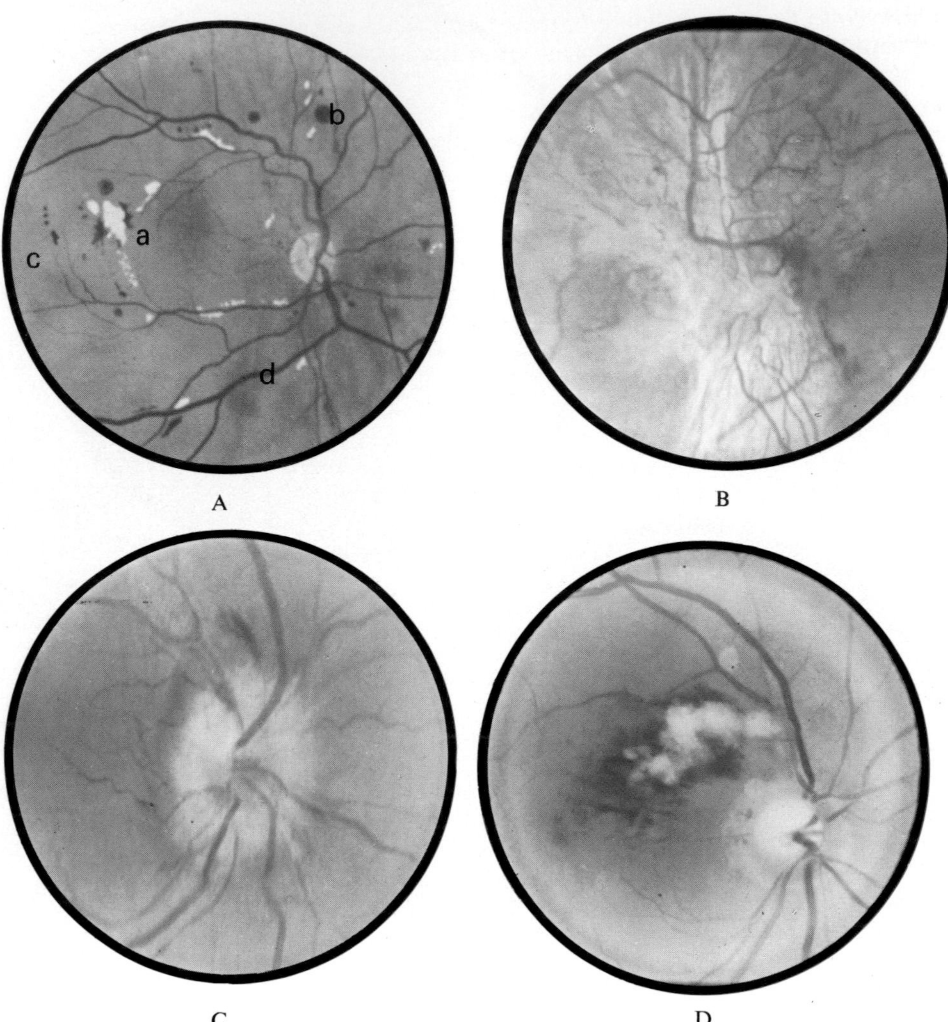


PLATE II

A. Painting of diabetic retinopathy; (*a*) exudates; (*b*) dot haemorrhages; (*c*) microaneurysms; (*d*) dilated veins. B. Photograph of advanced proliferative diabetic retinopathy. Heavily vascularised sheets of fibrous tissue are forming in the vitreous, mainly derived from the optic disc. C. Photograph of papilloedema. Note swelling of the disc and haemorrhages on or very near the disc. D. Photograph of thrombosis of the lower temporal branch of the central retinal vein. Note haemorrhages and exudates. There is also pathological cupping of the disc due to raised intra-ocular pressure which probably predisposes to retinal thrombosis.

*(By permission of Professor C. I. Phillips, Department of Ophthalmology, University of Edinburgh)*

*Facing page 531]*

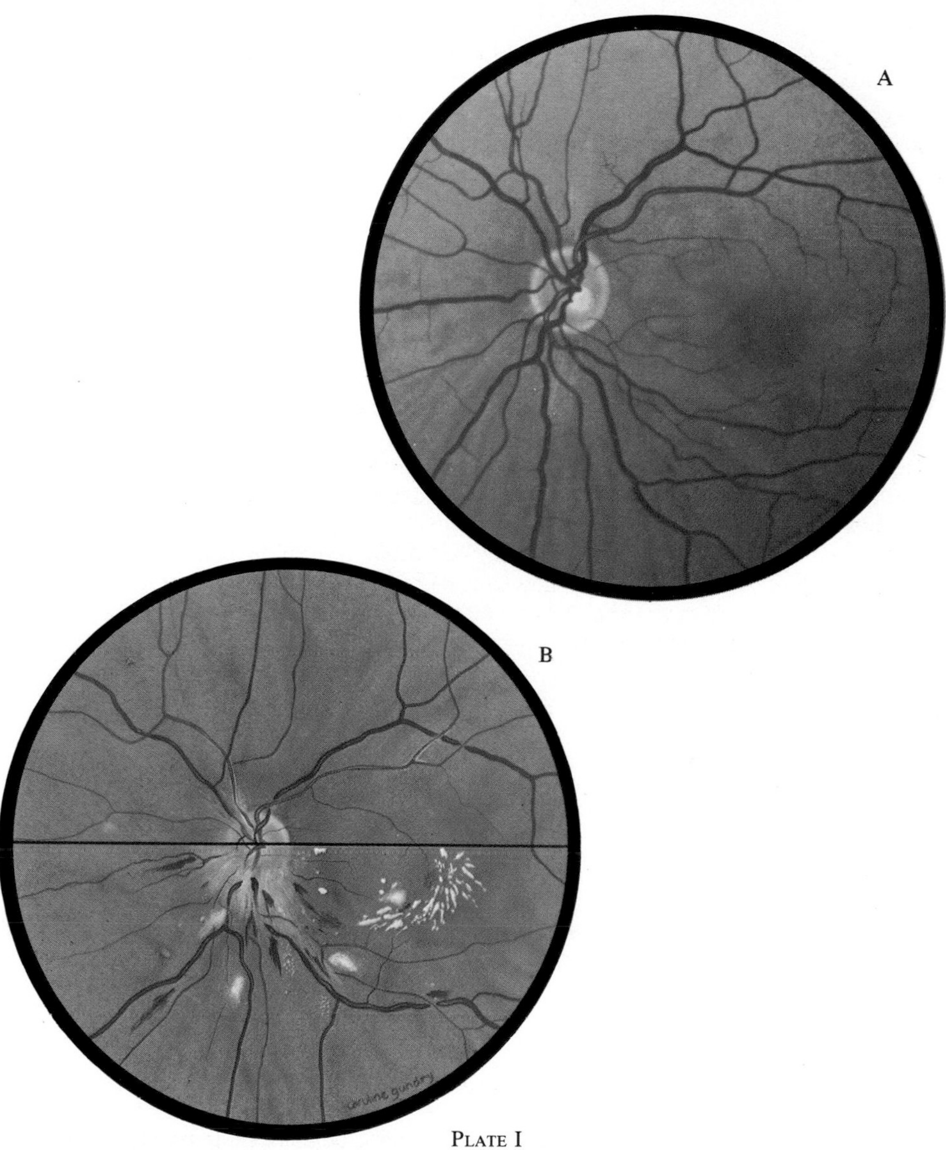


PLATE I

A. Painting of normal retinal vessels. B. Hypertensive retinopathy. The upper half of this painting shows the retinal blood vessels in hypertension of moderate severity. The arteriolar blood column is narrower than normal and a central white streak (light reflex) is visible or is more prominent than normal. Irregularity of breadth of the arteriolar blood column indicates an irregular lumen. Veins at arterial-venous crossings are narrowed ('nipping'), partly because of pressure by arterioles and also because opacity of the arterial wall obscures the venous blood column. The lower half of the painting shows severe hypertensive retinopathy. Haemorrhages and 'soft' exudates are added to the abnormalities seen in the upper half and these are also more marked.

*(By permission of Professor C. I. Phillips, Department of Ophthalmology, University of Edinburgh)*

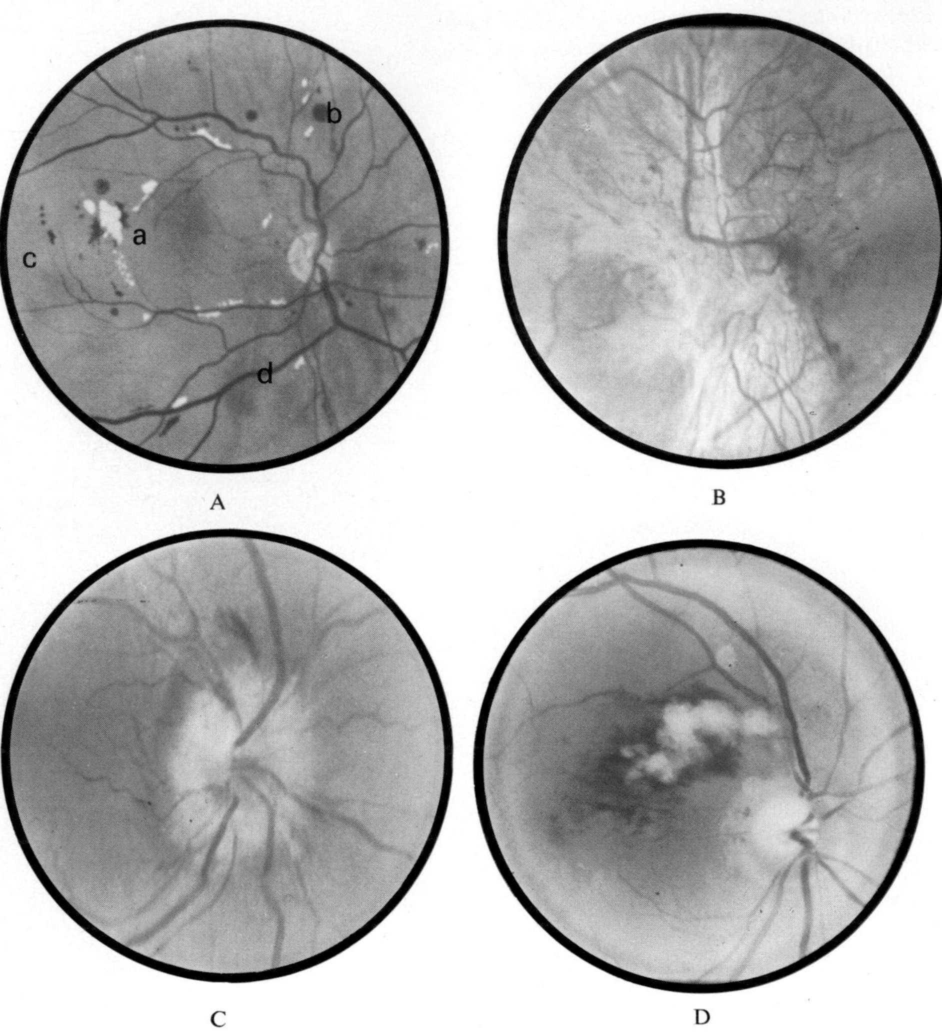


PLATE II

A. Painting of diabetic retinopathy; (*a*) exudates; (*b*) dot haemorrhages; (*c*) microaneurysms; (*d*) dilated veins. B. Photograph of advanced proliferative diabetic retinopathy. Heavily vascularised sheets of fibrous tissue are forming in the vitreous, mainly derived from the optic disc. C. Photograph of papilloedema. Note swelling of the disc and haemorrhages on or very near the disc. D. Photograph of thrombosis of the lower temporal branch of the central retinal vein. Note haemorrhages and exudates. There is also pathological cupping of the disc due to raised intra-ocular pressure which probably predisposes to retinal thrombosis.

*(By permission of Professor C. I. Phillips, Department of Ophthalmology, University of Edinburgh)*

*Facing page 531]*

*Carbohydrate*. Diabetes mellitus is by far the most frequent and important disorder of carbohydrate metabolism. Rare genetic errors lead to abnormalities in the metabolism of galactose (galactosaemia), fructose (fructosuria), and glycogen (glycogen storage diseases, such as von Gierke's disease.

*Amino Acids*. Inborn errors account for many relatively rare diseases such as cystinuria (p. 423) and the Fanconi syndrome (p. 423). Phenylketonuria is also rare but leads to mental retardation if not detected in the neonatal period and treated with a special diet.

*Purines*. Gout (p. 635) is a classical example of a metabolic disorder but in practice is best considered along with other causes of arthritis.

*Lipids* are complex mixtures among which cholesterol and triglyceride are the most useful indices for the detection and monitoring of hyperlipidaemia. Lipids circulate as lipoproteins, while free fatty acids are bound to albumin (p. 377). Analysis of fasting serum lipids and particularly of lipoproteins provides a useful classification of the hyperlipidaemias as devised by WHO, and based particularly on the work of Fredrickson (p. 533). In this classification there are five major types (I–V) of hyperlipidaemia due either to genetic defects in lipid metabolism or to environmental factors such as diet, alcohol and drugs, including oestrogens and corticosteroids. Measurement of lipoproteins is usually not necessary for management which can generally be determined by clinical observation along with measurement of fasting serum cholesterol and triglyceride.

## Primary Hyperlipidaemias

Patients with primary hyperlipidaemia can for most clinical purposes be classified into three groups. Two of these are metabolically heterogeneous but treatment can usually be allocated on a group basis.

*Group I* consists of those with hypercholesterolaemia (Fredrickson's Type IIa). The serum is clear, cholesterol concentration raised, triglyceride levels normal, and $\beta$ (low density) lipoproteins increased. Most patients have mild to moderate hypercholesterolaemia (7–10 mmol/*l*) and physical signs are usually absent although early arcus senilis or xanthelasma may be present. The disorder is relatively common in Britain and is a risk factor for ischaemic heart disease. It is usually weakly inherited and environmental factors, such as the dietary intake of saturated fat and cholesterol, are probably important in its aetiology.

About 5% of patients with hypercholesterolaemia have a more sharply defined disorder transmitted as an autosomal dominant and present from birth. Serum cholesterol levels range from 8–16 mmol/*l* in heterozygotes and from 16–32 mmol/*l* in the rare homozygotes. In this disorder clinical stigmata of hyperlipidaemia are frequent. Tendon xanthomas and arthritis (p. 627) are common. Arcus senilis and xanthelasma on the eyelids are often prominent and 50% have ischaemic heart disease by the time they are 50 years old.

*Group II* comprises those with predominant hypertriglyceridaemia (Fredrickson's Type IIb, III, IV and V). The serum is cloudy, triglyceride and pre-$\beta$ (very low density)-lipoproteins increased, and cholesterol may be normal or, if increased, the rise is usually less pronounced than that of triglyceride. Specific physical signs are uncommon although xanthomas can occur. Obesity, impaired carbohydrate tolerance and hyperuricaemia often coexist. There is a strong association with ischaemic heart disease and this group is also relatively common in Britain.

*Group III* is represented by Fredrickson's Type I. This is a rare disorder consisting of chylomicronaemia resulting from deficiency of extrahepatic lipoprotein lipase.

## Secondary Hyperlipidaemia

This occurs in association with diabetes mellitus, in hypothyroidism, the nephrotic syndrome, biliary obstruction and in pancreatitis.

**Treatment of Hyperlipidaemia.** Control of primary hyperlipidaemia always requires dietary measures. Obesity must be corrected in every case. The low calorie diet on page 900 can be appropriately modified in relation to the fat content.

Groups I and II should have a fat-modified diet in which the intake of cholesterol is restricted and the total fat intake is reduced to provide about 36% of the total calories. The intake of saturated fat is reduced, while the intake of polyunsaturated fat is increased to provide a polyunsaturated: saturated fat ratio of more than 1:1. A list of foods to be avoided is given on page 903. An abnormal sensitivity to carbohydrate and/or alcohol is responsible for inducing hyperlipidaemia in some of those in Group II who will require to restrict their consumption of sucrose and alcohol, even if they are not obese.

Group III patients improve dramatically with restriction of fat intake to about 25 g daily.

If dietary measures alone are insufficient to control the hyperlipidaemia, Group I patients should first be given cholestyramine. An incomplete response in these patients may be improved by the addition of nicotinic acid. Patients in Group II usually respond to nicotonic acid. Indications for the use of clofibrate came under scrutiny when two extensive clinical trials of this drug for the primary prevention of ischaemic heart disease revealed an increased mortality from ischaemic heart disease, cerebrovascular disorders and neoplasms, particularly of the respiratory and gastrointestinal tracts, among treated individuals. This excess mortality is unexplained but the use of clofibrate should be strictly confined to the few cases of severe hyperlipidaemia which have failed to respond to the measures outlined above and where the clinical benefit seems likely to be greater than the risk associated with medication. Those in this category are likely to include patients with the relatively uncommon Fredrickson's Type III hyperlipoproteinaemia (broad-$\beta$-band disease) which is associated with early-onset peripheral vascular disease and cardiac ischaemia and those with severe endogenous hypertriglyceridaemia (Frederickson's Type IV or V hyperlipoproteinaemia) where there is a risk of acute relapsing pancreatitis when the plasma triglyceride concentration exceeds 6–7 mmol/*l*.

Secondary hyperlipidaemia usually responds to treatment of the underlying condition when this is possible.

## Prospects in Diabetes

The scale of the clinical problem presented by patients with microangiopathy, the suggestion that good control of blood glucose may prevent or retard the development of diabetic complications, the introduction of better methods of assessing diabetic control and the realisation that at present good control is achieved in only a minority of diabetic patients, has led to a search for better methods of treatment.

Improved control has been reported with continuous subcutaneous and intramuscular infusion of insulin for periods of up to four months. In these systems insulin is delivered at fixed rates without reference to the blood glucose concentration.

'Artificial pancreas' systems consist of three basic components: a glucose sensor, an insulin delivery pump, and a computer controller which regulates the administration of insulin on the basis of blood glucose concentration. Ideally such a device should be small enough for implantation and measure blood glucose without consuming blood. Existing systems use blood and are large, extracorporeal, relatively unreliable and expensive. They have few clinical applications but have some use as an investigative tool.

Whole pancreas transplants have been uniformly unsuccessful in man. Work with isolated pancreatic islets is more encouraging but there are major problems in relation to both their supply and rejection following transplantation. The latter may be circumvented by implanting islets inside capillary tubes made from inert materials.

Human insulin has now been synthesised by recombitant DNA technology using genetically modified strains of *Esch. coli*. Supplies for clinical trial should be available in the near future.

JOYCE D. BAIRD

*Further reading about diabetes mellitus:*


Davidson, Sir Stanley, Passmore, R., Brock, J. F., Truswell, A. S. (1979). *Human Nutrition and Dietetics*, 7th edn. Edinburgh: Churchill Livingstone.

Irvine, W. J. (ed.) (1980) *The Immunology of Diabetes Mellitus* . Edinburgh: Teviot Scientific Publications.

Keen, H. & Jarrett, R. J. (1980) *Complications of Diabetes,* 2nd edn. London: Arnold.

Oakley, W. G., Pyke, D. A. & Taylor, K. W. (1978) *Diabetes and its Management,* 3rd edn. Oxford: Blackwell.

WHO Technical Report Series 646. (1980) WHO Expert Committee on Diabetes Mellitus. Second report. Geneva: WHO.


*Further reading about metabolic disorders:*


Beaumont, J. L., Carlson, L. A., Cooper, G. R., Fejfar, Z., Fredrickson, D. S. & Stasser, T. (1970) Classification of Hyperlipidaemias and Hyperlipoproteinemias. *Bulletin World Health Organisation*, **43**, 891. — This is a definitive classification agreed by a W.H.O. specialist committee.

Bondy, P. K. & Rosenberg, L. E. (1980) *Duncan's Diseases of Metabolism,* 8th edn. London: Saunders.

Lewis, B. (1976). *The Hyperlipidaemias. Clinical and Laboratory Practice*. Oxford: Blackwell.

Stanbury, J. B., Wyngaarden, J. B. & Fredrickson, D. S. (1978) *The Metabolic Basis of Inherited Disease*, 4th edn. New York: McGraw-Hill.

# 12. Diseases of the Blood and Blood-Forming Organs

## Blood Formation

Up to the fifth month of fetal life blood cells are formed both in the liver and the spleen. Thereafter normal formation of the red cells, the granular series of white cells and the platelets takes place increasingly in the medullary cavity of bones and from birth onwards is restricted to these sites. During childhood there is a progressive diminution in the amount of red haemopoietic marrow so that in the young adult it is confined to the heads of the femur and humerus, to flat bones such as the sternum, ribs and ilia and to the vertebrae, the rest of the marrow cavity being occuped by fat. The red marrow may extend into the shafts of the long bones, replacing the fat, when there is an increased demand for blood formation.

Blood cells have a finite life span and require to be continuously replaced. Newly formed cells are provided by actively proliferating cell systems derived from mesenchymal stem cells found in the marrow, spleen and lymph nodes. The morphology of the haemopoietic stem cells is uncertain but they probably resemble lymphocytes. A stem cell has two functions. The first is to provide a continuous supply of cells committed to becoming the mature cells of the blood by a process of proliferation, to produce numbers, and maturation to produce specificity. The second function is to replenish the stem cell compartment itself. Not all the daughter cells of stem cells proceed to maturation; some return to the stem cell compartment to maintain its size and integrity.

Stem cells probably exist at two levels; primary or pluripotential stem cells are capable of producing a secondary or unipotential series of stem cells committed to one or other of the mature cell systems. The secondary stem cells giving rise to the lymphocyte series probably appear at an earlier stage of differentiation of the pluripotential stem cells than those producing the erythrocytes, granulocytes and megakaryocytes.

Haemopoiesis is influenced by controlling mechanisms that enable it to respond to fluctuation in demand. These mechanisms are mainly humoral, although there may also be cell to cell interaction.

Of the three types of cell found in the blood, erythrocytes and platelets are truly blood cells; they differ from most cells in the body in that they have no nuclei. Leucocytes are a migratory population of cells which use the blood as a channel to move from the marrow or other production site to the tissues where some mature further and their main functions are performed. Thus, the white cells in the circulation at any one time form only a very small fraction of the total body white cell mass.

### The Red Blood Cells (Erythrocytes)

The earliest identifiable red cell precursor in the marrow is the pro-erythroblast, a large cell with a nucleolated nucleus and deeply basophilic cytoplasm. This cell undergoes a series of divisions rapidly so that the cell does not have time to regrow between divisions and becomes progressively smaller. At the same time maturation proceeds with the formation of haemoglobin in the cytoplasm. Early, intermediate and late normoblasts can be identified. Proliferation ceases at the intermediate normoblast stage and maturation is then completed with condensation of the nuclear chromatin and eventual ejection of the nuclear remnant. At this stage the cell still has the capacity to synthesize haemogolobin, due to the presence of ribosomes in the cytoplasm. This material (RNA) gives the cell a faintly bluish colour with Romanowsky stains. Supravital staining with cresyl blue causes condensation of the ribosomes to form reticular material which makes these cells easy to identify, and they can be counted as reticulocytes. The reticulocyte matures into an adult red cell in about three days and is released to the circulation about half way through this period. Under stress, marrow reticulocytes can be released sooner, raising the reticulocyte count without there necessarily being an increase in erythropoiesis. These marrow reticulocytes can be recognised as they have a much more dense central aggregate of reticulum with supravital staining.

The mature erythrocyte is an eosinophilic circular disc with a mean diameter of 7·2 microns. Its biconcave shape allows the cell considerable plasticity, enabling it to pass through capillaries and other structures of smaller diameter. The red cell membrane is a complex dynamic structure through which water, potassium and sodium ions are passed by active processes, the energy for which is supplied by glycolysis. The red cell membrane carries the blood group characteristics on its surface. After the first few days of life there are, in health, no nucleated red cells in the peripheral blood. The presence there of normoblasts indicates excessive or abnormal blood formation or irritation of the bone marrow by invasion with foreign elements. An increased number of reticulocytes reflects increased erythropoiesis.

The red cell has an excess of membrane. This is partly the reason for its biconcavity, but energy is also required. In various disorders the red cell may lose membrane and become progressively more spherical and rigid. As a result, it is more susceptible to destruction, particularly in the spleen where it fails to traverse fenestrations that are smaller than its diameter and through which it must pass. Thus the spleen is uniquely adapted to filtering out such cells.

Red cell production has specific requirements for substances such as iron for haemoglobin synthesis. A number of other factors influence erythropoiesis and these include vitamin $B_{12}$ (p. 548), folate (p. 551), thyroxine, vitamin C, androgens and possibly trace elements such as copper and manganese.

Erythropoiesis is controlled by a hormone, erythropoietin, produced mainly in the kidneys. There, cells which are probably located in the tubules, and which are responsive to tissue hypoxia, monitor the provision of oxygen to the tissues and respond to hypoxia by the production of erythropoietin. It acts mainly on the stem cell compartment stimulating increased activity. It also improves the speed and efficiency of erythropoiesis.

## Haemoglobin

The function of the erythrocytes depends on their content of haemoglobin which is formed as the red cells mature in the bone marrow. It is the oxygen transport mechanism of the blood and is also important in carbon dioxide transport because it buffers carbonic acid (p. 141). Haemoglobin is a complex molecule, being a conjugate of protein (globin) with a red pigment (haem), the latter being a combination of a porphyrin with ferrous iron. In normal adult haemoglobin (haemoglobin A) the molecule of globin consists of four paired polypeptide chains, two alpha chains of 141 amino acids and two beta chains of 146 amino acids. Haemoglobin F, the fetal haemoglobin, differs by having two gamma chains instead of beta chains. Haemoglobin A2, which is found in small amounts of between two to three per cent of the total haemoglobin in adults, has two delta chains instead of beta chains.

One molecule of oxygen is carried by each haem fraction of the haemoglobin molecule which is therefore capable of carrying four molecules of oxygen. Beta, gamma and delta chains are incapable of accepting oxygen to their haem pockets until the alpha chains have taken up oxygen. When this occurs a configurational change in the haemoglobin molecule prises open the haem pockets of the other chains, allowing them to accept oxygen. Thus the more oxygen the haemoglobin molecule has, the more easily it acquires further oxygen until saturated. In the tissues where oxygen is lost, the reverse occurs, initially easy loss becoming more difficult as the haemoglobin becomes desaturated. The haemoglobin molecule is thus complex but structured precisely for a specific purpose. Its function can be influenced further by a by-product of glucose metabolism, 2–3–diphosphoglycerate (2–3–DPG). The concentration of 2–3–DPG in the red cell affects the configuration of the molecule by reversible combination with deoxygenated haemoglobin and thus the avidity of the haemoglobin molecule for oxygen. 2–3–DPG decreases haemoglobin's oxygen affinity and improves release to the tissues. Under hypoxic conditions, 2–3–DPG levels in the red cells increase as a compensatory mechanism. This is the first step in acclimatisation at high altitude; it occurs within 24–48 hours, long before there is any increase in red cell numbers stimulated by increased erythropoetin production.

## The White Blood Cells (Leucocytes)

**The Granular Series** (*Polymorphonuclear Leucocytes*). These are so called because of the granules shown by Romanowsky stains in the cytoplasm of the more mature forms. Granulocytes are derived from stem cells in the bone marrow (Table 12.1), where their earliest recognisable precursors are myeloblasts which have large nuclei containing nucleoli and no cytoplasmic granules. Myeloblasts mature through promyelocyte, myelocyte and metamyelocyte stages with loss of nucleoli, coarsening of nuclear chromatin and development of cytoplasmic granules. The nucleus becomes kidney shaped and finally segments into lobes connected by thin chromatin strands characteristic of the polymorphonuclear leucocytes. The cells are classified as neutrophil, eosinophil or basophil, according to the staining reactions of their granules.

*Neutrophil granulocytes* are phagocytic cells which ingest bacteria and fungi. Their granules contain lysozyme which is discharged into the vacuole created by the ingestion of bacteria and which assists in the killing and digestion of the bacteria. The products of autodigestion from cells killed by organisms (pus cells) are potent stimulants of fresh neutrophil formation by the marrow. Pyrogens are also released. Apart from responding to infection, neutrophils also produce a vitamin $B_{12}$ binding protein; this explains the high levels of vitamin $B_{12}$ in the serum in conditions in which there is a greatly increased number of these cells, e.g. chronic myeloid leukaemia.

Mature neutrophil granulocytes account for more than 50% of the total leucocytes in the peripheral blood in a healthy adult; a huge reserve is held in the marrow and they are also present in large numbers in various organs and tissues. Physiological factors which increase their number in the peripheral blood include exercise, emotional stress and pregnancy.

Immature granulocytes, represented by metamyelocytes, are found when the pro-

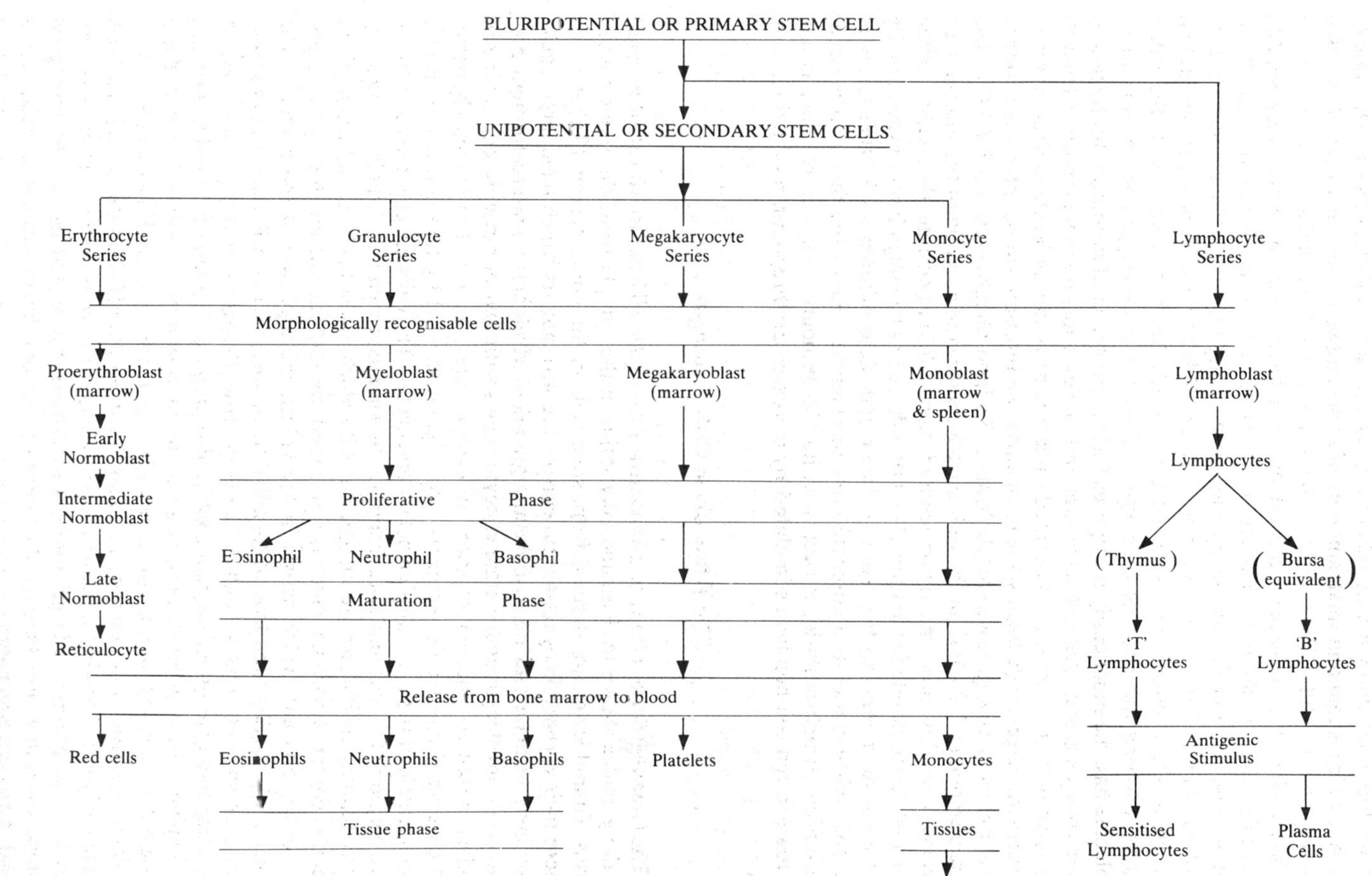


Table 12.1 Origin and development of blood cells.

duction of leucocytes is being stimulated by severe pyogenic infections and an increase in the cytoplasmic granulation may also be seen (toxic granulation). In adults the occurrence in the blood of more primitive forms such as myeloblasts and promyelocytes indicates a serious disturbance of marrow function as in leukaemia or invasion by metastases.

*Eosinophil granulocytes* are also phagocytic but less actively so than neutrophils. They ingest antigen-antibody complexes and are concerned in processes involving foreign proteins, such as hypersensitivity reactions and in association with parasitic infections.

The *basophil granulocytes* are poorly phagocytic; they possess IgE on their surface which, when activated by antigens, results in degranulation of the cell with the release of histamine. Basophils also contain heparin which may be released to participate in lipid metabolism.

**Lymphocytes** are mainly derived from stem cells in lymphoid tissue throughout the body though some are found in the bone marrow. The immature form, the lymphoblast, is a large cell with a nucleolated nucleus and so closely resembles a myeloblast that special staining methods and immunological techniques are required to differentiate them. Large and small lymphocytes, both of which are found in the peripheral blood and widely distributed throughout the body tissues, are derived from lymphoblasts. The majority of lymphocytes circulating in the blood are T lymphocytes (p. 24). About 20% are B lymphocytes. Both types respond to antigenic stimulus by transformation, in the case of B lymphocytes to immunoglobulin-producing plasma cells. T lymphocytes retain their lymphoid morphology and perform their immune functions themselves (cell-mediated immunity). Other lymphocytes, K (killer) cells, undertake cell destruction (p. 26).

**Monocytes** are formed from stem cells in the bone marrow. Monoblasts are large nucleolated immature forms, very similar to myeloblasts; they mature into cells with a lobulated nucleus in a cloudy blue cytoplasm containing numerous minute red granules. The monocytes are motile and phagocytic and migrate into the tissues where they develop into macrophages. There they remove debris as well as micro-organisms and collect and present antigenic material to lymphocytes (p. 25).

## The Platelets (Thrombocytes)

These are derived from megakaryocytes in the bone marrow. Megakaryocytes are very large cells containing multilobulated nuclei and granular cytoplasm from which the platelets are formed. Platelets are small (2–4 microns), hyaline, non-nucleated bodies with blue or purple granules.

## Normal Haematological Values

These are given in the appendix (p. 908).

## Blood Destruction

Destruction of all formed elements of the blood occurs in cells of the reticuloendothelial system. The survival time of the mature erythrocytes in the peripheral blood is approximately 110 to 120 days. This is the time as estimated by cross-transfusion experiments and represents the mean life span. A more practical technique is one in which red cells labelled with $^{35}Cr$ are transfused and the time taken for half of the radioactivity to disappear is estimated. By this method the half life of the radioactivity in the red cells is 25 to 35 days and is shorter than the true half life because of the elution of chromium from the cells. As red cells age their enzyme activity declines, the cells become defective and are removed from the blood and broken down in the reticuloendothelial system. The degradation of haemoglobin yields iron from haem which is mostly utilised by the marrow for fresh haemoglobin synthesis. The iron-free residual pigment, biliverdin, is converted to bilirubin and carried by the plasma to the liver for excretion. The globin is recycled.

The life span of the platelets is 9 – 11 days, but less is known about the survival of the leucocytes. The granulocytes probably last three to four days of which less than 24 hours is spent in the circulation. The life span of monocytes and lymphocytes is less certain. It appears that some small lymphocytes may re-enter the circulation at intervals for years (p. 25).

## Terms relating to Blood Disorders

*Microcytosis* means that the average size of the red cells is reduced and is commonly found in iron deficiency anaemia and other disorders of haemoglobin synthesis.

*Macrocytosis* means that the average size of the red cells is greater than normal. It is seen, for instance, in megaloblastic anaemias but its occurrence does not necessarily mean megaloblastic change in the marrow.

*Hypochromia* exists when the red cells contain less than the normal amount of haemoglobin. They stain less deeply and show central pallor in the blood film. The mean corpuscular haemoglobin concentration (MCHC) is lower than normal. Hypochromia is commonly associated with microcytosis and is the characteristic feature of iron deficiency anaemia.

*Anisocytosis* means inequality in the size of the red cells. It is found in many forms of anaemia but is most prominent in megaloblastic anaemia.

*Poikilocytosis* means marked irregularity in the shape of the red cells. It is never present without anisocytosis and usually reflects dyserythropoiesis.

*Elliptocytosis* means elliptical red cells; *ovalocytosis* refers to a less marked abnormality. Such cells are found in small numbers in a variety of disorders such as megaloblastic and hypochromic anaemias. When the majority of cells are oval or elliptical it indicates a hereditary disorder of Mendelian dominant type which is usually clinically benign. In less than 10% of cases with the hereditary disorder, a haemolytic state exists and may cause anaemia.

*Polychromasia and Reticulocytosis.* Young red cells when stained by the Romanowsky method have a faint bluish colour. A blood film in which such cells are present in increased numbers along with those of normal pink colour is said to show polychromasia. When stained supravitally by cresyl blue the young cells are slightly larger than adult erythrocytes and show up as reticulocytes. Polychromasia and reticulocytosis indicate increased production of new red cells by the bone marrow.

*Punctate Basophilia.* Pathologically damaged young red cells may show several deep blue dots in the cytoplasm with Romanowsky staining. Punctate basophilia may be found in any severe anaemia, but the presence of many of these cells is most commonly seen in $\beta$ thalassaemia and chronic lead poisoning where it may occur when the anaemia is slight.

*Nucleated red cells* are usually normoblasts and are found when erythropoiesis is very vigorous or more often when there is irritation of the bone marrow, as in leukaemia, or infiltration by secondary tumour.

*Leucocytosis* means an increase in the total number of white blood cells (over 11·0 × $10^9/l$ in adults). This may take the form of a polymorphonuclear leucocytosis in which the increase is due to the outpouring of many young neutrophil granulocytes, as occurs in the presence of pyogenic infections such as tonsillitis or pneumonia. Alternatively it may take the form of a lymphocytosis, as is frequently found, for example, in whooping cough. Infants commonly respond to infections by producing a lymphocytosis.

*Leucopenia* means a decrease in the total number of white cells below 4·0 × $10^9/l$ and usually involves a reduction only of the granulocytes (neutropenia). Leucopenia is found in tuberculosis, enteric fever, many acute viral infections and brucellosis. Occasionally a leucopenia is found in overwhelming infections and is a bad prognostic sign. In a small number of patients it may be constitutional and represent no threat to health.

*Eosinophilia* is the term used when the number of eosinophil granulocytes exceeds 0.4 × $10^9/l$. Eosinophilia is found most commonly in infections with worms, in allergic diseases, Hodgkin's lymphoma, polyarteritis nodosa and certain skin diseases.

*Monocytosis* refers to a monocyte count exceeding 0·8 × $10^9/l$ and is found for example in advanced tuberculosis, malaria and in some neutropenic states.

*Thrombocytopenia* means a diminution in the number of blood platelets and is significant only below a figure of 100 × $10^9/l$. Capillary bleeding tends to occur when the platelet count falls below 40 × $10^9/l$ but there is a poor correlation between the platelet count and a bleeding tendency.

*Leucoerythroblastic* is used to describe a blood picture in which primitive granulocytes and erythroblasts are simultaneously present in the peripheral blood. It is commonly but not necessarily associated with anaemia and reflects bone marrow irritation as in malignant infiltration of the marrow or disordered haemopoiesis as in myelofibrosis.

*Extramedullary haemopoiesis* means that production of blood cells takes place outside the normal sites. The term *myeloid metaplasia* is also used and refers particularly to the finding of blood cell precursors in the blood and extramedullary sites as seen in myelofibrosis. There is usually progressive enlargement of the spleen and liver and an accompanying leucoerythroblastic anaemia. Extramedullary haemopoiesis occurs not uncommonly in the first year of life when the available bone marrow space is insufficient to allow for an increased demand for blood formation.

## DISORDERS OF THE RED BLOOD CELLS

### The Anaemias

Anaemia may be defined as a state in which the level of haemoglobin in the blood is below that which is expected, taking into account both age and sex. At birth the haemoblobin is high (18 g/dl) because the fetus has lived in a relatively hypoxic environment. After birth, oxygenation of the baby's haemoglobin in the lungs is more effective and the haemoglobin level rapidly drops, partly by removal of effete red cells and partly by reduced production, reaching about half the birth level when the baby is three months of age. Thereafter the average level rises gradually until the child reaches puberty when a further rise occurs which is more marked in males than females. Adult males have haemoglobin levels on average 2 g/dl higher than adult females. This reflects the stimulus of androgens on erythropoiesis. It is possible therefore for a haemoglobin level of 12 g/dl to be regarded as anaemic in an adult male, but normal in an adult female. In practice, most adults who are otherwise in reasonably good health function satisfactorily if the haemoglobin is above 10 g/dl, provided this lower level has not appeared too quickly. The presence of symptoms related to anaemia depends partly on its severity but also on how quickly the anaemia has appeared. Thus a patient who has a reduction of haemoglobin from 13 g/dl to 8 g/dl in one week may have severe symptoms, while another patient whose anaemia has developed slowly to a similar level over months may be asymptomatic and unaware of the anaemia.

A useful approach to the elucidation of the cause of an anaemia is to keep in mind that the condition results from one or more of the following three factors:

1. Loss of blood, which may be either acute or chronic.
2. Inadequate production of normal red cells by the bone marrow.
3. Excessive destruction of red blood cells (haemolysis).

Most anaemias are multifactorial in their aetiology and many causes are relatively rare. The vast majority of anaemias are due to the failure of haemoglobin synthesis as a result of iron deficiency, the commonest reason for which is blood loss. This simple classification of the anaemias helps to guide the clinician in planning investigation.

## Classification of Anaemias

1. **Blood Loss**
   - (i) Acute (large volume over short period).
   - (ii) Chronic (small volumes over long period).

2. **Inadequate Production of Red Blood Cells**
   - (i) Deficiency of essential factors: iron, vitamin $B_{12}$, folate.
   - (ii) Toxic factors: inflammatory disease (infective and non-infective), hepatic and renal failure, drugs.
   - (iii) Endocrine abnormalities: hypothyroidism, hypoadrenalism, hypopituitarism, hypogonadism.
   - (iv) Invasion of bone marrow: leukaemia, secondary carcinoma, fibrosis.
   - (v) Disorders of developing red cells: sideroblastic anaemia, other idiopathic refractory anaemias, hereditary disorders of haemoglobin synthesis (thalassaemia).
   - (vi) Failure of stem cell compartment: aplastic anaemia, frequently drug induced.

3. **Excessive Destruction of Red Blood Cells (Haemolysis)**
   - (i) Intra-erythrocytic defect. (a) Hereditary: spherocytosis, haemoglobinopathies (abnormal haemoglobins and thalassaemias), disorders of glycolysis.
     (b) Acquired: red cells produced by dyserythropoietic states, e.g. vitamin $B_{12}$ and folate deficiency.
   - (ii) Extra-erythrocytic abnormalities. (a) Antibodies (autoimmune and isoimmune) (b) Physical trauma (prosthetic heart valve) (c) Chemical trauma (drugs) (d) Infections (malaria) (e) Toxic factors associated with inflammatory or neoplastic disease and metabolic failure.

**Clinical features of anaemia** are the direct consequences of diminished oxygen-carrying power of the blood on the tissues and organs of the body. Their occurrence and severity depend on the degree of anaemia and especially on the rapidity of its development, but are independent of its type. The symptoms of anaemia are fatigue, lassitude, breathlessness on exertion, palpitations, anorexia, dyspepsia, dizziness, dimness of vision, headache, insomnia and paraesthesiae in the fingers and toes. Myocardial anoxaemia causes angina pectoris, especially in older patients with coronary artery disease. There may be pallor of the skin and, much more significantly, of mucous membranes, tachycardia, cardiac dilatation, systolic murmurs and, in severe cases, oedema of the ankles.

## Anaemias Due to Blood Loss

**Acute Blood Loss.** A healthy adult can lose about half a litre of blood without ill effect. This makes it possible to provide a blood transfusion service using donors. When more than half a litre of blood is lost, compensatory mechanisms come into play; these reduce the blood flow to peripheral structures such as skin and muscle, and conserve the supply for central organs. The pulse rate rises and the blood pressure is maintained. The patient is pale, cold and sweaty and usually has to lie flat in order to maintain the cerebral circulation; hypovolaemic shock may ensue. At this stage the haemoglobin level of the blood is unchanged and in some cases it may even be higher than it was before the acute blood loss. If no further bleeding occurs, plasma production replenishes the volume, diluting the remaining red cells, and anaemia appears in about 24–36 hours. If blood loss is very severe, compensatory mechanisms fail and irreversible hypovolaemic shock supervenes, progressing to death. Anaemia may not have had time to appear.

In acute blood loss the primary problem is lack of blood volume which must be replaced by transfusion of whole blood, red cell concentrate, plasma or plasma substitutes. The anaemia which appears later if transfusion is not given or if plasma or plasma substitutes are used will be self correcting by increased red cell production over the ensuing few weeks unless the body iron stores are depleted. When acute blood loss is associated with other disease states, which themselves impair erythropoiesis, recovery of haemoglobin may be very slow and the anaemia may become chronic. Immediately after acute blood loss there may be a transient leuco-erythroblastic blood picture. After a few days a reticulocytosis of 5–10% develops, subsiding gradually as recovery of the haemoglobin level occurs. A rise in platelet count may also be observed and is usually transient unless the blood loss becomes chronic.

**Chronic blood loss** in contrast to the acute process, does not give rise to reduction in blood volume or to anaemia since the body has time to compensate by increased plasma and red cell production. Eventually, however, the continued loss of red cells causes depletion of iron stores and red cell production is impaired.

## Anaemias Due to Inadequate Production of Red Cells

### Iron Deficiency Anaemia

Iron deficiency is by far the commonest cause of anaemia in most parts of the world.

*Iron Metabolism.* Iron is essential for the synthesis of the haem fraction of haemoglobin. It is also present in myoglobin and other enzymes such as cytochrome. Iron in food is absorbed from the upper small intestine, mainly in the ferrous form, but can also be absorbed as haem from red meat. Much of the iron in food is unabsorbable because it is irreversibly bound to other substances, for instance phytates and phosphates. Also, iron readily takes the ferric form in which it cannot be absorbed. The low pH of the stomach contents helps to preserve the iron in the ferrous form and that process is assisted by binding of iron to sugars and amino acids which protect it from conversion to the ferric form. Haem absorption is uninfluenced by these factors and it is thus a very important source of dietary iron. Some foods, for example rice and bread, are rich in phytates and other substances which prevent iron absorption. Other foods, for example spinach, have a high iron content but almost none is absorbable.

All cells obtain iron by transfer across their membrane from the iron transport system (transferrin) in the blood. The intestinal mucosal cell is no exception but it also receives iron by absorption from the gut lumen. When body stores of iron are adequate and there is no unusual call for iron, the intestinal mucosal cell is well supplied with iron from the blood, and absorption from the gut is discouraged although not completely prevented. As iron enters the cell from the gut it goes into a labile pool within the cell from which iron may be directed to storage by the formation of a complex with apoferritin to form ferritin. It also goes to the mitochondria, or it may pass to the blood transport system with which the labile pool in the cell is in dynamic equilibrium. When erythropoietic demands for iron increase or the body stores are low, the mucosal cell becomes iron depleted and therefore avid for iron and absorption increases. Iron for erythropoiesis comes mainly from the iron transport system and almost all iron absorbed from the gut goes straight to the bone marrow and is used in erythropoiesis. Increased erythropoiesis associated with a variety of disorders may increase iron absorption even when iron stores are increased. Thus some forms of prolonged anaemia which are not due to blood loss or iron deficiency can be associated with excessive iron stores. Iron in the mucosal cells of the gut is lost with cell turnover. In this way unwanted iron is discarded. Otherwise iron loss from the body is minimal and occurs mainly from the skin and urinary tract. Total loss from these other sources amounts to about 1 mg a day. Haem that has been absorbed by the mucosal cell is split in the cell and the iron liberated. This iron is then made available to the general iron pool and treated in the same way as iron absorbed by other means. Iron obtained from the catabolism of haemoglobin is recycled either to the bone marrow, or if there is excess, to the iron stores. Iron is stored in cells in two forms, ferritin and haemosiderin. Iron is available from ferritin more readily than from haemosiderin; the latter as the more stable form constitutes the bulk of the iron identified by the Prussian blue reaction and is probably formed by degradation of ferritin. Various forms of ferritin exist depending on the tissue in which they are found.

**Aetiology.** Deficiency of iron may be caused in a number of ways. The diet may be inadequate in the amount of iron available for absorption. Disease of the gastrointestinal tract may give rise to malabsorption of iron. Most commonly iron may be lost from the body in amounts greater than can be balanced by absorption. This is usually due to blood loss but occasionally iron may be lost in the urine in the form of haemosiderinuria.

There are situations in which iron deficiency might be regarded as almost physiological. At birth the normal infant has a store in the form of a very high haemoglobin level and in addition some iron is available in the liver. This is adequate for erythropoietic requirements in the first few months of life. Thereafter a mild degree of deficiency appears since milk is a very poor source of iron. If weaning is delayed to as late as one to two years, as is the custom in certain parts of the world, the deficiency may become marked. If the child is weaned to a good diet, the deficiency is fairly quickly corrected. When prematurity and haemorrhage from the cord at birth deprive the infant of the normal store of iron, deficiency may appear sooner and be more severe.

In females menstruation causes an average loss of 30 mg of iron per month requiring approximately 1 mg a day absorption in addition to the normal needs. Although this loss disappears during pregnancy, the mother must find iron for the fetus, the placenta, her own increased red cell mass and blood loss at parturition. The requirements will be about 2·5 mg per day plus her own basic requirement of 1 mg a day giving a total of 3·5 mg a day. In practice, the need rises as pregnancy progresses and is therefore greatest in the second half of pregnancy. It follows that during the reproductive years iron deficiency is much more common in females than in males.

In adolescents, in whom a marked growth spurt occurs, iron requirements may outstrip absorption. Food fads are not uncommon at this age and may contribute.

Apart from the above, iron deficiency usually indicates either an inadequate diet or pathology in the patient. The best source of iron is red meat because haem can be absorbed as such. Vegetables have variable amount of absorbable iron. Soya bean is a rich source; spinach despite its high iron content is very poor, as the iron is so unabsorbable. Foods, e.g. bread, may be fortified with iron to improve their quality and greatly increase iron nutrition of thc lower economic group in which dietery inadequacy of iron is most common because the diet is generally poor in quality and regular meat cannot be afforded. Old people living alone, particularly men, run the risk of allowing their dietary habits to deteriorate with a low or absent meat content and then iron deficiency is not uncommon.

Absorption of iron is optimal where the pH of the gut contents is low keeping the iron in a ferrous state and is therefore most effective in the duodenum and upper jejunum. Reduction in gastric acid output, either by gastritis or resection raises the pH and reduces absorption. Reduction of exocrine secretions from the pancreas increases iron absorption because less bicarbonate is available to raise the pH in the lower duodenum and jejunum. Gastric operations which bypass the duodenum reduce iron absorption. Disorders of the small bowel mucosa, affecting mainly duodenum and upper jejunum, may cause severe malabsorption of iron as in coeliac disease.

In post menopausal women and adult men the commonest cause of iron deficiency is gastrointestinal bleeding. Erosions, ulcers, neoplasia, infective and non-infective inflammatory disease, parasitic infestations and varices, whether oesophageal or haemorrhoidal, may be the sources of blood loss. Hookworm infection is very common indeed and is the main cause of iron deficiency in many parts of the world.

*Anaemia of chronic disease.* Not all patients presenting with haematological findings of iron deficiency are iron deficient. The iron storage sites may show abundant iron which is unavailable for haemoglobinisation of the developing red cells. This is usually associated with chronic inflammatory or neoplastic disease in which there is an inhibition of mobilisation of iron from the body stores. The microcytic, hypochromic blood picture is associated with a low serum iron (p. 908) but also a normal or low iron binding capacity; the saturation of the iron binding capacity is usually less reduced than is found in iron deficiency anaemia with a similar level of serum iron. Saturation of the iron binding capacity below 15% almost always means iron deficiency. Iron can be observed in the storage cells in the marrow and virtually no sideroblasts (p. 547) are seen. Serum ferritin levels are normal reflecting the true state of the body stores.

**Clinical Features.** In many cases there are no symptoms and the deficiency may be discovered incidentally. In others vague symptoms of tiredness are insufficient to make the patient seek medical help. The symptomatology of iron deficiency is mainly that of anaemia (p. 542). However, some features are particularly associated with this state. Cracking of the corners of the mouth (angular stomatitis), sore tongue (glossitis) and brittle finger nails are relatively common. Dysphagia is rare. Pica, the eating of strange things, such as coal, earth, or foods in great excess, such as tomatoes or greens is more common than generally realised and may be revealed by the patient only if specifically asked.

On examination the signs of anaemia and of the particular complaint mentioned above may be observed. Flattening or concavity of the nails, (koilonychia), is sometimes seen in addition to the evidence of nail cracking. Sideropenic dysphagia (p. 319) is rarely encountered. Splenomegaly is not uncommon if the anaemia is severe but may reflect other disease such as portal hypertension, of which the iron deficiency is also symptomatic.

**Investigation.** The diagnosis that an anaemia is of an iron deficiency type is made mainly on laboratory findings. The first abnormality to appear is microcytosis. Later, hypochromia occurs due to a reduced saturation of haemoglobin in the red cells. As the deficiency becomes more severe, other evidence of red cell dysplasia in the form of misshapen red cells and poikilocytes is seen, although the finding of oval and elliptical forms occurs quite early. Some target cells may be found but often indicate other problems, and may be the signal to suspect beta thalassaemia minor, a hereditary defect of haemoglobin synthesis.

The blood count findings are, therefore, a reduced haemoglobin level with normal or slightly reduced red cell count, a low mean cell volume (MCV) of less than 76 fl., a reduced mean corpuscular haemoglobin concentration (MCHC) and the blood film appearances mentioned above. The white cell and differential counts are usually normal, although hypersegmentation of the neutrophils commonly occurs. The ESR is usually lower than would be expected for the degree of anaemia or associated disease.

Blood count indices vary according to whether they are produced by electronic counters such as the Coulter counter model S or by manual means. In the latter case, the MCV will not be satisfactory in many instances, as it depends on accurate red cell counting and the MCHC is then the index to use. Since the MCH, which is also dependent on an accurate red cell count, reflects both cell size and haemoglobin saturation, it is a less useful index.

The iron binding capacity of the blood reflects the level of the iron transport protein, transferrin, which is normally about one third saturated with iron. Saturation below 15% indicates iron deficiency and above 50%, iron overload, or failure to utilise available iron as in pernicious anaemia. Serum ferritin is present in minute quantities and is measurable only by radio-immunometric means. The range is wide in both sexes, mean values being higher in males. The levels, which correlate well with body iron stores, are very low in iron deficiency and raised in iron overload.

Bone marrow iron stores are found to be empty when stained by the Prussian blue technique.

DIAGNOSIS OF THE CAUSE OF IRON DEFICIENCY. Once it has been established that an anaemia is of an iron deficiency type, a cause should be sought. The direction of the investigations is influenced by the age and sex of the patient, the history and the findings on examination. Dietary histories are notoriously unreliable but evidence from relatives and friends may be helpful. In the absence of any clear lead it is reasonable to start by looking for evidence of gastro-intestinal blood loss with faecal occult blood tests, barium meal and enema and endoscopy. Negative barium studies should not be accepted as evidence of the absence of lesions. In patients in whom there is a known cause of intravascular red cell destruction, such as a prosthetic heart valve, the urine should be tested for haemosiderin. In tropical countries hookworm infection and schistosomiasis must be considered as likely causes but additional factors may require to be sought.

**Treatment.** It is self evident that the patient who is iron deficient requires iron. Almost all patients can be treated by the oral route and the cheapest preparation is ferrous sulphate given as a tablet containing 200 mg three times a day. A small proportion of patients develops indigestion, constipation or diarrhoea and then more expensive proprietary preparations may be tried. There are many of these and there is probably little to choose between them except that preparations employing a delayed release effect are to be avoided although they may give rise to less side-effects. This reflects the fact that they do not release the elemental iron at the best absorption site. Some proprietary preparations can be given once daily. For the patient who cannot swallow tablets, proprietary liquid preparations may be used and are generally palatable.

Evidence of a response to oral medication usually appears in under two weeks. When there is concomitant inflammatory or neoplastic disease, response may be much slower and oral therapy should not be discarded until two to three months have passed. If no response is seen, it may be that the patient is not taking the tablets for a variety of reasons. A check may be made by examining the stool which should be grey black if the patient is taking the tablets.

The rise in reticulocyte count associated with response to iron therapy is usually modest and seldom above 10%. After the haemoglobin level has returned to normal, iron should be continued for at least six months and in some cases a year in order to replenish iron stores. In cases of malabsorption, almost continuous therapy may be required or the parenteral route utilised.

*Parenteral Iron Therapy*. Commercial preparations of iron for injection should not be used except when one or other of the oral preparations cannot be tolerated or is found to be ineffective. The parenteral route of administration is suitable for the few patients who are genuinely unable to take iron by mouth because of pain, vomiting or diarrhoea, or who are unable to absorb iron because of some disorder of the gastrointestinal tract (p. 347). Iron given by injection has been used for the treatment of the anaemia of rheumatoid arthritis (p. 611), for the correction of severe anaemia in the late stages of pregnancy and following major operations.

The recommended single dose of iron-sorbitol is 1·5 mg of iron per kg of body weight given daily. It is assumed that about 250 mg of iron are required to increase the haemoglobin level by 1 g/dl of blood but the total dosage of iron should not exceed 2·5 g. Iron-sorbitol should be given by intramuscular injection and should never be given intravenously.

Iron-dextran is seldom given intramuscularly because of local irritation and since it has been shown to cause sarcomatous change in certain animals. It can be given intravenously by what is known as the 'total dose infusion method' in a suitable diluent. Alarming systemic anaphylactic reactions may occur (p. 30).

### Sideroblastic Anaemias

These are rare conditions in which red cell production is impaired by disordered iron metabolism.

The term *sideroblast* refers to a developing erythroblast which can be shown to have one or two iron granules in the cytoplasm. A *siderocyte* is a red cell containing iron granules. Both are normal findings. The iron granules are free in the cytoplasm and not associated with organelles. In certain pathological states iron accumulates in the mitochondria and appears as a ring of granules round the nucleus. These are called *ring sideroblasts* and are the characteristic cells of the sideroblastic anaemias. Pathological non-ring sideroblasts are cells in which there are excessive numbers of free iron granules in the cell cytoplasm. They occur in a number of conditions in which there is disordered erythropoiesis, for instance, untreated megaloblastic anaemia.

**Aetiology.** Sideroblastic anaemias occur in two forms: (1) A *hereditary* condition which usually shows a sex linked mode of inheritance, produces a microcytic, hypochromic blood picture very similar to that of iron deficiency, is unresponsive to iron therapy and is a benign disorder. (2) An *acquired* group of anaemias seen mainly in the elderly, many of which are idiopathic. Others are associated with a variety of disorders, including inflammatory disease, (e.g. rheumatoid arthritis), malignant disease, pernicious anaemia, myxoedema, ingestion of drugs such as isoniazid, and rarely pyridoxine deficiency. The blood picture in these cases does not resemble iron deficiency, the mean cell volume is usually slightly raised and hypochromic red cells are seen among mainly normochromic cells.

**Clinical features** are those of anaemia. Often an unsuccessful attempt has been made to treat the patient with iron, particularly in the hereditary form which mimics iron deficiency. Some patients with the idiopathic variety progress to develop acute myeloblastic leukaemia and the condition may be regarded as preleukaemic.

The diagnostic feature of all these conditions is the finding of ring sideroblasts within the bone marrow when stained by the Prussian blue reaction. In addition the marrow may be hypercellular and in the acquired group there may be dysplastic changes resembling a megaloblastic picture. Iron overload is often present. The serum iron is raised but saturation of the iron binding capacity is usually less than is seen in haemochromatosis.

**Treatment** includes the withdrawal of iron therapy. In some patients venesection may result in an improvement if iron overload is present. Any folate deficiency should be corrected. Rarely the disorder is caused by pyridoxine deficiency and then response will be observed to doses as small as 1 mg daily. Other cases that respond to pyridoxine require massive doses of up to 600 mg daily; improvement may be slow in appearing and treatment should not be abandoned in less than three months. When these measures are unsuccessful, transfusions with red cell concentrate may be required for the rest of the patient's life. In cases where the disorder is secondary to remediable disease, specific treatment usually corrects the sideroblastic disorder.

## The Megaloblastic Anaemias

Haemopoietic tissue is one of a number of rapidly proliferating tissues in which DNA synthesis is intense. Both vitamin $B_{12}$ and folate are essential for the synthesis of DNA and deficiency of one or both results in disordered cell proliferation. Haemopoiesis is particularly susceptible to deficiency of either of these vitamins and division of cells is delayed and eventually halted. Morphological changes appear in the marrow cells. In the red cell series these changes are described as megaloblastic because the cells appear abnormally large. Changes also occur in the granulocyte precursors and megakaryocytes and are not unique to haemopoietic tissue. Disordered morphology can be seen in other rapidly dividing cells such as those of the gastrointestinal tract. Similar changes occur in other rare anaemias in which the aetiology is obscure and commonly in patients who are receiving chemotherapy for neoplastic disease if the treatment schedule includes drugs which interfere with DNA synthesis (metabolic antagonists).

The production of megaloblasts reflects the continued RNA and protein production in cells in which DNA production is impaired. Normally in red cell production, cell division occurs rapidly. Between divisions the cells do not have time to regrow to their full size and a progressive reduction in cell size occurs. When DNA synthesis is reduced, the time between divisions is increased, more cell growth occurs and the cells become larger. In red cell precursors, haemoglobin production appears to be one of the factors limiting proliferation. Once a certain haemoglobin level has been reached, division stops. Thus in megaloblastic disorders not only do the red cell precursors have time to grow to a larger size, but they also undergo less divisions because there is no inhibition of haemoglobin formation. The end products are abnormally large and misshapen red cells which are well haemoglobinised.

As megaloblastic change becomes worse, increasing numbers of erythroblasts fail to mature and are destroyed in the marrow (ineffective erythropoiesis). Even in normal marrow a small proportion of developing cells suffer this fate but in advanced megaloblastic change the majority of the cells never mature to red cells. This massive destruction of cells in the marrow liberates large amounts of enzyme material and lactate dehydrogenase in the blood rises to very high levels. Eventually, in the absence of treatment, cell production fails. Excessive doses of metabolic antagonists have similar effects and may induce severe aplasia.

**Vitamin $B_{12}$** is a cobalt-containing porphyrin known as a cobalamin of which there are several. In man the assimilation of vitamin $B_{12}$ from the lower ileum is facilitated by gastric intrinsic factor which complexes with vitamin $B_{12}$. Absorption is at specific receptor sites in the ileum. Two forms of the vitamin are used in treatment. The first was cyanocobalamin but hydroxocobalamin is now preferred as it is less rapidly excreted in the urine and is therefore more effective.

*Deficiency of Vitamin $B_{12}$.* This vitamin is obtained mainly from animal foodstuffs. Vegetables alone are an inadequate source. Requirements of vitamin $B_{12}$ in the normal person amount to 1 – 2 $\mu$g daily. Deficiency takes at least 3 years to appear as there are large stores in the liver. It occurs because:

1. The diet may be inadequate (true vegans).
2. There may be intrinsic factor deficiency due to gastric atrophy as in pernicious anaemia, gastrectomy or, rarely, to congenital deficiency without gastric atrophy.
3. There may be disease of the terminal ileum reducing or eliminating the absorption site, e.g. Crohn's disease.
4. Vitamin $B_{12}$ may be removed from the gut either by bacterial proliferation in blind loops or fistulae, or by parasites such as the fish tapeworm (p. 867).

**Folate** metabolism is discussed on page 551.

## Addisonian Pernicious Anaemia

The term Addisonian pernicious anaemia should be limited to megaloblastic anaemia due to a failure in secretion of intrinsic factor by the stomach other than from surgery. This disease is rare before the age of 30, occurs mainly between 45 – 65 years and affects females more than males.

**Pathology.** The marrow shows the evidence of failure of DNA synthesis with extensive maturation arrest in the red cell precursors and disparity in the maturation of nucleus and cytoplasm. Granulocyte precursors are often diminished in number and giant metamyelocytes are seen. Megakaryocytes may also be reduced in number and show dysplastic changes. There is evidence of increased blood destruction — including unconjugated hyperbilirubinaemia and increased deposition of iron (haemosiderin) in the liver, spleen, kidneys and bone marrow. The gastric mucosa is thin and atrophic. In untreated or inadequately treated cases degenerative changes in the posterior and lateral tracts of the spinal cord may be found.

**Clinical Features.** The onset is insidious and the degree of anaemia is often great before the patient consults the doctor. In addition to the general symptoms of anaemia (p. 542) there may be intermittent soreness of the tongue and occasionally periodic diarrhoea.

The patient generally appears well nourished despite the fact that weight loss is a common feature. The skin and mucous membranes are pale and in severely anaemic cases the skin may show a faint lemon yellow tint. The surface of the tongue is usually smooth and atrophic, but sometimes it is red and inflamed. The spleen is sometimes palpable. In many cases paraesthesiae occur in the fingers and toes and occasionally there are signs of subacute combined degeneration (p. 726), which may rarely be found before the anaemia. Dementia may also occur. In the female there may be infertility. The urine contains excess of urobilinogen.

**Investigation.** Examination of the stained blood film shows a macrocytic blood picture. There is marked anisocytosis and poikilocytosis and in more advanced cases, fragmented red cells. Nucleated red cells sometimes show the features of megaloblastic change and can be found in the blood film, particularly if a 'buffy coat' preparation is made. This latter technique is useful if it is not possible to examine the bone marrow.

The reticulocyte count is usually low in absolute terms. Results expressed as a percentage must be assessed in relation to the reduced number of red cells. The absolute count is usually less than $100 \times 10^9/l$. Leucopenia is often present and is due to neutropenia. Hypersegmentation of the neutrophils is common. The platelet count is often within normal limits but may be reduced and occasionally severe thrombocytopenia is seen.

With modern counting equipment and the widespread availability of blood counts, this disorder is often diagnosed before anaemia appears as the result of the finding of a raised MCV. Consequently more florid, advanced cases are now seen less often.

Diagnosis is achieved in the first place by demonstrating that the patient has a megaloblastic anaemia, based on the finding of a macrocytic blood picture with the features mentioned above and a megaloblastic marrow. Thereafter a *Schilling test* will demonstrate that there is a failure of vitamin $B_{12}$ absorption due to a lack of gastric intrinsic factor. The fasting patient is given 1 microcurie of $^{57}$cobalt or $^{58}$cobalt labelled vitamin $B_{12}$ orally and at the same time 1000 micrograms of vitamin $B_{12}$ are administered intramuscularly. The injected material saturates the binding proteins in the patient's blood so that vitamin $B_{12}$ absorbed from the gut is lost in the urine. Urine is collected for 24 hours (48 hours if the patient has renal disease) and the radioactivity in the urine measured and related to the dose given orally. Normal subjects excrete more than 15% of the administered radioactivity in the 24 hour urine specimen. Patients with pernicious anaemia usually excrete less than eight per cent and very often less than one per cent of the administered dose in the urine. The test is then repeated adding intrinsic factor to the oral dose of labelled vitamin $B_{12}$. If the defect in absorption is corrected, it is reasonable to assume that the patient has a failure of intrinsic factor production. Uncommonly the correction is poor due to high levels of anti-intrinsic factor antibodies in the stomach contents and higher doses of intrinsic factor may be required. Alternatively poor correction may indicate disease in the ileum.

It is possible to conduct the Schilling test using both isotopes of cobalt, one labelling free vitamin $B_{12}$ and the other the vitamin $B_{12}$ bound to intrinsic factor. These are given simultaneously and the urine collected. The results are assessed on the ratio of the two isotopes appearing in the urine. The Schilling test can be used for diagnostic purposes, even after the patient has been treated and is in remission.

Other tests which contribute in making a diagnosis of pernicious anaemia are the finding of *intrinsic factor antibodies* (p. 31) in the plasma in 50% of cases and the demonstration of *pentagastrin fast achlohydria*, although often this unpleasant test is omitted if the results of the Schilling test are clear cut. *Parietal cell antibodies* are found in 80% of patients with pernicious anaemia but are diagnostically unhelpful as they are found in many patients who do not have pernicious anaemia.

**Treatment.** *General.* The decision to give a blood transfusion is based on general principles concerning the clinical state of the patient. When the haemoglobin level is so low as to endanger life, e.g. under 4 g/dl, it should be seriously considered. In all types of chronic anaemia of sufficient severity to require transfusion the blood should be given very slowly, preferably as red cell concentrate, because of the danger of producing cardiac failure. Frusemide should be given simultaneously by mouth or intravenously with the red cell concentrate.

*Specific.* Hydroxocobalamin should be given in a dosage of 1000 $\mu$g twice during the first week, then 1000 $\mu$g weekly until the blood count is normal.

Within 48 hours of the first injection of hydroxocobalamin the bone marrow shows a striking change from a megaloblastic to a normoblastic state. Within two to three days the reticulocyte count begins to rise, reaching a maximum between the fifth and tenth days. If there is co-existing inflammatory disease the response may be delayed. There is a brief peak of red cell output due to the maturation of the large number of cells held in maturation arrest by the vitamin $B_{12}$ deficiency. Reticulocyte counts may exceed 50%, the level depending on the initial erythrocyte count, but soon drop to below 10% as more normal production is resumed.

In some cases the rapid regeneration of the blood depletes the iron reserves of the body and recovery is halted. To prevent this occurring ferrous sulphate (200 mg t.i.d.) should be given soon after the commencement of treatment. A combined deficiency of vitamin $B_{12}$ and iron is recognised by the presence of macrocytosis and hypochromia. It is sometimes referred to as a dimorphic blood picture.

If a patient diagnosed as having pernicious anaemia fails to respond to the parenteral administration of adequate dosage of hydroxocobalamin, it suggests that the diagnosis is wrong or the preparation used is not potent. The patient may be suffering from one of the other types of megaloblastic anaemia which may be partially or completely refractory to hydroxocobalamin. Such cases may respond to folic acid.

*Maintenance.* The patient suffering from pernicious anaemia must be given regular doses of hydroxocobalamin indefinitely (1000 μg i.m. every three months). Theoretically the interval between doses may be longer but there is no merit in seeking the minimum effective dose. Blood counts should be done once every year and the assessment should never be made solely on clinical impression or on the haemoglobin level alone. With the maintenance of a normal blood count by adequate specific treatment the patient has a normal expectancy of life. There is, however, a statistically significant increase in deaths from gastric carcinoma in patients with pernicious anaemia.

### Other Causes of Megaloblastic Anaemia due to Vitamin $B_{12}$ Deficiency

*Dietary insufficiency* is rare except in countries where meat and other animal food stuffs are not eaten for religious or other reasons. The deficiency is readily corrected by the parenteral administration of vitamin $B_{12}$. Thereafter the vitamin may be given by mouth.

*Gastrectomy.* Total resection of the stomach induces a state indistinguishable from pernicious anaemia and patients should be treated in the same way as for that disease. Partial gastrectomy reduces vitamin $B_{12}$ absorption, in some cases to the point that vitamin $B_{12}$ deficiency occurs. Possibly gastritis may, in part, be responsible. The Schilling tests often demonstrates reduced absorption. One annual injection of 1000 μg of hydroxocobalamin is adequate prophylaxis for a patient who has had a partial gastrectomy.

*Disease of the terminal ileum* should be suspected if the Schilling test is not corrected by the addition of intrinsic factor in adequate amounts.

*Bacterial colonisation of the small intestine* (p. 348) results in an abnormal Schilling test, both without and with intrinsic factor; this is corrected by the administration of tetracycline.

### Megaloblastic Anaemias due to Folate Deficiency

**Folate** occurs in varying concentrations in many foodstuffs mainly in the form of polyglutamates. These are broken down to simpler forms by folate conjugase in the small intestinal lumen or mucosal cell. At some stage after absorption the enzyme dihydrofolate reductase produces reduced forms. Pteroylglutamic acid, also called folic acid, is the therapeutic agent mainly employed. Folate is available from both vegetable (foliage) and animal foodstuffs. Much is destroyed by cooking and body stores are relatively small, lasting only a few weeks.

*Deficiency of folate* arises from:

1. Inadequate Intake. Diets which totally lack fresh vegetables and meat or which consist of overcooked food, do not provide enough folate.
2. Disease of the upper small bowel, where folate is mainly absorbed. This may occur in coeliac disease or tropical sprue; very rarely extensive resection of the small bowel has a similar effect.
3. The body's demands exceeding intake. (a) When there is very active cell proliferation, e.g. haemolytic anaemia, leukaemias and other neoplastic disease, and during periods of acute or chronic infection.

   (b) Pregnancy, when the demands of the fetus and placental growth require

large amounts of folate. In this situation folate is taken by the fetus in amounts adequate for its needs, even when the mother is folate deficient. There is no evidence that the fetus is ever affected by folate deficiency in the mother although a female, deficient in folate, may be infertile.
4. Interference with the dihydrofolate reductase system. This enzyme system may be blocked by certain drugs, particularly methotrexate and pyrimethamine. In theory trimethoprim (p. 72) may also do this but a real danger appears to exist only in patients deficient in folate from another cause.
5. An unexplained mechanism. The anticonvulsant drugs phenytoin and primidone may cause folate depletion by an unknown mechanism not related to 4.

Approximately 60% of all cases of megaloblastic anaemia in Britain are due to folate deficiency. The majority of those suffering from vitamin $B_{12}$ deficiency have pernicious anaemia. In tropical countries most megaloblastic disease is due to folate deficiency associated with malnutrition, pregnancy and concomitant infection. Addisonian pernicious anaemia appears to be relatively uncommon in the tropics and in some areas is quite rare.

**Clinical features** are those of anaemia and of the underlying cause. Glossitis is less common than in vitamin $B_{12}$ deficiency. Neurological problems are very rare.

**Investigation.** The blood and bone marrow findings in megaloblastic anaemia due to folate deficiency are indistinguishable from those in vitamin $B_{12}$ deficiency as described for pernicious anaemia but serum and red cell folate levels are low. However, when the onset of folate deficiency has been recent and acute, the red cell folate, which reflects the patient's folate status over the previous three months, may still be within normal limits. Likewise, patients who have received folate therapy for a day or two will have a high serum folate level but may still show evidence of their past deficiency in the red cell folate. Serum folate should always be measured on a fasting specimen. The vitamin $B_{12}$ level in the serum may also be marginally reduced for reasons that are not clear. The Schilling test, however, is normal and the vitamin $B_{12}$ level returns to normal with folate therapy provided there is not a true vitamim $B_{12}$ deficiency from another cause.

**Treatment.** A daily dose of 5 mg of folic acid by mouth is sufficient; for maintenance therapy 5 mg once a week is almost always adequate. Folic acid must never be given, other than with vitamin $B_{12}$, in Addisonian pernicious anaemia or other vitamin $B_{12}$ deficiency anaemias, because of the risk of aggravating or precipitating neurological features of vitamin $B_{12}$ depletion. In pregnancy megaloblastic change due to vitamin $B_{12}$ deficiency is very rare indeed. It is therefore reasonable to give folate supplements to pregnant women. When a drug such as methotrexate inhibits dihydrofolate reductase, it is possible to employ folinic acid to overcome the metabolic block.

## Primary Idiopathic Aplastic Anaemia

This is a rare but grave disease of the stem cell compartment which fails to a varying degree, producing serious hypoplasia of the marrow elements.

**Clinical Features.** Men are affected more often than women. The disorder may occur at any age, the peak incidence being around 30 years. The onset is insidious and the clinical problems are due to the reduction or virtual absence of production of red cells, granulocytes and platelets. Infections and haemorrhage are the most troublesome complications and may prove lethal. Bleeding occurs in the skin and mucous membranes. Haematuria and epistaxis are common. Necrotic mouth and throat ulcers and monilia infections reflect the neutropenia.

**Investigation.** Known causes of hypoplastic and aplastic anaemia must first be excluded. Usually there is a pancytopenia. Neutropenia is the most marked aspect of the leucopenia, although it may not be the first to develop. The anaemia is normocytic, normochromic and often severe. Platelet production is often the most markedly affected and the last to recover. Studies with $^{59}Fe$ show poor clearance of the isotope from the blood, poor uptake and utilisation by the marrow and no extramedullary haemopoiesis.

**Treatment.** There are two aspects to the management. The first is supporting the patient by replacement therapy. This consists of maintaining a reasonable haemoglobin level and is the least of the problems because transfusion of red cell concentrate can be given regularly. Vigorous antibiotic therapy for infection and platelet transfusions for bleeding are required as outlined in the management of the ablative treatment for acute myeloblastic leukaemia (p. 573). Corticosteroids may be used to reduce bleeding.

The second aspect is an attempt to stimulate haemopoiesis and promote recovery. Androgenic steroids with a low virilising activity are employed; these include oxymetholone by mouth or nandrolone deconate intramuscularly. High doses of methyl prednisolone may also be used. Red cell production and to a lesser extent granulocyte production benefit most from these drugs which unfortunately have undesirable and troublesome side effects when used over long periods. This is particularly so in children in whom secondary sexual characteristics may be stimulated and premature fusion of epiphyses may occur if the treatment is not suitably curtailed. Androgens may also cause cholestasis. Fluid retention and prostatic enlargement may occur.

Bone marrow transplantation is now being advocated for this disorder in children and young adults and, in some centres, carries a better prognosis than when the disease is treated in a more conservative manner. In a few patients leukaemia supervenes and it is probable that these have been cases of leukaemia presenting in an aplastic or hypoplastic phase.

**Prognosis.** The course tends to be prolonged. Spontaneous improvement and recovery may occur and is one reason why treatment should be vigorous and prolonged. Androgens may be ineffective in the early phase of the disease but become effective later and should not be abandoned because of initial failure. The prognosis is undoubtedly poor and more than 50% of the patients die usually within the first year after diagnosis. Patients who survive longer than one year have a better chance of remission. Perhaps in some instances there is an immunological defect and, in the future, treatment directed towards this will prove to be of value.

**Secondary pancytopenia** may be due to: (1) Idiosyncrasy to certain drugs such as chloramphenicol, phenylbutazone, oxyphenbutazone, indomethacin, sulphamethoxypyridazine, tolbutamide and troxidone or to certain industrial chemicals and insecticides chiefly benzene and its derivities such as trinitrophenol, trinitrotoluene and gamma-benzene hexachloride. (2) The majority of drugs used in the chemotherapy of malignant disease. (3) X-rays and radio-activity. (4) Replacement of the bone marrow by abnormal cells such as tumour or by fibrous tissue. (5) Viral infections.

The clinical features and methods of diagnosis are the same as for primary idiopathic aplastic anaemia. The noxious agent is identified, and should be removed. Treatment is as for the idiopathic form except that little is known about the value of marrow transplantation.

## Anaemias due to Excessive Red Cell Destruction (Haemolytic Anaemias)

Red cell turnover is a normal physiological process, red cells having an average survival of 120 days. This means that all the red cells are replaced every four months. Various abnormalities either in the red cell or its environment may shorten its life span and require more rapid replacement. Anaemia develops when the marrow can no longer compensate. The increased output of new red cells causes a raised reticulocyte count which in part is due to shift of marrow reticulocytes into the blood. Under more extreme stress nucleated red cells may be released.

The catabolic pathways for haemoglobin degradation are unimpaired but overloaded. There is an increase in unconjugated bilirubin in the blood and increased reabsorption of urobilinogen from the gut, this then being excreted in the urine in increased amounts. Bile does not appear in the urine. The level of bilirubinaemia is not greatly increased and jaundice is mild (p. 588).

*Intravascular and extravascular haemolysis.* The latter occurs in the phagocytic cells of the spleen, liver, bone marrow and other organs. Intravascular haemolysis liberates haemoglobin into the plasma where it is bound mainly by an alpha-2 globulin, known as *haptoglobin*, to form a complex which is too large to be lost in the urine, but which is taken up by the liver and degraded. Some haemoglobin is bound to albumin to form methaemalbumin, and this is the basis for the *Schumm's test* for haemoglobin in the plasma. If all the haptoglobin has been consumed, free haemoglobin may be lost in the urine. In small amounts this is reabsorbed by the renal tubules where the haemoglobin is degraded and the iron stored as haemosiderin. Sloughing of the renal tubular cells gives rise to *haemosiderinuria* which always indicates intravascular haemolysis. When greater amounts of haemoglobin are lost through the kidneys *haemoglobinuria* occurs, giving the urine a black appearance.

Extravascular haemolysis may not result in much depletion of haptoglobin. Furthermore inflammatory disease increases haptoglobin levels as does steroid therapy. Ahaptoglobinaemia may occur as an inherited disorder. For these reasons estimation of the haptoglobin level in the blood is not always easily interpreted. Nevertheless absence of haptoglobin is a strong indicator of haemolytic disease.

*Blood and Marrow Findings.* The peripheral blood shows a moderate macrocytosis and polychromasia due to the reticulocytosis. Specific red cell abnormalities may give a clue to the type of haemolytic disease. There may be a polymorphonuclear leucocytosis. The marrow shows erythroid hyperplasia. Megaloblastic change may occur and usually reflects depletion of folate reserves.

Increased erythropoietic turnover in the marrow is associated with increased levels of lactic dehydrogenase in the blood, which, in the absence of any dyserythropoietic state such as megaloblastic change, closely follows the severity of the haemolytic disorder.

If necessary the survival of the red cells can be measured crudely by using radioactive chromium. Surface counting done at the same time over liver and spleen may give an indication of whether haemolysis is taking place. If transfusion has been given the patient's blood contains a mixed cell population which is not suitable for $^{51}Cr$ studies. In these circumstances cross matched donor cells should be used for labelling.

*Classification* of haemolytic anaemias is given on page 541.

## Haemolytic Anaemia due to Hereditary Abnormalities of the Erythrocyte

The principal disorders are hereditary spherocytosis, G6PD deficiency, haemoglobinopathies, such as sickle-cell disease and thalassaemia. G6PD deficiency and haemoglobinopathies are most common in Negroes and thalassaemia in the Mediterranean area. There has been a rise in the incidence of these disorders in other countries including Britain because of immigration.

### Hereditary Spherocytosis

The exact abnormality is unknown but there are metabolic defects in the red cell membrane with increased leak of sodium ions into the cell, giving the sodium pump excessive work. Membrane loss occurs and this gradually compels the cell to lose its biconcave structure and become spherical. Spherocytes are destroyed by the spleen. The red cell life span is thus reduced giving rise to varying degrees of haemolytic disorder, often enough to cause anaemia. The haemolysis is extravascular.

**Clinical Features.** Symptoms vary from none to those of fairly severe anaemia. Episodic jaundice may be noted. The spleen is often but not always palpably enlarged. The severity of the disorder tends to vary in any one patient with crises of haemolysis at times. Aplastic crises, which can occur in anybody following a viral infection, are noticeable in these patients because of the greatly increased red cell turnover which has become their normal state. There is an increased risk of pigment stone formation and cholecystitis may be the presenting event. Leg ulcers sometimes occur.

**Investigation.** The diagnosis is made by demonstrating a haemolytic state together with spherocytes in the blood film, increased osmotic fragility due to the spherocytes and the demonstration of the same disorder in other members of the family. The Coomb's test (p. 31) is negative. There is an excessive loss of urobilinogen in the urine. Red cell survival studies show destruction of red cells almost exclusively in the spleen. The differential diagnosis is from other causes of spherocytosis, particularly the various forms of immune haemolysis. Loss of membrane due to trauma to red cells in the circulation usually gives rise to many more schistocytes than are seen in hereditary spherocytosis.

**Treatment.** Splenectomy results in striking and usually permanent improvement both in the symptoms and in the anaemia. All authorities are agreed that operation should be advised when the anaemia causes persistent impairment of health, when severe haemolytic crises have occurred, when other members of the family have died from the disease, or where evidence of cholecystitis and cholelithiasis is present. Opinion differs as to the desirability of operation in mild cases with no resulting disability. The operation should be carried out during a period of remission, and in young children should be deferred until school age. Severe haemolytic crises require treatment by blood transfusion. Blood must be matched very carefully and administered by very slow drip, as gross haemolytic transfusion reactions are common in this disease. Iron is of no value. In this type of haemolytic anaemia treatment with corticosteroids is not indicated. Folic acid, 5 mg daily, should be prescribed.

### Glucose-6-Phosphate Dehydrogenase Deficiency

Glucose-6-phosphate dehydrogenase (G6PD) is the first enzyme in the hexose monophosphate shunt of the Embden Myerhof glycolytic pathway from which red cells derive most of their metabolic energy. The function of the hexose monophosphate shunt is to service the enzymes glutathione reductase and glutathione peroxidase which protect the red cells against damage due to oxidation. In the absence of G6PD this protective mechanism is crippled and certain drugs in sufficient concentration can seriously injure the red cell.

It is now known that the deficiency is inherited as an X-linked recessive disorder and has a high frequency among Negroes. In West and East Africa about 20% of males (hemizygotes) and about 4% of females (homozygous for the abnormal gene) are affected. A small number of heterozygous females are also deficient in G6PD. A similar deficiency occurs in Caucasian and Mongoloid races where it is usually more severe. *Favism* (haemolytic anaemia from ingestion of the broad bean, *Vicia faba*) is due to deficiency of G6PD of the severe Caucasian variety. In Negroes the activity of the enzyme is about 15% of normal, whereas in the others it is often less than 1% with consequently greater clinical effects. Recently some hitherto unexplained cases of haemolytic disease of the newborn in Caucasians have been found to be due to the same defect. Yet other types of G6PD biochemically different from the above may be associated with congenital nonspherocytic haemolytic disease and have been found in persons of pure British ancestry. In these cases it is important to realise that splenectomy is valueless.

Many drugs in common clinical use, e.g. some antimalarials and sulphonamides, are capable of precipitating haemolysis in individuals with this defect. Infections may also potentiate the haemolytic action of drugs such as acetylsalicylic acid, chloramphenicol, chloroquine, and phenacetin.

**Clinical Features.** Persons with G6PD deficiency normally enjoy good health but are liable to haemolysis if any of the incriminated drugs or foods is ingested. However the haemolytic effect is related to the dose and will not be clinically detectable if the amount does not exceed a critical level. It is thus often possible to employ doses which are not toxic. The anaemia, when it occurs, may be rapid in onset, becoming obvious between 2 and 10 days after exposure to the precipitating agent and may be sufficiently severe to cause haemoglobinuria as well as the other classical signs of haemolysis. In the Negro type of deficiency only cells of a certain age and over are involved so that the haemolysis is to some extent self-limiting even when the offending agent is continued. Young red cells do have some G6PD activity and remain viable until their enzyme complement decays when they become susceptible to haemolysis. Since in the Caucasian variety the enzyme deficiency is much more severe, destruction tends to be more disastrous. Anuria is an infrequent but serious complication.

**Investigation.** Diagnosis can be confirmed by estimating the G6PD activity of the red cell but this may not be entirely accurate if there is a considerable reticulocytosis. A number of screening tests are also available e.g. (1) the ascorbate cyanide test of Jacob and Jandl which monitors the whole glutathione regulating system of which G6PD is a fundamental part; (2) spot tests employing either the reduction of soluble tetrazolium compounds to insoluble purple formazan or the fluorescence of NADPH which is a biproduct of G6PD activity. This last test can be performed on aged blood or blood collected on filter paper and dried. The Jacob and Jandl test has the advantage of being cheap. These tests should always be performed alongside normal controls.

**Treatment** is by removal of the toxic agent. Recovery is usually rapid but if the anaemia is severe, transfusion of red cells with a normal enzyme complement may be required. Thereafter the patient should be advised to avoid drugs which may precipitate the disorder.

## The Haemoglobinopathies

The haemoglobinopathies can be classified into three subgroups. In the first there is an alteration in the amino acid structure of the polypeptide chains of the globin fraction of haemoglobin, commonly called the abnormal haemoglobins, although some function as normal variants. In the second subgroup the amino acid sequence is normal but polypeptide chain production is impaired or absent for a variety of reasons; these are the thalassaemias. In the third subgroup there is the persistence of haemoglobin, normal in early life, namely haemoglobin F, into adult life. The hereditary persistence of high fetal haemoglobin is a benign condition and can be advantageous to persons carrying the haemoglobin S gene with which it is allelomorphic.

### Sickle-cell Anaemia

Sickle-cell anaemia has been recognised among Negroes and to a lesser extent in other races since the beginning of the century. It is caused by the presence of the abnormal haemoglobin, haemoglobin S.

Abnormal haemoglobins are caused by amino acid substitutions in their polypeptide chains. These in turn reflect mutations in the structural genes controlling the production of these chains. There are four loci for these structural genes, all on autosomal chromosomes, active in postnatal life. They are designated alpha, gamma, beta and delta and are responsible for the production of the three main haemoglobins seen after birth, namely haemoglobins F, A and A2. Each of these haemoglobins contains in common two alpha chains and their differences reflect the possession of two gamma chains in the case of haemoglobin F, two beta chains in the case of haemoglobin A, and two delta chains in the case of haemoglobin A2. Thus the globin fraction of these three types of haemoglobin may be written $\alpha2\gamma2$, $\alpha2\beta2$ and $\alpha2\delta2$, respectively. Each chain in the globin fraction carries one haem moiety in its folds. It is convenient and practical to represent normal adult haemoglobins by the capital letter A and the abnormal haemoglobins by S, C and E and so on. As there are now well over 200 haemoglobin variants known, the letters of the alphabet do not suffice and for some years new variants have been given names, often of the towns or districts in which they were discovered. Sickle-cell haemoglobin is the most important but haemoglobin C, D and E are also significant in some parts of the world, particularly when inherited along with haemoglobin S or with beta thalassaemia (p. 561).

Modern nomenclature includes a statement of the site of the amino acid substitution and the substituting amino acid. Thus sickle haemoglobin may be defined as:

$$\text{Hb S } \beta^{6\text{GLU}-\text{VAL}} \text{ or Hb S } \beta^{\text{A3GLU}-\text{VAL}}$$

The second method is more accurate since it defines the helix or bend in which the substitution occurs.

Control of haemoglobin synthesis is inherited from both parents. Thus a normal adult can be depicted as having the haemoglobin genotype AA, sickle-cell trait by AS and sickle-cell anaemia or homozygous haemoglobin S disease by SS. The inheritance when both parents have sickle-cell trait can be shown thus:

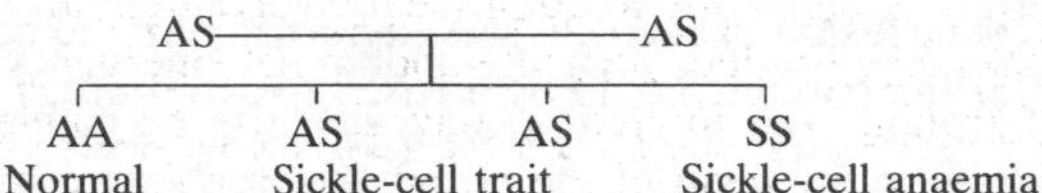


The patient with sickle-cell trait is relatively resistant to the lethal effects of falciparum malaria in early childhood. The high incidence of this deleterious gene in equatorial Africa is thus explained by the selective advantage for survival it confers in an environment of endemic falciparum malaria. Surprisingly, patients with sickle-cell anaemia do not have a greatly increased resistance to falciparum malaria.

**Pathogenesis.** When haemoglobin S is deoxygenated, the molecules of haemoglobin polymerise to form pseudo-crystalline structures known as 'tactoids'. These distort the red cell membrane and produce characteristic sickle-shaped cells. The polymerisation is reversible when reoxygenation occurs. The distortion of the red cell membrane, however, may become permanent and the red cell 'irreversibly sickled'. The greater the concentration of sickle-cell haemoglobin in the individual cell, the more easily tactoids are formed, but this process may be enhanced or retarded by the presence of other haemoglobins. Thus haemoglobin C participates in the polymerisation more readily than haemoglobin A, whereas haemoglobin F strongly inhibits polymerisation. In sickle-cell anaemia most of the red cells contain haemoglobin S and little else and are very prone to sickle even *in vivo* under normal conditions. This happens particularly in those parts of the microvasculature which are sinusoidal and where the flow is sluggish. Sickle cells increase blood viscosity, traverse capillaries poorly and tend to obstruct flow, thereby increasing the sickling of other cells and causing cessation of flow. Thrombosis may follow and an area of tissue infarction results causing severe pain, swelling and tenderness (pain crises). In addition these cells are phagocytosed in large numbers by the reticuloendothelial system, thus reducing their life span considerably and giving rise to haemolysis.

**Clinical Features.** The two major problems are chronic anaemia due to reduced red cell survival and episodes of tissue infarction.

*Anaemia.* Problems do not arise until the fourth month of life when haemoglobin F production gives way to haemoglobin containing beta chains. The anaemia is haemolytic in type, severe, the haemoglobin seldom rising above 10 g/dl and averaging approximately 8 g/dl. Secondary folate deficiency is common and exacerbates the anaemia. When persistent, growth retardation and delayed puberty may occur. Episodes of increased sequestration and destruction of red cells occur, sometimes for no apparent reason and may lead to a swift fall in haemoglobin with rapidly enlarging spleen and liver. Transient hypoplasia of red cell production associated with infection, as is seen in normal persons, is also liable to have exaggerated effects (aplastic crisis). The chronic anaemia is responsible for fatigue, reduced exercise tolerance, increased susceptibility to infection, cardiomegaly, leg ulcers and cholelithiasis. Hyperplasia of the marrow in the first year of life expands the marrow cavity producing bossing of the skull, prominent malar bones and protuberant teeth.

*Infarction crises* are characterised by episodes of severe pain and these punctuate the patients' lives. Commonly they occur in bones and spleen but no tissue is exempt. In the infant they classically affect the fingers and toes, producing large fusiform swellings (dactylitis). Metacarpal and tarsal bones may be affected and residual stigmata of shortening of digits due to epiphyseal involvement may occur. At any age mesenteric infarction may produce an acute abdominal emergency. The renal papilla is another site of trouble and infarction may give rise to painless haematuria. In adults aseptic necrosis of the head of the femur is a disabling complication.

Precipitating factors include dehydration, chilling and infection, but sometimes the attacks occur spontaneously. The onset is usually rapid, the pain excruciatingly severe in the first 24 hours, thereafter abating over the next few days. Fever, increasing jaundice and malaise are frequent concomitants and, if persistent, may suggest the establishment of infection in the infarcted site. Salmonella osteomyelitis is common.

Pregnancy is hazardous unless careful antenatal care is provided and towards the end of pregnancy, infarctive crises in the bones may liberate large amounts of fat and bone marrow emboli which cause diffuse microembolism of the lungs with pulmonary infarction, cor pulmonale and even death. These complications may also be seen in the less severe haemoglobin SC disease.

Sickle-cell anaemia should always be suspected in a patient who has had symptoms of anaemia since infancy and who belongs to a race which is often affected. In areas where sickle-cell anaemia is common, it should be considered in the differential diagnosis of many disorders. Patients must be adequately screened before major surgery and bloodless field surgery should never be employed, because infarction of the entire limb below the tourniquet may occur.

**Investigation.** Microscopic examination of the stained blood film will show some sickle-shaped red cells in patients with sickle-cell anaemia but these are not seen in patients with sickle-cell trait. The presence of haemoglobin S can be confirmed by the demonstration that the red cells will sickle within 20 minutes when mixed on a glass slide with a freshly prepared 2% solution of sodium metabisulphite under a cover slip. Controls should be set up at the same time. Alternatively solubility tests may be employed. If neither of these is available, a small drop of blood diluted in saline may be incubated under a sealed cover slip overnight when sickling will occur. A positive result indicates the presence of haemoglobin S but does not distinguish between sickle-cell trait, sickle-cell anaemia, haemoglobin SC disease, sickle-cell thalassaemia, etc.

When suspected, the diagnosis should be confirmed by electrophoretic analysis of the haemoglobin and, if necessary, by a family study to demonstrate the inheritance. In this way true sickle-cell anaemia can be differentiated from other diseases in which haemoglobin S is combined with thalassaemia or some other abnormal haemoglobin such as C or D.

**Treatment and Prevention.** There is no known method of changing the genetic constitution of an individual and therefore no means of curing this disease. Management is therefore aimed at alleviation of the symptomatology and the promotion of a lifestyle that will minimise the ill effects of the disorder. Basically this consists of the elimination of infections such as malaria and life-long antimalarials should be taken, if necessary. The patient should avoid becoming chilled or dehydrated. Regular folic acid supplements (5 mg daily) should be prescribed to support the greatly increased erythropoietic activity. Improvement of socio-economic circumstances is of considerable importance to the underprivileged and will go a long way to alleviating the serious results of this disease. However, acute episodes will occur whatever is done and these should be managed as follows.

Exacerbation of the chronic haemolytic anaemia is commonly associated with infections and these should be eliminated. The patient should be adequately hydrated but transfusion with red cell concentrate used only in exceptional circumstances. Most patients are habituated to a haemoglobin level of about 8 g/dl and should be transfused only when the haemoglobin drops below 5 g/dl. Clearly the circumstances in individual cases will vary so that transfusion may be needed at higher levels. Diuretics should be avoided unless cardiac failure supervenes when they should be used with caution.

The pain caused by tissue infarction crises can be extremely severe and the clinician is strongly tempted to use powerful analgesics. However, as the episodes will be recurrent, this should be avoided if at all possible and simple non-addictive analgesics such as aspirin, paracetamol and codeine used. Water and electrolyte depletion should be corrected as quickly as possible. Antibiotics will be necessary if there are infective complications such as osteomyelitis.

Many lines of prophylactic therapy of *in vivo* sickling have been tried but even those with a theoretical hope of success have proved disappointing. Sodium bicarbonate orally in large doses may help in altering blood pH but cannot be given for very lengthy periods.

**Prognosis.** It is probable that in Africa, without medical attention, few children with sickle-cell anaemia survive to adult life. With full medical facilities and improved social and economic circumstances many patients survive and, although subject to recurrent ill health, lead a fairly normal life but are unlikely to reach old age.

## Other Sickle-cell Diseases

**Sickle-Cell Trait.** Most patients who are carriers of the sickle gene lead healthy lives. However, under certain circumstances they may be liable to sickling. These include bloodless field surgery and flying at altitudes over 15 000 feet (4575 m) if pressurisation is inadequate. In addition these patients are liable to attacks of painless haematuria due to infarction of the renal papillae.

**Haemoglobin SC Disease.** This disorder behaves like a mild variety of sickle-cell anaemia. Episodes of infarction crises are less frequent and anaemia is either absent or less severe. Aseptic necrosis of the femoral head, retinal thrombosis and painless haematuria are not uncommon complications.

Pregnancy is the main hazard as the same complications already mentioned under sickle-cell anaemia occur. Treatment of these should be by heparinisation and if necessary by premature induction of labour or delivery by Caesarean section. Another risk is that the symptomatology may mimic closely other problems in pregnancy characterised by hypertension and proteinuria, but the treatment as for these may be lethal. Sedatives should be avoided. Careful antenatal and postnatal care are required and folic acid supplements will be needed and also iron if there is a deficiency.

**Haemoglobin C Disease.** This is a benign haemoglobinopathy which, in its homozygous form, is not associated with much morbidity but may cause megaloblastic anaemia in pregnancy and considerable splenomegaly in adult life. It requires no specific treatment other than folic acid supplements in pregnancy.

## The Thalassaemias

Thalassaemia is an inherited impairment of haemoglobin synthesis, in which there is partial or complete failure to synthesise a specific type of globin chain. The exact nature of the defect is not yet understood but it is probable that a number of different faults occur along the pathway which translates the genetic information into a polypeptide chain. The gene itself may be deleted. Beta chain synthesis is most commonly affected. When the abnormality is heterozygous, synthesis of haemoglobin is only mildly affected and little disability occurs. When the patient is homozygous, synthesis is grossly impaired and severe anaemia results.

### Beta Thalassaemia

Failure to synthesise beta chains ($\beta$-thalassaemia) is the commonest type and is seen in highest frequency in the Mediterranean area. Heterozygotes have what has been called *thalassaemia minor*, a condition in which there is usually mild anaemia and little or no clinical disability. Homozygotes (*thalassaemia major*) are unable to synthesise haemoglobin A and, after the neonatal period, have a profound hypochromic anaemia associated with much evidence of red cell dysplasia and increased red cell destruction. Haemoglobin F ($\alpha 2\gamma 2$) production normally ceases in the neonatal period, but because of the severe anaemia some production persists to provide much of the circulating haemoglobin. Thus these patients attempt to supply their requirements with haemoglobins that normally comprise only 3% of the total. At best they usually manage little more than 30 to 50% of the normal adult complement of haemoglobin.

**Clinical Features.** The anaemia is crippling and the possibility of survival for more than a few years without transfusion is poor. Bone marrow hyperplasia early in life may produce head bossing, prominent malar eminences and other changes giving a Mongoloid appearance. The skull radiograph shows a 'hair on end' appearance and general widening of the medullary spaces which may interfere with the development of the paranasal sinuses. Development and growth are retarded and folate deficiency may occur. Splenomegaly is an early and prominent feature. Hepatomegaly is slower to develop but may become massive especially if splenectomy is undertaken. Transfusion therapy inevitably gives rise to haemosiderosis. Cardiac enlargement is common and cardiac failure, in which haemosiderosis may play a part, is a frequent terminal event.

There are several types of $\beta$-thalassaemia and a great variety of clinical manifestations which present a broad spectrum of disease. For further study the reader is referred to publications dealing with this subject in greater detail (p. 602).

**Diagnosis.** Thalassaemia minor is often detected only when iron therapy for a mild hypochromic anaemia fails. The demonstration of microcytes, increased resistance of red cells to osmotic lysis and a raised haemoglobin A2 fraction, together with evidence of the same abnormalities in other members of the family, establishes the diagnosis. In contrast haemoglobin A2 levels are diminished in iron deficiency states.

The diagnosis of thalassaemia major is made by the finding of profound hypochromic anaemia associated with evidence of severe red cell dysplasia, erythroblastosis, and the absence or gross reduction of the amount of haemoglobin A, raised levels of haemoglobin F and evidence that both parents have thalassaemia minor.

**Treatment.** Transfusion is the mainstay in the treatment of homozygous $\beta$-thalassaemia and if possible the haemoglobin levels should be maintained between 10 and 12 g/dl. The intraperitoneal route may be used in young children to conserve veins. Iron therapy is strongly contraindicated but folic acid supplements should be given. Attempts to remove iron by the administration of chelating agents such as desferrioxamine should be employed but fail to keep pace with the iron deposition from transfusion therapy until the patient has been transfused with over 100 units of red cells when the level of iron overload becomes considerable and chelating agents more effective as a result. Splenectomy may be required for mechanical reasons or for hypersplenism. The later this can be done the better. Intercurrent infection must be treated vigorously with appropriate antibiotics.

### Alpha Thalassaemia

The reduction or absence of alpha chain synthesis is found mainly in South-east Asia. There are probably at least two inherited abnormalities, one associated with severe, and the other with mild inhibition of alpha chain production. Heterozygotes of either abnormality are at little disadvantage since $\alpha$-chain production is adequate. A slight excess of gamma chain production at birth may form tetramers $\gamma 4$ (haemoglobin Bart's) and this can be demonstrated by electrophoretic techniques. The combination in the patient of a mild and a severe $\alpha$-thalassaemia disorder results in a deficiency of $\alpha$-chain production which is less than absolute, so that some normal haemoglobin is formed. There is an excess of beta chains and these form tetramers $\beta 4$ (haemoglobin H) and this may explain the syndrome of haemoglobin H disease. The inheritance of the severe $\alpha$-thalassaemia abnormality from both parents is incompatible with life and such offspring are stillborn (hydrops fetalis).

## Autoimmune Haemolytic Disease

In this disorder autoantibodies are formed against red cell antigens and cause inappropriate destruction of the cells (p.31). There are two main types categorised on the basis of the thermal characteristics of the antibody. 'Warm' antibodies have a thermal optimum of 37°C, this being characteristic of most immune antibodies. The majority are IgG. 'Warm' type autoimmune haemolytic anaemia has antibodies of this type and these can almost always be shown to have rhesus specificity. In some cases IgA and IgM antibodies are also seen, and complement binding may also be demonstrated in quite a proportion of cases, either with or without evidence of specific antibodies. 'Cold' antibodies have a thermal optimum of 4°C, but often a thermal range of up to 37°C. Naturally occuring antibodies tend to be of this type and most are IgM.

### 'Warm' Type Autoimmune Haemolytic Anaemia

Many cases are idiopathic but some occur in association with chronic lymphatic leukaemia, lymphoma and systemic lupus erythematosus. Treatment with methyldopa may induce this type of haemolytic disorder and it is the commonest form of drug induced haemolytic anaemia in Britain.

**Clinical Features**. Patients of all ages are affected with a slight preponderance of females. Symptoms vary with the severity of the disease and its cause and are mainly those of anaemia. In addition, in severe cases there may be fever, vomiting and prostration. Splenomegaly and sometimes hepatomegaly is present.

**Investigation**. The diagnosis is established by demonstrating evidence of antibody attack on the red cells by the direct antiglobulin test (Coomb's test p. 31). Antibody in the plasma may be shown by the indirect antiglobulin test. Elution of antibody from the red cells allows investigation of specificity against a panel of cells. The rhesus antibody, anti-e is the commonest. Identification of specificity is useful in obtaining blood for transfusion as blood which does not carry the specific antigen can be chosen. The blood film almost always shows polychromasia and spherocytosis.

**Treatment** should be with prednisolone 60 mg daily for three to four weeks, the dose thereafter being slowly reduced. Response to treatment can be monitored with reticulocyte counts and haemoglobin estimations. If relapse occurs at a lower dose, the dosage should be raised and maintained for a further three weeks, when reduction may be tried again. If treatment fails from the beginning or, if after six months of steroid therapy the patient still has active haemolytic disease, splenectomy should be considered. If splenectomy fails, immune suppression with drugs such as azathioprine may be tried. However, disease that behaves in this way usually turns out to be chronic. Blood transfusion should be avoided unless an antibody has clearly been identified and antigen free blood is available. In life threatening situations blood may be given even though there are problems about complete compatibility, together with high doses of prednisolone.

### 'Cold' Type Antibodies (Cold Agglutinin Disease)

Idiopathic cold agglutinin disease occurs mainly in the elderly and the symptoms reflect a tendency of the red cells to agglutinate and sludge in the microvasculature of the extremities where the blood is cooled. Raynaud's phenomenon is usually present and also acrocyanosis. A low grade chronic haemolytic anaemia occurs. All these problems are worse in cold weather. Investigations demonstrate an increased red cell turnover and a 'cold' antibody in enormously high titres. The antiglobulin test is almost always positive and reflects complement binding.

Treatment consists of keeping the extremities warm. Transfusion should be avoided if possible. Steroids and splenectomy are of little value but immunosuppressive therapy may decrease antibody levels in severe cases.

**'Cold' Agglutinin Disease Secondary to Other Disorders**. Paroxysmal cold haemoglobinuria may be associated with syphilis or be idiopathic and have the Donath Landsteiner IgG antibody. 'Cold' antibody-type disease may also occur in association with *Mycoplasma pneumoniae* infection and infectious mononucleosis and then the haemolysis is usually self limiting. If seen in lymphoma the haemolysis is usually more chronic.

*Paroxysmal nocturnal haemoglobinuria* is a very rare disease sometimes found in aplastic anaemia and leukaemia. The red cells have acquired susceptibility to antibodies which are normally present in the blood and are most active against red cells at acid pH. Thrombocytopenia is common and haemosiderinuria occurs. The disorder may be fatal.

## Isoimmune haemolytic disease

### Haemolytic Disease of the Newborn

This disease, previously called erythroblastosis fetalis, occurs in either sex at birth or within the first 2 to 3 days. The first-born child in the family is usually healthy, but in successive children the severity of the disease increases and later children may be born dead. Hydrops fetalis is the most severe form, death occurring *in utero*; icterus gravis neonatorum is a dangerous illness but compatible with survival; haemolytic disease of the newborn is the mildest form.

It appears that in most cases the rhesus (Rh) factor is the sensitising agent or antigen. The majority (85%) of people, men and women, have red cells which contain the Rh antigen, D, and these people are said to be Rh-positive. Some of the children of an Rh-positive father and an Rh-negative mother are Rh-positive, since the factor is inherited as an autosomal dominant. The Rh-negative mother becomes sensitised by the Rh-positive substance contained in the fetal red cells. The maternal agglutinins (antibodies to Rh-positive factor) thus produced, penetrate the placental barrier and cause haemolysis of the fetal erythrocytes.

In about 1 pregnancy in 10 the mother is Rh-negative and the fetus Rh-positive. However haemolytic disease of the fetus is very rare in first pregnancies (provided the mother has not previously been sensitised by transfusion) and, fortunately, sensitisation does not occur as often as might be anticipated even in subsequent pregnancies. Indeed the risk of an Rh-negative woman having a baby with haemolytic disease of the newborn in any pregnancy other than the first is about 1 in 22.

If a mother is Rh-negative and her husband Rh-positive, the maternal serum must be tested for antibodies between the 32nd and 36th week of each pregnancy. If they are found, delivery should be carried out in hospital. If no antibodies are detected the infant will probably escape the disease, but nevertheless the cord blood should be tested for antibodies. If they are present, preventive treatment can be instituted.

Very occasionally an antigen other than D is responsible for the development of haemolytic disease of the newborn.

It must be remembered that an Rh-negative mother who has had an Rh-positive fetus may be sensitised to Rh-positive blood. If she receives a transfusion and Rh-positive blood is given a haemolytic reaction may occur. Consequently all women of child-bearing age or under and all pregnant women who may require transfusion must have their blood typed for Rh factors as well as for the main blood groups.

**Clinical features** of haemolytic anaemia of the newborn are those of severe haemolytic anaemia with oedema and enlargement of the liver and spleen. Clinical jaundice is usually absent for 24 hours after birth. Thereafter deep jaundice leading to kernicterus (p. 719) may occur. The severity of the jaundice is largely due to the immaturity of the fetal liver which is unable to conjugate the large amounts of bilirubin with which it has to deal. The blood picture is very striking. The haemoglobin level, which should normally be about 18 g per 100 ml at birth, falls rapidly. Enormous numbers of nucleated red cells and a reticulocytosis of 10 to 50% are found in the peripheral blood.

In the severe cases the mortality is 70 to 80% without treatment, death occurring within 2 weeks, but with exchange transfusion the mortality is low. Spontaneous recovery occurs in the mild cases.

**Treatment**. Exchange transfusion should be given to all severely affected infants, as this is the only method of treatment that will overcome heart failure in the very anaemic infant and prevent deep jaundice and kernicterus in others. Delay of even a day may prove fatal and hence early diagnosis is essential. Antenatal prediction from tests of the maternal serum for antibodies gives the infant the best chance. In mild cases simple transfusion will be sufficient, and in some instances no treatment is required.

It is now believed that the most common cause of primary Rh immunisation may be transplacental haemorrhage during the third stage of labour. The likelihood of an Rh-negative woman developing anti-Rh antibodies is related to the number of Rh-positive red cells present in her circulation immediately after delivery. The injection of gamma globulin containing a high titre of anti-D immunoglobulin into the mother shown to have such cells should be carried out within 72 hours of delivery. This will destroy the infant cells that have leaked into the mother's circulation and will prevent the development of antibodies in the mother and haemolytic disease in later babies.

## Haemolytic Anaemia due to Other Abnormalities

**Physical Trauma to Red Cells.** Prosthetic heart valves, bacteria and intravascular fibrin formation associated with disseminated intravascular coagulation may all traumatise the red cells reducing their life span. Fragmented cells may be seen in the blood film.

**Drugs**, e.g. sulphasalazine or dapsone, may stress the metabolic processes of the red cells to the point of destruction even though the red cell is not enzyme deficient. Antigen-antibody reactions due to drugs acting as haptens may damage red cells directly or indirectly (p. 36).

**Haemolytic Anaemia due to Malaria.** Haemolysis always accompanies malaria and in severe or prolonged attacks very considerable anaemia may ensue. Generally the degree of anaemia is related to the severity of the parasitaemia but the destruction of red cells is always in excess of that due to parasitised cells and sometimes considerably so. During an acute attack of malaria the reticulocyte count may be low but, as the patient recovers, a brisk outpouring of young red cells occurs. Recuperation may be embarrassed by deficiency states, especially of folate and iron, or by other infection. Where these occur anaemia will be more severe and prolonged.

Immunity to malaria is greatest where the infection rate is highest and lowest where there is a low rate of infection or the patient is non-immune. Furthermore acquired immunity may be prejudiced by pregnancy, prolonged antimalarial therapy, splenectomy, lymphoma and allied disorders. Splenomegaly and anaemia diminish with increasing immunity but are universally found in young children. Splenectomy in patients exposed to malarial infection should be done with caution and only if lifelong prophylaxis against malaria can be ensured, otherwise disastrous levels of parasitaemia can develop and the patient die of cerebral malaria.

**Inflammatory and neoplastic disease** shortens the life span of the red cell. The mechanisms are complex and not completely understood. Excessive erythrophagocytosis by macrophages occurs. Red cells are damaged as they pass through affected tissue and drugs used in treatment may also harm them.

## Transfusion with Incompatible Blood

Transfusion with incompatible blood may arise: (1) with clerical errors leading to the wrong blood being given; (2) when the infused red cells are of the wrong main blood group due to careless typing of the bloods; (3) when the blood of recipient and donor are of compatible main groups but incompatible subgroups. Direct cross-matching of recipient's serum against donor's cells greatly reduces this risk; (4) from the transfusion of Rh-positive blood to a sensitised Rh-negative recipient.

Symptoms usually begin after only a few millilitres of blood have been given, and if the transfusion is immediately stopped there may be no serious consequences. In severe reactions the patient complains of shivering and restlessness, nausea and vomiting, precordial and lumbar pain. There is a cold, clammy skin with cyanosis. The pulse and respiration rates increase and the temperature rises to 38–40°C. The blood pressure falls and the patient passes into a state of shock. There is haemoglobinaemia, and possibly even haemoglobinuria; oliguria may occur with renal failure due to acute tubular necrosis. Jaundice appears after a few hours. In severe cases the anuria persists and uraemia develops, from which the patient may die. In others diuresis occurs even after several days and the patient recovers. In the majority the acute features subside in 24 to 48 hours.

Prophylaxis involves great care in the typing of blood and direct cross-matching before administration. The first 50–100 ml of any transfusion should be given very slowly and the transfusion stopped at once if any untoward symptoms develop. The patient should be under continuous observation during transfusion especially if unconscious.

Treatment of the established reaction involves giving hydrocortisone (100 mg i.v.), inducing a diuresis with mannitol and dealing with shock. If acute tubular necrosis occurs the measures recommended on page 448 must be instituted at once.

## Erythrocytosis, Polycythaemia and other Myeloproliferative Disorders

There are three states in which the numbers of red cells are increased above normal: 1. When there is a physiological response to a physiological stimulus, as in hypoxia, when the production of erythropoietin is increased. Hypoxia may be due to altitude (p. 805), pulmonary disease or congenital heart disease with cyanosis or where there are abnormal haemoglobins with a high oxygen affinity. The white cells and platelets are unaffected and there is no splenomegaly.

2. When there is a physiological response to a pathological stimulus. In this group the red cells respond to the production of abnormal substances with erythropoietic activity; this is occasionally found with certain benign and malignant tumours, e.g. of the kidney, liver, bronchus, uterus and cerebellum (haemangioblastoma) and with renal cysts. As in the first group the white cells and platelets are usually normal and there is no splenomegaly. However, the blood counts may be affected by the underlying disease.

3. When there is a pathological proliferation of red cells without erythropoietin stimulus. This is true polycythaemia (polycythaemia vera).

### Polycythaemia Vera

Polycythaemia vera is one of a group of disorders of the pluripotential stem cells that include myeloid metaplasia, myelofibrosis and thrombocythaemia. The group is known as the myeloproliferative disorders. These are overlapping conditions with features in common and they may progress from one form to another. All carry the risk of terminating as acute leukaemia.

**Clinical Features**. Polycythaemia vera occurs mainly in patients over the age of 40 and is more common in males than females. There may be no symptoms and the patient is diagnosed incidentally. A number, mainly males, present with peripheral vascular disease. Common symptoms among the majority of patients are lassitude, loss of concentration, headaches, dizziness and blackouts, pruritus and indigestion. The patients often have a high colour and the spleen is palpable in 75% of cases at diagnosis. Thrombotic complications may occur and peptic ulceration is common.

**Investigation**. The diagnosis is made by accumulation of evidence. The haemoglobin level is greater than 18 g/dl in males and 16 g/dl in females with an associated elevation of white cell count and platelet count in many but not all cases. The bone marrow is hypercellular with erythroid hyperplasia, very active granulopoiesis and increased numbers of megakaryocytes. Iron depletion of the marrow is usual. The red cell mass is greatly increased as is the plasma volume giving a very high total blood volume. The neutrophil alkaline phosphatase score is normal or raised and urate levels are often elevated. Whole blood viscosity is increased. In some patients the above results may be marginal and the diagnosis uncertain.

**Treatment**. Venesection is the simplest therapeutic measure and the best to use if the diagnosis is in doubt; 500 ml of blood (less if the patient is elderly) may be removed and this venesection repeated within a day or two if necessary. Venesection should continue until the haematocrit reading is reduced to 45%. Clinical improvement occurs rapidly with the reduction of blood viscosity. Iron deficiency appears, if not already present, but generally iron is not prescribed as its deficiency curbs erythropoiesis. It may be given with other methods of treatment. Venesection should be used with caution when the platelet count is very high because of the risk of thrombosis.

Radioactive phosphorus may be used when the diagnosis is certain and is an excellent form of treatment (5 mCi. of $^{32}P$ i.v.). The full effect will not appear for three months but the white cell count and platelets respond more quickly. Further doses may be necessary in time.

Chemotherapy with busulphan (2–4 mg/day), or melphalan (2–4 mg/day) until the disease is brought under control is equally effective but requires more supervision and more frequent blood counts than radioactive phosphorus. It carries a slightly greater risk of severe marrow depression. Pyrimethamine may be used if no other treatment is available but can be associated with drug-induced ill health.

**Prognosis**. The average life span after diagnosis exceeds 10 years. Some survive more than 20 years. Progress to a refractory state with anaemia, myelofibrosis or acute leukemia eventually occurs if the patient does not succumb to intercurrent disease.

**Stress or Spurious Polycythaemia**. Haemoglobin and red cell count measurements are not always true indicators of red cell mass. Some patients with a high haemoglobin are found to have a red cell mass which is normal or even subnormal. The cause is a reduced plasma volume. This disorder tends to occur in middle-aged males who carry heavy responsibility or who are stressed for other reasons. It is often associated with hypertension and vascular disease. A change in lifestyle, tranquillisers or $\beta$-blockers sometimes have beneficial effects with recovery of normal blood values.

## Myeloid Metaplasia and Myelofibrosis

Myeloid metaplasia is the appearance of precursors of red cells, granulocytes and platelets in abnormal sites such as the liver and spleen, and is usually associated with a leucoerythroblastic blood picture. This is not a phenomenon compensating for loss of marrow activity but is evidence of disordered behaviour by the precursor cell lines. Myeloid metaplasia is seen in myelofibrosis. Early in myelofibrosis the marrow may have little or no fibrous tissue but as the disease progresses this increases and may eventually fill most of the marrow space.

**Clinical features** are very variable. Most patients suffer lassitude, weight loss, night sweats and some intolerance of heat. The spleen may be greatly enlarged in myelofibrosis and splenic infarcts may occur. Rarely splenomegaly is absent. Peptic ulceration is common and there is an increased incidence of gastrointestinal bleeding.

**Investigation**. Anaemia, sometimes macrocytic, is common. The white cell count varies with a diminution or increase of granulocytes and usually a leucoerythroblastic blood picture. The red blood cells show very characteristic tear drop poikilocytes. The platelet count may be very high, normal or low and giant forms are seen in the blood film. The neutrophil alkaline phosphatase score is frequently raised as are urate levels. The marrow is often difficult to aspirate and the trephine biopsy shows an excess of megakaryocytes and increased reticulin and fibrous tissue replacement. Folate deficiency is very common.

**Treatment** is largely supportive with blood transfusion, folic acid, and non-virilising androgen therapy. Corticosteroids may be helpful in some patients. Cytotoxic therapy should be used very cautiously. Splenectomy may be required if the grossly enlarged spleen is causing distress or because transfusion requirements are excessive but the outcome is unpredictable. Prognosis is generally rather poor. The disease is progressive with steady deterioration.

## Essential Thrombocythaemia

This is a rare disorder of the elderly associated with a tendency both to bleed and to have thrombotic episodes. The platelet count is usually in excess of $1000 \times 10^9/l$ with an excessive number of megakaryocytes in the marrow. It responds well to radioactive phosphorus. Aspirin in small doses may help to counteract the thrombotic tendency. While it may alleviate vascular insufficiency by discouraging platelet aggregation there is the danger that excess may interfere with production of the natural anticoagulant prostacyclin (p. 590).

# DISORDERS OF THE WHITE BLOOD CELLS AND THE RETICULO-ENDOTHELIAL SYSTEM

## Agranulocytosis

This serious disease is characterised by marked leucopenia with severe reduction or absence of neutrophil granulocytes.

**Aetiology and Pathology.** In most cases the cause is an idiosyncrasy or sensitisation to, or poisoning by, a variety of drugs, notably amidopyrine, chlorothiazide, chlorpromazine, chlorpropamide, imipramine, phenindione, phenylbutazone, oxyphenbutazone, streptomycin, various sulphonamides and the thiouracil derivatives. Exposure to insecticides should also be considered.

Agranulocytosis may follow excessive irradiation or the use of cytotoxic drugs or antimetabolites and it is found as an integral part of pancytopenia, leukaemia and some cases of hypersplenism.

Agranulocytosis occurs, rarely, in severe infections, while in some cases there is no discoverable cause — idiopathic agranulocytosis.

In most cases the bone marrow shows virtual disappearance of the granular cells and their precursors. In some the marrow contains many early myelocytes, with few mature forms — an arrest of maturation. In others the appearance is that of the underlying blood disease.

**Clinical Features.** There may be a history of exposure to one of the agents mentioned above. The onset may be either sudden or gradual. In the acute and severe cases the condition begins with sore throat, fever and often rigors which may be followed by great prostration. There is rapidly advancing necrotic ulceration in the throat and mouth, with little evidence of pus formation. In fulminating cases the patient dies in a few days from toxaemia and septicaemia. In less acute cases there may be a preliminary period of malaise and weakness.

A chronic type has been described in which there is a persistent or recurring leucopenia with granulopenia. Rarely the neutropenia occurs in cycles of three to four weeks (*cyclic neutropenia.*) In such cases the symptoms are chiefly malaise, low grade fever and sore throat often without ulceration.

**Investigation.** Blood examination may show little alteration in the haemoglobin or red cell count. There is marked leucopenia, usually below $2{\cdot}0 \times 10^9/l$ falling to $0{\cdot}5 \times 10^9/l$ or less. The percentage of granulocytes falls rapidly until none may be found.

Rarely severe agranulocytosis may occur as an inherited disorder of Mendelian dominant type. In these cases there is a compensatory monocytosis. The marrow shows a maturation arrest at the myelocyte stage. Such patients can produce neutrophils in the face of severe infection.

**Prevention and Treatment.** All the drugs mentioned at the beginning of this section should be regarded as potentially dangerous and must be employed carefully. The patient should be warned to report unusual symptoms, fever or a sore throat.

The most important measure in treatment is removal of the offending agent if it can be identified. The patient is at risk from septicaemia. Blood culture should be done and the patients managed in the same way as those with agranulocytosis that follows ablative chemotherapy used for acute myeloblastic leukaemia (p. 573). If the patient survives the acute phase, the outlook is fairly good, with recovery in many cases.

## Infectious Mononucleosis (Glandular Fever)

This is a benign, acute infective disease due to the Epstein Barr (E.B.) virus, a herpes virus which also causes Burkitt's lymphoma and nasopharyngeal carcinoma. It occurs chiefly in adolescents and young adults of either sex, sporadically or in epidemics. It is mildly infectious and often spread by direct oral contact — the 'kissing disease'. The incubation period is about a week to ten days.

**Clinical Features.** The most common presenting features are tiredness, malaise, headache, anorexia, fever and enlargement of superficial lymph nodes, particularly the posterior cervical. Petechial haemorrhages at the junction of the hard and soft palate may occur early and be followed by sore throat with or without exudate. A maculopapular rash often appears during the first ten days in adults. Patients who have been given ampicillin for the sore throat develop a skin eruption due to the drug in over 90% of cases. Epigastric and right subcostal tenderness is common and reflects hepatitis. The spleen is often palpable. It is usually soft and not tender. Pain in the right iliac fossa may result from mesenteric adenitis. Rarely there may be signs of meningitis or encephalitis.

**Investigation.** There is usually no anaemia and in the early stages the white cell count may be normal or low. A mild neutrophil leucocytosis is often present in the first few days, thereafter being replaced by an increase in the characteristic atypical mononuclear cells and lymphocytes. The proportion of the atypical cells varies greatly from case to case. The total white cell count is commonly raised to between 10 and $20 \times 10^9/l$. Another herpes viral infection, that due to cytomegalovirus and also toxoplasmosis (p. 821) may cause lymphadenopathy and changes in the blood similar to infectious mononucleosis.

Heterophil antibodies develop in the serum of patients with infectious mononucleosis. After the first week the Paul-Bunnell reaction becomes positive in titres of 1:200 or more in over 80% of cases and may remain positive for weeks. The 'Monospot test' is widely used as a screening procedure. It is a simple slide test which is quick and more sensitive than the Paul-Bunnell. The Wasserman reaction may be falsely positive.

**Treatment** is symptomatic. The patient should be rested during the acute phase, if necessary in bed. Although recovery is invariable some patients suffer prolonged illness, debility, with intermittent fever, sweating, inability to concentrate and depression. These symptoms may respond dramatically to corticosteroid therapy. Rarely thrombocytopenia or autoimmune haemolytic anaemia may occur; in most cases these also respond to corticosteroids.

## The Leukaemias

In these disorders there is an abnormal proliferation of the leucopoietic tissues throughout the body; this is usually associated with an increase in the number of white blood cells of one type in the peripheral blood, among which immature forms occur. Leukaemia is a progressive and fatal condition causing death from anaemia, haemorrhage or intercurrent infection, although its course may vary from a few weeks to several years.

**Aetiology.** The cause of leukaemia is unknown. The uncontrolled proliferation of cells and the development of foci of leucocyte formation in organs other than the bone marrow, spleen and lymph nodes leads to its classification as a neoplastic disorder. However, the cells show no truly invasive properties and the process appears to start as a generalised cellular disturbance. Chromosomal abnormalities, such as may be produced by exposure to ionising radiation, can be found in some leukaemic cells and irradiation may be an aetiological factor in the disease. In some animals and birds, viruses are known to cause leukaemia and it is recognised that these agents can transform cells of the lymphocyte series. Though the possibility of a viral aetiology of leukaemia in man continues to attract attention there is no direct evidence that the disorder is caused by such an infection.

**Clinical and Haematological Features.** The terms acute and chronic, when applied to leukaemias reflect the clinical behaviour of the two main types of the disease. In acute leukaemia the history is often brief and life expectancy, without treatment, short. In chronic leukaemias the patient may have been unwell for years and survival is measured in years. These differences are mirrored in the haematological findings. The general rule that in neoplastic disease the more acute the clinical course, the more primitive or undifferentiated the cell type, holds true. Thus in acute leukaemia the most primitive blast cells are characteristic whereas in the chronic forms differentiation to mature types of cell is seen.

Not all leukaemias are associated with an increased white cell count or even the appearance of abnormal cells in the blood. The term *subleukaemic* is used when the white cell count is within or below normal limits but abnormal cells are seen in the blood. *Aleukaemic* is used when there are no abnormal cells to be seen in the blood. In these cases the white cell count is usually subnormal. The diagnosis is made from the marrow. Almost all cases which present subleukaemic or aleukaemic forms are acute leukaemias. Sometimes the acute leukaemia presents as an apparent aplastic anaemia and declares itself later. Some of these cases also have paroxysmal nocturnal haemoglobinuria.

**Classification.** The leukaemic process affects either the precursors of the lymphocytes or the granulocyte-monocyte series. Thus acute leukaemias may be classified as lymphoblastic and non-lymphoblastic (myeloid, myelomonocytic or monocytic). Each of these can be sub-classified.

*Acute lymphoblastic leukaemia* can be divided into types in which the T and B receptors can be recognised by specialised techniques and a third in which the cells are receptor 'silent' but can be recognised by reaction to antisera raised against acute lymphoblastic leukaemia cells. A small fourth group exists in which the cells are completely undifferentiated. This sub-classification is of major clinical significance since it is the receptor silent type which constitutes 70% of all cases; these respond well to treatment and carry a very real chance of long-term remission. When immunological techniques are not available, acute lymphoblastic leukaemia may be recognised with some certainty on the basis of Romanowsky stains, together with special staining techniques such as the PAS reaction and staining with Sudan black.

*Acute non-lymphoblastic or myeloid leukaemia* may also be subclassified into at least eight varieties. These cannot all be detailed here but the subclassification reflects the variable and common involvement of the monocyte series with the granulocytic series and also the involvement of the erythroid and megakaryocytic elements. In some, a degree of differentiation to the promyelocyte and even to the myelocyte stage can be seen and in the latter may be associated with a more chronic course. In these cases the term 'subacute' is sometimes used. It is also true that not all cases pursue an acute course even though the morphology of the disease would appear to indicate that they should. They may 'smoulder'. One relatively chronic form is known as 'refractory anaemia with an excess of blasts'.

*Chronic leukaemias* are similarly divided into lymphocytic and non-lymphocytic (granulocytic or myeloid). There may be a chronic monocytic leukaemia but this is probably related to the myeloid type, since it usually terminates in acute myeloblastic leukaemia.

## Acute Leukaemias

Acute leukaemias are disorders in which there is a failure of maturation. Proliferation of cells which do not mature leads to an ever increasing accumulation of useless cells which take up more and more of the space required for normal marrow function. Eventually this proliferation spills into the blood. The cells in acute leukaemia proliferate more slowly than normal haemopoietic tissue, a fact that is useful in treating these patients.

Acute myeloblastic leukaemia is the most common type of acute leukaemia, except in young children in whom the lymphoblastic variety is more frequently found. In adults the incidence of acute leukaemia rises with age.

**Clinical Features.** The disease may begin insidiously but the clinical onset is usually abrupt. There is fever, malaise and a rapidly advancing anaemia. Epistaxis, spongy bleeding gums or other haemorrhagic manifestations including purpura are common and are due largely to thrombocytopenia. Sore throat and ulcers in the mouth or pharynx are frequent, due to reduction in normal polymorphonuclear leucocytes. Hypertrophy of the gums is often noted in monoblastic leukaemias. Muscle and joint pains may occur. The spleen and often the liver are enlarged in the later stages. There may be cervical lymphadenopathy secondary to pharyngeal sepsis but in the lymphoblastic form increase in the size of these and other lymph nodes is a common early feature.

**Investigation.** Blood examination usually shows a profound and increasing anaemia of normochromic type. The MCV is often raised. The total white cell count may vary from a very low count of less than $1 \times 10^9/l$ to as high as $500 \times 10^9/l$ or more, but in the majority the count is less than $100 \times 10^9/l$. The blood film appearances are usually diagnostic of acute leukaemia since blast cells and other primitive cells are to be found, but sometimes marrow examination is required in aleukaemic forms before the nature of the disease is understood. Severe thrombocytopenia is usual but not invariable. The marrow is involved in all cases and study of it is the most important investigation. It is usually hypercellular with replacement of the normal marrow elements by leukaemic blast cells in varying degrees. However, in some cases marrow is impossible to obtain by aspiration. Trephine biopsy is a poor substitute but should then be done. Special staining techniques and immunological procedures are used to subclassify these diseases. The presence of Auer rods in the cytoplasm of the blast cells indicates a non-lymphoblastic type of leukaemia.

**Treatment.** Accurate sub-classification of the acute leukaemias is of great importance as treatment of the lymphoblastic and non-lymphoblastic varieties is very different. Chemotherapy is the major element in both, with radiotherapy being used in a secondary role.

The first decision must be whether to treat specifically or not. In the very elderly it may be unreasonable to subject the patient to unpleasant therapy which stands only a small chance of success for a brief period. In such cases supportive treatment should be given and this often alleviates distress for a while. However, with the considerable improvement in the results of treatment, the view is taken that an attempt to achieve remission should be made in most patients.

SPECIFIC THERAPY is designed to clear the leukaemic tissue and allow the recovery of the normal haemopoietic cells. In *acute lymphoblastic leukaemia* it is fortunate that this can be achieved in the majority of patients using a combination of vincristine and prednisolone, a regime which is almost non-toxic to normal cell lines. Regrowth of the normal cells occurs as the leukaemic tissue regresses and the patient goes rapidly into remission. This phase of treatment is known as *induction*. A phase of *consolidation* follows in which other drugs including daunorubicin, mercaptopurine, cytarabine and methotrexate are used and intrathecal therapy is given using the last two drugs, together with irradiation of the cranium to eradicate disease in the central nervous system which may have survived the initial chemotherapy. Finally a *maintenance* phase of treatment is given in which the patient receives a repeating cycle of the above drugs until two or three years have been completed in remission. Active treatment is then withdrawn because the patient probably stands more chance of death as the result of treatment than from the disease itself. Unfortunately, patients with the T or B cell types of acute lymphoblastic leukaemia tend to relapse within a year after initial good response. If relapse occurs in any patient the chances of achieving long-term remission are remote.

*Acute non-lymphoblastic (myeloblastic) leukaemia* must be managed rather differently. The three more useful drugs are daunorubicin, cytarabine, and thioguanine. All these are drugs that are very toxic to the normal as well as leukaemic cells. In addition daunorubicin is cardiotoxic. In order to clear the leukaemic tissue, a phase when the normal tissues are severely depressed must be accepted. During this phase of 'ablation' the patient may be gravely at risk from infection and bleeding as there will be severe neutropenia and thrombocytopenia. Young patients tolerate this aggressive management better than old. Treatment is generally given in 'pulses'. A pulse of chemotherapy is a brief period of treatment between which there is an interval when no treatment is given. A number of pulses make up a course of therapy. Assessment of progress is made on blood and bone marrow findings. Once the marrow has been cleared of blast cells the normal haemopoietic tissue may be allowed to repopulate the marrow. The advantage of the more rapid proliferation of normal haemopoietic tissue is seen at this stage. As neutrophil production resumes, the patient rapidly feels better. Infections come under more effective control. Bleeding problems disappear as the platelet count rises.

At best only 50 – 60% of patients treated for acute non-lymphoblastic leukaemia achieve a remission. In the others the disease is to a greater or lesser extent refractory. Once the disease is seen to be refractory to specific therapy there is no point in giving more as this merely makes the patient more ill. If stopped, the patient may have a few weeks of quite good life, with suitable support.

When remission is achieved and the bone marrow recovers the patient should receive *maintenance therapy*. There are many regimes but most employ the same drugs as are used for induction, except that daunorubacin must be used very frugally or not at all as its cardiotoxic side effects are cumulative.

*Bone marrow transplantation* by the intravenous route from matched siblings, preferably of the same sex, is now being used to treat acute leukaemia and some measure of success is being obtained. This is done when a good initial remission is achieved, and is a form of therapy likely to develop further in the near future.

SUPPORTIVE THERAPY. The specific treatment of acute leukaemia, particularly the acute non-lymphoblastic form, would be difficult if not impossible without intensive supportive therapy. The easiest problem to deal with is the *anaemia* and transfusions of red cell concentrate are given to maintain an adequate haemoglobin level, preferably above 10 g/*l*. Bleeding is due mainly to thrombocytopenia and is exacerbated by infection. Platelet transfusions are required. Platelets are harvested from six freshly collected blood packs and pooled to provide one donation for the patient. Two or more such donations may be required in a 24 hour period to control bleeding. Platelets may also be used for prophylaxis if bleeding is anticipated.

*Infection*, particulary septicaemia, is a serious and frequent problem. An infection can arise very rapidly within hours and it is necessary to act quickly when it occurs. Unexplained fever over 38°C, lasting more than six hours, should be regarded as septicaemia until proven otherwise, if the patient is severely neutropenic (absolute neutrophil count less than $0{\cdot}2 \times 10^9/l$.). Parenteral antibiotic therapy using gentamicin and ticarcillin (p. 74) with corticosteroid supplements should be administered. If a staphylococcal lesion is suspected, cloxacillin or flucloxacillin may replace the ticarcillin. In 50% of patients the blood culture is sterile and the cause of the pyrexia remains unknown. When antibiotic therapy fails to control fever and there is severe neutropenia, white cell transfusion may be given. The preparation is usually obtained from a compatible adult relative donor, whose white cells are harvested for four to five hours, irradiated to kill any cells which might transplant to the recipient, and then administered. The effect can be dramatic with rapid resolution of the fever. Patients with chronic granulocytic leukaemia and a high white count make excellent donors for these problems. The leucapheresis is also of benefit to the donor by reducing the unnecessarily high white count.

Management of infection other than septicaemia should be along standard lines, always keeping in mind, however, that any infection may give rise to a septicaemia. Candidiasis in the mouth, gastrointestinal tract and elsewhere tends to be intractable during periods of severe neutropenia, or if the patient is on steroid therapy and requires treatment with nystatin (p. 317).

A reduction of risk of infection may be achieved in several ways. The patient may be regularly bathed in antiseptic baths (povidone-iodine) and may be nursed in a protected environment, of which there are many kinds. The gut, which is a major source of infection, may be 'sterilised' using mainly unabsorbable antibiotics, and procedures such as brushing teeth or doing rectal examinations should be avoided.

*Psychological support* of the patient is of great importance. Most patients will rapidly discover their diagnosis if not told. It is usually better therefore to give the patients the opportunity to find out what they want to know and avoid telling them any untruths. In this way the patients' trust and confidence are retained and they understand why they must cooperate in an extremely trying period of treatment. This is a delicate area of doctor–patient relationship and requires tact, sensitivity, and an understanding of the psychology of the individual. The quality of the nursing service is also important and a team of nurses familiar with the specialised management of leukaemia is required if the best results are to be obtained.

Isolation, which may be necessary because of the risk of infection, can be psychologically very disturbing to some patients. Others prefer it. Patients are at less risk of infection with resistant organisms at home than in hospital and should be discharged whenever possible if the home circumstances permit and they are sufficiently fit. Often treatment can be given on an out-patient basis. Cranial irradiation causes almost total epilation. The prospect can be devastating, especially for women. Restyling of the hair, the choice of a good wig and the firm promise that the hair will grow in again go a long way to alleviate the patient's distress.

**Prognosis.** At the time of diagnosis it is difficult to give a clear prognosis other than to say that without treatment it is very poor. It is wise to explain that a clearer idea of the outlook can be given after the effects of induction therapy have been observed. The outlook for most cases of acute non-lymphoblastic (myeloid) leukaemia is poor, the majority dying within a year. Patients with acute lymphoblastic leukaemia of the common 'null' cell variety, can be encouraged to hope that they may have the prospect of long-term remission. For those that generally do not have a particularly good outlook, hope should never be dashed, as even in some of these cases the outcome of treatment may occasionally be better than anticipated.

### Chronic Myeloid Leukaemia

The disease occurs chiefly between the ages of 35 and 60 years and is equally common in males and females.

**Pathology**. There is an extension of the marrow through the long bones. The marrow is grey and gelatinous and is crowded with myelocytes and young polymorphonuclear leucocytes. Leukemic infiltrations occur in the liver, spleen and lymph nodes and in most organs throughout the body.

**Clinical Features**. The onset is insidious and the manifestations varied. There may be slowly advancing anaemia with loss of weight, prominence of the abdomen and dragging discomfort in the left upper quadrant due to great splenomegaly. Attacks of acute left upper abdominal pain may develop when infarction occurs in the spleen. Epistaxis or other haemorrhages may occur in the later stages. A hypermetabolic state may result in sweating, intolerance of heat and weight loss. Priapism is sometimes the presenting symptom. Secondary gout may also occur.

The spleen is usually considerably enlarged and in occasional patients may reach the symphysis pubis. It is firm, smooth and painless but if infarction has occurred, it may be exquisitely tender and a friction rub may be heard over it. The liver may also be enlarged but lymph nodes are not usually involved.

**Investigation**. Examination of the blood shows an anaemia, usually normochromic, normocytic in type which increases as the disease progresses. The white cell count is usually considerably increased to between 50 and 500 $\times 10^9/l$ and occasionally more. A blood film demonstrates the full spectrum of granulocyte precursors from myeloblasts to mature neutrophils, the more mature forms being the most numerous. Myeloblasts usually number less than 10% of the total. There is also an increase in eosinophils and basophils. In the later stages, the appearance of an increasing number of myeloblasts may indicate the approach of a terminal acute phase and confirmation of this may be obtained from the bone marrow. The relative number of basophils also increases as the disease progresses. The platelet count is often high initially but with treatment usually comes down to normal levels, although high counts are sometimes seen at the time of transformation to an acute phase.

The peripheral blood is more useful diagnostically than the bone marrow but the latter should be examined in order to obtain material for chromosome analysis and to exclude other conditions causing a leucoerythroblastic blood picture. The neutrophils of chronic myeloid leukaemia are usually deficient in alkaline phosphatase. Normal neutrophils stained for this enzyme can be scored and usually give a result of between 20 and 100. In chronic myeloid leukaemia, the score is usually less than 5. However, a result within the normal range does not exclude the diagnosis. If initially low the score often rises to normal with treatment. In almost all cases the chromosome analysis demonstrates the presence of the Philadelphia chromosome (p.9).

**Treatment.** *Chemotherapy*. Effective palliative treatment can restore most patients to a period of symptom-free life. The method of choice is by chemotherapy using the alkylating agent busulphan. It is given orally in a commencing dose of 4 mg daily and can bring about a temporary but satisfactory clinical and haematological remission in a high proportion of cases, with marked reduction in splenomegaly. Generally no response is seen in the first two weeks. Thereafter the count falls and the results plotted on semi-logarithmic paper against time give a straight line allowing prediction of the point at which the dose of busulphan may require reduction or withdrawal. On average between twelve and eighteen weeks are required to achieve a normal count, but rarely the count falls more rapidly and, unless dosage is stopped, severe and even lethal aplasia of the marrow may result. For this reason it is customary to stop the busulphan when the white cell count is between 10 and 20 $\times$ $10^9/1$ and wait until it shows signs of rising before reintroducing the drug. Regular blood counts are of the utmost importance at this stage. Maintenance dosage of busulphan is generally 1–2 mg daily, but variation of the dose should be based on regular blood counts and should be tailored to suit the individual patient.

Alternatively a combination chemotherapy regime employing a smaller dose of busulphan, 2 mg daily and either mercaptopurine 50 mg daily or thioguanine 80 mg daily may be used. Allopurinol influences the effective dose of mercaptopurine but not of thioguanine. If allopurinol is not being given the dose of mercaptopurine should be 100 mg daily. This regime is given five days per week and results in a very much more rapid reduction in white cell count, taking on average 4–6 weeks, with correspondingly quicker induction of remission. Despite this, the regime does not carry so great a risk of inducing severe aplasia as the count tends to plateau in the normal range of white cell counts. Dosage can be modified by varying the number of days per week the standard dose is given. Patients find this arrangement the easiest to handle. Reduction in dose should be introduced when the count reaches normal levels.

A further and satisfactory way of using busulphan is to give the drug in large doses, 50–100 mg in single doses spaced two to three weeks apart. Remission is induced more quickly than by the single agent daily dose method and appears to be safe. Busulphan produces minor degrees of pulmonary fibrosis in most patients. In a few, however, this may assume serious proportions and is known as 'busulphan lung'. The main symptom is severe breathlessness. If this occurs the drug should be stopped and never used again. Alternative drugs which are satisfactory include hydroxyurea, melphalan, chlorambucil and dibromomanitol. Mercaptopurine and thioguanine are effective but when used alone are rather difficult to control. Radiotherapy to the spleen can also be used and is effective in inducing control of the disease. However, it has been shown to be inferior to busulphan therapy.

*Other Therapy*. Splenectomy has been shown to be of little value; it does not appear to delay transformation to an acute phase. However, patients who present with massive splenomegaly and who run the risk of even more massive and disabling splenomegaly in the terminal phase of the disease, may benefit from splenectomy. This is done, once the patient has achieved a good remission, in order to avoid the distressing end phase.

A novel approach to the treatment of this disease, in which survival has not been significantly altered by treatment, has been to store the chronic leukaemia phase cells in liquid nitrogen. When the transformation stage appears, the patient is prepared by chemotherapy and radiotherapy as for transplantation, and seeded with his or her own chronic phase cells. The intention is to reintroduce a second chronic phase of the disease. When this type of management is planned, the spleen should be removed as early as possible once the disease has been brought under control. In some cases an encouraging extension of life has been obtained, although there have been problems and it remains to be seen if it will become established as a satisfactory form of management.

Very high platelet counts may be seen, especially after splenectomy, but appear to carry less danger of thrombotic complications than in other myeloproliferative disorders and may be well tolerated by the patient. The platelets are ineffective and may not be haemostatically adequate for major surgery, when platelet concentrates should be given postoperatively. If this is not done, there is a risk of intractable bleeding.

**Prognosis**. On average patients with Philadelphia chromosome positive disease survive three and a half years from the time of diagnosis. Philadelphia chromosome negative varieties, which are rare, carry a much poorer prognosis, the majority dying within one year. Long survival of up to ten years or more occurs in a small proportion of patients.

In the majority the disease transforms sooner or later, either to an acute leukaemic phase, which may be either myeloblastic or lymphoblastic, or to the chronic refractory phase, with marrow fibrosis and an excess of basophils and blast cells. Unless the transformation is to acute lymphoblastic leukaemia, the outlook is extremely poor as this phase is very unresponsive to therapy. Sometimes the patient is diagnosed at the stage of transformation and this may account for cases of acute leukaemia with the Philadelphia chromosome.

**Eosinophil leukaemia** is a rare variant of chronic myeloid leukaemia and shows features of the hypereosinophilic syndrome in which cardiomyopathies and endomyocardial fibrosis occur, leading to severe cardiac failure. Treatment is difficult.

### Chronic Lymphatic Leukaemia

This is the commonest variety of leukaemia. It occurs more frequently in males than in females and the majority of patients are over the age of 45. The disease is very rare in the Chinese and other mongoloid races.

**Pathology**. There is moderate enlargement of lymph nodes and other lymphoid tissues throughout the body, the normal structure being replaced by a mass of lymphocytes. The histology is that of diffuse well-differentiated lymphocytic disease, nodular histology being rare. The spleen and liver are moderately enlarged and show lymphocytic infiltration. The bone marrow becomes progressively infiltrated with lymphocytes which eventually replace the erythropoietic and myeloid tissue.

In this disease lymphocytes which would normally respond to antigenic stimulae by transformation and antibody formation, fail to do so. An ever increasing mass of immuno-incompetent cells accumulate to the detriment of immune function and bone marrow proliferation. The receptor profile of the lymphocytes almost always demonstrates a B cell type of disease. T cell disease occurs rarely. Immunoglobulins produced by B cells tend to be either $\varkappa$ or $\lambda$ (p. 27) indicating in the majority of cases, a monoclonal expansion of cells. The disease is closely related to and indeed overlaps with well-differentiated lymphocytic lymphoma.

**Clinical Features**. The onset is very insidious. Tiredness and vague ill health are common although some patients are symptom free and the disorder is found incidentally. In contrast to chronic myeloid leukaemia the development of anaemia tends to be much slower and the presenting feature is usually the finding of firm rubbery, discrete and painless lymph nodes in the cervical, axillary and inguinal regions. The spleen is usually palpable but is smaller than in chronic myeloid leukaemia. The liver may also be enlarged. As a result of immunosuppression there is an increasing tendency to recurrent infections.

**Investigation**. Peripheral blood examination usually shows a mild but gradually increasing anaemia. Haemolytic anaemia may occur and is usually autoimmune in type. The white cell count may be greatly increased up to $1000 \times 10^9/l$ but in the majority of cases it is between $50–200 \times 10^9/l$. Of these cells about 95% or more are lymphocytes which are predominantly of the small variety. A large lymphocyte variety also occurs. Lymphoblasts are rare but may increase in number in the terminal stages. The platelet count is either low, normal or only mildly reduced.

Bone marrow examination both by aspiration and trephine should be done to assess the degree of marrow involvement. Dysplastic changes in the erythroblasts suggestive of folate deficiency may be noted and folate levels should be measured. Estimations of total proteins and immunoglobulin levels should be undertaken to establish the degree of immunosuppression which is common and progressive. In some patients immunoglobulin levels may be raised and there may be a monoclonal band. Urate levels are seldom raised as cell turnover is low.

STAGING

The disease may be staged according to the following criteria:

*Stage 0*: Lymphocytes, $15 \times 10^9/l$ or more in the blood, 40% or more of cells in the marrow. No enlarged lymph nodes, spleen or liver. Hb equal to or greater than 11 g/dl, platelets equal to or greater than $100 \times 10^9/l$.

*Stage I*: As in stage 0 but with enlarged lymph nodes.

*Stage II*: As in stage 0 but with enlarged spleen, liver or both. Lymph nodes need not be enlarged.

*Stage III*: As in the above stages, but with a haemoglobin less than 11 g/dl.

*Stage IV*: As in all the above stages, but platelet count less than $100 \times 10^9/l$.

**Treatment**. Specific treatment is usually not required until stage III or IV of the disease is reached. General measures to maintain good health, adequate rest, good food and exercise should be advised. The patient should be told that although the disorder is incurable it should be possible to live with it and that it may give little trouble for many months. Eventually specific treatment may be required and regular supervision by a haematologist or physician may be necessary. Patients with stage III and IV disease will require specific and supportive therapy. Folate deficiency should be corrected. Anaemia may require transfusion with red cell concentrates. If the bone marrow is severely overrun, initial treatment with prednisolone 40 mg daily and oxymetholone 25–50 mg daily, for several weeks before starting cytotoxic drugs, may rescue the haemopoietic element and allow more vigorous treatment.

There is disagreement about whether treatment should be by gentle single agent therapy employing chlorambucil, either continuously in doses between 2 and 5 mg daily, or intermittently at higher doses, or by more vigorous combination chemotherapy. The latter induces more convincing remissions judged by investigational findings, but has yet to be shown to improve the well-being or the survival of the patient in the long-term; the former method of treatment is therefore recommended. Combination therapy usually includes cyclophosphamide, doxorubicin, vincristine and prednisolone. Some believe doxorubicin is the most important of these drugs, but like daunorubicin it is cardiotoxic.

Alternatively radiotherapy may be used. Total body irradiation with a very small total dose of only 150 rads, spread over five weeks in ten treatments, 15 rads being given two times a week, can be very effective and may induce satisfactory remission with a minimum of upset to the patient. Whichever treatment is used, dosage should be controlled by accurate blood counts, the absolute neutrophil count and the platelet count being the most important.

Infections must be treated with appropriate antibiotics. If there is severe depression of immunoglobulins, gammaglobulin intramuscularly may reduce the frequency and severity of infections. When the platelet count is low, the use of intramuscular immunoglobulin may not be possible and can be replaced by fresh frozen plasma given intravenously weekly. Gammaglobulin concentrate should not be given intravenously, as it may induce severe reactions. Splenectomy may be required for autoimmune haemolytic anaemia which has proved unresponsive to corticosteroid therapy.

**Hairy cell leukaemia** is a variant of chronic lymphatic leukaemia now recognised to be more common than was previously thought. It is a disease of adult life affecting males four times more frequently than females. The mean age is 50 years. Patients usually present with general ill health and troublesome infections especially in the skin and are found to have considerable splenomegaly, severe neutropenia, monocytopenia and the characteristic hairy cells in the blood and bone marrow. These cells appear to be a cross between a B lymphocyte and a monocyte. The diagnostic test is to show that the acid phosphatase staining reaction in the cells is resistant to the action of tartrate. The neutrophil alkaline phosphatase score is usually high. Splenectomy is the best treatment. Corticosteroids may help but cytotoxic chemotherapy is seldom successful and is generally to be avoided. The prognosis varies between very poor and very good.

**Prolymphocytic leukaemia** is another variant of chronic lymphatic leukaemia found mainly in males over the age of sixty. There is massive splenomegaly with little lymphadenopathy and a very high white cell count, often in excess of $400 \times 10^9/l$. The characteristic cell is a large lymphocyte with a prominent nucleolus. Treatment is generally unsuccessful and the prognosis very poor.

# The Lymphomas

This group of disorders is divided into two main types: Hodgkin's lymphoma and non-Hodgkin lymphoma.

## Hodgkin's Lymphoma (Lymphadenoma)

This disease is characterised by progressive painless enlargement of lymphoid tissues throughout the body. It occurs in both sexes, often in adolescence and early adult life, but it may be found also in older people. The pathogenesis is unknown and the condition is usually regarded as a form of malignant disease related to other neoplastic processes of haemopoietic tissue.

**Pathology.** Microscopic examination of involved tissue, usually lymph nodes, shows damage to the normal structure, with proliferation of lymphoid cells. Giant cells, known as Reid-Sternberg cells, are seen classically with paired mirror imaged nuclei and prominent nucleoli; unless they are found it may be difficult to make a histological diagnosis. In addition there may be an increase in eosinophils, neutrophils and plasma cells in the tissue. The numbers of well-differentiated lymphocytes vary from many to few and the degree of lymphocyte depletion forms the basis for the main pathological classification of the disease. In some cases the fibrous stroma is increased. Caseation and necrosis are most unusual. Infiltration with greyish areas of Hodgkin's tissue causes enlargement of the spleen and liver. The bone marrow, lungs, kidneys and alimentary tract may also be involved although deposits in the nervous system are rare.

The disease is divided into four main histological types. These show a relationship to the degree of lymphocytic depletion that is found. This in turn demonstrates a crude but useful correlation with the aggressiveness of the disease clinically. The four types are (1) lymphocyte predominant, (2) nodular sclerosing, (3) mixed cellularity and (4) lymphocyte depleted. The nodular sclerosing variety is the most commonly encountered with the mixed cellularity type coming second, lymphocyte predominant third and lymphocyte depleted the least often seen.

**Clinical Features.** The onset is insidious, usually with enlargement of one group of superficial nodes. While the cervical nodes are often the first to be involved, the disease may also appear to start in the mediastinal and axillary nodes and more rarely in abdominal, pelvic and inguinal areas. Involved lymph nodes are usually painless, discrete and rubbery, though tenderness does occur in some cases, particularly when the nodes have enlarged rapidly. The overlying skin is freely mobile. Extension of the disease from the lymph nodes to adjacent tissues may occur, and is found particularly in the mediastinum. Pressure by node masses on neighbouring structures may cause a variety of problems, such as dysphagia, dyspnoea, venous obstruction, jaundice and paraplegia. Splenomegaly is uncommon at the outset and even when present does not always signify involvement. Absence of splenomegaly does not exclude involvement of this organ. Rarely the disease may be limited to the spleen.

General features may include progressive weakness and loss of weight. Fever may be present and in some instances is of a low grade irregular type while in others there are bouts of pyrexia with the temperature rising to 39°C and above for several days, alternating with apyrexial periods (Pel-Ebstein fever). In many cases, however, fever does not occur until the terminal stages. Pruritus is a troublesome symptom in about

10% of cases. Some patients experience discomfort at the site of a lesion shortly after an alcoholic drink.

**Investigation.** Anaemia is fairly common and progressive. It is usually normochromic and normocytic but occasionally there may be a haemolytic component. There is no diagnostic change in the white cells although a modest eosinophilia occurs in about 10–15% of cases. The total white cell count may be normal but sometimes it is considerably raised and there is a neutrophil leucocytosis. Lymphopenia, when it occurs, is a bad sign and an indicator of lymphocyte depletion. In the terminal phases there may be leucopenia and thrombocytopenia which may be as much a reflection of treatment as of the disease. Bone marrow involvement demonstrated by marrow aspiration and trephine biopsy is very uncommon at the time of diagnosis but may be found later in the disease. The diagnosis can be established with certainty only by tissue biopsy, usually of a lymph node. Liver biopsy may provide the diagnosis in cases with hepatic enlargement.

STAGING. Hodgkin's disease is thought to arise in one area and spread from there to others. It is of the utmost importance to establish the extent of the disease at the time of diagnosis, if at all possible. Clinical staging largely determines the therapeutic approach. To this end the patient requires intensive investigation including chest radiographs, bipedal lymphangiography, marrow trephine and aspirate. In some instances it is necessary to undertake laparotomy with splenectomy and biopsy of liver and various abdominal lymph nodes since lymphangiography does not demonstrate the nodes around the coeliac axis, porta hepatis and mesenteric vessels. The use of ultrasound, $^{67}$Gallium scanning and computed tomography, if available, can add to the delineation of the extent of the disease and may be important in a patient in whom a laparotomy would be inadvisable. In time these non-invasive procedures may come to replace the need for laparotomy.

There are four clinical stages based primarily on the extent of the disease:

*Stage I:* Involvement of a single lymph node region (I) or extralymphatic site ($I_E$).

*Stage II:* Involvement of two or more lymph node regions (II) or an extra-lymphatic site and lymph node regions on the same side (above or below) the diaphragm ($II_E$).

*Stage III:* Involvement of lymph node regions on both sides of the diaphragm with ($III_E$) or without (III) extra-lymphatic involvement or involvement of the spleen ($III_S$) or both ($III_{SE}$).

*Stage IV:* Diffuse involvement of one or more extra-lymphatic tissues, e.g. liver or bone marrow. The lymphatic structures are defined as the lymph nodes, spleen, thymus, Waldeyer's ring, appendix and Peyer's patches.

Each stage is sub-divided into 'A' or 'B' categories, according to whether they have systemic symptoms or not. The symptoms that place a patient in the 'B' category are: (1) unexplained weight loss of more than 10% of the body weight in the previous six months, (2) unexplained fever above 38°C, and (3) night sweats.

**Differential diagnosis** is from other conditions producing enlargement of lymph nodes and of the spleen namely (1) tuberculous lymphadenitis, which is usually confined to the neck, in which the nodes may become matted together and may show caseation and sinus formation, and there is no splenomegaly; (2) chronic pyogenic lymphadenitis (chiefly also of the neck) in which the nodes are small and tender, a source of infection can be found and there is no splenomegaly; (3) lymphatic leukaemia in which the examination of the blood and bone marrow reveal the characteristic changes; (4) infectious mononucleosis in which the lymph node and the splenic enlargement is transient and the blood examination and a positive Paul Bunnell or monospot test are diagnostic; (5) other types of malignant lymphoma which can be distinguished only by microscopic examination of an excised node; (6) secondary syphilis with generalised lymph node enlargement in which the swelling is transient, a rash is common and serological reactions are positive; (7) sarcoidosis in which the histology should differentiate.

**Treatment.** There are two main methods of treatment, radiotherapy and chemotherapy. Megavoltage radiotherapy can eliminate the disease in a high proportion of patients provided the disease is localised. For this reason radiotherapy is chosen for most cases of stage I and II disease. Exceptions are when structures such as the lung are involved when chemotherapy may be used to shrink the lesion to dimensions suitable for radiotherapy. Moreover radiotherapy should not be used in stage II if three or more areas are involved, particularly if the patient has 'B' symptoms because such patients tend to suffer relapse after this form of treatment; chemotherapy should be employed instead. As a generalisation patients with stage III or IV types of disease are treated with chemotherapy. However, stage III A patients in whom only nodes in the upper abdomen are involved do well with radiotherapy.

*Radiotherapy* consists of treatment of the node areas. For disease above the diaphragm a 'mantle' treatment is used and includes nodes in the neck, axillae and mediastinum. In some cases, if the mediastinum is involved this field is later extended downwards to include the para-aortic region. Disease below the diaphragm is given an 'inverted Y' distribution of irradiation which includes the coeliac, para-aortic, iliac and groin nodes and follows roughly the bifurcation of the aorta. If splenectomy has not been performed the spleen should also be irradiated. In female patients the 'inverted Y' distribution of irradiation causes severe damage to the ovaries and if a staging laparotomy has been done the opportunity is usually taken to place the ovaries behind the uterus where they may be more protected.

*Combination chemotherapy* has revolutionised the treatment of advanced Hodgkin's disease. The classical combination is nitrogen mustard, a vinca alkaloid such as vincristine or vinblastine, together with procarbazine and prednisolone, given in two week pulses (p. 573) with two to four week intervals between. Five pulses are given after all objective evidence of disease has gone. The minimum number of pulses is six and it is seldom necessary to give more than twelve. If the patient relapses during treatment, usually about the time of the third course, the disease is resistant to these drugs and treatment should be changed to an alternative combination.

Nitrogen mustard is very unpleasant for patients and must be given intravenously. In most patients nausea and vomiting occur and can be severe, usually starting two to four hours after the injection and lasting from twelve to twenty four hours in some cases. Antiemetics such as chlorpromazine or metoclopramide or both, given parenterally in liberal doses, are helpful.

Cyclophosphamide, which is a phosphorylated nitrogen mustard, may be substituted in the regime, replacing nitrogen mustard. Little advantage is gained as regards side effects as it is a potent epilator and also may cause haemorrhagic cystitis.

Chlorambucil, also a nitrogen mustard analogue, has been used successfully in this regime in place of nitrogen mustard and has the advantage that it can be given by mouth and is well tolerated. Patients can easily be managed on an out-patient basis. Nitrogen mustard and its analogues are all severely myelotoxic.

The vinca alkaloids, vincristine, vinblastine and vindesine are relatively less toxic to the bone marrow. In particular vincristine has this advantage but is more neurotoxic than vindesine which in turn is more neurotoxic than vinblastine. Numbness and paraesthesiae in the fingers and toes is very common and can usually be tolerated. Paralysis of muscle groups or burning pains may force the discontinuation of the drug. Patients complain of severe constipation. This may be avoided by the use of high roughage diet and gentle aperients, if necessary. Most of these symptoms improve with time although full recovery may not occur.

Procarbazine is a myelotoxic drug which is under suspicion as possibly the most oncogenic of the drugs in this combination.

Prednisolone is almost useless in this disease on its own but has been shown to play an essential role in combination with other agents. Antituberculous chemotherapy should be used if there is evidence of old untreated disease. Exacerbation of peptic ulceration can be controlled by cimetidine. It is generally kinder to the patients to wean them off prednisolone over three days at the end of each pulse. In many instances prednisolone is a euphoriant and helps the patient to tolerate the side effects of the other drugs in the combination. Insomnia troubles some and hypnotics may be required.

Other combination chemotherapy regimes exist but none has been shown to be as effective as the one outlined above. However, they do provide an alternative chemotherapeutic regime when there is resistance to the classical combination.

Chemotherapy carries a fairly high risk of inducing sterility in males and this may be permanent. To a lesser extent it occurs in females, in whom evidence of premature menopause may appear. Since many of these patients are young, the males in particular may require counselling about the effect of chemotherapy in this respect.

**Prognosis.** If the patient is not treated the disease is fatal. With stage $I_A$ disease the five year survival rate in patients treated with radiotherapy exceeds 90% and in stage $II_A$ disease is greater than 70%. In more advanced disease the results of chemotherapy are very satisfactory and more than 50% of patients remain disease free after five years. Just how effective combination chemotherapy is, remains to be seen since many patients who were treated in this way are still alive. The prognosis so far as histological type is concerned seems to matter less when chemotherapy is used. The prognosis is relatively poor when evidence of resistance to treatment appears and very few of such patients survive thereafter for five years.

## Non-Hodgkin Lymphoma

In this group of disorders there is a monoclonal neoplastic proliferation of lymphoid cells, usually identifiable as B cells. Occasionally T cells are affected. Non-Hodgkin lymphomas merge with the lymphoblastic and lymphocytic leukaemias with which they have many features in common.

**Pathology and Classification.** This group of lymphomas has always proved difficult to classify. At present the most widely used classification is that of Rappaport. This system has major defects but it is easily understood and used and it has not been superseded, internationally, by any classification developed since.

The first and most important division is between lymphomas in which a nodular (follicular) structure can still be seen and those in which this structure has been replaced by a diffuse sheet of cells. These two groups are known as nodular (follicular) and diffuse respectively. In both, the lymphoid cells may be either well-differentiated lymphocytic, poorly-differentiated lymphocytic, mixed lymphocytic-histiocytic or histiocytic. In general nodular lymphomas carry a better prognosis than diffuse.

One defect of this classification is that it uses the term 'histiocytic'. It is now known that true histiocytic lymphomas are very rare and that the majority which are called histiocytic are large B cell lymphomas, consisting of primitive blast cells. Another defect is the inability to place in this classification certain lymphomas, such as Burkitt's lymphoma (p. 801).

Unlike Hodgkin's lymphoma the disease in non-Hodgkin lymphoma is frequently widespread at the time of diagnosis, often involving not only lymph nodes, but also bone marrow, spleen and other tissues. Early involvement of bone marrow is typical of nodular lymphoma. Extra-lymphatic tissue involvement at the time of presentation is more common and almost every organ or tissue in the body may be the site of initial disease. In gastrointestinal lymphomas the stomach is most frequently and the rectum least frequently involved. Thyroid lymphomas tend to be associated with gastrointestinal involvement. Some skin lymphomas are T cell in type, e.g. mycosis fungoides. Most lymphomas involving extra-lymphatic tissues are of the diffuse variety and therefore carry a rather poor prognosis unless well localised.

**Clinical Features.** These lymphomas occur at all ages, are rare under two years and become more frequent with increasing age. Males are more frequently affected than females. Nodular lymphomas occur mainly in adults between the ages of thirty and sixty.

Lymph node enlargement is the most common presenting finding, and is usually painless unless it has developed very quickly. The nodes are discrete and firm. The patient usually complains of tiredness, lassitude, loss of drive, loss of weight and occasionally fever and sweating. When the presentation is extra-lymphatic the symptoms will reflect the tissues involved. Quite often the diagnosis of lymphoma comes as a surprise at laparotomy or during other investigative procedures. Weakness of the legs progressing to paraplegia may be due to an extradural lymphoma compressing the cord. Pressure effects in other areas may cause dysphagia, breathlessness, vomiting, intestinal obstruction or ascites. Pain is the main symptom of bone involvement which may present with a pathological fracture.

Physical examination often reveals more widespread node involvement than the patient has noticed. Unexplained lymphadenopathy which fails to resolve spontaneously within a few weeks should always be suspect. Moreover lymphomatous nodes may wax and wane in size and the shrinkage of nodes does not exclude a diagnosis of lymphoma. Splenomegaly usually indicates that the spleen is involved in the neoplastic process.

**Investigation.** Diagnosis is based primarily on histological findings from biopsy of a lymph node or other involved tissue. In some cases a clinical suspicion of lymphoma is not confirmed initially when reactive hyperplasia is seen in the biopsy. Further biopsies may eventually reveal a lymphoma.

The staging process is similar to that adopted for Hodgkin's disease except that laparotomy is seldom necessary although it may be required for diagnostic purposes when only retroperitoneal nodes are involved. Bone marrow aspiration and trephine biopsy should be done early in the investigation since involvement is common and when present indicates stage IV disease. Blood counts usually show normal values unless there is splenomegaly with hypersplenism or a complicating autoimmune haemolytic anaemia when a reduced haemoglobin level, reticulocytosis and positive direct antiglobulin test (Coombs' test) will be found. In some cases a slight excess of lymphocytes may be present. Thrombocytopenia is uncommon. Moderate degrees of anaemia may be also present if there is considerable bone marrow involvement.

An evaluation of the receptor characteristics of the peripheral blood and lymph node lymphocytes is helpful, particularly in cases in which the diagnosis is in doubt, but this has to be done in specialised laboratories. The demonstration of a monoclonal expansion of the B lymphocyte population is characteristic. These techniques also assist in the identification of the rare cases of T cell lymphoma. For this reason a second biopsy of lymph nodes may be required for proper evaluation of the type of disease. Patients accept this readily if they understand why it is being done. An assessment of immune competence is also important and immunoglobulin levels should be measured. In some cases a monoclonal band may be found.

**Treatment**. In the case of the more benign non-Hodgkin lymphomas, such as the nodular lymphocytic and even diffuse well-differentiated lymphocytic varieties, no specific therapy may be necessary if the disease is not advanced. Some patients can be watched for years before active measures are indicated.

*Radiotherapy*. When treatment is required localised disease is best managed, as in Hodgkin's disease, with radiotherapy and this may be curative. Non-Hodgkin lymphoma is often at stage III or IV when diagnosed and in these cases chemotherapy is generally the treatment of choice. However, where there are pressure problems the local disease may be treated with radiotherapy in combination with chemotherapy (combined modality treatment). The more benign types of disease may also respond very well to total body irradiation, a form of radiotherapy that employs very small doses of only 150 rads over a period of five weeks in ten divided doses of 15 rads. This is very suitable for elderly patients as it is relatively free of side-effects.

*Chemotherapy*. Most cases of nodular lymphoma, with the exception of the histiocytic variety, do very well with gentle, single agent chemotherapy and chlorambucil is the drug usually chosen. More dramatic results in terms of remission induction may be achieved with combination chemotherapy but there is as yet no evidence that this is of long-term benefit to the patient and it may cause considerably greater morbidity. Chlorambucil may be given as continuous therapy at a dose of 5 mg daily initially, reducing to 2 mg daily as indicated by blood count. This may be given over many months in order to induce control of the disease. Alternatively the drug may be given intermittently in higher doses. Combination with prednisolone may be useful, especially at the start of treatment when the bone marrow may be heavily involved with lymphoma. The steroid therapy may be started before as described for chronic lymphatic leukaemia (p. 579). Oxymetholone therapy may also help to rescue the bone marrow. Long-term steroid therapy should be avoided.

Combination chemotherapy is indicated for the more aggressive diffuse lymphomas of poorly differentiated lymphocytic, mixed cell or histiocytic variety. The diffuse histiocytic type should always receive the most aggressive chemotherapy as a number of these cases apparently become free from disease for long periods with this treatment. Radiotherapy does not appear to be able to achieve as good results. If these patients survive a year without relapse they have a chance of long-term remission. There are a number of regimes but most physicians employ a combination of cyclophosphamide, doxorubacin, vincristine, bleomycin and prednisolone. Alternatively the combination chemotherapy regime described for Hodgkin's disease may be given.

Rather less aggressive management has been used for the diffuse poorly differentiated lymphocytic variety and accordingly cyclophosphamide, vincristine and prednisolone with or without doxorubicin is generally prescribed. All these combination regimes are given as pulses (p. 573) with variable periods of rest for bone marrow recovery between each pulse. The number of pulses is usually between six and twelve in any one course. Once the disease has become resistant to the standard drugs, second line chemotherapy usually produces only brief benefit and the value of achieving this at the expense of the patient's wellbeing has to be evaluated in each case. It may be better to deal with troublesome disease as it arises with short courses of radiotherapy. This palliative approach can be quite successful.

As a generalisation patients over seventy years do not tolerate aggressive chemotherapy well. Adolescents who present with an undifferentiated lymphoma which is often initially in the mediastinum should be managed in the same way as patients with acute lymphoblastic leukaemia. Some patients with well-differentiated lymphocytic lymphoma progress to chronic lymphatic leukaemia and should be managed as for that disorder.

The treatment of these diseases consists of balancing the prospects of killing off the disease with those of destroying the patient. The effect on the patient's normal tissues is usually monitored by watching the blood count. In this respect the white cell count, the absolute neutrophil count and the platelet count are the most useful. As the absolute neutrophil count drops below $1 \times 10^9/l$ infection with bacteria or fungi becomes an increasing risk. Similarly, bleeding is increasingly likely to occur as the platelet count drops below $50 \times 10^9/l$ although many patients tolerate very low levels for long periods without serious bleeding. Dosage of myelotoxic drugs must be reduced once these figures are approached and some physicians would reduce the dose at higher levels. The effect of drugs may continue after they have been withdrawn and this should be kept in mind. Regular blood counts are absolutely essential for the satisfactory management of these patients.

*Surgery*. In lymphomas of extra-lymphatic tissue surgical excision may be employed and is usually supplemented with radiotherapy, with or without chemotherapy thereafter.

*Supportive therapy*. General supportive measures such as blood transfusion with red cell concentrate should be used for anaemia when necessary. Infections should be treated promptly with antibiotics or other agents. A watch should be kept for the development of monilia infection in the mouth of patients who have developed neutropenia or are on steroids. Severe heartburn may indicate oesophageal thrush.

**Prognosis**. The mean survival of patients with diffuse lymphomas is in the region of two years and those with the histiocytic variety who do not respond well to treatment often survive less than one year. Patients with nodular lymphomas or lymphocytic or mixed cell type have a mean survival of seven to eight years and in the histiocytic variety of about three years.

## Multiple Myeloma (Myelomatosis)

This is a neoplastic disorder of plasma cells.

**Immunopathology**. Normal plasma cells are derived from B lymphocytes by transformation after exposure to antigenic stimuli, and individual plasma cells manufacture only one type of immunoglobulin. The finding that in myeloma, and in other related malignant disorders of B lymphocytes, all the malignant cells produce the same immunoglobulin indicates that the tumour is derived originally from one cell by cloning; the disease is therefore monoclonal. The immunoglobulin is called a paraprotein and appears on electrophoretic strips as a clear cut band. Each of the five normal types of immunoglobulin (IgG, IgA, IgM, IgD, and IgE) has light chains of either lambda or kappa varieties (Fig. 2.3). In myeloma the paraprotein produced belongs to one of these immunoglobulin types and has one or other of the two light chains. In some cases only part of the immunoglobulin molecule is produced by the tumour cells, most commonly the light chains. These appear in the urine as Bence Jones proteinuria and if myeloma is associated only with light chains it is known as *Bence Jones myeloma.*

In just over half of the patients with myeloma an IgG paraprotein is produced. About 20% are IgA producing and a similar percentage are of the Bence Jones variety. IgD, IgM and IgE myelomas are rare and together amount to only 2% of cases. Patients with IgG and IgA myelomas may, in due course, develop light chain proteinuria, so called 'Bence Jones escape'. This usually indicates an accelerated phase of their disease.

In the majority of patients the bone marrow is heavily infiltrated with atypical plasma cells which are usually larger and paler staining than normal plasma cells and contain nucleoli. Some cells may be multinucleated. Progressive replacement of the marrow occurs with eventual reduction of the normal cell lines, inducing anaemia, leucopenia and thrombocytopenia. Bone osteoclasts are stimulated and absorption of bone occurs, producing diffuse osteoporosis. Local tumour formation by the myeloma causes punched out translucencies in the bone radiograph. Rarely the disease may present as a solitary plasmacytoma either in bone or soft tissue.

Excessive production of the myeloma paraprotein is associated with progressive reduction in normal immunoglobulin levels and impairment of immune function.

**Clinical Features**. The disease is very uncommon under the age of thirty. It becomes increasingly frequent with age, having its peak incidence between sixty and seventy years. Males are affected rather more frequently than females and Negroes two to three times more often than Caucasians. There is a long pre-clinical phase, in some instances as much as twenty-five years. The disorder may be discovered incidentally by laboratory tests during this phase and the patient may thereafter be observed for years before symptoms appear.

Symptoms usually reflect bone involvement, impairment of immune function, renal damage, anaemia or hyperviscosity. The diffuse osteoporosis and local erosion of bone by myeloma result in stress pain and eventual pathological fracture. The stress pain is often wandering, difficult to locate and described as 'rheumatics'. On the other hand the first intimation of trouble may be the sudden onset of acute localised and referred pain due to pathological fracture. These symptoms arise mainly in weight bearing bones, the vertebrae, pelvis and femur being particularly susceptible. Collapse of vertebrae is common and produces nerve root pressure symptoms and shortening of stature. Patients are often severely crippled. Weight lifting may also cause pain in the arms. Similar lesions in the skull seldom give rise to pain. Whatever the cause, pain is often severe, prolonged and very exhausting.

The progressive impairment of immune function due to the deficiencies of normal immunoglobulins and the excess of abnormal immunoglobulins renders these patients susceptible to infections, particularly of the respiratory tract. Pneumonia is quite frequently the presenting illness and infection very often the cause of death.

The excessive production of light chains which are lost in the urine may damage tubular cells and block the tubular lumen. Amyloidosis (p. 436) may occur. Mobilisation of calcium from the skeleton may be excessive and cause hypercalcaemia, which may result in nephrocalcinosis (p. 451). High calcium levels may also cause lethargy, drowsiness and eventually coma if untreated.

Patients often complain of tiredness which may be due to anaemia. Bleeding and bruising problems are seldom presenting features but may be troublesome terminally and are due both to thrombocytopenia and hyperglobulinaemia. Hyperviscosity is a problem in some patients with very high levels of paraprotein. It may impair the circulation, notably in the central nervous system, causing headaches, vertigo, dizziness, somnolence and stupor progressing to coma.

Clinical examination may reveal tender areas in the bones, kyphoscoliosis, muscle spasm and impaired mobility, particularly with vertebral involvement. Retinal haemorrhages, exudates and gross dilatation of the retinal veins, with periodic constrictions giving a 'string of sausages' appearance, suggest hyperviscosity.

**Investigation**. Assessment of myeloma is very dependent on laboratory findings. The degree of bone marrow involvement is reflected in the haemoglobin level, the white cell count and the platelet count and can be assessed directly with bone marrow examination. A high ESR is very characteristic but is not always present. Rarely myeloma cells appear in the blood as a plasma cell leukaemia.

The level of paraprotein production is evaluated using electrophoresis and measurement of the monoclonal band, the level being expressed in grams per litre. This measurement should be used to follow progress. Immune impairment can be assessed from the electrophoretic strip and the immunoglobulin levels. The raised level of the specific immunoglobulin involved is not a good measurement for monitoring the paraprotein level. Renal function should be assessed by blood urea and creatinine clearance. Plasma calcium should always be evaluated. Plasma alkaline phosphatase is usually within normal limits despite the bone involvement unless there has been a fracture when a transient rise may occur. Plasma urate levels should also be known.

Diagnosis depends on finding at least two of the characteristic features of the disease. The bone marrow may be pathognomonic but it is not always so. A sure diagnosis may depend on the demonstration of a monoclonal paraproteinaemia and bone destruction in the radiographs. Reactive plasmacytosis in the marrow can mimic myeloma but the increased immunoglobulins are polyclonal. Paraprotein bands may be found in lymphomas, macroglobulinaemia and so called 'benign monoclonal hypergammaglobulinaemia'; they may also be associated with a wide range of inflammatory, neoplastic and autoimmune disease. In these cases the level of paraprotein does not significantly increase with time and is usually less than 10 g/*l*.

**Treatment**. Local skeletal problems should be treated with radiotherapy and the general disease with chemotherapy. Melphalan is the drug of choice, although cyclophosphamide is probably as effective.

Patients in the pre-clinical phase generally do not require treatment. In the clinical phase melphalan may be given either alone as low dose continuous therapy, 2 mg daily or as high dose intermittent therapy (0·25 mg/kg/d for four days) in combination with prednisolone (2·0 mg/kg/d for four days), weaning off over the following three days. Such treatment should be administered in pulses every four to six weeks. The dosage of melphalan should be adjusted according to the white cell, absolute neutrophil and platelet count. In most patients the disease is slowly brought under control. Progress should be evaluated by measuring the levels of paraprotein in the blood. When this has reached a plateau, chemotherapy may be stopped. A small proportion of patients are resistant to treatment and the disease is progressive.

In patients with the more rapidly advancing forms of myeloma more aggressive therapy may be required, with combination chemotherapy regimes. Those who present with anaemia, hypercalcaemia, evidence of renal damage and in whom there is Bence Jones proteinuria require urgent management with alkalinisation of the urine with oral bicarbonate, high fluid intake, corticosteroids and possibly mithramycin to reduce calcium levels. Careful transfusion with red cell concentrate is also required unless the haemoglobin is above 10 g/dl. Specific treatment under such circumstances should be with combination chemotherapy, bearing in mind that dose reductions may be required because of renal failure the management of which is described on page 439. In this situation cyclophosphamide is contra-indicated. Vincristine, doxorubicin and prednisolone form a useful combination.

Despite good control of the general disease, further episodes of bone pain and fracture may occur and require radiotherapy. Prophylactic irradiation of eroded vertebrae may be warranted before crush fracture has occurred. Fractures of femur and humerus require orthopaedic surgery with pinning of the bone, followed by radiotherapy. Bed rest should be minimised to avoid further loss of calcium from the skeleton. Hyperviscosity problems may require plasmapheresis.

Maintaining the morale of patients in the face of crippling and painful disease may be difficult but they should be encouraged to look forward to gradual improvement. Given time and good management many can return from a bed-ridden state to active lives.

**Prognosis**. Without treatment the disease progresses relentlessly to death. With treatment the outlook for the majority of patients is considerably improved and a few may survive for many years. Bad signs at the time of diagnosis are a haemoglobin level of less than 7 g/dl, severe hypoalbuminaemia and renal failure. The presence of Bence Jones proteinuria is also indicative of more serious disease. Prognosis should be guarded in any individual until the response to treatment has been assessed; this may take six months or more.

**Waldenström's macroglobulinaemia** is a rare disease of the elderly, more common in males than females. There is a monoclonal IgM paraproteinaemia and a tendency to develop a hyperviscosity syndrome. The marrow is infiltrated with neoplastic lymphocytes. Untreated, the progress is often slow with eventual immune deficiency and susceptibility to infection. Chlorambucil on a long term low dose basis, such as 2 mg daily, may control the lymphocyte proliferation and the advance of the disease. Some patients are unresponsive. Plasmapheresis may then be required. The majority of patients survive two to five years and some live considerably longer.

## Hypersplenism

This term is used to describe the depression of leucocyte and platelet counts in the peripheral blood which is often encountered in a wide variety of conditions in which splenomegaly is a prominent feature, such as portal hypertension (p. 404). The cause of the leucopenia and the thrombocytopenia is not fully understood but it may in part be due to the sequestration of leucocytes and platelets in the enlarged spleen.

Another important effect of splenomegaly is, for reasons unknown, an increase in total plasma volume. This dilutes the red cell mass which remains normal in total amount but the dilution gives a low haemoglobin reading, as low as 8 g/dl in some patients. The apparent anaemia can be identified by measurement of the red cell mass and plasma volume and is corrected only by splenectomy which may also improve leucopenia and thrombocytopenia.

# HAEMORRHAGIC DISORDERS

This heading comprises conditions characterised by an abnormal tendency to bleed.

## Pathophysiology

The mechanism concerned in the arrest of haemorrhage can be divided into three stages. The first is spasm of damaged small blood vessels. The second is formation of platelet plugs on the damaged areas of vascular endothelium by aggregation of platelets. The third is the coagulation of blood which is the end product of a chain reaction involving many coagulation factors.

**1. The Vascular Factor**. Spasm of small arterioles and capillary sphincters in response to injury constitutes an essential feature of natural haemostasis. It is the first reaction, slowing the blood loss and allowing other factors to operate. Eventually the spasm relaxes and if the platelets and coagulation factors have not carried out their functions, secondary bleeding develops.

**2. The Platelet**. Normal platelets do not adhere to the vascular endothelium when it is intact. The natural anticoagulant, prostacyclin, (p. 599) produced by the vascular endothelial cells from arachidonic acid, possibly helps to prevent platelet adhesion and aggregation. Platelets adhere readily to collagen under the vascular endothelium when it is exposed by injury. They also adhere to each other under the influence of adenosine diphosphate (ADP) released in damaged tissue. A platelet aggregate forms – primary aggregation. At this stage it is possible for the platelets to break off into the circulation as small emboli which usually disintegrate rapidly. This probably happens inside blood vessels when injury is minimal. When the injury is such that the full effects of the haemostatic mechanism is required, primary aggregation is followed by a shape change in the platelets. An irreversible stage of aggregation is reached, promoted by thromboxane $A_2$ which is formed in platelets from arachidonic acid through endoperoxide intermediates $PGG_2$ and $PGH_2$ (Fig. 12.1). Another factor involved in the irreversible phase is ADP. Platelet granules release numerous substances including fibrinogen, platelet factors 3 and 4, prostaglandins and thromboxane $A_2$. These participate in the formation of fibrin and in the establishment of a stable haemostatic plug which differs in structure from a thrombus.

Capillary bleeding can be stopped by platelet plug formation and does not require the coagulation mechanism. This is why the bleeding time is normal in haemophilia. The platelet plug is inadequate for blood vessels larger than capillaries, because the blood pressure in them is too great and without the support of fibrin formation the platelet plug is expelled when the vessel spasm relaxes. However, when the injury is slight the full train of the haemostatic mechanism will not proceed as it will be inhibited by antithrombin III and other anticoagulant factors in the blood. In this way blood flow can be maintained in blood vessels where the injury is not sufficient to require the cessation of flow. Thrombocytopenia leads to capillary bleeding because the platelet provides the main means of stopping this type of bleeding.

**3. Coagulation of the Blood**. The end point of the clotting mechanism is the formation of fibrin from fibrinogen. Haemostasis, initiated by vascular spasm and platelet plug formation, is strengthened by the laying down of a fibrin mesh. The fibrin then contracts and consolidates the initial repair by binding the tissues together.

This mechanism can be activated in two ways: (1) by an *intrinsic system* in the blood vessels which is activated by contact with collagen exposed by injury to the

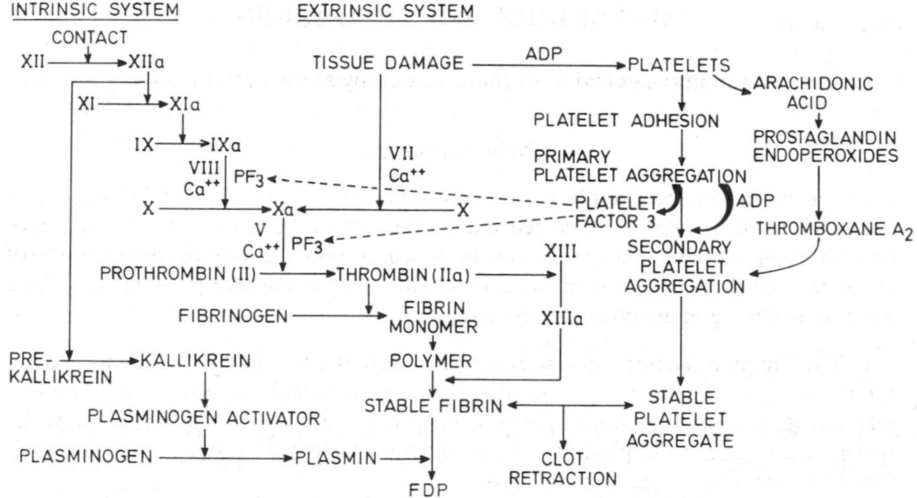


Fig 12.1 Interaction of blood coagulation, fibrinolytic, kallikrein and platelet systems. ADP = adenosine diphosphate. FDP = fibrin degradation products. a = activated.

vascular endothelium and (2) by an *extrinsic system* activated by tissue fluid. The intrinsic system is more potent but there appears to be interaction between the two. It is possible that the extrinisic system activates factor X which in turn generates the production of thrombin from prothrombin. Thrombin at this stage then acts as an enhancer of the intrinsic system.

Thirteen main coagulation factors have been named. It is now recognised that factor III (thromboplastin) and factor VI do not exist as distinct biochemical entities. Thromboplastin probably represents the co-operative activity of several factors. The term, factor VI, is no longer used.

The coagulation mechanism is a biological amplifier, a cascade of activated enzymes assisted by co-enzymes. Precursor substances or factors circulating in the blood are activated and in turn activate other factors and so on. Ionised calcium is absolutely essential at several points in the mechanism. Anticoagulation *in vitro* can be achieved by chelation of the ionised calcium as by using acid citrate dextrose (ACD) or citrate phosphate dextrose (CPD) to prevent the coagulation of blood for transfusion purposes.

In the intrinsic system the trigger that initiates the cascade is contact with water-wettable surfaces such as collagen. This activates factor XII which activates factor XI which in turn activates factor IX (Fig. 12.1). Activated factor IX (IXa) in the presence of factor VIII, platelet factor 3 (phospholipid) and calcium ions activates factor X. The precise role of the other platelet factors is uncertain.

The extrinsic system of activation is initiated by tissue damage and tissue factors activate factor X in the presence of factor VII. Factor X is the point at which the intrinsic and extrinsic systems meet and is the start of the final common pathway.

Activated factor X together with factor V, platelet factor 3 and calcium ions activates prothrombin to thrombin and this digests the fibrinogen molecule to fibrin. The effect of the amplification of the biochemical reaction is so powerful that conversion of fibrinogen to fibrin is almost instantaneous. Fibrin is formed sufficiently quickly to prevent it being flushed away by further bleeding.

Thrombin also activates factor XIII (fibrin stabilising factor) which stabilises the chemical structure of the polymerised fibrin. Subsequent contraction of the fibrin is dependent on adequate numbers of platelets being involved in the clotting process. When there is thrombocytopenia, retraction of the clot is poor.

*Factor VIII (antihaemophilic globulin)* is deficient in haemophilia. It is a molecule formed by the combination of two fractions, (1) a coagulant fraction which is genetically sex linked and (2) a fraction which can be recognised antigenically and is produced by an autosomal gene (factor VIII related antigen or VIII RAg). The coagulant fraction is measured by assay of its activity in the coagulation mechanism and the factor VIII related antigen by the use of heterologous antiserum.

*Factor XII* is the only one of the coagulation factors, a deficiency of which is not associated with a tendency to bleed. Deficiency of this factor is more likely to be associated with a liability to thrombosis due to failure of activation of the fibrinolytic mechanism through the kallikrein system (Fig. 12.1).

**The fibrinolytic system** functions in much the same way as the coagulation mechanism. Plasminogen, an inert precursor, can be activated to form plasmin which digests fibrin to give soluble degradation products. In excess, it will also digest fibrinogen and other coagulation factors. This system comes into play when there is a threat of widespread intravascular coagulation and prevents the deposition of fibrin in the blood vessels. An increase in fibrin degradation products is found when disseminated intravascular coagulation does occur (p. 601). Plasminogen is closely bound to fibrinogen and fibrin and is slowly activated after normal clotting to cause digestion of the fibrin clot. This process can be accelerated artificially with streptokinase and this therapeutic substance is used sometimes in the lysis of thrombi.

**Coagulation Inhibitors**. The tendency of the coagulation mechanism to function is counterbalanced by inhibitory factors in the blood. These substances neutralise the activated factors rapidly. In blood vessels activation of the coagulation mechanism is minimal and these inhibitors can cope. At the point of an injury, however, the activation of the coagulation mechanism is so powerful that the inhibitors are overwhelmed. One important inhibitor is antithrombin III which inactivates thrombin (factor II) and activated factors IX, X, XI, and XII. It is required for the action of heparin. Without it heparin is useless. Patients who are deficient of antithrombin III are very liable to thrombosis.

**Investigation of Bleeding Disorders**. If there is a suspicion that a patient has a bleeding disorder a basic screen of haemostatic function should be performed. Blood should be taken for a blood count, including platelet count and blood film and for basic coagulation investigations. A bleeding time should be done by the Ivy method. It is an excellent test of capillary and platelet function but does not reflect coagulation defects.

Coagulation investigations should include a prothrombin time to evaluate the activity of factors II, VII and X and their function in the final common pathway and the extrinsic system. A partial thromboplastin time with kaolin (the latter being used to activate the contact factors) will detect problems of significance in the intrinsic pathway or the presence of inhibitors to this pathway. A thrombin time may be done to monitor heparin-like activity. This may be produced by the presence of excessive levels of fibrin degradation products. The fibrinogen level should be measured, particularly when depletion is anticipated. If an abnormality is detected, more detailed investigation follows with factor assays, platelet function tests and tests of fibrinolysis.

The results of such investigations do not explain all the phenomena observed in patients who are bleeding. For example a prolonged bleeding time due to thrombocytopenia is not associated with insuperable haemostatic problems at a major surgical procedure such as splenectomy although haemostasis is abnormal. Equally, although the bleeding time is normal in haemophilia, major surgery would be haemostatically impossible if special control was not undertaken (p. 597). An intact extrinsic clotting system does not compensate for a defective intrinsic system as seen in haemophilia. It would seem that the platelets are essential for controlling bleeding due to minor trauma and the coagulation mechanism for bleeding due to major trauma. Thus when platelets are deficient, capillary bleeding predominates and when the coagulation mechanism is faulty more serious deep seated bleeding occurs. These observations may explain what may appear to be anomalies in the clinical findings associated with various defects in the haemostatic mechanism.

### Classification of Haemorrhagic Disorders

1. **Due to Defect of the Blood Vessels**

(i) The vascular purpuras: (a) Infections, e.g. typhus, typhoid, meningococcal meningitis, measles, infective endocarditis, septicaemia, smallpox.
(b) Chemical agents, e.g. aspirin, ergot, frusemide, indomethacin, iodides, phenobarbitone, phenylbutazone, phenytoin, quinine and snake venom.
(c) Anaphylactoid purpura (purpura simplex and Henoch-Schönlein purpura p. 624).
(d) Metabolic purpura (uraemia, p. 437 hepatic failure p. 397).
(e) Scurvy (p. 108).
(ii) Hereditary haemorrhagic telangiectasia.

2. **Due to Disorders of Blood Platelets**

(i) Reduced numbers of platelets: idiopathic and secondary (symptomatic) thrombocytopenic purpura.
(ii) Increased numbers of platelets: thrombocythaemia.
(iii) Defective platelets: hereditary and acquired thrombasthenia.

3. **Due to Defects of the Clotting Mechanism**

(i) *Hereditary* (a) Haemophilia (factor VIII deficiency) or haemophilia A.
(b) Christmas disease (factor IX deficiency) or haemophilia B.
(c) Von Willebrand's disease (also shows abnormalities of capillary and platelet function).
(d) Deficiency of clotting factors other than factor XII or those listed at (a) and (b) (all rare).
(ii) *Acquired:* (a) Deficiency of certain coagulation factors due to vitamin K deficiency.
(b) Oral anticoagulant therapy.
(c) Advanced liver disease.

## Haemorrhagic Disorders due to Defect of the Blood Vessels

Most of these disorders are discussed with the primary cause noted above.

### Hereditary Haemorrhagic Telangiectasia

This rare disease is transmitted as an autosomal dominant. It is characterised by bleeding from multiple telangiectases which consist of localised collections of non-contractile capillaries. The first and frequently the only symptom may be epistaxis but haematemesis, haemoptysis or bleeding elsewhere may occur. Telangiectases are not usually prominent till after the age of 20 and may be found on the face or hands, or in the mucous membrane of the nose or mouth. Treatment of bleeding areas is sometimes difficult, but cauterisation of the nose may be helpful. Continuous iron therapy is usually required, sometimes with parenteral supplements. Oestrogens may reduce bleeding from mucous membranes in some patients.

## Haemorrhagic Disorders due to Abnormalities of Blood Platelets

Thrombocytopenia occurs either because (1) platelets are consumed or destroyed almost as soon as they are made (consumption thrombocytopenia), or (2) because they are not being produced (production thrombocytopenia). In the first, megakaryocytes are found in normal or increased numbers in the marrow. In the second, megakaryocytes are absent from the marrow or, if present, are incapable of platelet production because they are functionally abnormal, in which case they are usually part of a neoplastic process and are morphologically abnormal. In some diseases there is both a production and a consumption problem and it may prove difficult to know which is the greater.

### Idiopathic Thrombocytopenic Purpura

This is a disease of unproved aetiology, characterised by a quantitative deficiency of platelets; in some instances it may be due to an antigen-antibody reaction. The disease occurs most commonly in children and young adults. In the former it frequently follows a viral infection and the disease usually runs a brief, self limiting course with spontaneous remission in two to three weeks. In a few it progresses to a more chronic form. In adults, spontaneous remission is less frequent and the chronic phase more common.

**Clinical Features.** There is purpura and bleeding from mucous membranes; haematuria and gastrointestinal bleeding may occur. Intracranial haemorrhage is the greatest risk but is uncommon, particularly in children; headache, dizziness and confusion are symptoms that should warn of the risk of intracranial bleeding. In the chronic phase the severity is usually variable with remissions and relapses.

Diagnosis is established by finding severe thrombocytopenia with normal and increased numbers of megakaryocytes in the bone marrow. It is therefore mainly a consumption thrombocytopenia although production may be inhibited by antibody attack on the megakaryocytes. Demonstration of anti-platelet and anti-megakaryocyte antibodies is possible in only a few patients although an immune basis for the disorder is suspected in most. There may be an associated iron deficiency anaemia.

**Treatment.** In young children acute idiopathic thrombocytopenic purpura following viral infection seldom requires treatment unless there is evidence suggestive of intracranial bleeding. In adults, prednisolone (60 mg/d) should be given until the platelet count rises to normal levels when the dose should be cautiously reduced until the drug is withdrawn. Relapse may require reintroduction of a higher dose for a longer period but if this fails or if there has been no response to prednisolone in three to four weeks, splenectomy should be considered. The spleen should be removed under corticosteroid cover and platelet concentrates given, if required, only after the splenic artery has been clamped. Splenectomy is successful in about 50% of patients, giving lasting remission. In the others a chronic phase of the disorder occurs with remissions and exacerabations that may require periodic corticosteroid therapy. Elderly patients generally respond poorly to corticosteroids. Surprisingly, some patients survive chronic thrombocytopenia for years with remarkably little disability.

**Secondary or symptomatic thrombocytopenic purpura** occurs in association with pancytopenia, leucopenia, hypersplenism, multiple neoplastic deposits in the bone marrow, from excessive exposure to X-rays or radioactive substances, and occasionally in very severe fevers. It may be found in megaloblastic anaemia and in systemic lupus erythematosus and can follow massive blood transfusion.

Thrombocytopenia may be part of a general pancytopenia or occur alone because of sensitivity to drugs, such as chlordiazepoxide, chlorothiazide, chlorpropamide, frusemide, indomethacin, phenylbutazone, oxyphenbutazone, certain sulphonamides and tolbutamide. Here the prognosis is much better, provided the drug is withdrawn and transfusion given as required. Platelet concentrates are available in some centres.

The name '*onyalai*' has been given to a form of thrombocytopenic purpura of unknown origin which occurs sporadically in Africa. Large haemorrhagic bullae on the tongue and buccal mucosa are a conspicuous feature.

### Thrombocythaemia and Thrombasthenia

*Thrombocythaemia* is a pathologically raised number of platelets in the blood usually in excess of $1000 \times 10^9/l$ which may result in a bleeding diathesis as well as a tendency to thrombosis. This is rectified by reduction of the platelet count to normal levels (p. 568).

*Thrombasthenia* is a state in which the platelets, although normal in quantity, are defective in function. A number of very rare hereditary defects of platelets occur and are known as primary thrombasthenias. Acquired thrombasthenia is much more common and is seen in severe uraemia and after exposure to certain drugs, of which aspirin is probably the most commonly used. The platelets in chronic myeloid leukaemia are ineffective and may not be adequate for major surgery.

## Haemorrhagic Disorders due to Defects in the Clotting Mechanism

### Haemophilia (Factor VIII Deficiency)

Of the various factors in normal plasma concerned with the clotting mechanism the most important from a clinical point of view is the anti-haemophilic factor (factor VIII, AHF or AHG), a deficiency of which leads to haemophilia. This factor is normally present in the globulin fraction of plasma.

Haemophilia is a hereditary disorder of blood coagulation, characterised by a life long tendency to excessive haemorrhage and a greatly prolonged coagulation time. The haemophilia gene is transmitted as an X-linked recessive character (p. 15). It follows that the sons of a haemophilic man do not suffer from haemophilia and do not transmit the trait to their descendants. The daughters of a haemophilic man all carry the trait. There is a 50% chance that sons of female carriers will suffer from haemophilia and a 50% chance that daughters will be carriers. In many instances no family history can be obtained and may reflect the fact that the disorder has been handed down on the female side for several generations. Alternatively there may have been a genetic mutation.

**Clinical Features.** The most common manifestation is haemorrhage into joints and in severe haemophiliacs these haemarthroses may occur frequently. They usually develop spontanously and are associated with pain, which may be severe, with swelling, warmth and muscle spasm. With appropriate treatment the lesion settles in a few days as the blood is reabsorbed. Repeated episodes cause damage to the joint with wasting of the related muscles, leading to deformity and crippling. These effects can be minimised by proper management. The knee joints are most frequently affected, but ankles, hips, shoulders, elbows and wrists are also common sites. Haemorrhage into the musculature and soft tissues is also a frequent and potentially disabling complication. Intra-abdominal bleeding may present diagnostic problems and haemorrhage from the gastrointestinal tract is relatively common and can be serious.

Superficial trauma gives rise to uncontrolled bleeding which will continue unless adequately treated. Intracranial haemorrhage may occur but is relatively uncommon unless related to trauma. Surgical procedures are not possible without replacement therapy. Tooth extraction will also promote prolonged bleeding.

The severity of haemophilia varies. In severe cases the factor VIII coagulant activity is usually less than 2% of normal. Cases with activity of between 2–5% are usually only moderately affected while those with levels above 5% have problems only with major trauma. The higher the factor VIII coagulant activity the less the clinical problem. A small number of haemophiliacs, varying between 5–15% of all cases, have factor VIII inhibitors in the serum. This greatly complicates their management.

**Investigation.** Diagnosis is based on the patient's sex, as the patient is almost certain to be a male, a family history if present, the clinical picture and the demonstration of deficiency of factor VIII coagulant activity in the absence of any other haemostatic defect. Female haemophiliacs are extremely rare, requiring the marriage of a haemophiliac to a carrier female. Haemophilia must be distinguished from Christmas disease (p. 597) and Von Willebrand's disease (p. 597).

Efforts have been made to detect carriers by demonstrating a disparity between the levels of factor VIII coagulant activity and factor VIII related antigen (VIII RAg). The factor VIII RAg level is higher than would be expected from the coagulant activity. However, it is hoped that immunoradiometric assay used to determine the antigenic determinant of the coagulant fraction of factor VIII will prove to be a more useful test for the carrier state. It is low in haemophilia and has been shown to be low in the haemophiliac fetus *in utero*.

**Treatment** is based on adequate replacement of the deficient factor. Factor VIII concentrate and cryoprecipitate (which contains factor VIII and is more easily prepared) are the main sources of material, both being obtained from freshly donated blood. Factor VIII concentrate used also to be prepared from animal material but was extremely antigenic. Unfortunately factor VIII has a short biological half-life of eight hours so that repeated administration is necessary. The aim should be to maintain factor VIII activity above a level which is necessary to achieve haemostasis and the initiation of healing. For a haemarthrosis or for muscle and soft tissue bleeding a level of factor VIII above 30% of normal is usually adequate. Haematuria and retroperitoneal haemorrhage require levels above 50%, while tooth extraction and major surgery require levels approaching 100%. In practice six or twelve packs of cryoprecipitate are usually given to the patient, with further administrations as required. Cryoprecipitate should always be of the correct blood group unless the patient is group O when cryoprecipitate from any donor can be given.

Teeth can be extracted under the cover of aminocaproic acid or tranexamic acid, both of which inhibit fibrinolysis, and this may greatly reduce the need for factor VIII. Dental procedures should always be done in hospital. When inhibitors are present very large amounts of factor VIII may be required to overwhelm the inhibitor. Unfortunately this causes a very rapid rise in inhibitor levels and is likely to be useful only for a few days. Blood transfusion may be given when there has been much blood loss. For open wounds, topical application of a thrombogenic agent, such as thrombin, is generally helpful but does not provide a satisfactory substitute for lack of factor VIII.

Haemarthroses and muscle bleeds require initial rest for the first 24–36 hours with splinting, followed by early mobilisation to minimise the risk of contractures, muscle wasting and deformity. Analgesics should be given when pain is severe but aspirin should be avoided as it may cause gastric bleeding. Addictive analgesics should not be used if possible. If aspiration is required for an extremely tense joint the procedure should be done before replacement therapy is started. Because haemophiliacs are repeatedly exposed to blood products, the incidence of hepatitis B and liver disease is relatively high. The patients are also at risk of developing drug addiction as they require analgesics frequently.

**Prevention.** Severely affected patients should avoid trauma while at the same time leading as normal a life as possible. Home therapy, where the patient has a supply of factor VIII and can inject himself immediately bleeding occurs, has considerably improved the outlook for some patients. Regular administration to prevent bleeding in very severe haemophiliacs, although expensive as regards materials, may be worthwhile. All haemophiliacs should be referred to a haemophilia centre for supervision and advice, not only in relation to their treatment, but also for help with the social and educational implications of their disorder.

### Christmas Disease (Haemophilia B)

This is due to deficiency of factor IX and, like haemophilia A, is sex linked. Haemophilia is ten times more common than Christmas disease. All that has been said about haemophilia applies to Christmas disease, except that replacement therapy is with factor IX concentrate. This has a longer half life and requires to be given less frequently.

### Von Willebrand's Disease

This is a rare disorder which is inherited as an autosomal dominant and is seen in both sexes equally. It is not dissimilar to haemophilia with which it may be confused. The laboratory findings are variable but there may be defects in all three components of the haemostatic mechanism, the capillaries, platelets and coagulation mechanism. There is deficiency of the plasma factor called the Von Willebrand's factor and also of factor VIII. The bleeding time varies from being greatly prolonged, to normal and can alter from time to time in an individual patient.

**Clinical Features.** There is excessive bleeding from cuts or other injuries. Patients who have very low factor VIII levels may develop bleeding episodes similar to those described for haemophilia.

**Investigation.** The diagnosis is established by family studies, the finding of a prolonged bleeding time, a normal platelet count, failure of aggregation of platelets by ristocetin, impaired adherence of platelets to glass beads, deficiency of the Von Willebrand's factor, and a depressed factor VIII level which can be shown to be due to a deficiency of both factor VIII related antigen and the coagulant fraction. Finally, infusion of plasma or cryoprecipitate causes a prolonged rise in factor VIII levels in excess of that due to infused factor VIII, a phenomenon never seen in haemophilia and thought to be due to an increase in the Von Willebrand's factor. The Von Willebrand's factor also corrects the platelet defects.

**Treatment.** Fresh frozen plasma or cryoprecipitate should be given for troublesome bleeding or surgical procedures. Very superficial trauma will usually respond to simple pressure.

## Deficiency of the Vitamin K Dependant Factors

Factor II (prothrombin) and factors VII, IX and X require vitamin K (p. 107) for synthesis by the liver and may be deficient if the absorption of the vitamin is impaired or if there is severe liver disease. When anticoagulation is required, drugs, particularly warfarin, are used to alter the synthesis of these factors: proteins are produced which are antigenically similar to factors II, VII, IX and X but do not have their procoagulant properties.

**Clinical Features.** Patients with simple vitamin K deficiency or overdosage with oral anticoagulants are liable to excessive bruising, gastrointestinal haemorrhage, haematuria, epistaxis and excessive menstrual loss. When deficiency is associated with severe liver disease the clinical and haemostatic problems are more complex because of the addition of other factor deficiencies, thrombocytopenia and toxic damage to the vasculature.

*Haemorrhagic disease of the newborn* is due to an exaggeration of the normal hypoprothrombinaemia which occurs 24–72 hours after birth when there is no bacterial formation of vitamin K in the gut.

**Treatment.** In simple vitamin K deficiency, whatever the cause, parenteral administration of phytomenadione (vitamin $K_1$) corrects the factor deficiency within 24 hours. Treatment of anticoagulant overdosage is given on page 600.

The management of the bleeding problems of severe liver disease is complex and will depend on the identification of the coagulation factor deficiencies, the platelet count and the degree to which fibrinolysis has been stimulated. Vitamin K is seldom deficient although it may be administered in the hope of producing some improvement. Fresh frozen plasma, platelets and blood transfusion may all be given. It is risky to give concentrates of factors II, VII, IX and X as these tend to induce disseminated intravascular coagulation (p. 601) unless the concentrates contain heparin. Generally, replacement therapy is best reserved for acute haemorrhage as its effects are short lived.

## Thrombosis

**Aetiology.** In health, blood is kept in a fluid state by various mechanisms (p. 592) which may be upset in favour of thrombus formation in certain circumstances. A thrombus may be defined as an abnormal mass formed inside a blood vessel and consisting of various components of blood which have reacted together in ways similar to, but not identical to, what occurs in the normal process of haemostasis. There are two types of thrombus: (1) the white thrombus which occurs in arteries. It is formed by platelet adhesion and aggregation, with fibrin deposition in layers and may in time occlude the artery; (2) the red thrombus which consists of large amounts of fibrin and red cells and relatively few platelets. It forms mainly in veins or behind a white thrombus and is similar to the clot formed by blood in a tube. A red thrombus is soft and friable and in veins may easily be detached to cause pulmonary embolism.

The factors which predispose to the formation of thrombi in blood vessels fall into three main groups: 1. Abnormalities of blood vessel walls due to (i) *atherosclerosis*; (ii) *trauma* (e.g. needles, cannulas, irritant infusions and endothelial damage over a myocardial infarction) (iii) *loss of venous tone*, e.g. varicosities; and (iv) *infiltration* of the vessel wall by neoplastic disease.

2. Abnormalities of blood flow due to (i) *stasis* occuring mainly in veins although it may develop in the auricles of the atria in atrial fibrillation. Stasis may also be due to lack of muscular activity as in general anaesthesia, to external pressure on veins (e.g. in pregnancy or neoplasia) or to venous pooling as occurs in cardiac failure; (ii) *hyperviscosity* either (a) because of an increase in the cellular components of blood as in polycythemia or leukaemia or (b) because of an increase in the protein levels as in myeloma or Waldenström's macroglobulinaemia; (iii) *turbulence*, caused for instance, by kinking of arteries forcing platelets on to the vessel walls.

3. Abnormalities of the blood due to (i) *thrombocytosis* occuring in disorders such as polycythaemia vera; (ii) *hypercoagulable states* from an increased activation of clotting factors during and after surgery, from decrease in the activity of the fibrinolytic mechanism as in factor XII deficiency and when there is a decrease in coagulation inhibitors in the blood, for instance antithrombin III deficiency.

*Prostacyclin.* The vascular endothelium synthesises a substance, prostacyclin, from prostaglandin endoperoxides produced from arachadonic acid by the enzyme cyclo-oxygenase. Prostacyclin is an unstable compound with a half life of two to three minutes; it inhibits platelet aggregation, promotes platelet disaggregation and causes vasodilatation. These effects are the opposite of those caused by thromboxane $A_2$ produced from the same precursors in platelets. It is thought that prostacyclin production is of major importance in inhibiting thrombus formation in blood vessels. Prostacyclin can also be produced in the lungs from which it perfuses the circulation. Levels of thromboxane $A_2$ are low in people eating a seafood diet, e.g. Eskimos who are observed to have a low incidence of thrombosis. This may be because the diet reduces the thrombogenic side of the mechanism by giving rise to an alternative form of thromboxane (thromboxane $A_3$).

Aspirin inhibits cyclo-oxygenase and hence reduces the production of thromboxane $A_2$ in platelets. However, by the same action, but in larger doses, it also probably reduces the production of prostacyclin by the cells of the vessel walls. This may explain why aspirin has been less effective in the prevention of thrombosis than was expected but the optimum dose of aspirin for this purpose has not yet been settled.

**Clinical Features.** Thrombosis in both arteries and veins is a major cause of morbidity and mortality. In arteries the occlusion is often crippling, if not lethal, depending on the tissue affected and whether there is a good anastamotic circulation e.g. in coronary (p. 186), cerebral (p. 689) and mesenteric thrombosis (p. 371). On the venous side the local effects are usually less damaging to health but deep venous thrombosis producing pulmonary emboli can be lethal (p. 199). The disability is likely to be severe in thrombosis of the cavernous and other venous sinuses, (p. 700) or of the renal veins, (p. 436).

**Treatment and Prevention.** The indications for the use of anticoagulant and other forms of therapy are discussed with the individual lesions.

HEPARIN THERAPY. Heparin is a natural, biologically produced anticoagulant. It acts by accelerating the activity of antithrombin III (p. 592) The effect is virtually instantaneous. Heparin has a half life of 60 – 90 minutes and disappears rapidly from the circulation. It is administered either by intermittent intravenous injection every six hours, by continuous intravenous infusion in a small volume or by intermittent (usually b.d.) subcutaneous injection. When given by continuous intravenous infusion the level of anticoagulation may be monitored by thrombin times or partial thromboplastin times with kaolin or, if necessary, by the whole blood clotting time. Heparin is seldom used for more than two weeks. Prolonged treatment can cause osteoporosis. It is often combined with oral anticoagulants, the heparin being used to initiate anticoagulation until the oral anticoagulants can exert their function; heparin is then withdrawn. Overdosage may be treated either by stopping administration or, when there is haemorrhage, by giving protamine sulphate in a dose based on laboratory tests.

ORAL ANTICOAGULATION. Warfarin is the drug of choice. Indanedione derivatives such as phenindione are much more likely to produce hypersensitivity reactions. Anticoagulation should be initated carefully as some patients require lower doses than others, and indeed the dose of 20 mg of warfarin on the first day and 10 mg on the following day, which is routinely given in many centres, will be excessive in a significant number of patients. It is better to give 10 mg of warfarin on the first day and then increase the dose in those who can tolerate the drug. The maintenance dose varies widely from 2–20 mg daily. Rarely enormous doses are required in patients who metabolise the drug in an abnormal manner.

Therapy is usually monitored by the so called ‘prothrombin time’, preferably corrected to a standard ratio to make results comparable between centres. This does not reflect factor IX deficiency and the thrombotest which does, is regarded by some as preferable. Since many drugs interfere with the binding of warfarin to albumin or induce enzyme activity in the liver, thereby increasing warfarin metabolism, introduction or withdrawal of drugs should be under medical supervision and the patient advised that such changes may have serious effects unless monitored. Transient illness also affects liver function and may require dosage alteration.

Patients should carry a card indicating that they are receiving warfarin. They should be advised specifically not to take aspirin or proprietary preparations containing aspirin, but to use paracetamol for headaches and other minor discomforts.

In the treatment of overdosage withdrawal of the anticoagulant may be sufficient. If reversal of anticoagulation is required phytomenadione (vitamin $K_1$) should be used. The disadvantage is that unless dosage is small it will be difficult to re-establish oral anticoagulation for some time. Alternatively fresh frozen plasma or blood may be administered if there is a need to correct the defect quickly. Concentrates of factor II, VII, IX and X may also be used in urgent situations and will correct the defect almost immediately. Such preparations usually contain a small dose of heparin to prevent the induction of disseminated intravascular coagulation. The heparin will not be enough to cause serious anticoagulation in the patient.

OTHER MEASURES. Lysis of thrombi with fibrinolytic therapy using streptokinase or urokinase has been used but is very expensive and potentially dangerous, especially postoperatively. Streptokinase is antigenic so that it can be given only for a limited period. This type of treatment is rarely used for longer than two days and is followed by anticoagulation therapy.

In the prevention of thrombosis low molecular weight dextrans have been used widely in surgical practice. Attempts to counteract the adhesive and aggregating properties of platelets with a variety of drugs such as aspirin and dipyridamole are being evaluated.

Efforts are being made to produce a stable analogue of prostacyclin in the hope that it will prove to be a useful agent in the prevention of thrombosis.

## Disseminated Intravascular Coagulation

This is a deranged state in which coagulation and lysis of fibrin produced by coagulation proceed simultaneously in the blood. It is a reflection of other problems, not a disease in itself.

The trigger is something that initiates intravascular coagulation. This may be transient or ongoing. Transient liberation of thrombogenic substances into the blood is seen classically in association with the end of pregnancy and parturition. Amniotic fluid embolism is potently thromboplastic and similar effects are seen in abruptio placentae, eclampsia and when there is a dead fetus *in utero*. Other triggers include malignancies, hepatic disease, severe trauma, anaphylaxis, hypoxia, venoms and sepsis. Bacterial endotoxins act indirectly through mediators such as granulocytes, platelets and damaged vascular endothelium.

Whatever the trigger, the effect is a threat to the circulation and the fibrinolytic mechanism responds, sometimes dramatically, to lyse fibrin as it is formed. This compensatory response may overshoot, and excess plasmin produced by the fibrinolytic system digests fibrinogen and other factors as well as the fibrin, causing a severe haemorrhagic state. The disseminated intravascular coagulation itself depletes, by consumption, the clotting factors. This depletion is then further exacerbated by the overactivity of plasmin. The fibrin degradation products produced themselves lead to bleeding by an uncertain mechanism.

Specific clinical findings are present only in severe cases. Bleeding occurs at all venepuncture sites, from mouth, nose, ears and other orifices. This is due to lysis of fibrin clots wherever they have been laid down. There is massive purpura with ecchymoses. The patient is usually gravely ill. Sometimes excessive fibrinolysis may occur locally at the site of severe trauma, such as brain operations and prostatectomy. No evidence of this phenomenon is then seen systemically.

Diagnosis of disseminated intravascular coagulation is by laboratory investigation. It is necessary to show depletion of coagulation factors and platelets and evidence of an increase in the products of fibrinolytic activity (fibrin degradation products). A full coagulation investigation with platelet counts and measurement of FDPs is required. When disseminated intravascular coagulation is severe, replacement of coagulation factors may be necessary. Heparin may be used when there is an ongoing stimulus to coagulation as in malignant disease, and antifibrinolytic drugs such as aminocaproic acid given when fibrinolysis appears to be the major problem.

In practice very severe disseminated intravascular coagulation is rare and in most cases the process is contained and excessive depletion of coagulation factors does not occur. In such cases the treatment is that of the underlying disorder.

## Prospects in Haematology

For many years haematology has had a firm base in blood film and marrow morphology. This has determined the classification of many of the blood diseases. Electron microscopy has extended this base by demonstrating the ultrastructure of the cells. More recently immunological techniques have brought a new dimension to the subject. Dynamic concepts have appeared and resulted in new ideas about classification particularly in the field of lymphomas and leukaemias. Cells are now recognised to have characteristics not evident from light or electron microscopy. Antigens originally thought to be tumour related are now known to be characteristic of certain stages in the differentiation of cells. This is a rapidly expanding field of knowledge and further contributions to our understanding of the nature of these diseases will undoubtedly come.

The chemotherapy of acute lymphoblastic leukaemias has proved to be highly successful in obtaining long remissions, even in adults. The same degree of success has not been obtained in the myeloblastic leukaemias or in the lymphoblastic leukaemia of T and B cell type. Here there is room for improvement as new drugs become available. The use of bone marrow transplantation in the treatment of acute leukaemia holds out hope for younger patients who have disease that is unlikely to be eliminated by chemotherapy. Improvements in the management of the chronic leukaemias have been awaited for a long time and while no obvious answers to the problems of these diseases can be foreseen it is possible that bone marrow transplantation may have something to offer.

In the field of coagulation problems the understanding of the role of the prostaglandins in platelet and vascular endothelial function opens up the prospect of new therapeutic techniques to deal with the problems of intravascular thrombosis. The development of antisera to the coagulant fraction of factor VIII will hopefully improve the measurement of that factor, assist in the identification of female carriers and enable the investigator to discover at the fetal stage whether a male offspring has the disease. Perhaps similar development will also occur in relation to factor IX deficiency.

N.C. Allan
R.H. Girdwood

*Further reading:*

Bagshawe, K.D. (1975) *Medical Oncology*. London: Blackwell.— For more detailed information on investigation and management of leukaemias and lymphomas.

Biggs, R. (1978) *The Treatment of Haemophilia A and B and von Willebrand's Disease*. London: Blackwell.— For detailed information on the management of these coagulation disorders.

Dacie, J.V. & Lewis, S.M. (1970) *Practical Haematology*, 4th edn. Edinburgh: Churchill Livingstone.— For information regarding investigative procedures.

de Gruchy, G.C. (1978) *Clinical Haematology in Medical Practice*, 4th edn. London: Blackwell.— An excellent reference volume with a clinical bias.

Girdwood, R.H. (1979) *Clinical Pharmacology*. London: Balliere Tindall.— For information about haematinics, anticoagulants and drugs used in malignant disease.

Hardisty, R.M. & Weatherall, D.J. (1974) *Blood and its Disorders*. London: Blackwell.— A reference volume particularly useful for its section on haemoglobinopathies and thalassaemias.

Hirsh, J. & Brain, E. (1979) *Hemostasis and Thrombosis: A Conceptual Approach*. Edinburgh: Churchill Livingstone.— An excellent and clearly understood introduction to coagulation.

Nilsson, I.M. (1974) *Haemorrhagic and Thrombotic Diseases*. London: Wiley.
Thompson, R.B. (1977) *Disorders of the Blood*. Edinburgh: Churchill Livingstone.— Very useful for further reading.
Wintrobe, M.M. (1974) *Clinical Haematology*, 7th edn. London: Kimpton.— Probably one of the best comprehensive reference volumes.

# 13. Diseases of Connective Tissues, Joints and Bones

Rheumatology, a major sub-speciality within general medicine, deals with a heterogeneous group of disorders of connective tissues, joints and bones. The 'rheumatic diseases' are conditions in which pain and stiffness of some part of the musculoskeletal system are prominent. It is convenient, if rather arbitrary, to group these disorders according to whether the basis for the connective tissue pathology is primarily inflammatory, metabolic or degenerative. Inflammatory diseases of connective tissue include rheumatoid arthritis and other types of inflammatory and infective arthritis, the spondyloarthritides and the diffuse connective tissue diseases. Metabolic disorders include the crystal deposition diseases, gout and chlondrocalcinosis, while the predominantly degenerative disorders are osteoarthrosis, spondylosis and a number of painful syndromes of the soft connective tissues.

Until recently these conditions have not received the attention of clinicians, medical teachers and researchers commensurate with their frequency and morbidity. Rheumatic diseases affect people of all sexes, ethnic groups and ages. Their frequency increases with age so that as many as 40% of persons over the age of 65 years have some rheumatic complaint. In Britain 20 million people experience a rheumatic disorder each year. Five million suffer from osteoarthrosis, 500 000 have rheumatoid arthritis and there are 10 000 children with chronic juvenile arthritis. Eight million people consult their general practitioner annually with rheumatic complaints, amounting to 18% of all consultations in general practice. Rheumatic diseases are the most important cause of physical impairment in the community. The lives of more than one million persons are so impaired and one-fifth of these are severely disabled. In 1971 rheumatic disorders were responsible for the loss of 44 million working days and for almost £500 000 000 in lost productivity.

## Rheumatoid Arthritis

In its typical and complete form rheumatoid arthritis is a chronic inflammatory, destructive and deforming polyarthritis associated with systemic disturbance, a variety of extra-articular lesions and the presence of circulating antiglobulin antibodies (rheumatoid factors). While the pattern of joint involvement is characteristically symmetrical and peripheral and its course typically prolonged, with exacerbations and remissions, atypical, asymmetrical and incomplete forms are not uncommon and give rise to difficulties in diagnosis.

**Epidemiology.** Rheumatoid arthritis occurs throughout the world in all climates and all ethnic groups. The overall prevalence in developed countries is about 3% with a female to male ratio of 3:1. There is an annual incidence of 0·3% so that over the age of 65 years 16% of the female population and 5% of males are affected. The disease commences most commonly in the 3rd and 4th decades but the age of onset follows a normal distribution curve and no age group is exempted. Prevalence is higher than expected in twins and 1st degree relatives but not in spouses suggesting a fairly weak genetic predisposition. This has been confirmed by tissue typing studies which show a modest but significant increase in the histo-compatibility antigen HLA-DR4 in patients and their families. Higher prevalence in urban than in rural Africans of the same ethnic origin suggests that environmental factors are important.

The disease appears to be more severe though not more frequent where the climate is cold and damp.

**Aetiology and Pathogenesis**. The cause of rheumatoid arthritis remains obscure. It is widely believed that an infection is the initiating factor although no causative organism has been identified. Nevertheless current concepts suggest that the disease results from altered immune reactivity and persistent antigenic stimulation in genetically predisposed persons. There is a good deal of evidence for persistent immune overactivity, autoimmunity and the presence of immune complexes at sites of articular and extra-articular pathology, namely: (1) The presence of circulating IgM, IgG and IgA serum antiglobulins (rheumatoid factors) as well as anticollagen and antinuclear antibodies. (2) The presence of self associating IgG and IgG-IgM immune complexes within the phagocytic cells of synovial effusions. (3) Depression of synovial fluid complement components in inflamed joints associated with activation of both the classical and alternate pathways (Fig. 2.4). (4) Increased numbers of plasma cells, lymphocytes and monocytes in the synovial membrane associated with local production of rheumatoid factors and lymphokines (p. 25). (5) The presence of serum factors which inhibit suppressor T lymphocyte activity (Fig. 2.2). (6) Amyloidosis complicating some cases of rheumatoid arthritis of long duration.

The importance of lymphocytes in the pathogenesis of the disease is confirmed by the striking remission of activity which follows lymphocyte depletion by thoracic duct drainage or cytotoxic drug therapy.

Thus rheumatoid arthritis is considered to be both an extravascular immune complex disease (p. 32) and a disorder of cell-mediated immunity (p. 33) in which the following sequence of events leads to inflammation, granuloma formation and joint destruction: (1) Localisation of unidentified antigen in joint. (2) Local synthesis of antiglobulin antibodies. (3) Formation of immune complexes and activation of the complement pathway. (4) Stimulation of neutrophil chemotaxis, cytolysis, lymphokine production and macrophage neutral protease secretion by biologically active complement components (p. 32). (5) Neutrophil and macrophage phagocytosis of immune complexes following IgG and C3 receptor recognition. (6) Release of mediators of acute inflammation—vaso-active amines, proteases, polypeptides, prostaglandins and slow reacting substances. (7) T lymphocyte infiltration and production of lymphokines. (8) Macrophage and chondrocyte activation, pannus formation and enzymatic destruction of articular cartilage and bone by collagenase and neutral proteinases.

The severity of erosive damage is related to joint movement and physical stress showing that mechanical factors are also important in pathogenesis.

**Pathology**. The earliest change is swelling and congestion of the synovial membrane and the overlying connective tissue, which becomes infiltrated with lymphocytes, plasma cells and macrophages. Effusion of synovial fluid into the joint space takes place during the active phase of the disease. Subsequently, hypertrophy of the synovial membrane occurs. Inflammatory granulation tissue (pannus) is formed, spreading over and under the articular cartilage which is progressively destroyed. Later, fibrous adhesions may form between the layers of pannus across the joint space and fibrous or bony ankylosis may occur. Muscles adjacent to inflamed joints atrophy and there may be focal infiltration with lymphocytes.

Subcutaneous nodules have a characteristic histological appearance. There is a central area of fibrinoid material consisting of swollen and fragmented collagen fibres, fibrinous exudate and cellular debris, surrounded by a palisade of radially arranged proliferating mononuclear cells. The nodule is surrounded by a loose capsule of fibrous tissue. Similar granulomatous lesions may occur in the pleura, lung, pericardium and sclera. Lymph nodes are often hyperplastic and show many lymphoid follicles with large germinal centres. Plasma cells are numerous in the sinuses and medullary cords.

**Clinical Features.** ONSET. In the majority of patients the onset is insidious with joint pain, stiffness and symmetrical swelling of a number of peripheral joints. Initially pain may be experienced only on movement of joints, but rest pain and especially early morning stiffness are characteristic features of all kinds of active inflammatory arthritis. In the typical case the small joints of the fingers and toes are the first to be affected. Swelling of the proximal, but not the distal, interphalangeal joints gives the fingers a 'spindled' appearance and swelling of the metatarsophalangeal joints results in 'broadening' of the forefoot. As the disease progresses, with or without intervening remissions, there is a tendency for it to spread to involve the wrists, elbows and shoulders in the upper limbs, and the knees, ankles, subtalar and midtarsal joints in the legs. The hip joints are affected only in the more severe cases but neck pain and stiffness from cervical spine involvement is common. The mandibular, acromioclavicular and sternoclavicular joints are sometimes affected as indeed is every synovial joint. In some patients the onset is 'palindromic' with recurrent acute episodes of joint pain and stiffness in individual joints lasting only a few hours or days. In about a third of such cases the disease sooner or later evolves into a more typical polyarthritis. In 10% of patients the onset of disease is as an acute polyarthritis with severe systemic symptoms including fever, weight loss, profound fatigue and malaise.

PROGRESSION. As the disease advances, pain, muscle spasm and progressive joint destruction result in limitation of joint motion, joint instability, subluxation and deformities. At first deformities are correctable, but later permanent contractures develop and the joints may become completely disorganised. Characteristic deformities include flexion contractures of the small joints of the hands and feet, the knees, hips and elbows. In the hands anterior subluxation of the metacarpophalangeal joints is common with ulnar deviation of the fingers. Other finger deformities lead to more loss of hand function. These include the 'swan neck' deformity (hyperextension at the proximal inter-phalangeal joints and fixed flexion at the distal interphalangeal joints), the Boutonnière or 'button-hole' deformity (fixed flexion of the proximal inter-phalangeal joint and extension of the terminal interphalangeal joint) and a Z deformity of the thumb. Dorsal subluxation of the ulnar styloid at the wrist is common and may contribute to rupture of the fourth and fifth extensor tendons when these are already the site of tenosynovitis. In the forefoot, subluxation of the metatarsophalangeal joints is followed by clawing of the toes, callosities over the exposed metatarsal heads and a painful sensation of 'walking on pebbles'. In the hind foot eversion deformities at the subtalar joint are common.

EXTRA-ARTICULAR FEATURES. Rheumatoid arthritis is a systemic disease. Anorexia, weight loss, lethargy, myalgia and malaise occur commonly throughout its course and may precede the onset of articular symptoms by weeks or months. *Raynaud's phenomenon* (p. 215) is common in the prodromal period and throughout the course of the disease. *Lymphadenopathy* is a frequent finding. Although it is particularly a feature of nodes draining actively inflamed joints, more generalised lymphadenopathy is not uncommon and can give rise to diagnostic confusion when arthritis is minimal or quiescent. The nodes are discrete and not tender. Histology shows a reactive hyperplasia which can occasionally be confused with giant follicular lymphoma. *Osteoporosis, muscle weakness and wasting* also occur adjacent to inflamed joints and more diffusely as part of the systemic disturbance. They are seen early in the course of the disorder and often progress to become prominent features in very active or advanced cases. *Tenosynovitis and bursitis* are frequent accompaniments of active arthritis as tendon sheaths and bursae are also lined with synovium. 'Triggering' of the fingers may be associated with nodules in the flexor tendon sheaths which can progress to permanent flexion contractures or tendon rupture if left untreated. *Popliteal cysts* (Baker's cysts) communicate with the knee, but fluid is prevented from returning to the joint by a valve-like mechanism. The high pressure generated by flexion of the knee, especially when effusions are present, can result in gradual extension or sudden rupture of the cyst into the calf. Rupture is accompanied by calf pain, swelling, tenderness, pitting oedema and a positive Homan's sign. Diagnostic confusion with deep vein thrombosis can usually be avoided by careful consideration of the history but a venogram, joint scan or arthrogram are occasionally required to establish the correct diagnosis. *Subcutaneous nodules* appear at some time in the course of the disease in about 20% of patients. They are usually seen at the sites of pressure or friction such as the extensor surfaces of the forearms below the elbow, the scalp, sacrum, scapula and Achilles tendon as well as on the fingers and toes. Ulceration and secondary infection are not uncommon. Their presence is almost invariably associated with positive tests for rheumatoid factor. Rarely they are found in visceral organs.

OCULAR MANIFESTATIONS. *Episcleritis* is a fairly common and benign feature in patients with nodular seropositive disease. The intermittent inflammation of the superficial sclera is usually painless. It is not associated with visual disturbance and requires no specific therapy. *Scleritis* is a rarer but more serious condition. The eye is red and painful with inflammatory changes throughout the sclera and uveal tract. The pupil may be irregular from adhesions (synechiae) which can cause secondary glaucoma and visual impairment. Scleritis often requires systemic corticosteroid therapy as well as local measures. *Scleromalacia* or thinning of the sclera may follow episodes of scleritis and is seen as a blue discolouration of the white of the eye. Progression to perforation very rarely occurs. *Scleromalacia perforans* follows necrosis of a scleral rheumatoid nodule and may require enucleation of the eye. *Keratoconjunctivitis sicca* occurs in 10% of patients. Lack of lacrimal secretion results in symptoms of grittiness, dryness, burning or itching associated with sticky mucous threads. The diagnosis can be confirmed by the Schirmer tear test and slit lamp examination following Rose Bengal staining. There may be associated dryness of the nose and mouth (xerostomia) as part of Sjögren's syndrome.

*Sjögren's syndrome* is the association of xerostomia and keratoconjunctivitis sicca with a connective tissue disorder. In the majority of cases this is rheumatoid arthritis but the syndrome may be associated with systemic lupus erythematosus, mixed connective tissue disease, polymyositis, myasthenia gravis, progressive systemic sclerosis, autoimmune liver disease and thyroiditis.

Keratoconjunctivitis sicca and xerostomia can occur in the absence of identifiable associated connective tissue disorder when the term *sicca syndrome* is applied. Patients with the sicca syndrome are more likely to have more widespread and more serious manifestations which can include: salivary gland enlargement; dysphagia and dyspareunia; severe dental caries; Raynaud's phenomenon or vasculitis; lymphadenopathy, leucopaenia and hepatosplenomegaly; hyperglobulinaemic purpura; macroglobulinaemia; renal tubular acidosis or glomerulonephritis; pneumonia and diffuse interstitial pulmonary fibrosis and extra and intrasalivary lymphoreticular malignancies.

Patients with Sjögren's syndrome may have a wide range of organ-specific and non-organ-specific autoantibodies including salivary duct and thyroid antibodies, antimitochondrial and smooth muscle antibodies, rheumatoid factors and antinuclear factors. An antibody to an extractable nuclear antigen, SS-B is characteristic of sicca syndrome. The characteristic pathological feature which can be detected in the minor salivary glands on a simple lip biopsy is intense infiltration with lymphocytes and plasma cells. A fall in IgM levels may herald the development of malignancy.

Treatment is usually limited to scrupulous oral and ocular hygiene and the instillation of artificial tears (hypromellose eye drops). Drug hypersensitivity is sometimes a problem.

CARDIOVASCULAR MANIFESTATIONS. Asymptomatic pericarditis is a rather common and benign feature of seropositive rheumatoid arthritis. Pericardial effusions, tamponade and constrictive pericarditis occur much more seldom. Nodules and granuloma formation rarely lead to heart block, cardiomyopathy, coronary artery occlusion or aortic regurgitation.

*Vasculitis*. Diffuse necrotising vasculitis is relatively common in patients with nodules and positive tests for rheumatoid factor. Clinical manifestations vary with the size and site of the vessel involved. Small vessel disease of the terminal digital arteries or capillaries is often associated with no more than nail fold infarcts, leg ulcers or purpura. Large areas of skin necrosis or digital gangrene have more sinister prognostic significance and may herald the onset of *'malignant' rheumatoid disease*. These patients are often febrile with severe systemic disturbance. They have multiple extra-articular manifestations of rheumatoid disease such as anaemia, scleritis, pleurisy and pericarditis. Mononeuritis multiplex follows occlusion of vasa nervorum and a larger vessel arteritis, histologically resembling polyarteritis nodosa, may result in catastrophic mesenteric, renal, cerebrovascular or coronary artery occlusion. Such patients frequently have evidence of circulating immune complexes, cryoglobulins and hypocomplementaemia.

PULMONARY MANIFESTATIONS. *Pleurisy or pleural effusions* occur in about 25% of men with classical rheumatoid arthritis. Diagnostic aspiration should be undertaken to exclude other causes. Characteristically the fluid has a high protein content, high cell count (mononuclear or polymorphonuclear) and low glucose. Pleural biopsy may show evidence of granuloma formation. Pleural or pulmonary nodules may require excision to exclude other pathology. *Caplan's syndrome* (p. 296) and *chronic interstitial pulmonary fibrosis* are rare manifestations of rheumatoid arthritis. The latter differs in no way from idiopathic fibrosing alveolitis which is associated with positive tests for rheumatoid factor in 30% of cases. *Obliterative bronchiolitis* is also a rare complication. Dyspnoea, from non-inflammatory small airways obstruction, begins suddenly and progresses rapidly to respiratory failure.

NEUROLOGICAL MANIFESTATIONS. *Entrapment neuropathies* result from compression of peripheral nerves by hypertrophied synovium. Median nerve compression in the carpal tunnel is the most common and may be an early clinical manifestation of the disease. *Peripheral neuropathy* is usually symmetrical and limited to symptoms and signs of mild 'glove and stocking' sensory loss. In patients with vasculitis sudden palsies of major peripheral nerves may be manifestations of mononeuritis multiplex (p. 733) but physical entrapment must be carefully excluded. *Cervical cord compression* may result from subluxation of the cervical spine at the atlanto-axial joint or at a subaxial level. Atlanto-axial subluxation is a common finding in long-standing rheumatoid arthritis which can easily be diagnosed from lateral radiographs of the cervical spine taken in full flexion when the distance between the odontoid and the anterior arch of the atlas is greater than 4 mm. Although usually associated with no more than neck pain radiating to the occiput and requiring no specific treatment, it can result in cord transection and sudden death if the neck is manipulated inadvertantly under an anaesthetic. Less dramatic cases of progresssive cervical myelopathy may present with limb weakness, difficulty in holding up the head and quadraparesis. These lesions occur more often at the subaxial level and frequently require operative decompression and fixation. Severe disease of the cervical spine may also give rise to nerve root compression, vertebro-basilar insufficiency and spinal artery occlusion.

HAEMATOLOGICAL MANIFESTATIONS are very common in active rheumatoid disease. A normochromic normocytic anaemia of chronic disease (p. 544) characterised by a low serum iron and iron binding capacity which does not respond to oral iron can often be complicated by true iron deficiency secondary to gastrointestinal blood loss from treatment with analgesic anti-inflammatory drugs. Much less frequently there may be a macrocytic anaemia associated with folate deficiency. Thrombocytosis is a feature of active disease.

*Felty's syndrome* is the association of splenomegaly and neutropaenia with rheumatoid arthritis; it tends to occur in patients with seropositive, long-standing, advanced but inactive arthritis. Other clinical features include anaemia, thrombocytopaenia, lymphadenopathy, weight loss, skin pigmentation and vasculitic leg ulcers. Susceptibility to recurrent bacterial infections occurs in about half of those affected but does not appear to be directly related to the neutrophil count. The mechanism for the neutropenia remains uncertain but a wide range of immunological abnormalities include granulocyte specific antinuclear antibodies, antibodies directed against leucocyte surface antigens and polymorph phagocytosis of immune complexes. Treatment with corticosteroids is generally unsatisfactory. Splenectomy is reserved for patients with troublesome recurrent infections and is followed by prolonged remission in about 60% of cases.

AMYLOIDOSIS (p. 436) may be a true complication of prolonged active disease. Evidence of amyloid is found in 25 – 50% of cases at autopsy making rheumatoid arthritis a leading cause of secondary amyloidosis. Clinical manifestations are however usually limited to mild proteinuria with only very few patients going on to the nephrotic syndrome or renal failure.

**Investigation.** Active disease is associated with a raised ESR and C-reactive protein. The plasma protein profile shows increased globulin and fibrinogen and decreased albumin.

IMMUNOLOGICAL TESTS. IgM rheumatoid factors are detected by testing the ability of serum to agglutinate carrier particles coated with IgG. Polystyrene particles coated with human IgG are used in the latex slide test. Sheep or human erythrocytes coated with rabbit anti-erythrocyte antibody are used in the Rose Waaler sheep cell agglutination test (SCAT), the human erythrocyte agglutination test (HEAT) and the differential agglutination test (DAT). The latex fixation test is simple and sensitive but less specific so that it is frequently used as a screening test. The erythrocyte tests are less sensitive and more specific. Significant titres which exclude 95% of the normal population are: SCAT 1 : 32; DAT 1 : 16; latex 1 : 20.

The Rose Waaler test is positive in 70% of patients with rheumatoid arthritis but may not become so until 18 months have elapsed. Positive tests are also found in: Sjögren's syndrome (100%); systemic lupus erythematosus (30%); mixed connective tissue disease (30%); scleroderma (30%); chronic juvenile arthritis (15%); chronic liver disease: sarcoidosis; myeloma and other paraproteinaemias and in chronic infections (infective endocarditis, tuberculosis, syphilis, malaria and leprosy).

Up to 30% of patients with rheumatoid arthritis have positive tests for antinuclear factor.

RADIOLOGY. In the early stages of the disease radiographs are normal or show no more than soft tissue swelling and periarticular osteoporosis. Progression to cartilage and bone destruction is seen as narrowing of the joint spaces and the development of marginal erosions. Very severe destructive changes ('*arthritis mutilans*') are associated with 'cup and pencil' deformities and massive bone resorption. Marginal sclerosis and osteophyte formation are indications of secondary osteoarthrosis.

**Diagnosis** presents no difficulty when symptoms and signs of inflammatory arthritis are associated with the typical pattern of joint involvement, a raised ESR, positive tests for rheumatoid factor and evidence of erosions on X-ray. The absence of one or more of these features makes the diagnosis less certain unless characteristic nodules are present.

*Examination of synovial fluid* can be of great value when the diagnosis is in doubt. Infection is excluded by microscopic examination of a Gram stained smear, culture and gas liquid chromatography. In inflammatory joint disease the synovial fluid is of low viscosity, turbid, clots on standing and contains many cells. By contrast fluid from joints affected by traumatic or degenerative joint disease is clear, viscid, does not clot and contains few cells. Examination of the spun sediment by polarising light microscopy will reveal crystals of monosodium urate or calcium pyrophosphate dihydrate in patients with acute gout or pseudogout. Measurement of synovial fluid total haemolytic complement (CH50) activity can help to distinguish rheumatoid arthritis from other forms of inflammatory arthritis. Local depression of CH50 in synovial fluid is seldom seen except in seropositive rheumatoid arthritis.

*Arthroscopy and synovial biopsy* are occasionally required to exclude tuberculosis, pigmented villonodular synovitis and synovial tumours.

**Treatment.** Since the aetiology of rheumatoid arthritis is unknown treatment is empirically directed towards the relief of symptoms, the suppression of active and progressive disease and the conservation and restoration of function in affected joints. To a greater or lesser extent these aims can be achieved by combining treatment of the patient by the judicious use of drugs, rest, physiotherapy and surgery with the modification of the environment by paying critical attention to housing, occupation, transport, the provision of aids and appliances, and statutory social benefits. In a chronic and progressive disease which may have exacerbations and remissions over many years as well as systemic, psychiatric and social complications, both the general practitioner and rheumatologist have a special responsibility: (1) to educate the patient to understand the nature of the disease and to develop a positive but realistic approach; (2) to develop a relationship of continuing trust and support without creating a situation of undue dependence; (3) to co-ordinate a team of orthopaedic surgeons, occupational therapists, physiotherapists, nurses, social workers and other allied health professionals in an integrated rehabilitation programme and (4) to improve the patient's general health.

In a disorder which is as complex and changeable as rheumatoid arthritis there is a need for repeated medical, functional and social reassessment if patients are to maintain their maximum physical, psychological, social and vocational potential.

GENERAL TREATMENT IN THE ACTIVE PHASE. Physical rest, anti-inflammatory drug therapy and maintenance physiotherapy are the cornerstones of treatment for exacerbations of rheumatoid disease. Admission to hospital may become necessary when widespread active polyarthritis is associated with signs of constitutional disturbance and there has been no response to rest at home and optimum doses of non-steroid, analgesic, anti-inflammatory drugs (NSAID). In most patients the rest from physical and emotional stress provided by two to three weeks of hospitalisation is sufficient to induce a marked remission of symptoms without recourse to strict bedrest. The time in hospital allows for detailed assessments by all members of the arthritis team. It ensures that the programme of medical and physical treatment best suited to the individual's needs can be started under supervision and it provides an opportunity to plan the solution of outstanding functional and social problems with appropriate aids and social services. In a few patients a period of complete bedrest may be required to induce a remission. In these circumstances it is essential to prevent the development of 'bed deformities'. The mattress should be firm or fracture boards inserted beneath it. A back rest with the minimum number of pillows should be in position during the day and only one firm pillow used at night. Pillows behind the knees must be avoided and a bed cage with padded footrest provided. The patient should be persuaded to spend an hour each day lying flat with a small pillow under the lumbar spine and two periods of 30 minutes prone lying will go a long way to prevent the development of flexion contractures of the hips. Foot and quadriceps exercises should be performed daily by all patients confined to bed along with maintenance exercises for muscle groups in unaffected limbs and in the thoracic, gluteal and abdominal regions.

Therapy with oral iron is indicated when true iron deficiency complicates the anaemia of chronic disease (p. 544). The normochromic normocytic anaemia which is resistant to oral iron may partially and transiently respond to parenteral injections but induction of disease remission is the best remedy. Rarely folic acid is required for a macrocytic anaemia.

LOCAL MEASURES IN THE ACTIVE PHASE. *Corticosteroids.* Where one or more joints continue to be extremely painful and inflamed, intra-articular injection of a suspension of hydrocortisone acetate, methylprednisolone acetate or triamcinalone hexacetonide will often bring symptomatic relief lasting weeks or months. The dose should be 50 – 100 mg of hydrocortisone for large joints such as the ankle or knee and 5 – 10 mg for small joints, or the equivalent doses of the longer acting synthetic steroids. Repeated injections at short intervals should be avoided, particularly in the case of weight-bearing joints. Local injection of hydrocortisone is also the treatment of choice for alleviating symptoms of median nerve compression in the carpal tunnel when this occurs during the course of an exacerbation of rheumatoid arthritis.

*Rest splints* can be very useful for stabilising a particularly painful joint, such as the knee or wrist, but are usually indicated only if general rest, non-steroidal anti-inflammatory drugs and intra-articular steroid injections fail to bring symptomatic relief. Splints are also used to prevent or correct flexion deformity especially at the knee.

ANALGESIC AND ANTI-INFLAMMATORY DRUGS are the mainstay of therapy for active inflammatory arthritis. They can be very effective in relieving pain and stiffness in optimal anti-inflammatory doses but they do not alter the course of the disease and the margin between effective and toxic doses is often small. *Aspirin* is widely regarded as the drug of first choice but only 50% of patients are able to tolerate adequate doses over prolonged periods. For anti-inflammatory, as opposed to simple analgesic, effect it needs to be given in doses of 4 – 6 g daily. It should be prescribed as soluble aspirin (the cheapest) or as enteric coated tablets when dyspepsia or occult gastrointestinal blood loss is a problem. Alternative drugs (NSAID) are listed in Table 13.1, with standard doses and leading side effects. Aspirin, indomethacin and phenylbutazone are more effective but more toxic than the newer propionic acid derivatives which should be tried if aspirin is not tolerated. Phenylbutazone should never be the drug of first choice because of the risk of agranulocytosis and aplastic anaemia. The 'second generation' propionic and acetic acid derivatives have few, if any, advantages over the first, but the 'third generation' drugs have the added convenience of long duration of action, so reducing the number of tablets that have to be taken and making once or twice daily dosage a possibility.

Inhibition of prostaglandin synthesis appears to be a major pharmacological action of all these agents. There is little to suggest that combinations are more effective or are less toxic than optimal doses of single drugs. Additional simple analgesics such as paracetamol can be given when pain relief is inadequate. Paracetamol dextropropoxyphene combinations are very widely used for this purpose. Although safe in moderate doses propoxyphene does have narcotic properties. In general centrally acting narcotic analgesics have no place in the management of rheumatic diseases. A number of combinations of aspirin and paracetamol are marketed.

SLOW ACTING ANTIRHEUMATIC DRUGS. The use of a 'second line' or 'disease-modifying' drug should be considered in all patients where symptoms and signs of active inflammatory arthritis have persisted for six months despite adequate general measures and optimal doses of NSAID.

*The antimalarials* chloroquine phosphate (250 mg daily) or hydroxychloquine sulphate (200 mg b.d.) may be used as an adjunt to basic therapy in such circumstances. Clinical benefit is noted in about half the patients in 4–12 weeks and the drug should be discontinued if there is no effect by six months. Occasional side-effects include nausea, diarrhoea, rashes, haemolytic anaemia, ototoxicity and neuromyopathy as well as a small risk of ocular toxicity after more than a year of therapy. Deposits of the drug in the cornea may produce disturbances of vision which tend to disappear when the drug is withdrawn. More rarely retinopathy can result in permanent visual impairment. If the drug is effective it is advisable to have a thorough ophthalmological assessment after one year and at six monthly intervals thereafter. In order to reduce the risks of ocular toxicity it is conventional to give the drug for only 10 months in each year. In some the dose can be halved without exacerbation of symptoms. Antimalarials do not retard the progression of radiological changes.

*Penicillamine and gold* are slow acting suppressive antirheumatic drugs which have been shown to decrease the progression of erosive changes as well as reduce the activity of the disease in 50–60% of patients. Because of a high incidence of toxic effects, treatment with these agents should be considered only in the following circumstances as an adjunct to basic therapy: (1) patients with active progressive disease developing erosions and/or deformities; (2) patients with nodules and/or high titres of rheumatoid factor who have persistently active disease after six months treatment with optimal doses of anti-inflammatory drugs; (3) patients with trouble-

Table 13.1 Non-steroid analgesic anti-inflammatory drugs (NSAID)

| Drug | Usual dose | Side-effects |
|---|---|---|
| Aspirin | 900–1200 mg q.i.d. | Tinnitus; deafness; dyspepsia; GI haemorrhage |
| Phenylbutazone | 100 mg t.i.d. | Dyspepsia; GI haemorrhage; fluid retention; agranulocytosis aplastic anaemia |
| Oxyphenbutazone | 100 mg t.i.d. | |
| Indomethacin | 25 mg t.i.d. | Dyspepsia; GI haemorrhage; headaches |
| *Propionic Acid Derivatives* | | |
| Ibuprofen | 400 mg q.i.d. | Occasional dyspepsia and GI haemorrhage |
| Ketoprofen | 50 mg q.i.d. | Occasional dyspepsia and GI haemorrhage |
| Fenoprofen | 600 mg t.i.d. | Occasional dyspepsia and GI haemorrhage |
| Naproxen | 250 mg mane<br>500 mg nocte | Occasional dyspepsia and GI haemorrhage |
| *Second Generation Propionic and Acetic Acid Derivatives* | | |
| Flurbiprofen | 50 mg q.i.d. | Occasional dyspepsia and GI haemorrhage |
| Sulindac | 100 mg b.d. | Minimal |
| Diclofenac | 50 mg q.i.d. | Occasional dyspepsia and GI haemorrhage |
| Fenclofenac | 400 mg t.i.d. | High incidence of rashes |
| Tolmetin | 400 mg t.i.d. | Occasional dyspepsia and GI haemorrhage |
| *Third Generation Propionic Acid Derivatives* | | |
| Piroxicam | 20 mg daily | Occasional dyspepsia and GI haemorrhage |
| Fenbufen | 600 mg daily | Occasional dyspepsia and GI haemorrhage |
| *Fenamates* | | |
| Mefenamic Acid | 500 mg t.i.d. | Diarrhoea; occasional renal insufficiency; dyspepsia |
| Flufenamic Acid | 200 mg t.i.d. | Diarrhoea; occasional renal insufficiency; dyspepsia |
| *Enolic Acids* | | |
| Azapropazone | 300 mg q.i.d.<br>or 600 mg b.i.d. | Occasional dyspepsia and GI haemorrhage; fluid retention |
| Feprazone | 200 mg t.i.d. | Dyspepsia and occasional GI haemorrhage; fluid retention; high incidence of rashes. |
| *Fourth Generation Propionic Acid Derivatives* | | |
| Benoxuprofen | 600 mg daily | Occasional rashes<br>Heliosensitivity<br>Onycholysis |

some extra-articular features; (4) patients who have failed to respond to antimalarial drugs; (5) patients whose symptoms are only controllable with unacceptably high doses of corticosteroids; (6) patients with palindromic onset rheumatoid arthritis who are having frequent attacks or developing persistent inflammatory arthritis.

*Penicillamine* is marginally preferable to gold unless there is a previous history of severe dyspepsia because it can be given orally and because the side-effects, though numerous and potentially serious, are usually more predictable and manageable. Treatment is commenced with a single evening dose of 125–250 mg and dosage is increased by no more than 250 mg/month to a maximum of 1 g/day. Clinical benefit is noted several weeks after an effective dose has been achieved and reaches a maximum only after 4–6 months. Early side-effects include rashes, loss of taste, nausea, vomiting and a serious febrile reaction. Later side-effects include mouth ulcers, proteinuria and nephrotic syndrome and more rarely diseases resembling systemic lupus erythematosus, myasthenia gravis, pemphigus and Goodpasture's syndrome. Thrombocytopaenia and pancytopaenia may occur at any time and are potentially the most serious toxic effects. Patients must be monitored by regular urinalyses and full blood counts including platelets at first at weekly intervals. Proteinuria and mild thrombocytopaenia are indications for temporary cessation of therapy followed by reintroduction of the drug at lower dosage if the abnormalities disappear. It is advisable to withdraw penicillamine altogether if the side-effects recur. Febrile reactions and pancytopaenia are absolute indications for drug withdrawal.

*Chrysotherapy* is given as weekly intramuscular injections of 50 mg sodium aurothiomalate, after a test dose of 10 mg, until a response is obtained, usually at about 2–3 months. The intervals between injections are progressively increased provided the remission is maintained and the drug is continued indefinitely. The course of gold injections should be terminated if there has been no clinical benefit after 6 months. Side-effects include pruritic skin rashes, mouth ulcers, enterocolitis, proteinuria and nephrotic syndrome, thrombocytopaenia, agranulocytosis and aplastic anaemia, all of which are potentially serious and preclude further therapy. Monitoring should include a routine urinalysis and full blood count including platelets initially prior to each injection.

Pruritus may respond to antihistamines and exfoliative dermatitis, thrombocytopaenia, agranulocytosis and nephropathy to corticosteroids. Patients with agranulocytosis almost invariably recover if they can be protected from serious infection; those with aplastic anaemia have a more serious prognosis. Dimercaprol (BAL) combines with heavy metals to form a stable compound which is rapidly excreted in the urine. 3 mg/kg body weight should be administered intramuscularly 6 hourly for 3 – 4 days in patients with aplastic anaemia who have not responded to withdrawal of gold injections after 4–5 days.

CORTICOSTEROIDS AND CORTICOTROPHIN have a very potent anti-inflammatory activity but do not possess the 'disease modifying' properties of the slow acting antirheumatic agents. Doses required to maintain adequate symptomatic relief on a long term basis are accompanied by an unacceptable level of side effects so their use is justified only in exceptional circumstances when other therapy is ineffective. The main indications for their use are: (1) in exceptionally severe exacerbations which are not remitting with rest, intra-articular injections of corticosteroids and non-steroidal anti-inflammatory drugs; (2) when all other measures fail to control persistently disabling symptoms in breadwinners or young mothers who have to return to work; (3) in some elderly patients when acute disease is threatening to render them bedbound; (4) life or sight threatening visceral disease such as severe pericarditis, polyarteritis or scleritis.

In each of these circumstances a suppressive slow acting antirheumatic agent is commenced simultaneously with a view to tailing off corticosteroid therapy once a remission is obtained.

*Prednisolone* is the corticosteroid of choice. It should ideally be administered as a single morning dose of no more than 7·5 mg/day to minimise suppression of the hypothalamo-pituitary-adrenal axis. In practice an evening dose of 5 mg is sometimes more useful in overcoming intractable early morning stiffness. Enteric coated tablets or small doses of corticotrophin may be preferred in patients with severe dyspepsia or a previous history of peptic ulceration. In other circumstances any possible advantages of ACTH seem to be outweighed by the disadvantages, namely the need for injections, the difficulty in knowing the dose of steroid being effectively administered and the high prevalence of mineralocorticoid side-effects.

IMMUNOMODULATION. Since rheumatoid arthritis is associated with evidence of both overactivity of humoral immunity and suppression of some facets of cell mediated immunity both 'immunosuppressive' and 'immunostimulant' drugs have been considered for management of the disease. Increasing understanding of the complexity of regulation of the immune system and the 'immunopharmacology' of cytotoxic and immunostimulant drugs makes it clear that these agents may have variable and even opposing effects on the expression of immune responses depending on the dosage, the timing of administration and the subpopulation of cells predominantly affected. For example, immune stimulation may result from treatment with a drug which predominantly inhibits a suppressor cell population while functional immunosuppression can follow use of an immuno-stimulant which selectively activates these cells.

In practice a number of cytotoxic and immunostimulant agents have been found to have both symptomatic and slow acting 'disease modifying' activity in rheumatoid arthritis. The effects, which are empirical, may be mediated as much by 'anti-inflammatory' as by the 'immunoregulatory' activity and their usefulness is very strictly limited by immediate and potential long term toxicity.

The indications for the use of these agents are limited at the present time to: (1) treatment of life threatening extra-articular manifestations which have failed to respond to corticosteroids or second line agents; (2) treatment of patients with severely active symptomatic and progressive joint disease who have failed to respond to all other forms of therapy; (3) treatment of patients receiving unacceptably high doses of corticosteroids in whom steroid dose reduction has not been possible.

*Azathioprine* is a purine analogue and antimetabolite. Both high dosage (2·5 mg/kg) and low dosage (1·25 mg/kg) have been shown to be effective. The dose must be reduced to 25% in patients receiving allopurinol since azathioprine metabolism is via xanthine oxidase. Side-effects include nausea, vomiting, stomatitis, diarrhoea, hepatitis and particularly bone marrow suppression and susceptibility to infection. Monitoring is with fortnightly or monthly full blood counts.

*Cyclophosphamide* is an alkylating agent which has been shown to be effective in daily doses of 1–2 mg/kg. Side-effects include alopecia, azoospermia, anovulation and bladder toxicity as well as gastrointestinal disturbance, susceptibility to infection, bone marrow suppression and teratogenesis. Monitoring is with fortnightly or monthly full blood counts and routine urinalysis.

Both agents are believed to carry a significant risk of carcinogenesis.

*Levamisole* is an antihelminthic which has been shown to augment T lymphocyte responses as well as polymorph and macrophage chemotaxis and phagocytosis in certain circumstances. It can be effective in patients with rheumatoid arthritis in doses of 150 mg once weekly. Side-effects include febrile reactions, nausea, vomiting, urticarial and vasculitic rashes. A high risk of agranulocytosis even with weekly monitoring of blood counts precludes its use routinely.

*Plasma exchange* and *thoracic duct drainage* have both been shown to be effective in inducing remissions of disease but have no place in its practical management.

SURGICAL TREATMENT AND REHABILITATION. In the overall management of patients with severe and progressive rheumatoid arthritis there are many circumstances when orthopaedic surgical procedures are required to relieve pain and conserve or restore locomotor function. Cosmetic operations are seldom if ever indicated.

Surgical decompression and synovectomy of the wrist and tendon sheaths of the hands are often needed when non-steroidal anti-inflammatory drugs, local injections of corticosteroids and simple physical measures have failed to relieve a carpal tunnel syndrome or flexion contractures of the fingers resulting from fibrosis and nodule formation. Flexor and extensor tendon synovectomy, the latter often accompanied by resection of a subluxated ulnar styloid, can be important measures in preventing tendon ruptures. Synovectomy of joints will not prevent disease progression but may be indicated for pain relief when drug therapy, local rest, intra-articular injections and $\beta$ emittor isotopes (yttrium silicate) have failed to provide symptomatic relief. At a later stage, when tendons, cartilage and bone have been eroded and the mechanics of joints disturbed, reconstructive tendon surgery, osteotomy, arthrodesis and a variety of arthroplasties with or without prostheses play a major part in the rehabilitation of the patient. Forefoot pain resulting from subluxation of the metatarsophalangeal joints and clawing of the toes can be effectively relieved by excision of the heads and necks of the metatarsals if insoles and moulded shoes have failed to provide symptomatic relief. Hip arthroplasty can be remarkably effective in relieving incapacitating pain and restoring ambulation in patients with severely damaged joints. Total hip replacement is now the most frequent major elective operation undertaken in Britain where over 30 000 are performed annually. Resurfacing and total condylar arthroplasties of the knee are less consistently successful but nevertheless performed in preference to osteotomy and arthrodesis in rheumatoid patients with intractable pain and disability. Arthrodesis is however still the best solution when severe hind foot pain is associated with destruction and subluxation of the ankle and subtalar joints. A number of 'salvage' and reconstructive operations are also available for relieving pain and restoring function in the upper limbs. Stabilisation or wrist arthrodesis, excision arthroplasty of the metacarpo-phalangeal joints with insertion of silastic spacers and arthrodesis of the PIP joints of the fingers are all procedures in appropriate circumstances to relieve pain and improve power grip. Pinch grip may be restored by arthrodesis of the interphalangeal joint of the thumb in patients with Z deformities. Radial head excision is a simple but effective procedure which will relieve the severe pain experienced on supination and pronation when the superior radioulnar joint is the major site of destructive changes. Relief of pain and restoration of function to patients with advanced shoulder and elbow destruction is however still a major problem. Suitable prosthetic surgery for these joints is still very much in the developmental phase.

If surgical treatment is to be successful it is very important that the aims and consequences of each operation are carefully considered as part of an integrated programme of management and rehabilitation. This is often best achieved where physicians and surgeons with special experience work together in a combined rheumatology/orthopaedic clinic with other allied health professionals. Assessment of motivation, social support and environment are no less important than careful consideration of the patient's general health and detailed assessment of the extent of disease in other joints, the integrity of the cervical spine, the presence or absence of infection, arteritis or osteoporosis. In particular it must be appreciated that whereas many patients with slowly progressive disease can be maintained mobile and functionally independent by a series of major joint replacements carried out over a number of years, it is seldom possible to mobilise a patient, who has been chair or bed-bound for a long period, by multiple joint replacement during a single lengthy hospital admission. In these and other circumstances pain relief and functional independence are better served by provision of a suitable wheelchair, home adjustments, physical aids and social services.

When a patient cannot return to a former occupation it may be necessary to suggest a change of employment where less strain will be thrown on the damaged joints. Although disablement resettlement officers, industrial rehabilitation units and government retraining centres are sometimes helpful in such cases, it should be emphasised that patients have the best chance of returning to active work with their former employers. It cannot be stressed too strongly that adequate treatment in the early stages and throughout the course of the disease enables most patients to return to some form of wage earning activity. Disabilities of all kinds can be reduced even in the 25% of patients running a severe progressive course.

**Prognosis.** The course and prognosis in rheumatoid arthritis is very variable. In those patients with disease of such severity as to require admission to hospital, review after 10 years shows that: 25% will have a complete remission of symptoms and remain fit for all normal activities; 40% will have only moderate impairment of function despite exacerbations and remissions of disease; 25% will be more severely disabled; 10% will be severely crippled. If the many patients in the community are considered whose symptoms are never of such severity as to require admission to hospital the overall prognosis is much better.

A poor prognosis may be associated with: (1) high titres of rheumatoid factor; (2) insidious onset of disease; (3) more than a year of active disease without remission; (4) early development of nodules and erosions and (5) extra-articular manifestations.

## Spondyloarthritis

This is a group of diseases in which an inflammatory arthritis, characterised by persistently negative tests for IgM rheumatoid factor, is variably associated with a number of other common articular, extra-articular and genetic features.

The seronegative spondyloarthritides are: ankylosing spondylitis; Reiter's syndrome and reactive arthritis; psoriatic arthritis; enteropathic arthritis associated with ulcerative colitis and Crohn's disease; Behçet's syndrome; Whipple's disease and juvenile chronic arthritis.

The features held in common by the seronegative spondyloarthritides are: (1) an asymmetrical, inflammatory seronegative oligoarthritis; (2) sacroiliitis and/or spondylitis in some cases; (3) a tendency to develop inflammatory lesions of tendinous attachments to bone (enthesopathy); (4) anterior uveitis in some cases; (5) familial association in some cases and (6) a higher prevalence of the histocompatibility antigen HLA-B27.

Current concepts of the aetiology of these disorders suggests that they may arise as an abnormal response to infection in genetically determined persons carrying the

HLA-B27 antigen. In some, an inciting organism has been identified as in Reiter's syndrome which can follow bacterial dysentery, or in the reactive arthritis following infection with *Yersinia enterocolitica*. In the others the infectious agent remains obscure. It is uncertain whether possession of HLA-B27 predisposes towards disease because: (1) it is merely a marker for an immune response gene; (2) susceptibility to infection is increased as a result of cross reactivity between an HLA-B27 determined host gene product and an antigen carried by the invading organism (molecular mimicry) or (3) the inciting organism modifies HLA-B27 positive cellular receptors in such a way as to initiate an autoimmune reaction or render the cells more susceptible to cytotoxic lymphocytes.

## Ankylosing Spondylitis

In its typical form this is a chronic inflammatory arthritis with a predilection for the sacroiliac joints and spine and characterised by progressive stiffening and fusion of the axial skeleton.

**Epidemiology.** Typically this is a disease of young men with a peak onset in the second and third decades and a male to female ratio of 9 : 1. About one in 250 adult Caucasian males are affected but incomplete forms may be more common and the overall sex ratio more equal. It occurs much more frequently in the Haida Indians of British Columbia and rarely in Negroes and Orientals. There is a greatly increased prevalence in the 1st degree relatives of patients with psoriatic arthritis, inflammatory bowel disease and Reiter's syndrome as well as in those with the disease itself. More than 90% of affected persons carry the histocompatability antigen HLA-B27. Chronic prostatitis is more common than would be anticipated but it has not been possible to isolate infectious organisms from prostatic fluid. Faecal carriage of some Klebsiella species is increased in ankylosing spondylitis and this may be related to exacerbations of the disease.

**Pathology.** Biopsy material from peripheral joints shows changes similar to those found in rheumatoid arthritis. Bony ankylosis, however, occurs more frequently. The characteristic *enthesopathy* comprises multiple foci of inflammation with lymphocytes and plasma cells at ligamentous attachments with adjacent erosion of bone. Healing of similar lesions at the junction of the vertebral bodies and annulus fibrosus of the intervertebral discs leads to the new bone formation (syndesmophytes) which is the hallmark of the disease.

**Clinical Features.** The onset is usually insidious with recurring episodes of low back pain and stiffness sometimes radiating to the buttocks or thighs. Characteristically the symptoms are worse in the early morning and following inactivity. Occasionally the onset may be acute, resembling a lumbar disc protrusion but on examination all movements of the lumbar spine are restricted, there is pain on sacroiliac compression and there are no associated symptoms or signs of nerve root compression. A few patients present with symptoms referable to the dorsal or cervical spine but such cases usually reveal evidence of previous sacroiliitis and lumbar spine involvement. Chest pain aggravated by breathing results from involvement of the costovertebral joints. Plantar fasciitis, Achilles tendinitis and tenderness over bony prominences such as the iliac crest, ischial tuberosity and greater trochanter are typical. 25% of patients have an attack of acute anterior uveitis during the course of the disease and this may be the presenting feature in a few cases. In 10% a peripheral joint is first affected and in a further 10% symptoms begin in childhood as one variety of pauciarticular juvenile chronic arthritis (p. 623). Early signs include failure to obliterate the lumbar lordosis on forward flexion, pain on sacroiliac compression, and restriction of movements of the lumbar spine in all directions. As the disease progresses stiffness increases throughout the spine and chest expansion frequently becomes restricted. Severe spinal fusion and rigidity occurs in only a minority and in most of these is not associated with much deformity. A few develop kyphosis of the dorsal and cervical spine which can be incapacitating especially when associated with hip involvement.

Extra-articular features of ankylosing spondylitis include non-granulomatous anterior uveitis; aortic regurgitation and conduction defects; apical pulmonary fibrosis; amyloidosis; osteoporosis and myelopathy associated with atlanto-axial subluxation.

**Investigation.** The ESR is usually raised but may be normal. Tests for rheumatoid factor and antinuclear factor are negative and synovial fluid complement levels are not depressed.

*Radiographs* in the early stages may be normal. Radiological signs of sacroiliitis begin in the lower parts of the joints with irregularity and marginal sclerosis eventually progressing to fusion. In the lumbar spine there may be 'squaring' of the vertebrae owing to ossification of the anterior longitudinal ligament, syndesmophyte formation, erosion and sclerosis at the anterior corners of the vertebrae and facetal joint changes. Progressive ossification results in the typical 'bamboo spine'. Erosive changes may be seen in the symphysis pubis, the ischial tuberosities and peripheral joints. Osteoporosis and atlanto-axial dislocation can occur.

*Radionuclide bone scanning* may reveal evidence of sacroiliitis or spinal involvement when radiographs are negative but the increased uptake of technetium polyphosphate or diphosphonate is non-specific and reflects bone blood flow and turnover.

**Differential diagnosis** is usually from prolapsed lumbar intervertebral discs and other traumatic lesions leading to low back pain or from other types of spondyloarthritis. Degenerative joint disease occurs in an older age group and is not accompanied by systemic symptoms. The radiological appearances are usually distinct although benign senile hyperostotic spondylosis can cause confusion when new bone formation is extensive and uniform. In osteoarthrosis the osteophytes extend horizontally from the edges of the vertebral bodies, there is frequently associated narrowing of the disc spaces and the sacroiliac joints are usually intact. When ankylosing spondylitis commences in a peripheral joint all other causes of seronegative inflammatory arthritis must be considered. Involvement of the MTP joint of the great toe can occasionally be mistaken for gout, pseudogout or an infective arthritis.

**Treatment.** The principles are to relieve pain and stiffness, maintain a maximal range of skeletal mobility and avoid the development of deformities. Early in the disease patients should be trained in regular exercising at home and encouraged to take up active non-contact sports like swimming. Poor bed and chair postures must be avoided . NSAID (p. 613) are used to relieve symptoms but do not themselves alter the course of the disease. Although aspirin, propionic acids, the enolic derivatives and indomethacin should be tried first, many patients with spondylitis find phenylbutazone the most effective drug. It can usually be given safely over prolonged periods provided a daily dose of 300 mg is not exceeded. Radiotherapy is occasionally indicated if the response to drug therapy is unsatisfactory. It does not affect the course of the disease and earlier regimes of treatment, when excessive radiation was employed, were associated with a tenfold increase in the risk of developing leukaemia. Local corticosteroid injections can be helpful for plantar fasciitis and the management of other manifestations of enthesopathy. Systemic steroids are sometimes required for treatment of acute iritis. Hip disease may require surgery and total hip arthroplasty has largely obviated the need for difficult spinal surgery in those with advanced deformity.

75% or more of patients with ankylosing spondylitis are able to remain in employment without significant loss of time from work. Restriction of chest movements does not predispose to pulmonary infection but systemic complications and especially hip involvement carry a worse prognosis.

## Reiter's Syndrome

Classically this is the triad of non-specific urethritis, conjunctivitis and arthritis that follows bacterial dysentery or sexual exposure. Incomplete forms are frequent and include the commonest variety of inflammatory arthritis seen in young men. When arthritis alone follows sexual exposure or enteric infection with salmonella, shigella, yersinia or campylobacter the term '*reactive arthritis*' is frequently used.

**Epidemiology.** 1–2% of patients with non-specific urethritis seen at clinics for sexually transmitted diseases have Reiter's syndrome and there is a similar incidence following outbreaks of shigellosis. A male with HLA-B27 runs a 20% risk of getting the disease following an attack of shigella dysentery. Although predominantly a disease of young men, the apparent 50:1 male to female ratio is spuriously high as urethritis is frequently ignored in women and children.

**Clinical Features.** The onset is typically acute with the simultaneous development of urethritis, conjunctivitis and an inflammatory oligoarthritis affecting the weight bearing joints of the lower limbs, 1–3 weeks following sexual exposure or an attack of dysentery. There may be considerable associated systemic disturbance with fever, weight loss and vasomotor changes in the feet. Equally often the onset is more insidious and many patients present with no more than monoarthritis of a knee or an asymmetrical inflammatory arthritis of some interphalangeal joints. Symptoms and signs of urethritis or conjunctivitis may have been minimal or forgotten. In such cases, heel pain, Achilles tendinitis or plantar fasciitis are valuable clues while the presence of circinate balanitis or the rash of keratodermia blenorrhagicum can clinch the diagnosis even in the absence of the classical triad and without an overt history of sexual promiscuity or dysentery. The skin lesions can vary from mild macules, vesicles and pustules on the hands and feet to marked hyperkeratosis with plaque-like lesions spreading to the scalp and trunk. These may be associated with severe nail dystrophy and massive subungual hyperkeratosis.

Ocular involvement is normally limited to mild bilateral conjunctivitis which subsides spontaneously within a month. In 10% of patients acute anterior uveitis occurs at the outset. It is distinguished from simple conjunctivitis by injection of the ciliary vessels around the cornea, by a constricted irregular or unreactive pupil and by cells in the anterior chamber on slit lamp examination. Unlike the conjunctivitis it requires urgent treatment. Chronic iridocyclitis may lead to glaucoma and blindness.

The urethritis is usually associated with minor dysuria and a clear sterile discharge. Sometimes it is asymptomatic and detected only by finding mucoid threads in the first voided specimen of early morning urine. Unusually there may be severe dysuria, haematuria and suprapubic discomfort from an associated acute haemorrhagic cystitis and prostato-vesiculitis.

Initially the arthritis appears to be self limiting with spontaneous remission of symptoms within 2–3 months of onset. There is however a recurrence rate of about 15% per annum not necessarily related to further overt exposure to infection. Low back pain and stiffness from sacroiliitis are common and 15–20% of patients develop spondylitis. Other rare extra-articular features include neurological complications, e.g. meningo-encephalitis, and peripheral neuropathy and cardiopulmonary sequelae e.g. pericarditis and pleurisy.

**Investigation.** The ESR is often greatly raised during the acute phase and may remain so for long after joint symptoms have settled. Polymorphonuclear leucocytosis and an anaemia of chronic disease are further indications of active systemic disturbance. The synovial fluid has the characteristics of a low viscosity inflammatory effusion with leucocyte counts as high as 50 000/cu.mm but it is sterile on culture. Giant synovial macrophages can be seen but synovial fluid complement levels are not depressed as they are in seropositive rheumatoid arthritis. Serum tests for rheumatoid factor and antinuclear factor are negative. Tissue typing reveals HLA-B27 in more than 70% of cases.

*Radiology*. Periarticular osteoporosis, reduction of joint space and erosive changes can be seen when there is prolonged or recurrent inflammatory arthritis. The changes reflect the asymmetry of joint involvement and are often accompanied by marked periostitis especially in the metatarsal and phalangeal bones. Periosteal reaction around the pelvis gives a characteristic appearance of 'whiskering' and there may be large and 'fluffy' calcaneal spurs. Sacroiliitis is indistinguishable from that seen in ankylosing spondylitis but the spinal changes include early isolated bony spurs and paravertebral ossification also found in psoriasis but not in ankylosing spondylitis.

**Treatment** is mainly symptomatic and supportive. Rest and NSAID (p. 613) are required during the acute phases together with judicious aspiration of joints and intra-articular or other local steroid injections. Systemic corticosteroids are very occasionally required. Anterior uveitis may be a medical emergency requiring topical, subconjunctival or systemic corticosteroids. Severe progressive arthritis and intractable keratodermia blenorrhagicum very occasionally warrant cytotoxic drug therapy. The non-specific urethritis is usually treated with a short course of tetracycline but there is little evidence that it is effective and no evidence that it alters the course of the rest of the disease.

10% of patients have evidence of active disease 20 years after the onset. Spondylitis, chronic erosive arthritis, recurrent acute arthritis and uveitis are the major causes of long-term morbidity.

## Psoriatic Arthritis

This is a seronegative inflammatory arthritis found in patients with psoriasis, a past or family history of psoriasis or with characteristic changes in the nails.

**Epidemiology.** Psoriatic arthritis occurs in about 1 out of 1000 of the general population and in 7% of patients with psoriasis. 20% of all patients with seronegative polyarthritis have psoriasis while the prevalence of psoriasis in seropositive rheumatoid arthritis is no higher than that in the general population, suggesting that the association of the skin disease with seronegative arthritis does not arise by chance alone. The onset is usually between the ages of 25–40 years and the sex incidence is equal except in those with spinal involvement where males are found to predominate.

**Clinical Features.** Five distinct clinical patterns of psoriatic arthritis are recognised: (1) An inflammatory arthritis involving the distal interphalangeal joints not usually affected in rheumatoid arthritis is seen in 15% of patients who almost invariably have associated nail changes. (2) An asymmetrical inflammatory oligo-arthritis affecting the small joints of the hand and feet is the most common clinical pattern and accounts for 70% of all cases. (3) A symmetrical but persistently seronegative inflammatory polyarthritis clinically indistinguishable from 'seronegative rheumatoid arthritis' accounts for 15% of cases. (4) Arthritis mutilans with extensive bone resorption and telescoping digits occurs in less than 5% of cases. (5) Sacroiliitis and spondylitis essentially indistinguishable from classical ankylosing spondylitis can occur alone or in association with any of the clinical patterns of peripheral arthritis.

Extra-articular features are limited to (1) Skin lesions which may be widespread scaling lesions typically over extensor surfaces or insignificant and confined to such areas as the scalp, natal cleft and umbilicus where they are easily overlooked. (2) Nail changes including pitting, onycholysis, subungual hyperkeratosis and horizontal ridging and (3) Anterior uveitis.

**Investigation.** The ESR is usually only moderately raised and there may be a mild normochromic normocytic anaemia in active cases. Tests for rheumatoid factor and antinuclear factor are negative. Asymmetrical disease, terminal I.P. joint involvement and relatively little peri-articular osteoporosis may help to distinguish psoriatic arthritis from rheumatoid arthritis radiologically. The changes in the axial skeleton resemble those in ankylosing spondylitis.

**Treatment.** NSAID are usually all that are required to control symptoms. Gold therapy can be used in persistently symptomatic progressive cases without exacerbation of the psoriasis but the antimalarials, chloroquine and hydroxychloroquine must be avoided. Immunosuppressive drugs are given very occasionally to try and control progressive arthritis mutilans or extensive incapacitating skin disease. Splints and prolonged rest are best avoided because of the increased tendency to fibrous and bony ankylosis but intra-articular steroid injections can be used with good effect in persistently active and symptomatic joints. Prognosis is better than for rheumatoid arthritis with the exception of those rare cases with arthritis mutilans.

### Other Seronegative Spondyloarthritides

**Enteropathic Arthritis.** Two patterns of seronegative inflammatory arthritis are associated with ulcerative colitis and Crohn's disease.

*Enteropathic Synovitis.* An acute, often migratory, non-erosive oligo-arthritis occurs in the course of the disorder in 12% of patients with ulcerative colitis and 20% of those with Crohn's disease. The knees, ankles and other weight-bearing joints are most commonly affected but the wrists and small joints of the fingers and toes can also be involved. The arthritis, which tends to follow exacerbations of the underlying bowel disease, sometimes in association with aphthous mouth ulcers, uveitis and erythema nodosum, ceases to be a problem following total colectomy in cases of ulcerative colitis. The higher prevalence in Crohn's disease may reflect the greater difficulty in eradicating the bowel problem.

*Sacroiliitis* (16%) and *ankylosing spondylitis* (6%) are also seen in the course of these disorders, but they pursue an independent course and often precede the bowel disease. Spinal changes which are indistinguishable from classical ankylosing spondylitis are associated with a high prevalence of HLA-B27 while the enteropathic synovitis is not.

In enteropathic synovitis treatment is directed at the bowel problem. The response to corticosteroids and colectomy is remarkable in such cases although the arthritis is never of such severity as to be itself an indication for these measures.

**Behçet's syndrome** was originally characterised by the triple complex of recurrent oral and genital ulceration and relapsing iritis. Other systemic manifestations have been incorporated into the present classification of this disease.

The major criteria are recurrent aphthous stomatitis; skin lesions; iridocyclitis and genital ulceration. The minor criteria are inflammatory arthritis of large joints, intestinal ulceration, epididymitis, thrombophlebitis and neuropsychiatric problems. In the presence of all four major criteria the syndrome is said to be 'complete'; in the presence of three, 'incomplete'. The arthritis is mono-articular or oligo-articular and non-erosive. It most frequently involves the knees, ankles, wrists and elbows. Occasionally the sacroiliac joints are affected. Treatment is symptomatic with NSAID; corticosteroids and immunosuppressive therapy are reserved for the more serious systemic manifestations.

**Whipple's disease** is a rare disorder characterised by diarrhoea, abdominal pain, malabsorption and arthritis. The pattern of the non-erosive arthritis can resemble the migratory oligo-articular enteropathic arthritis but sometimes it is symmetrical and polyarticular. Joint symptoms, most commonly affecting the knee or ankle, may precede other clinical manifestations by months or years and sacroiliitis and ankylosing spondylitis may occur. The diagnosis is confirmed by demonstrating the presence of PAS positive macrophages in a small intestinal biopsy. Unidentified rod shaped organisms have been detected by electron microscopy in the lamina propria and synovial membrane. Treatment is with prolonged antibiotic therapy, usually tetracycline 1 g daily for one year. Arthralgias and arthritis settle within a month of starting treatment.

## Juvenile Chronic Arthritis

A number of patterns of chronic arthritis commence in childhood before the age of 16 years.

**Systemic Onset Juvenile Chronic Arthritis (Still's disease).** In 20% of children with juvenile chronic arthritis the disease begins with a profound systemic disturbance. Lymphadenopathy, hepatosplenomegaly, pleurisy, pericarditis and a high intermittent fever are associated with myalgias, arthralgias and eventually polyarthritis. Weight loss and retardation of growth may be striking and there is often a characteristic but non-specific evanescent macular rash which tends to appear at times when the temperature is raised. This pattern of disease can occur in children of any age. In addition to a raised ESR and an anaemia of chronic disease, there may be a polymorphonuclear leucocytosis. Tests for rheumatoid factor and antinuclear factor are negative. Remission of systemic symptoms usually occurs within six months of onset but half the children have recurrent systemic attacks and one-quarter go on to develop a severe chronic polyarthritis.

**Polyarticular Juvenile Chronic Arthritis.** In half the children, usually girls, four or more joints are affected. The inflammatory arthritis may begin acutely or insidiously and large joints are most commonly first affected; in some there is more widespread polyarthritis. Inflammatory arthritis in the proximity of growing epiphyses may result in growth acceleration or arrest. Early fusion and growth arrest in the cervical spine and mandible give rise to the short stiff neck and receding chin very characteristic of adults who have had juvenile chronic arthritis. Systemic features are usually mild. Tests for rheumatoid factor are negative but the antinuclear factor is positive in 25% of cases. The overall prognosis is good and only 10–15% have severe destructive arthritis.

**Seropositive polyarticular disease** occurs in 10% of children with juvenile chronic arthritis. Girls are more frequently affected than boys and the onset is usually after the age of 8 years. The disease resembles severe adult onset rheumatoid arthritis with progressive erosive joint changes in more than half of those affected. Extra-articular features include nodules and vasculitis as well as low grade fever and an anaemia of chronic disease. Antinuclear factor tests are positive in 75% but these children do not get iridocyclitis.

**Pauci-articular juvenile chronic arthritis** accounts for the remaining 20% of children affected. Four or less joints are involved and two distinct subsets can be identified:

1. *Young girls* with mono or pauci-articular arthritis affecting knees, ankles, elbows or occasionally a small joint of the hand or foot. There are seldom any constitutional symptoms and the ESR is frequently normal. Positive tests for antinuclear factor appear to be a marker for chronic iridocyclitis which can occur in up to half of this group of children. Regular three monthly slit lamp examinations are required if this complication is to be detected and treated early enough to preserve normal vision.
2. *Older boys* with mono or pauci-articular arthritis affecting hips, knees or ankles. Sacroiliitis is common and there is frequently a family history of uveitis, ankylosing spondylitis or another spondyloarthritis. 75% of these boys are HLA-B27 positive and in many the disease gradually evolves into spondyloarthritis in early adult life.

**Differential diagnosis** of acute arthritis in childhood includes bacterial, viral and reactive arthritis as it does in adults and also rheumatic fever (p. 172) and osteomyelitis (p. 643).

*Henoch Schönlein* (anaphylactoid) purpura is associated with abdominal pain and an acute arthritis affecting one or more joints for a few days at a time. There may be an erythematous or urticarial rash as well as non-thrombocytopenic purpura which may be seen only in areas of pressure such as over the buttocks. The disease frequently follows an upper respiratory infection in the early spring. It is a self limiting form of arthritis which usually lasts for less than three months. Intussusception, rectal bleeding and haematuria are features of more severe cases and a few children have a more chronic or relapsing course with evidence of an immune complex glomerulonephritis. Serum IgA levels are raised in half the cases.

**Treatment.** The principles of management in juvenile chronic arthritis do not differ from those in adult rheumatoid arthritis but special consideration has to be given to maintaining the child's education and helping parents to develop a sensible, vigilant but not overprotective approach to the child's disease. Bedrest may be essential during acute phases but care must be taken to avoid development of flexion deformities of the hips and knees by regular prone lying and appropriate lightweight splints. Whenever possible the child should be kept mobile and ambulant and daily physiotherapy is given throughout to maintain a good range of joint movements and muscle strength. Hydrotherapy in a warm pool is particularly useful. Aspirin is the drug of choice in children who appear to tolerate salicylates better than adults. Naproxen (5mg/kg) is safe and effective in children. Chloroquine, hydroxychloroquine, gold salts and penicillamine can be used provided the same precautions are taken as in the treatment of adult rheumatoid arthritis. Corticosteroids are reserved for children with severe systemic disease, those with chronic iridocyclitis not responding to local therapy and a few cases where very active joint disease does not respond to other measures. Corticotrophin or alternate day corticosteroids are always considered as daily doses of prednisolone as low as 3 mg/day can inhibit growth in children under the age of 5. Older children can be taught to give their own injections of corticotrophin if this has to be continued for any length of time. Corticosteroids do not arrest the progression of disease. Immunosuppressive drugs are used only in children with amyloidosis and persistently active disease. Surgery is usually limited to the rehabilitation of children with deformities. Soft tissue release operations may be helpful in eliminating difficult flexion contractures and osteotomies may be required when joints have been allowed to fuse in poor positions. Total hip arthroplasty can be considered for severely destroyed joints as soon as growth has ceased.

## Infective Arthritis

Septic arthritis can accompany septicaemia throughout life. *H. influenzae* is the common causative organism in infancy; staphylococcal and streptococcal infections are normally responsible in older children and adults. Other organisms which may be implicated are gonococci, pneumococci, meningococci, *Esch. coli*, *Pseudomonas* and *Proteus*. Important predisposing factors include debilitating illnesses, diabetes mellitus, immunodeficiency disorders and immunosuppression. Joint trauma, surgery, penetrating injury and intra-articular injections may lead to bacterial joint infections and may complicate rheumatoid arthritis and other established arthritides.

**Clinical Features.** Characteristically septic arthritis has an abrupt onset with severe pain and swelling of a single joint associated with a swinging fever, severe malaise and a polymorphonuclear leucocytosis. Large joints are most frequently affected and the joint is hot, tender and swollen with an effusion; there is marked limitation of movement. The diagnosis may be missed when more than one joint is involved, in patients with rheumatoid arthritis or when the presentation is less acute in patients receiving corticosteroids or immunosuppressive drugs. It is essential to try to establish the diagnosis early by joint aspiration and blood culture where there is any suspicion of bacterial joint infection. The synovial fluid is typically turbid with a high polymorphonuclear cell count. Organisms may be easily and immediately identified on Gram stain of a film but special culture techniques may be required especially for gonococci and anaerobic organisms. Radiographs show no more than soft tissue swelling initially. Later there may be periarticular osteoporosis, joint space narrowing, periostitis and articular erosions. In more longstanding infections the joint margins have a peculiar 'rubbed out' appearance.

**Treatment.** In all cases where bacterial infection is suspected treatment should be commenced with high parenteral doses of broad spectrum antibiotics as soon as joint aspiration and blood cultures have been completed and until the responsible organism and its sensitivity have been established. Appropriate antibiotics must then be administered for 4–6 weeks. Antibiotics readily cross the inflamed synovial membrane so that there is no need to inject them intra-articularly. The joint should be rested and immobilised with a splint and daily joint aspiration undertaken until no more fluid reaccumulates. If the fluid becomes loculated or too thick for aspiration, surgical drainage is required. The prognosis for recovery without joint damage should be excellent and is directly related to the speed with which antibiotic therapy is instituted.

**Gonococcal Arthritis** is more common in females than males and not infrequently commences at the time of a menstrual period within 2–3 weeks of genital infection. Joint involvement is usually asymmetrical and polyarticular with an acute or subacute, migratory polyarthralgia, or polyarthritis. Tenosynovitis, an 'additive' as opposed to 'flitting' pattern of joint involvement and a macular, vesicular or pustular rash are important diagnostic clues even in the absence of overt genital gonorrhoea. The diagnosis can be established by cultures of synovial fluid, blood, skin lesions or from the genital tract. There is a dramatic response to penicillin, 1 mega unit daily for 3–4 days, but treatment should be continued for two weeks.

**Meningococcal infection** can be associated with (1) an acute transient polyarthritis that is seen simultaneously with the characteristic petechial rash, (2) a purulent monoarthritis which usually occurs after 5 days or (3) a flitting polyarthralgia in patients with chronic meningococcaemia. Penicillin is the treatment of choice.

**Brucellosis** (p. 62) is characteristically associated with polyarthralgia or transient polyarthritis. Much more rarely there may be a destructive, septic arthritis of a large joint or a characteristic spondylitis. Destructive lesions in one or more contiguous vertebrae lead to severe back pain, disc narrowing, marginal proliferation of osteophytes with early bony fusion of vertebrae. Chronic bursitis and osteomyelitis may also occur. The diagnosis is established by blood and synovial fluid cultures coupled with rising titres of agglutinating antibodies. Treatment is given on page 63.

**Tuberculosis of joints** is usually secondary to an established focus in the lungs or kidneys. Since the eradication of bovine tuberculosis in Britain, articular infection is seen mainly in debilitated, malnourished, socially deprived, elderly or immigrant groups. The organism is carried to the synovium or subchondral bone by the blood stream or lymphatic spread. In more than three-quarters of all cases a single large joint is affected. Joint pain, stiffness, swelling and restriction of movements are associated with anorexia, weight loss, night sweats and malaise.

The ESR is usually only moderately raised. In the early stages radiographs show only periarticular osteoporosis and soft tissue swelling. Later there is narrowing of the joint space, bony erosion and collapse of subchondral bone with little associated periosteal reaction. The tuberculin skin test is strongly positive and diagnosis can sometimes be made by joint aspiration and synovial analysis. In other cases synovial biopsy is required. After antibiotic control has been established (p. 259), synovectomy is often undertaken in those with extensive disease.

**Viral infections** are commonly associated with arthralgia and transient polyarthritis, as in some cases of hepatitis B, mumps, chickenpox, infectious mononucleosis, adenoviral and enteroviral infections.

*Arborviral* infections (p. 842) are also frequent causes of arthritis and arthralgia. *Lyme arthritis* is an intermittent pauciarticular inflammatory arthritis which is associated with a characteristic rash (erythema chronicum migrans). It is assumed to be a tick borne viral disease.

*Rubella.* Arthritis follows 1–7 days after the rash or 2–6 weeks after vaccination in 30–40% of adults. A symmetrical inflammatory polyarthritis may be associated with symptoms of carpal tunnel compression or tenosynovitis. Joint pain, stiffness and swelling, which may be severe, usually settle in 1–4 weeks but the condition may grumble on with intermittent arthralgia for some months. Posterior cervical lymphadenopathy and a high lymphocyte count in the synovial fluid may be helpful in diagnosis. The latex test for rheumatoid factor and the ESR are often transiently raised.

## Miscellaneous Disorders of Synovial Joints

*Acromegaly* is associated with a symmetrical arthropathy in 50% of cases. The small joints of the hands, wrists and knees are particularly affected as is the spine. Hypertrophy of synovium and articular cartilage are characteristically associated with periosteal new bone formation, osteophytosis, 'tufting' of the terminal phalanges and premature osteoarthrosis and hypertrophic spondylosis.

*Primary amyloidosis* (p. 436) can be associated with carpal tunnel compression and a polyarthritis superficially resembling rheumatoid arthritis. The synovium is infiltrated with amyloid tissue and the diagnosis can be made by finding fragments of amyloid tissue in the synovial fluid.

*Hyperlipidaemia.* Type II (p. 531) can be associated with a migratory polyarthritis, and widespread xanthomas with tendon deposits. Type IV hyperlipoproteinaemia can be associated with arthralgia and morning stiffness and also hyperuricaemia and gout.

*Sarcoidosis.* Two distinct patterns of inflammatory arthritis may be seen. Erythema nodosum and hilar lymphadenopathy are frequently associated with a symmetrical non-destructive inflammatory arthritis especially affecting the knees, ankles and wrists. A more specific asymmetrical destructive arthritis affects similar joints especially in Negroes. Biopsy of the synovium in such cases shows evidence of non-caseating granulomata. Radiologically there may be 'punched out' cystic bone lesions and also 'cortical erosions' and joint destruction.

## Systemic Lupus Erythematosus (SLE)

This is a multisystem connective tissue disorder characterised by the presence of numerous autoantibodies, circulating immune complexes and widespread immunologically determined tissue damage.

**Epidemiology.** SLE affects individuals throughout the world but occurs more frequently in the United States and the Far East. American blacks are particularly susceptible, with a prevalence as high as 1 in 250 among Negresses. The increasing use of sensitive tests for antinuclear antibodies suggest that mild and incomplete cases are much more frequent than previously thought. The onset is most commonly in the 2nd and 3rd decades, with a female/male ratio of 9:1. In children and the elderly the sex incidence is more equal.

**Aetiology and Pathogenesis.** Although the cause of SLE remains obscure, current concepts suggest that this is a multifactorial disorder in which there is profound disturbance of immune regulation. A defect of suppressor T lymphocytes is associated with polyclonal B lymphocyte activation and the uncontrolled production of a variety of autoantibodies and immune complexes (Table 13.2). To what extent the cellular defect is primary or secondary to the production of lymphocytotoxic antibodies is uncertain. Evidence for *genetic factors* in the aetiology of the disease includes: (1) Its occurrence in monozygotic twin pairs; (2) A higher than expected prevalence of SLE, other connective tissue diseases, antinuclear antibodies and immune complexes in related family members; (3) Inherited deficiency of isolated complement components, notably C2 in some patients; (4) Increased prevalence of the histocompatibility antigens HLA-B8 and DR3.

Evidence for the influence of *environmental factors* includes: (1) The provocative effect of sunlight in many cases; (2) The induction of lupus erythematosus by many drugs; (3) The importance of oestrogens as determinants of disease expression. Exacerbations commonly occur in pregnancy and the puerperium and prevalence is increased in fertile women, those taking oral contraceptives and men with Klinefelter's syndrome.

In animal models of SLE there is clear evidencé of *viral infection* but in humans the findings are inconclusive.

*Immunologically mediated tissue damage* results from at least two different mechanisms in SLE: 1. Direct antibody (and complement) mediated cytotoxicity (Type II reactions). Brain damage and abortion may be a consequence of direct antibody mediated cytotoxicity by cold reactive lymphocytotoxic antibodies which cross react with renal and trophoblast tissues.

2. Immune complex (and complement) mediated (Type III reactions). The renal and vascular lesions of SLE appear to be a consequence of deposition of circulating DNA — Anti DNA and other complexes in tissues.

**Clinical Features**. *Arthritis,* arthralgia and fever are the commonest presenting features, frequently accompanied by tiredness, anaemia, and malaise. There may be a previous history of migraine, depression or other psychiatric disturbance. Unlike other types of inflammatory arthritis, symptoms may begin during pregnancy and there may be a past history of spontaneous abortions. The arthritis can be transient and migratory or a more persistant seronegative polyarthritis. Chronic inflammatory arthritis and tenosynovitis may lead to deformities and contractures but erosive changes are very uncommon.

Table 13.2 Immunological abnormalities detectable in blood of patients with systemic lupus erythematosus

| | |
|---|---|
| Anti-nuclear Antibodies | Antibodies against erythrocytes, leucocytes and platelets |
| Anti-DNA-histone (and LE cells) | Circulating anticoagulants |
| Anti-DNA (single strand) | Anti-thyroid (and other organ specific autoantibodies) |
| Anti-DNA (double strand) | Rheumatoid factors |
| Anti-RNA | Biological false positive tests for syphilis |
| Anti-SM | Cryoglobulins |
| Anti-RNP | Circulating immune complexes |
| Anticytoplasmic Antibodies (Ro and La) | Depression of $CH_{50}$ and C3 and C4 |
| Lymphocytotoxins | |

*Skin lesions* are seen in more than two-thirds of cases. In addition to the classical, photosensitive erythematous 'butterfly' rash across the face, there may be lesions of discoid lupus, a less specific maculopapular eruption or a vasculitic rash. The last may present as purpura or periungual erythema with 'chilblain-like' lesions or digital infarcts. Livedo reticularis and Raynaud's phenomenon are common while bullous eruptions and panniculitis ('lupus profundus') occur more rarely. Alopecia can be a useful diagnostic pointer and is seen in more than 50% of cases. Painful oral or nasopharyngeal ulcers are rather less common.

*Cardiopulmonary features* include pericarditis, pleurisy, fibrosing alveolitis and acute lupus pneumonitis as well as a 'shrinking lung syndrome' with progressive elevation of the diaphragms and linear scars from recurrent pulmonary infarction. Lung function tests reveal impairment of ventilation and diffusion in these and many patients without overt clinical or radiological evidence of pulmonary involvement. Verrucous (Libman – Sachs) endocarditis is a common finding at autopsy but is rarely diagnosed during life.

*Renal involvement* occurs in half the patients and carries the worst prognosis. It may result in the nephrotic syndrome and acute or chronic renal failure. It may be limited to insignificant proteinuria or the presence of red cells or casts. Renal biopsy is a guide to therapy and prognosis. Subendothelial dense deposits on electron microscopy and 'lumpy - bumpy' basement membrane deposits of C3 and IgG on immunofluorescence are early signs of significant immune complex disease. A diffuse proliferative glomerulonephritis on light microscopy is often associated with a bad prognosis and is an indication for vigorous treatment with corticosteroids and/or immunosuppressive drugs. Membranous glomerulonephritis may be associated with a prolonged nephrotic syndrome but the eventual outlook is usually good. Focal proliferative changes and mesangial or 'minimal change' glomerulonephritis are seldom associated with progressive renal disease.

*Central nervous system* involvement is seen in up to half the patients. In the majority this is limited to mild psychiatric disturbance, migraine or epilepsy but in a few there may be severe depression, dementia, organic psychosis, cranial nerve lesions, hemiplegia, transverse myelitis, chorea, cerebellar ataxia or peripheral neuropathy. The more severe manifestations are associated with a poor prognosis.

*Other manifestations*. Gastrointestinal symptoms are frequent but non-specific. Abdominal pain can be due to peritonitis, perisplenitis, pancreatitis or vasculitis. Gastric or duodenal perforation may be complications of corticosteroid therapy; colonic or gall bladder perforations are more likely to be a consequence of necrotising arteritis. Lymphadenopathy is found in half the patients and a moderately enlarged spleen in 20–30%. Ocular findings include kerato-conjunctivitis sicca, episcleritis and retinal vasculitis and hard exudates.

**Investigation**. The ESR is usually raised in active disease but the C reactive protein rarely so in the absence of infection. Haematological findings may include a normocytic normochromic anaemia of chronic disease, a Coombs positive haemolytic anaemia, leucopenia, thrombocytopenia or evidence of a circulating anticoagulant.

*Antinuclear antibodies* can be detected in the serum of more than 90% of patients but positive tests for ANF are often found in rheumatoid arthritis, juvenile chronic arthritis, Sjögren's syndrome, fibrosing alveolitis and progressive systemic sclerosis. Chronic liver disease, thyroiditis, Addison's disease, myasthenia gravis, leukaemia and other connective tissue diseases can all be associated with a positive ANF as can therapy with a variety of drugs. Positive tests in low titre have no clinical significance and are frequently found in normal elderly persons. *The LE cell test* is less sensitive, very time consuming and hardly more specific.

Antibodies to undenatured double stranded DNA have much greater specificity but are present in the serum in significant amounts in only about half the patients at any one time. High levels of anti-DNA antibodies coupled with depressed total haemolytic complement ($CH_{50}$) activity and low C3 and C4 complement components suggest that there is activation of the classical complement pathway by active immune complex disease (Fig. 2.4). Further evidence for circulating immune complexes may be obtained by finding a cryoprecipitate or by using one of a number of tests for CIq binding. Tissue evidence for immune complex deposition comes from detection of complement components and immunoglobulins by immunofluorescence at the dermoepidermal junction of normal skin or in organ biopsies.

**Treatment**. Acute and life threatening manifestations of SLE require systemic corticosteroid therapy, often initially in doses of 40–60 mg prednisolone or equivalent daily. With remission of disease careful attempts are made to withdraw steroids or maintain patients on very low doses or alternate day regimes of steroid therapy. Articular symptoms and less severe inflammatory manifestations should be managed with NSAID therapy wherever possible. Anti-malarials are particularly useful in the management of patients with troublesome skin and joint lesions and they can reduce the frequency of severe exacerbations of disease.

Immunosuppressive drugs are reserved for patients with severe diffuse proliferative glomerulonephritis who are not responding adequately to corticosteroids and for those requiring maintenance steroid doses so high as to cause severe side-effects. The combination of plasma exchange and immunosuppressive drug therapy may be useful in some patients with serious steroid resistant exacerbations.

**Prognosis** for life appears to have improved dramatically in SLE over the last 30 years so that overall 5 year survival should now be better than 90% with careful monitoring and the judicious use of corticosteroid and immunosuppressive drugs. Much of this apparent improvement in prognosis is, however, attributable to the detection of milder cases as a result of heightened clinical awareness and the availability of the sensitive ANF test for diagnostic purposes. Patients with severe renal, neurological and pulmonary involvement remain those at greatest risk but infection is an important cause of morbidity and mortality particularly in patients receiving high doses of corticosteroids and immunosuppressives. Pregnancy is not contra-indicated provided the disease is in reasonable remission and renal, cardiac and cerebral functions are intact.

**Chronic discoid lupus erythematosus** is probably more common than SLE. The skin lesions are characterised by photosensitivity, erythema, scaling, follicular plugging and telangiectasia. In the majority of patients the disease is limited to the skin. ANF tests are positive but anti-DNA antibodies are not usually found and complement levels are normal. SLE may occasionally supervene.

**Drug Induced Lupus**. Positive tests for antinuclear factor are frequently encountered in patients receiving procainamide, hydrallazine, anticonvulsants, oral contraceptives and phenothiazines. Much more rarely a syndrome resembling SLE develops. Fever, polyarthritis, skin lesions, lymphadenopathy, serositis and pulmonary infiltrates are frequent, but renal disease and neurological manifestations are rare. Complement levels are usually normal and antibodies to double stranded DNA absent.

Slow acetylators of hydrallazine and those with the HLA-DR3 histocompatibility antigen appear to be particularly at risk. Remission usually follows drug withdrawal. Occasionally a short course of corticosteroids is required.

**Mixed connective tissue disease** (MCTD) is characterised by clinical features resembling systemic lupus erythematosus, progressive systemic sclerosis (see below) and polymyositis (p. 633) in association with very high titres of a circulating antinuclear antibody with specificity for a ribonuclease sensitive extractable nuclear antigen (ENA) identified as a nuclear ribonucleoprotein (RNP). Women are affected four times more commonly than men. The onset is usually in the 3rd or 4th decade but may be at any age. Raynaud's phenomenon with 'sausage' swelling of the fingers, skin changes resembling dermatomyositis or scleroderma and a mild inflammatory polyarthritis are typically associated with proximal muscle weakness and tenderness, abnormal oesophageal motility and minor systemic disturbance. Diffuse interstitial pulmonary fibrosis is not uncommon but cardiac, renal and central nervous system involvement are very rare. There may be a mild anaemia of chronic disease, leucopenia or thrombocytopenia. The ESR and muscle enzymes are usually moderately raised. The condition is further characterised by an excellent prognosis and a good response to low dosage steroid therapy.

## Progressive Systemic Sclerosis

This is a generalised disorder of connective tissue characterised by fibrosis and degenerative changes in the skin and many internal organs. Although its aetiology is unknown, it is believed to be at one end of the spectrum of diffuse connective tissue diseases where immunologically determined inflammation is followed by intimal thickening of small blood vessels and excessive production and cross-linking of collagen. It is less common than SLE but is seen throughout the world. Its prevalence appears to be increased among miners and others occupationally exposed to silica dust, but in general women are affected four times more frequently than men.

**Clinical Features**. The onset is most frequently in the 30–50 year age group although persons of all ages may be affected. Severe, classical Raynaud's phenomenon is usually the presenting complaint and may precede other features by months or years.

*Skin Changes*. Initially there is often well demarcated non-pitting oedema and induration associated with 'sausage' swelling and restriction of movement of the fingers. Later the skin becomes shiny with loss of cutaneous appendages, atrophy and ulceration of the finger tips with or without associated calcinosis. The skin of the face, limbs and trunk is variably affected and there may be striking pigmentation and telangiectasia. As the disease advances, the face may become taut and 'mask-like' with 'beaking' of the nose and difficulty in opening the mouth. Tightening of skin over bony prominences results in flexion contractures and liability to trauma.

*Musculo-skeletal* manifestations include early arthralgia and a mild non-erosive inflammatory arthritis often characterised by 'leathery' crepitus in affected tendon sheaths or joints. Muscle weakness and wasting result from both disuse atrophy and low grade myositis.

*The gastrointestinal tract* is involved in the majority of cases. Reflux oesophagitis associated with a sliding hiatus hernia is a common problem and loss of oesophageal peristalsis on recumbent barium swallow examination is often detected even in the absence of dysphagia. Dilatation of segments of large and small bowel occur less frequently, causing intermittent abdominal pain, constipation, distention and obstruction; there may be diarrhoea and malabsorption secondary to bacterial overgrowth. Scleroderma may be associated with primary biliary cirrhosis and with Sjögren's syndrome.

*Pulmonary fibrosis* occurs in the majority of patients. In many it is limited to a symptomless defect in gaseous diffusion. In others progressive fibrosis is accompanied by increasing dyspnoea on exertion, a restrictive pattern of impaired lung function and reticulation and 'honeycomb' changes in the lower zones on a chest radiograph. Pulmonary involvement can be complicated by pulmonary hypertension and right ventricular failure, or by alveolar cell or bronchiolar carcinoma. Aspiration pneumonia may be a consequence of oesophageal involvement.

*Other manifestations*. Cardiac involvement is usually secondary to systemic rather than pulmonary hypertension but pericarditis, cardiomyopathy, heart block and aortic valve lesions can also occur. Renal involvement may develop at any stage of the disease and is an important cause of morbidity and mortality. Characteristically it is associated with a clinical picture indistinguishable from malignant hypertension. Cranial or peripheral nerve lesions occur rarely.

**Investigation**. In the early stages there may be a mild normochromic, normocytic anaemia and moderately raised ESR. The ANF is positive in about 50% of patients with a nucleolar or speckled staining pattern. Antibodies to single stranded RNA with uracil specificity are characteristic. Anti-DNA antibodies are not detected and complement levels are normal. Tests for rheumatoid factor and anti-nRNP antibodies may be positive but usually in low titre.

**Differential Diagnosis and Related Syndromes.** *The CRST or CREST syndrome* comprises a subset of patients whose disease is limited to calcinosis, Raynaud's phenomenon, oesophageal (esophageal) involvement, sclerodactyly and telangiectasia. An antinuclear antibody with specificity for a component of the chromosomal centromere is present in the serum.

*Morphoea and linear scleroderma* are localised forms of disease limited to characteristic, well demarcated lesions of the skin and subcutaneous connective tissues. Serological findings are similar to those of systemic sclerosis and very occasionally systemic features do occur.

*Eosinophilic fasciitis* is a scleroderma-like condition characterised by pain, swelling and tenderness of the hands, forearms and feet where induration of the skin and subcutaneous tissues is not associated with Raynaud's phenomenon or systemic sclerosis. Carpal tunnel compression may be an early feature and the onset frequently follows abnormal exercise. Eosinophilia and hyperglobulinaemia are characteristic and the diagnosis is confirmed by finding an inflammatory cell infiltrate with prominent eosinophils in association with marked fibrosis of the subcutaneous fascia. Eosinophilic fasciitis responds to corticosteroids but is usually self-limiting.

*Pseudoscleroderma*. Other conditions which may give rise to induration or brawny oedema of the skin that must be considered in the differential diagnosis of scleroderma are scleredema, scleromyxoedema, amyloidosis, acromegaly, carcinoid syndrome, phenylketonuria and porphyria.

**Treatment**. No form of drug therapy has been proved to be effective in arresting the course of systemic sclerosis. Corticosteroids may produce some symptomatic benefit in early cases where inflammatory oedema or associated myositis and/or arthritis are prominent features but great care must be taken not to aggravate or precipitate hypertension. Penicillamine and colchicine have been shown to inhibit collagen cross-linking and procollagen to collagen conversion respectively, but are disappointingly ineffective in the management of the disease. Attention should be paid to protecting the limbs from cold, the urgent treatment of chest infections and hypertension and therapy for oesophagitis, dysphagia, cardiac, respiratory and renal failure. Articular symptoms should be managed with NSAID. Episodes of steatorrhoea often respond to a short course of a broad spectrum antibiotic.

The outlook appears to be worse in those with late onset disease, widespread skin involvement of the trunk and early renal, cardiac or respiratory system disease. The overall 5 year survival is about 70%.

## Polymyositis and Dermatomyositis

These are diffuse connective tissue disorders in which muscle weakness and inflammatory changes in muscle and skin are the predominant features. They are relatively rare but occur throughout the world in all races and at all ages.

**Clinical Features.** It is possible to define the following 4 rather arbitrary subsets: *Adult Polymyositis* (Type I) occurs three times more frequently in women than men. The onset is usually insidious in the 3rd to 5th decade. The patient may experience difficulty in climbing stairs or rising from a low chair and on examination there is weakness of the pelvic and shoulder girdle muscles. Sometimes the onset is more abrupt with rapid progression of muscular weakness. Involvement of pharyngeal, laryngeal and respiratory muscles can lead to dysphagia, dysphonia and respiratory failure within a few days. In the majority of cases progression is less rapid and profound. Spontaneous remissions are followed by some return of muscle strength but there may be atrophy, calcinosis and fibrosis in damaged muscles leading to flexion contractures. Muscle pain and tenderness are unusual except in very acute cases. Mild arthralgia or inflammatory arthritis, Raynaud's phenomenon and atypical erythematous rashes on the elbows and knuckles are frequent associated features.

*Adult Dermatomyositis* (Type II) is also more common in women. Acute or subacute muscle weakness is accompanied by periorbital oedema and a characteristic purple 'heliotrope' rash on the upper eyelids. In addition, there may be a photosensitive, erythematous, scaling rash on the face, shoulders, upper arms and chest with red patches over knuckles, elbows and knees. Muscle pain, tenderness, weight loss and malaise are common as are arthralgia and mild inflammatory polyarthritis.

*Inflammatory Myositis associated with Malignancy (Type III)* is less common than was previously thought. It is seen only after the age of 40 and occurs more frequently in men than women. The onset of symptoms is usually insidious and the clinical picture does not differ from that of typical polymyositis or dermatomyositis. The associated neoplasm, which is usually a carcinoma of the bronchus, prostate, ovary, uterus, breast or colon, may not become apparent for 2–3 years. Resection of the neoplasm is sometimes associated with remission of the myositis.

*Childhood Dermatomyositis* (Type IV) most commonly affects children between the ages of 4 and 10. Muscle weakness is usually accompanied by the typical rash of dermatomyositis. Muscle atrophy, contractures and subcutaneous calcification may be widespread and severe. Recurrent abdominal pain due to vasculitis is also a feature.

**Investigation.** Active disease is often associated with a normochromic normocytic anaemia, a polymorphonuclear leucocytosis and a raised ESR. Serum transaminases, aldolase and creatine phosphokinase are usually raised and can be useful guides to the activity of the disease. Tests for rheumatoid factor and ANF are often positive and there may be antibodies to an extractable nuclear antigen (PM-I). Electromyography may show characteristic changes which can be very helpful in distinguishing polymyositis from other types of primary muscle disease. Muscle biopsy shows necrosis and regeneration in association with an inflammatory cell infiltrate.

**Treatment.** Prednisolone in doses of 40–60 mg daily is used initially to induce a remission. Muscle enzyme levels may fall before clinical improvement is noted. The steroid dose is then gradually reduced whilst continuing to monitor muscle strength and serum enzyme levels. Doses of 10–15 mg prednisolone daily are often needed to maintain the remission. Immunosuppressive therapy is occasionally used when there is no response to corticosteroids. The use of splints and physiotherapy to prevent contractures should not be neglected.

Prognosis is closely related to the age of onset and the presence or absence of associated malignancy. The four year survival is 80% when the disease begins before the age of 20; 60% for those under the age of 40 and 33% for older patients.

## Arteritis

Vasculitis which occurs as part of rheumatoid arthritis, systemic lupus erythematosus, progressive systemic sclerosis and childhood dermatomyositis has been described in the relevant sections.

Polyarteritis nodosa (p. 214), Takayasu's arteritis (p. 215) and cranial arteritis (p. 215) are diffuse connective tissue disorders in which immunologically determined vasculitis is the cause of the pathology. Polymyalgia rheumatica is related to cranial arteritis.

### Polymyalgia Rheumatica

This is a relatively common condition in elderly Caucasians, especially women. Pain and stiffness in the shoulder and pelvic girdles of at least one month's duration, are characteristically associated with a raised ESR and a dramatic response to low dosage corticosteroids.

**Clinical Features.** The onset is often abrupt with severe pain and stiffness in the neck, back, shoulders, upper arms and thighs, often worse in the morning. There may also be fever, weight loss, malaise and depression. Physical signs are usually limited to slight tenderness. Occasionally there may be evidence of a mild inflammatory arthritis in a more peripheral joint. The muscles themselves usually show no evidence of tenderness or atrophy and examination of the peripheral arteries is usually normal. However, up to one-third of patients at some time develop symptoms of cranial arteritis (p. 215) and are at risk of blindness from arteritic involvement of a branch of the ophthalmic artery.

The ESR is markedly raised in the majority of cases and there may be a mild normochromic normocytic anaemia of chronic disease. Temporal artery biopsy shows evidence of giant cell arteritis in about 40% of cases but the true frequency of arteritis is probably much higher.

**Treatment.** The response to low dosage corticosteroid therapy is dramatic. The diagnosis must be reviewed if there is no striking remission of symptoms within 4–5 days of starting prednisolone 15 mg once daily. The ESR frequently takes longer to fall. Two to three weeks after starting therapy the dose of prednisolone is gradually reduced over several weeks. Most patients can be maintained in remission with 5–7·5 mg prednisolone daily. High dosage corticosteroids (prednisolone 40–60 mg/day) are reserved for patients with clinical features of cranial arteritis.

The natural history is for remission to occur in 6 months to 2 years although relapses are not uncommon and occasional patients have a more prolonged chronic disease. The need for maintenance corticosteroids should be reviewed by an attempt at gradual steroid withdrawal every six months.

## Crystal Deposition Diseases

### Gout

Gout is not a single disease. The term is used to describe a number of disorders in which crystals of monosodium urate monohydrate derived from hyperuricaemic body fluids give rise to inflammatory arthritis, tenosynovitis, bursitis or cellulitis, tophaceous deposits, urolithiasis and renal disease.

Hyperuricaemia is a necessary but not a sufficient prerequisite for clinical manifestations of gout.

**Epidemiology.** Gouty arthritis is predominantly a problem of post pubertal males and is seldom seen in women before the menopause. Its overall prevalence in Britain is about 0·6%. Asymptomatic hyperuricaemia is ten times more common. Serum uric acid concentrations are distributed in the community as a continuous variable and are determined by a number of demographic factors of which age, sex, body bulk and genetic constitution are the most important. Serum uric acid levels are higher in urban than in rural communities and are positively correlated with intelligence, social class, weight, haemoglobin, serum proteins and a high protein diet. Hyperuricaemia is arbitrarily defined as a serum uric acid level greater than two standard deviations from the mean i.e. above 0·42 mmol/litre in adult males and 0·36 mmol/litre in adult females (p. 907).

**Aetiology of Gout and Hyperuricaemia.** A number of genetic and environmental factors lead to hyperuricaemia and gout by decreasing the excretion of uric acid, increasing its production or by a combination of both mechanisms (Table 13.3).

IMPAIRED EXCRETION OF URIC ACID is the problem in more than 75% of patients with gout. In most of these there appears to be an as yet undefined genetically determined defect in fractional urate excretion.

EXCESSIVE PRODUCTION OF URIC ACID is at least partly responsible for hyperuricaemia in 20–25% of gout patients. In the absence of significant renal impairment such patients are hyperexcretors of uric acid.

SPECIFIC ENZYME DEFECTS resulting in an increase in *de novo* purine synthesis should be suspected: (1) In the absence of disorders resulting in increased turnover of purines (Table 13.3); (2) If gout develops at an unusually early age; (3) If there is a family

Table 13.3 Factors predisposing to hyperuricaemia and gout

| Diminished renal excretion of uric acid | | Increased production of uric acid |
|---|---|---|
| Renal failure | | *Increased turnover of purines:* |
| Drugs: | Lactic Acidaemia: | Myeloproliferative disorders e.g. polycythaemia vera |
| Diuretics | Alcohol | |
| Pyrazinamide | Excercise | Lymphoproliferative disorders e.g. chronic lymphatic leukaemia |
| Low doses aspirin | Starvation | Psoriasis–severe, exfoliative |
| Lead poisoning | Vomiting | *Increased purine synthesis de novo*: |
| Hypertension | Toxaemia of pregnancy | HGPRT deficiency |
| Hyperparathyroidism | Type 1 Glycogen Storage Disease | Glucose-6-Phosphatase deficiency |
| Myxoedema | | PRPP synthetase overactivity |
| Down's syndrome | | Idiopathic |

history of gout commencing at an early age; (4) If uric acid lithiasis is the first presenting feature.

*Deficiency of hypoxanthine-guanine-phosphoribosyl transferase* (HGPRT). The Lesch-Nyhan Syndrome is a rare X-chromosome linked inborn error of metabolism in which gout and severe overproduction of uric acid are associated with choreoathetosis, spasticity, a variable degree of mental deficiency and compulsive self-mutilation. The enzyme defect can be detected in red cell lysates; female carriers can be identified from skin fibroblast cultures or hair root analysis and prenatal detection can be undertaken using amniotic fluid cells. The elucidation of the mechanism whereby this deficit in purine salvage enzyme leads to primary purine overproduction has been a key to the understanding of purine metabolism and the development of allopurinol in the prevention of gout.

*Phosphoribosyl pyrophosphate (PRPP) sythetase overactivity.* Severe gouty arthritis and uric acid lithiasis is seen from an early age in families with inborn errors of metabolism resulting in increased activity of this enzyme. The defect can be detected in red cell lysates.

*Glucose-6-phosphatase deficiency.* Children with glycogen storage disease type 1 (von Gierke's disease) who survive to adult life develop severe gout and hyperuricaemia as a consequence of impaired uric acid excretion secondary to lactic acidosis and increased purine synthesis *de novo*. The enzyme defect can be detected only in liver, kidney or intestinal mucosa.

*Idiopathic.* The enzyme defect(s) responsible for most cases of gout with increased synthesis of purines *de novo* remain to be discovered.

**Clinical Features.** *Acute gout.* The metatarsophalangeal joint of a great toe is the site of the first attack of acute gouty arthritis in 70% of patients; the ankle, the knee, the small joints of the feet and hands, the wrist and elbow following in decreasing order of frequency. The onset may be insidious or explosively sudden, often waking the patient from sleep. The affected joint is hot, red and swollen with shiny overlying skin and dilated veins; it is excruciatingly painful and tender. Very acute attacks may be accompanied by fever, leucocytosis and a raised ESR and are occasionally preceded by prodromal symptoms such as anorexia, nausea or a change in mood. If untreated, the attack lasts days or weeks but it eventually subsides spontaneously. Resolution of the acute attack may be accompanied by pruritus and local desquamation. Some patients have only a single attack, or suffer another only after an interval of many months or years. More often there is a tendency to have recurrent attacks. These increase in frequency and duration so that eventually one attack may merge into another and the patient remains in a prolonged state of subacute gout. Acute attacks are occasionally polyarticular and tenosynovitis, bursitis or cellulitis may be the presenting feature.

Acute attacks may be precipitated by sudden rises in serum urate following dietary excess, alcohol, severe dietary restriction or diuretic drugs or by sudden falls following initiation of therapy with allopurinol or uricosuric drugs. Acute attacks may also be provoked by trauma, unusual physical excercise, surgery or severe systemic illness.

*Chronic gout.* First attacks of gouty arthritis are seldom associated with residual disability but recurrent acute attacks are followed by progressive cartilage and bone erosion in association with deposition of tophi and secondary degenerative changes. Severe functional impairment and gross joint deformities may be associated with chronic tophaceous gout. Tophi are frequently found in the cartilage of the ear, bursae and tendon sheaths. Rarely they may give rise to compression of the median nerve in the carpal tunnel, paraplegia or heart block.

*Urate urolithiasis* occurs in about 10% of patients with gout attending British hospital clinics. The incidence is much higher in hot climates. The formation of urate calculi is also favoured by (1) hyperuricosuria; (2) purine over production; (3) excessive purine ingestion; (4) uricosuric drugs and defects in tubular reabsorption of uric acid and (5) low urine pH e.g. chronic diarrhoeal diseases or following ileostomy.

*Chronic urate nephropathy* results from a combination of renal tubular obstruction, tophus formation, hypertension, glomerulosclerosis and secondary pyelonephritis. It is rare and hardly ever occurs in the absence of well-established chronic gouty arthritis. It may occasionally be familial (autosomal dominant) without evidence of an inborn error of metabolism.

Minimal renal insufficiency is found in up to 50% of patients with gout but is largely age related. Proteinuria is found in 25% and is mild and non-progressive. Renal failure accounts for 25% of deaths in patients with gout. Most are, however, from unrelated causes and overall life expectancy is not reduced.

*Other manifestations.* Gout and hyperuricaemia are frequently associated with obesity, type IV hyperlipoproteinaemia, impaired glucose tolerance, hypertension and ischaemic heart disease. Hyperuricaemia itself does not, however, appear to be a risk factor for vascular disease or diabetes mellitus.

**Investigation.** The serum urate level is usually raised but it is important to realise that this does not prove the diagnosis as asymptomatic hyperuricaemia is very common. Whenever possible synovial fluid should be aspirated and examined under polarising light. Acute attacks of gout can occur when the serum urate level is normal. This is usually seen in patients who have received treatment with allopurinol, a uricosuric agent or NSAID with uricosuric side effects such as phenylbutazone. Joint radiographs are seldom useful in establishing the diagnosis. Although they may show characteristic punched-out erosions associated with the translucent soft tissue swelling of urate tophi, occasionally flecked with calcium, the diagnosis will be clinically apparent in such cases and in others the erosions are indistinguishable from those seen in other forms of inflammatory arthritis.

**Treatment.** *Acute attack.* NSAID are the agents of choice. It is important to start treatment as early as possible, to use adequate doses and to avoid salicylates and diuretics. Patients known to have gout should keep a supply of NSAID with which they are familiar so that an acute attack can be aborted as soon as the first symptoms are noticed. Indomethacin (50mg), phenylbutazone (200mg), azapropazone (600mg) 6 hourly or naproxen 250 mg t.i.d. are given until the acute attack subsides. Treatment is then continued with lower doses for 7–10 days. Colchicine is highly effective but causes vomiting and diarrhoea in many patients in the doses that need to be used (1mg stat followed by 0·5mg 2 hourly).

**Prevention.** Prolonged administration of drugs which lower the serum urate level should be considered following the resolution of the acute attack in patients with: (1) recurrent acute attacks of gouty arthritis; (2) tophi or evidence of chronic gouty arthritis; (3) associated renal disease; (4) gout and markedly raised serum urate.

*Allopurinol* is the drug of choice for long-term prophylaxis because of its convenience and low incidence of side-effects. It lowers serum urate primarily by inhibiting xanthine oxidase which is responsible for the conversion of xanthine and hypoxanthine to uric acid. Treatment is commenced with 300 mg once daily together with colchicine 0·5 mg b.d. to avert the acute attacks of gouty arthritis which frequently follow initiation of hypouricaemic drug therapy. It is important not to commence treatment with allopurinol until several weeks have elapsed after the last acute attack and to continue concurrent administration of colchicine for several months. The dose of allupurinol may have to be adjusted in the range of 300–900 mg daily to bring the serum urate within the normal range.

*Uricosuric agents* can also be very effective in lowering the serum urate level, reducing the frequency of acute attacks of gout and decreasing the size of tophi. Probenecid 0·5–1 g b.d. or sulphinpyrazone 100 mg t.d.s. are given with colchicine 0·5 mg b.d. Salicylates must be avoided as they antagonise the uricosuric effects of these drugs. Uricosuric drug therapy is contraindicated: (1) in gout with over production of uric acid and gross uricosuria; (2) in patients with renal failure (ineffective); (3) in patients with urate urolithiasis.

*Diet.* There is no need for severe dietary restrictions but grossly excessive purine intake and alcohol excess should be avoided. Gradual weight loss is encouraged in obese patients and is associated with a fall in serum urate. Severe calorie restriction must be avoided as it causes lactic acidosis and a rise in serum urate.

*Surgery* is occasionally required to deal with large or ulcerating tophi.

*Asymptomatic hyperuricaemia* does not require prophylactic treatment in the absence of a history, family history or clinical evidence of gout. A search should be made for causes of secondary hyperuricaemia (Table 13.3). Obese subjects should be encouraged to lose weight gradually and blood pressure and renal function should be monitored annually.

## Chondrocalcinosis and Pseudogout

### *Pyrophosphate arthropathy: Calcium pyrophosphate dihydrate deposition (CPPD)*

In this variety of crystal deposition disorder, pyrophosphate crystals are deposited in fibrous and articular cartilage where they are associated with degenerative changes. Shedding of crystals into the joint space provokes an acute attack of synovitis — 'pseudogout'. Autopsy and radiological surveys indicate that chondrocalcinosis is a common age related finding often unassociated with symptoms of articular disease. The menisci and articular cartilage of the knee are the commonest sites.

**Aetiology.** Chondrocalcinosis and pseudogout are clearly not a single disease. The majority of cases are sporadic and no underlying cause can be found. Genetic factors are important in some families. A variety of metabolic disorders clearly predispose to chondrocalcinosis, namely hyperparathyroidism, haemochromatosis, hypothyroidism, gout, hypomagnesaemia and hypophosphatasia. No common determinant, comparable to the hyperuricaemia of gout has been identified but pyrophosphate concentrations are increased in synovial fluids. This, coupled with the association with hypophosphatasia, has suggested that the disease may be a consequence of defective pyrophosphatase activity.

**Clinical Features.** Pyrophosphate arthropathy can mimic many other conditions. Six clinical patterns of disease are described. Type A: Pseudogout. As with gout the affected joint becomes suddenly painful, warm, swollen and tender. The knee is the site of more than half of all attacks, the duration of which can vary from a few days to four weeks. Subacute or 'petite' attacks are not uncommon and there may be polyarticular clustering of acute attacks. Men are affected more frequently than women. Type B: Pseudo rheumatoid arthritis. In a few patients there is a subacute inflammatory polyarthritis which may last for several months. Type C: Pseudo osteoarthritis with superimposed acute attacks. Type D: Pseudo osteoarthritis without acute attacks. Types C and D account for nearly half the patients. Women are more frequently affected. Prominent involvement of the wrists and MCP joints clearly distinguishes pseudo osteoarthritic chondrocalcinosis from primary generalised osteoarthrosis. Type E: Lanthanic (asymptomatic) is the most common pattern. Type F: Pseudo neuropathic. Severe destructive changes resembling those of Charcot joints can occur in the knee and shoulder in the absence of any neurological defect.

**Investigation.** Acute attacks may be accompanied by fever, mild leucocytosis and a raised ESR. Radiographs show CPPD in articular cartilage, the menisci of the knees, the labrum of the acetabulum and glenoid cavity, the triangular cartilage of the wrist and the symphysis pubis. Examination of synovial fluid under polarising light microscopy allows CPPD crystals, which are positively birefringent, to be distinguished from monosodium urate crystals. X-ray diffraction techniques are however required for its precise identification and distinction from other forms of calcium phosphate and calcium hydroxyapatite which have been described in the synovial fluids of patients with degenerative joint disease.

**Treatment.** Joint aspiration and intra-articular injection of corticosteroids are the most effective means for treating acute attacks of pseudogout. Colchicine and NSAID are less effective than in classical gout.

## Osteoarthrosis

Osteoarthrosis (OA) is not a single disease. Rather it is the end result of a variety of patterns of joint failure. To a greater or lesser extent it is always characterised by both degeneration of articular cartilage and simultaneous proliferation of new bone, cartilage and connective tissue. The proliferative response results in some degree of remodelling of the joint contour.

**Epidemiology.** Radiological and autopsy surveys show a steady rise in degenerative changes in joints from the age of 30. By the age of 65, 80% of people have radiographic evidence of osteoarthrosis although only 25% may have symptoms. Males and females are both affected but OA is more generalised and more severe in older women. Geographical surveys show differences in both the prevalence of OA and the pattern of joint involvement. OA of the hips is much more frequent in Caucasians than in Negroes or Chinese. It is particularly common in men in the north of England. Cold, damp climates are associated with more symptoms but not with greater radiological prevalence.

**Aetiology and Pathogenesis.** OA is classified as primary if the aetiology is unknown and secondary when degenerative joint changes occur in response to a recognisable local or systemic factor (Table 13.4). Developmental abnormalities are currently believed to be of major importance in the aetiology of OA of the hip in the vast majority of cases. Abnormal surface contacts and weight bearing alignments are thought to arise from minor degrees of acetabular dysplasia, epiphysiolysis, altered femoral neck shaft angles etc. leading to increased local mechanical stress and wear. Post traumatic malalignment or incongruity of joints is well established as an important predisposing cause of premature OA. Metabolic diseases lead to cartilage degeneration by very different mechanisms. In alkaptonuria (ochronosis) the genetically determined defect of homogentisic acid oxidase results in the accumulation of a pigmented polymer that binds to cartilage collagen, rendering it brittle and prone to mechanical degradation. It has been suggested that there may be other inborn errors of metabolism where unknown colourless metabolites may induce changes in the biochemical composition of cartilage matrix in a similar way and so predispose to OA. Crystal deposition of calcium pyrophosphate dihydrate or hydroxyapatite may alter cartilage matrix properties directly and low grade crystal inflammation may play a part in pathogenesis.

It is uncertain whether the degenerative joint disease seen in acromegaly (p. 627) is a consequence of joint incongruity following cartilage overgrowth or whether the endocrine disturbance results in a mechanically defective matrix. Paget's disease, Gaucher's disease and the various diseases associated with aseptic necrosis result in subchondral bone pathology, and altered stresses on the overlying articular cartilage.

Current concepts of the pathogenesis of OA are based on the assumption that whatever the provoking cause, the final pathway of changes in articular cartilage will be identical. Two mechanical hypotheses merit consideration. The first suggests that the initiating event is fatigue fracture of the collagen fibre network. This is followed

Table 13.4 Causes of secondary osteoarthrosis

| | |
|---|---|
| *Developmental* | Perthes' disease, slipped capital femoral epiphysis, epiphysiolysis, hip dysplasis, epiphysial dysplasias, intra-articular acetabular labrum. |
| *Traumatic* | Intra-articular fracture, menisectomy, occupational e.g. elbows of pneumatic drill workers, hypermobility e.g. Ehlers Danlos syndrome, long leg arthropathy. |
| *Metabolic* | Alkaptonuria (ochronosis), haemochromatosis, Wilson's disease, chondrocalcinosis. |
| *Endocrine* | Acromegaly. |
| *Inflammatory* | Rheumatoid arthritis, gout, septic arthritis, haemophilia. |
| *Aseptic Necrosis* | Corticosteroids, sickle cell disease, caisson disease, SLE and other collagenoses. |
| *Neuropathic* | Tabes dorsalis, syringomyelia, diabetes mellitus, peripheral nerve lesions. |
| *Miscellaneous* | Paget's disease, Gaucher's disease. |

by increased hydration of the articular cartilage with unravelling of the proteoglycans and loss of proteoglycans into the synovial fluid. There is no evidence of augmented neutral protease or collagenase activity and collagen is simply lost as a result of mechanical attrition.

The alternative hypothesis suggests that the initial lesions are microfractures of the subchondral bone following repetitive loading. Healing of the microfracture leads to significant stiffening of the subchondral bone which in turn creates a shear stress gradient in the adjacent articular cartilage. As the process evolves, the cartilage surface becomes fibrillated and deep clefts appear with reduplication and proliferation of chondrocytes within them. Simultaneous proliferative changes commence at the joint margins with formation of osteophytes. Eventually articular cartilage is lost altogether in areas of maximum mechanical stress exposing the hardened, eburnated underlying bone. Cysts may form but bony ankylosis does not occur.

**Clinical Features.** The joints most frequently involved are those of the spine, hips and knees. In the majority of patients the disease is confined to one or only a few joints. The symptoms are gradual in onset. Pain is at first intermittent and aching. It is provoked by use of the joint and relieved by rest. As the disease progresses, movement in the affected joint becomes increasingly limited, initially as a result of pain and muscular spasm, but later because of capsular fibrosis, osteophyte formation and remodelling of bone. There may be repeated effusions into joints especially after minor twists or injuries. Crepitus may be felt or even heard. Associated muscle wasting is an important factor in the progress of the disease, as in the absence of normal muscular control the joint becomes more prone to injury. Pain arises from trabecular microfractures, traumatic lesions in the capsule and periarticular tissues, and a low grade synovitis. Nocturnal aching may be attributable to hyperaemia of the subchondral bone.

*Nodal osteoarthrosis* is a clinically distinct form of primary generalised OA which occurs predominantly in middle-aged women. Characteristically it affects the terminal IP joints of the fingers with the development of gelatinous cysts or bony outgrowths on the dorsal aspect of these joints (Heberden's nodes). The onset is sometimes acute with considerable pain, swelling and inflammation. Although these lesions may be associated with a good deal of deformity they seldom cause disability. Similar lesions may affect the proximal IP joints and the disorder also frequently involves the carpometacarpal joints of the thumbs, the spinal apophyseal joints, the hips and knees. A strong family history of Heberden's nodes is usual in such cases and though the existence of multigeneration families with the disorder appears to suggest a single autosomal dominant gene, careful family studies suggest polygenic inheritance in both nodal and non-nodal primary generalised osteoarthrosis.

**Investigation.** The blood count and ESR are characteristically normal in osteoarthrosis. Synovial fluid is viscous and has a low cell count. Apatite crystals can be detected on rare occasions. Radiographs show loss of joint space and formation of marginal osteophytes. Subchondral bone sclerosis, bony remodelling and cyst formation are seen in more advanced cases.

**Treatment.** Although the pathological changes of osteoarthrosis are irreversible much can be done to alleviate symptoms particularly in the early stages. Periods of rest and avoidance of undue trauma and physical stress to affected joints are essential. This may involve such measures as the fitting of rubber heels to reduce jarring and minimise the risk of slipping, the provision of built-up shoes to equalise leg lengths, weight loss in obese patients with OA of the knee or hip and the provision of a suitable walking stick. Occasionally patients may have to be advised to change their occupation, transfer to lighter work or give up unduly strenuous hobbies.

NSAID can be used to relieve pain and stiffness but are often disappointingly ineffective in osteoarthrosis.

Occasional intra-articular or periarticular corticosteroid injections can be very helpful especially in the knee. Hydrotherapy may be useful for patients with OA of the hip associated with pain and muscle spasm. Hip or knee arthroplasty may be necessary in advanced cases. Arthrodesis of a knee is occasionally considered if the knee is the only joint involved.

## Miscellaneous Lesions of Connective Tissue

Musculo-skeletal aches and pains are extremely common and become more frequent with increasing age. More than one-third of all 'rheumatic' complaints cannot be attributed to defined diseases of the spine, peripheral joints or connective tissues. Many are trivial, self limiting and cause little disability. Others can be more troublesome. The neck, shoulder girdle, back and gluteal regions are the common sites for many of these complaints. Muscular spasm of reflex origin is a prominent feature and must be differentiated from limitation of movement due to structural damage. Absence of signs of systemic illness and a normal ESR will help to distinguish them from the inflammatory connective tissue diseases.

Certain factors may be of importance in precipitating attacks in susceptible individuals. Exposure to cold and damp has always been suspected as a cause of non-articular 'rheumatic' complaints. Unaccustomed physical effort, undue fatigue, minor injuries and poor posture have also been incriminated. Any reduction in muscular efficiency will render an individual more prone to sprains of tendons, ligaments and extra-articular soft tissue structures. Loss of resilience and elasticity of the intervertebral discs can occur long before radiological evidence of disc degeneration becomes apparent and the interfacetal joints of the spine may be more exposed to strains and sprains. Pain arising from such deep structures is poorly located and referred diffusely to the overlying skin. Pain may be referred from the cervical intervertebral joints to the occipital region, shoulder girdle and arm. 'Lumbago' and 'sciatic pain' (p. 731) without signs of root pressure may be caused by minor disc injury. More often they appear to be associated with acute or chronic 'sprain syndromes'. Although poor posture, flabby muscles and obesity may be predisposing causes, occupational factors may be of great importance. Sickness absence attributable to 'rheumatic' complaints is much higher among miners, dockers and foundry workers than it is among clerks or employees in light industry. Up to 10% of the population may have abnormally lax joints and ligaments without the stigmata of major connective tissue disorders such as the Marfan or Ehlers Danlos syndrome. Such persons are particularly prone to recurrent sprains, dislocations and arthalgia — the '*hypermobility syndrome*'.

Diffuse muscular pain and stiffness is common in certain infections, particularly of viral origin, such as influenza, rubella and measles. Localised pain occurs in epidemic myalgia (Bornholm disease p. 298). Many anxious and depressed people complain of aches and pains, particularly in the region of the neck, shoulders or lower back.

*Shoulder pain* is frequently a consequence of extra-articular traumatic, degenerative or inflammatory lesions of the capsule and 'rotator cuff' of tendons. *Supraspinatus tendinitis* is characterised by a 'painful arc' on arm abduction which can be abolished by external rotation. There is localised tenderness over the greater tuberosity of the humerus and a radiograph may show calcification in the supraspinatus tendon. Rupture of calcific material into the subacromial bursa occasionally results in acutely painful 'gout-like' attacks of inflammatory *subacromial bursitis*. Fluid aspirated from the bursa beneath the acromion contains crystals of calcium hydroxyapatite. Local injection of hydrocortisone is used to give symptomatic relief. *Bicipital tendinitis* can be recognised by pain and tenderness over the bicipital groove aggravated by resisted shoulder flexion. '*Frozen shoulder*' is the name given to a common and disabling condition in which severe spontaneous shoulder pain is associated initially with capsular tenderness and painful restriction of all shoulder movements and later with painless restriction of movements alone. A frozen shoulder may be a late consequence of a rotator cuff lesion and sometimes follows myocardial infarction, hemiplegia, herpes zoster, breast or thoracic surgery. Treatment is with analgesics and local corticosteroid injection in the early phase and mobilising exercises after the pain has resolved. The natural history is for slow but complete recovery, the complete cycle sometimes taking as long as two years.

In the *shoulder-hand syndrome* restricted shoulder movements are associated with a painful swollen hand. The condition is characterised by burning pain, vasomotor changes and severe limitation of movements of the hand. A radiograph of the hand shows patchy osteoporosis after some weeks or months. It may be a sequel to the same disorders that precede a frozen shoulder but epilepsy, barbiturates and antituberculous drugs can also be predisposing factors. Not infrequently these patients have an hysterical personality. Treatment is aimed at mobilising the affected limb. Analgesics, short courses of systemic corticosteroids, sympathetic nerve block and physiotherapy each have their advocates in this difficult situation. The prognosis for complete recovery is less certain than in frozen shoulder.

'*Tennis elbow*' appears to follow partial tears of the origin of the extensor muscles at the lateral epicondyle. Local tenderness and pain on active wrist extension are characteristic. '*Golfer's elbow*' results from similar lesions in the origin of the common flexor tendon at the medial epicondyle. Local corticosteroid injections relieve both conditions.

## Diseases of Bone

### Infections

**Osteomyelitis** is most commonly encountered in children under the age of 12. The onset is abrupt with fever, nausea, malaise and severe pain at the site of bone infection. When this is close to a joint there may be a 'sympathetic' effusion and diagnostic confusion with septic arthritis may occur. Isotope scanning and careful delineation of the site of bone tenderness can be helpful in establishing the correct diagnosis but radiographic changes do not occur for some days or weeks. Multifocal sites of bone infection are not uncommon. Staphyloccoci are the most frequent organisms responsible and in about half the cases evidence can be found for haematogenous spread from a boil or superficial infection. Hypogammaglobulinaemia, malnutrition or debilitating illness may all be predisposing factors and salmonella bone infections are a characteristic complication of sickle cell anaemia.

An antibiotic e.g. sodium fusidate (p. 77) must be commenced after taking blood for culture as soon as the diagnosis is suspected, and continued in adequate doses for long enough to eliminate the infection. Delay in starting treatment or inadequate therapy may result in chronic indolent bone infection (*Brodie's abscess*) with sequestrum formation. Surgical exploration and decompression are required if there is not an immediate response to antibiotics.

*Tuberculous osteomyelitis* has become much less common in Britain since the elimination of bovine tuberculosis but there is some evidence of a recent increase in the elderly population and immigrant communities. 50% of cases of skeletal tuberculosis affect the spine. Typically the infection starts at the margins of vertebral bodies and invades the disc space, narrowing of which and destruction of bone leading to vertebral collapse with kyphosis. A paraspinous 'cold' abscess may form and track to the thigh, chest wall or neck. The hip, knee, ankle or wrist joint may be affected by spread from adjacent bone. Tuberculous dactylitis and sacroiliitis are unusual but characteristic lesions. The treatment of tuberculosis is described on page 259.

## Paget's Disease (Osteitis Deformans)

This is a disease of unknown aetiology characterised by softening, enlargement and bowing of bones. It is uncommon before the age of 40 years but increasingly frequent thereafter. Histologically there is increased osteoblastic and osteoclastic activity resulting in a high rate of bone turnover and increased local blood flow. This is reflected in abnormal isotope bone scans and radiological evidence of localised bone enlargement, altered trabecular pattern and alternating areas of rarefaction and increased density.

**Clinical Features**. Men are more commonly affected and there may be a family history of the disease. Often the condition is symptomless and detected only when radiological examination is made for some other reason. In others there is pain of a deep aching character often aggravated by weight bearing. The pelvis, femur, tibia, lumbar spine and skull are common sites of bone involvement. The increased vascularity may cause warmth of the affected part on palpation; rarely widespread arteriovenous shunting causes high output cardiac failure. Deformity of bones develops when the condition is advanced. Bowing of the femur and tibia is characteristic and Paget's disease may predispose to secondary osteoarthrosis of the hip. Fractures may occur spontaneously or after minor trauma but they usually heal normally. Skull involvement may result in headache, progressive enlargement of the cranium and deafness from compression of the auditory nerves. Paraplegia can follow involvement of the base of the skull. Osteogenic sarcoma is an uncommon late complication. The serum calcium and phosphate are usually normal with high levels of alkaline phosphatase and increased hydroxyproline excretion during phases of active disease.

**Treatment.** Calcitonin (p. 479) is used for the treatment of severe bone pain not controlled by analgesics. A daily subcutaneous self-administration of 0·5 mg of human calcitonin can be continued for six months and recommenced if pain recurs. Mithramycin and diphosphonates, which reduce bone turnover, are less satisfactory alternatives.

Confinement to bed may be followed by rapid mobilisation of calcium with hypercalcaemia, hypercalciuria and formation of renal calculi. Such patients must be carefully monitored, given a high fluid intake and measures must be taken to lower the serum calcium if it becomes dangerously high. Secondary degenerative joint disease is treated with NSAID. Hip arthroplasty is occasionally required. Osteogenic sarcoma is treated with early surgery but has a poor prognosis.

## Metabolic and Endocrine Diseases

Rickets (p. 102), osteomalacia (p. 105), osteoporosis (p. 106), hyperparathyroidism (p. 480), renal osteodystrophy (p. 438) and Cushing's syndrome (p. 438) are important causes in decrease in bone mineral content and pathological fracture.

## Neoplastic Disease

Malignant neoplasms of bone are important causes of diffuse skeletal aches and pains that are not infrequently dismissed as being 'rheumatic'.

*Metastases* from carcinomas of the bronchus, breast or prostate, are the commonest tumours of bone. Secondary deposits from most primary tumours appear typically as osteolytic areas on radiological examination and are frequently associated with a rise in serum alkaline phosphatase. Only prostatic metastases are commonly osteosclerotic and associated with a rise in serum acid phosphatase. Metastatic deposits can often be localised by skeletal isotope scans before radiological changes are apparent and widespread bone metastases can occur even in the absence of symptoms. A number of malignancies are hormone dependent and useful remissions can sometimes be obtained following hypophysectomy or administration of androgens to patients with metastatic breast cancer, or dienoestrol to those with prostatic metastases. Local radiotherapy and cytotoxic chemotherapy can occasionally be helpful in symptomatic management.

*Multiple myeloma* (p. 586) may also present with skeletal aches and pains associated with 'punched-out' osteolytic lesions on radiological examination. Unlike metastatic carcinoma these deposits usually fail to take up bone seeking isotopes and the serum alkaline phosphatase is normal.

*Primary bone tumours* are less common. Ivory *osteomas* are benign tumours which occur most frequently in the vault of the skull and are not usually associated with symptoms. Cancellous osteomas (osteochondromas or exostoses) are slender outgrowths of bone which arise from the metaphyses of long bones or from the flat bones of the pelvis and scapulae. They may give rise to pressure symptoms and most frequently present during adolescence. Diaphyseal aclasis (multiple exostosis) is a rarer inherited disorder seen in younger children.

*Primary osteosarcomas* occur most frequently in the lower end of the femur, the upper end of the tibia or the upper end of the humerus. These are tumours of young people rarely seen after the age of 20. Swelling with or without vague aching are the presenting symptoms and the bone may be tender and warm. Radiographs show a characteristic increase in radiolucency associated with bone expansion, triangular areas of new bone formation at the periosteal margin and a 'sun-ray' appearance due to new bone formation. Early blood-borne metastases to the chest are common and the 5 year survival is less than 10% despite treatment with radiotherapy and amputation.

*Fibrosarcomas* are of two types. Endosteal fibrosarcomas arise within bones and give rise to destructive lesions as they grow out. They metastasise to both the local lymph nodes and the lungs and are associated with a poor prognosis. Despite treatment with radiotherapy or amputation the 5 year survival is only 25%. Periosteal fibrosarcomas seldom invade bone or metastasise to distant sites. Treatment is with local excision and this can be repeated in the event of local recurrence.

*Benign chondromas* arise from cartilage within the long bones or small bones of the fingers. Multiple enchondromatosis is an unusual disorder of childhood in which multiple chondromas give rise to unsightly swellings attached to bones. Malignant change is very rare in chondromas. *Chondrosarcomas* occur in the long bones, pelvis or scapulae of adults between the ages of 20 and 50. Pain and swelling are the presenting features and bone radiographs show only loss of bone density associated with some speckled calcification. Amputation is the treatment of choice and the 5 year survival is better than 50%.

*Ewing's tumour* is a highly malignant bone neoplasm which affects children between the ages of 5 and 15. It probably arises from the marrow endothelium and has characteristic radiographic features. Areas of osteolytic bone destruction are surrounded by layers of periosteal new bone formation giving the lesions an 'onion skin' appearance. Pain, swelling and tenderness may be associated with fever and leucocytosis so that these tumours can easily be mistaken for osteomyelitis. The 5 year survival is virtually nil despite radiotherapy and amputation.

*Giant cell tumours* of bone may be benign or malignant. They usually occur in young adults between the ages of 20 and 40 and present with pain and swelling of a long bone in the neighbourhood of a joint. Radiographs show a typically eccentric tumour with a 'soap-bubble' appearance. The prognosis is relatively good even for malignant tumours. Local excision is the treatment of choice.

*Osteoid osteoma* is a rare cause of severe bone pain which is characteristically worse at night and relieved by NSAID. The condition occurs between the ages of 10 and 30 in any bone except the skull. There may be warmth, swelling and tenderness on palpation and radiographs show some increase in sclerosis with a characteristic area of translucency surrounding a central nidus. Excision of the nidus cures the symptoms and these lesions do not recur.

## Skeletal dysplasia

The skeletal dysplasias form a large and heterogeneous group of conditions which can be important causes of bone and joint deformity. Those with predominant epiphyseal involvement such as multiple epiphyseal dysplasia may be associated with premature osteoarthrosis. Those with predominant metaphyseal involvement such as achondroplasia are associated with short-limbed dwarfism (p. 464). There are disorders such as osteogenesis imperfecta, idiopathic juvenile osteoporosis and the hereditary osteolyses in which decreased bone density, fractures and bone loss are prominent features and others such as osteopetrosis and sclerosteosis where increased bone density occurs. Skeletal abnormalities are prominent in a number of hereditary disorders of connective tissue such as the Marfan syndrome or neurofibromatosis as well as in inborn errors of metabolism such as the mucolipidoses, and homocystinuria. The reader is referred to Fairbank's *Atlas of General Affections of the Skeleton* and to McKusick's *Hereditable Disorders of Connective Tissue* (p. 468) for details of all these groups of conditions.

## Prospects in Rheumatology

The outlook for patients with rheumatic diseases has substantially improved over the last 30 years. In particular, the remarkable developments in prosthetic surgery have transformed the lives of patients with advanced and crippling rheumatoid arthritis and osteoarthrosis of the hip. Continuing collaboration between bioengineers and orthopaedic surgeons is gradually overcoming the technical problems involved in developing suitable prostheses for severely damaged knees, elbows, ankles, shoulders and hands so that some practical advances can be expected. Progress along these lines is however likely to be progress with diminishing returns. In many ways the anatomy of the hip joint makes it uniquely suited for total joint replacement; a similar degree of success is unlikely in other joints. Already waiting lists for hip arthroplasty are many years in length and it is calculated that Britain would require one new 300-bedded hospital annually just to cope with this single operation. As numbers of patients with replaced joints increases so does the problem of loosening and infection of prostheses, particularly in those with multiple joint replacements. Future efforts must clearly be directed towards controlling or curing these disorders as well as improving salvage surgery.

In some respects the prospects in these directions look hopeful. The development of new anti-inflammatory drugs which suppress the cellular phase of the inflammatory process rather than acting as prostaglandin inhibitors may bring better control of inflammation coupled with less gastrointestinal side effects. Gold salts, antimalarials, penicillamine and immunomodulating drugs have all been shown to have significant practical value in slowing the progress of rheumatoid arthritis. The prospects for developing drugs with similar effects, but less formidable toxicity, look hopeful.

Advances in diagnostic immunological tests have allowed the more accurate definition of sub-sets of patients with diffuse connective tissue disorders and improved diagnosis, empirical treatment and prognosis. Most encouraging of all, however, are the developments in understanding the genetic and biochemical basis for regulation of the immune system and the macromolecular composition of articular cartilage.

Thirty years ago gout was a crippling disorder every bit as bad as rheumatoid arthritis or osteoarthrosis. Advances in understanding the biochemical basis for the disease were rapidly followed by rational and effective drug therapy for both the treatment and prevention of the disorder. The prospects for similar advances in understanding the aetiology of rheumatoid arthritis, the diffuse connective tissue diseases and even degenerative joint diseases are beginning to look more promising.

J. N. McCormick
G. Nuki

*Further reading:*

Hughes, G. R. V. (1977) *Connective Tissue Diseases.* Oxford: Blackwell. — Concise clinical monograph on the diffuse connective tissue diseases. Includes information on clinical applications of immunological tests.

Huskisson, E. C. & Hart, F. D. (1978) *Joint Disease: All the Arthropathies*, 3rd edn. Bristol: Wright. — Thumb nail sketch of more than 180 conditions associated with arthritis or arthralgia.

Kelley, W. N., Harris, E. D. Jun., Ruddy, S. & Sledge, C. B. (eds.) (1981). *Textbook of Rheumatology.* Philadelphia: Saunders. — Major new international textbook with comprehensive basic science and clinical coverage.

Lawrence, J. S. (1977) *Rheumatism in Populations.* London: Heinemann. — Source book of information on epidemiology of rheumatic diseases.

McCarty, D. J. (1979) *Arthritis and Allied Conditions*, 9th edn. London: Kimpton. — Standard American textbook. More detailed, with a little more emphasis on basic science and a little less on clinical aspects than the British equivalent.

McKusick, V. A. (1979) *Hereditable Disorders of Connective Tissue*, 5th edn. St Louis: Mosby. — Classical monograph.

Nuki, G. (1980) *The Aetiopathogenesis of Osteoarthrosis.* London: Pitman. — Up-to-date set of research reviews.

Panayi, G. S. & Johnson, P. M. (1979) *Immunopathogenesis of Rheumatoid Arthritis.* London: Reed Books. — Comprehensive set of research reviews.

Scott, J. H. S. (1979) In *Clinical Examination* 5th edn., ed. Macleod, J. Edinburgh: Churchill Livingstone. — Gives an account of the examination of the locomotor system.

Scott, J. T. (1978) *Copeman's Text Book of the Rheumatic Diseases*, 5th edn. Edinburgh:

Churchill Livingstone. — Standard British text book. Excellent and comprehensive source of information on all aspects of clinical rheumatology.

Wright, V. & Moll, J. M. H. (1976) *Seronegative Polyarthritis*. Oxford: Elsevier North Holland. — Comprehensive clinical monograph on all aspects of spondyloarthritis.

Wyngaarden, J. B. & Kelley, W. N. (1976) *Gout and Hyperuricaemia*. New York: Grune and Stratton. — Comprehensive clinical and biochemical monograph.

Wynne-Davies, R. & Fairbank, T. G. (1976) *Fairbank's Atlas of General Affections of the Skeleton*, 2nd edn. Edinburgh: Churchill Livingstone. — Concise and beautifully-illustrated introduction to skeletal dysplasias and other general disorders of bone.

# 14. Diseases of the Nervous System

The approach to patients presenting neurological problems must follow a logical course starting with the history and followed by the physical examination. The latter reveals neurological signs which reflect disordered neural function. The nature and distribution of these signs depend on the anatomical localisation of lesions within the central nervous system. It is a fundamental error to relate particular signs to specific pathological processes. Paralysis of one side of the body, hemiplegia, may equally well arise from a stroke or from a cerebral tumour since both lesions may similarly interrupt motor pathways. It is the history of the neurological illness which indicates the nature of the pathological process involved. A careful chronological assessment of the way in which a neurological disability has developed is essential if a diagnosis is to be made. Attention to the symptoms and signs which indicate loss of function of particular parts of the nervous system then follows for purposes of localisation.

Lesions which suddenly affect the nervous system, cause maximal disability within a few hours and after a static period of days or weeks then show a tendency to improve are usually due to vascular disturbances and sometimes to trauma. Disabilities of insidious onset and slow but inexorable progression are often due to degenerative disorders or to tumours of the central nervous system. A remittent history, wherein episodes of disability are followed by periods of improvement, with later recurrence of symptoms elsewhere in the nervous system, is characteristic of multiple sclerosis. Inflammatory lesions such as infections often develop rapidly, but less acutely than traumatic or vascular catastrophes and the recovery phase is also usually rapid. Some conditions are characterised by paroxysmal short-lived disorders of function, followed by rapid and complete recovery. A history of this type may be due to epilepsy or migraine or to transient ischaemic attacks. These general principles are a useful guide but atypical presentations occur. Sometimes a neoplasm may produce very rapid deterioration and occasionally repetitive, minor vascular lesions give rise to a progressive, 'step-wise' deterioration of function.

Some diseases cause systematised affection of cells or fibres of similar type; these conditions, of which motor neurone disease is a good example, usually result in bilateral and symmetrical dysfunction. Tumours produce progressive involvement of adjacent neural structures causing clinical disabilities which may later be accompanied by symptoms resulting from the occupation of space by the tumour within the confines of the skull or the spinal canal.

A neurological diagnosis is achieved by the integration of all the information gained from the patient's history, the general medical examination and the neurological examination.

## Anatomy and Physiology

### The Motor System

Movements, whether voluntary or involuntary, are the result of the contraction or controlled relaxation of groups of muscles and never of only a single muscle. They are effected by contraction of muscles which act as prime movers and reciprocal relaxation of their antagonists. The action of the prime movers is provided with a firm base by contraction of synergists which stabilise the joints, and by appropriate adjustments of posture. The postural adjustments are largely under the control of the extrapyramidal motor system and the vestibular and spinal reflexes. Voluntary movements require the participation of the precentral gyrus of the cerebral cortex ('motor area') and the timing and degree of contraction or relaxation of the muscles of the synergy are coordinated by the cerebellum, especially when a movement involves more than one segment of a limb. The activities of the upper motor neurones from the motor area of the cortex, the extrapyramidal motor system and the cerebellum influence, directly or indirectly, the cells of the anterior horn of spinal grey matter or motor cranial nuclei from which the lower neurone runs to a group of muscle fibres ('motor unit'). Thus the lower motor neurone is the 'final common path' for all efferent impulses directed at the muscle and the groups of anterior horn cells may be considered to 'represent a muscle' in the same sense as the cells of the motor cortex 'represent a movement'. This distinction is vital to an understanding of the signs and disorders of the motor system.

**Upper Motor Neurone.** The fibres arise from cells in the precentral gyrus ('motor area'). These initiate movements of different parts of the opposite side of the body, the parts being represented in the following order from below upwards — tongue, face, hand, forearm, arm, trunk, thigh, leg, foot and perineal areas with considerable overlap. The cortical area representing movements of each of these parts is proportional to its functional importance rather than to its anatomical size. The projections of the upper motor neurones through the corticospinal (pyramidal) tracts to the contralateral motor nuclei of the brain stem and anterior horn of the spinal cord are shown in Figure 14.1.

A destructive lesion of the lateral corticospinal tract above its decussation causes a loss of some voluntary movements of part of the opposite side of the body, according to the fibres involved, but automatic associated movements, such as the stretching of a paralysed arm when yawning, may persist and other voluntary or reflex movements using the same lower motor neurones and muscles may be preserved. This is the essential difference between paralysis of upper motor neurone type and that due to a lower motor neurone lesion. For the same reason stretch reflexes are retained but these are usually of heightened activity. This indicates that the upper motor neurone normally carries fibres which are inhibitory to the stretch reflex. The pattern of cutaneous protective reflexes also changes, causing the emergence of an extensor plantar reflex. There are thus two types of disturbance, a negative one due to loss of a particular activity, and a positive one due to the release of lower levels from control. Hughlings Jackson considered this to be a principle of general application in the nervous system and the concept is important in understanding the signs of upper motor neurone disease. Another type of positive symptom results from irritative lesions (usually incomplete damage to a nerve cell or its fibre) which cause spontaneous activity of the affected neurones. Spontaneous activity in upper motor neurones causes involuntary movements as in focal epilepsy (p. 677).

SIGNS OF A LESION OF THE UPPER MOTOR NEURONE are:

1. Weakness or paralysis of movements of part of one side of the body.

2. Increase of tone of spastic type. This is characterised by an increased resistance to passive movement, which is maximal at the beginning of movement, smoothly sustained, and suddenly lapses as passive movement is continued ('clasp-knife re-

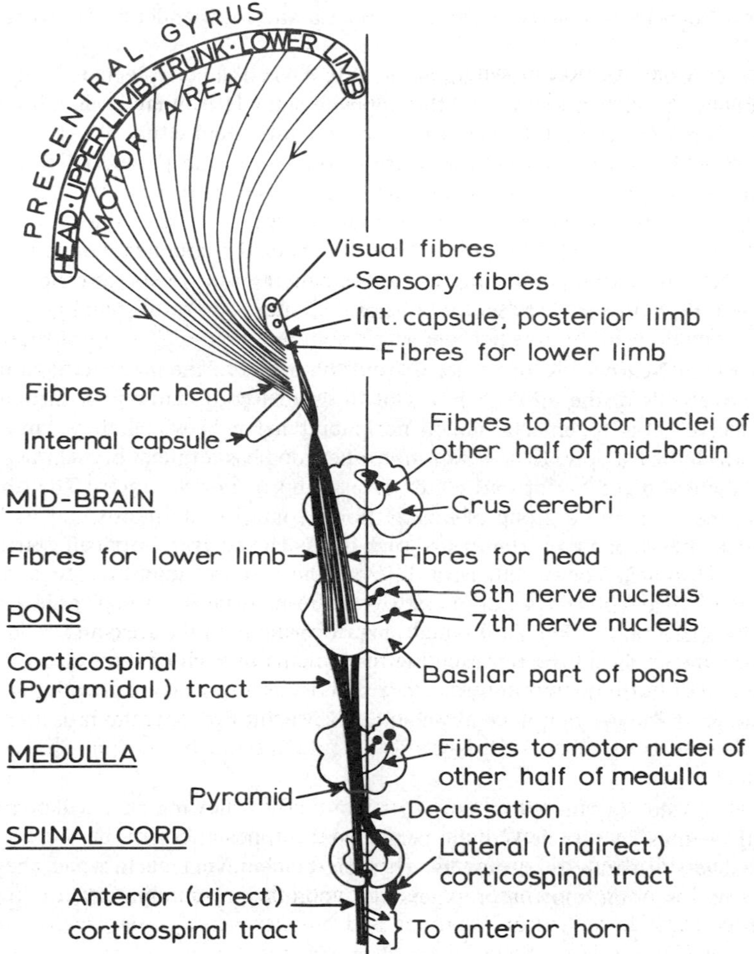


Fig. 14.1 The motor pathways

sponse). It occurs predominantly in flexor muscles in the upper limbs and extensor muscles in the lower limbs (the antigravity muscles).

3. Increase in amplitude of tendon reflexes: clonus may be present.
4. Loss of the abdominal reflexes.
5. An extensor plantar response (Babinski reflex).
6. No muscle atrophy apart from slight wasting which may occur as a result of disuse.
7. Normal electrical excitability of the involved muscles (p. 652).

These signs occur with disease involving any part of the upper motor neurone from the cortex down, but the exact level at which the lesion lies may be determined by the upper level of increased reflexes and by associated features.

*Cortex*. Localised paralyses, affecting for example, one limb only, are characteristic of lesions at the cortical level. The upper motor neurones are spread over a wide area and only very large lesions could cause a hemiplegia. There may be associated evidence of cortical dysfunction such as dysphasia and focal epileptic fits sometimes occur.

*Internal Capsule.* As the fibres here are closely packed, a hemiplegia is likely, with involvement of face, arm and leg on the opposite side. There may be hemihypoaesthesia and hemianopia from damage to adjacent sensory and visual fibres.

*Brain Stem.* Lesions in this area are rarely confined to the pyramidal tract. One presentation comprises affection of one or more cranial nerves on the side of the lesion and signs of an upper motor neurone lesion on the opposite side.

*Spinal Cord.* The pyramidal pathways may be affected bilaterally. The level of the lesion in the cord is often delineated by accompanying lower motor neurone signs, sensory disturbance or loss of tendon reflexes.

**Lower Motor Neurone.** Axons emerge from the nuclei of the motor cranial nerves and from the cells of the anterior horns of the spinal cord. They pass through the anterior nerve roots to enter a mixed peripheral nerve in which they run to the muscles which they supply. Each lower motor neurone has terminal branching so that it is distributed to the motor end-plates of a group of muscle fibres. The anterior horn cell, the axon and a group of muscle fibres comprise the motor-unit and each muscle is composed of a large number of such units. The anterior horn cell is activated by impulses from the corticospinal tracts, from the extrapyramidal tracts, and from some afferent fibres of the posterior nerve root responsible for spinal reflexes. The lower motor neurone is thus an integral part of the spinal reflex arc and is the final common pathway for all motor impulses, involuntary or voluntary, directed to a muscle. Normal nutrition of a muscle appears to depend on its contact with the spinal cord through the lower motor neurone since, if it is interrupted, the muscle rapidly wastes.

SIGNS OF A LESION OF THE LOWER MOTOR NEURONE. The following signs will be present only in those muscles supplied by the particular neurones affected:

1. Weakness or paralysis of muscles. This affects all movements in which they take part whether as prime movers or synergists, voluntary or involuntary, or in reflex contractions.
2. Loss of tone on passive movement (flaccidity).
3. Wasting of the affected muscles which appears within two or three weeks of an acute lesion (atrophy).
4. Absence of reflexes subserved by the affected neurones. Abdominal and plantar reflexes remain normal unless the neurones to the appropriate muscles are damaged and then these reflexes cannot be elicited.
5. Single fibres contract spontaneously when they are no longer influenced by their associated lower motor neurone. This phenomenon, called fibrillation, is detectable by electromyography but is invisible through the skin. Lower motor neurones which are damaged but still able to conduct impulses may give rise to spontaneous contractions of bundles of fibres in the muscles supplied. Such contractions (fasciculation) may be visible, e.g. in motor neurone disease.
6. Contractures of muscles due to replacement by fibrous tissue and 'trophic' changes such as dryness and cyanosis of the skin, and brittleness of the nails, partly due to impaired circulation.
7. The electrical excitability of the peripheral nerves and muscles is altered. These tests may be combined with electromyography to confirm that a weak and wasted muscle is denervated. Lesions of peripheral nerves short of complete interruption may cause slowing of conduction.

If lower motor neurones are damaged in the cord or nerve roots the muscles and reflexes affected in the ways described above will be those supplied by one or more segments of the spinal cord. If the neurones are damaged more peripherally after they have been redistributed in the nerve plexuses, the paralysis will occur in the territory supplied by the appropriate peripheral nerve and it is probable that there will be similar damage to the sensory fibres with which they are associated in the mixed nerve.

**Extrapyramidal System.** This is a complex neuronal network, extending from the cortex to the medulla, from which emerge descending spinal pathways whose influence on lower motor neurones modifies voluntary motor activity. Interspersed in this latticework of fibres are areas of grey matter. Some of these are only loose aggregations of nuclei in the reticular formation of the brain stem, but there are also several well defined nuclear masses called the basal ganglia, which include the corpus striatum (caudate nucleus and putamen), the globus pallidus or pallidum, the substantia nigra and the subthalamic nucleus.

There are rich interconnections between the constituents of the basal ganglia and thence via the ventrolateral nucleus of the thalamus to the extrapyramidal areas of the cortex and to the medullary reticular formation. The normal functions of the extrapyramidal system are ill-understood.

SIGNS OF AN EXTRAPYRAMIDAL LESION. *Disturbance of Voluntary Movements.* There is not true paralysis in extrapyramidal disease, but rather slowness of movement and poverty of movement in that spontaneous gestures, changes in facial expression, and associated movements for postural adjustment, such as swinging the arm when walking, are lost on the side opposite to the lesion.

*Disturbance of Tone.* Tone may be increased as in parkinsonism or decreased as in chorea. Increase in tone, of extrapyramidal type, has characteristic features. It is present throughout the whole range of passive movement; it affects opposing muscle groups equally; it may be smooth and plastic ('lead-pipe rigidity') or intermittent ('cog-wheel rigidity') which is more common.

*Involuntary Movements.* There are many varieties, notably the tremor of parkinsonism (p. 716), choreiform movements (p. 720) and athetosis (p. 720).

**Cerebellum.** This is the most important part of the nervous system for the coordination of movement and the muscular contractions required to maintain posture. The cerebellum receives impulses from many sources, principally the proprioceptive end-organs, the skin, the vestibular nuclei and the cerebral cortex. The pontine nuclei and the inferior olive relay fibres from the cerebral motor cortex and basal ganglia respectively to the cerebellar cortex of the opposite side. The cerebellar cortex integrates this information about body posture, limb position and motor intention and sends efferent fibres via the cerebellar nuclei to the reticular formation, red nucleus and vestibular nucleus of the opposite side, whence fibres descend to influence motor cells in the anterior horns of the spinal cord; as these descending fibres cross again each cerebellar hemisphere controls the ipsilateral side of the body. Efferent fibres from the cerebellum also ascend to the contralateral thalamus through which the cerebral cortex is influenced. The cerebellum is therefore a great coordinating centre controlling the synergistic action of muscles during voluntary and automatic movements as well as adjusting posture.

SIGNS OF A CEREBELLAR LESION. The effects of disease of the cerebellum are best seen in acute lesions, for in chronic lesions considerable compensation occurs so that the deficit is less than might be expected. A lesion of the cerebellar hemisphere produces all its effects on the same side of the body. The principal signs are:

*Hypotonia.* The muscles show diminished resistance to passive movement and, when an outstretched limb is suddenly displaced, it makes a greater excursion than usual and oscillates before resuming its posture.

*Disturbance of Tendon Reflexes.* The reflexes are either diminished or pendular as when the knee jerk is followed by a series of diminishing oscillations.

*Disturbance of Posture and of Gait.* The head may be tilted towards the side of the lesion and the patient leans or may even fall towards that side. The gait is reeling with a tendency to stagger to the side of the lesion.

*Disorders of Movement.* Incoordination, hypotonia and the fact that muscular contraction is unregulated by the muscle spindles cause ataxia which manifests itself in different ways:

1. Dysmetria. Movements are not accurately adjusted to their object, so that the finger may overshoot or fall short of the object it is required to touch. If a movement is attempted with the eyes closed the finger overshoots towards the side of the cerebellar lesion ('past-pointing').
2. Dyssynergia. Movements which involve more than one joint are broken up into their component parts. When severe this leads to a decomposition of movement which resembles the jerky movements of a marionette.
3. Intention tremor. A combination of dyssynergia and dysmetria causes faulty correction of the badly directed limb movement so that it approaches the target in a zig-zag manner. The coarse irregular tremor increases as the target is approached. It is not increased when the eyes are closed. The contraction of muscles necessary to maintain a posture may be similarly affected so that tremor at rest occasionally occurs in cerebellar disorders.
4. Dysdiadochokinesis. The arrest of one movement and its immediate replacement with the opposite movement requires accurate coordination of the various muscles of the synergy. Rapidly alternating movements are therefore disturbed and carried out in a clumsy, irregular, jerky fashion.
5. Rebound phenomenon. For the same reason a strong contraction cannot be arrested when resistance is suddenly removed, whereupon the limb shoots beyond the normal range.
6. Disorders of articulation and phonation. Articulation is irregular, slurred and explosive as the volume of sound is poorly controlled. A rarer form of dysarthria is 'scanning-speech' in which the syllables tend to be separated from each other.
7. Disturbance of eye movement. Jerking nystagmus in the horizontal plane is commonly seen. It is a defect of postural fixation involving conjugate gaze (p. 669). In a unilateral cerebellar lesion the movements are greater in amplitude and slower in rate when the eyes are deviated to the side of the lesion.

## The Sensory System

*Superficial sensation* which arises from the skin has four primary components, touch, pain, warmth and cold. *Deep sensations* arising from subcutaneous structures are deep pain, pressure and proprioception which enables the recognition of movements of joints and the position of the parts of the body relative to one another. Vibration is a sensation due to rhythmical stimulation of groups of deep and superficial touch receptors. Some of the afferent impulses carried in 'sensory' nerve fibres do not reach consciousness but convey impulses directly or indirectly to motor neurones for reflex functions or to the cerebellum for purposes of coordination, e.g. many impulses from muscle and tendon receptors. All sensory impulses arise in the sensory receptors or end-organs which are widely distributed throughout the body. It is probable, though debatable, that specialised receptors respond to specific types of stimuli. Stimulation of an end-organ causes impulses to pass along the first sensory neurone to the spinal cord. This neurone has its cell body in a dorsal root ganglion but does not synapse until it reaches a second order neurone in the spinal cord or brain stem.

On entering the cord by the posterior nerve root, fibres subserving proprioception, vibration and a proportion of touch sensation turn medially and ascend in the posterior column of the same side to the lower part of the medulla oblongata to synapse with cells in the gracile and cuneate nuclei (Fig. 14.2). From there, the second order neurone crosses to the other side of the medulla and ascends in the medial lemniscus to the main sensory nucleus of the thalamus.

Fibres subserving pain, warmth, cold and the remainder of touch sensation synapse in the posterior horn of the spinal cord soon after entering it. Most of the second order neurones cross at the same level, or one or two segments higher, to reach the anterolateral column where they ascend to the thalamus as the spinothalamic tract.

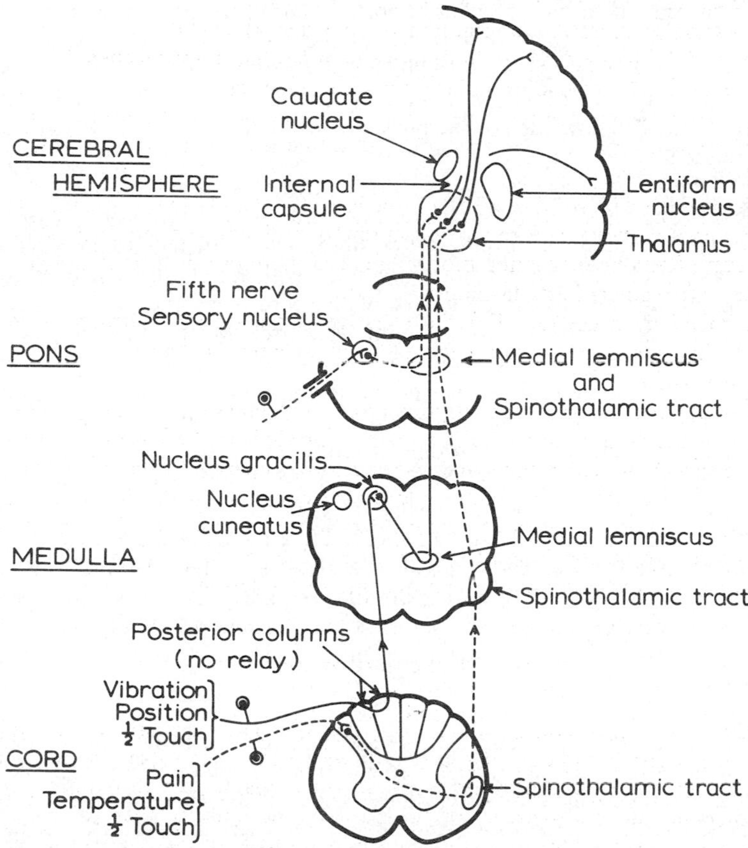


Fig. 14.2 The sensory pathways.

Some of these fibres do not cross but enter the ipsilateral spinothalamic tract. As it ascends through the brain stem the tract gradually intermingles with the medial lemniscus and terminates along with it in the main sensory nucleus of the thalamus. Third order neurones, maintaining their functional specificity, are then relayed from the thalamus to the sensory area of the cortex which is situated in the postcentral gyrus.

Areas of the sensory cortex representing the different parts of the body are arranged in a similar manner to the motor cortex. Some appreciation of sensation is possible at the thalamic level but the cortical projection is necessary to allow discrimination of the intensity and pattern of stimulation. From the postcentral gyrus further connections are made with other parts of the cortex, particularly in the parietal lobe where the information derived from superficial and deep sensation is integrated so that judgement of the size, shape, weight, texture and pattern of objects is possible. This sensory information is also integrated with information derived from the special senses to provide a mental picture of the body (body image). This synthesis is mainly carried out in the non-dominant parietal lobe. The corresponding part of the left cerebral hemisphere is important for other mental functions in which recurrent patterns of stimulation achieve the status of symbols and so are used for the receptive and interpretative aspects of speech functions. For this reason it is usually called the dominant or major hemisphere (in some left-handed people speech is mainly represented in the right hemisphere). This important part of the parietal lobe is connected with the lower part of the motor cortex of the same side so that patterns of lip, tongue, respiratory and finger movements may be used to convert ideas into motor symbols, the motor side of speech. An understanding of the link between symbol and meaning requires a knowledge of the physiological basis of the mind which we do not have at present.

Most of the afferent signals entering the central nervous system never reach consciousness. Some are used for spinal reflexes and make contact directly or through interneurones with motor neurones. Other fibres which originate in muscle receptors end at the base of the posterior horn in contact with second order neurones. These neurones turn laterally to the periphery of the cord to ascend in the anterior and posterior spinocerebellar tracts to the cerebellar cortex. Most of these ascend without crossing but some second order neurones cross to the opposite anterior spinocerebellar tract. These fibres carry some of the proprioceptive information required to enable the cerebellum to coordinate limb movements. Still other sensory fibres, which do not carry 'sensation' in the ordinary sense, are extremely important for the maintenance of consciousness. These are collateral branches of the main spinothalamic pathways and of the special sensory tracts which turn medially into the upper part of the reticular formation in the midbrain. Here there is a chain of short neurones with intimate interconnections which also receives neurones from most parts of the cerebral cortex. It is therefore an important integrating centre. At its upper end it communicates with the non-specific nuclei of the thalamus which relay impulses to all areas of the cortex. Activity in this system is considered to be essential for the conscious state and may be important in some mental functions in collaboration with the cerebral cortex.

Disease of the sensory system may be accompanied by positive phenomena such as pain or paraesthesiae due to spontaneous activity or irritation of sensory neurones, or by negative phenomena in which there is loss of the ability to appreciate some modality of sensation (anaesthesia and analgesia). These symptoms occur only with disorders of the first or second order neurones, i.e. from the end-organs to the thalamus. Suprathalamic lesions show certain differences. Paraesthesiae may occur with irritative lesions of the sensory cortex but anaesthesia does not. Instead there is a loss of sensory discrimination and of the spatial and quantitative aspects of sensation.

SIGNS OF SENSORY LESIONS. *Peripheral Nerve.* With a complete lesion all forms of sensation are lost in the area supplied by the affected nerve, but the zone of anaesthesia may be limited by the fact that neighbouring nerves overlap into its territory, the extent varying from person to person. The resistance of different types of fibres to disease need not be the same so that it is common for one type of cutaneous or deep sensation to be more affected than another and indeed some may be spared. If the afferent fibres of a reflex arc are affected, as for instance in the sciatic nerve in the ankle jerk, the reflex concerned is lost. Some neuropathies do not affect individual nerves but rather damage fibres selectively. As a general rule the longest fibres are most susceptible and so the sensory and motor disturbance is first noticed at the tips of all the toes and fingers, irrespective of nerve supply, and spreads proximally as the advancing disease involves progressively shorter fibres. This produces a 'glove and stocking' distribution of sensory loss.

*Posterior Root.* The different forms of sensation are affected by a posterior root lesion in the same way as for a peripheral nerve but the distribution of the loss follows a dermatomal pattern. The overlap from adjacent roots may be so great that no anaesthesia can be detected. When the root is irritated pain and paraesthesiae are experienced in the full dermatomal distribution of the root and pain may also be experienced in the deep structures such as muscles and ligaments which are supplied by the root. These structures do not necessarily underlie the dermatome. Any reflex subserved by the involved root is also lost, for example, the ankle jerk where the S1 posterior root is damaged by a prolapsed intervertebral disc.

*Posterior Column.* A lesion confined to the posterior column of the spinal cord will cause loss of position and vibration sense on the same side, but the sensations of pain, touch, warmth and cold will be preserved (Fig. 14.3). The loss of the sense of position causes sensory ataxia since the patient is unable to control movements by awareness of the position achieved at each instant. Sensory ataxia differs from cerebellar ataxia in that it is more marked when the eyes are closed, because vision can compensate to a certain extent for loss of proprioceptive information. Thus there is unsteadiness in the finger-nose test which is greater when the eyes are closed but

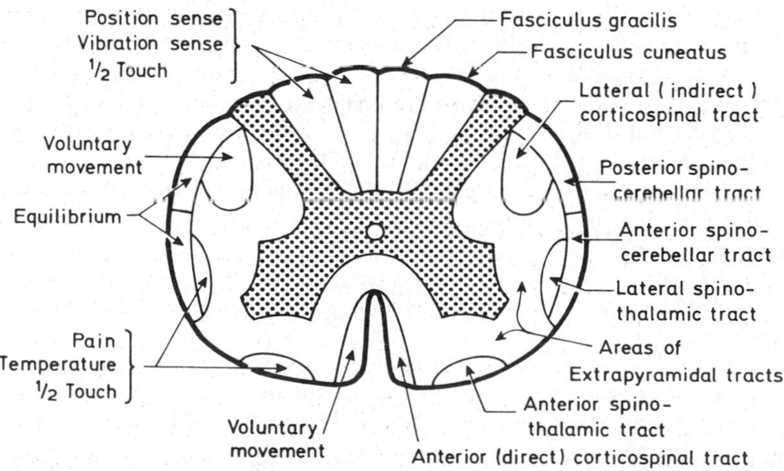

Fig. 14.3 Cross-section of spinal cord

without the marked tremor of cerebellar ataxia. The gait is ataxic and the patient walks with a broad base to provide a firmer foundation and steps high to make sure that the feet clear the ground which cannot be felt with certainty. If the eyes are closed it is not possible to stand with the feet close together without swaying (Romberg's test). Vibration sense is abolished below the level of the lesion ipsilaterally. The same symptoms will be found if the first order neurones of the proprioceptive nerve fibres are damaged peripherally but they will then be associated with other signs of peripheral nerve disease.

*Spinothalamic Tract.* Lesions of the anterior and lateral spinothalamic tracts in the anterolateral columns of the cord or their continuation through the brain stem cause impairment of the ability to appreciate pain, warmth and cold on the contralateral side of the body below the level of the lesion. Touch is usually modified (it feels 'different') but not abolished because of its alternative pathway in the posterior columns. This is the situation produced by the operation of anterolateral cordotomy for the relief of intractable pain.

*Brain Stem.* Since the spinothalamic tract and medial lemniscus run close together and eventually intermingle, lesions of the upper brain stem usually affect all forms of sensation on the contralateral side of the body. With midbrain lesions the hemihypoaesthesia will extend to the face, but with pontomedullary lesions the second order neurones from the trigeminal sensory nucleus or the nucleus and descending tract of the fifth nerve may be damaged so that sensory loss will be on the same side of the face as the lesion but on the contralateral side of the rest of the body (Fig. 14.2).

*Thalamus.* Lesions of the main sensory nuclei in the lateral part of the thalamus may cause spontaneous pain of most unpleasant quality in the opposite side of the body. The threshold for pain is raised on the opposite side of the body but when it is exceeded the resulting pain is exquisite and has the same unpleasant quality which often causes considerable emotional reaction.

Loss of other modalities of sensation occurs on the opposite side of the body.

*Sensory Cortex.* Lesions above the thalamus do not abolish any form of sensation though the threshold may be raised. There is impairment of position sense, of two-point discrimination, of the ability to localise touch and to recognise objects in the palm of the hand (astereognosis) since shape and texture cannot be identified though the patient is able to feel the object. Disturbance of the spatial aspects of sensation is greatest when the parietal lobe is involved, and especially in lesions of the 'minor' hemisphere this may cause disturbance of the body image and of spatial orientation. For instance the patient may be unable to recognise part of his own body on the side opposite to the lesion or may feel that it is distorted. He may ignore one side of external space or of his own body (though he is capable of feeling it) and this is most evident if the unaffected (ipsilateral) side of his body, or visual field, is stimulated simultaneously. When presented with this 'perceptual rivalry' his brain 'ignores' the stimulus on the side contralateral to the affected parietal lobe though a stimulus applied to that part alone would be recognised immediately. Lesions of the dominant hemisphere in the region where parietal, temporal and occipital lobes meet (angular and supramarginal gyri) are associated with receptive dysphasia (p. 661). This is a special case of the failure to analyse the temporal and spatial aspects of sensory stimuli.

### The Reflexes

Certain functions are economically catered for by the nervous system by means of reflexes, which are short chains of neurones (the reflex arc) connecting a receptor to an effector organ such as muscle or gland, so that an appropriate stimulus invariably leads to a specific response. The quantity but not the nature of the response may be modified by other stimuli or by supraspinal influences from the cortex, extrapyramidal system or the cerebellum. There are two main categories of reflex — postural and protective. The appropriate stimuli for postural reflexes are muscle stretch and vestibular impulses. Protective reflexes are evoked by stimuli to pain receptors. They are usually superficial (cutaneous or corneal); the protective 'spasm' of muscles around a painful lesion is similar in nature.

**Tendon (Stretch) Reflexes.** A basic postural reflex depends on the stimulation of muscle spindles when a skeletal muscle is stretched. The afferent fibre enters the cord by a posterior nerve root and communicates directly or via a chain of interneurones with the anterior horn cells which control the stretched muscle, thus causing it to contract and so resist the displacement. A sudden tap to a tendon results in a sharp but brief contraction of the muscle. This activity may be increased by certain manoeuvres such as clenching the teeth or pulling the interlocked hands apart. This is termed reinforcement of the reflex and a tendon jerk should not be declared absent until reinforcement has failed to make it visible. The stretch reflex is inhibited by receptors in the tendon if muscle tension rises too high, thus risking the integrity of its fibres. This may happen when the reflex is exaggerated by withdrawal of a normal inhibitory effect of the corticospinal tract so that the contraction is abruptly stopped. This is the mechanism of the 'clasp-knife' response. There are also supraspinal facilitatory and inhibitory influences from the extrapyramidal system and cerebellum so lesions of these systems may abolish the reflexes.

An example of a monosynaptic stretch reflex is a knee jerk. A tap on the patellar tendon activates stretch receptors in the quadriceps muscle giving rise to impulses in first order sensory neurones which pass directly to the lower motor neurones to the quadriceps muscle making it contract. A lesion anywhere along this path will cause loss of the reflex; hence it is important in the localisation of disease to know through which spinal segment each reflex passes. The common tendon reflexes are the brachioradialis or supinator (C 5–6), the biceps (C 5–6), the triceps (C 7), the knee (L 3–4) and the ankle (S 1).

**Superficial Reflexes.** These are polysynaptic reflexes originating from stimuli to superficial structures. The interneurones may connect with motor neurones at several segmental levels and so the response may be a coordinated movement, usually designed to withdraw the stimulated part from a potentially dangerous stimulus. There are very many of these reflexes, some of which are conflicting. For example, stimulation of the sole of the foot evokes both flexion and extension reflexes. Which reflex will predominate is determined by higher influences. The nature of this influence is unknown but is believed to require the corticospinal (pyramidal) tract and damage to this tract will cause a change in the predominant reflex pattern.

*Plantar Reflex.* When the outer border of the sole of the foot is stroked in normal people after infancy, there is plantar flexion of the great toe. In 1896 Babinski pointed out that when the upper motor neurone was damaged the same stimulus caused dorsiflexion of the toe. (Anatomically this is described as an extensor plantar response though physiologically it is part of the flexion withdrawal reflex.) When the reflex is well developed it can be elicited from the medial side of the sole of the foot or even from the lower part of the leg and the hallux response is accompanied by dorsiflexion and abduction or fanning of the other toes and even withdrawal of the limb. The fundamental importance of the extensor plantar or Babinski response as a sign of loss of function of the upper motor neurone is widely accepted but it may occur in transient form during temporary states such as coma or after an epileptic fit and need not indicate permanent damage. It is often extensor in normal infants during the first year of life.

*Abdominal Reflexes.* When the skin on one side of the abdomen is stroked with a pin, there is a reflex contraction of the underlying muscles, a reflex for protection of the viscera. This may be lost on the affected side in disease of the upper motor neurone though the sign is less reliable than the plantar reflex. For instance the abdominal reflexes may be lost early in multiple sclerosis yet retained despite severe pyramidal tract damage in motor neurone disease. The abdominal reflexes may not be obtained on either side in elderly, obese or multiparous patients and may be lost where operative incisions have severed the nerves concerned. The abdominal reflexes are served in their peripheral course by the intercostal nerves arising from segments T 8 to 12.

*Corneal Reflex.* A light touch on the cornea provokes a blink of the eyelids on both sides. The afferent path for this reflex is the first division of the trigeminal nerve and the efferent path is the facial nerve. Loss of both corneal reflexes is a valuable indication of a deepening level of unconsciousness from any cause but should be elicited with discretion to avoid accidental damage to the cornea.

## Nervous Control of the Bladder and Rectum

**Bladder.** The nerve supply to the bladder is derived from three sources:

1. Sympathetic, from the first and second lumbar segments via the inferior hypogastric plexus and hypogastric nerves, which relax the bladder wall and contract the sphincters.

2. Parasympathetic, from segments S 2, 3, 4 via the pelvic nerves (nervi erigentes) which contract the bladder wall and relax the internal sphincter.

3. Somatic, from segments S 2, 3, 4 via the pudendal nerves, which contract the external sphincter of the urethra.

Afferent impulses from the bladder wall travel via the pelvic nerves and from the sphincters via the pudendal nerves. Distension of the bladder activates stretch receptors in the bladder wall and stimulates the parasympathetic fibres by means of a reflex arc through the upper sacral segments of the spinal cord; for example in the infant the bladder empties automatically when distension reaches a certain degree. Subsequently two descending pathways from higher levels assume control, one which inhibits the automatic reflex emptying, and the other which relaxes the inhibition when appropriate. The expression of urine is then promoted by contracting the abdominal and relaxing the pelvic muscles.

Interruption of the sacral reflex arc leads to retention of urine. This is accompanied by loss of bladder sensation if the lesion is on the afferent side of the arc, as in tabes dorsalis. Damage to the anterior sacral nerve roots causes an atonic bladder without loss of sensation ('lower motor neurone paralysis'). Lesions in the spinal cord above the sacral segments may damage the inhibitory fibres, causing urgency, precipitancy or incontinence of urine, or damage to the facilitatory fibres may cause hesitancy or retention. If the higher control is completely lost there is a period of retention with overflow from a passively dilating atonic bladder until the sacral reflex begins to function as in infancy, restoring automatic bladder emptying. The bladder is hypertonic ('upper motor neurone paralysis') and may shrink if this is not prevented. Cerebral lesions at the vertex near the motor or sensory areas may also give rise to incontinence or retention, and with frontal lobe lesions the intellectual disturbance may be associated with failure to inhibit reflex emptying.

**Rectum.** This has a dual nerve supply from the sympathetic (inhibitory) and the parasympathetic (facilitatory) systems. Disturbances of function similar to those in the bladder occur, but are less severe and more transient (p. 370).

## Speech

Speech employs verbal symbols to communicate thoughts and information. Coherent speech requires the formulation of propositions, which are translated into conventional symbols, earlier acquired and readily accessible, which then reach external expression by means of an efficient vocalising apparatus. Disease processes may interrupt this sequence at various levels to produce different types of speech defects.

*1. Intellectual Impairment.* Speech is deranged as a result of a generalised deficit of intellectual function which prevents the organisation of meaningful propositions. Such a disturbance reflects a diffuse impairment of cortical function which may be a temporary phenomenon in toxic confusional states (delirium) or permanent in dementia.

*2. Dysphasia* comprises disturbances of the symbolic aspects of language and these arise as a result of damage in or near the cortex of the dominant hemisphere. The nature of the defect varies with the site of the lesion. In *expressive or motor dysphasia* the patient can formulate thoughts in appropriate words (i.e. internal speech is preserved) but is unable to translate them into corresponding sounds. This occurs despite an intact articulatory system and represents a specialised form of apraxia (p. 664) which results from lesions in the posterior part of the inferior (3rd) frontal convolution. Impaired comprehension of language is called *receptive or sensory dysphasia*. The patient fails to understand or carry out spoken instructions. Internal speech is disturbed and hence there is also impairment of the patient's external speech. This is an agnosic deficit (p. 664) and results from lesions of the posterior part of the upper temporal convolutions and the angular gyrus of the parietal lobe.

In clinical circumstances all the speech areas of the major hemisphere are often injured together, which results in combined receptive and expressive dysfunctions. This picture, called *'global or central dysphasia'*, is usually due to occlusion of the internal carotid or middle cerebral arteries which supply all the regions concerned with speech.

*3. Dysarthria.* Imperfect articulation of speech is called dysarthria. Precise enunciation of words requires normal function and coordination of lips, tongue and palate. Any abnormality thereof results in slurring and distortion of speech. Dysarthria may be due to mechanical derangements such as cleft palate or ill-fitting false teeth. Lesions of muscles, myoneural junctions, or lower motor neurones of lips, tongue or palate will also result in dysarthria as will upper motor neurone and extrapyramidal affections of these structures.

When normal monitoring of speech is disturbed by deafness, dysarthria may ensue. This is particularly liable to occur when auditory feedback is distorted by impaired hearing in early childhood.

*4. Dysphonia.* Reduced volume of speech, often accompanied by hoarseness, results from dysfunction of the phonating mechanism. This may be due to weakness of respiratory movements so that air flow across the vocal cords is reduced or to malfunction of the vocal cords. The causative lesion may be in the respiratory musculature, in the peripheral nerves, or in central structures. Thus, for example, bilateral palsies of the recurrent laryngeal nerves cause aphonia. Dysphonia may be part of the picture of a bulbar palsy or it may result from extrapyramidal disease, such as parkinsonism.

## The Visual Pathway

The optic nerve carries second order neurones, the first order neurones being very short fibres within the retina. For much of its length it is surrounded by a protrusion of the meningeal membranes into which cerebrospinal fluid can pass, especially if intracranial pressure is raised. For these reasons the optic nerve is liable to suffer from different pathological states than other nerves.

The visual pathway is illustrated in Figure 14.4. Sensory impulses from the retinae pass along the optic nerves to the optic chiasma where the fibres from the temporal halves of the retinae continue posteriorly in the lateral angle of the chiasma into the optic tracts on the same side. Fibres from the nasal halves of the retinae decussate so that the optic tract carries fibres from that part of each retina which receives light from the contralateral half of the visual field of each eye (the light rays crossing in the refractory media of the eyes). In the same way the light rays from the upper part of the visual field stimulate the lower part of each retina and the fibres arising there remain inferior throughout their further path to the cortex. The optic tracts continue to the lateral geniculate bodies where the fibres concerned with vision synapse and the impulses are relayed along the optic radiations to the calcarine area of the occipital cortex. The uppermost fibres which carry impulses derived from the superior quadrants of each retina (lower quadrants of visual fields) pass directly through the parietal lobe, whereas the lowermost fibres which relay impulses from the lower quadrants of the retina (upper quadrants of visual fields) sweep downwards and forwards round the temporal horn of the lateral ventricle in the temporal lobe before passing to the occipital cortex. Throughout the whole of the visual pathway fibres from the various parts of each retina maintain approximately the same relationship with each other.

Some fibres originating in the retina and passing centrally in the optic nerve form the afferent limb of the light reflex arc of the pupils. These bypass the lateral geniculate bodies and pass medially to the superior colliculi of the midbrain where they synapse with neurones which pass to the nuclei of the third cranial nerves on each side. From these nuclei arise the efferent limbs of the light reflex (direct and consensual) to the sphincter muscles of the pupils. No visual stimulus is required for the accommodation 'reflex' of the pupil which is more properly an associated contraction related to the movement of convergence of the eyes. This is believed to involve an unidentified cerebral path and a midbrain nucleus which controls the pupillomotor cells of both third nerve nuclei. This explains the dissociation between the light reflex and the convergence reflex which may occur in neurosyphilis and other diseases.

### Clinical Manifestations of Lesions of the Visual Pathway

*The Optic Nerve.* A complete lesion of the optic nerve produces total loss of vision in the affected eye. There is no light reflex, direct or consensual, when that eye is illuminated but both pupils contract normally when the unaffected eye is illuminated. The pupil may be slightly larger in the blind eye. If the lesion is only partial, islands

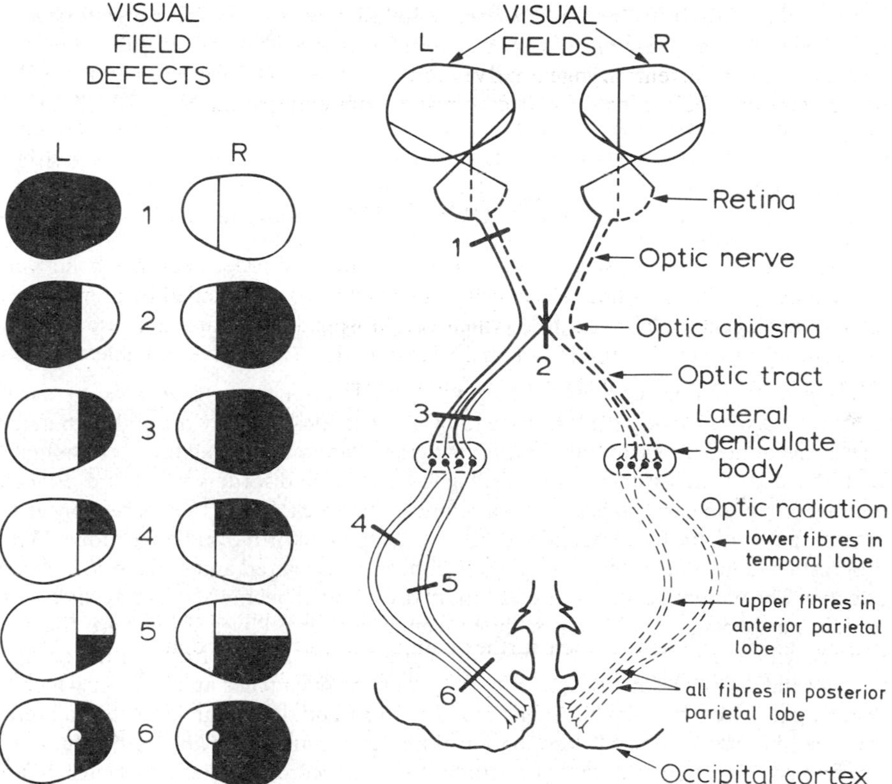


Fig. 14.4 Visual pathways and field defects

of loss of vision (*scotomas*) of various shapes occur in the field of the affected eye. When the fibres originating in the macular area are damaged there is a loss of visual acuity (*amblyopia*) which cannot be corrected by lenses. Direct and consensual light reflexes are depressed or absent when the amblyopic eye is stimulated but the convergence pupil response is unaffected.

*The Optic Chiasma.* A lesion of the central portion of the chiasma involves the decussating fibres from the nasal halves of both retinae and so gives rise to bitemporal hemianopia. In practice such lesions are rarely symmetrical and hence the degree of involvement of the visual fields of each eye is often unequal. A pituitary tumour first compresses the lower fibres and so the bitemporal hemianopia begins in the superior quadrants, whereas a suprasellar cyst compresses the chiasma from above so that field loss starts in the lower quadrants.

*The Optic Tracts.* A lesion of an optic tract gives rise to a homonymous hemianopia, the lost half of the field of vision of each eye being on the side opposite to the lesion. The involvement of the two fields is often unequal ('incongruous'), being slightly greater in the field of the eye on the side of the lesion.

*The Optic Radiation.* The effects of a lesion of the optic radiation depend on its exact site. A lesion of the temporal lobe involves the lower fibres only and gives rise to a homonymous defect involving mainly the upper quadrants of the visual fields

(Fig. 14.4). A lesion in the anterior part of the parietal lobe causes a homonymous hemianopia mainly affecting the lower quadrants as it affects fibres from the upper part of the retinae. A lesion at the posterior part of the parietal lobe, where both groups of fibres are again adjacent, gives rise to a total homonymous hemianopia.

*The Occipital Cortex.* A destructive lesion of one occipital cortex gives rise to a complete (and congruous) homonymous hemianopia if it is extensive, or to a scotoma which is present in the fields of both eyes. Irritative lesions, as in the ischaemia caused by migraine, cause hallucinations of flashing lights which are referred to the contralateral field of both eyes.

## The Localising Signs of Cerebral Disease

*The prefrontal lobe* comprises the frontal lobe anterior to the precentral gyrus. It is concerned with some aspects of psychological reactions, notably the ability to make intelligent anticipations of the future, and the emotional correlations of thought. Disturbances of these functions cause vague psychiatric disorders which are difficult to diagnose in the early stages. The patient loses appreciation of the consequences of actions, fails to take forethought and becomes apathetic or morbidly facetious. With progressing dementia, memory and intellect become impaired and social sense is also affected. The patient becomes careless about dress and appearance and may micturate in public or become incontinent without seeming to care. Physical signs are few but there may be generalised convulsions and a grasp reflex may be found in the contralateral hand. With this reflex, the patient involuntarily clutches at an object which is drawn lightly over the palm between the index finger and the thumb. The contralateral arm may be ataxic if the frontopontine fibres connecting with the cerebellum are interrupted. Expanding lesions of a frontal lobe may compress the underlying olfactory nerve causing unilateral loss of the sense of smell (anosmia, p. 666). These signs may be missed in a routine examination. It is important, therefore, to search for them when confronted with a patient with early mental changes.

*The Precentral Gyrus.* Lesions in this region give rise to unequivocal signs. Jacksonian epilepsy (p. 677) occurs and monoplegia readily develops. A lesion such as a meningioma arising from the falx cerebri involving the superior ends of both 'motor areas' may give rise to signs of an upper motor neurone lesion in both lower limbs, the upper limbs being spared. When a lesion in the dominant hemisphere extends forwards from the inferior end of the precentral gyrus it gives rise to dysphasia of expressive type.

*The Parietal Lobe.* Lesions of this area may also present with Jacksonian epilepsy, but of sensory type, and in addition there is disturbance of the integrative and localising aspects of sensation on the opposite side of the body.

Lesions situated more posteriorly in the parietal lobe may cause:

1. Spatial disorientation — lack of the patient's ability to find his way about.
2. Apraxia — loss of the ability to perform a pattern of movements though the patient understands its purpose and has no motor or sensory deficit.
3. Agnosia — loss of the ability to recognise a previously familiar object though the patient has good vision and sensation.
4. 'Sensory inattention' or 'perceptual rivalry' — the patient tends to ignore a cutaneous or visual stimulus on the contralateral side presented simultaneously with one on the same side as the lesion, though it is perceived if presented alone. This is most prominent in disease of the non-dominant hemisphere.
5. Receptive dysphasia — lesions of the angular and marginal gyri or the posterior

temporal-parietal junction cause receptive dysphasia which may be predominantly for written or spoken speech. There may be specialised types of dysfunction such as the loss of ability to count or to recognise parts of the body such as a particular finger.

6. Homonymous hemianopia — deep posterior lesions in the parietal lobe may involve the optic radiation and so cause a contralateral homonymous hemianopia.

*The Occipital Lobe.* Irritative lesions cause crude visual hallucinations such as flashing lights, while destructive lesions cause a contralateral homonymous hemianopia.

*The Temporal Lobe.* Irritative lesions in the posterior temporal lobe may cause visual sensations which are more elaborate than with occipital lobe irritation. Patterns of moving colours or hallucinatory pictures may be experienced by the patient. A similar lesion of the anterior part of the temporal lobe may cause auditory hallucinations (superior temporal gyrus), gustatory and olfactory hallucinations (uncus) or misinterpretations (illusions) of auditory and visual sensations. These are often associated with altered states of consciousness such as dreamy states, automatic behaviour, temporary upsets of memory (*déjà vu* p. 677) or brief amnesia. In affections of the dominant hemisphere there may be dysphasia of receptive type. An important sign easily overlooked is a homonymous upper quadrantanopia due to destruction of the lower fibres of the optic radiation which sweep down into the temporal lobe (Fig. 14.4).

## The Cerebrospinal Fluid

The cerebrospinal fluid (CSF) is secreted by the choroid plexuses in the lateral, third and fourth ventricles. It leaves the ventricular system through apertures in the roof of the fourth ventricle and flows through the cerebral and spinal subarachnoid spaces. It is returned into the venous sinuses by the arachnoid villi. In health, the fluid is clear and colourless. The pressure in the lumbar subarachnoid space with the patient lying on one side is 50–150 mm of cerebrospinal fluid. A lumbar puncture should not be performed in the presence of raised intracranial pressure.

The CSF provides useful information in a number of conditions and is invaluable in the diagnosis of acute and chronic inflammatory diseases of the nervous system. A large number of polymorphonuclear leucocytes is found in bacterial meningitis and a smaller number in the earliest stages of tuberculous and viral meningitis. A lymphocytosis accompanies viral meningitis and encephalitis, tuberculous meningitis and neurosyphilis.

A rise in the total protein content of the CSF is a non-specific finding in many neurological diseases. Very high values are associated with a complete block within the subarachnoid space, with neurofibromas and with Guillain-Barré polyneuropathy. A rise in the IgG fraction of the CSF protein is a feature of multiple sclerosis, neurosyphilis and connective tissue disorders. A rise in the glucose content of the CSF reflects the hyperglycaemia of diabetes. Glucose is absent or very low in pyogenic meningitis and reduced in tuberculous and carcinomatous meningitis. Appropriately stained smears and cultures of the CSF often define the infecting agent in cases of meningitis.

**Hydrocephalus** denotes an excessive amount of CSF within the cranial cavity. It may be a consequence of atrophy of the brain parenchyma, which results in passive dilatation of the ventricles; it is then called compensatory hydrocephalus.

Hydrocephalus may, rarely, result from oversecretion of CSF due to a papilloma of the choroid plexus. Much more commonly it is caused by obstruction to CSF circulation or to a failure of absorption. Obstruction may occur anywhere within the ventricular system due to an intraventricular tumour or from extrinsic compression due to a space-occupying lesion or oedema. The narrow channels in the third ventricle, aqueduct and fourth ventricle are particularly likely to be occluded. Inflammatory exudate may block the foramina in the fourth ventricular roof or occlude the subarachnoid space. Absorption through the arachnoid villi may be prevented by thrombosis of the sagittal sinus.

Of particular interest is normal pressure (normotensive or low pressure) hydrocephalus. In this condition the ventricular system is dilated. The dilatation initially results from an obstruction to flow due to trauma, meningitis, or other cause. The initial lesion subsides. It is postulated that the force exerted outwards on the brain is proportional to the surface area of the ventricles. These having been dilated the force exerted on the brain, by fluid at normally innocuous pressure, is increased. The brain atrophies and the conditions for progressive ventricular dilatation and cerebral atrophy are established. Dementia and ataxia result. An operation which reduces CSF pressure by a shunt from a lateral ventricle to the superior vena cava sometimes improves the patient's dementia and ataxia.

## DISEASES OF THE CRANIAL NERVES

The cranial nerves are frequently involved in generalised disease of the nervous system. In addition, there are specific conditions affecting a single cranial nerve.

### The First Cranial Nerve

The olfactory nerve arises from olfactory receptors in the nasal mucosa. The fine first order fibres pass through the cribriform plate in the floor of the anterior fossa of the skull. They synapse in the olfactory bulb and second order neurones run to the olfactory area of the brain (the anteromedial part of the temporal lobe) and higher autonomic centres by the olfactory tract which lies under the orbital surface of the frontal lobe. Thus tumours of the frontal lobe may compress this tract and cause loss of the sense of smell (anosmia) on one side of the nose. The fragile fibres passing through the cribriform plate are readily damaged by head injuries.

### The Second Cranial Nerve

The anatomy and central connections of the optic nerve are described on page 662 and the visual field defect caused by a lesion of the nerve on page 663.

**Papilloedema** means swelling of the optic nerve head (optic disc). The main disorders causing papilloedema are: 1. Increased intracranial pressure due to lesions within the cranial cavity such as cerebral tumour, cerebral abscess, or meningitis. The rise in pressure of the cerebrospinal fluid causes distension of the subarachnoid space round the optic nerve and compresses the venous drainage of the retina.

2. Obstruction of the venous drainage from the orbit by thrombosis of the central vein of the retina, cavernous sinus thrombosis or, rarely, an orbital neoplasm.

3. Lesions of the optic nerve itself, some of them inflammatory, may also cause swelling of the optic disc which is usually then referred to as *papillitis*.

4. Diseases of the retinal arteries such as cranial arteritis.

5. Extracerebral conditions such as malignant hypertension and severe chronic respiratory failure.

The earliest manifestation of papilloedema is engorgement of the retinal veins, followed by an intensified pink colouration of the optic disc and blurring of its margin which usually begins on the nasal side. As swelling proceeds the physiological cup is obliterated and the whole optic disc may be elevated. If the papilloedema is severe and particularly when it is of rapid development, there may be accompanying haemorrhages abutting on to the disc (Plate II p. 531). If papilloedema is of long standing the disc becomes progressively paler as optic atrophy develops.

Often it is of clinical importance to differentiate the swelling due to raised intracranial pressure from that due to lesions of the optic nerve which present indistinguishable ophthalmoscopic appearances. The visual acuity is usually well preserved when papilloedema is due to raised intracranial pressure whilst optic neuritis usually causes marked loss of visual acuity. Papilloedema due to raised pressure gives rise to early enlargement of the blind spot; chronic severe papilloedema may be accompanied by peripheral constriction of the visual field. Optic neuritis is accompanied by a central scotoma.

**Optic neuritis** encompasses inflammatory, demyelinating and some vascular diseases of the optic nerve which, in common, cause loss of vision. In many cases pain in the eye, aggravated by movement and tenderness over the eye, precedes or accompanies the visual disturbance. There is loss of central vision and the direct reaction to light is impaired whilst the consensual light reflex is preserved. When the lesion lies anteriorly in the nerve there may be swelling of the optic disc (papillitis). Where the ophthalmoscopic appearances are normal, the lesion lies posteriorly and is called a *retrobulbar neuritis*. A light flash or a moving, patterned visual stimulus evokes potentials over the occipital lobe which can be recorded using an averaging computer. These *visual evoked responses* (V.E.R.) are delayed when there is optic neuritis and the prolonged latency persists, providing evidence of an earlier optic neuritis.

Optic neuritis is most commonly due to demyelination, itself usually a manifestation of multiple sclerosis, and in this condition recovery of vision within four to six weeks is usual. Rarer causes include vitamin deficiencies, syphilis and toxins, such as methyl alcohol.

The optic neuritis associated with vitamin $B_{12}$ deficiency and that accompanying excessive smoking of strong pipe tobacco (*tobacco amblyopia*) may have a common pathogenesis. Tobacco smoke contains cyanide which experimentally has been shown to cause demyelination. Hydroxocobalamin, derived from vitamin $B_{12}$, plays an important part in the detoxification of cyanide. If the intake of vitamin $B_{12}$ is low and cyanide ingestion is high, demyelination of the optic nerve is liable to occur. This is an important observation since tobacco amblyopia may effectively be treated by large doses of hydroxocobalamin.

*Nutritional amblyopia* is a progressive failure of vision due to a retrobulbar neuropathy which may occur in severe malnutrition. Sometimes in West Africans and West Indians the visual failure is associated with lesions of the spinal cord (p. 726).

**Optic Atrophy.** Loss of fibres in the optic nerve is followed by reactive gliosis and reduced vascularisation. These pathological changes are manifest clinically by pallor of the optic disc and may result from many causes including (a) optic neuritis from the various causes listed above; (b) pressure on the optic nerve by glaucoma, tumours, aneurysms etc.; (c) long-standing papilloedema; (d) thrombosis of the central retinal artery; (e) trauma.

## The Third, Fourth and Sixth Cranial Nerves

The *third nerve (oculomotor)* supplies all the external ocular muscles except the lateral rectus and the superior oblique. It also supplies the levator palpebrae superioris, the constrictor of the pupil, and the ciliary muscle. It may be involved in multiple sclerosis, meningovascular syphilis, diabetes mellitus, and cerebral aneurysms which may compress the nerve at several sites. The manifestations of a third nerve palsy are ptosis, diplopia, external deviation of the eye (divergent strabismus) due to the action of the unopposed lateral rectus muscle and defective ocular movement in the directions in which the muscles supplied by the third nerve move the eye. The patient complains of double vision but in a long-standing lesion one of the images is suppressed. A complete lesion of the third nerve also paralyses the constrictor of the pupil; consequently the pupil is large and fails to react to light (by the direct or consensual path) or on convergence.

The *fourth nerve (trochlear)* supplies the superior oblique muscle. A lesion of the nerve gives rise to defective movement and diplopia which is maximal when the patient attempts to look down with the eye turned inwards. The pupils are not affected. An isolated lesion of the nerve is rarely encountered, as usually there is also involvement of either the third or sixth nerve.

The *sixth nerve (abducent)* supplies the lateral rectus muscle of the eye. A lesion of the nerve causes diplopia due to inability to abduct the eye, and deviation of the eye medially (convergent strabismus) due to the unopposed action of the medial rectus muscle. The sixth nerve may be involved by pressure from an aneurysm in the cavernous sinus. Downward displacement of the brain stem due to raised intracranial pressure may stretch the nerve causing a lateral rectus palsy. The causal lesion may lie at a distance from the sixth nerve whose involvement in this manner constitutes a false localising sign.

### Squint

Squint (strabismus) may be paralytic or concomitant.

*Paralytic squint* is due to weakness of one or more of the extraocular muscles. Defective movement of the eye can be seen when the patient uses the weak muscle to move the eye, and this usually causes diplopia. The rules for identifying the paretic muscles causing diplopia or squint are:

1. The separation of the images is greatest when the patient attempts to look in the direction to which the paretic muscle should move the eye.
2. In this position, the most peripheral image is the 'false image' from the affected eye. It is identified by covering one eye with a green glass and the other with a red one.

*Concomitant squint* ('lazy eye') is due to failure to maintain the correct posture of an eye which is so defective in vision that its image is suppressed by the brain. There is no muscle paresis and both eyes are capable of full movements in all directions. The most common cause is an error of refraction during childhood. If recognised and properly treated with suitable spectacles the squint can be prevented, though a 'latent squint' often remains.

## Nystagmus

Nystagmus is a series of involuntary, rhythmic oscillations of one or both eyes. It may be manifest in horizontal or vertical planes or as a series of rotations of the eye about its central axis (rotatory nystagmus). The oscillations may be equal in speed and amplitude in both directions of movement (pendular nystagmus) or movement in one direction may be faster than in the other (jerking nystagmus). When there are fast and slow components, the direction of the nystagmus is arbitrarily defined by the direction of the fast component. When severe, nystagmus may be present on looking to the side opposite to the fast component — this is a measure of severity, not an indication of nystagmus to both sides. It may occur spontaneously or be induced in response to a stimulus such as rotation of the head. When testing for nystagmus it is important to keep the visual fixation point within the field of binocular vision. Some normal people show sustained fine jerking nystagmus at the extremes of lateral gaze, especially when fatigued.

Voluntary conjugate movements of the eyes depend on pathways descending from centres in the frontal lobe to brain stem structures which then relay impulses to the nuclei of the extraocular muscles.

### Types and Causes of Nystagmus

Pathological nystagmus results from impairment of the mechanisms controlling conjugate eye movements, namely gaze, fixation, vestibular, cerebellar and peripheral mechanisms.

*Gaze Nystagmus.* Voluntary conjugate movements of the eyes depend on pathways descending from centres in the frontal lobe to brain stem structures which then relay impulses to the nuclei of the extraocular muscles. Gaze nystagmus is usually due to lesions of the brain stem. The nystagmus is of jerking type. There is no nystagmus when the eyes are in the central position but it appears on deviation of the eyes laterally. The faster component is always in the direction of gaze.

A special form of gaze nystagmus involves only the abducting eye on conjugate lateral deviation of the eyes. This is called *ataxic nystagmus* and results from lesions of the medial longitudinal bundle in the pontine region. The ocular movements are dissociated. On looking to one side, the abducting eye shows coarse nystagmus. The other eye fails to adduct fully and if it exhibits nystagmus this is of smaller amplitude. This type of nystagmus is common in multiple sclerosis but also occurs in brain stem gliomata and Wernicke's encephalopathy.

*Fixation Nystagmus.* Reflex mechanisms enable the object of interest continuously to be viewed by the macular area of each eye even when the object is moving. These reflexes are mediated through pathways which run from the eye to the cortex of the occipital lobe and adjacent parietal lobe and to the superior colliculi of the brain stem. Fixation nystagmus is usually present when the eyes are in the mid position, i.e. gazing straight ahead. A common cause of fixation nystagmus (often called ocular nystagmus) is defective central vision which usually gives rise to pendular movements. Congenital visual defects produce this type of nystagmus. Rarely fixation nystagmus is associated with diffuse brain stem lesions.

*Vestibular Nystagmus.* Reflex adjustments enable the retinal images to be stabilised, even when the head is being moved in space: they are evoked by impulses arising in the semicircular canals of the labyrinth and these are relayed to the central vestibular systems via the vestibular nerve. Vestibular nystagmus may arise from lesions of the labyrinth or the vestibular nerve.

1. Disorders of the labyrinth. Imbalance between labyrinthine stimuli from the two ears leads to jerking movements of both eyes. If the lesion involves the end-organs in the semicircular canals or their central connections, nystagmus is precipitated by sudden movements of the head. Lesions of the otolith organs or their central connections cause nystagmus which occurs when the head is in a particular position.

Spontaneous nystagmus is present with acute lesions of the labyrinths but tends to subside in a few days or months. This tendency to adaptation may be seen during testing, as nystagmus, brought on by movement of the head or by caloric stimulation, is not maintained. It may be difficult to elicit again if the test is repeated. It is often associated with vertigo (p. 673) and this is also brief. Cochlear function is usually affected, causing tinnitus or deafness. Labyrinthine nystagmus may be caused by inflammatory diseases (serous or purulent labyrinthitis), degenerative middle ear disease, hypertension, atherosclerosis of the internal auditory artery, head injury and Ménière's syndrome.

2. Lesions of the vestibular nerve. Nystagmus due to lesions of the eighth nerve has the same features as labyrinthine nystagmus. It may be due to an acoustic neuroma or neuronitis. The latter is a short-lasting disease.

*Lesions of the Central Vestibular Systems and Cerebellum.* Spontaneous nystagmus, or nystagmus induced by head position or head movement may be found with brain stem lesions affecting the vestibular nuclei. Spontaneous nystagmus unaffected by head position and maximal on looking to the side of the lesion is found with some cerebellar lesions. The cerebellum also participates in the coordination of eye movements, as it does in the coordination of limb movements.

Central nystagmus often occurs without vertigo, but when nystagmus is present it tends to persist and neither the nystagmus nor the vertigo shows the adaptation which is a feature of a peripheral lesion. Central nystagmus and vertigo often occur without cochlear symptoms, and may be associated with other brain stem symptoms, such as diplopia, or with asynergia of the limbs or dysarthria if the lesion involves cerebellar connections. The nature of the nystagmus may be like that of peripheral vestibular lesions, but vertical nystagmus, or nystagmus which affects each eye differently, is always central in origin. It may be caused by multiple sclerosis, vascular lesions such as occlusion of the posterior inferior cerebellar artery, pontine and cerebellar tumours, encephalitis, syringobulbia, or as the result of toxic states of which alcoholism is the most common.

Postconcussional vertigo and nystagmus may be peripheral or central in type, and they are often precipitated by a particular posture of the head. Indirect disturbances of the vestibular nuclei may occur when the intracranial pressure is raised. Nystagmus is then a 'false localising sign'.

*Nystagmus Due to Muscle Paresis.* All the above mechanisms need an efficient effector apparatus and hence peripheral lesions of nerve or muscle may also lead to nystagmus. This common cause of nystagmus is often overlooked. If one or more of the extraocular muscles are weak, then the affected eye will manifest jerking nystagmus when it is moved by the weakened muscles. Thus a partial sixth nerve palsy will result in nystagmus in the affected eye on attempted abduction.

## The Fifth Cranial Nerve

The trigeminal nerve has an extensive sensory distribution through its three branches, the ophthalmic, maxillary and mandibular divisions. It supplies the skin of the face (excluding the angle of the jaw), the cornea, the sinuses, the mucous membrane of the nose, the teeth, the tympanic membrane and common sensation (but not taste) to the anterior two-thirds of the tongue. The motor division of the nerve innervates the temporal, masseter and pterygoid muscles which are responsible for the closure and opening of the jaw. The nerve fibres and nuclei may be involved within the brain stem by conditions such as syringobulbia and thrombotic lesions, and the peripheral nerve by localised pressure such as occurs in cerebral aneurysms in the region of the cavernous sinus, and by tumours of the cerebellopontine angle. The ganglion of the nerve may also be involved by herpes zoster, giving rise to the characteristic shingles lesion over the skin of the face and causing ulceration of the cornea when the ophthalmic division is involved.

## Trigeminal Neuralgia (Tic Douloureux)

This is a condition of unknown aetiology and without recognised histopathology which usually affects elderly people.

**Clinical Features.** Pain, usually paroxysmal and sharp, is the characteristic feature. It is confined to the distribution of the fifth nerve. The maxillary or mandibular divisions of the nerve are usually first involved and spread from one to the other is common but the ophthalmic division is rarely affected. Each paroxysm lasts for only a few seconds but the stab of pain may be followed by a dull ache, or frequent attacks following one another may make the pain appear to be of longer duration. The pain is precipitated by touching localised 'trigger zones' on the affected side of the face. A cold wind blowing on the face, washing the face, chewing or even talking may be sufficient to bring on an attack. Paroxysms may continue for days or weeks, after which a remission of equal or longer duration may follow, but remissions become shorter and less frequent as the disease progresses. The agonising pain commands the patient's full attention. It may provoke a spasm of the facial muscles. No abnormalities of fifth nerve function can be detected on examination.

When a typical history is volunteered by an elderly patient the diagnosis is obvious. If similar symptoms occur in a young person the possibility of multiple sclerosis needs to be considered. Facial pain, mimicking trigeminal neuralgia may rarely be a manifestation of basilar aneurysm or cerebral tumour, particularly of a neurofibroma of the fifth nerve itself. When the fifth nerve is implicated in disease processes, the pain is often continuous and there are usually signs of fifth nerve dysfunction; there may be associated disturbances of other cranial nerves or neural pathways.

**Treatment.** Carbamazepine (200 mg t.i.d.) is the most effective drug. Phenytoin (100 mg t.i.d.) is also useful and may with advantage be combined with carbamazepine. Either or both of these drugs will reduce the frequency and severity of the pain in the majority of patients. Clonazepam (1–2 mg t.i.d.) is a useful alternative. Long remissions may occur. If pain persists and remissions are rare or of short duration it is necessary to interrupt the central passage of pain impulses by injection of phenol or alcohol into a branch of the nerve, if neuralgia is localised, or into the Gasserian ganglion. Section of the sensory part of the fifth nerve or its descending root in the medulla has the disadvantage of requiring intracranial operation but permits sparing of corneal sensation which is difficult to achieve with injection of the ganglion. These procedures secure permanent relief but the face becomes anaesthetic. Loss of sensibility from the cornea demands that special care must be taken to avoid trauma with its danger of subsequent corneal ulceration.

## The Seventh Cranial Nerve

The facial nerve innervates the muscles of expression of the face and, through its chorda tympani branch, carries taste fibres from the anterior two-thirds of the tongue. Paralysis of the facial muscles may be due to: (1) lesion of the fibres of the upper motor neurones concerned with voluntary movement, (2) lesion of the fibres of the upper motor neurones concerned with emotional movement, (3) lesion of the lower motor neurones.

1. Upper motor neurone fibres originating in the lower part of the precentral gyrus are distributed to the part of the opposite facial nucleus subserving the muscles of the lower part of the face, and to the parts of the facial nuclei on both sides of the pons which supply the upper parts of the face. Accordingly, a lesion of the upper motor neurones affects more severely the voluntary movement of the lower part of the face, contralaterally. Weakness of the upper part (the orbicularis oculi and frontalis muscles) may occur transiently but is often absent because the lower motor neurones to the upper facial muscles are supplied by upper motor neurones from both hemispheres. The patient is unable to retract the angle of the mouth on command, but in smiling and talking the mouth may move well because emotional movement is controlled by upper motor neurones which are not those concerned with voluntary movement of the face.

2. Upper motor neurones concerned with emotional movement of the face take origin further forward in the frontal lobe and so may be damaged by a lesion which spares the fibres for voluntary movement of the face. Involvement of these fibres is revealed by defective movement of the angle of the mouth when the patient smiles, with preservation of the ability to retract the angle of the mouth on command.

3. Since the lower motor neurone is the final common pathway, complete damage to the facial nucleus or nerve abolishes both voluntary and emotional movements equally in upper and lower parts of the face. Lower motor neurone paralysis restricted to part of the facial muscles can occur only when the lesion is distal to the branching of the nerve, e.g. with disease of the parotid gland, through which the nerve passes, or in leprosy.

The most common cause of damage to the nerve proximal to its branching in the parotid gland is Bell's palsy but it may be damaged by disease of the brain stem, by an acoustic neuroma, or by inflammation during its passage through the middle ear.

### Bell's Palsy

This term should be restricted to cases of isolated facial paralysis of unknown cause. Bell's palsy is accompanied by oedema of the facial nerve within the facial canal. It has been suggested that the swelling may be due to a viral infection since minor epidemics of the condition occasionally occur. Swelling within the rigid facial canal results in pressure on the nerve causing paralysis of function and sometimes Wallerian degeneration.

**Clinical Features.** The condition occurs in both sexes at any age. The first symptom is often an ache in the region of the stylomastoid foramen which may persist for a few hours or 1 or 2 days. A unilateral facial paralysis then develops. The eye on the affected side cannot be closed and the mouth is drawn over to the opposite side so that often it may appear to the patient that there is a spasm of the normal side. Saliva and fluids may escape from the angle of the mouth. Food may collect between the teeth and the paralysed cheek when the patient is eating. The patient often complains that the affected side feels 'numb', but there is no objective impairment of sensation of the skin. In most instances the lesion is distal to the chorda tympani and facial paralysis is the only feature. In a minority of cases when the lesion lies proximal to the chorda tympani there will be loss of taste on the anterior two-thirds of the tongue and diminished salivation. When the lesion is proximal to the nerve to the stapedius, hyperacusis on the affected side is an additional complaint.

Physical examination reveals paralysis of the upper and lower parts of the affected side of the face. The lines of expression are flattened, the patient is unable to wrinkle the brow or whistle or retract the angle of the mouth. The eye on the affected side cannot be closed, and on attempting to do so the eyeball rolls upwards

**Treatment and Prognosis.** ACTH or oral steroids, if started early, increase the rate of recovery, maximum benefit being obtained if they are given within 48 hours of the onset of the palsy. Dexamethasone (2 mg t.i.d.) for five days is a suitable treatment. Recovery occurs in over 90% of patients, usually after 2 or 3 weeks and is complete after 2 to 3 months. Approximately 5% of patients have permanent loss of function and develop facial contractures and involuntary spasms of the facial muscles. Complete recovery is virtually certain if there is any return of voluntary movement within a week after the onset and is probable if recovery of function begins within a month. A guide to the prognosis is given by electrodiagnostic studies. If the voltage required to produce a contraction on the abnormal side is more than twice that on the normal side, Wallerian degeneration has probably occurred. This indicates a poor prognosis. However, a good response after stimulation of the facial nerve within a week of the onset indicates that there is merely a conduction block and complete recovery is likely. Recurrence of Bell's palsy is unusual.

## The Eighth Cranial Nerve

The auditory nerve has two components, the cochlear nerve which is concerned with hearing and the vestibular nerve which is concerned with the appreciation of the position of the head and its movement in space. It is impossible without special tests to differentiate lesions involving these nerves from lesions confined to their end-organs in the inner ear. Irritative lesions of the inner ear or of the cochlear nerve cause *tinnitus*, and destructive lesions *deafness*. Thus, tinnitus is often due to aural causes but it may be an early symptom of a neuroma of the eighth nerve (acoustic neuroma) which is the most important destructive lesion of the eighth nerve. It may also be damaged in meningitis, and by the toxic effects of streptomycin and kanamycin.

Irritative lesions of the vestibular part of the eighth nerve cause *vertigo* which is a subjective feeling of movement of the external environment or of the head. The movement may be rotatory or a feeling of displacement in one direction. Vertigo is accompanied by a disturbance of balance which usually causes the patient to seek support and, if sudden and severe, may throw him to the ground.

The most important causes of vertigo are:

1. *Cerebellar Lesions*. Vertigo may occur when the cerebellovestibular connections are involved but this symptom is not invariable.
2. *Brain-stem Lesions*. Atherosclerosis of the basilar artery, medullary infarction or syringobulbia may cause severe vertigo when they involve the vestibular nuclei. The vertigo may be produced by particular positions of the head.

3. *Lesions of the Vestibular Nerve*. An acoustic neuroma may damage the nerve and cause vertigo. Vestibular neuronitis is a more common cause; it is a benign short-lasting condition of unknown aetiology which may occur in epidemics.
4. *Aural lesions* of many kinds, including otitis media and Ménière's syndrome, cause vertigo. The labyrinth may be damaged in a head injury and the vertigo may then be most severe when the head is in a certain position, usually backwards and to one side. A similar type of positional vertigo may occur in brief paroxysms. It is a benign condition which may disappear after a few months. The labyrinth may be damaged by mumps and by drugs such as streptomycin, quinine and salicylates. Hearing is almost invariably affected when the lesion is labyrinthine rather than in the nerve or central connections.
5. *Ocular Lesions*. Diplopia may be accompanied by vertigo because the false projection of one image causes confusion regarding position in space.

### Ménière's Syndrome

Ménière's syndrome is characterised by recurrent paroxysms of vertigo associated with tinnitus and progressive nerve deafness. The cause is unknown but the condition is associated with dilatation of the endolymphatic system due to increase in the amount of endolymph. Many patients also give a history of migraine.

**Clinical Features.** The most common initial symptoms are progressive deafness and tinnitus which are frequently slight at the onset. Sooner or later vertigo occurs and is characterised by suddenness of onset and severity. It may develop so suddenly that the patient may fall, and at the height of the attack may be unable to stand. There is often accompanying nausea and vomiting, and there may be sweating, weakness and faintness. Deafness and tinnitus may be intensified during the attack which may last for a few minutes to several hours. Examination during an attack shows rotatory nystagmus and ataxia. Between attacks there is only nerve deafness with impaired vestibular function as shown by caloric tests. The frequency of attacks tends to decrease as deafness increases but the disease may last many years.

**Treatment.** No treatment will abort an episode of vertigo; during severe attacks the patient should lie still and may be helped by an intramuscular injection of 50 mg of chlorpromazine. Treatment is aimed at preventing or reducing the number of attacks and includes cinnarizine (15 mg t.i.d.), prochlorperazine (5 mg t.i.d.) and betahistidine (8 mg t.i.d.). All of these drugs are sometimes effective but none is consistently so. If attacks are frequent and disabling, destruction of the labyrinth by surgery or ultrasonics may be required.

## The Ninth, Tenth and Eleventh Cranial Nerves

These nerves are grouped together because isolated lesions of one nerve alone are rarely encountered. The glossopharyngeal nerve (IX) transmits taste and common sensation from the posterior one-third of the tongue and motor fibres to the pharynx; the vagus nerve (X) is the parasympathetic nerve for the viscera of the thorax and upper part of the abdomen and also supplies somatic motor fibres to the soft palate and the larynx; the spinal accessory nerve (XI) supplies the trapezius and sternomastoid muscles. Unilateral lesions disturb their somatic functions but do not appreciably affect visceral function. These nerves or their nuclei may be involved by disease of the medulla such as syringobulbia or in their course across the posterior fossa by neoplasms and basal meningitis. Lesions at the jugular foramen, such as thrombophlebitis of the internal jugular vein following suppuration in the skull or neck, may involve all three nerves as they emerge from the skull. Glossopharyngeal neuralgia is described on page 686.

## The Twelfth Cranial Nerve

The hypoglossal nerve supplies motor fibres to the muscles of one side of the tongue. Upper motor neurone lesions cause spastic contraction of the muscle fibres. The tongue is small and pointed but not atrophic. Articulation is defective (spastic dysarthria) especially for the lingual sounds. There is rapid recovery of function after a unilateral lesion of upper motor neurone type, but bilateral lesions cause permanent dysarthria. This may occur in motor neurone disease or in pseudobulbar palsy (p. 693). Lower motor neurone lesions cause wasting and fasciculation of the affected part of the tongue and, when protruded, the tongue deviates to the side of the lesion. It may be seen in motor neurone disease.

The lower cranial nerves may be involved by carcinoma of the nasopharynx spreading to the base of the skull so otolaryngological examination is necessary. All cranial nerves, but particularly those emerging from the base of the skull, may be affected by bone disease in that area, particularly by Paget's disease.

## The Cervical Sympathetic Fibres

The higher centres for autonomic functions in the hypothalamus are connected with some areas of the cortex, notably the orbital surface of the frontal lobe and the insula. From the hypothalamus sympathetic fibres descend through the brain stem and spinal cord to their lower neurones in the small lateral horn of the thoracic region of the spinal cord from which they pass into the anterior spinal roots from T1 to L2. Fibres destined for the head and neck emerge mainly through the first thoracic anterior root, and ascend in the cervical sympathetic chain, reaching their final destination by means of the plexuses in the walls of blood vessels. Stimulation of the cervical sympathetic fibres causes dilatation of the pupil, protrusion of the eye-ball and elevation of the upper eyelid; conversely paralysis of these fibres results in pupillary constriction, enophthalmos and ptosis (*Horner's syndrome*). In addition, sweating is impaired on that side of the face. These signs may occur in lesions of the brain stem such as syringobulbia and thrombosis of the posterior inferior cerebellar artery, in lesions of the cervical part of the spinal cord such as syringomyelia, and in lesions at the thoracic outlet such as bronchial carcinoma at the apex of the lung.

# THE EPILEPSIES

*Generalised Seizures (grand and petit mal); Focal or Partial Fits (temporal lobe and Jacksonian epilepsy); Status Epilepticus.*

An epileptic fit may be defined as a brief disorder of cerebral function, usually associated with a disturbance of consciousness, and accompanied by a sudden, excessive, electrical discharge of cerebral neurones. The electrical activity recorded by the electroencephalogram (EEG) is of high voltage relative to the background and results from an unphysiological, synchronous discharge of an aggregation of neurones.

The basic mechanism of epilepsy depends on a population of abnormal, hyperexcitable nerve cells. Such susceptible neurones are subject to excitatory and inhibitory influences from other sources. Excitatory chemical transmitters released from connecting nerve terminals tend to depolarize epileptic neuronal membranes; inhibitory transmitters lead to hyperpolarization of membranes. The discharge of the abnormal group of cells is governed by the balance at a given time between these two opposing factors. Acetylcholine is an excitatory transmitter. Gamma-aminobutyric acid (GABA) is an inhibitory transmitter and hence has anticonvulsant properties.

Epilepsy may be generalised (grand and petit mal) or focal (partial).

In *generalised seizures* loss of consciousness is accompanied by symmetrically synchronous EEG discharges. It has been suggested that generalised fits originate in midline diencephalic areas; the site of the abnormal discharge could be in the cortex and the generalised manifestations occur because of rapid spread to brain stem structures leading to loss of consciousness and then to the secondary evocation of bilateral discharges over the hemispheres.

In *focal (partial) fits* consciousness may be retained to some extent. The discharge arises in a localised area of the cortex; it may remain circumscribed or spread to adjacent cortical regions, to the opposite hemisphere via the corpus callosum or to the brain stem. In the latter case sequential activation of both hemispheres may result so that a fit, initially focal, may become generalised.

**Aetiology.** In many, perhaps the majority, of cases, epilepsy arises from causes which at present cannot be identified. This large category of cryptogenic or idiopathic epilepsy includes many cases in which generalised fits first occur in children whose relatives are similarly affected but also includes many other cases without a family history or with atypical fits.

Any intracranial disease may give rise to epilepsy, either as a manifestation of an active pathological process or as sequel thereof. Important causes of 'symptomatic' epilepsy include cerebral tumours, head injuries and cerebrovascular disease.

Fits may occur as a result of disease elsewhere than in the brain. Hypoglycaemia, hyperglycaemia, uraemia, heart block, ingestion or sudden withdrawal of alcohol or drugs are but a few of the conditions which may evoke seizures. About 5% of patients with epilepsy are sensitive to light, e.g. flicker, and, in many of these, attacks are induced by television.

**Clinical Features.** GRAND MAL (Tonic-clonic seizures). These fits conform to a stereotyped clinical pattern in which several stages may be recognised: (1) a *prodromal phase*, lasting hours or days, may warn the patient that an attack is impending. This is an occasional phenomenon and usually takes the form of a change of mood. (2) An *aura*, which is uncommon in grand mal fits. When it does occur, it is brief, usually being no more than an apprehension that a fit is about to happen or a 'feeling' in the epigastrium. (3) The *tonic stage*, which is an invariable part of a grand mal attack. At the onset of this stage the patient loses consciousness and, if upright, falls to the ground. A sustained, tonic spasm of all the musculature occurs and involves the respiratory muscles, so that air is forcibly expired through the partially closed glottis giving rise to a sound or 'cry'. This phase lasts 20 to 30 seconds and during this time respiratory movements are suspended so that cyanosis occurs. (4) A *clonic phase* in which the sustained tonic spasm gives place to interrupted powerful jerking movements of face, body and limbs. The movements of jaw and tongue cause saliva to froth in the mouth. This stage, also, lasts about half a minute. During the tonic and clonic stages the patient may bite and chew the tongue and may be incontinent of urine and, less often, of faeces. (5) The *stage of relaxation*: After movements cease, the patient lies in a flaccid comatose state which evolves into normal sleep. This phase often lasts only a few minutes but may be prolonged for half an hour or more. After regaining consciousness there is often a phase of variable duration wherein the patient is confused and may suffer from headache.

PETIT MAL. This term is often used imprecisely. It is best restricted to those cases showing a characteristic EEG pattern, namely bilaterally synchronous spike and slow wave complexes occurring at a frequency of three per second. This pattern occurs with three types of clinical manifestation:

1. The most common variety of attack takes the form of a transient loss of consciousness. The patient interrupts whatever he is engaged in and may stare blankly ahead. The whole episode usually lasts only 10 or 15 seconds, and is so brief and undramatic that it may pass unnoticed. Such 'absences' may occur very frequently in childhood. Petit mal invariably starts in childhood but may persist into adult life. Sometimes the attacks cease during adolescence or give place to grand mal fits.
2. Less commonly the brief loss of consciousness is accompanied by myoclonic jerking of the arms.
3. The least common type of attack is the akinetic seizure in which the patient falls to the ground unconscious but recovers consciousness, and is able to rise again, almost immediately.

FOCAL OR PARTIAL EPILEPSY. Since there are many neuronal regions from which epileptic discharges may originate there are many clinical variations of focal fits. Any focal discharge may spread to become generalised, and initially localised clinical disturbances may progress to mimic a grand mal fit. It is important, therefore, to establish the nature of the phenomena which occur at the onset of any form of seizure since these indicate the site of origin.

1. The *temporal lobe* is the commonest site of focal epilepsy. Most characteristic of the clinical manifestations are hallucinations of smell though these are uncommon; hallucinations of taste, hearing or sight also occur. Also indicative of temporal lobe fits are disturbances of memory including the *déjà vu* phenomenon. This refers to the patient's sensation of reliving an experience or a feeling of great familiarity with the environment. Sometimes these features are associated with intense emotional or mood changes.

In temporal lobe attacks consciousness is usually disturbed but not necessarily lost. The patient often maintains some contact with the surroundings but feels remote from them, often likening the experience to a dream-like state. Occasionally the patient during this state will carry out well-coordinated and apparently purposeful motor acts, even of a violent or antisocial nature, without any memory of such activity thereafter (*automatism*). Temporal lobe discharges do not always give rise to such distinctive clinical features and an EEG may be required in order to reveal the temporal lobe origin of seizures.

2. *Jacksonian epilepsy* is a term best restricted to fits in which clinical disturbance of function, initially confined to a circumscribed part of the body, spreads to involve adjacent areas. There is a relatively slow 'march' of clinical events which reflects the spread of the electrical discharge to nearby cortical areas. Motor seizures usually take the form of involuntary twitching or clonic movements which begin in part of a limb, spread to involve the whole limb, then perhaps the whole of one side of the body or the involvement may even eventually become bilateral. The extent of the spread is highly variable. Consciousness may or may not be lost. Sometimes after recovery

from a Jacksonian fit, the parts affected remain paralysed. This is called a *Todd's palsy* and if prolonged for more than an hour or two suggests that there is a structural lesion in or near the cortical representation of the paralysed part.

**Diagnosis.** Observation of an episode by a trained person is the best and most certain method of diagnosis, but is rarely possible. A good description by, and cross-examination of, an eyewitness furnishes useful, and often conclusive evidence. The patient's own account of the attacks and the circumstances attendant upon them will sometimes give diagnostic information. The EEG is not a substitute for this type of clinical assessment nor can an EEG, recorded between attacks, alone establish or refute a diagnosis of epilepsy. The EEG may be helpful in supporting a clinical diagnosis and may be of great value in localising a cerebral cause of symptomatic epilepsy.

After the diagnosis of epilepsy has been established the next stage is to assess its cause. In practice the most important aspect of this process is to recognise patients whose epilepsy is due to a structural or progressive lesion. Fits of recent onset, of focal nature, occurring in patients of middle age, would obviously suggest an underlying lesion, perhaps a tumour. Accompanying headache and neurological signs would strengthen such a suspicion. Fits occurring for the first time in the elderly are often due to cerebrovascular disease. They may be the result of infarction, but some are due to cerebral ischaemia secondary to cardiac arrhythmias in such conditions as the sick sinus syndrome (p. 156) which can be demonstrated by prolonged cardiac monitoring and controlled by the insertion of a pacemaker.

The history and examination will in most cases furnish pointers to the aetiology of fits and hence to the need for special investigations. An EEG and skull radiographs should be obtained in all cases. Before embarking on more traumatic investigations, the need for such tests should be appraised in the light of the clinical features. In many instances repeated observation of patients over a period is the most valuable and least distressing course of action.

**Treatment.** The care of the patient comprises social and psychological as well as pharmacological aspects. Patients and their relatives and too many of the general public believe that epilepsy bears a stigma. Many patients are more socially disabled by feelings of bitterness and aggression engendered by society's rejection than by their fits. Simple, rational explanations of the nature and causes of seizures should be given.

Restrictions should be kept to a necessary minimum. Children, in particular, are often in danger of being overprotected by their parents but until fits are well controlled it is unwise for children to cycle on public roads; nor should they swim alone at sea. An epileptic child should be educated at a normal school unless there is an intellectual deficit. An adult should be guided into an occupation in which neither the patient nor the community is put at risk by a propensity to fits. Exposure to moving machinery and work at heights should be avoided. The legal restrictions about driving should be explained to patients. In Britain no one who has suffered from fits may drive a motor vehicle until free of attacks during waking hours for 3 years. Continued treatment with anticonvulsants and the occurrence of nocturnal fits do not debar the patient from driving.

Note should be made of factors which precipitate attacks. Some patients have fits only during sleep, or when they are pyrexial. Others recognise that certain sensory stimuli, such as flickering light, or emotional disturbances trigger their seizures.

*During a fit* the patient should be protected from injury. It will rarely be possible to break the fall during a grand mal attack because the warning is too short. The patient should be moved away from fires and sharp and hard objects. A padded gag should be inserted between the teeth if this can be accomplished without force. The incident should be treated with a minimum of fuss. Embarrassment because of public attention is usually the most distressing aspect of a fit from the patient's viewpoint.

*Anticonvulsant drugs* will usually be needed to control fits. Phenytoin, phenobarbitone, primidone and carbamazepine are all effective in grand mal and focal epilepsy. The dosage needs to be tailored to the individual needs and responses of patients. Phenytoin and phenobarbitone have half-lives which are greater than twenty-four hours and can be given once daily. Carbamazepine and primidone should be given in divided doses twice or thrice daily. An average daily dose, for an adult, of phenytoin is 200 to 400 mg, and of phenobarbitone 60 to 120 mg daily. Primidone is given in a dosage between 750 and 1500 mg daily and carbamazepine between 600 and 1800 mg daily. Hepatic metabolism of these varies because of genetic differences, and when possible, drug levels in the blood should be monitored so that the patients can be adequately treated and toxic levels avoided. It is better to use one drug, rather than a combination; only if a single drug does not control fits should a further anticonvulsant be added. Phenytoin may be combined with phenobarbitone or carbamazepine, though, because of induced hepatic enzymes the serum level of phenytoin may be reduced when it is given concurrently with carbamazepine. Primidone and phenobarbitone should not be given together, since primidone is partially converted into phenobarbitone.

All of these drugs may cause drowsiness; they may also cause osteomalacia (p. 102) and folate deficiency resulting in megaloblastic anaemia. All have some teratogenic effect, which is probably most marked with phenytoin. Phenytoin also gives rise to gingival hyperplasia in children and coarsening of features in adults. Rarer toxic effects of phenytoin include lymphadenopathy and a syndrome mimicking systemic lupus erythematosus.

None of the above drugs is useful in the treatment of petit mal. Ethosuximide is probably the most useful drug in this condition in a dose between 750 and 1500 mg daily. Effective treatment should be guided by serum levels of the drug when possible. Ethosuximide occasionally causes nausea, drowsiness and rarely, leucopenia.

Sodium valproate differs in chemical structure from other anti-epileptic drugs. It seems to act, in part, by inhibiting the enzymatic breakdown of gamma-aminobutyric acid (GABA) and hence increasing its level within the brain. Sodium valproate is useful in the treatment of grand mal epilepsy, and is particularly effective in petit mal attacks but is of little value in focal epilepsy. It does occasionally cause potentially fatal liver necrosis and accordingly it would seem wise to restrict the use of sodium valproate to those patients who have mixed grand mal and petit mal attacks, and to those patients with petit mal who have not responded to ethosuximide.

Other drugs, such as diazepam, nitrazepam and clonazepam can also be used in the treatment of epilepsy.

*Status epilepticus* refers to a continuous succession of fits occurring without any period of recovery. It may be fatal if not rapidly controlled. It is commoner in childhood and in patients who have intracranial lesions but it may occur in all types of epilepsy if medication is irregular or is suddenly withdrawn.

Treatment should be prompt and energetic since status epilepticus constitutes a grave emergency. Adequate respiration must be maintained and the fits suppressed. Intravenous diazepam is probably the most useful drug for the control of status epilepticus. Initially 20 mg should be injected intravenously and this should be repeated at five minute intervals until the fits are controlled; thereafter the drug is given by slow intravenous infusion for as long as necessary. In those rare instances where diazepam does not control status epilepticus, chlormethiazole can be given intravenously. Thiopentone and clonazepam are also used for the control of status epilepticus; the intravenous use of these anticonvulsants should be restricted to those situations where facilities for artificial respiration are available.

### Narcolepsy

This is characterised by irresistible attacks of sleep from which, however, the patient can be aroused immediately. The patient may go to sleep at work, and several attacks may occur in a day. Narcolepsy is associated with three other phenomena; *cataplexy*, in which, as a result of a sudden emotion, power is lost from the limbs, though consciousness is preserved; *sleep paralysis*, in which on waking or falling asleep the patient is unable to move though mentally wide awake; *hallucinatory states*, in which vivid and terrifying hallucinations occur, often just as the patient is falling asleep. This combination of symptoms may be associated with disease in the region of the hypothalamus. In most cases no abnormality can be demonstrated in the nervous system. Amphetamine sulphate (5–10 mg b.d.) or methylphenidate hydrochloride (10 mg b.d.) reduce the frequency and intensity of narcolepsy. Cataplexy often responds dramatically to treatment with a tricyclic antidepressant such as imipramine (50 mg t.i.d.). However, tricyclics and amphetamines should not be given together. Which drug is used will depend on whether narcolepsy or cataplexy is the patient's principal disability.

## CEREBRAL TUMOURS

Intracranial tumours account for 2% of deaths at all ages. Neoplasms classified histologically as malignant and benign occur but the implications of these categories differ from those in other sites. Since they grow within the rigid confines of the skull all types of neoplasm may cause disability and death by impinging on and displacing the cranial contents. The clinical features produced by an intracranial tumour depend primarily on its site of origin and its rate of growth. The histological characteristics of tumours offer a guide to rapidity of growth and to the possibility of complete removal.

**Pathology.** Malignant cerebral tumours rarely give rise to extracerebral metastases, but approximately a half of all brain tumours are secondary deposits from carcinoma elsewhere, particularly in bronchus and breast.

Of primary cerebral tumours those derived from glial cells are the commonest. These vary in cellular type, in degrees of malignancy and in rates of growth. An astrocytoma Grade 1 is a slow-growing, infiltrative tumour which may spread widely throughout the brain, sometimes for years, before causing serious disability. A Grade 4 astrocytoma (also called a glioblastoma multiforme) is a highly malignant, fast-growing tumour causing rapid clinical deterioration. Other glial tumours such as oligodendroglioma and ependymoma are graded from 1 to 4 as the degree of malignancy increases. Medulloblastoma occurs most commonly in children, arises usually in the cerebellar vermis, and is almost always highly malignant. The various types of glioma account for a quarter of all cerebral tumours. They can rarely be completely excised.

Meningiomas comprise approximately one-fifth of intracranial tumours. They are almost always benign, encapsulated, attached to the dura mater and, in the majority of instances, completely removable. Their common sites of origin are the convexities of the hemispheres, the sphenoidal ridges, the suprasellar region and the olfactory groove.

Other less common tumours arise within the cranial cavity. Craniopharyngiomas (p. 461), adenomas of the pituitary gland (p. 461) and neuromas from the sheaths of the eighth and fifth cranial nerves are benign and potentially curable. Cerebral lesions resembling tumours also occur in cysticercosis, as hydatid cysts, in schistosomiasis and rarely in other helminthic infections.

Intraventricular tumours are rare but colloid cysts of the third ventricle and papillomas of the choroid plexus can cause raised intracranial pressure and are removable.

**Clinical Features.** Primary brain tumours occur at all ages with a maximal incidence in the fifth decade. Medulloblastomas are commonest in children. Acoustic neuromas usually present in the third and fourth decades. Glioblastomas and meningiomas are commonest in middle life. In general brain tumours in children are situated in the posterior fossa and in those over thirty, supratentorial tumours account for 85% of cerebral neoplasms.

Cerebral tumours produce symptoms and signs by their local effects and by causing alterations in intracranial pressure and hydrodynamics.

FEATURES DUE TO LOCAL INVOLVEMENT. The local effects of a tumour on adjacent cerebral tissue may cause paralysis of function and/or excitatory effects. The neural deficits produced by a neoplasm are dependent on the site of origin of the tumour. Lesions in the various lobes of the brain can cause the types of dysfunction outlined on pages 664 – 665. Vascular lesions affecting these same structures cause similar disturbances but those produced by tumours are characterised by the time course of their development. In general the focal disabilities produced by a tumour are of slow onset and are progressive. The rate of this progression is highly variable and depends on the rate of growth of the tumour and its nearness to neural structures whose interruption evokes clinical signs. Occasionally localised oedema in the brain tissue surrounding a tumour will cause a rapid progression of paralytic symptoms and the picture thus produced may mimic a cerebrovascular lesion. Sometimes, too, the initial manifestations of a metastatic tumour are of sudden onset, followed by a period of improvement. Rarely, haemorrhage into a tumour causes an acute presentation of signs and symptoms which resembles a stroke.

In addition to local paralytic effects the infiltration by tumour cells of an area of cerebral cortex often evokes excitatory responses in neighbouring cerebral neurones. Thus a discharging epileptic focus may be a manifestation of a cerebral tumour. The nature of the fit produced is variable and depends on the site of origin of the epileptic discharge and the extent of its propagation. Focal epilepsy beginning in adult life should always suggest the possibility of a tumour.

Headache is a common, but not invariable manifestation of cerebral tumour. The tumour mass tends to distort and exert traction on nearby arteries, venous sinuses or meninges which are pain sensitive structures. Headache is often localised to one area of the cranium and its site offers a rough guide to the location of the tumour. In general headache is felt on the same side as the neoplasm. Tumours which lie in the anterior and middle cranial fossae are often attended by headaches situated in front of a line joining the ears. Posterior fossa tumours usually cause headaches which are felt over the occiput or nuchal area. There are many exceptions to these generalisations. Headache commonly accompanies an increase in intracranial pressure; its features are discussed below.

FEATURES DUE TO INCREASED INTRACRANIAL PRESSURE. Since cerebral tumours occupy space within the rigid skull they may cause an increase in pressure within the cranium. The liability of tumours to do this varies and several mechanisms may be involved. The mass of the tumour itself, if large enough, will cause a rise in pressure due to relative incompressibility of the brain. Slowly growing tumours may achieve large size before there is any rise in pressure whereas a highly malignant and rapidly growing tumour, though relatively small, may cause early changes. Raised intracranial pressure may also result from obstruction to the flow of cerebrospinal fluid. Subtentorial tumours are particularly liable to do this but even supratentorial lesions may cause obstruction to the foramina of Monro and tumours of the temporal lobe may compress the third ventricle. Tumours lying within the ventricles themselves may cause a sudden rise in intracranial pressure in the absence of focal neurological abnormalities. Increased pressure may also occur as a result of cerebral oedema or from obstruction of the cerebral venous system by malignant tissue impairing the absorption of CSF. Whichever of these mechanisms is operative the end result is a rise in pressure within the skull causing similar clinical features.

*Headache* is an almost invariable accompaniment of increased intracranial pressure; the pain is felt diffusely over the head and is aggravated by manoeuvres which cause a further rise in intracranial pressure. The headache is intensified by bending, coughing and straining at stool. Such headaches often tend to be particularly troublesome on waking in the morning when the patient is lying flat and to be relieved to some extent when the patient stands upright and moves about since this causes a fall in intracranial pressure.

There is often *clouding of consciousness*, varying in degree from listlessness and drowsiness to deep coma, depending both on the level of the raised pressure and the rapidity of its attainment. During the early stages of this alteration in consciousness there may be behavioural and personality changes with apathy and irritability, or withdrawal and inattention, predominating.

*Generalised epileptic fits* are commonly produced by raised intracranial pressure from tumours at any site.

Many patients with increased intracranial pressure complain of *dizziness* which may take the form of true rotatory vertigo or of sensations of light-headedness or unsteadiness. Such feelings of instability are often produced or aggravated by head movement.

*Papilloedema* is one of the most significant signs of raised intracranial pressure (p. 666). It may be of insidious onset and slow progression but equally often a sudden rise in pressure due to cerebral oedema or obstructive hydrocephalus causes the rapid development of papilloedema attended by haemorrhages radiating out from the optic disc. The amount of visual disturbance produced by papilloedema is variable. Often there is little change in the visual acuity but the production of transient blurring of vision when the patient stoops or bends is characteristic. Swelling of the optic nerve head is usually bilateral but may be unilateral in the early stages. When the underlying lesion has caused optic atrophy in one eye papilloedema occurs only in the other eye. Such is the case sometimes with tumours of the inferior surface of a frontal lobe which compress the adjacent optic nerve causing optic atrophy; as the tumour grows in size raised intracranial pressure supervenes and papilloedema occurs in the other eye. This is known as the *Foster Kennedy syndrome*.

*Vomiting* and progressive *bradycardia* occur as the intracranial pressure continues to rise.

*Complications.* The rise in intracranial pressure does not necessarily occur evenly over the whole of the cerebral contents and sudden alterations in pressure relationships within the skull may lead to displacement of parts of the brain. Large supratentorial lesions may cause herniation of the hippocampal gyrus and the upper brain stem downwards through the incisura of the tentorium. This not only causes damage to the hippocampal gyrus itself but may also lead to compression of the cerebral peduncles, occlusion of the posterior cerebral artery and stretching of cranial nerves, particularly the sixth nerve.

These developments themselves cause signs which may lead to erroneous localisation of the cerebral tumour. They are called *false localising signs*. Commonest of these is a sixth nerve palsy occurring on the side of the lesion or bilaterally. The third nerve may similarly be involved and occasionally the fourth nerve is also implicated. The cerebral peduncle on the side opposite the tumour may be compressed giving rise to pyramidal tract signs on the side of the lesion. Compression of the posterior cerebral artery may lead to a homonymous hemianopia or quadrantanopia. Very rapid downward movement of the brain stem may lead to haemorrhage in the mid-brain with coma and death.

Another form of herniation or 'pressure cone' is the downward movement of the cerebellar tonsils so that they impact within the foramen magnum thus compressing the medulla. This may lead to further aggravation of raised intracranial pressure since the onward passage of cerebrospinal fluid into the spinal subarachnoid space is blocked. Such an event is often manifest by loss of consciousness and the rapid development of palsies of the sixth and third nerves with dilatation of the pupil on the side of the lesion being followed by dilatation on the opposite side. Frequently when a medullary pressure cone has occurred the patient takes up a decerebrate posture, at first intermittently. These developments almost invariably lead to death.

Such brain displacements and pressure cones may occur spontaneously because of increased cerebral oedema or some other alteration in cerebral haemodynamics caused by the tumour's growth but are particularly liable to be produced if the closed CSF system is disturbed by lumbar puncture.

**Investigation** of cerebral tumours should, in most instances, begin with simple and non-traumatic procedures which may obviate the need for more specialised techniques or indicate which would be the more apposite to a particular case.

*Radiography.* A chest radiograph may reveal a bronchial carcinoma and hence enable the metastatic nature of a cerebral tumour to be inferred.

A skull radiograph will rarely give definitive information about cerebral tumours but should never be omitted since occasionally it will reveal very significant abnormalities. Some slow growing tumours in the brain calcify and hence are visible on a radiograph of the skull. Erosion or thickening of the skull bones may point to an underlying malignant tumour or a meningioma respectively. A calcified pineal gland may be displaced from the midline by a tumour. Raised intracranial pressure may give rise to erosion of the clinoid processes which may also result from tumours arising near the pituitary. The pituitary fossa may be expanded by an adenoma therein.

*Computed Tomography.* The sensitivity of the method enables a clear distinction to be made between grey matter, white matter and CSF within the ventricular system, as well as between pathological changes in the brain. Lesions are seen as alterations of normal density. Increased density is produced by meningiomas, low grade astrocytomas, calcium in the walls of aneurysms and blood clot. Density is lowered below normal levels in tissue necrosis (e.g. infarction), oedema, cysts and haemorrhage before clotting has occurred. The density of some lesions, notably tumours, may be enhanced by the intravenous injection of substances containing large atoms (such as sodium iodothalamate). Computed tomography is of particular value in the diagnosis of dementia by distinguishing between cerebral atrophy, hydrocephalus and cerebral tumour.

*Electroencephalography*. Abnormally slow waves may localise a tumour in the cerebral hemispheres. Diffuse slowing may arise as a result of raised intracranial pressure from tumours situated above or below the tentorium.

*Echoencephalography*. Ultrasonic waves are reflected back from midline structures in the brain and displayed on a cathode ray tube. Displacement of these structures can be shown and hence space-occupying lesions can be lateralised. The procedure is simple and rapid in execution and can be carried out at the bedside.

*Radioisotope Scanning*. Isotope-encephalography depends for its effectiveness on a concentration, greater in cerebral tumours than in normal brain tissue, of an isotope (usually technetium) given intravenously. It is particularly successful in meningiomas, less accurate in gliomas and least effective in metastatic tumours and those tumours situated in the posterior fossa.

*Cerebrospinal Fluid*. Lumbar puncture should rarely be carried out if there is evidence of raised intracranial pressure and never in such circumstances unless neurosurgical help is rapidly available. If there is clear evidence of a space-occupying lesion in the brain, examination of the CSF is usually unnecessary and unhelpful. Where a meningitic picture is present and no tumour mass can be demonstrated the diagnosis of carcinomatosis of the meninges may be made by examination of the CSF, whose sugar content is reduced and which may contain tumour cells.

*Arteriography*. The intracranial vessels, outlined by a radio-opaque dye injected into the carotid or vertebral arteries, may be displaced in the region of a tumour, and the appearance of the vessels may indicate the pathological nature of the lesion. The procedure is relatively safe and does not upset the balance of intracranial pressure as does pneumoencephalography.

**Treatment.** *Medical treatment* of tumours can never be anything more than temporary or palliative. Medical measures for relief of raised intracranial pressure are often demanded in circumstances when surgery is not available or when the patient's life is threatened before investigation has revealed the diagnosis. This can best be achieved by the administration of dexamethasone 4 mg four times daily, initially given by injection and later by mouth; striking improvement in a patient's conscious level is often produced and sometimes regression of focal disabilities. The use of intravenous hypertonic solutions has largely been supplanted by treatment with dexamethasone but the intravenous administration of 50% sucrose or of a 15% solution of mannitol or of a 30% solution of urea can produce marked but short lived reduction of intracranial pressure.

Cytotoxic drugs, such as cyclophosphamide, administered either systemically or through a carotid artery, offer little more than temporary palliation.

*Surgery* is the definitive treatment of intracranial tumours. When possible the whole of a tumour should be excised but complete removal of the tumour depends on a number of factors. The tumour may be inaccessible and thus its exposure may be attended by unacceptable brain damage. It may invade areas where excision of small amounts of tissue may cause major disability as is particularly likely to happen in the brain stem or in areas of the dominant hemisphere.

In general, benign tumours such as meningiomas and neuromas offer the best prospects for complete removal without unacceptable damage to vital structures. Meningiomas can usually be totally excised and rarely is there any recurrence. Meningiomas of the olfactory groove, those in the suprasellar area and those over the convexity of the hemispheres have a particularly favourable prognosis. Often, meningiomas of the inner part of the sphenoidal ridge and within the cerebellopontine angles cannot be completely removed but their partial excision results in long continued improvement. Even after a successful removal of a meningioma, a number of patients may develop recurrent fits.

Craniopharyngiomas can sometimes be completely removed but often the closeness of the hypothalamus prevents total excision. Pituitary adenomas can usually be extirpated and even when only incomplete excision is possible further visual loss is prevented.

Colloid cysts of the third ventricle and other intraventricular neoplasms can often be removed but sometimes their complete excision is technically very difficult.

Malignant gliomas cannot be removed completely though favourably situated tumours may benefit markedly for a time from partial removal.

Less malignant slow growing tumours such as Grade 2 astrocytomas and oligodendrogliomas, though they can rarely be completely excised, may benefit for many years from partial removal. The prognosis for cystic astrocytoma is particularly good if the cyst is drained and as much as possible of the tumour removed. Medulloblastoma of the cerebellar vermis, found in childhood, cannot be completely excised and surgery produces little improvement.

There is a place for palliative surgery even when complete excision of a tumour cannot be attempted. Partial removal or drainage of a cyst is often of benefit. Decompression and hence relief of raised intracranial pressure may be produced by removing part of the tumour, excising normal brain tissue in the frontal or temporal lobes. Removal of part of the skull vault is also effective in reducing pressure. Internal hydrocephalus may be relieved by a short-circuiting procedure in which a drain is placed in one of the lateral ventricles and led into the cisterna magna.

**Prognosis.** The precise surgical approach and the prognosis for a cerebral tumour can be assessed only in the light of its site, its pathological nature, its blood supply and the degree of disability it causes. Early treatment is particularly important for those tumours which are susceptible to complete removal and which menace life or sight. Early diagnosis of acoustic neuromas and pituitary tumours markedly improves the outlook for their treatment.

Death is inevitable if a malignant tumour cannot be removed though it may be postponed by palliative decompression; even so, the average expectation of life is less than six months in the case of the more malignant growths. Benign tumours can be removed completely if they grow in an accessible part of the brain, as can gliomas, or even a solitary metastatic tumour, when they are in a part of the brain such as the frontal lobe or cerebellum which can be sacrificed with relative impunity.

## Headache

Headache is a term which literally describes pain felt anywhere in the head. Custom usually restricts its usage to pains in the region of the cranial vault; facial pain and nuchal aches are excluded, but the lines of demarcation are vague and overlapping.

Headache poses certainly the commonest, probably the most ambiguous and sometimes the most difficult clinical problem in medicine. It has a multiplicity of causes but is produced by relatively few mechanisms. In the vast majority of cases the cause is trivial and reversible but in a few patients headache presages sinister intracranial disease.

The extracranial coverings and arteries are sensitive to pain. Within the cranial cavity there are few pain sensitive structures. The brain parenchyma, pia-arachnoid, ventricular linings and choroid plexuses are insensitive. Pain can be evoked from the venous sinuses, the arteries and the dura mater at the base of the brain. Displacement and distortion of these structures, particularly if rapid, cause headache. The fifth, ninth and tenth cranial nerves contain pain fibres and direct compression of these nerves produces pain.

**Clinical Features.** Pain in the head may be due to lesions in nearby structures, such as the eye and ear, causing referred headache; it may be due to the cranial neuralgias, meningeal irritation, vascular disturbances, traction and distortion of intracranial structures, or to psychogenic causes.

*Referred Headaches.* Eye diseases such as glaucoma and iritis cause frontal headache. Ciliary spasm induced by some errors of refraction may cause pain but 'eye strain' is certainly not a common cause of headache. Nasal and sinus disease causes pain in the malar, nasal and frontal areas which responds to vasoconstriction in the form of nasal drops. Dental and aural conditions may cause pain spreading far beyond the area of primary pain. Occipital headaches occasionally result from severe cervical spondylosis. A cold stimulus on the soft palate in some people evokes a dull, frontal headache (ice-cream headache).

*Cranial Neuralgias.* The episodic, lancinating pain of trigeminal neuralgia (p. 671) and the continuous, burning pain of postherpetic neuralgia (p. 711), both occurring within the distribution of the fifth cranial nerve, present well-defined and usually easily-recognised entities. Less common is *glossopharyngeal neuralgia* in which pain, usually of a stabbing character, is felt in the pharynx and deep in the ear. The pain occurs in bouts and may be triggered by swallowing and talking. It responds to treatment similar to that given for trigeminal neuralgia. There are a number of facial neuralgias and pains which present inconsistent and vague patterns of affection. *Temporomandibular neuralgia* arises as a result of derangement of the temporomandibular joint secondary to an alteration of the bite caused by loss of teeth, ill-fitting dentures or habitual overclosure of the jaws because of tension. Pain which varies from a dull ache to intense stabs may radiate from the region of the affected joint to the temporal and frontal areas, the cheek, lower jaw and occasionally to the neck. In malocclusion, a prosthetic device to prevent overclosure of the jaw is a simple and usually effective treatment.

Other types of atypical facial pains of variable characteristics occur, particularly in the elderly. They defy categorisation and some patients present individual patterns of discomfort over long periods which are resistant to all forms of treatment.

*Meningeal Irritation.* Headache is an almost invariable accompaniment of encephalitis and meningitis. It is probable that meningeal inflammation lowers the pain threshold of the pain-sensitive structures at the base of the brain so that minor mechanical stimuli produce headache. The headache is usually generalised though it may be more intense in the occipital region, is of a continuous aching or boring character and is frequently associated with photophobia and drowsiness. The pain is increased by exertion and even by minor movements of the head; the accompanying pyrexia and neck stiffness usually make the diagnosis obvious.

Blood in the CSF due to subarachnoid haemorrhage produces headaches and neck rigidity similar to those of meningitis, but the pain in this condition is characteristically of abrupt and even explosive onset and may be accompanied by loss of consciousness.

*Vascular headaches* are almost always described as throbbing in character and are aggravated by head movements. They may arise from dilatation of the intracranial or extracranial arteries in 'hangovers', fever and the hypercapnia of respiratory failure. Severe arterial hypertension may cause headaches in the early morning. In the elderly localised temporal headache may be due to cranial arteritis.

The commonest form of vascular headache is migraine (p. 688). A migrainous variant, *'cluster' headache*, presents a distinctive picture, which is unilateral, intense and brief. Many attacks occur in quick succession during a period of a few hours or a few days, and then there is often a prolonged period of freedom, hence the name 'cluster'. The pain is usually severe and burning, primarily involves the frontal region and the eye but often spreads to the face and sometimes to the neck. It occurs most commonly in young males, characteristically wakes patients from sleep and is often accompanied by flushing of the skin, rhinorrhoea and injection of the conjunctival vessels. It is thought to be due to histamine sensitivity and attacks can sometimes be precipitated by the subcutaneous injection of 0·3 mg of histamine. Patients sometimes respond to treatment with antihistamines and to the measures used in the treatment of classical migraine.

Rare causes of vascular headaches include saccular aneurysms and arteriovenous malformations (p. 695).

*Headaches Due to Traction on Intracranial Structures.* Headaches may occur in the presence of an expanding intracranial lesion such as cerebral tumour or subdural haematoma whether or not there is a generalised rise in intracranial pressure.

Traction headache due to reduced CSF pressure may occur after lumbar puncture; patients tend to develop their symptoms when standing or sitting and a recumbent posture produces rapid relief. Traction headaches whether produced by raised or lowered intracranial pressure are usually aggravated by bending, straining at stool and coughing.

Sometimes traction headache may be produced in patients who have raised intracranial pressure, unassociated with a space-occupying lesion, in the syndrome of *benign intracranial hypertension*, a rare condition usually occurring in obese women.

*Psychogenic Headache.* Rarely headache may be a feature of psychotic illness such as schizophrenia and it may occur in conversion hysteria. Most commonly, however, psychogenic headaches are associated with anxiety and depression, and other manifestations of these affective disorders may be present concurrently. Most patients suffering from psychogenic headache describe it as of 'pressing' character. Pain tends to be localised to the front of the head or to the vertex or it may involve the whole head. It is usually not prominent on waking in the morning and in most instances tends to get worse as the day wears on. It is often described as severe, continuous and unrelieved by analgesics.

**Investigation and Treatment.** The extent and nature of investigations to be employed are determined by the history. Non-traumatic procedures such as radiographs of chest and skull and computed tomography should precede more traumatic investigations. A detailed history followed by a meticulous examination will help not only to clarify the diagnosis but will also be therapeutic in patients suffering from psychogenic headache. Reassurance and explanation after careful clinical assessment of these patients is often more effective than analgesics.

## Migraine

Migraine is characterised by periodic headaches which are typically unilateral and are often associated with visual disturbance and vomiting.

**Aetiology.** The condition is believed to be due to a disturbance in the carotid or vertebrobasilar vascular tree. An initial phase of vasoconstriction causes symptoms of local cortical or brain stem ischaemia and this is followed by vasodilatation. These changes affect both intra- and extracranial arteries and it is dilatation of the extracranial vessels which causes pain by stretching the pain nerve endings in the arterial wall. Pain may be prolonged by secondary muscular contraction.

There is a genetic predisposition; approximately three-quarters of patients who suffer from migraine have close relatives similarly affected.

Migrainous attacks may be precipitated by a variety of factors such as menstruation, flashing lights, stress and anxiety. Cheese, chocolate, sherry and red wine are common precipitants and are all rich in tyramine; experimental ingestion of tyramine will often promote an attack. Reserpine, which liberates 5-hydroxytryptamine (serotonin) in the brain, can also cause migraine. It is of interest that some serotonin antagonists are helpful in treatment. The significance of these findings is not clear but it seems likely that, in some and perhaps many instances, migraine is mediated by one or more biochemical disturbances.

**Clinical Features.** The condition usually starts after puberty and continues until late middle life. Headaches occur in paroxysms and are often related to emotional stress. Attacks occur at intervals which vary from a few days to several months. The first symptom is due to vasospasm. This is commonly a sensation of white or coloured lights, scintillating spots, wavy lines, or defects in the visual fields. Paraesthesiae or weakness of one half of the body may be experienced or there may be numbness of both hands and around the mouth. These symptoms may last up to half an hour, and are followed by headache which usually begins in one spot and subsequently involves the whole of one side of the head; this may be the same or the side opposite to the visual or sensory symptoms. The side affected is not constant with each attack and the headache often becomes bilateral. The pain is usually severe and throbbing and is associated with vomiting, photophobia, pallor, sweating and prostration which may necessitate the patient taking to bed in a darkened room. The attack may last from a few hours to several days and it leaves the patient weak and exhausted. In rare cases the cerebral changes may last for several days, particularly if the motor area is involved (*hemiplegic migraine*).

Rare cases of headache resembling migraine are caused by a cerebral aneurysm or angioma ('symptomatic migraine'). In these cases the pain is unilateral and usually associated with focal signs.

**Treatment.** An attentive physician, a carefully recorded history and a meticulous examination followed by a full explanation of the nature and phenomena of migraine often relieves the patient's anxiety about the possibly sinister significance of the headache. These simple measures are themselves effective therapy as is the physician's continuing interest in the patient's well-being.

Neither the patient's personality nor the stresses and strains of life can be altered, but such trigger factors as flashing lights and dietary precipitants can be avoided.

If the patient suffers only occasional attacks of headache at intervals of months, it is probably unnecessary to embark on drug treatment. For those whose lives are disrupted by migraine, treatment should include prophylaxis together with appropriate treatment to abort the headaches.

There are numerous prophylactic treatments; all are inconsistently successful. Phenobarbitone, diazepam or pizotifen given thrice daily often reduces the frequency of headaches. Occasionally other drugs, such as monoamine oxidase inhibitors and tricyclic antidepressants are helpful. Methysergide, a serotonin antagonist, is sometimes effective but is prone to produce peripheral vasoconstriction and, rarely, retroperitoneal fibrosis; it should be used only in those patients who have not responded to simpler measures and whose attacks are very frequent, severe and disabling.

Treatment of a migrainous episode is based on the use of ergotamine, which should be given as early as possible during the premonitory stages either as ergotamine tartrate (1 mg) held under the tongue or in aerosol form. Unfortunately, all the oral methods of administration of ergotamine frequently produce nausea and vomiting. In such circumstances ergotamine suppositories are sometimes helpful and if the patient is capable of self-injection, ergotamine tartrate (0·5 mg) given subcutaneously or intramuscularly may effectively halt an attack. Too frequent use of ergotamine may, rarely, cause peripheral vasoconstriction. It should not be given during pregnancy, nor to patients with ischaemic heart disease or hypertension.

## CEREBROVASCULAR DISEASE

Intracranial vascular lesions are the third commonest cause of death in Western countries. The pithy and commonly used term 'stroke' describes the sudden neurological defect that often ensues. The annual incidence of strokes of various types is more than 1% in those over 65 years old. In every 1000 of the population in any one year, two people will suffer an initial stroke and one will die from a stroke. The high morbidity caused by cerebrovascular disease in the elderly is reflected in the large number of hospital beds occupied by such patients.

Despite the prevalence of the problem and its high cost in economic terms as well as human disability, cerebrovascular disease claimed, until recently, less attention and study than some rarer conditions. Diagnoses of 'cerebrovascular accident' or 'stroke' without specification are still common. Such imprecision in assessment leads to vagueness about prognosis and apathy in treatment. Conversely, attempts rigidly to link patterns of clinical disability to blockage of individual cerebral arterial branches have been shown to be simplistic and often misleading as well as therapeutically unrewarding.

Knowledge of the natural history of intracranial vascular disease is still incomplete. Cerebrovascular disease may be due to lesions of veins and capillaries as well as arteries but the latter are much the commonest. Arterial lesions can logically be divided into two main groups: (1) Ischaemic cerebral lesions due to reduced perfusion of brain tissue by blood and often resulting in infarction. (2) Haemorrhagic lesions in the brain or in the spaces between the brain and skull.

This division into ischaemic and haemorrhagic lesions is pathologically clear and although clinical differentiation is often difficult the two processes should be discussed separately.

### 1. Ischaemic Cerebral Lesions

**General Considerations.** Approximately a fifth of the cardiac output normally passes through the carotid and vertebral arteries to supply intracranial structures. A reduction in total cerebral blood flow to less than half of normal will impair cerebral function.

Occlusion of a cerebral artery usually, but not necessarily, leads to infarction in the tissue it normally supplies. A system of anastomoses and collateral channels affords a safety mechanism. The circle of Willis usually provides wide connecting channels between the two carotid arteries and the vertebrobasilar system. Perforating branches from the major cerebral arteries and from the circle of Willis pass through the brain to anastomose with capillaries derived from other branches of the anterior, middle and posterior cerebral arteries which ramify over the surface of the hemispheres and penetrate through the cortex. A similar anastomosis between centrifugal and centripetal twigs is found in the brain stem where the vertebral and basilar arteries give off penetrating and circumferential branches. At the junctions between their respective areas of supply the anterior cerebral artery anastomoses with the middle cerebral artery which in turn anastomoses with posterior cerebral branches. There are also collateral channels between the internal and external carotid circulations through their orbital branches.

These alternative routes of blood supply to the brain mean that the effects of impaired cerebral flow are determined by complex factors. Systemic hypotension tends first to produce ischaemia in the border zones between the anterior, middle and posterior cerebral arteries. Variations in this pattern occur if, in addition to generally reduced brain perfusion, there is a superimposed local blockage in one of the branches of the three major vessels.

If one internal carotid artery is occluded in the neck there is an immediate increase in flow through the other carotid artery. Young adults who sustain a blockage within one of the four major arterial trunks may manifest no ill-effects. However, the occlusion of one of these arteries in the neck in the presence of widespread arterial disease (a likely accompaniment in the elderly) may give rise to extensive infarction. The compensatory mechanisms are less effective more distally and occlusion of one of the deep penetrating branches arising from the circle of Willis often produces infarction of predictable extent.

The effects of any arterial obstruction depend, in part, upon the rate of its development. Sudden blockage is more likely to produce infarction than is the gradual reduction of an arterial lumen which allows time for the opening up of collateral channels.

Reduced blood flow is often attributed to arterial spasm. Cerebral vasoconstriction occurs in young people and is responsible for transient cerebral dysfunction in migraine and may, in this condition, rarely lead to infarction. Spasm also occurs if cerebral arteries are manipulated during operations and as a result of irritation during angiography and after a subarachnoid haemorrhage. Ischaemia may result from vasoconstriction due to hypertensive encephalopathy or to the concurrent ingestion of tyramine and monoamine oxidase inhibitors. There is, however, no evidence that arterial spasm plays any significant part in the production of ischaemia in elderly patients suffering from cerebrovascular disease.

Atherosclerosis is by far the commonest cause of reduced blood flow and arterial occlusion. Other causes are embolism and arteritis.

### Cerebral Atherosclerosis

Atheromatous changes in cerebral arteries are almost invariable findings in people over 60 years old, but even quite extensive atheroma is commonly symptomless.

Atheromatous plaques may cause narrowing (stenosis) or may lead to thrombosis and occlusion of arteries. Fibrin, platelet and lipid emboli may arise from such plaques in the proximal vessels including the aorta and be carried distally in the cerebral circulation eventually to impact in small vessels. These mechanisms can cause localised ischaemia or infarction or a generalised, progressive loss of brain tissue.

**Aetiology.** There is an association between cerebrovascular disease and ischaemic heart disease. In those patients who suffer an attack of transient cerebral ischaemia more people die from myocardial infarction than from cerebral infarction. Atheroma and thrombosis are related to both conditions. Despite this association the risk factors of cerebrovascular disease are not as well understood as those in myocardial ischaemia (p. 183) and there are notable discrepancies between the two. Genetic predisposition, hyperlipidaemia and diabetes seem to be much less important factors in cerebral than in myocardial infarction. Cigarette smoking and obesity have been clearly linked to an increased incidence of coronary arterial disease but not to liability to strokes. Hypertension is a factor which seems strongly to predispose to both.

**Clinical Features.** Symptoms are rare before the age of 40, and uncommon before 50. The clinical presentations comprise (1) a 'stroke', i.e. the rapid development of focal cerebral dysfunction, due to infarction, (2) a relatively slow, or stepwise, extension of an infarct — sometimes called a stroke-in-evolution, (3) transient ischaemic attacks wherein neural disability presents suddenly and recovers completely within 1 hour, (4) progressive, diffuse loss of cerebral functions. More than one of these patterns may be manifest in a single patient. After a series of transient ischaemic attacks a patient may present with a completed stroke which may also supervene during the course of progressive, diffuse cerebral atherosclerosis.

(i) STROKE. Haemorrhage and occasionally cerebral tumour, as well as infarction, may sometimes be the cause. When due to infarction, there are often premonitory features such as mild headache or malaise during the few days preceding a stroke.

The onset of focal disability may occur at any time. The patient may awake with an established lesion. Very frequently the deficit evolves during a period of 1 or 2 hours. Rarely the maximal level of disability will be attained within a few minutes and occasionally impairment will progress for 1 or 2 days. Loss of consciousness at the onset occurs in a minority of cases though drowsiness is common. Severe headache is unusual. Epileptic fits, sometimes of the focal type, occasionally occur at the beginning or during the extension of a stroke.

The neurological picture presented depends on the site of infarction. The area supplied by the middle cerebral artery is most commonly involved so that a hemiplegia involving the face, arm and leg on the side opposite the lesion is a frequent presentation.

If the paralysis develops very rapidly it may initially be of flaccid type, but spasticity and hyperreflexia are soon manifest and usually are detected from the onset. There may be loss of the visual half fields and hemianaesthesia on the side of the hemiplegia. If the infarct lies in the dominant hemisphere dysphasia may supervene. This familiar stroke pattern reflects the frequency of infarcts in the brain territory supplied by the middle cerebral artery but it should not be assumed that the causal lesion lies within this artery. In more than half of cases presenting this picture the primary lesion lies in the internal carotid artery or in more proximal vessels.

Other clinical presentations occur. An infarct within the area normally supplied by the anterior cerebral artery often causes a hemiplegia in which the leg is weaker than the arm and which may be accompanied by disturbance of micturition, apraxia or motor dysphasia. Lesions in the posterior cerebral territory usually lead to contralateral homonymous hemianopia with macular sparing and occasionally, if the thalamus is involved, diffuse, burning pain on the opposite side of the body. This thalamic syndrome may also result from infarcts in the area served by the anterior choroidal artery.

Approximately a tenth of infarcts involve the brain stem where they are more commonly accompanied by severe headaches than are those within the hemispheres. Vertigo, ataxia and vomiting, double vision and nystagmus are common features. A crossed paralysis, with ipsilateral affection of one or more cranial nerves and contralateral long tract (usually pyramidal) signs are characteristic of brain stem infarction.

(ii) STROKE-IN-EVOLUTION. The temporal pattern of a stroke is sometimes extended. Disability may increase by step-wise progression; sudden deteriorations are interspersed with static intervals. Less commonly there is slow uninterrupted progression; the deficit spreads and intensifies. The full extent of the patient's lesion may not be exhibited for 3 or 4 days; occasionally the disability may extend for 1 to 2 weeks. This type of clinical presentation, which suggests the diagnosis of a cerebral tumour, may be associated with occlusion of an internal carotid artery.

(iii) A TRANSIENT ISCHAEMIC ATTACK is a sudden deficit followed, within the hour, by complete recovery of function. Most such episodes last only a few minutes. If symptoms persist for more than 1 hour infarction has probably occurred. Symptoms depend on the site of ischaemia. Transient loss of vision in one eye and a hemiparesis or sensory disturbance affecting the contralateral half of the body are due to ischaemia in the carotid territory. Ischaemia affecting the area supplied by the vertebral and basilar arteries may cause vertigo, diplopia, hemiparesis or loss of consciousness.

The duration and frequency of transient ischaemic attacks are variable. Some patients suffer many attacks daily for periods of a week or more; attacks then cease and may not recur for months or years. Other patients have only occasional episodes at intervals of months. The attacks in an individual patient are usually stereotyped, the pattern and duration of dysfunction being repeated several times.

Many transient ischaemic attacks are due to emboli which arise from atheromatous plaques, are carried distally, lodge in and block small arteries and then break and disperse. In other cases flow through a stenotic artery may be reduced because of hypotension and may cause transient cerebral ischaemia. Occasionally, in patients suffering from cervical spondylosis, neck rotation leads to pressure on, and reduced flow through, a vertebral artery causing ischaemia in the brain stem.

An uncommon cause of transient cerebral ischaemia is the '*subclavian steal syndrome*'. This may arise if the subclavian artery is stenosed proximal to the origin of the vertebral artery. The increased blood flow needed when the arm on the affected side is exercised may be met by blood from the unaffected subclavian artery via the two vertebral arteries. Blood destined for the basilar artery from the vertebral artery on the normal side is diverted down the other vertebral artery by vasodilatation in the muscles of the arm being used. The brain stem is thus rendered ischaemic. Such symptoms as diplopia or ataxia, produced by use of an arm, should suggest the possibility of 'subclavian steal'. A significant difference between the blood pressures measured in each arm, and a bruit audible over the supraclavicular fossa on the affected side, are distinctive signs of the syndrome.

Some episodes labelled as transient 'ischaemic' attacks may be due to small intracerebral haemorrhages.

(iv) DIFFUSE CEREBRAL ATHEROSCLEROSIS. Gradual reduction in cerebral blood flow leads to progressive brain atrophy which is reflected in a clinical picture of blunted intellectual function and multiple motor deficits. Increasing dementia may predominate but is usually accompanied by features of bilateral lesions of the pyramidal tracts, notably supranuclear bulbar palsy (*pseudobulbar palsy*). These defects cause lability of emotional expression, dysarthria and dysphagia as well as a reduction in spontaneity, drive and movement which mimics parkinsonism. In some cases true parkinsonian features accompany bilateral pyramidal tract signs.

Sudden accelerations of disability, or transient episodes of neural deficit, usually differentiate this type of vascular disease from other causes of progressive cerebral atrophy and dementia.

**Diagnosis and treatment** are discussed on pages 696 and 698.

## Cerebral Embolism

The role of cerebral embolism in the production of cerebral ischaemia and infarction is consistently underestimated. Post-mortem studies have shown that at least half of cerebral infarcts can be attributed to embolisation from the heart or from atheromatous plaques in the large arteries in the neck and thorax. Transient ischaemic attacks are frequently the result of emboli from these same sources. The disability produced by the lodgement of an embolus in a cerebral artery may be of very sudden onset. However, in many instances the picture produced by cerebral infarction due to thrombosis and that due to cerebral embolism are indistinguishable in terms of the time, course and nature of the neural picture presented. A firm diagnosis of embolism demands evidence of a source of emboli and the presence of multiple sites of impaction. In many cases of cerebral embolism both criteria — and particularly the latter requirement — are absent. Arrhythmia, particularly atrial fibrillation associated with rheumatic or ischaemic heart disease, may lead to the presumptive diagnosis of cerebral embolism. In contrast evidence of an embolic source within large proximal arteries is often difficult to obtain.

Direct evidence of embolisation is occasionally provided by ophthalmoscopy. Emboli, composed mainly of platelet aggregations, can sometimes be seen in the retinal vessels of the affected eye during an attack of transient monocular blindness. The likelihood of embolic infarction may be inferred if there is a history of earlier transient ischaemic attacks. The presence of an embolic site is suggested by a bruit localised to the region of the carotid bifurcation.

More cerebral emboli arise in the heart than in any other site. Thrombus following old or recent myocardial infarction is the commonest source of emboli; rheumatic valvular lesions, cardiomyopathy, infective and thrombotic endocarditis and atrial myxoma are other potential causes of cerebral embolism. A large embolus of cardiac origin may block the internal carotid artery at its origin. Smaller emboli often lodge at the trifurcation of the middle cerebral artery. Embolism at these sites is usually followed by thrombosis and complete occlusion.

A meticulous exploration of the possibility of embolic ischaemia should be made in all cases of occlusive cerebrovascular disease since the patient's management may thus be significantly influenced (p. 699).

### Arteritis

A completed stroke or multifocal, minor cerebral lesions or a toxic confusional state may be a manifestation of arteritis due to systemic lupus erythematosus or polyarteritis nodosa. Associated systemic features will usually suggest the diagnosis. Cranial arteritis (p. 215) is a frequent cause of arterial inflammation in the elderly and occasionally the disease causes cerebral infarction.

Cerebral infarction may be the presenting feature of meningovascular syphilis and the possibility should always be considered when a stroke occurs in a relatively young person. Occasionally tuberculous arteritis, associated with meningitis, may cause multiple small cerebral infarcts. Rarely a disabling stroke may be the predominant feature of tuberculous meningitis.

## 2. Haemorrhagic Cerebral Lesions

### Primary Intracerebral Haemorrhage

Intracerebral haemorrhage is strongly associated with hypertension. In malignant hypertension there is fibrinoid necrosis of arterioles, and vessels so affected rupture to cause bleeding into the brain. Patients with long-standing hypertension develop hyaline changes in the muscular and elastic arterial layers which give rise to small aneurysms that are also liable to rupture. The penetrating branches of the middle cerebral artery, notably the lenticulostriate arteries, are particularly prone to develop such aneurysms and the majority of intracerebral haemorrhages occur in the region of the internal capsule.

An intracerebral haemorrhage usually presents abruptly when the patient is awake and is prone to occur whilst engaged in physical exertion. There may be premonitory severe headache and in over a half of patients there is loss of consciousness, sometimes accompanied by an epileptic fit. Since the internal capsule is so frequently involved, a hemiplegia commonly supervenes and initially may be of the flaccid type. When the haemorrhage is massive and bleeding persists, intracranial pressure is raised; coma deepens and papilloedema develops. Haemorrhages frequently extend into the lateral or third ventricles and sometimes there is rupture through the surface of the brain into the subarachnoid space so that in many cases of initially intracerebral haemorrhage, blood is found in the cerebrospinal fluid. A massive haemorrhage accompanied by loss of consciousness has a grave prognosis; approximately a half of patients die within a few days. Smaller haemorrhages occurring in any part of the brain may present a clinical picture indistinguishable from infarction.

Haemorrhage into the pons usually produces rapid loss of consciousness, pinpoint pupils and periodic respiration; often there is bilateral involvement of cranial nerves and pyramidal pathways. Hyperpyrexia is sometimes a feature.

Cerebellar haemorrhage is frequently of abrupt onset and is usually ushered in by occipital headache, vomiting, vertigo and ataxia. Consciousness is often lost after a few hours at which time the patient frequently develops pupillary constriction and a contralateral hemiplegia.

### Subarachnoid Haemorrhage

Haemorrhage into the subarachnoid space results from rupture of a vascular malformation, notably a saccular aneurysm, from trauma, from extension of an intracerebral haemorrhage or from a bleeding cerebral tumour.

The onset of subarachnoid haemorrhage is often marked by severe and sudden headache, which is sometimes followed by impairment or loss of consciousness. There may be focal features whose nature depends on the site of the lesion; diplopia or other cranial nerve lesions, hemiparesis and aphasia occur. Signs of meningeal irritation, i.e. neck stiffness and a positive Kernig's sign, develop. Ophthalmoscopy may reveal unilateral or bilateral haemorrhages between the retina and the hyaloid membrane. The shape of these subhyaloid haemorrhages is determined by gravity so that if the patient is sitting upright the upper border is horizontal. If the subarachnoid haemorrhage is extensive and continuous, papilloedema may occur.

The outlook for subarachnoid haemorrhage due to an extension of intracerebral bleeding is similar to that of the primary condition. If subarachnoid haemorrhage is due to the rupture of a saccular aneurysm bleeding is liable to recur within 6 to 8 weeks.

**Saccular Aneurysm.** The first manifestation of an intracranial aneurysm is often a subarachnoid haemorrhage, but sometimes aneurysms present focal features before rupture. The nature of these depends on the site of the aneurysm. An aneurysm of the internal carotid artery within the cavernous sinus usually causes pain or paraesthesiae in the distribution of the ophthalmic division of the fifth nerve and a third nerve palsy sometimes accompanied by palsies of the fourth and sixth nerves. Rarely, an aneurysm of the internal carotid artery will rupture into the cavernous sinus, forming a caroticocavernous fistula. This causes severe pain in and around the eye, pulsatile exophthalmos, papilloedema and complete ophthalmoplegia. A loud bruit can usually be heard over the affected eye.

Aneurysm of the supraclinoid part of the internal carotid artery may compress the optic nerve, chiasma or tract leading to impaired visual acuity and a variety of scotomata and visual field defects. These visual disturbances may be accompanied by paralysis of the third nerve.

Aneurysms on the middle cerebral artery tend to present with bleeding, but occasionally their presence will be heralded by focal epilepsy and occasionally by a progressive hemiparesis. Anterior communicating and anterior cerebral aneurysms may compress the optic chiasma from above, resulting in bilateral loss of the inferior part of the visual fields.

Posterior communicating aneurysms often lead to an isolated third nerve palsy. Aneurysms of the posterior cerebral artery may compress the cerebral peduncle and the adjacent third nerve causing an ipsilateral third nerve palsy and contralateral pyramidal tract signs.

**Arteriovenous Malformation.** A subarachnoid haemorrhage without antecedent clinical features is the commonest presentation of an arteriovenous malformation. Some present with focal epilepsy accompanied later by progressive focal signs and others cause recurrent localised headaches of throbbing character which superficially may resemble migraine. A bruit can often be heard through the skull overlying a large arteriovenous malformation.

## Extradural and Subdural Haematoma

*Extradural haematomas* are produced by skull fractures involving the branches of the middle meningeal artery. Symptoms usually develop a few hours after the injury. Coma rapidly ensues with an obvious hemiparesis. Later there are signs of tentorial herniation which often rapidly causes death so that operation should be undertaken urgently.

*Subdural haematoma* may occur as an acute complication of a head injury resulting from venous haemorrhage into the subdural space. The picture then resembles that of an extradural haematoma.

A *chronic subdural haematoma* may follow a minor head injury especially in an elderly person. Often the injury is so slight that the patient has no memory of it. After an interval of weeks or months the patient may present with headache, a confusional state, or the development of focal neurological signs such as hemiparesis. Characteristically, as the subdural haematoma increases in size, there is fluctuation in the level of consciousness, and, later, signs of raised intracranial pressure may be manifest. The progressive changes may closely mimic a cerebral tumour and require investigation along similar lines. Exploratory burr holes in the skull may confirm the diagnosis and produce dramatic benefit in the case of a haematoma.

## Diagnosis of Cerebrovascular Disease

**Clinical Features.** The diagnosis and assessment of a patient suffering from cerebrovascular disease ideally comprises four stages. Firstly, the nature of the patient's disabilities are defined and the site and extent of the lesion inferred. Secondly, other possible causes of the disturbance of function are excluded. Thirdly, the nature of the vascular pathology is determined. Fourthly, the state of the systemic circulation is investigated and associated diseases delineated.

The time course of a completed stroke will usually suggest the correct diagnosis. Occasionally patients suffering from a cerebral tumour will present with a rapidly developing disability. Multiple sclerosis and demyelinating encephalopathies present acutely but in most instances the age of onset, multiple lesions affecting the spinal cord as well as the brain and a characteristic earlier history will distinguish these conditions from cerebrovascular disease. The progression of a stroke-in-evolution may closely imitate the features of a rapidly growing cerebral tumour.

Transient ischaemic attacks may need to be distinguished from epilepsy and migraine. Consciousness is unimpaired in most transient ischaemic attacks. Migraine rarely presents after the age of 50 years whilst transient ischaemic attacks usually occur after this age. Transient ischaemic episodes are rarely accompanied or followed by headaches.

Progressive, diffuse, cerebral atherosclerosis may be difficult to distinguish from other forms of senile and presenile dementia and the diagnosis should not be made too readily. The occurrence of acute focal disabilities, interrupting otherwise steady deterioration, is in favour of diffuse cerebral atherosclerosis as is circumstantial evidence such as accompanying hypertension, peripheral vascular disease or myocardial ischaemia. In most instances the history and clinical findings will differentiate cerebrovascular disease from other intracranial pathologies. In a minority of instances special investigations will be required to confirm the diagnosis.

The elucidation of the type of cerebrovascular disease is sometimes difficult. It is important rapidly to define those conditions which require life-saving, urgent or specific treatment. The history of trauma and the clinical features are distinctive in extradural and acute subdural haematoma. The diagnosis of chronic subdural haematoma can occasionally be made with confidence on clinical grounds but the possibility of this condition should be considered and investigated particularly in an elderly patient manifesting a progressive cerebral deficit accompanied by headache.

Signs of meningeal irritation indicate a subarachnoid bleed which can be confirmed by lumbar puncture. Arteritis will often be diagnosed because of accompanying systemic clinical features and by the results of simple investigations such as a raised ESR, positive ANF or positive serology for syphilis.

An attempt should be made to distinguish between patients with cerebral infarction and those who have bled into the brain. A history of transient ischaemic attacks favours a diagnosis of infarction rather than haemorrhage. The development of neural disability during sleep is likely to be due to infarction; onset during exertion suggests a haemorrhage. Blood in the CSF obviously indicates intracranial bleeding. A source of emboli is in favour of arterial occlusion rather than rupture. Hypertension is frequently associated with both infarction and haemorrhage but severe hypertension, particularly in young patients, predisposes to haemorrhage. Though these clinical hints are generally valid they do not provide firm criteria for differentiating thrombosis, embolism and haemorrhage.

The cerebral circulation cannot be considered in isolation. In any patient who suffers from cerebrovascular disease the status of heart, blood pressure, blood vessels and blood should be carefully appraised. The heart should be examined to define the presence or absence of arrhythmias, valvular or myocardial lesions and heart failure. Peripheral limb vessels and the arteries in the neck should be palpated and auscultated to detect changes in the walls and the presence of stenoses. Recordings of the blood pressure are mandatory. Abnormalities of the blood, particularly anaemia, polycythaemia and thrombocytopenia should be sought.

**Investigation.** The extent to which diagnostic investigations should be pursued depends on individual circumstances.

*Computed tomography* will not only reveal tumours but in many instances will define the nature of cerebrovascular lesions. Intracerebral bleeding gives high density abnormalities so that even very small haemorrhages are detected. Intraventricular, subarachnoid and subdural haemorrhages are readily distinguished and sequential scanning will monitor the subsequent organisation and resolution of intracerebral haematomas. Ruptured aneurysms can be differentiated from primary intracerebral haemorrhage in almost all instances and the site of the aneurysms predicted with fair accuracy.

Cerebral infarction leads to low density abnormalities which may be detectable within a few hours of onset. Some infarcts are not revealed by computed tomography but even in these cases the confident exclusion of tumours and haemorrhage enables a firm presumptive diagnosis to be made.

*Other investigations* are less informative. The EEG usually shows marked abnormalities after infarction or haemorrhage and serial recordings demonstrate progressive improvement. Similar EEG abnormalities due to tumour persist and become more marked. Echoencephalography may reveal a shift of the midline echo. A marked shift suggests the presence of haemorrhage rather than infarction. Facial thermography may indicate reduction of flow through a carotid artery. Cerebral angiography should be undertaken only if surgery is likely to be required. It should be performed if there is evidence of a tumour, vascular malformation, subdural haematoma or extracranial vascular disease in a young patient which might be amenable to surgical treatment.

### Treatment of Cerebrovascular Disease

The management of patients suffering from cerebrovascular disease should be approached in a logical sequence. Initially patients may need to be protected from the dangers of unconsciousness and immobility. The causal lesion should be treated if possible and measures to improve functional recovery instituted. Patients who survive but are left with residual disability need support and rehabilitation. Finally, progression and recurrence of cerebrovascular lesions should, as far as possible, be prevented.

*General Measures.* An adequate airway should be established in those patients whose consciousness is impaired. The patient's fluid and nutritional intake should be maintained, employing a nasogastric tube or intravenous infusion if necessary. Pressure sores should be prevented by frequent alteration of the patient's posture, the use of pads and massage of vulnerable areas of skin. Catheterisation may be needed because of urinary incontinence. Rapid cleaning is required for the patient who is incontinent of faeces. Passive movement of limbs should be started early and the patient should be moved from bed and sat in a chair for periods during the day as soon as possible. Intercurrent urinary or respiratory infections should be treated with appropriate antibiotics.

*Specific Medical Treatment.* A minority of patients have treatable underlying conditions. Hypertension should be controlled. Those with meningovascular syphilis should bc given a course of penicillin (p. 706). Those suffering from temporal arteritis or a connective tissue disorder may need steroids. Polycythaemia or anaemia should be treated appropriately.

*Neurosurgery.* Early operation is required for patients who have bled from a ruptured aneurysm. The neck of the aneurysm should be clipped if this is technically possible. The wall of the aneurysm may be reinforced by plastic or muscle. If such a direct attack is impracticable carotid ligation may reduce the liability to further bleeding from the aneurysm. Surgical drainage of extradural and subdural haematomas usually produces dramatic and rapid improvement.

*Stroke.* Little can be done to reverse the effects of infarction or haemorrhage. In a very few instances blood flow has rapidly been restored through an occluded carotid artery by surgical removal of thrombus. This is effective only when the affected artery is accessible and when the operation is carried out within a few hours of the onset of the symptoms. These conditions very rarely obtain. Treatment is aimed at minimising the extent of brain death. Around the margins of an infarct or haemorrhage there is potentially viable tissue whose function can be restored if an alternative supply of blood is available. Attempts to provoke cerebral vasodilation have not been effective and it is likely that the promotion of generalised cerebral vasodilation could be harmful by 'stealing' blood from the damaged area. Low-molecular-weight dextran has been employed in the expectation that its effects in decreasing the aggregation of platelets and blood viscosity would improve cerebral circulation. Five hundred ml of a 10% solution of dextran in dextrose is given intravenously as early as possible after the onset of symptoms and repeated at 12–hourly intervals for three days. There is evidence that this treatment reduces the early death rate from severe strokes but there is no long-lasting benefit.

Dexamethasone (4 mg t.d.s.) reduces cerebral oedema and may help those patients with cerebral infarction or haemorrhage who develop deepening coma. There is little evidence that it improves the long-term prognosis. Anticoagulants have no place in the treatment of an established stroke. Thrombolytic agents such as streptokinase are ineffective. There is thus as yet no specific medical treatment available which significantly and consistently improves the outlook for patients who have suffered a stroke.

*Stroke-in-evolution.* The early use of anticoagulants has been advocated to halt progression in an evolving stroke. There is some evidence that this treatment does help but there is a danger that anticoagulants may cause haemorrhage and before they are used in this situation an intracerebral haemorrhage must be excluded by investigation. There may be a place for the use of low-molecular-weight dextran in the treatment of a stroke of gradual development.

*Transient Ischaemic Attacks.* Anticoagulants (p. 600) seem to reduce the incidence of future strokes. Inhibitors of platelet aggregation have also been employed, namely aspirin 150 mg b.d. dipyridamole 25 mg four times daily or sulphinpyrazine 200 mg four times daily. Their efficacy has not yet been fully assessed.

*Cerebral Embolism.* Anticoagulants should be given, provided other conditions do not contraindicate their use.

*Rehabilitation.* A large number of patients are left with residual deficits as a result of cerebrovascular lesions. Much can be done to mitigate disabilities so that patients can live a largely independent life in the community. Early institution of treatment is essential. In the period immediately following a stroke, passive movements of limbs should be practised. Supervised exercises and encouragement should later aim at the development of mobility. Few, if any, patients, no matter how severe their original hemiplegia, cannot be taught to walk again. Later the patient should be guided in the performance of the activities of everyday living. Modifications of dress, housing, baths, lavatories and kitchen equipment may enable the patient to cope at home.

Throughout the period of rehabilitation communication should be encouraged, using, if appropriate, the skills of the speech therapist. The degree and extent of paralysis is less of a bar to successful rehabilitation than are disorders of perception, spatial disorientation, dysphasia and, particularly, dementia. Active cooperation between physicians, nurses, physiotherapists, occupational therapists, speech therapists and social workers improves the end result of the physical and social rehabilitation of patients who have had a stroke. The recruitment and education of relatives enables them to continue rehabilitation at home.

*Prevention of Recurrence.* Some of the treatments outlined above, such as anticoagulant therapy and inhibitors of platelet aggregation, are preventive measures. The most important prophylactic factor is the control of hypertension by appropriate drugs (p. 196). It has been shown conclusively that early, effective and continued reduction of high blood pressure significantly improves the outlook for both occlusive and haemorrhagic cerebrovascular disease.

**Prognosis** for an individual suffering from a cerebrovascular lesion depends on complex factors. There are some general guidelines. In one well-studied series of strokes the mortality within the first month after infarction was roughly 30%. From proven intracerebral haemorrhage the mortality in the same period was 80%. After a subarachnoid haemorrhage 65% died within 1 month. This investigation emphasised the poor prognosis after large haemorrhagic lesions. Many epidemiological studies have stressed the general tendency of clinicians to overestimate the incidence of cerebral haemorrhage. Data from death certificates suggest that haemorrhage is twice as common as infarction whereas careful clinical differentiation of the two types of lesion indicates that infarction is at least five times commoner than haemorrhage and in those over 75 years of age, 20 times more frequent.

Signs of a poor outlook for a stroke, whether due to infarction or haemorrhage, are impairment of consciousness, defects in conjugate gaze and a severe hemiplegia.

Of those who survive an initial stroke life expectancy is roughly halved. Approximately 10% suffer a second stroke within 1 year of the first and 20% within 5 years. Many patients who initially present with stroke die from myocardial infarction.

The prognosis in patients who suffer transient ischaemic attacks is difficult to ascertain because of difficulties of definition. A subsequent stroke is to be expected in approximately one-third of patients who have transient ischaemic attacks and is most likely to occur within 3 years of the first attack. In 50% of patients attacks cease within 1 to 3 years of their onset. Transient ischaemic attacks are attended by a worse prognosis (in terms of survival) in people below the age of 65 than in those over that age when compared with the rest of the population.

Much further work is needed to define the factors which influence the prognosis of cerebrovascular disease.

## Diseases of Intracranial Veins and Venous Sinuses

Occlusion by thrombosis is the principal lesion which may affect the cerebral veins or venous sinuses. The thrombus may be infected or aseptic. Infection may spread to the veins or sinuses from a source of infection on face or scalp, in dental roots, middle ear or air sinuses; it may also follow fracture of the skull, meningitis or septicaemia. Complications such as leptomeningitis, suppurative encephalitis or brain abscess may ensue.

Aseptic thrombosis is also relatively rare. It may occur in water and salt depletion, polycythaemia, malaria and marasmus. Occasionally a cerebral venous thrombosis occurs in the puerperium or in women using oral contraceptives.

**Clinical Features.** *Superior Sagittal Sinus Thrombosis.* Severe headache, accompanied by papilloedema, may be the principal feature. However, in most cases thrombophlebitis spreads to the adjacent cortical veins; the motor or sensory areas of one or both hemispheres may thus be infarcted. Characteristically there is a paraparesis, though often one leg is affected more than the other. Occasionally a hemiplegia results. Less commonly there are hemianopia and aphasia. At the onset there is occasionally a generalised epileptic seizure.

*Transverse Sinus Thrombosis.* Generalised headache and vomiting are common. There may be associated papilloedema and drowsiness. At the onset there are usually few signs of focal cerebral infarction but extension to involve the superior petrosal sinus and veins draining the lower part of the precentral gyrus may give rise to faciobrachial paresis, hemiparesis or hemianopia, and spread to the superior sagittal sinus may give rise to a paraparesis. Occasionally the thrombosis spreads into the jugular veins, sometimes leading to paralysis of the lower cranial nerves.

*Cavernous sinus thrombosis* nearly always follows an infection such as a boil on the face. Usually the patient is gravely ill, and before antibiotics were available few patients survived. Headache and fever are marked and there is a neutrophil leucocytosis. Occlusion of the ophthalmic veins causes proptosis, chemosis and oedema of the eyelids. There are almost always complete palsies of the third, fourth and sixth nerves as well as pain in and above the eye and diminished sensation over the forehead. Papilloedema in the affected eye is common. The condition is usually initially unilateral but often becomes bilateral within 2 to 3 days.

*Thrombosis of Cortical Veins.* Initially there is usually localised headache or an epileptic seizure followed by focal neurological deficit whose nature depends on the area of cortex involved. Monoparesis or hemiparesis may occur, and sometimes extension of thrombosis to neighbouring veins causes progressive neural disability.

**Treatment.** The administration of antibiotics has markedly improved the outlook for infected thromboses such as occur in the cavernous sinus. Surgical drainage of pus in adjacent sinuses may be necessary. Anticoagulants are unhelpful.

## INFECTIONS OF BRAIN, MENINGES AND SPINAL CORD

### Suppurative Encephalitis and Intracerebral Abscess

**Aetiology and Pathology.** Direct infection may occur following a compound fracture of the skull or there may be local spread by suppurative thrombophlebitis from an infected ear, paranasal sinus or scalp. Metastatic infections may occur from the lungs or from infective endocarditis.

The initial infection causes a suppurative encephalitis. The pus is slowly localised by a surrounding wall of gliosis which in a chronic abscess may form a tough capsule. Multiple abscesses, communicating or discrete, occur, particularly with metastatic spread.

**Clinical Features.** There are three main types of presentation:

*Acute Encephalitis.* Soon after head injury or otitis media (in which aural discharge may be temporarily suppressed) the patient develops headache, vomiting and drowsiness passing to coma. Focal cerebral signs may be present and the temperature is raised.

*Subacute or Delayed Encephalitis.* Head injury, cranial infection or infected embolism may be followed after weeks or months of apparent recovery by symptoms of encephalitis or of a chronic space-occupying lesion. During the latent interval there may be minor headache, irritability, malaise and intermittent pyrexia. These features should lead to a search for a focal cerebral lesion in patients with infections such as otitis media or bronchiectasis.

*Chronic abscess.* This may follow one of the previous types of onset or there may be nothing to suggest that the lesion is infective. The chronic abscess causes focal symptoms of a cerebral lesion (p. 664) and those of raised intracranial pressure which are indistinguishable from those of cerebral tumour. The temperature is usually normal or even subnormal.

**Diagnosis.** The possibility of an abscess should be considered if there is a progressive, focal, intracranial lesion. The likelihood is increased if there are signs of infection, such as pyrexia, leucocytosis or a raised ESR but these may be absent if there is a chronic abscess. The EEG may show focal abnormalities. The CSF may show a pleocytosis or a raised protein but often is normal and should not be examined if there are signs of raised intracranial pressure. CT scanning should be performed whenever the suspicion of an abscess arises. Contrast enhanced CT scanning will define the vast majority of intracranial abscesses.

**Treatment.** High dosage antibiotics are given as for pyogenic meningitis (p. 702). When a collection of pus has been demonstrated it should be aspirated surgically and appropriate antibiotics instilled into the cavity. This procedure may need to be repeated on several occasions. After the infection has been controlled excision of the abscess is often necessary. It is important to treat the underlying cause if possible, especially middle ear and sinus infections which can cause repeated abscesses.

### Spinal Epidural Abscess

This condition usually arises as a metastasis from infection elsewhere, often a boil, which may be so trivial as to be easily overlooked. Pain of root distribution is severe. It develops acutely and is followed by progressive loss of sensation and power in the lower limbs with sphincter disturbance. The signs are those of transverse myelitis (p. 727) but the local root irritation is the clue to the true cause. The temperature may be only slightly raised, but a polymorphonuclear leucocytosis is found in the blood. There may be radiological evidence of localised osteomyelitis of the spine. Paraplegia will become complete and irreversible if treatment is delayed. Large doses of antibiotics such as benzylpenicillin 600 mg 4 hourly should be given immediately and the patient transferred to the care of a neurosurgeon without delay.

## Meningitis

**Aetiology and Pathology.** Inflammation of the pia and arachnoid membranes may be sterile or infective.

*Sterile.* Blood in the CSF as in subarachnoid haemorrhage causes severe meningeal inflammation (p. 694). Meningeal irritation (*'meningism'*) without inflammatory reaction occurs in acute specific fevers, otitis media and pneumonia in childhood. Cellular reaction (lymphocytic) may be associated with symptoms and signs of meningeal irritation in poliomyelitis (p. 710) and acute encephalomyelitis (p. 708). Carcinomatosis of the meninges is a rare cause.

*Infective.* Formerly the most common meningeal infections were due to the meningococcus or pyogenic organisms. These types of meningitis have become rare since the introduction of the antibiotics, and for similar reasons, tuberculous meningitis is now seldom seen in Britain. The most common infection is now viral. In endemic areas other causes are leptospirosis, relapsing and typhus fevers and amoebic infections (p. 795).

The pia-arachnoid is congested and infiltrated with inflammatory cells. A thin layer of pus forms and this may later organise to form adhesions. These may cause obstruction to the free flow of CSF leading to hydrocephalus, or may damage the cranial nerves at the base of the brain. The CSF pressure rises rapidly, the protein content increases and there is a cellular reaction which varies in type and severity according to the nature of the inflammation and the causative organism. The sugar content of the CSF is decreased in bacterial infections and in carcinomatosis of the meninges. If the patient is not kept in electrolyte balance the chloride content may be reduced due to loss by sweating and vomiting.

**Clinical Features.** Signs of meningeal irritation are present:

*Neck Rigidity.* The patient complains of neck stiffness and the examiner is unable to put the patient's chin on the chest by passive flexion of the neck. Spasm may be so severe, particularly in children, as to cause head retraction.

*Kernig's Sign.* If the patient's thigh is flexed to 90 degrees from the abdomen, it is then impossible to straighten the knee passively owing to spasm of the hamstring muscles. This manoeuvre stretches the roots of the sciatic nerve which are inflamed at their exits from the spinal theca.

**Treatment** is directed at the primary cause.

*Acute pyogenic meningitis.* Early and vigorous specific treatment is needed. Ideally the appropriate antibiotics are determined by the sensitivities of the infecting organisms but whilst awaiting this information benzylpenicillin should be commenced. Initially 12–20 mega units (7 to 12 g) should be given intravenously. In mild cases a single intravenous dose should suffice and treatment should be continued intramuscularly. In severe cases intravenous therapy should be maintained until clinical improvement occurs in about 7 to 10 days. For *pneumococcal meningitis*, which has a high mortality, benzylpenicillin should also be given intrathecally in a dose of 10 000 units (6 mg) daily for ten days.

In meningitis due to *H. influenzae*, ampicillin (2 g four hourly) is most effective. In appropriate circumstances, gentamicin, cloxacillin and co-trimoxazole may be administered. Intrathecal antibiotic therapy is often effective but is necessary only in fulminating conditions and should be used only after careful consideration and establishment of the dosage and method of administration.

*Meningococcal meningitis*. Treatment is discussed on page 63.

## Tuberculous Meningitis

**Aetiology and Pathology.** The usual source of infection is a caseous focus in the meninges or brain substance adjacent to the cerebrospinal fluid pathway. The focus arises as a result of spread by the blood stream from a site elsewhere. The condition occurs most commonly shortly after a primary infection in childhood or as part of miliary tuberculosis.

The brain is covered by a greenish, gelatinous exudate especially around the base, and numerous scattered tubercles are found on the meninges.

**Clinical Features.** In children the onset of tuberculous meningitis is so insidious that it may be weeks before the parents realise that the illness is serious. At first there is merely lassitude, loss of interest in toys and in play, unwillingness to talk, anorexia and constipation. Headache, at first slight, gradually becomes worse but meningeal signs may not appear for days or weeks. In adults the malaise, headache and meningeal signs usually progress more rapidly. There may be vomiting. The temperature is intermittently raised during the period of ingravescence but remains raised, though rarely to high levels, once meningeal signs appear. The condition then progresses more rapidly, and in untreated cases cranial nerve palsies, hemiparesis or other signs of cerebral damage, hydrocephalus with drowsiness, coma and moderate papilloedema may occur. In miliary tuberculosis choroidal tubercles may be seen.

The CSF is under increased pressure. It is usually clear or slightly turbid but, when allowed to stand, a fine clot may form. The fluid contains up to 400 cells per cmm predominantly lymphocytes (the count must be made on a fresh specimen before it forms a clot). There is a slight rise in protein and a marked fall in glucose. Detection of the tubercle bacillus in a smear of the centrifuged deposit from the CSF may be difficult, the clot being the most likely place to find it. Inoculation of CSF into a guinea-pig is valuable for confirming the diagnosis if this cannot be done from smears or cultures of the CSF but as the outcome will not be known for six weeks, treatment must be started without waiting for confirmation.

**Treatment and Prognosis.** Chemotherapy should be started as soon as the diagnosis is made using one of the regimes described on page 261, together with pyrazinamide (p. 259). All patients should also receive prednisolone, 10 mg four times daily. If subsequent lumbar punctures suggest the development of a spinal subarachnoid block, then hydrocortisone hemisuccinate should be injected intrathecally each day in a dose of 1 mg/kg body weight. If obstructive hydrocephalus develops in spite of treatment with corticosteroids, surgical methods for ensuring continuous ventricular drainage must be adopted. During the acute stage of the illness skilled nursing is essential and measures must be taken to maintain adequate hydration and nutrition.

The intensive regime of drug treatment should be continued for eight weeks and be followed by a continuation phase (p. 261). Prednisolone is then reduced to 20 mg daily and stopped after about three months.

Untreated tuberculous meningitis is fatal in a few weeks but complete recovery is the rule with modern treatment if it is started before the appearance of focal signs or stupor. When treatment is started at a later stage the recovery rate is 60% or less and the survivors may be mentally deficient, epileptic, deaf, blind or show some other permanent deficit.

### Viral Meningitis

Acute lymphocytic choriomeningitis and other forms of viral meningitis are described on page 708.

## Neurosyphilis

An old and frequently reiterated neurological aphorism says that neurosyphilis may mimic any neurological disease. As a corollary it is emphasised that neurosyphilis must be included in the differential diagnosis of all neurological problems.

Neurosyphilis may present as an acute or chronic process and may involve, singly or in combination, the meninges, blood vessels and parenchyma of brain and spinal cord. Though the clinical manifestations produced are diverse, certain general observations are pertinent.

*Pupillary abnormalities*, described by Argyll Robertson, may accompany any neurosyphilitic clinical syndrome. The pupils are small, irregular and unequal. They do not react to light but respond to convergence and show an impaired response to mydriatics. The irises may be atrophied. In relatively few instances will all of these features be present. The complete picture of Argyll Robertson pupils is most frequently seen in tabes dorsalis and is distinctly uncommon in general paresis wherein some pupillary changes occur in about half of the cases. The observation of any discrepancy between the pupillary response to light and convergence even when other manifestations are lacking, should always suggest the possibility of neurosyphilis.

*Serological tests for syphilis* (p. 66) are usually positive. In general paresis it is almost always so in both blood and cerebrospinal fluid, as it is in about 90% of cases of meningovascular syphilis. In a fifth of tabetic patients, the Wassermann reaction in the CSF is negative and 10% show negative serology in the blood. The FTA and TPI (p. 66) are more specific tests for the detection of neurosyphilis.

*Examination of the CSF* reveals abnormalities in the vast majority of cases of neurosyphilis. An increase in the cell count, usually lymphocytic and of moderate degree is almost invariably present when the disease is active. A moderate rise in the protein content is usual and the gamma globulin fraction thereof is often increased.

### Meningovascular Syphilis

The essential lesion is endarteritis obliterans which may lead to arterial thrombosis and to the formation of a granuloma or gumma. The meninges may be covered by an exudate which damages cranial nerves. Lesions may predominantly affect arteries or meninges or both structures may be involved. Clinical manifestations usually occur within five years of the primary infection.

*Intracranial Lesions*. Occlusion of a cerebral artery may be due to syphilis which should be considered as a possibility in cases of stroke, particularly when cerebral infarcts occur in young people.

Basal gummatous meningitis may present with cranial nerve palsies. Meningitis over the surface of the hemispheres may give rise to headaches and fits in addition to focal signs of cortical dysfunction. Rarely, a single large gumma may present as a slowly growing cerebral tumour.

*Spinal Lesions*. Thrombosis of the anterior spinal artery gives rise to lower motor neurone signs at the level of the lesion. Below the affected segments, pyramidal tract disturbance is usually manifest and there may also be impairment of pain and temperature sensation though the latter is often transient.

Thickening of the dura mater in the cervical region — called *hypertrophic pachymeningitis* — gives rise to lower motor neurone lesions in the arms and upper motor neurone lesions in the legs.

Meningitis accompanied by myelitis in the dorsal region causes 'girdle' pains and leads to progressive cord damage.

## Parenchymal Disease

### General Paralysis of the Insane

The principal pathological changes are seen in the cortex. There is degeneration of cortical neurones giving rise to atrophy, particularly marked over the anterior part of the hemispheres. The meninges are thickened and infiltrated with lymphocytes. General paralysis of the insane usually presents 5 to 15 years after the primary infection. Men are much more often affected than women.

**Clinical Features.** The initial and most characteristic feature is dementia, often of insidious onset and slow progression. Relatives or workmates usually first recognise the patient's intellectual deficit and, later, deteriorating social adaptation. Delusions of grandeur occur only in a minority of cases. Signs of upper motor neurone lesions, usually bilateral and initially mild, are usually present and tremors of the head and lips are often manifest. Less common features include epileptic fits and transient episodes of focal cerebral disturbance such as hemiplegia, hemianopia or dysphasia.

### Tabes Dorsalis

The primary lesion is a degeneration of first order sensory neurones, central to the dorsal root ganglia, in the lower thoracic and lumbar nerve roots. Obvious macroscopic wasting affects the dorsal columns but all modalities of sensation may be impaired. Males are more often affected than females, usually 5 to 20 years after the primary infection.

**Clinical Features.** Sensory disturbances are the most common initial symptoms. 'Lightning' pains of severe, lancinating nature occur in paroxysms. They are most common in the legs. Pains radiating around the trunk in a 'girdle' distribution also occur. Paraesthesiae often affect the feet.

Other disabilities may accompany these sensory manifestations or may be presenting features. Ataxia, of sensory type, due to proprioceptive loss is often prominent. Sphincter disturbance, particularly retention of urine, may be accompanied by impotence. Failing vision or diplopia may be symptoms. Perforating, painless ulcers of the feet and swollen, unstable joints (Charcot's joints) are sometimes found. Visceral crises may cause acute symptoms and the disturbance in function of a viscus may point to disease in the affected organ rather than in its innervation. Most common are gastric crises which give rise to abdominal pain and vomiting. Less common are laryngeal crises causing stridor, the strangury of vesical crises and tenesmus due to rectal crises.

The signs of tabes are mostly explicable on the basis of posterior root lesions. Tendon reflexes are lost, due to interruption of the reflex arcs, first at the ankles, then at the knees and later in the upper limbs; hypotonia with resultant hyperextensibility of the joints appears. The pain fibres are affected early with delay in or impairment of the response to pin prick over a characteristic distribution. The classical areas of loss are around the nose, the trunk from the angle of the sternum to the costal margin, the inner border of the forearms and the ring and little fingers, the perineum and the distal part of the lower limbs. Deep pain appreciation is also impaired so that the tendo calcaneus, calf muscles and testes become insensitive to pressure. Vibration and position sense in the feet are also lost early, but light touch is not affected until a later stage. The combination of loss of position sense and hypotonia gives rise to severe ataxia, so that the patient walks on a wide base lifting the feet high and stamping them down in an irregular and forceful manner. Romberg's test (p. 658) is positive. The plantar responses remain flexor, but may be absent as a result of sensory loss.

Bilateral ptosis with compensatory wrinkling of the forehead and Argyll Robertson pupils constitute a typical tabetic facies. Less constant clinical manifestations also include pallor of the optic discs, defects in external ocular movement, distension of the bladder, and trophic changes such as ulcers or painless arthropathy.

### Combined Neurosyphilitic Lesions

It is emphasised that the clinical syndromes outlined above represent only the commoner presentations of neurosyphilis. Combinations of pathological lesions also occur and give rise to mixed clinical pictures. Tabetic manifestations sometimes accompany those of general paralysis of the insane and the hybrid (*taboparesis*) may lead to cases of dementia accompanied by ataxia, lightning pains or areflexia; patients presenting with visceral crises may be found to have extensor plantar responses.

### Treatment of Neurosyphilis

The essential part of the treatment of neurosyphilis of all types is the injection of procaine benzylpenicillin, 1 g daily for three weeks. The aim of treatment is to arrest the disease and restore the blood and CSF to normal. Further courses of penicillin must be given if symptoms are not relieved, the condition continues to advance, or the CSF continues to show signs of active disease. The first abnormality to regress is the increase in cells but these may not return to normal until three months after treatment has been completed. The elevated protein takes longer to subside and the

Wassermann reaction may never revert to normal. Lumbar puncture should be repeated at 6 monthly intervals for 2 years and further courses of penicillin given so long as signs of activity remain. Evidence of clinical progression at any time is an indication for renewed treatment.

## Viral Infections

Some viruses have a propensity for invasion of nerve cells and are called 'neurotropic'. The affinity may be specially marked for one type of nerve cell; the zoster variant of the varicella virus particularly involves sensory neurones and the anterior horn cells are vulnerable in poliomyelitis. Though these viruses most commonly invade their sites of predilection they may also sometimes involve the nervous system more widely; the virus of poliomyelitis often gives rise to a meningoencephalitis and the zoster virus may rarely cause motor disability. Many viruses which usually cause diseases of other systems may sometimes implicate the nervous system. The many varieties of echo and Coxsackie viruses, which are common enteric pathogens, fairly often cause neurological disease as well as more widespread manifestations in other systems. The viruses of herpes simplex and mumps, among many others, may occasionally invade the nervous system. About 1% of infants in developed countries are infected with cytomegalovirus *in utero* and about 10% of these have gross brain damage.

Some neurological diseases, of which encephalitis lethargica is one, are presumed to be of viral origin because of their epidemiological, clinical and pathological features though the causal agent has not been identified.

Neurological disorders are sometimes indirectly associated with viral diseases. In these instances abnormal immunological responses, evoked by the virus, cause damage to neural tissue without any viral invasion of neurones. The demyelinating encephalomyelitis (p. 715) which may follow any of the exanthemata is such an entity.

**Slow viral infections** may cause chronic or relapsing neurological disease. These infections exhibit a latent period of many months or years between the initial infection and the subsequent clinical illness which, once manifest, tends to run a protracted course.

*Kuru* is a disease which occurs only in the members of one cannibalistic New Guinea tribe. It can, however, be transmitted to chimpanzees and there is much evidence to suggest that kuru is a slow viral infection transmitted by the eating of the infected brains of dead tribal members. There is degeneration of grey matter, most marked in the cerebellum, causing a progressive ataxia.

*Creutzfeldt-Jakob disease* is a subacute encephalopathy characterised by presenile dementia, epilepsy, extrapyramidal and motor neurone signs and can also be transmitted from man to chimpanzees.

A slow viral infection has been adduced as a possible cause of a number of chronic neurological diseases, including motor neurone disease and multiple sclerosis.

### Viral Meningitis

Viral infections of the central nervous system such as encephalitis and poliomyelitis may be associated with meningitis. Viral meningitis can also occur alone, without clinical manifestation of parenchymal involvement of the nervous system, in acute lymphocytic choriomeningitis and infection by echo or Coxsackie viruses. Thirdly, meningitis may develop as a complication of viral infections primarily involving other organs, e.g. mumps, measles, infectious mononucleosis, herpes zoster and hepatitis.

**Acute lymphocytic choriomeningitis** is caused by a virus endemic in house mice. The condition occurs mainly in children and young adults. The onset is acute and evidence of meningeal irritation develops rapidly. Focal neurological signs are usually absent. There may be a high pyrexia which gradually reverts to normal in 5 to 7 days. The CSF is under increased pressure. It is usually clear but may be turbid as there is an excess of lymphocytes which may persist long after clinical cure. There may be a slight increase in the protein but the sugar and chloride levels are normal.

Lymphocytic choriomeningitis has to be differentiated from pyogenic meningitis in which the turbid CSF contains an excess of polymorphonuclear leucocytes and the causative organism can be isolated. Tuberculous meningitis may be difficult to distinguish owing to the technical difficulties of isolating the tubercle bacillus. A normal level of sugar in the CSF is in favour of a diagnosis of acute lymphocytic choriomeningitis. If there is any serious doubt as to the diagnosis, it is better to start treatment for tuberculous meningitis while awaiting further bacteriological reports.

There is no specific treatment for lymphocytic choriomeningitis. The patient is kept at rest in bed on symptomatic measures until the temperature has returned to normal. Complete recovery is the rule.

## Viral Encephalitis

All of the viruses which cause meningitis may also give rise to an encephalitis. Encephalitic features may predominate or a combined picture of meningo-encephalitis may occur. More specific types of viral encephalitis occur in epidemic forms, such as Japanese-B encephalitis (p. 847). Sporadic cases occur fairly commonly but often the causative virus is not isolated though influenza and herpes simplex viruses are fairly frequently implicated.

**Pathology.** The distribution and extent of lesions vary to some extent with the type of infecting virus. There is usually diffuse damage to cells in the cortex, basal ganglia and brain stem. Inclusion bodies are often present in neurones and glial cells. There is usually infiltration between neurones and in the perivascular spaces by polymorphonuclear cells initially and later by lymphocytes and mononuclear cells. There is accompanying neuroglial proliferation. Herpes simplex encephalitis tends particularly to affect the temporal lobes and in encephalitis lethargica the substantia nigra, midbrain and basal ganglia are most prominently involved.

**Clinical Features.** An acute onset of headache, often accompanied by fever, is the usual clinical presentation common to all types of viral encephalitis. Disturbance of consciousness, varying from mild drowsiness to deep coma, usually supervenes early and may sometimes advance dramatically. Epilepsy of focal or generalised type is common. A variety of focal signs such as aphasia, hemiplegia or tetraplegia, cranial nerve palsies and sensory disturbances may occur but sometimes there are none. The clinical features usually do not enable a firm diagnosis of the causal agent to be made but some types of encephalitis present distinctive manifestations as follows:

*Herpes Simplex Encephalitis*. The onset is usually acute and commonly is marked by behavioural disturbance and a confusional state resembling a psychosis. This often lasts 2 or 3 days before other features develop. Fits are very common. Papilloedema and variable focal neurological signs may be present. Progression over a few days to coma is common.

*Brain-stem encephalitis* is presumed to be of viral origin but the causal agent has not been defined. There is usually an antecedent history of mild upper respiratory infection. The onset, attended by headache, is often marked by double vision and dysarthria. Later there is increasing drowsiness and progressive cranial nerve involvement.

*Encephalitis lethargica* occurred in epidemic form during the 1920s and sporadic cases still occur. The illness varies markedly in severity. Headache and double vision may be the only features but sleep disturbances, pyramidal and extrapyramidal signs may be manifest. Oculogyric crises or parkinsonism may develop during the early stages of the illness or may be a sequel.

*Epidemic myalgic encephalomyelitis* is a condition which is presumed, though not proven, to be of viral origin. It occurs in closed communities such as schools and hospitals. Common features are headaches, diffuse muscle pains, exhaustion, low grade pyrexia, lymphadenopathy, paraesthesiae and marked mood disturbances which may recur over long periods.

*Subacute sclerosing panencephalitis* is thought to be due to infection by a myxovirus which is either measles virus or a closely related agent. It occurs in children and adolescents. The onset is usually an insidious intellectual deterioration, apathy and clumsiness accompanied later by myoclonic jerks and other involuntary movements. The EEG is distinctive, showing bursts of triphasic slow waves. As the disease progresses, rigidity and dementia supervene.

*Rabies* presents a distinctive clinical picture described on page 848.

*Progressive multifocal leucoencephalopathy* is a rare condition occurring late in the course of an antecedent disease, e.g. lymphoma or carcinoma. The pathological findings comprise widely disseminated demyelinating lesions in the brain together with distinctive changes in the glial cells suggestive of invasion by one of the papova group of viruses. It is a condition of rapid and progressive nature usually leading to death within a few weeks or months of its being manifest. The clinical picture varies widely. Hemiparesis is the commonest disability but dysphasia, dysarthria and hemianopia are also frequent. Dementia may occur, as may convulsions.

**Diagnosis.** These various forms of viral encephalitis should first be distinguished from other intracranial diseases such as cerebral tumour or abscess, from encephalopathies and from demyelinating encephalomyelitis (p. 715). Thereafter the type of viral infection should, if possible, be determined. The differential diagnosis depends on the nature of the clinical features and the attendant circumstances. When the predominant features are progressive, focal affection of one hemisphere accompanied by headache and drowsiness, the picture may strongly suggest a space-occupying lesion and intensive investigation may be needed to exclude such conditions as cerebral abscess. When the illness is mild, neurological signs indefinite and there are attendant general signs of viral infection the diagnosis will often be made presumptively after the patient improves.

Investigations are more helpful in excluding other lesions than in confirming the diagnosis of viral encephalitis. In a minority of instances the CSF is normal. Usually the CSF pressure and protein content are moderately raised and there is a lymphocytic pleocytosis. The sugar content is normal. The EEG is usually altered. There is a diffuse slowing of the rhythms but the findings are nonspecific except in subacute sclerosing panencephalitis.

Occasionally in herpes simplex encephalitis a cerebral scan will show areas of increased uptake in one or both temporal lobes. This condition is potentially treatable so that it is important to establish the diagnosis when the patient's illness is severe and progressive. In such circumstances a biopsy of the temporal lobe may be justified.

Serological tests and culture may identify the infecting virus but the results of such tests are usually available too late to guide treatment.

**Treatment and Prognosis.** The management of most cases of viral encephalitis consists of nursing care and the prevention of intercurrent infections. When a positive diagnosis of herpes simplex encephalitis has been made, an antiviral agent such as vidarabine (p. 79) may be used.

Most patients survive and may recover completely but persisting focal defects are frequent. A significant number (perhaps 10–30%) die. The outlook is particularly poor in herpes simplex encephalitis and in subacute sclerosing panencephalitis. Brain-stem encephalitis has a good prognosis; complete, if sometimes slow, recovery is almost invariable.

## Poliomyelitis

**Aetiology and Pathology.** The disease is caused by one of three related polioviruses which comprise a subdivision of the group of enteroviruses. It is becoming much less common following the widespread use of prophylactic immunisation by oral vaccines. Infection usually occurs through the nasopharynx.

The virus is particularly liable to affect the grey matter of spinal cord, brain stem and cortex and has a particular propensity to damage anterior horn cells especially those within the lumbar segments. There is often accompanying infiltration of the meninges with lymphocytes.

**Clinical Features.** The incubation period is 7–14 days. At the onset there is usually mild pyrexia and headache which improves after a few days. Many cases do not progress beyond this stage. In other instances, after a period of well-being lasting approximately a week, there is a recurrence of pyrexia and headache accompanied by neck stiffness and signs of meningeal irritation. Paralysis may occur later. The extent is variable. Weakness of one muscle group may progress to widespread paresis. Respiratory failure may supervene if intercostal muscles are paralysed or the medullary motor nuclei are involved.

The CSF shows a lymphocytic pleocytosis, a rise in protein and a normal sugar content.

**Treatment and Prognosis.** In the early stages bed rest is imperative. At the onset of respiratory difficulties a tracheostomy and intermittent positive pressure respiration are required. Subsequent treatment is by physiotherapy and orthopaedic measures.

Epidemics vary widely in their incidence of abortive and nonparalytic cases and in mortality rate. Death occurs from respiratory paralysis. Paralysis is greatest at the end of the first week of the major illness. Gradual recovery may then take place for several months but any muscle showing no signs of recovery by the end of a month will not regain useful function. It is difficult to make a more definite prediction about the extent of permanent disability until three to six months after the onset. Second attacks are very rare.

Prevention is by oral vaccination (p. 49).

### Herpes Zoster (Shingles)

Invasion of posterior root ganglia by the varicella/zoster virus causes pain followed by a rash over the cutaneous distribution of the affected nerve. Zoster is believed to be due to reactivation of a previous infection by chickenpox virus which has lain dormant in the body. Chickenpox may be contracted from a patient with zoster. The frequency and severity of zoster increases with age and in patients with lymphoma or leukaemia whose immune defences are impaired.

**Clinical Features.** The first symptom is usually severe continuous pain in the distribution of the affected nerve root. After three or four days the skin in the painful area becomes reddened and vesicles appear which dry up over the course of 5 or 6 days, leaving small scars. The pain of zoster usually subsides as the eruption fades, but occasionally, especially in old people, it may be followed by a persistent and intractable neuralgia which may last for months.

Any dorsal root ganglion may be infected, most commonly those supplying the trunk where two or three adjacent dermatomes on one side only are often involved. Infection of the trigeminal ganglion usually involves the ophthalmic division; the vesicles appear on the cornea and may lead to corneal ulceration with the danger of scarring and impairment of vision (*ophthalmic herpes*).

Segmental muscle wasting may occur sometimes from involvement of the motor root. The virus occasionally invades the spinal cord or the brain, giving rise to myelitis or encephalitis.

**Treatment.** Idoxuridine (p. 79) may be applied to the skin in a 5% solution in the early stages of the evolution of the rash; 0·1% drops are used for corneal infections. The treatment of post-herpetic neuralgia is difficult. Analgesics should be continued, but addictive ones, such as morphine must be avoided.

## DEMYELINATING DISEASES

Loss of myelin sheaths occurs with many disorders of the central and peripheral nervous systems but there is a particular category with certain clinical and pathological features in common in which loss of myelin is considered to be the primary change and the axis cylinders may be spared or, if affected, are damaged secondarily. The lesions are almost entirely confined to the white matter of the central nervous system. They are initially inflammatory in type but differ from lesions known to be caused by direct viral infection and so they are grouped separately from viral encephalitis.

### Multiple Sclerosis

Multiple sclerosis, also known as *disseminated sclerosis*, is the commonest of the demyelinating diseases. It affects about 1 in 2000 of the population in Britain.

**Aetiology.** The cause of the disease is unknown but there is much information about its prevalence and about the factors associated with its development. Incidence varies widely in different geographical areas. It is very low in the tropics and high in the temperate zones of both northern and southern hemispheres. Migrants from a high to a low prevalence area have a reduced risk of developing multiple sclerosis. Those who migrate from a low to a high prevalence area are at greater risk than had they remained in their original environment. These effects apply only to those who move before the age of 15 years. Migrants at a later age bear the same liability to the disease as do the people of their country of origin.

A genetic susceptibility is suggested by an increased frequency of HLA-A3, B7 and DW2/DRW2 and particularly of the B cell alloantigen, BT101, in patients with multiple sclerosis. There is also a greater occurrence of the disease in close relatives of sufferers than in the general population.

The part played by an autoimmune mechanism, possibly induced by a slow viral or a persistent measles infection, is also being studied but the results are inconclusive. One theory is that in genetically susceptible individuals the disease follows a dormant viral infection, either directly or via an immunological mechanism.

**Pathology.** The acute lesion consists of a circumscribed area in which the myelin sheaths have undergone destruction while the axis cylinders show only irregular swelling. The plaque has a swollen pinkish appearance as blood vessels are dilated, but there is little infiltration with inflammatory cells. Reactive gliosis follows, so that the chronic lesion becomes a glial scar with a shrunken greyish appearance. The lesions are widely scattered in the white matter of the brain, especially round the ventricles, in the spinal cord, and in the optic nerves. Despite the disseminated distribution there is a tendency for spinal cord and brain stem lesions to occur in symmetrical situations.

**Clinical features** are diverse. It is impossible to outline a 'typical' history. Characteristic features are a relapsing and remittent course and widespread lesions which result in varied symptomatology.

The first manifestation may occur at any age but onset before puberty or after the age of 60 years is rare. Initial symptoms present between 20 and 40 years of age in the majority of cases. Women are affected about one-and-a-half times as often as men.

Weakness of one or more limbs developing acutely is probably the commonest presentation. Unilateral retrobulbar neuritis is also a frequent mode of onset as are paraesthesiae affecting a limb or felt in a girdle distribution around the trunk. Diplopia, vertigo and ataxia are also common initial features. Less frequent are epilepsy, aphasia, hemiplegia, facial palsy and bouts of facial pain resembling trigeminal neuralgia.

In most instances the symptoms and signs of the initial manifestation recover completely within 1 to 3 months of the onset. A period of well-being follows and after a very variable interval there is a recurrence. In a few instances there is no remission; the initial disability progresses and more widespread deficits develop. A minority of patients suffer three or four further exacerbations during the year following the onset. Another small group remains well for more than 10 years after the first disturbance. In many cases neural deficits recur within 2 years of the first incident. The outlook for the second and subsequent manifestations is variable. Some patients continue to show exacerbations with virtually complete recovery for many years. In other instances successive relapses are attended by diminishing degrees of improvement. Eventually half of the sufferers enter a chronically progressive stage with persisting and increasing disability.

The signs depend on the site of the demyelinating lesion. Pallor of one or both optic nerve heads is common and is particularly prominent over the temporal halves of the discs even in patients who give no history of an earlier retrobulbar neuritis. Patients who develop diplopia show affection of the third or sixth cranial nerves.

Nystagmus is often found and is usually of cerebellar or ataxic type. Signs of motor dysfunction are usually found at some stage, particularly involving the pyramidal pathways. The abdominal reflexes are often absent early in the course of the disease and remain so. Pyramidal tract signs in the early stages may be unilateral but usually become bilateral as the disease progresses. Later pyramidal signs in both upper and lower limbs become more marked. Spasticity and paraplegia in flexion and flexor spasms ensue. In people who develop the disease in middle age the only manifestation is often a slowly progressive, moderate paraparesis without remission but without severe exacerbations.

Cerebellar signs include the staccato, interrupted rhythm of scanning speech, ataxia and intention tremor; they are usually found during the progressive stage of the disease and are especially disabling.

Motor deficits are often temporarily but strikingly aggravated after a hot bath.

Sensory symptoms are almost invariable at some time during the course of the disease. Paraesthesiae of varying type and distribution occur. Objective impairment of superficial sensation is usually less prominent than would be anticipated from the intensity of symptoms. A distinctive symptom is a tingling or 'electric shock-like' sensation which radiates into the arms, down the back, or into the legs when the patient flexes the head. This is sometimes called the 'barber's chair' sign. It is most commonly due to multiple sclerosis but is not diagnostic thereof since it may occur in other diseases of the cervical spinal cord such as compression, syringomyelia or vitamin $B_{12}$ deficiency. Localised muscle wasting, parkinsonian tremor and choreoathetotic movements are rare and it is unusual for the spinothalamic tracts to be involved to such an extent as to cause painless burns and trophic lesions. As the disease progresses sphincter disturbances occur, notably frequency and urgency of micturition or hesitancy and retention.

A number of patients exhibit a sustained euphoria. This is by no means invariable; some patients are fully aware of their disabilities and become depressed. Late in the course of the disease there is often significant intellectual impairment.

**Diagnosis** of multiple sclerosis depends clinically on the demonstration of lesions occurring at different times and at different sites in the central nervous system. Sometimes the occurrence of multiple lesions may not be apparent clinically but delayed cerebral evoked potentials (p. 667) after visual, auditory or somatosensory stimulation may indicate the presence of earlier lesions.

There is no specific test which will confirm the diagnosis. A raised gammaglobulin in the CSF in the presence of a normal total protein is present in approximately 70% of patients suffering from multiple sclerosis. More sophisticated tests, utilising the electrophoresis of CSF protein, have shown that oligoclonal bands of IgG are present in 80 to 90% of patients with multiple sclerosis and in approximately 40% of patients suffering from a variety of infections of the central nervous system.

In some cases the diagnosis of multiple sclerosis has to be achieved by a process of exclusion. It is important in all patients to eliminate potentially curable conditions. The appropriate investigations, and the lengths to which they should be pursued, depend on the particular clinical syndrome presented. In cases of slowly progressive spastic paraparesis, as commonly occurs in late onset multiple sclerosis, a myelogram may be needed to exclude compression of the spinal cord. The possibility of syphilis or vitamin $B_{12}$ deficiency should be excluded.

**Treatment.** There is no curative treatment but much can be done to support the patient during the course of the illness. Corticosteroids promote more rapid and complete recovery during acute exacerbations; 2 mg of dexamethasone given orally three times daily, for five days, is an adequate course of treatment. There is no evidence that prolonged administration of corticosteroids significantly alters long-term prognosis. A variety of other treatments has been tried, including immunosuppression and transfer factor, but the results have been disappointing.

Spasticity may become severe in multiple sclerosis and baclofen in a dose of 20 to 60 mg daily is sometimes helpful. Severe, painful flexor spasms may be relieved by the intrathecal injection of phenol in glycerine. Spinal cord stimulation is an interesting but ill-understood method of treatment. Electrodes are inserted into the epidural space and the dorsal columns are repetitively stimulated. In some series more than half of patients so treated have shown improvement, particularly in sphincter control.

Of prime importance in the management is encouragement and support of patients and their relatives. Regular medical supervision contributes to this end. Patients with motor disabilities should avoid gain in weight. Periods of physiotherapy help the disabled patient. Assisted and passive movements and walking exercises improve gait as well as the patient's morale. In general the patient should be advised to avoid long periods in bed during intercurrent infections. Pressure sores should be prevented by advice about changes in posture and skin care; should they occur they must be treated early and vigorously in hospital.

Walking aids such as tripod supports or frames and the provision of wheel-chairs and motor vehicles together with the advice of an occupational therapist may enable the patient to function more easily at home and at work and to enjoy some form of social life. Nurses and social workers should regularly visit patients at home to assist in their care and to ensure that all the help which the community can provide is made available.

The care of the bladder is particularly important. Infections should be treated with an appropriate antibiotic. Male patients suffering from incontinence, urgency and frequency can be relieved by continuous drainage, through a tube attached to the penis, into a portable urinal strapped to the thigh. In some patients bladder neck resection is helpful. Various appliances are now available which help incontinent female patients. A permanent in-dwelling catheter, changed at intervals of a month or two, often makes life more comfortable and helps to prevent pressure sores.

**Prognosis** is variable. Multiple sclerosis does not inevitably lead to immobility and a chair-bound or bedridden existence. Approximately 5% of patients die within 5 years of the onset of the disease but a rather larger proportion remain well and retain unrestricted mobility for 20 years. The disease may run a progressive, disabling course, or may be relatively benign. It is not possible to predict the outlook with confidence in any individual patient though there are some useful indicators.

A favourable course often follows when retrobulbar neuritis is the initial manifestation, particularly when it occurs unaccompanied by any other neural deficit. A long gap between the presentation and the next recurrence often presages a fairly good prognosis, and particularly so if both manifestations recover completely. If motor function is only slightly impaired during the early years of the disease, crippling disability is usually long delayed. Repeated episodes of purely sensory deficit with complete recovery point to a benign course. Those whose initial manifestation is relatively late have usually a better prognosis. In those who show the so-called middle-aged spinal form the disease remains confined to a very slow progressive paraparesis.

Males generally seem to be more severely affected than females. An onset in the late teens or early twenties is often attended by a bad prognosis. Incomplete recovery from the initial attack is a sinister feature. Early recurrence, within 6 months of the initial manifestation, also suggests that relapses are likely to be frequent and disability rapidly progressive. Early manifestations of motor disability or brain stem and cerebellar dysfunction usually forecast a poor outlook. However, at any stage of the disease striking improvement may follow sudden deterioration.

### Acute Demyelinating Encephalomyelitis

This is a group of related acute disorders occurring without obvious cause about a week after diseases such as measles and chickenpox or following vaccination. There are areas of perivenous demyelination widely disseminated throughout the brain and spinal cord probably due to an immunological reaction.

Headache, vomiting, pyrexia, delirium and signs of meningeal irritation are presenting features. Fits or coma may occur. Flaccid paralysis and extensor plantar responses are common but sensory loss is unusual. Cerebellar signs may be present especially when the disorder follows chickenpox. The CSF may be normal or show a small increase of mononuclear cells and protein.

*Neuromyelitis optica* is a restricted form of the disease characterised by massive demyelination of the spinal cord and both optic nerves.

ACTH 80–120 units by injection or prednisone 60 mg by mouth daily for several days followed by a maintenance dose for 2 to 3 weeks is beneficial. These drugs must be used with caution in chickenpox if encephalitis develops before the rash has subsided as it may become confluent and haemorrhagic. The usual care of the paralysed and incontinent patient is required.

The mortality rate is high in neuromyelitis optica and in postvaccinial encephalomyelitis but is low in the postexanthematous cases. If the patient survives, the recovery may be remarkably complete and second attacks are very rare.

## DISEASES OF THE EXTRAPYRAMIDAL SYSTEM

In diseases of this system voluntary movement is disturbed, involuntary movements appear and muscle tone is altered.

### Parkinsonism

Parkinsonism is the name given to a clinical syndrome comprising impairment of voluntary movement (hypokinesis), rigidity and tremor. Its incidence is approximately 1 in every 1000 of the population rising to about 1% in those over 60 years.

**Aetiology.** Parkinsonism is caused by lesions in the basal ganglia and is associated particularly with damage to the interconnecting system between the substantia nigra and the corpus striatum. The nigrostriatal pathways utilise dopamine as a neurotransmitter, and parkinsonism is associated with dopamine deficiency. The precise pathophysiology and the interdependent biochemical abnormalities in parkinsonism are incompletely defined.

The commonest entity, accounting for perhaps three-quarters of cases, is paralysis agitans (also called idiopathic parkinsonism or Parkinson's disease) which is of unknown origin. It has been suggested that a slow viral infection might cause paralysis agitans. Parkinsonism is a recognised sequel of encephalitis lethargica and rarely results from other encephalitides caused by such viruses as Coxsackie type B and Japanese B. Parkinsonism is frequently — and usually wrongly — attributed to cerebral atherosclerosis. Many patients suffering from parkinsonism also show signs of cerebral atherosclerosis, but it is probable, in most instances, that the two conditions — both common in the elderly — occur coincidentally. Discrete cerebrovascular lesions affecting the substantia nigra may, very occasionally, cause parkinsonism.

Of the known causes, drugs are the commonest, and notably those of the phenothiazine group. Parkinsonism may occasionally follow a single head injury and is often a sequel of repeated head trauma in the 'punch-drunk' syndrome. There are other infrequent causes of parkinsonism, namely cerebral tumours, notably those causing midbrain compression, parasagittal and sphenoidal ridge meningiomas, meningovascular syphilis, carbon monoxide poisoning, manganese poisoning and copper deposition in Wilson's disease.

**Pathology.** In parkinsonism the most consistent histological change is cellular loss and depigmentation of the substantia nigra. In paralysis agitans the characteristic pathological changes accompanying loss of cells are Lewy bodies (hyaline masses of cytoplasm and sphingomyelin) in the central areas of the substantia nigra. In postencephalitic parkinsonism the cell depletion affects the whole substantia nigra and is usually more severe than in paralysis agitans. Other changes, such as atrophy of the globus pallidus and patchy cortical atrophy, are inconstant.

**Clinical Features.** Two-thirds of patients first develop symptoms in the fifth or sixth decades. Initial manifestations are usually so slight and develop so insidiously that a gap of 2 or 3 years may elapse between the onset of the condition and its diagnosis. Occasionally the presentation is acute and progression is rapid; this is particularly likely in postencephalitic or drug-induced cases.

Tremor is usually the feature which causes the patient to seek advice. It first involves the fingers and spreads to proximal parts of the arm; it may later extend to the tongue and legs. The tremor is slow and in the earliest stages involves rhythmical movement of the thumb towards the fingers. The fully developed movement comprises a combination of adduction and abduction of the thumb, flexion and extension of the interphalangeal and metacarpophalangeal joints as well as pronation and supination of the wrists. The tremor is present at rest and often is lessened during purposive activity. Stress and embarrassment aggravate the tremor's amplitude. These factors are operative during clinical testing so that requested movements may be accompanied by increased, rather than reduced tremor. Head tremors are rare in parkinsonism. Tremor may never be present during the course of the condition and often diminishes as rigidity progresses.

Rigidity is usually detectable early. Resistance to passive movement is increased throughout the range of movement of a joint. Concurrent tremor may lead to the 'cog-wheel' phenomenon — a superimposed jerky sensation. Profound rigidity is accompanied by fixed abnormalities of posture. The patient is flexed at neck, hips, elbows and knees. The hands are flexed at the metacarpophalangeal joints and hyperextended at the interphalangeal joints; these deformities, accompanied by adduction of the thumb across the palm, present a characteristic picture.

Hypokinesis, comprising delay in initiation of movement together with paucity, slowness and lack of precision of movements, is the most disabling feature. Of insidious onset it may first be manifest by a gradual reduction in size and legibility of a patient's handwriting. Other fine movements, such as fastening buttons and laces, are impaired, and later feeding and even turning over in bed become difficult. There is often difficulty in rising from a chair and in starting to walk. Loss of normal arm swinging when the patient walks is a very early sign of hypokinesis. Later the gait displays characteristic features. Steps are short and shuffling. Walking is usually slow but is sometimes accompanied by periods of uncontrolled acceleration when walking downhill. This phenomenon, called festination, causes the patient to take ever more rapid, smaller and smaller steps as he chases his own centre of gravity. Falls often result.

Normally pliant emotional movements of the face are slow in starting, reduced in amplitude and prolonged in their accomplishment. Blinking is usually reduced but spontaneous blepharospasm is an occasional feature, particularly in postencephalitic parkinsonism.

Impaired pupillary accommodation is a common finding in all types of parkinsonism. Sustained, involuntary, conjugate deviation of the eyes, usually upwards, called oculogyric crises, may last for minutes or hours; they occur in postencephalitic and drug-induced parkinsonism.

Speech is often affected. Some loss of voice volume is almost invariable. Delayed initiation and dysarthria are common. The cadence is slow; inflection is restricted so that speech becomes monotonous.

Hypokinesis may be overcome for short periods under the influence of a strong emotional drive such as fear or anger. Though the defects in voluntary movement are often striking and disabling, power is well preserved.

Pyramidal tract signs are not found in uncomplicated paralysis agitans, but they may be detected if there is accompanying cerebral atherosclerosis; they commonly accompany postencephalitic and post-traumatic parkinsonism and are found in those rare instances where parkinsonism is due to a cerebral tumour.

**Differential Diagnosis.** Physiological tremor often is exaggerated in the elderly and by anxiety, alcoholism and thyrotoxicosis. It is much faster than parkinsonian tremor, tends to occur only in one plane and lacks the abduction/adduction movement of the thumb.

Cerebellar atrophy is of fairly frequent occurrence in elderly patients who manifest intention tremor. Such a tremor is relieved when an affected limb is supported and relaxed and increases as the limb approaches a target.

Depressed and hypothyroid patients are often apathetic and lack normal facial expressiveness so that their appearance may suggest a diagnosis of parkinsonism.

Atherosclerotic dementia, with its attendant apathy, is often associated with increased tone due to bilateral pyramidal tract signs and may mimic parkinsonism. Other clinical features such as an exaggerated jaw jerk, increased tendon reflexes and spasticity rather than rigidity differentiate this condition from parkinsonism.

**Treatment.** Ideally, this should be aimed at the cause. The drug-induced condition is the only type which is both relatively common and curable if the offending drug is discontinued. In the majority of parkinsonian patients the cause is not known and treatment is designed to ameliorate disability. The most effective treatment now available is a combination of an anticholinergic preparation together with levodopa plus a dopadecarboxylase inhibitor.

Anticholinergic drugs produce modest improvement in parkinsonism. There are a number of synthetic preparations, such as benzhexol hydrochloride (2 mg or 5 mg), benztropine (2 mg) and orphenadrine (50 mg). One of these drugs is introduced in small amounts, such as one tablet twice daily, and the dose is increased until dryness of the mouth or blurring of vision supervene. The dose is then reduced slightly to obviate these effects.

Levodopa has strikingly improved the treatment of parkinsonism. Given by mouth in doses varying from 2 to 8 g (average 5 g daily) levodopa reduces disability in more than two-thirds of patients and is particularly effective in relieving hypokinesis. The drug causes many side-effects, some of which develop early, e.g. nausea, vomiting, and cardiac arrhythmias; these are reduced if the drug is given together with a dopadecarboxylase inhibitor.

More than 90% of an orally ingested dose of levodopa does not reach the brain and is metabolised in extracerebral tissues. Selective inhibition of extracerebral dopadecarboxylase reduces the amount of levodopa required to produce a therapeutic effect and also diminishes the side-effects caused by peripheral breakdown of levodopa. Preparations are available which combine levodopa with extracerebral dopadecarboxylase inhibitors, e.g. 250 mg of levodopa and 25 mg of carbidopa. One such tablet is equivalent in its therapeutic effect to 1 g of levodopa. This combined therapy, like levodopa itself, must be introduced in small amounts (half of a tablet twice daily) and increased gradually by a further half tablet every 4 or 5 days.

The long-term and centrally determined side-effects of levodopa are not reduced by combined therapy. Induced involuntary movements and psychiatric disturbances are very troublesome and may demand reduction or temporary cessation of treatment. Particularly disabling is the so-called 'on/off' effect which develops in patients who have been treated, often with considerable success, for more than 2 years. Manifestations of this phenomenon include unsteadiness of gait, hypotonia, anxiety and, commonly, akinesis. These disabilities tend to develop and regress suddenly. Accompanying the 'on/off' effect in some patients and persisting between the acute manifestations are unusual defects in higher cerebral function, including disinhibition, aphasia, apraxia and memory impairment. It seems likely that the frequency of occurrence of these distressing phenomena increases as treatment becomes more prolonged. Their alleviation requires withdrawal of levodopa therapy for several weeks, after which patients will often again tolerate and derive benefit from the drug.

Alternative treatment includes dopamine agonists of which the most useful is bromocriptine. An initial dose of 2·5 mg twice daily is gradually built up to 30 to 40 mg daily. The drug may be given alone or in combination with levodopa. Amantadine hydrochloride (100 mg b.d.) produces some effects both therapeutic and untoward, resembling those of levodopa but less in degree; improvement is maintained for only a few months in most cases. Other drugs, notably amphetamine and tricyclic antidepressants, have mild antiparkinsonian properties. Monoamineoxidase inhibitors should not be given to patients taking levodopa.

Stereotactic thalamotomy is now rarely employed; however, for those occasional patients whose disability is unilateral tremor unresponsive to medical treatment, it may be helpful.

**Prognosis.** There are extreme variations in the rate of progression and the degree of disability produced. Twenty per cent of patients suffering from parkinsonism at any given time cannot cope independently with the normal activities of living. The mortality of patients suffering from parkinsonism is three times that of the general population of similar age. Levodopa, though it ameliorates disability, does not affect the progress of the basic pathology.

## Hepatolenticular Degeneration (Wilson's Disease)

**Aetiology.** This is a rare autosomal recessive disorder of copper metabolism. Copper is normally absorbed in small amounts from the gut as a loose complex with albumin and carried to the liver. There some of it is re-excreted in the bile but a fraction enters the general circulation. In the liver some of the blood copper is transferred to globulin to which it is more firmly bound, forming caeruloplasmin. This copper-globulin is an oxidase enzyme but its physiological role is unknown.

In Wilson's disease copper is absorbed in excess but the transfer from the albumin-bound to the globulin-bound complex is defective, thus the serum caeruloplasmin level is low. Some of the extra copper absorbed is excreted in the urine while the rest is deposited in the tissues, particularly in the brain, liver, kidney and in Descemet's membrane in the eye. These organs may be damaged either by enzymatic poisoning by the heavy metal or by cellular necrosis followed by fibrosis (or gliosis in the brain).

**Clinical Features.** The biochemical abnormality of Wilson's disease is present from birth, but clinical evidence does not appear until adolescence. There are two main clinical types depending on whether the cerebral or hepatic signs are more evident.

In the cerebral type necrosis and sclerosis of the corpus striatum cause basal ganglion syndromes in adolescence. Most common is choreoathetosis, but parkinsonism may be caused according to the site mainly affected. There is usually cortical involvement leading to progressive dementia in which loss of emotional control is a feature.

In the hepatic type (p. 410) episodes of jaundice, fulminant hepatic failure, active chronic hepatitis or a well-compensated cirrhosis may occur.

In both types copper deposition in Descemet's membrane of the eye causes a golden-brown, yellow or green ring round the cornea. This Kayser-Fleischer ring is pathognomonic of Wilson's disease.

The urine contains excess copper and often excess amino acids. Renal tubular damage by copper may upset excretion of uric acid, sugar and phosphates. Caeruloplasmin is deficient in the blood (p. 386).

**Treatment.** This disorder was previously progressive and fatal within a few years after the appearance of clinical signs. It can now be arrested by giving copper-binding drugs (chelating agents) which mobilise copper from the tissues and promote its excretion in the urine. The most valuable of these is penicillamine, 300 mg t.d.s. orally. If it is not available or too expensive, dimercaprol or disodium calcium versenate may be given but either is a less satisfactory substitute. Hepatic and cerebral symptoms are treated symptomatically with diet and antiparkinsonism drugs.

Siblings should be examined as clinical or biochemical evidence of Wilson's disease may be detected at a stage where treatment, if started promptly and continued throughout life, may prevent the appearance or progression of clinical features.

## Kernicterus

Kernicterus is a disorder of the basal ganglia and auditory nuclei occurring in association with neonatal jaundice, particularly in premature infants. It may be caused by haemolytic disease of the newborn (p. 564), but any severe neonatal jaundice may be followed by this complication, and prematurity is more important than Rh incompatibility.

Premature babies have a functional immaturity of the glucuronyl transferase enzyme system of the liver, and, as a result, unconjugated bilirubin formed by haemolysis is not conjugated. When the infant is born it is deprived of its placental excretion route, and unconjugated bilirubin rapidly accumulates in its blood to toxic levels which depress oxidative metabolism of brain cells, and in particular those of the basal ganglia. The danger decreases rapidly about 10 days after the birth in normal full-term infants when the liver enzyme system matures, but the premature baby is in danger for a longer period.

Convulsions, coma, opisthotonos and rigidity may be early manifestations but athetoid movements or spastic paralysis, deafness of nuclear type, and mental deficiency may not appear until the baby is several months old.

Prevention depends on the early detection of haemolytic jaundice, especially in the premature child, and its prompt treatment by exchange transfusion. There is no treatment for established kernicterus and the future management is that of the child with cerebral palsy.

## Chorea

Choreiform movements are irregular, jerking, ill-sustained and unpredictable, easily recognised when fully developed. In milder forms the condition may seem to be no more than restlessness or fidgeting. Often chorea is accompanied by athetoid movements.

**Sydenham's chorea** (St. Vitus' dance) occurs in adolescents and is commoner in girls. It often follows a streptococcal throat infection. The onset may be abrupt or insidious. Choreiform movements are usually generalised and are accompanied by emotional lability so that often the condition is thought initially to be psychogenic. Pregnancy may precipitate a recurrence of chorea.

Because of the agitation, the patient, in all but the mildest cases, should be admitted to hospital and preferably nursed in isolation. Diazepam or haloperidol should be prescribed. An initial course of penicillin should be given.

Most patients recover within a month, though more prolonged illnesses occur and relapses are common. Since many patients later develop valvular heart disease their future observation and management should be as for rheumatic fever.

**Huntington's chorea** is of autosomal dominant inheritance and usually first presents in the thirties. Choreiform movements, often particularly prominent in the face, are accompanied by progressive dementia. The movements may be well controlled by tetrabenazine (50–200 mg/d) which is usually tolerated in this condition. The mental deterioration is untreatable and institutional care may be needed as the disease progresses.

## Ballism and Athetosis

Flinging limb movements of wide amplitude are called *ballismic movements*. They resemble chorea but are much more violent. It is sometimes an arbitrary decision whether one calls movements severe chorea or ballism. Usually they suddenly affect one side of the body (hemiballism or, if less dramatic, hemichorea) as a result of a vascular lesion in elderly patients. Spontaneous improvement usually occurs over a period of weeks and during this time tetrabenazine may mitigate the disability. When hemiballism persists it can effectively be treated by stereotactic thalamotomy.

*Athetoid movements* are relatively slow, confluent, writhing movements, usually most prominent at the periphery of the limbs. They are often accompanied by choreiform movements and by forced axial rotations of the trunk and neck (torsion dystonia). Athetosis usually results from cerebral hypoxia or trauma at birth or during the neonatal period and from kernicterus. Drug treatment is usually ineffective, though tetrabenazine, haloperidol or diazepam occasionally produce improvement in mild cases. Stereotactic procedures, indicated only in severe disability, sometimes help.

**Differential Diagnosis.** The involuntary movements of chorea, athetosis and ballism must be distinguished from *tics* which in most cases are not due to organic disease of the nervous system. Tics are usually rapid, repetitive, co-ordinated and stereotyped movements, most of which can be mimicked. Their pattern varies widely but an individual's tic tends to be reproduced faithfully. Common mild tics, including blepharospasm, sniffing, and shrugging movements, may be irritating but rarely need treatment. When well established in an adult they are virtually irremediable. In contrast, many children develop tics, often elaborate facial movements which cause much parental concern but which almost always disappear.

In adults, tics of recent development may be induced by drugs. Amphetamine addiction leads to repeated, rapid chewing movements of the jaws. Complex tongue, mouth, and cheek movements may result from taking phenothiazines or levodopa. Withdrawal of the causal drug usually leads to rapid cessation of the movement.

*Spasmodic torticollis* is a form of tic which comprises involuntary turning of the head to one side and starts most commonly in the thirties. Initially rapid and correctable rotating movements may give place to long-sustained and later to fixed deviation of the neck.

## CONGENITAL AND DEGENERATIVE DISEASES

In many diseases of unknown cause, there is clinical and pathological evidence of damage which is confined to a special type of neurone, e.g. motor neurone disease. Although no causative factors have been identified, it seems probable that many of the following disorders will ultimately be classified together as being due to 'biochemical lesions'. The metabolic functions of the neurone are controlled by its cell body but when any gradual failure of any of these processes occurs the effect is first seen at the end of its axon, so that there occurs a progressive 'dying back' of the neurone from its termination towards the cell body, associated with loss of nucleoprotein in the cell (chromatolysis). This will be seen to be the typical feature of the pathology of the congenital and degenerative disorders.

### Motor Neurone Disease

This rare disorder is the paradigm of a systematised neurological disease.

**Aetiology and Pathology.** The cause is unknown. Metallic poisoning, particularly by aluminium, has been implicated. As in all progressive neurological disorders autoimmune and slow viral aetiologies have been postulated. The latter possibility at present seems particularly attractive since Creutzfeldt-Jakob disease (p. 707) is of proven slow viral origin and shows some features in common with motor neurone disease.

Loss of motor neurones and gliosis can be demonstrated in the motor cortex, in the motor nuclei of the brain stem and in anterior horn cells of the spinal cord. In the cord, there is also loss of myelinated corticospinal fibres.

**Clinical Features.** Motor neurone disease is characterised by the insidious onset and uninterrupted progression of combinations of lesions of upper and/or lower motor neurones. Fasciculation (p. 652) is common. Motor neurone disease is twice as frequent in males and is rare before 40 years of age. The commonest age of onset is in the sixth decade. Some patterns of evolution are frequently manifest and are usefully categorised because they offer a guide to prognosis.

*Progressive bulbar palsy* comprises dysarthria, dysphonia and dysphagia. Impaired articulation is usually the earliest feature but difficulty in swallowing, hoarseness and loss of voice volume supervene. There are signs of true, as well as supranuclear, bulbar palsy. Wasting and fasciculation of the tongue are accompanied by spasticity thereof and a pathologically brisk jaw jerk. Features of bulbar palsy eventually develop in the later stages of the other types listed below.

*Amyotrophic lateral sclerosis* is probably the commonest mode of presentation and is characterised by lower motor neurone signs in the upper limbs and pyramidal tract signs in the legs. Wasting and weakness of the small muscles of the hands, usually the earliest manifestation, are accompanied by spasticity of thc legs and extensor plantar responses. Wasting and fasciculation spread to the proximal arm muscles and the leg musculature; increased tendon reflexes in the arms may later indicate involvement of the upper motor neurones.

*Progressive muscular atrophy* implicates only lower motor neurones for long periods. It usually presents with foot drop, which is often initially unilateral but eventually becomes symmetrical. Wasting and weakness of the hands, proximal spread of lower motor neurone affection in the limbs and the addition of pyramidal tract involvement occur after an interval of years.

*Course*. These labelled entities are frequently recognised but variant patterns are common. As the disease progresses the pictures of the different categories merge so that the final picture usually includes severe bulbar palsy as well as upper and lower motor neurone signs in all four limbs.

**Diagnosis**. Some aspects of the clinical features of motor neurone disease, irrespective of the particular type of natural history, are useful in diagnosis. There are no sensory signs. Sensory symptoms, with the exception of pain, are rare. Aches caused by the use of weakened muscles and painful cramps in the legs are fairly common. Paraesthesiae, unless clearly attributable to a coincidental cause, are not a feature of motor neurone disease and their presence should lead to critical reappraisal of the diagnosis. Fasciculations, though not pathognomonic of the condition, are seen almost invariably in motor neurone disease in which they are usually more obvious and more widespread than in any other disease. Though the initial manifestations of motor neurone disease are commonly unilateral, they usually become bilateral, and indeed symmetrical, in the vast majority of instances, within a few months.

In few other conditions do severely wasted muscles subserve pathologically brisk tendon reflexes. This phenomenon, sometimes called tonic atrophy is common to all types of motor neurone disease other than progressive muscular atrophy during its early stages. Defects in external ocular movements and sphincter disturbances are extremely rare. Full awareness and normal intellectual abilities are usually preserved intact throughout the course of the illness. The CSF is almost always normal.

Three pathological processes which are potentially treatable may closely mimic motor neurone disease and should always be excluded. (i) An occult carcinoma (particularly of the bronchus) may produce systematised motor neurone lesions. A chest radiograph should always be obtained in patients presenting the features of motor neurone disease, and if there are indicative clinical features further investigations should be performed. (ii) Diabetic amyotrophy (p. 735) may resemble motor neurone disease and accordingly diabetes mellitus must be excluded. (iii) Meningovascular syphilis can present a picture similar to that of motor neurone disease and syphilitic serology is therefore an essential investigation.

**Treatment and Prognosis.** No medical treatment improves the outlook in motor neurone disease. Management includes the provision of walking aids and wheel-chairs and the maintenance of morale. Physicians have a duty to support patients and their relatives and to relieve distress in the disease's terminal stages.

Motor neurone disease is inexorably progressive and invariably fatal. Death usually results from pneumonia and respiratory failure and within 2 years of the onset of bulbar palsy. Amyotrophic lateral sclerosis is compatible with 4 or 5 years of life from the initial manifestation. Progressive muscular atrophy runs the most prolonged course; death usually occurs in 8 to 10 years from the onset.

The final state, of anarthria, aphagia and widespread limb weakness in a patient fully aware of the position is extremely distressing for the patient and the family.

## The Hereditary Ataxias

This is a group of related hereditary or familial disorders in which the systems of neurones which 'die back' (p. 721) are mainly the spinal and brain stem tracts leading to the cerebellum, the corticospinal tracts, and the optic nerves. Different combinations of these elements form recognisable clinical pictures, which usually 'breed true' in a family, but it may be impossible to differentiate the different types during life. The group forms a link with hereditary disorders of the peripheral nerves such as peroneal muscular atrophy (p. 734) and with neurofibromatosis (p. 725) and these may occur in association with the hereditary ataxias either in one individual or in the same family. Congenital deformities, particularly pes cavus, are also commonly present.

Cerebellar degeneration commencing in later life may be due to cacinomatous neuropathy (p. 742).

**Clinical Features.** The onset may be any time from infancy to middle life. Symptoms are slowly progressive. Where cerebellar or spinocerebellar neurones are involved there is progressive ataxia of gait, followed by intention tremor of the arms, dysarthria of explosive type and, in some types, nystagmus. Where the main lesion is in corticospinal tracts there is a hereditary spastic paraplegia. Optic atrophy and loss of bladder reflexes may occur.

*Friedreich's ataxia* is the most common type, usually familial but occasionally sporadic. Unaffected members of the family as well as the patients may show pes cavus. There is degeneration of the spinocerebellar and corticospinal tracts, and of the posterior columns. There is therefore very severe ataxia. Tendon jerks are lost at an early stage, the ankle jerks first, then the knee jerks but finally all tendon jerks may be absent. Muscle tone is decreased. The plantar reflexes are extensor. Muscle, joint and vibration senses are impaired as the posterior column degeneration progresses. Scoliosis and pes cavus are almost invariable and other congenital abnormalities such as spina bifida and conduction defects in the heart, giving rise to ECG abnormalities, are common.

**Treatment and Prognosis.** There is no specific treatment. Co-ordination exercises and occupational therapy will help the patient to overcome the disability in the early stages but a wheel-chair life becomes inevitable later. Scoliosis and pes cavus may require appropriate appliances or orthopaedic surgery. All diseases of this group are progressive but compatible with a long life.

## Syringomyelia

Cavities, filled with fluid and surrounded by glial tissue, lying near to the centre of the spinal cord, are the characteristic pathological lesions in syringomyelia.

**Aetiology.** The most important factor is failure of development of the foramina of Magendie and Luschka. Cerebrospinal fluid cannot escape into the subarachnoid space from the fourth ventricle since its roof is imperforate. Pressure rises within the closed ventricular system and is communicated to the central canal of the cord which expands along irregular paths of least resistance. The expanding cavity usually disrupts second order spinothalamic neurones (p. 655), often interrupts the lateral columns and may extend laterally to damage anterior horn cells. Clinical signs predictably reflect the interruption of function of these neural structures; this is usually maximal in the lower cervical region.

Dilatation of the central canal of the cord may result from increased pressure in the canal associated with congenital malformations of the brain in the region of the foramen magnum, e.g herniation of parts of the cerebellum through the foramen magnum (*Arnold-Chiari syndrome*) and cysts.

**Clinical Features.** Symptoms are of insidious onset, and slow progression. Patients usually present in the third or fourth decade but signs may be detectable much earlier. Most characteristic sensory feature is 'dissociated' sensory loss, i.e. loss or depression of pain and temperature sensation with preservation of the modalities of touch, vibration and position. The patient often recognises this sensory loss and seeks advice because of it. Less commonly, when pain fibres are irritated, pain in the arms is a presenting feature. Loss of protective sensory functions leads to trophic lesions such as painless burns and ulcers on the hands and sometimes painless, disorganised joints (Charcot's joints) in the upper limbs.

Wasting of the small muscles of one or other hand is often manifest early. Loss of one or more reflexes in the arms is almost invariable. Characteristically there are pyramidal tract signs in the legs. Hyperreflexia in the legs and extensor plantar responses are common. Upward extension of the cavities to involve the lower brain stem (*syringobulbia*) leads to dissociated sensory loss on the face, palatal palsy, Horner's syndrome and nystagmus. Kyphoscoliosis, pes cavus and spina bifida are often found.

Investigations should be aimed at defining potentially treatable anomalies around the foramen magnum. Radiographs of this area may show bony malformations. CT scanning or myelography demonstrates cysts or malformations of the medulla.

**Treatment and Prognosis.** Where causative congenital lesions are demonstrated early, surgical treatment is indicated. Decompression of the foramen magnum, opening the roof of the fourth ventricle, aspiration of the cavity in the cord and occlusion, by muscle, of the upper end of the central canal, may prevent progression of the disease. If surgical treatment is not feasible, management is directed towards preventing injury and relieving pain, when present, by radiotherapy aimed at the cavity. If untreated the condition is slowly progressive, and worsens if the brain stem is involved.

### Neurofibromatosis (von Recklinghausen's Disease)

This is an autosomal dominant disorder in which tumours are derived from the neurilemmal sheath of the peripheral nerves, nerve roots or cranial nerves. Cutaneous fibromas, which are pedunculated tumours named *mollusca fibrosa*, are considered to be of similar origin. Tumours such as gliomas, meningiomas and phaeochromocytomas may also be associated with neurofibromatosis.

**Clinical Features.** A patient may show only one or many of a wide range of cutaneous or of peripheral or central neurological abnormalities. Some of the more common are *café-au-lait* patches of skin pigmentation, cutaneous fibromas and benign tumours of peripheral nerves which are discrete, movable lumps arranged along lines of nerves. The nerve trunks may be thickened or there may be a diffuse plexiform growth. Solitary neurofibromas may occur on a spinal nerve root or on a cranial nerve, especially the eighth. The tumours may also occur within body cavities, in the eyes and within the bones where they cause cystic change or kyphoscoliosis. New tumours gradually appear throughout life but the progress is slow. Any tumour may become malignant (sarcoma) but the chances of it doing so are small.

Biopsy of a tumour is rarely necessary. With intracranial and intraspinal types the protein level of the CSF is very high. Radiology may show that an internal auditory meatus or intervertebral foramen is widened if it contains a neurofibroma.

**Treatment.** No treatment is required unless there is cerebral or spinal compression, or sarcomatous change, when operative removal of the tumour is necessary.

## NUTRITIONAL NEUROLOGICAL DISEASE

Malnutrition may cause lesions in a number of sites in the central nervous system. Deficiencies, particularly of the B vitamin group, are important causes but there are often multiple contributory factors and vitamin deficiencies may be combined with protein deficiency and toxins, notably alcohol. The various neurological syndromes that ensue are best considered on an anatomical basis.

**Lesions of the Cerebral Cortex.** Vitamin $B_{12}$ deficiency may cause a toxic confusional state and, if the deficiency is prolonged, may result in dementia.

Pellagra (p. 114) gives rise to marked impairment of higher cerebral function often associated with dysarthria, dysphagia, and diarrhoea. There are usually upper motor neurone signs and characteristic skin changes. Treatment is given on page 115. An isolated deficiency of pyridoxine (p. 117) occasionally occurs in infants and causes irritability and epileptic fits.

Alcoholics may develop a slowly progressive dementia with cerebral atrophy due in part to a direct toxic effect but associated multiple vitamin deficiencies also contribute.

**Brain Stem Lesions.** Rapidly developing, severe deficiency of thiamin may cause Wernicke's encephalopathy (p. 112). Pathologically there are petechial haemorrhages in the brain stem and widespread patchy necrosis of neurones. Clinically there are disorders of ocular movement with nystagmus often accompanied by memory defect and confabulation (Korsakoff's psychosis). The condition, if untreated, may be fatal but thiamin (p. 112), if started early enough, produces dramatic improvement.

Central pontine myelinolysis occurs in alcoholics. There is widespread destruction of myelin in the pons involving all the long tracts. The picture usually develops suddenly with tetraparesis, dysphagia and anarthria and is often terminal.

**Cerebellar Lesions.** Ataxia of gait and of leg movements with little affection of the arms is due to degeneration of the anterior superior vermis of the cerebellum in alcoholics; if the patient continues to drink alcohol more widespread cerebellar dysfunction develops. The contributions of dietary deficiency and the toxic effect of alcohol are not clearly defined but withdrawal of alcohol and giving vitamins result in marked improvement.

**Spinal Cord Lesions.** VITAMIN B12 DEFICIENCY: This condition is also called *sub-acute combined degeneration of the spinal cord* and is characterised by demyelination affecting particularly the posterior columns and corticospinal tracts of the spinal cord. There is usually involvement of the peripheral nerves.

The condition is associated with Addisonian pernicious anaemia (p. 549) and rarely follows gastrectomy. It usually develops gradually in the middle aged. The most common presenting symptoms are paraesthesiae of the toes and, later, of the fingers. Motor symptoms, notably weakness and ataxia, become progressively more severe as the spinal cord is more extensively involved.

The physical signs depend on the degrees of involvement of the peripheral nerves and of the posterior and lateral columns of the spinal cord. Glove and stocking impairment of superficial sensation is almost invariable. Calf tenderness is often increased. Position and vibration sense are usually markedly impaired in the legs. The tendon reflexes may be brisk but commonly the ankle jerks are lost. The plantar responses are usually extensor. Occasionally there may be an associated toxic confusional state. It responds to treatment, but without treatment, dementia follows.

The diagnosis should be considered whenever a patient presents with symmetrical paraesthesiae or with unexplained dementia. Associated features such as glossitis, megaloblastic anaemia and achlorhydria will strongly support the diagnosis but need not be present. Diagnosis should be confirmed by the estimation of vitamin $B_{12}$ in the serum.

The treatment of vitamin $B_{12}$ deficiency comprises large doses of hydroxocobalamin, 1000 micrograms daily for a week, weekly for three months and monthly thereafter. The response to treatment depends on the stage at which it is initiated. The signs due to a peripheral neuropathy often recover completely; ataxia may markedly improve; severe spasticity and dementia often persist.

TROPICAL SPINAL ATAXIA occurs mainly in West Africa. In most cases the picture is one of sensory spinal ataxia but sometimes there is upper motor neurone involvement and amblyopia with optic atrophy. This type of spastic paraparesis seems in most cases to be due to chronic exposure to excess dietary cyanide in those who live largely on a diet of cassava which is rich in cyanide. A similar type of spastic paraparesis with amblyopia occurs in West Indians, but the nature of the aetiology in these cases is ill-defined.

LATHYRISM. The consumption of lathyrus peas, a common constituent of Indians' diets, may produce a slowly progressive spastic paraplegia. Lathyrus seeds contain a neurotoxin. A similar type of spastic paraplegia was described in European prisoners of war in the Far East. This was probably due to multiple vitamin deficiencies though the precise agent was not identified.

**Peripheral Nerve Lesions.** Deficiencies of one or more of the vitamins of the B complex lead to neuropathy. Thiamin, pantothenic acid, nicotinic acid and pyridoxine deficiencies may cause a symmetrical, mixed sensory-motor neuropathy (p. 735). In many instances, particularly in alcoholics, there are combined deficiencies of these vitamins. If treated early, nutritional polyneuropathy responds well to a mixed diet and generous doses of the vitamin B complex.

The *burning feet syndrome* is due to a mild but painful sensory neuropathy. It was found in European prisoners in the Far East during the Second World War and now occurs among the elderly who subsist on an inadequate diet. The cause is deficiency of the B group of vitamins. Patients complain of severe, lancinating or burning pains in the feet and distal parts of the legs, particularly in bed at night. Signs of polyneuropathy are sparse or absent. The response to vitamin B complex, given orally, is usually good.

# DISEASES OF SPINAL CORD AND PERIPHERAL NERVES

## Compression of the Spinal Cord or Nerve Roots

**Aetiology and Pathology.** The more important causes of spinal cord compression are: 1. *In the vertebral column*: crush fracture of a vertebral body; posterior protrusion of an intervertebral disc; secondary carcinoma (from breast, prostate, bronchus or other sites); myelomatosis and tuberculous disease of the spine.

2. *In relation to the spinal meninges*: epidural abscess; tumours (meningioma, neurofibroma; infiltration with lymphomatous and leukaemic deposits); syphilitic meningitis.

3. *In the spinal cord*: tumours (gliomas, ependymoma and metastatic deposits).

Tumours, disc protrusions and trauma account for the majority of cases of spinal cord compression. It is convenient in practice to divide the tumours into those arising outside the spinal cord (extramedullary), which constitute about 80%, and those arising within (intramedullary).

A space-occupying lesion within the spinal canal may involve nerve tissue directly by pressure, or indirectly by interfering with the blood supply. Oedema from venous obstruction impairs the function of the neurones. Ischaemia from arterial obstruction leads to necrosis of the spinal cord. The earlier stages are reversible but severely damaged neurones do not recover so it is most important to diagnose and treat spinal compression without delay.

**Clinical Features.** The onset of symptoms of spinal cord compression is usually slow but it may be acute with trauma or metastases, especially if there is arterial occlusion. Pain localised over the spine or in a root distribution is the most common initial symptom. It may be aggravated by spinal movement or by coughing, sneezing or straining at the toilet which cause temporary elevation of spinal fluid pressure. Paraesthesiae and numbness or cold sensations may also develop early, especially in the lower limbs. Motor symptoms, which usually appear later, consist of heaviness, stiffness or weakness of a limb, Urgency or hesitancy of micturition, leading eventually to urinary retention is usually a late manifestation.

The signs found on examination vary according to the structures involved. There may be a local kyphosis if there is vertebral disease, and local tenderness may be present with this or with extradural abscess. A bruit may be heard with a stethoscope over the site of the vascular tumour (angioma). Involvement of the posterior roots gives rise to hyperaesthesia and later to sensory loss over the appropriate dermatome. When the anterior roots are affected there are signs of a lower motor neurone lesion at the corresponding level. Interruption of ascending fibres in the spinal cord causes sensory loss below the level of the lesion which may be of superficial sensation or of proprioceptive sense, according to which tracts are mainly involved (Fig. 14.3). Light touch, however, is often affected early. Interruption of descending fibres gives rise to upper motor neurone signs below the level of the lesion and control of the sphincters may be lost. If damage is confined to one side of the cord the *Brown-Séquard syndrome* results. On the side of the lesion there is a band of hyperaesthesia with below it loss of proprioceptive sense and upper motor neurone signs. On the other side there is loss of spinothalamic sensation (pain, warmth and cold) as fibres of that tract decussate soon after entering the cord.

The distribution of these signs varies with the level of the lesion. Lesions above the fifth cervical segment give signs of an upper motor neurone lesion and sensory loss in upper and lower limbs (tetraplegia); a lesion between the fifth cervical and first thoracic segments gives signs of a lower motor neurone lesion and segmental sensory loss in the upper limbs and signs of an upper motor neurone lesion in the lower limbs; a lesion in the thoracic cord causes a spastic paraplegia with sensory loss having a horizontal upper level on the trunk; a lesion in the lumbosacral cord gives signs of a lower motor neurone lesion in the appropriate segments of the lower limbs and sensory loss. Spinal lesions lower than the first lumbar vertebra cannot damage the spinal cord but may damage the roots of the cauda equina.

Examination of the CSF is of great value but withdrawal of fluid may alter the pressure balance above and below the lesion in the cord and lead to rapid exacerbation of compression. For this reason, if lumbar puncture confirms the diagnosis, the patient should be referred without any delay to a neurosurgeon and if the diagnosis is highly probable on clinical grounds the puncture should be postponed until it is convenient to operate on the patient. Queckenstedt's test may reveal the features of a partial or complete block but a normal result does not exclude the diagnosis. The cell content is normal but there is a great excess of protein and xanthochromia is present (*Froin's syndrome*). Radiological examination of the spine may reveal abnormalities at the site of the lesion but often myelography is required.

**Diagnosis.** Pain, which is so often a presenting symptom of spinal cord compression, may be wrongly attributed to such conditions as pleurisy, cholecystitis or 'rheumatism', but a careful examination will reveal signs of organic nervous disease. It is insufficient to be content with eliciting the tendon reflexes, as motor signs may be delayed long after sensory signs are present. If there is indisputable evidence of spinal cord damage it is essential to decide the site of the primary lesion. A general examination may reveal evidence of disease elsewhere making it likely that the lesion in the cord is secondary to this. A search should be made for a primary tumour in another organ, enlargement of lymph nodes, the cutaneous signs of neurofibromatosis and the presence of sepsis which could lead to extradural abscess. An abscess should always be considered if pain is severe and signs of cord disease develop rapidly as immediate treatment is imperative.

If the lesion causing compression arose initially in the spinal cord it is necessary to distinguish it from conditions such as multiple sclerosis, syringomyelia, motor neurone disease and subacute combined degeneration. Multiple sclerosis appearing for the first time in middle-aged people may present as a slowly progressive lesion of the spinal cord. The differentiation from spinal cord compression is, however, so difficult and of such importance that there should be no hesitation in seeking expert advice.

**Treatment and Prognosis.** Surgical relief of the compression is a matter of great urgency since recovery from severe paralysis is unlikely. A delay of even a few hours may be critical in extradural abscess. Exploration is also often required to ascertain the pathological nature of the lesion. If a benign extramedullary tumour is found, it may be removed. In malignant tumours, leukaemic infiltration, and in most intramedullary lesions decompression helps little if at all. Radiotherapy may halt the course of the disease and may be of help in the relief of pain.

Prognosis depends on the severity and duration of the compression before it is relieved. In addition, the nature of the cause must be taken into account. Thus decompression for a malignant lesion may be undertaken though it will be of only temporary benefit.

## Paraplegia

Paraplegia may result from many causes, e.g. tumours, trauma and other forms of spinal compression (p. 727), multiple sclerosis, subacute combined degeneration of the cord and, in India, lathyrism.

**Treatment** must be directed to the cause but management of the paraplegia itself is most important if complications which may in themselves lead to death are to be avoided. Pressure sores, urinary infections, renal calculi, faecal impaction and contractures are complications which can be prevented.

*Skin.* The skin is liable to be damaged with the formation of pressure sores because of the loss of sensation, diminished blood supply and the immobility of the patient. The patient must be nursed on a specially made rubber mattress and every two to four hours should be turned and nursed in such a position as will avoid pressure on bony prominences such as the sacrum and heels. This is most easily done by nursing the patient in a Stryker frame. The skin must be kept dry and clean. If a pressure sore forms, the patient must not lie on the affected side and scrupulous asepsis must be observed until healing takes place. Skin grafting may be required. Nutrition must be maintained by a well-balanced diet containing adequate amounts of protein, vitamin C and iron. Blood transfusions may be required in individual cases.

*Bladder.* If retention occurs, aseptic intermittent catheterisation must be carried out. An indwelling catheter may then be inserted and attached to a water-seal drainage bottle. It should be clipped and allowed to drain at regular intervals to establish reflex emptying of the bladder. As the rhythm becomes established the catheter is withdrawn and the patient trained to micturate reflexly at fixed times. Emptying of the bladder should be assisted by manual compression of the lower abdomen by patient or nurse. It is not advisable to give antibiotics prophylactically but if infection develops it must be treated promptly. An adequate consumption of fluid should be ensured. Frequent turning and early ambulation where possible are the best measures for reducing the dangers of urinary stagnation and calculus formation.

*Bowel.* Constipation must be prevented by suitable diet and laxatives. If it occurs it must be relieved by enemas; otherwise the faeces will become hard and impacted and may require to be removed manually.

*Paralysed Parts.* Spasticity readily leads to the development of flexor spasm and contractures in the limbs. This danger can be reduced by regular passive movement of the limbs and by nursing the patient in such positions as will discourage flexion of the joints. The weight of the bedclothes should be taken from the lower limbs by a cradle to reduce reflex stimulation and prevent drop-foot deformity. If there is no hope of recovery, flexor spasms may be abolished by intrathecal injection of phenol in glycerine or by section of anterior nerve roots.

*Rehabilitation.* When the cause of paraplegia is not progressive, a great deal can be done by rehabilitation. Patients may learn to walk with calipers or to use a wheel-chair. They may thus be able to care for themselves and may even follow a suitable occupation and take part in a variety of recreational activities.

## Cervical Disc Herniation and Cervical Spondylosis

Degenerative changes occur in the cervical intervertebral discs in the same manner as in the lumbar region (p. 731) and may lead to herniation. This may affect one disc only, most commonly that between the sixth and seventh cervical vertebrae, or there may be involvement of several discs with secondary osteoarthrosis. The latter changes (cervical spondylosis) are especially liable to interfere with the blood supply to the spinal cord, and thus lead to further damage.

The clinical syndromes of acute cervical disc protrusion and chronic cervical spondylosis may occur at different times in the same patient, depending on the anatomical relation of disc protrusions and osteophytic outgrowths to the nerve roots and spinal cord, and on secondary postural or traumatic factors. Acute herniation is usually laterally situated and causes compression of a nerve root but does not involve the spinal cord. The chronic degeneration of discs is associated with midline herniation and so spinal cord compression may result.

**Acute Protrusion of a Cervical Intervertebral Disc.** This may occur at any age, usually without apparent trauma to the neck. The patient complains of attacks of pain in the neck. In severe attacks pain is referred to the skin segmental area of one of the lower cervical nerve roots and to the muscles, bones and joints which it supplies. Hyperaesthesia and hyperalgesia may be found in the affected segment but sensory loss sometimes occurs. Depression of tendon reflexes utilising the affected root is common and lower motor neurone paresis of root distribution is also an occasional finding. The neck is held stiffly, and pain is produced by its movement.

**Cervical Spondylosis.** This term is usually reserved for the disorder resulting from chronic cervical disc degeneration. The highest incidence is in the decade 60 to 70. The symptoms are of two types depending on whether the protrusion is lateral or dorsomedial.

(1) Lateral herniation of discs, with secondary calcification and osteophytes encroaching on the intervertebral foramina, causes radicular symptoms like those of the

acute disc syndrome just described, but the onset may be subacute or insidious and involvement of more than one root on one or both sides is common.

(2) Dorsomedial herniation of discs which become calcified results in transverse bars which cause pressure on the spinal cord and on the anterior spinal artery which supplies the anterior two-thirds of the cord. The onset is insidious. Upper motor neurone weakness involves one or more limbs and the legs may be spastic before the upper limbs are involved. Sensory loss is most common in the upper limbs where it has a dermatome pattern. Involvement of the spinothalamic tracts may cause disturbance of pain and temperature sensation in the lower limbs, and in some cases muscle-joint sense is also defective. Pain and limitation of movement of the neck are not marked features unless a particular posture causes nipping of a nerve root.

**Investigation.** Radiological examination shows narrowing of the disc spaces and osteophyte formation with loss of the normal cervical lordosis. Oblique views show encroachment by osteophytes on the intervertebral foramina. Queckenstedt's test (p. 728) should be performed while the neck is flexed and extended, as a complete or partial block may be present when the head is in one or other of these positions. The fluid is normal unless its circulation is obstructed, when the protein may be raised. It may be necessary to confirm the diagnosis by myelography.

**Treatment.** The acute syndrome is treated by rest in bed or by intermittent neck traction followed by immobilisation of the neck in a light metal or plastic collar. Some form of immobilisation should be maintained for at least three months. It is important to watch for progressive cervical cord compression but decompressive surgery is rarely required.

### The Lumbago-Sciatica Syndrome

Lumbago is pain in the lower part of the back; sciatica is pain in the distribution of the sciatic nerve. They are not, therefore, disease entities but symptoms and they are often associated.

**Aetiology and Pathology.** The most common cause is herniation of an intervertebral disc. Other causes are much rarer but important to recognise. They include spinal tumour (neurofibroma and meningioma), ankylosing spondylitis, malignant disease in the pelvis, and tuberculosis of the vertebral bodies or of the sacroiliac joint. Degenerative changes in the intervertebral discs may appear as early as 20 years of age, but herniation is often precipitated by trauma such as twisting the spine, lifting heavy weights while the spine is flexed or during childbirth. The nucleus pulposus may bulge or rupture the annulus fibrosus, giving rise to lumbago by pressure on nerve endings in the spinal ligaments and by producing changes in the vertebral joints, and to sciatica by causing congestion of, or pressure on, the nerve roots.

**Clinical Features.** The onset may be sudden or gradual, and may follow closely upon trauma to the back. Attacks of lumbago may precede sciatica by months or years. Lumbago is characterised by sudden severe low back pain when the patient is bending, preventing him from straightening. The sciatic pain is felt in the buttock and radiates down the posterior aspect of the thigh and calf to the outer border of the foot. It is exacerbated by coughing or sneezing which raises the pressure in the veins and the spinal subarachnoid space. Paraesthesiae and later numbness may be felt over the distribution of the involved nerve root, most often the first sacral. In severe cases, weakness of the calf muscle or foot-drop may occur, according to which roots are involved. The signs associated with prolapse of an intervertebral disc may be divided into two groups.

*Signs due to altered mechanics of the lumbar spine.* Muscle spasm causes flattening of the lumbar curve and scoliosis at the level of the prolapsed disc. Tenderness may be found when pressure is applied to the side of the vertebral spines in the region of the affected disc.

*Signs due to pressure on the nerve root.* Involvement of the *first sacral* root causes loss of the ankle jerk, weakness of eversion and plantar flexion of the foot, and sensory loss over the outer border of the foot. The glutei may be wasted on the affected side. Involvement of the *fifth lumbar* root causes weakness of dorsiflexion of the toes and sometimes foot-drop. Sensory loss occurs on the dorsum of the foot and the lateral aspect of the leg over the fifth lumbar dermatome. The ankle jerk is not affected. Involvement of the *fourth lumbar* root causes weakness of inversion of the foot and of the quadriceps muscle and loss of the knee jerk. Sensory loss is over the medial aspect of the leg.

A valuable sign of root pressure is limitation of flexion of the thigh on the affected side if the straight leg is raised (Lasègue's sign).

**Investigation.** Other causes of sciatic pain can be excluded by pelvic examination and by radiological examination of the lumbosacral spine. There may be no apparent radiological change in acute disc herniation, or there may be narrowing of the disc space with osteophyte formation at the margins of the vertebral bodies. Myelography is required only if the diagnosis is in doubt or for purposes of localisation before operation. Intraspinal neoplasm as the cause should be suspected if the CSF protein is raised.

**Treatment.** The initial treatment in all cases is rest in bed on a firm mattress supported by fracture boards. Rest must be absolute with prohibition of the sitting position. Compromise in this respect and permission to leave bed for toilet purposes are the usual reasons for failure of this treatment. The roots most commonly involved are the first sacral and the fifth lumbar, in which case the patient should be kept supine and no rotation of the spine permitted; but in disc protrusion involving the fourth lumbar root the lateral position with flexion of the hips is best suited to relax tension on the affected root and hence to relieve pain. Bed rest is continued for two to four weeks, after which gradual mobilisation with back-strengthening exercises is carried out over a further period of 10 to 14 days. For middle-aged or elderly patients with chronic residual backache and a tendency to acute attacks of lumbago, a spinal support may be of great value. Cases which do not respond to rest, or in which there have been recurrences, may require surgery.

## Peripheral Neuropathy

The cells of origin of peripheral nerves lie in the anterior horns of the spinal cord and the dorsal root ganglia. Axons represent elongated processes of these cells. They are enveloped by a series of Schwann cells, forming the fatty myelin sheath. Pathological processes which primarily affect cell bodies may first manifest themselves at the distal ends of axonal processes.

Many diseases affect peripheral nerves whose pathological reactions may be

(1) parenchymal where the lesion affects (a) nerve cells and their axons, or (b) the myelin sheath; (2) interstitial where the pathological process primarily affects the connective tissue or blood vessels of nerves. Although these rather stereotyped reactions do not lead to distinctive clinical features, a knowledge of the pathological nature of a neuropathy is helpful in assessing its prognosis. The clinical classification of peripheral nerve lesions comprises (1) involvement of one or more individual peripheral nerves or (2) a generalised polyneuropathy.

## Mononeuropathy

This term refers to affection of a single nerve. *Trauma* is a common cause. Sustained pressure or stretching of nerve occurs in a variety of situations. The radial nerve is implicated as, for instance, in the 'Saturday night' palsy which results from bizarre sleeping postures caused by drunkenness. The ulnar nerve at the elbow and the common peroneal nerve at the head of the fibula may be compressed. The signs are those of lower motor neurone paresis and sensory loss in the distribution of the respective nerves. Complete recovery of function in four to six weeks is almost invariable.

*Entrapment Neuropathy*. Nerves may be compressed whenever they pass through or near rigid anatomical structures, particularly fibro-osseous tunnels; this is one of the most frequent affections of peripheral nerves. Compression of the median nerve in the carpal tunnel is the commonest example. It occurs most frequently in middle-aged women and is then usually unaccompanied by other disease. It may also be a complication of pregnancy, myxoedema, acromegaly or rheumatoid arthritis. The patient complains of pain, numbness, tingling or an 'electric shock' feeling in thumb and fingers supplied by the median nerve, especially after using the hand or in bed at night when it may waken the patient from sleep. There is sometimes objective sensory loss of the radial three and a half digits and there may be weakness and wasting of abductor pollicis brevis and opponens pollicis muscles. The condition is often bilateral. Rest and splinting at night should be tried. Local injection of hydrocortisone is sometimes effective if there is no muscular wasting. Thyroxine therapy relieves the carpal tunnel syndrome in myxoedema. The syndrome occurring in pregnancy usually disappears in the puerperium but until then may be relieved by the use of diuretics. If these measures are unsuccessful the condition can be relieved by surgical decompression of the nerve in the carpal tunnel.

The lower trunk of the brachial plexus may be compressed at the thoracic outlet, especially if there is a cervical rib. Nocturnal pain in the arm and sensorimotor disturbance in the C8–T1 distribution are relieved by rest and physiotherapy. Operative treatment is rarely necessary.

The lateral cutaneous nerve of the thigh may be entrapped at the inguinal ligament giving rise to paraesthesiae and pain over the anterolateral aspect of the thigh (meralgia paraesthetica).

*Diabetes*, particularly if insulin dependent, is a common cause of an acute mononeuropathy affecting a peripheral (or cranial) nerve. Recovery is usually complete in 4 to 8 weeks.

## Mononeuritis Multiplex

In this condition several spinal nerves are damaged concurrently or serially. Clinically signs are limited to discrete neural territories. Leprosy is a common cause of this picture in some geographical areas (p. 795). Polyarteritis nodosa, rheumatoid arthritis (p. 608) and other connective tissue disorders, diabetes mellitus and sarcoidosis may also give rise to multiple peripheral nerve lesions.

### Localised Radiculopathy

**Neuralgic Amyotrophy.** Demyelination of a localised group of nerve roots sometimes follows vaccination or inoculation; an immunological mechanism may be responsible. It may also occur after infection, injuries or operations.

The patient complains of severe pain over one shoulder girdle, sometimes spreading up the neck or down the arm. Simultaneously, or two or three days later, paralysis develops in the painful muscles. These are usually supplied by the fifth and sixth and less commonly the seventh cervical roots so that the deltoid, spinati, and serratus anterior muscles are usually involved, and frequently also the muscles of the upper arm. The tendon jerks disappear in the affected limb and wasting is rapid. Sensory loss is slight or absent. If present it is usually on the outer aspect of the upper third of the affected arm. The brachial plexus is often tender. Sometimes paralysis of single nerves of the upper limb occurs and occasionally both shoulder girdles are involved. Constitutional symptoms are mild or absent. The CSF is normal or shows only slight lymphocytosis.

Pain usually subsides in one to two weeks. Recovery from paralysis is slow. It usually takes several months, but eventual complete recovery after two or more years is usual. Recurrent attacks of neuritis in the same or the opposite shoulder rarely occur. Corticosteroids may be tried in the early stages.

### Generalised Polyneuropathy

When the causal lesion lies in the nerve cell body the first manifestations are at the distal end of the longest nerves. This gives rise to the typical picture of a generalised polyneuropathy with distal paraesthesiae first affecting the feet and later the hands, and progressing proximally up the limbs. These sensory symptoms are associated with diminution of superficial sensation over 'stocking' and 'glove' areas. There is also distal weakness with diminished or absent tendon reflexes. There are variations of this stereotyped picture, e.g. neuropathies due to peripheral segmental demyelination, such as the Guillain-Barré syndrome (p. 736). In all cases the approach to the diagnosis must be preceded by a definition of the type of peripheral neuropathy; it should be noted whether the affection is primarily distal, whether it is symmetrical, and whether or not sensory and motor functions are equally affected.

**Aetiology.** There are a large number of causes; some of the most important are listed:

GENETICALLY DETERMINED NEUROPATHIES: peroneal muscular atrophy; progressive hypertrophic polyneuritis; hereditary sensory neuropathy.

DEFICIENCY NEUROPATHIES: deficiencies of vitamins $B_1$, $B_2$, $B_6$ and $B_{12}$; folate deficiency.

TOXIC NEUROPATHY: lead, arsenic, mercury, triorthocresylphosphate; a variety of organic chemicals such as carbon tetrachloride, acrilamide and aniline dyes; a large number of drugs including chloroquine, phenytoin, nitrofurantoin, and vincristine.

NEUROPATHIES ASSOCIATED WITH INFECTIONS: leprosy is true infective neuropathy; polyneuropathy may complicate a number of infections including influenza, measles, and typhoid fever; some neuropathies are due to exotoxins notably diphtheritic polyneuropathy; acute post-infection polyneuritis.

CONNECTIVE TISSUE DISORDERS: polyarteritis nodosa; rheumatoid arthritis, systemic lupus erythematosus and occasionally giant cell arteritis.

METABOLIC NEUROPATHIES: diabetes mellitus; renal and hepatic failure; acute intermittent porphyria.

MALIGNANT DISEASE: carcinoma of the bronchus and other malignant tumours.

Descriptions of the many neuropathies listed above would be repetitive. Diabetic neuropathies illustrate the various clinical patterns of the polyneuropathies and acute post-infection polyneuropathy is a relatively common and life threatening disease. These conditions will be discussed in more detail.

## Diabetic Polyneuropathy

Peripheral neuropathies of various types are commonly associated with diabetes mellitus. Conversely diabetes is a very common cause of peripheral neuropathy. In general, diabetic neuropathies occur more commonly in older diabetics and their incidence increases when control of diabetes is poor. However, diabetic neuropathy can occur at any age and does occur in well-controlled diabetics. It used to be thought that most cases of diabetic neuropathy were due to vascular changes in the nerves but it is probable that metabolic factors also cause neural damage in diabetes though the nature of the biochemical lesion has not been defined.

**Distal, symmetrical, mixed sensori-motor polyneuropathy** is a common form of diabetic neuropathy. It occurs most frequently in elderly, long-standing diabetics. Distal, symmetrical paraesthesiae are the commonest presenting features. There is usually glove and stocking sensory loss and distal weakness with loss of ankle jerks. Exacerbations may occur when control of the diabetes is inadequate but this type of distal neuropathy occurs in well-controlled diabetics and responds poorly to treatment.

**Motor neuropathy (diabetic amyotrophy)** is an asymmetrical, predominantly motor and proximal form of neuropathy. It often occurs in elderly diabetics and is sometimes the presenting feature in patients who have no other symptoms of diabetes. There is usually asymmetrical wasting of the quadriceps with diminution or loss of knee reflexes. With good control of diabetes, complete recovery is usual though resolution may take one or two years.

**Sensory neuropathy** is a distal, symmetrical, sensory neuropathy. Patients complain of numbness and paraesthesiae of the feet spreading up the legs and later involving the fingers. Glove and stocking sensory loss is common. As the condition progresses there is loss of position sense and vibration sense in the legs with the development of spinal ataxia. Trophic lesions such as ulcers and Charcot joints may supervene. Since many patients with diabetes have pupillary abnormalities due to recurrent attacks of uveitis this picture may resemble tabes dorsalis and indeed is sometimes called diabetic pseudotabes.

**Autonomic neuropathy.** Impotence is probably the most frequent symptom of autonomic diabetic neuropathy. There is sometimes accompanying diarrhoea which is usually nocturnal or postprandial. Impaired cardiovascular reflexes are found in

20% of diabetics but symptomatic postural hypotension is uncommon. Other manifestations are tachycardia and disturbances of sweating and micturition.

These categories of diabetic neuropathy are not mutually exclusive, and mixed pictures are common.

### Acute Post–Infection Polyneuropathy (The Guillain–Barré Syndrome)

Approximately one-half of the patients who develop this type of neuropathy give a history of a viral illness one to four weeks prior to the onset of the neuropathy. The presenting clinical features vary. There may be tingling affecting the distal part of the limbs and ascending proximally. In about 50% of patients motor symptoms predominate, with weakness which may be profound and rapidly progressive and which often affects proximal more than distal limb musculature. Facial muscles are commonly involved. The most striking findings on examination are diffuse weakness and widespread loss of reflexes. The rate of spread is variable. Occasional patients will develop tetraparesis with respiratory failure within a few hours of the initial symptoms. In other cases there will be a progression for one to two weeks.

The protein content of the cerebrospinal fluid is markedly raised in most patients at some time during the illness though it may be normal during the first ten days. There is usually no rise in cells.

The most important aspect of the management of patients with the Guillain-Barré syndrome is the maintenance of respiration. During the initial stages of the illness careful monitoring of respiratory function is essential. A deterioration in respiratory function tests or subjective feelings of dyspnoea should lead to early tracheostomy and the institution of intermittent positive pressure respiration.

The prognosis is good providing respiration is maintained. Approximately 90% of patients will recover completely within 3 to 8 weeks; 5% will die and 5% will be left with residual paralysis.

*Acute intermittent porphyria* may cause a neuropathy similar to that of postinfection polyneuritis. Acute intermittent porphyria is characterised by attacks of unexplained colicky abdominal pain, constipation and psychiatric disturbances, notably confusion and emotional lability. Tachycardia and hypertension are frequent. The condition is due to a hereditary deficiency of an enzyme in the pathway of haem biosynthesis and an attack may be precipitated by phenobarbitone, oral contraceptives, sulphonamides, pentazocine, methyldopa, chlorpropamide, alcohol and other drugs. The diagnosis is confirmed by the finding of porphobilinogen in the urine (p. 427).

### Diagnosis, Prevention and Treatment of Polyneuropathy

The clinical picture will usually localise the lesions to the peripheral nerves. Nerve conduction velocities will, in most cases, confirm the presence of impaired conduction in nerve trunks. This will be gross in most cases of peripheral segmental demyelination and relatively minor in lesions affecting nerve cell bodies. Occasionally, particularly in those with interstitial neuropathies, a sural nerve biopsy will establish the cause. Sometimes the pattern of the clinical picture, as in the Guillain-Barré syndrome, will indicate the likely cause. Although the presence of a polyneuropathy is easily established clinically, the definition of a cause may be difficult. The presence of associated diseases, drug ingestion or exposure to toxic chemicals should be sought in each case. The possibility of diabetes should always be excluded.

If the constellation of findings from the history or clinical signs does not indicate a likely aetiology then it may often prove impossible to establish a cause for a peripheral neuropathy.

Any new drug which is liable to cause neuropathy must be used with care and industrial hazards should be avoided by protective clothing, exhaust ventilation and other techniques advised by the industrial medical officer. When polyneuropathy has developed as a result of exposure to a toxic substance the first step is to remove the patient from further exposure. When the cause is nutritional every effort should be made to restore the original body weight; plenty of protein is desirable supplemented by generous doses of the vitamin B complex. If the cause is metabolic the appropriate treatment must be initiated without delay, e.g. for diabetes.

In severe cases bed rest is essential since the nervous control of the heart may be defective and cardiomyopathy is sometimes associated. The limbs should be supported in the optimum position, and passive movements carried out several times a day. A cage should protect the feet from the weight of the bed-clothes. Respiratory insufficiency may require tracheostomy or institution of intermittent positive pressure respiration (p. 236). When recovery begins, active movements should be carried out under the supervision of a physiotherapist.

## Myasthenia Gravis

This condition is characterised by undue fatiguability of muscles.

**Aetiology.** HLA B8 is associated with myasthenia gravis particularly in young women. In middle-aged and elderly males who develop the disease HLA A2 is often present. Circumstantial evidence for immunological dysfunction is provided by the greater than chance association of myasthenia gravis with a number of autoimmune diseases, notably systemic lupus erythematosus, rheumatoid arthritis, thyrotoxicosis, Hashimoto's disease, pernicious anaemia and diabetes mellitus. T cell abnormalities have been demonstrated, resulting in hyperactivity of B cells (p. 25) and the production of autoantibodies culminating in the destruction of acetylcholine receptors on the muscle cell. Other immune mechanisms may be implicated and the basic cause of myasthenia gravis may be a genetically determined defect in the regulation of the immune system.

**Clinical Features.** The disease usually appears between the ages of 15 and 50 and females are more often affected than males. It tends to run a remitting course especially during the early years. Relapses may be precipitated by emotional disturbances, infections, pregnancy and severe muscular effort. The cardinal symptom is abnormal fatiguability of muscles; movement, though initially strong, rapidly weakens. Intensification of symptoms towards the end of the day or following vigorous exercise is characteristic. The first symptoms are usually intermittent ptosis or diplopia but weakness of chewing, swallowing, speaking or of moving the limbs also occurs. Any muscle of a limb may be affected, most commonly those of the shoulder girdle, so that the patient is unable to undertake work above the level of the shoulder, such as combing the hair, without frequent rests. Respiratory muscles may be involved and respiratory failure is a not uncommon cause of death. Asphyxia occurs readily as the cough may be too weak to clear foreign bodies from the airways. Muscle atrophy may occur in long-standing cases. There are no signs of involvement of the central nervous system.

An invaluable diagnostic aid is the increase in muscle strength produced by an intravenous injection of a short-acting anticholinesterase, edrophonium hydrochloride. An initial dose of 2 mg is injected and a further 8 mg given half a minute later if there are no undesirable reactions such as fasciculation, sweating and colic. Improvement in muscle power occurs within 30 seconds of the injection and usually persists for 2 or 3 minutes. Ptosis or defects in eye movements are the most convenient parameters of improvement but diminution of dysarthria or increase of power in the limbs can also demonstrate a response to edrophonium.

**Treatment** is based on the administration of anticholinesterase drugs of which neostigmine and pyridostigmine are the most widely used. The dose of either of these drugs varies between individuals. Fifteen mg of neostigmine given orally four times daily is sometimes sufficient but in some patients 30 mg every 2 hours is needed. Pyridostigmine gives less prompt relief than neostigmine but has a more prolonged action. It is particularly useful when given late in the evening when it preserves muscle power during sleep. Sixty mg of pyridostigmine is equivalent in its effect to 15 mg of neostigmine. Anticholinesterase drugs frequently cause bowel colic and sometimes diarrhoea and excessive salivation. These side-effects may be controlled by propantheline (15 mg t.i.d.) or, on occasion, by the parenteral administration of atropine (0·6 mg). When the patient is unable to swallow and during pre- and postoperative periods neostigmine may be given intravenously (0·5–1 mg hourly). One mg of neostigmine intravenously is equivalent to 15 mg given orally.

There is a danger of overdosage with anticholinesterase drugs, and this is perhaps particularly likely when long acting preparations are used since their effect tends to be cumulative. Excessive dosage of anticholinesterases can cause permanent depolarisation block at the neuromuscular junction. This is sometimes referred to as a *cholinergic crisis*. Warning signs of overdosage are fasciculations, pallor, sweating, persistently small pupils and excessive salivation.

Overdosage can be prevented by 'titrating' the dose according to the reaction to intravenous edrophonium. If the limit of anticholinesterase dosage has been reached then edrophonium will increase muscle weakness. Some muscle groups may be overdosed while others are still responsive to neostigmine. It is, therefore, important to observe the effect of an injection of edrophonium on respiration rather than on ocular or limb movement.

Sudden exacerbations of myasthenia or cholinergic block may require intermittent positive pressure respiration to save life.

Some patients benefit markedly from thymectomy. The operation should always be performed if a thymoma is demonstrated and if disability progresses despite medical treatment. It is particularly indicated if bulbar muscles are involved. The best results follow thymectomies carried out on young women whose disease has been present for less than 3 years.

Steroid treatment may be used in those who have responded poorly to thymectomy either in a short course of high dosage or in longer low dosage. A few days after the introduction of steroids there may be a marked exacerbation of myasthenic symptoms which may cause respiratory failure; accordingly steroids should be started only in a hospital where facilities for artificial respiration are available. As an alternative when steroids have failed, prolonged treatment with azathioprine (p. 39) has been shown to be beneficial. Remissions can also be achieved by plasma exchange.

**Prognosis** is variable. Remissions sometimes occur spontaneously. When myasthenic affection is confined to the eye muscles prognosis for life is normal and disability slight. Rapid progression of the disease more than 5 years after its onset is uncommon. Thymectomy, perhaps followed by high dosage steroid treatment, often leads to marked improvement so that disability is minimal and life expectancy normal. When the disease is associated with a thymoma, even though this is removed, the outlook is markedly worsened.

# DISEASES OF MUSCLE

Diseases of muscle are not diseases of the nervous system, but as some of their manifestations may be readily confused with neurological conditions some relevant examples are described here. There are obvious exceptions, but it is a useful generalisation that muscular disease affects mainly the proximal muscles of the limbs whereas neuropathic disease (polyneuropathy or motor neurone disease) affects mainly the distal muscles.

## Myopathy

Myopathy is a generic term comprising all primary diseases of muscle. It may be subdivided into genetically determined, congenital, metabolic and drug induced myopathy. Inflammatory myopathy (polymyositis) is described on page 733.

### Genetically Determined Myopathy

**Progressive muscular dystrophy** is a group of hereditary disorders characterised by progressive degeneration of groups of muscles without involvement of the nervous system. The wasting and weakness are symmetrical, there is no fasciculation, tendon reflexes are preserved until a late stage and there is no sensory loss. Several clinical types have been described; from a prognostic viewpoint there are three major groups.

The *Duchenne type* is transmitted by an X-linked recessive gene and occurs almost exclusively in males (p. 15). The disease usually appears within the first three years of life, beginning in the pelvic girdle and lower limbs and later spreading to the shoulder girdle. About 80% of cases show an initial pseudohypertrophy involving the calf muscles, quadriceps, glutei, deltoids and infraspinati. Contractures are common. The affected muscles are larger and firmer than normal, but are nevertheless weak. The weakness gives rise to a characteristic waddling gait, and when rising from the supine position, the child rolls on to his face and then uses his arms to push himself up. Death occurs from inanition or respiratory infection by the middle of the second decade.

*Limb girdle type* (Juvenile scapulohumeral type of Erb). The gene carrying this disorder is inherited as an autosomal recessive, affecting both sexes. It usually appears in the second or third decade. It starts in either the shoulder or pelvic girdle and later spreads to involve both. The rate of progression is variable; it may be slow, with long periods of arrest, but severe disablement usually occurs within 20 years and the patient does not survive to middle age.

*Facio-scapulo-humeral type* (Landouzy-Déjerine). This type is inherited by an autosomal dominant gene so that several siblings of both sexes may be affected. It appears at any age, first in the facial muscles and then in the shoulder girdle. After many years the pelvic girdle may also be involved. The disease progresses very slowly with periods of arrest and is compatible with a long life.

The *diagnosis of muscular dystrophy* is readily confirmed by electromyography

(EMG) or muscle biopsy. Aldolase, or creatine kinase and other enzymes which are usually intracellular, are increased in the serum, especially in the rapidly advancing Duchenne type. Serum enzyme changes may be found before other clinical signs, enabling early detection of the disease in siblings. Less severe changes of the same type are found in women who carry the abnormal gene of the Duchenne type.

*Treatment*. No effective treatment is known. Deterioration may occur with excessive confinement to bed. Physiotherapeutic and orthopaedic measures may be required to counteract deformities and contractures.

**Myotonic Dystrophy.** Myotonia consists of slow relaxation of muscles due to hyperexcitability of the muscle cell membrane.

*Myotonia congenita* (Thomsen's disease) is inherited as an autosomal dominant and appears in early childhood. The only symptom is the slow relaxation of a muscle if it is contracted voluntarily or by mechanical stimulation. The patient may be unable to relax the grasp or to open the eyes if they have been closed tightly. The muscles may be unusually powerful in early life.

*Myotonia atrophica* is also autosomal dominant and appears between the ages of 20 and 30. There is wasting of the facial and temporal muscles, sternomastoids, shoulder girdle, forearms, quadriceps and leg muscles, and all these and the tongue show myotonia after voluntary contraction or after percussion of the muscle. Ptosis is prominent. Unlike most muscular diseases, distal muscles are more severely affected than proximal. There is also cataract, frontal baldness and gonadal atrophy leading to impotence and sterility in men and amenorrhoea in women.

*Treatment*. There is no treatment for the muscular dystrophy, but if myotonia is troublesome it can be relieved by procainamide, 0·5–1·0 g q.i.d., quinine sulphate 300–600 mg t.i.d., or diphenylhydantoin 100 mg t.i.d.

## Congenital, Metabolic and Drug Induced Myopathy

**Congenital myopathies** are rare and present in infancy with muscular weakness and limpness. Serum enzymes tend to be normal or slightly raised. The EMG is usually myopathic. The mode of inheritance is variable. They are named according to the type of structural abnormality found in the skeletal muscle fibres. Most cases are non-progressive or only slowly progressive.

**Metabolic Myopathy.** *Thyrotoxic Myopathy*. Mild weakness of the proximal muscles of the limbs is a common feature of thyrotoxicosis. In a few patients muscular wasting and weakness predominate, and the other manifestations of hyperthyroidism may not be obvious.

*Corticosteroid Myopathy*. Weakness of the pelvic girdle may occur in Cushing's syndrome and as a result of treatment with corticosteroid hormones.

*Familial periodic paralysis* is characterised by attacks of profound weakness, lasting for several hours and often occurring after exertion or after a heavy carbohydrate meal. In the common variety the attacks of weakness are accompanied by a fall in the serum potasssium level.

**Drug Induced Myopathy.** A wide variety of drugs may cause disorders of muscle. Often muscle cramps and mild weakness are the first symptoms. Lithium, cimetidine and salbutamol may cause mild symptoms which disappear when the drug is withdrawn. Clofibrate may cause the acute onset of muscle necrosis, with pain and weakness and markedly elevated serum levels of creatine phosphokinase. Withdrawal of the drug is followed by a gradual improvement. $\beta$-blockers sometimes cause generalised muscle weakness and rarely lead to a severe, proximal myopathy. Alcohol may cause a spectrum of muscle diseases varying from a mild, proximal weakness to severe muscle necrosis with myoglobinuria.

## Neurological and Myopathic Complications of Carcinoma

Cerebral invasion or spinal compression may be the presenting feature of a metastasis from an unsuspected primary neoplasm or may augment the disability already caused by tumours arising elsewhere in the body, particularly in bronchus and breast. More than half of all cerebral tumours are secondary deposits and this high incidence emphasises the need for a careful search for a primary neoplasm in those patients who present with an intracranial space-occupying lesion.

Neurological complications may arise at a distance from a primary carcinoma in the absence of metastases. The relationship between the underlying malignant process and the neurological manifestations remains obscure in most instances. Neural disturbances may occur at any stage during the development of the primary lesion and frequently antedate the symptoms directly attributable to the carcinoma by weeks or months and occasionally by as much as two or three years. At the time of neurological presentation the primary carcinoma often cannot be defined even by radiological techniques. Nor does the course of the neurological complication consistently parallel the development of the carcinoma. Immunological mechanisms, conditioned nutritional deficiencies and the direct effects of toxins produced by tumours have all been adduced as explanations of attendant neurological dysfunction but there is little supporting evidence for any of these hypotheses. Investigations have suggested the possibility that tumours may produce an alteration in protein metabolism which in turn interferes with the synthesis of enzymes and hence causes neural dysfunction. It is likely that progressive multi-focal leucoencephalopathy (p. 709) results from viral infection when immunological responses are impaired by malignant disease.

The neurological features evoked by distant carcinoma are protean; they may affect singly, or in combination, muscles and peripheral nerves as well as central neural structures and the brain. The syndromes presented are most conveniently categorised anatomically.

**Myopathy, Myositis and Myasthenia.** A proximal weakness of late onset, usually first affecting the legs may be due to a lesion of muscles secondary to a distant carcinoma. Histologically the muscles may show changes of a non-specific myopathy or there may be collections of inflammatory cells, characteristic of polymyositis. Sometimes the myopathic weakness is markedly exacerbated by exertion producing a myasthenic syndrome. Weakness and fatiguability most often affect the legs, and less commonly the arms; bulbar and ocular affections are uncommon in contrast to myasthenia gravis. Fatiguability of muscle may sometimes be improved by an intravenous injection of edrophonium hydrochloride but this response is inconstant and is often poorly sustained. The electromyographic picture in these carcinomatous myasthenic syndromes differs from that produced by myasthenia gravis. Guanidine (40–50 mg/kg body weight) sometimes improves muscle power in carcinomatous myasthenia.

**Peripheral neuropathy** is probably the commonest of the distant neurological complications of carcinoma. Clinically the neuropathy is usually of mixed sensori-motor type (p. 735). The cerebrospinal fluid protein content is often raised. Much less commonly a pure sensory neuropathy may be manifest, almost always in association with a bronchial carcinoma of oat-cell type. Pathological lesions in this rare condition are mainly situated in the dorsal root ganglia where there is degeneration of the sensory neurones.

**Spinal Cord Affection.** Carcinomata may produce a picture which resembles motor neurone disease with loss of anterior horn cells, accompanied sometimes by upper motor neurone signs. Uncommonly this picture, which mimics amyotrophic lateral sclerosis, may be accompanied by a bulbar palsy. Necrosis affecting the cells and the tracts of the spinal cord, maximal in the thoracic segments, is a rare complication of carcinoma.

**Subacute degeneration of the cortical layers of the cerebellum** is an uncommon manifestation of distant carcinoma. Ataxia, affecting upper and lower limbs, is a consistent presenting feature; dysarthria too is often found but nystagmus is present in only a minority of cases.

**Encephalopathy** has occasionally been found in patients suffering from carcinoma particularly of the bronchus, breast and uterus. The most common presentation is an insidious and progressive dementia with memory disorder and sometimes mood disturbance. These psychiatric and mental symptoms may occasionally be accompanied by features of brain stem involvement such as double vision or bulbar palsy and often there are accompanying pyramidal tract signs.

**Treatment** of the neurological complications is that of the primary lesion. Improvement, and occasionally complete remission, of a myasthenic-myopathic syndrome may occur with removal of the primary tumour but this is by no means invariable. Carcinomatous motor neurone disease often tends to halt its progress despite the fact that the primary carcinoma continues to grow. Clearly the treatment for the underlying malignancies is imperative but the response of the neurological complications is unpredictable.

## Prospects in Neurology

In the last edition of this book the most exciting diagnostic prospect was the development of computed tomography. This technique has contributed enormously to the diagnosis of structural intracerebral lesions. A new approach to cerebral imaging is positron-emission tomography. This uses radionuclides which emit positively charged electrons which are recorded to build up a three-dimensional picture of cerebral events. Metabolic substrates are labelled with radioisotopes and their ingress, egress and distribution in the brain can be measured. This affords a means of studying the dynamics of metabolism and cerebral circulation which complements the structural information gained from computed tomography.

Evoked electrical potentials (p. 667) are increasingly used in diagnosis. Refinements of these techniques should provide non-invasive means of demonstrating impaired function and localising lesions. The impact of immunological studies is being increasingly felt in neurology. Much information about multiple sclerosis and myasthenia gravis is already available. The treatment of myasthenia gravis is already being guided, to some extent, by the demonstration of different types of HLA antigens in patients.

The use of electrical stimulation of parts of the nervous system offers an intriguing, if rather mysterious, approach to treatment. Spinal cord stimulation is employed to help patients with multiple sclerosis. Analogous methods are being used to treat chronic, painful conditions and are being explored in the treatment of epilepsy. It will be interesting to see if these prosper.

C. MAWDSLEY
J.A. SIMPSON

*Further reading*:

Adams, R. A. & Sidman, R. L. (1968) *Introduction to Neuropathology*. New York: McGraw-Hill.— Though it deals in considerable detail with pathological processes this book is particularly valuable because of its extensive discussion of the correlation of pathological lesions and clinical features.

Brain, Lord & Walton, J.N. (1977) *Diseases of the Nervous System*, 8th edn. London: Oxford University Press.— See next reference.

Elliot, F. A. (1971) *Clinical Neurology*, 2nd edn. Philadelphia: Saunders.— Both of these are comprehensive texts written for postgraduate students but they are suitable reference works for undergraduates.

Jennett, W.B. (1977) *An Introduction to Neurosurgery*, 3rd edn. London: Heinemann.— A succinct and clearly written introduction to surgical neurology.

Matthews, W. B. & Miller, H. (1979) *Diseases of the Nervous System*, 3rd edn. Oxford: Blackwell.—A concise, readable account of neurological disorders intended for undergraduates.

Mawdsley, C. (1979) In *Clinical Examination*, 5th edn, Macleod, J. Edinburgh: Churchill Livingstone.—Contains an account of the examination of the nervous system designed to be read in conjunction with this chapter.

Walton, J. N. (1975) *Essentials of Neurology*, 4th edn. London: Pitman Medical.— A short but authoritative textbook, designed for undergraduates and packed with accurate information.

# 15. Psychiatry

Psychiatry is the study and treatment of disorders of the mind and of behaviour. The mind, or psyche, is usually defined as the part of the person consisting of the thoughts, the feelings and the function of willing. Psychiatric disorder, therefore, can be viewed to occur whenever there is an impairment of thinking (cognition), feeling (affect) or willing (volition). In a paranoid reaction, for instance, the patient wrongly thinks he is being persecuted by an ill-intentioned acquaintance; in depressive psychosis the patient is incapacitated by a persistent feeling of intense gloom; and in schizophrenia some patients are inactive, ineffectual and lacking in volition.

Psychiatry is the proper concern of all doctors, not only of psychiatrists. Only a small proportion of the psychiatric illness in the community is seen and can be treated by psychiatrists. In a country with as many doctors as Britain only 1 in 20 cases of psychiatric disorder is treated by psychiatrists. The epidemiological evidence makes it clear that the great proportion of psychiatric morbidity falls in the clinical domain of non-psychiatrists: general practitioners mainly but also physicians, surgeons, obstetricians and gynaecologists. Neurologists should also be singled out, for they treat many psychiatric patients

Patients with emotional disorders tend to consult their doctors more often than patients with physical diseases and complain of a wider variety of symptoms. As a result, they are often referred to a succession of clinics for specialist investigation and commonly undergo minor or major surgery without avail. This involves a waste of both doctors' and patients' time, which could be avoided if the psychological disorder had been recognised at an earlier stage. Another reason for requiring all doctors to be psychiatrically informed and skilled is that psychiatric disorder and physical illness frequently occur in the same patient.

It follows that the priority is to ensure that psychiatric knowledge and skills, and professional attitudes appropriate to adequate provision of psychiatric care, are part of the clinical equipment of all doctors. They must know the symptoms, signs and syndromes in psychiatry, and they should all be aware of the psychological, pharmacological and physical treatments that are effective in psychiatric illness.

The basic skills are the ability to take a psychiatric history and to examine the mental state; such technical competence enables the doctor to elicit the clinical features of psychiatric disorder presented by the patient. This constitutes the psychiatric examination which is described on page 750.

## MENTAL HEALTH

As a basis for understanding the abnormal, all doctors must know what constitutes mental as well as physical health. Before defining this it is necessary to consider the development of personality and the mechanisms of psychological defence.

**Personality Development.** Personality is socially acquired, given its genetic basis, over the course of time. The individual arrives at an adult psychological state after passing successively through a series of maturational stages. A baby is born into a family, which provides immediate social support and responses. From the start the baby's 'personality' consists of the totality of its actions, but also of the reactions made particularly to the caring parent. At first the baby is helpless and receptive, dependent utterly on succour; such total care occurs as a result of nurturing impulses in the mother, fostered from the first days by the relationship and the interactions which develop in the nursing couple. The baby's cries, its smiles after some weeks, its need of nourishment and the relative satisfaction or distress deriving from its alimentary experiences, its fear of strangers from 8 months, all combine to bring out the protectiveness of the parental family. During this *oral stage*, the baby is perforce relatively passive; its needs are for care and nourishment.

During the *anal stage*, from 9 months to 18 months of age, the infant comes to gain sphincter control and to become more socialised as a member of the family in other ways also, starting to learn the language and its usage, and coming to grasp the rules of the parental household.

The *genital stage* extends from 2 to 6 years of age. One of its characteristics is that the child now has sufficient awareness of family interactions and social norms to want to become informed about such matters as the difference between the sexes, where babies come from and how they are made. Boys begin to imitate and assimilate aspects of their father's behaviour and character, while girls also become less concentrated in their attachment to the mother; they can show the most intense affection for their fathers, a passion that apparently needs recognition and an affectionate response for proper personality growth between 2 and 6 years.

During the *oedipal phase* (as this period is called in the psychoanalytic literature), the child is often intensely frustrated by diminutive size, puny powers and subservience to the powerful parents at a time when perception, knowledge and mastery of its environment evolve rapidly as physical and mental abilities develop.

At 6 years, the child enters the *latency period,* which will last to puberty. The child is socially obliging, very actively adapting to school life and is becoming increasingly an independent personality, able to be away from the parents for substantial portions of the day. If the parents are not seriously deficient as culture carriers, through neurotic illness or crippling social handicaps, the child now comes closely to grips with the norms, the roles, the stereotypes and the obvious and prevailing cultural values. The child is extremely impressionable, as advertisers on television well know, eager to add to personality and experience by observing and borrowing from the behaviour and ideas of others.

At *puberty* the child's personality can enter a period of relative flexibility, when it may be given 'a second chance' and can set aside some trait patterns and in their place substitute new attitudes and beliefs. With the bodily and sexual changes of this period come demands for new orientations and relationships; a special requirement is for a friend. Children, just before entering their teens, either do succeed in achieving a close friendship or else they may suffer from a sense of unpopularity or loneliness.

The early teenage years are when *identity formation* either occurs or else fails to happen, when identity diffusion will result. Then the youngster continues in a state of not knowing what he wants to be, what his capacities and potential allow him to aim for. The boy may be timid and lacking in confidence, or compensatorily brusque and hostile; the girl may inwardly bewail her female state, be perturbed at having menstrual periods and feel uncertain and wretched in social relationships especially as these relate to the future prospect of being courted. When identity formation does occur successfully, the young person decides on life goals and works towards them more or less hopefully, while feeling common cause with enough age-mates to be a member of a group.

At about 18 years, the late adolescent becomes capable of *intimacy*, able to regard the welfare of another loved person as no less important than one's own. Young adulthood follows, with the capacity for *generativity*, with the intention and the potential to provide responsibly and reliably for others.

When the question of psychological normality of a patient is at issue, this chronological and subjective progression through biographical epochs has to be borne in mind. Psychological theory holds that each of these different stages is not obliterated by the one succeeding it but, like layers of an onion, one developmental phase superimposes the challenges (and the person's solutions to them) over and around the earlier solutions achieved. The residues of past developmental periods persist to give individuality to the person. When particularly upsetting setbacks (psychologically traumatic experiences) are encountered, a *fixation* may result, the person not negotiating oral, or anal, or genital challenges but instead remaining unduly preoccupied with the issues of that earlier life epoch. Often the facts about the psychic trauma are not remembered, as when a small child is parted from his parents for a surgical operation he does not comprehend. Jean Piaget was a pioneer in discovering that intellectual development also proceeds in stages, and that in the early years of life unrealistic thinking prevails. Only in middle childhood, from 7 or 8 years onwards, does the child acquire logical thinking, and even then abstract thinking and reasoning is not possible until about 13 years of age. Thus the first three stages of emotional development described above take place in parallel with magical, prelogical modes of thought. This knowledge makes it clearer why there are infantile psychic remnants in the thinking of many disturbed adults. Although knowledgeable about sex, a girl can fear she is pregnant despite intercourse not having occurred; a man can be distressed that he 'caused' the death of his mother by behaving harshly to her when she was terminally ill. Thinking that departs from reality or distorts it is often related to early demands which the child found unmanageable, or to distress which was intolerable emotionally at that time of life, such as the loss of a parent through death, or the family breaking up.

The adult, when handicapped by a persistence of immaturity, need not constantly manifest distortion of thinking or feeling in his behaviour. Only when a fresh setback occurs in adult life may he decompensate in behaviour and *regress* to act in extreme variance from his everyday demeanour, for example with dependency and passivity (as when confronted by major surgery), or with obstinacy or hostility.

**Mechanisms of Defence.** As a consequence of excessive strains occurring early in life with which the personality was insufficiently mature to cope, the person can make use of psychological devices, 'mental tricks', to alter the inner environment or the surrounding reality and create an illusion of safety and predictability. A girl, unable to clarify sexual issues at the age of 5 years, perhaps lacking a reassuring relationship with a kindly father, may use *denial* excessively: there are women who remain unaware of their sexual impulses and behave like school-girls forever: 'pregenital' personalities, some writers name them. A person may *overcompensate*: a timid, insecure boy setting out to acquire the outward characteristics of a tough male when he reaches adulthood. A boy who copes with upsetting homosexual desires at puberty by means of *repression*, in later life can be in greater emotional difficulty should he use the mechanism of *projection*: if psychotic, such a man may have an auditory delusion that other people are alleging he is a homosexual. A sexually deprived single woman, using the same mechanisms, may be profoundly distressed, in the course of a paranoid reaction, by her erroneous beliefs that neighbours view her as sexually promiscuous: her own suppressed wishes are not admitted to her awareness but are exteriorised so that she believes others falsely suspect her of immorality.

There are other psychological mechanisms in the range of distortions and evasions to which troubled people can have recourse in extremity. By *reaction formation* we imply that an individual gives forth the opposite of facts he cannot acknowledge about himself: the son dominated by his father often becomes not a domineering adult himself, but a timid, ingratiating, subservient adult — perhaps hen-pecked by an intimidating wife. However, such a man can change character drastically (the 'return of the repressed' is a term applied) and turn on his oppressor; the bedroom is the commonest setting for matrimonial murder when the victim is the wife; the husband dies often in the kitchen.

Of course, psychological defence mechanisms rarely present so dramatically, and for clinical purposes more precise observation of smaller cues is required. We all use defence mechanisms at times of great stress: the surgeon's matter-of-fact manner is sometimes seen as necessary suppression of sympathetic emotions which could impair his competence, and his *selective inattention* to pathetic life circumstances may be altogether appropriate in an emergency. A civilian disaster is not the time for anguish over the human condition, if one is a surgeon with an operation to carry out. The defences which a person assumes psychologically, therefore, can be of much social value to others. A latently homosexual youth leader may be a boon to a neighbourhood — until his *sublimation* no longer serves, perhaps if he drinks excessively and loses his customary mental controls. School teachers and clergymen who interfere sexually with boys are in this category, and some doctors who become sexually involved with patients. In the course of clinical work, we judge a patient to assess whether he or she is spontaneous and unconstrained, or whether in contrast the patient when troubled denies mental conflict and imaginatively but unknowingly distorts surrounding reality in order to gain psychological relief.

## Psychological Normality

In common with medical practice generally, individuals are often considered psychiatrically normal if no evidence of disorder is clinically evident. An epidemiologist doing a population survey may use an *empirical definition of normality* and regard as normal everybody who has not seen a psychiatrist nor consulted a general practitioner for any nervous ailment during the preceding year.

Another concept of normality at times invoked is an *ideal norm*, conveying an aspiration towards a desired state of well-being (such as is expressed in the preamble to the World Health Organisation constitution), devoutly to be wished but not to be found in this world: 'Health is a state of complete physical, mental and social well-being and not merely the absence of disease or infirmity'.

Psychiatrists occasionally write about normality, or aspects of it, in such inspirational terms that only too evidently they are not describing people as they are but as they would be, if a theoretical schema or 'mental health' blueprint were to become actual.

The third concept is a *statistical norm*, implying the state of most people contained in the community of which the patient is a member. In this sense, without straining after the ideal, we can indicate features characteristic of psychiatric normality in mature adults. Each of these can be readily identified, especially when the doctor has additional background information from prior acquaintance with the patient or members of his family.

A person who has successfully negotiated the sequence of stages in personality development is *appropriately autonomous*; he can manage his own affairs and tasks without undue reliance on others and can be depended on to meet obligations and to discharge responsibilities appropriate to his occupation, social circumstances and interests. The statement that a mature person can work, love and play perhaps reflects this capacity for autonomy.

A second feature of normality is *accurate self-perception*, the person not overestimating nor belittling his abilities. A third characteristic is correct *reality-testing,* the environment being perceived in an undistorted way. A fourth feature is *adjustment,* the person taking things as they are and making the best of them. The final two qualities of maturity are *integration* (relative coherence of the parts of the personality in contrast to gross self-contradictions), and *achievement*, the person using his skills and interests in such a way that his efforts are productive.

## DIAGNOSTIC DECISION-MAKING

The doctor's first consideration when examining a patient for psychiatric disorder, is to question whether the patient may be suffering from a psychosis, one of the serious disorders to which the term 'insanity' used to be applied. The psychoses are the serious illnesses which interfere with a patient's perceptions, thinking and feelings so profoundly that, at times, what he says to his fellow-men no longer makes sense to them and he is regarded as insane. The doctor scans the understanding he has obtained by means of history-taking and examination of the mental state, perhaps augmented—when the patient is uncooperative—by information from a relative or other informant. He judges whether the syndrome presenting indicates an illness of psychotic quality and severity. Syndrome identification is of course possible only if the doctor has knowledge about the signs and symptoms of the two main classes of psychoses; the organic psychoses due to cerebral impairment, and the functional psychoses presumed to be related to an as yet undiscovered disturbance of cerebral biochemistry.

### The Major Disorders (The Psychoses)

**Organic Psychoses.** In these organic brain syndromes the functioning of the brain is impaired either by a physical lesion (trauma, tumour or infection) or by a toxic or degenerative process. Organic brain syndromes when acute are known as *delirium*. Examples are the toxic confusional states occurring with brain trauma, cerebral anoxia, infection, or intoxication with barbiturates, amphetamines or alcohol.

The chronic psychoses, where an irreversible brain lesion has occurred, are the *dementias*. The most common are those associated with ageing — atherosclerotic and senile dementia. Mild degrees of dementia make the patient forgetful, easily confused, irritable and emotional; more severe dementia results in disorientation, gross loss of memory and deterioration in personal habits.

**Functional psychoses** are the major psychiatric illnesses occurring without brain disease or impairment. It is postulated that a neurophysiological or neurochemical aetiology will be found, resulting from the operation of complex causes. The two most common forms are *manic-depressive psychosis*, in which the principal symptom is a profound disturbance of the patient's mood, and the *schizophrenias* in which the patient's thoughts become bizarre and disorganised, so that he loses contact with his fellows and with his surroundings.

The major disorders are discussed further on pages 755 to 761.

## The Minor Disorders

The second step in the decision-making process towards a psychiatric diagnosis, having excluded the presence of psychosis, is for the doctor to determine whether the patient suffers from a 'minor' psychiatric disorder. The following forms of minor disorder are differentiated:

**The Psychoneuroses.** Clinical recognition of one of the forms of psychoneurosis depends on the doctor knowing the signs and symptoms of each syndrome and of being able to elicit the relevant clinical data from the patient. The psychoneuroses are the most common forms of psychiatric illness encountered in general medical practice. They are subdivided into *anxiety, hysterical, obsessive, depressive* and *phobic psychoneurosis.*

**Personality Disorder.** This term is used to describe patients whose personalities differ markedly from the normal population.

The third diagnostic rule, after the presence of possible psychosis or of psychoneurosis has been considered, is to make an appraisal of the personality of the patient. An individual's personality is regarded as normal if his actions and reactions are not grossly different from customary behaviour in society; when a personality is diagnosed as disordered, the implication is that the person deviates observably in behaviour, presenting a type of abnormal personality which is well recognised clinically. The abnormal personality manifests in recurrent disturbance in relationships with other people. In addition to their social difficulties, such people can be recognised to have traits (e.g. hostility, passivity) not found to the same degree in the personalities of normal people. Patients with moderate degrees of personality disorder are distressed by their inability to get on constructively with others and often seek treatment; otherwise they do so when they are further disabled by psychoneurosis or psychosomatic illness. Those with gross degrees of disorder (sociopathy) interfere disruptively in the lives of their relatives and associates and may come into conflict with the law; they may not regard themselves as abnormal and reject any efforts to treat them.

It is by no means unusual, indeed it is usual, for psychiatric illness and personality disorder to coexist. When the associated illness is of psychotic dimensions, the symptoms may so distort behaviour that a reliable estimate of the pre-illness personality will be possible only after recovery from the insanity. When the illness is a neurotic reaction, however, functioning personality remains sufficiently intact for a personality diagnosis to be made at the same time as the illness is appraised. A personality disorder may also be associated with sexual deviation, alcoholism, drug dependency or psychosomatic illness.

**Sexual Deviation.** People not conforming sexually to the prevailing norm most often consult (or are brought to) their doctor only when their abnormality has become seriously disturbing to their relatives or has put them into conflict with the law. Some, however, are themselves distressed by their deviation and may on occasion need psychiatric treatment for complicating psychiatric disorder, such as a depressive illness or paranoid reaction. Now that sexual relations between consenting adult males is no longer a crime in many countries, homosexuals are less vulnerable socially.

**Alcoholism and Drug Dependency.** An alcoholic is an excessive drinker who is unable to stop although to do so has become necessary because of health impairment, marital strife or difficulties at work. An addict is physically or psychologically dependent on a drug which is used repetitively, and suffers distressing side-effects when deprived of it.

**Psychosomatic illnesses** are the extremely common illnesses, such as some cases of asthma, peptic ulcer, dermatitis or ulcerative colitis, which emotional factors help to precipitate or to prolong.

The 'minor' disorders are discussed further on pages 761 to 778.

### Mental Handicap

The fourth and final diagnostic decision is to be clear about a patient's intellectual status. Mental subnormality is an impairment of the intellect present from birth or an early age, unlike psychiatric illnesses which supervene after a more or less normal psychological development. Two categories are distinguished:

*Mild mental retardation* (I.Q. 50 to 70). Although the intelligence level is below normal (I.Q. 85 to 115), the child may benefit from special teaching and social training.

*Severe mental retardation* (I.Q. 49 and below) refers to those so handicapped that they require very considerable attention and support and are incapable of leading an independent existence. The most common single cause of severe subnormality is Down's syndrome. A definite cause of subnormality is found only in a minority of cases, and then various clinical conditions can be responsible, e.g. phenylketonuria or hypothyroidism. Patients who are mentally subnormal may also suffer from other mental illnesses. They may, for example, become depressed or schizophrenic, but when this happens the symptoms of their mental illness will be modified by their basic handicap of mental retardation.

## The Psychiatric Examination

It must be emphasised that attention should be paid to the patient's emotional state not only when a frank psychiatric illness is suspected, but in the course of any thorough clinical examination. Psychiatric disturbances can be elicited while taking the history and while examining the patient's mental state. The procedures for conducting these two aspects of the psychiatric examination are described in *Clinical Examination* (p. 780) and will be indicated only briefly here.

**The Psychiatric History.** Taking a psychiatric history is one of the chief clinical skills in psychiatry. The technique differs from history-taking in general medicine, being rather less directive, the doctor to a greater extent, perhaps, allowing the patient to raise apparently unconnected subjects and expand in directions initiated by the patient rather than the clinician. In general medicine the doctor may have a course of enquiry which he wants to have pursued; this is also so with psychiatric history-taking, but inevitably the patient will have personal information to give which may be unexpected. Hence the clinician is well advised to be especially receptive and to encourage disclosures which the patient initiates. The following areas need to be explored in the course of taking the history:

(i) The date of the examination and the reason why the patient is seeking help.
(ii) The presenting complaints and the patient's detailed account of the present illness.
(iii) The patient's parental family: an account of father, mother, each brother and sister (with the patient's birth order in the sibship), and the home atmosphere.
(iv) The personal history, including early childhood; schooling and other education; sexual development and experience; work record; friendships; marriage.
(v) Previous illnesses, physical and psychiatric.
(vi) The personality before illness, with an account of the patient's interests, social activities, traits and such other information about subjective experiences and life events as the patient can provide.

Taking the history is the first therapeutic step. Psychological treatment begins the moment that the patient and doctor meet. The doctor's attitude to the patient and to his illness should be powerful therapeutic factors which operate immediately. If history-taking is done patiently, thoroughly and objectively the patient feels interest is being taken in his case and that his problem is being understood. A spontaneous account of the illness by the patient should be encouraged. Too systematic an approach to the history often results in a mass of facts being obtained, but the real problem, from the patient's aspect, may be entirely overlooked.

**Examining the Mental State.** As the interview proceeds, the doctor already is observing the patient's current mental functioning. The examination of the mental state is carried out in a systematic manner, paying attention in turn to the separate aspects of observable behaviour which disclose the state of mind.

*Appearance and Behaviour.* The appearance of the patient may be immediately informative, a dejected posture suggesting depressive illness; if the gestures the patient makes are tense and restless, clues may be provided which guide the doctor to enquire after further evidence of anxiety.

*Mood.* Whether the patient feels cheerful or depressed, confident or fearful, suspicious or bewildered, will become evident when the doctor asks the appropriate questions. 'How do you feel in yourself?' may be enough, but many patients need some help before they can unburden themselves of fears, anxieties or feelings of intense unhappiness. Some patients are ashamed to mention emotional disturbances, such as a phobia, i.e. unreasonable intense anxiety experienced in certain settings, e.g. in open or confined spaces. The patient may show a lack of emotional response; a very marked loss of rapport should also alert the doctor to the possibility that the patient may be schizophrenic.

*Thought Processes.* The way a patient thinks is evident in the patient's talk, which may be abnormal through incoherence, changes of topic, or bewildering shifts from one topic to another: all these can be features of schizophrenia. The patient may speak very rapidly, with puns and rhymes, as occurs in mania. Talk may be laboured, slow and flat and indicate a depressive state. Repetitive thoughts characterise obsessional psychoneurosis, an important feature of which is an *obsession*, a persistent idea which the patient cannot get rid of; the repetitiveness may be extremely distressing even when the patient recognises the idea as absurd — e.g. a girl may ponder whether she could be pregnant, although she knows perfectly well she has not had sexual intercourse.

*Perceptions of Environment.* The doctor next ascertains if the patient's perceptions are accurate. He may be unduly sensitive to glances or chance remarks. He may suffer from *illusions*, misinterpretations of sensations arising from real stimuli: a patient with delirium tremens may misinterpret furniture as menacing persons. *Hallucinations* are sense perceptions, such as visions, which occur in the absence of any kind of external stimulus. *Delusions* are false beliefs, such as that one is being slowly put to death, to which the patient adheres even when demonstrably wrong; a man with a hypochondrial delusion, e.g. a depressed patient convinced he has venereal disease, persists in his morbid notion despite evidence to the contrary. A schizophrenic may be firmly of the belief that he has changed sex. These are signs of major illness.

*Intellectual Functions.* While listening to what he tells us, we can at the same time pick up clues about the patient's intellectual level from his choice of words and from the ease or difficulty with which he expresses himself. The best clues to the basic intellectual level are given by the patient's scholastic record and by the type of job which he has been able to perform in adult life. If there is reason to suspect that he may be intellectually impaired, one can test his general information by posing simple questions, such as asking him to name the head of state, the capitals of the larger countries in Europe, or to perform simple sums of mental arithmetic. We note whether he knows the date and time of day, and recognises where he is and to whom he is talking: this tests his orientation for time, place and person. Impairment of mental function is commonly shown by inability to concentrate, to 'take things in', and hence to remember recent events. This may become apparent during the interview or it may be elicited by asking the patient to remember a name and address or a telephone number and then asking him to repeat it after an interval of 1 or 2 minutes. The final step in the mental state examination is an assessment of the patient's degree of insight into his condition; that is, does he recognise that he is ill or is he wrongly convinced that it is his environment and his fellows that are at fault?

When the history has been taken and an examination of the mental state completed, a thorough *physical examination* should be carried out and, following this, appropriate investigations when required. Such intervention needs to be handled well. Investigations which are necessary must be carefully planned, and quickly executed, and then a halt must be called. The pernicious habit of 'just having one more test' must be avoided as it undermines the confidence of the patient in the certainty of the diagnosis; the practitioner must be able to decide how much evidence is required to elucidate the nature and the cause of the disorder and, having obtained it, must act upon it.

**Diagnosis and Formulation.** The doctor is now in a position to make a formal *diagnosis*, deciding from which psychiatric syndrome the patient suffers, i.e. whether the patient's illness falls in the general class of neurosis, personality disorder, functional psychosis or organic mental illness.

The next step is the *formulation*, a brief statement in which the doctor summarises his understanding of the disorder and the person suffering from it, including the main setbacks or conflicts with other people, in the sequence in which they occurred.

## Psychiatric Interviewing

When the clinician undertakes to see the patient for a series of interviews, particularly when psychoneurosis or a personality disorder is present, a more detailed investigation of the psychological state is embarked upon. To do so, the clinician must acquire the necessary skills by receiving training in psychiatric interviewing, and must gain theoretical understanding of the common developments which occur as the therapeutic relationship is established and progressively extended. The clinician has available four well-documented theoretical approaches to interviewing on which to base his own style and approach; at times a combination of approaches is best suited to a particular patient.

1. *The descriptive approach* is most akin to medical history-taking and examination and leads to syndrome identification. As in other branches of medicine, it is appropriate in psychiatry to think in terms of disease entities, that is, to assume that the patient is suffering from a particular disease with its specific aetiology, pathology, signs and symptoms, which can be elicited by history-taking and examination.

2. The *analytical approach* enables the doctor to elicit any relevant complexes or pathogenic ideas of which the patient may be partially or totally unaware; Charcot, the nineteenth century French neurologist who was the first modern doctor to treat emotional disorder with individual psychotherapy, spoke of a 'psychic lesion' and described '. . . those remarkable paralyses which have been designated physical paralyses, paralyses depending on an idea, paralyses by imagination'. He gave the name 'dissociation' to the process by which distressing thoughts, memories or ideas disappeared from awareness, and then reappeared in disguised form as a dream or a physical symptom. The minor psychiatric disorders are usually associated with bodily discomfort and patients naturally consult their doctors about these complaints; many medical-sounding names have been coined, like anorexia nervosa or globus hystericus or cardiac neurosis. As a result it is easy to assume that each such diagnostic term refers to a separate disease process. Here, however, the 'disease-orientated' model can be misleading. In addition to their symptoms, patients suffering from these conditions can also be found to have disturbances in the relations with people close to them. These self-defeating patterns of behaviour in personal relationships have been learned by life experience; the early life of the neurotic or psychosomatic patient has included some painful, frustrating or damaging experiences which disturbed his peace of mind and continue to interfere with his performance. Moreover, the minor psychiatric disorders differ from diseases by being biographically meaningful. We can often understand why that person became ill in that way at that particular time as we come to understand the course of his life and to comprehend his dilemma in relation to the people of importance to him. A psychoneurosis, in this sense, symbolises a personal predicament of the patient.

3. A third interview procedure is the *interpersonal approach*, the doctor now exploring a patient's significant interpersonal relationships; much psychiatric illness, as we shall see, accompanies difficulties the patient currently has in his associations with the people most important to him.

4. Finally, the *phenomenological approach* is the method whereby the doctor, by an effort of imagination, uses his own life experience to enable him intuitively to grasp what the patient is suffering; such empathic perception of the patient's present predicament in living calls on the clinician to attempt a feat of fellow-feeling by which he can extend his understanding of the patient derived from the other three approaches.

## Professional Attitudes of the Doctor

Three habits of mind, or mental sets, are relevant to psychiatric work, in addition to those clinical attitudes which are necessary for the practice of medicine in general.

First, the clinician needs, for purposes of comprehensive interviewing, to surrender temporarily the relative detachment and authority appropriate to the practice of internal medicine, and instead to adopt a more receptive, less directive, clinical style. Much of the patient's experiences relevant to the psychiatric illness are locked up in the patient and get disclosed only if security, trust and some hope of being helped can be aroused in the patient. A paranoid patient who believes that there is a plot against him may conclude the doctor is part of the plot, unless by warmth and encouragement the doctor reassures the patient and brings him out of himself; a phobic patient may consider a fear of open spaces too ridiculous to disclose to the doctor, especially if already that doctor seems abrupt and critical.

Michael Balint wrote, in *The Doctor, His Patient, and the Illness* (1968), that medical training handicaps many clinicians for psychological work. He had in mind that when a person becomes a doctor he sets aside to some extent the innate perceptiveness, readiness to be informed by the patient and to be led by him into unexpected avenues. The question-and-answer interviewing technique in medicine, and the professional status as the expert who knows what course the clinical discussion should take, often constrains the patient. The 'small but necessary personality change' the doctor has to make, for purposes of psychiatric interviewing, is to be more passive, less decided in advance about matters to be explored, and more ready to receive private disclosures from the patient. Indeed, at first the patient often imparts a 'cover story', a version of his illness and his personal troubles which he hopes will not offend the doctor; only when he confirms for himself that the doctor is not censorious and remains open to receive further revelations will the patient give utterance to more distressing facts.

The second professional attitude of importance in psychiatric work is related to a skill which has already been indicated. The doctor must practise minimal intervention and allow the patient to be the more active.

Third, the doctor doing psychiatric work requires an orientation of self-scrutiny, reflecting constantly on the impact exerted on the patient and asking oneself whether the patient is being influenced as intended. A readiness continuously to study one's own personality in clinical action and the responses made to patients enables the doctor progressively to increase knowledge about the life experiences of others, skills for alleviating personal distress, and capacity for gaining self-knowledge. The doctor's personality is the chief clinical tool. It is always in this personal capacity that the psychiatrically ill patient will respond, over and above the clinical expertise the doctor exercises when engaged on the exploration, diagnosis and management of any disorder of the patient's mind or personality.

# PSYCHIATRIC DISORDERS

## Classification of Psychiatric Disorders

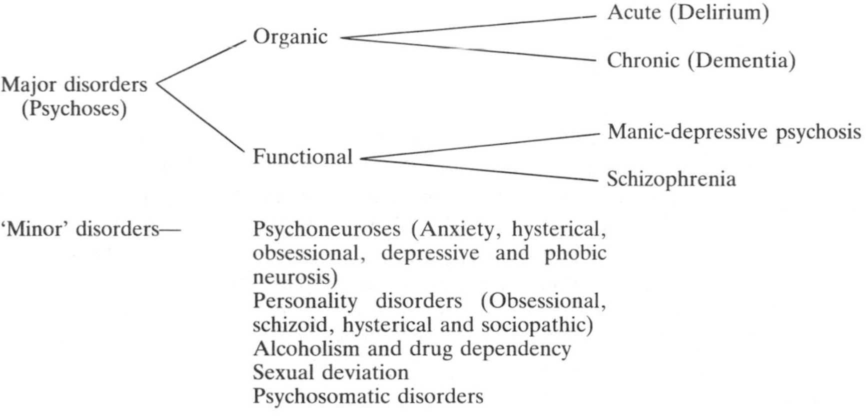


Mental handicap (mental retardation)

## The Organic Psychoses

Psychiatric symptoms may arise in the course of physical illnesses which either primarily or secondarily affect the brain. The mental symptoms of general paresis or the occurrence of delirium during the course of febrile illnesses are two well-known examples. It is important to recognise certain mental symptoms which occur in organic mental syndromes, since their presence should lead to the search for physical factors which may not otherwise have declared themselves. The organic psychoses can be divided into two groups: *delirium*, which is an acute disorder, and *dementia* which is a chronic disorder. Generally speaking the acute form is potentially recoverable, being the result of temporary effects on the brain from toxic processes or disorders of metabolism, while the chronic form is the expression of more severe and progressive tissue changes in the brain and is thus not reversible. The mental symptoms of each of these organic syndromes are not specific to the causative disease and will be the same whatever may be the underlying physical disorder producing the delirium or dementia.

### Delirium

This acute syndrome may be produced by such varied conditions as (i) drug intoxication (alcoholism, LSD), (ii) physical disease such as infections (encephalitis, typhoid fever); (iii) diseases of the brain, (iv) electrolyte imbalance and metabolic disorders (hepatic failure, uraemia), (v) vitamin deficiency (Wernicke's encephalopathy), and (vi) cerebral hypoxia (severe respiratory or heart failure).

In addition to the physical symptoms appropriate to the primary disorder there are often found slurred speech, tremor, nystagmus, diplopia and sluggish pupillary reactions. The characteristic mental symptoms are: insomnia and restlessness; disorientation; impairment of the sensorium (clouding of consciousness) so that alertness and attention are diminished; confusion; hallucinations, particularly in the visual sphere;

ideas of persecution (paranoid ideas); and a feeling of fear or terror. All the symptoms and particularly the level of consciousness are variable. The patient may be in a state of restlessness varying from simple tossing and turning to such activities as aimlessly searching in the bedclothes or agitation. He may appear orientated for time and space and be able to recognise visitors at one moment, only to be quite confused soon after. The patient will often give the easiest answer to a question without regard to the truth and may supplement his faulty memory and perception by invention (confabulation), as when he describes in detail a large meal which he says he has just had, when in fact he has eaten nothing. Visual hallucinations are characteristic of delirium, and are usually vivid and may be terrifying. Many are based on illusional misinterpretations of objects seen in the room; thus patterns on the wallpaper may become an advancing army of hideous and menacing reptiles. Hallucinations of other senses may occur. Doubt and suspicion are readily induced by the impaired mentality leading to misinterpretations and may blossom for a short time into transient and rather ill-defined delusions of persecution. Such an acute organic syndrome is commonly precipitated by withdrawal of alcohol or of barbiturates, from patients who have become habituated to taking them in substantial amounts. When the syndrome is due to alcoholism it is known as delirium tremens, but its features do not greatly differ from those of delirium from other causes.

The course and prognosis of delirium depend, of course, on the underlying physical disease, and treatment of this in most cases clears up the mental symptoms completely. Sometimes, however, delirium may be an episode in a progressive dementia.

**Treatment.** The use of chlorpromazine (25 mg t.i.d. by mouth or 100 mg i.m.) has transformed the management of acute delirium, enabling the majority of patients to be cared for in a side-room of the medical or surgical ward where their primary disease is being treated. Thioridazine in similar doses has less hypotensive effect. In all these conditions the patient can be helped by explanations and friendly support; patients who are frightened and bewildered tend to regress to a state of childlike dependency and welcome a firm reassurance from someone whom they are willing to trust. They cannot, however, be kept calm if staff changes expose them to many strange faces or if they are bewildered by too many novel events. Some patients have catastrophic reactions following operations on the eyes, when they must submit to being blindfolded for some time, and others have reacted adversely to the accompaniments of cardiac resuscitation or renal dialysis. These acute psychoses contain an element of panic. Nitrazepam (5–10 mg) or dichloralphenazone (1–4, 650 mg tablets) are suitable hypnotics.

## Dementia

This chronic organic syndrome may be caused by a wide variety of diseases of the brain. The most common of these are cerebral atherosclerosis and atrophy. Other important causes include cerebral trauma, inflammations (neurosyphilis, encephalitis), multiple sclerosis, intoxications and deficiency disorders (chronic alcoholism, pellagra, vitamin $B_{12}$ deficiency), prolonged hypoglycaemia, carbon monoxide poisoning, cerebral neoplasm, and degenerative disorders such as Huntington's chorea. It will be seen that some of these conditions (encephalitis, alcoholism, vitamin deficiencies) may also cause delirium. The cerebral changes brought about at first by these factors result in delirium and can be reversed by treatment, but if they are allowed to continue unchecked too long, permanent cerebral damage occurs, giving rise to dementia.

The clinical picture of dementia varies to some extent with the cause, the previous personality of the patient, the age of onset, and the rate of progression, but in all cases the mental symptoms are seen to involve the intellect, memory, emotions and behaviour, although the actual degree of impairment depends on the factors mentioned above. Insomnia is often an early symptom and may lead to nocturnal restlessness and confusion as the disease advances. Judgement and reasoning are involved early, and the disability caused by this will depend on the extent to which these faculties are utilised in the patient's daily life and work; it will be more noticeable in a teacher than in an unskilled labourer. Impairment of memory is the most prominent finding, particularly in relation to recent events, and in the later stages this may combine with defective perception to produce disorientation in space and time. Impairment of higher control leads to emotional instability and outbursts of violence or sexual aberrations at variance with the patient's previous character. There may be wide fluctuations of mood with euphoria or depression but finally, as mood flattens, the patient sinks into apathy. Delusions are common, and may be either centred on the patient himself, when they are grandiose or self-condemnatory and hypochondriacal according to the mood, or centred on others, when they tend to be paranoid. As the structure of the personality disintegrates, the patient neglects his appearance, becomes lax in personal cleanliness, and careless incontinence occurs. Focal neurological signs may be found, e.g. dysphagia, apraxia, agnosia, hemiplegia, and epileptic attacks, either focal or generalised.

Dementia in the elderly is usually due either to cerebral atherosclerosis or is of senile type. Table 15.1 shows the differences between the two syndromes.

## Functional Psychoses

### Depressive Psychosis

Depression is a mood which all of us experience from time to time, usually as a result of some distressing circumstance. In contrast, patients suffering from depressive psychosis complain of a prolonged dejected state. They seem to have become ill for no reason they can identify, their low spirits and subjective misery causing them to feel altogether different as people. Such patients are suffering from depressive psychosis known also as endogenous depressive illness. They are often individuals who

Table 15.1 Dementia in the elderly

| | *Atherosclerotic* | *Senile* |
|---|---|---|
| Sex | Commoner in women | Commoner in men |
| Age of onset | From 45 onwards | After 65 |
| Impairment of intellect | Late in illness | Early |
| Deterioration of personality | Late | Early |
| Course | Steplike | Progressive |
| Brain damage | Focal | Global |
| Physical symptoms | Present | Absent |
| Physical signs | Present | Rare and late |
| CT scan | May show multiple infarcts | Cortical shrinkage and dilatation of ventricles |

have been subject previously to mood swings or who have over-scrupulous rigid personalities following too strict upbringing. Depressive psychosis may be induced by physical illness such as influenza or by drugs, notably antihypertensives, corticosteroids and oral contraceptives. Like the less severe psychoneurotic depressive reaction (p. 769), depressive psychosis may be precipitated by external events particularly those which impart a sense of loss, separation or disappointment. Much more often it arises without detectable external influences. Depressive psychosis is commoner in patients of middle age or older, but certainly does occur in the young and also in children.

**Clinical Features.** In addition to a mood varying from mild depression to black despair the manifestations are: insomnia of a type characterised by early waking after 2 to 3 hours sleep; diurnal variation of mood, in which the depression often lifts considerably towards evening; slowness of thought, and inability to make decisions; ideas of guilt, unworthiness and self-blame which are often delusional in intensity, i.e. they are impervious to reasoned argument or demonstration of their falsity; and various somatic manifestations such as loss of appetite, loss of weight, amenorrhoea, pressure headache, backache, constipation, retardation of physical activity (more rarely aimless over-activity or agitation), and hypochondriacal delusions. Such a patient may sit bowed and immobile on the edge of a chair obviously in the depths of misery, weeping silently, and answering questions in slow monosyllables; but in the earlier stages the physical appearance is much less striking and the diagnosis depends on the doctor's ability to elicit the symptoms described above.

Severe depressive psychosis, especially when associated with restlessness and agitation, with delusions of unworthiness and preoccupation with thoughts of death, is an extremely distressing condition and fraught with risks of suicide. This is the main hazard and the risk is often greatest at the onset of depressive psychosis or when treatment begins to relieve the depression and reduce the accompanying psychomotor retardation. Severe cases should be admitted to psychiatric care in hospital.

*In manic-depressive psychosis* the patient, apart from depressive attacks, can suffer from morbid elation and hyperactivity. He looks excessively cheerful, speaks rapidly, shifting from one idea to another, often joking, teasing, making puns and paying poor attention to his environment. He is overconfident, over-optimistic and overimportant. He may suffer from grandiose delusions and behave in an extravagantly spendthrift way. He ususally does not realise he is ill, and may react with violence if crossed or restrained. Failure to diagnose mania can have very serious consequences for a patient, who can run up vast debts or jeopardise his social position drastically by ill-judged, embarrassing or boisterously inappropriate and undesirable behaviour.

**Treatment.** The first task after diagnosing depressive psychosis is to proceed without delay to treat the patient with one of the potent antidepressant drugs. One has to bear in mind, however, that these do not take effect until after some 6 to 14 days.

There are two principal groups of antidepressant drugs:

1. Tricyclic drugs (e.g. imipramine, amitriptyline and trimipramine), the monoamine reuptake inhibiting drugs (MARI).

2. The monoamine oxidase inhibitor (MAOI) drugs (e.g. phenelzine, mebanazine and tranylcypromine).

1. *Tricyclic drugs* are indicated for the treatment of endogenous depressive illness. In order to be effective, they have to be given in sufficient dosage. It is usual to prescribe 25 mg t.i.d. for one week, and 50 mg or more t.i.d. subsequently. Trimi-

pramine may be given as a single dose (50–100 mg) at night. Amitriptyline is also available in 50 or 100 mg sustained-release tablets for use at night.

Tricyclic drugs give rise to some disagreeable anticholinergic effects, for example on the eyes, causing difficulty in focussing. Imipramine may make the patient feel even more on edge and restless during the first few days and it may also cause some difficulty in micturition. Amitriptyline tends to make some patients feel uncomfortably drowsy and causes dryness of the mouth. These side-effects usually recede with continued use and become quite easily tolerated once the patient begins to experience a lifting of the mood and a return of former energy. A course of tricyclic drugs should be taken for 3 to 6 months; if they are stopped too soon the symptoms of depression may recur. A patient who fails to respond to one drug, may benefit from another.

2. *The monoamine oxidase inhibitor drugs* are especially helpful in the treatment of 'atypical' depressions (or prolonged phobic symptoms), occurring in patients with good previous personalities. Patients on MAOI drugs should be warned not to partake of substances rich in tyramine (such as cheese, chianti and some types of beer) because these may interact with the drug to provoke a hypertensive crisis, with splitting headaches and a risk of subarachnoid haemorrhage. The MAOI drugs also potentiate other drugs, including pethidine, opiates, barbiturates, phenothiazines, amphetamine and alcohol, all of which should be avoided while a patient is taking this form of antidepressant. Caution is needed when changing from a MAOI drug to a tricyclic or vice versa : a drug-free interval of a week is advisable.

*Electroconvulsive therapy* administered under intravenous anaesthesia and modified by muscle-relaxant drugs may be indicated if the patient's suffering is not relieved after antidepressant medication for 2 to 3 weeks.

*Lithium carbonate* is effective in controlling manic-depressive states. The patient needs to be in hospital at the start of treatment. It may also prevent the recurrence of manic attacks when used as maintenance therapy, in daily doses of 750–1500 mg, out-patients returning for weekly estimation of plasma lithium and a check on adverse effects which include hypothyroidism.

As a general rule, it is wise to postpone any practical decisions about business, change of work or domestic matters until the patient has regained a normal frame of mind. Once the patient's mood has responded to drugs or ECT it is essential to review personal circumstances and to help make plans to cope with the difficulties which may have precipitated the illness. Moreover, the patient may need to know that the psychosis sometimes takes a recurring form and that advice must be sought if symptoms return. However, depressive psychosis, once of gloomy prognosis, is now eminently treatable, and with appropriate care few such patients become chronic hospital inmates.

## Schizophrenia

Schizophrenia is the illness with symptoms corresponding most closely to the popular conception of madness. The personality becomes disintegrated, and detached from the social environment. The mental life becomes split up. The cardinal features are: disorder of thinking, which becomes incoherent, disjointed and rambling; incongruity of emotion; impulsive actions and utterances; and hallucinations (most commonly, in the form of threatening or unfriendly voices). Patients express bizarre delusions with little or no appreciation of why it is that their ideas are unacceptable to those around them.

Both delusions and hallucinations may occur in other forms of mental illness, such as severe depressive illness, mania, or delirium, but certain other features are especially suggestive of schizophrenia. These include (1) *passivity feelings*, in which the patient is convinced that his actions are controlled by some alien power, (2) *thought insertion* and *thought broadcasting*, in which he feels that other people put thoughts into his mind, and are able to read his thoughts and (3) *paranoid delusions* in which he believes that he is surrounded by hostile forces which watch him and secretly intervene to do him harm. Patients with depressive illness may also develop paranoid ideas, but these are coloured by their all-pervading feelings of guilt. For example, a depressed patient may believe that he is being watched by secret police because they have found out that he has committed a terrible crime. The paranoid schizophrenic, on the other hand, is quite sure that it is his unseen enemies who are the villains of the piece, and he their innocent victim.

Schizophrenic patients tend to have little insight into the fact that they are ill and in need of treatment. When their behaviour is becoming alarming, it may be necessary, in their own interests, to admit them compulsorily to hospital. In Britain application is made by the patient's nearest relative supported by two medical recommendations by the patient's family doctor and a psychiatrist. The patient's case must be reviewed after 28 days. In many cases he will continue in hospital voluntarily. A mentally ill patient who is a danger to himself or others may also be admitted compulsorily as an emergency for 3 days in England and Wales and 7 days in Scotland. This certificate is signed by only one doctor and can be used when the patient is already in hospital.

These are the more florid manifestations of schizophrenia. Milder signs are less easy to recognise. These include instances of unexpected rudeness or tactlessness, abrupt and inexplicable behaviour with a marked withdrawal from ordinary social contacts. Such persons may be considered awkward or unsociable and it is only when they reveal quite bizarre ideas, shout back at their hallucinatory voices, or otherwise behave in a conspicuously strange manner, that one realises that they are not merely eccentric, but mentally ill.

**Treatment.** Phenothiazine drugs such as chlorpromazine, and the butyrophenones (e.g. haloperidol) have changed the prognosis of schizophrenia but it should be remembered that even before there was any specific drug treatment for this illness, many cases made a spontaneous recovery from the acute stage of the psychosis in the course of 3 to 9 months. These drugs offer symptomatic relief of the patient's delusions, hallucinations and alienation from reality, rather than a radical cure of this little-understood disease. There is abundant evidence that the way in which the patient is treated, in hospital and in the community, will influence both the degree of recovery and the probability of a subsequent relapse.

Putting it briefly, it may be said that schizophrenic patients do badly if they are allowed to withdraw too completely from social contacts and practical activities; but they also do badly if they are involved in emotionally demanding relationships, to which they are unable to respond. Many, if not most, schizophrenics must be regarded as having particularly vulnerable personalities and many emerge from the acute stage of their illness with some residual defects ('end states'). They are best able to cope with their handicap if they can be helped to come to terms with their limitations. These patients are not necessarily intellectually impaired — they may be highly intelligent — but they are seldom able to cope with positions of responsibility, particularly when they are required to supervise, or interact with other people. Hence such partially recovered patients do best in tasks in which they can work on their own, with only rather formal contacts with their fellows. Nowadays the great majority of schizophrenic patients are treated at home, taking their prescribed drugs for at least the first year or two after discharge from hospital. The doctor should be ready to enlist the help of a community nurse or of a social worker if patients appear to be having difficulties either at work or in their domestic relationships.

During the acute stage of the illness, chlorpromazine and thioridazine are in general use, 150–1000 mg being given each day in divided doses. About 60% of patients with acute schizophrenic symptoms can be expected to improve significantly within a matter of weeks. A suitable maintenance dose for a schizophrenic in remission is 100 mg thrice daily. Chlorpromazine is also given by intramuscular injections (50–100 mg) in order to control stages of agitation or over-excitement. Postural hypotension is an important side-effect which is more marked with elderly patients, who should be given smaller doses. Haloperidol intramuscularly or by mouth may be substituted for chlorpromazine.

A long-acting phenothiazine, fluphenazine decanoate (12·25–25 mg each 2–4 weeks) can be given intramuscularly on a maintenance basis for chronic schizophrenics treated as out-patients who are unreliable with oral medication. All the phenothiazines can have adverse extrapyramidal effects, and anti-parkinsonian drugs (p. 717) may also have to be taken. Restlessness and dystonia of the jaw and neck can occur. Another drug effect is tardive dyskinesia, continuous movements of the head and tongue, which may persist for years.

When the schizophrenic psychosis is of acute onset, and the previous personality relatively sociable and well-adapted, the outcome is better. It is important for doctors to know about the condition and recognise it when it occurs, because competent and early treatment can spare the patient and the relatives extreme harm, through social catastrophe or accident.

## The Psychoneuroses

There are two conditions to be met before the doctor can regard an illness as psychoneurotic. First, one of the typical syndromes (to be described below) must be in evidence. Second, the person must have experienced a recent setback, usually a disturbance in his relationship with a person or persons important to him. Often, when the first condition applies, the doctor may need to act on the basis of his clinical diagnosis without having elicited the biographical corroboration, but he must know that the omission exists and needs to be remedied, otherwise serious mistakes can happen. Symptoms resembling those of neuroses, e.g. hysterical states, can occur with cerebral trauma or disease or in a functional psychosis.

The interpersonal or social setback preceding the onset of psychoneurotic illness need not be a gross one. However, it will be highly charged emotionally, in the context of the patient's biography, sometimes fitting as a key does into a lock with an earlier similar setback. It then seems understandable that the recent miscarriage of a relationship (the dynamic cause, or the process event) has disorganised the adaptation of a person previously sensitised by an earlier emotional trauma (the predisposing cause). A woman who becomes ill with psychoneurosis when afraid that she may be deserted on discovering that her husband has become attracted to another woman, may be found by further questioning to have lost her loved father through his death before her teens. The threat of the present loss is more understandably distressing in relation to the earlier deprivation.

Psychoneurosis, one of the 'minor' disorders, is an illness taking the form of one of the well-described syndromes in this category of disability: anxiety, hysterical, obsessional, depressive or phobic neurosis.

With all these characteristic syndromes the patient will be only partially disabled, many aspects of personality and social competence being unaffected. The man or woman can often cope with work and household responsibilities, and hence usually be treated as an out-patient. Reality testing is not impaired in any gross way, i.e. the misperceptions of the human and material environment characterising psychotic illness do not occur. The patient has only partial energy available for everyday activities.

There is a great amount of psychoneurotic illness in every community, for psychoneurosis is much the most common psychiatric disorder. Many individuals will be mildly disturbed and may not need medical treatment. The presence of a psychiatric syndrome does not of itself necessarily require intervention. A man with a fear of heights is not disabled if he works on the ground in a community made up of low houses; the same man who moves for postgraduate work to New York, for example, where he may have to attend seminars in skyscrapers, can become seriously impaired. On the other hand, flying phobia developing in any member of aircraft personnel is instantly incapacitating.

Given the much greater amount of psychiatric disability in all countries than there are facilities for treatment, the doctor may decide to treat those psychoneurotic patients in whom there is both a clinical syndrome and also fairly conspicuous incapacity. The presence of psychoneurosis of itself does not necessarily call for treatment. Subjective distress on the patient's part is the indication that therapeutic intervention is needed.

Not all patients, of course, will accept with equanimity a diagnosis of psychoneurosis when their preferred concept of their illness is a physical one. This will often be evident from the initial reluctance with which some patients accept advice for psychiatric referral. A sickness of one's body is not regarded as a matter for which one is culpable (although Samuel Butler in *Erehwon* fancifully developed the opposite notion—that physical illness could be one's own fault). In contrast, a disturbance of one's mind could be regarded as an affliction of one's very self, and therefore a weakness in one as a person. The early neurologists, such as Head and Holmes, in discussing the body schema or body image, indicated the extent to which a person regards his body as somehow intermediate between the self and the outside world.

It has been demonstrated that the higher the social class of the patient, the more prepared he is to accept a psychiatric diagnosis. The same correlation between socioeconomic disadvantage and somatisation is evident in transcultural psychiatric studies: in the East and in Africa, patients in much greater numbers than in developed countries present psychogenic illness in the form of physical complaints. Indeed, as university health service experience with medical and other students has shown, even sophisticated patients often tend to complain first about somatic symptoms such as headache or stomach discomfort (and many doctors are more receptive about physical illnesses), and only afterwards proceed to relate a personal problem or to describe emotional distress.

The most important clinical rule is the need not only to elicit any psychoneurotic syndrome which may be present, but also to uncover the intrapersonal subjective tension preceding the onset of the illness; it usually consists of an upset in an important personal relationship (e.g. with a wife, another relative or a work associate).

### Anxiety Neurosis

Anxiety is a state of fear, occurring with a feeling of inner tension and somatic manifestations such as tense muscles, sweating, tremor and tachycardia. Anxiety neurosis is the most common form of psychoneurosis. Although anxiety is a symptom of many psychological disorders, in this syndrome it dominates the clinical picture and other symptoms such as depression are but minor features of the total illness.

**Aetiology.** Hereditary factors play a part, although a relatively small part, in the genesis of anxiety neurosis, manifestations of anxiety being found in 15% of parents and siblings of patients, which is more than in the population as a whole (5%). Twice as many women as men are affected.

In addition to the genetic trait, even more important aetiologically are emotionally disturbing experiences during the early formative years. These traumatic experiences need not be highly distressing nor need they be single events such as early loss of the mother. An isolated trauma is therefore not to be expected as a frequent predisposing cause in early life. More often it is found that the patient's early years were attended by prolonged insecurity. For example, a parent may have been so burdened by problems that the child felt unloved, if not unwanted; a brother or sister may have seemed to get preferential treatment; or a mother's own exaggerated anxieties may have imparted an excessive timidity to her child, profoundly undermining the child's self-confidence.

This emotional trauma may not be apparent for several years, particularly if the experiences of school life and early adolescence prove free from alarming or painful incidents: but a setback in early adult life may precipitate adult emotional illness. Painful events, such as a bereavement, a reverse in a love affair, disappointment in one's career, being obliged to contend with disagreeable or frankly hostile people at work, or being involved in prolonged domestic strife, may cause a vulnerable individual to succumb to feelings of anxiety which interfere materially with the ability to cope with the daily routine. The adult setback will often be found to have been similar in quality to the earlier childhood emotional trauma.

**Clinical Features.** The illness may take many forms. It may occur as an acute anxiety attack, often severe in intensity, appearing against a relatively normal background, or a chronic anxiety state, present since adolescence in mild degree, but subject to periodic exacerbations occurring at the time of social setbacks, disappointments in close relationships, or work stresses.

The oustanding feature of the illness is anxiety, with its accompanying feeling of inner tension and unpleasant anticipation. Sometimes the anxiety is fear of a potential danger but often it is a diffuse dread. (A *phobia* implies that anxiety is associated with a specific form of activity such as travelling in a bus or train, and so much may this be dreaded that the patient is eventually house-bound through being unable to travel at all.) The fear and foreboding fluctuate in intensity, being sometimes a mild feeling of tension or nervousness, at other times a state of panic, in which the patient may be overwhelmed by a feeling of terror, which is no less disturbing because the reason for it is not apparent to the patient.

The state of anxiety gives rise to other symptoms. The ability to concentrate is impaired and decisions are difficult to make. There may be a continuous state of restlessness or extreme irritability. The patient may fear becoming insane or committing suicide though, in fact, both are extremely rare in anxiety neurosis. Preoccupation with bodily functions and fear of serious illness (*hypochondriasis* and *cancerophobia*) are frequently manifested. Continued stress exhausts the patient who, lacking energy and perseverence, may be unable to continue at work.

Somatic symptoms are also prominent. There is a general tenseness of muscles, with hyperactivity, especially the hands. A fine tremor of the fingers is often present and profuse perspiration, especially of the palms and forehead, is common. The pulse rate is raised, the blood pressure labile and overactivity of smooth muscle is commonly manifest by frequency of micturition or of defaecation. Breathing is often rapid and feelings of nausea and flatulence occur; headaches of tension type, dizziness and unsteadiness are frequent. The patient sleeps badly, finding it difficult to get off to sleep and being easily disturbed. Appetite is poor, and loss of weight may be a pronounced feature. Disturbances of menstruation are common.

Not uncommonly the patient omits mention of the distressing emotional state and complains to the doctor only of the somatic accompaniments of anxiety; unnecessary special investigations can be initiated or diagnostic errors made if the doctor omits to ask about the state of the patient's mood.

**Diagnosis.** Medical illnesses that produce symptoms resembling those of anxiety neurosis include cardiac arrhythmias, angina pectoris, hyperthyroidism, phaeochromocytoma and parathyroid disease.

It is scarcely surprising that some patients who know that they suffer from physical disease, e.g. diabetes, angina, peptic ulceration, renal failure or other forms of chronic disease, undergo episodes of severe anxiety which is in part at least related to the real threat to their lives. These patients with psychological complications of organic disease have to be distinguished from those who are crippled by an unjustified conviction that they have just such diseases (*hypochondriasis*). Not only will there be a negative physical examination, but when the patient has been helped to give free expression to fears a positive diagnosis of anxiety neurosis can be made. Differentiation from other psychiatric illnesses is less difficult.

Though hysterical, obsessive or depressive symptoms may also be present in anxiety states, the diagnosis can usually be made on the totality of the picture: anxiety often occurs in attacks and its accompanying somatic manifestations dominate the clinical presentation. It is rarely difficult to distinguish an acute anxiety state from a case of depressive psychosis with severe agitation and restlessness.

**Treatment.** When the formulation of the case indicates that emotional factors are prominent, some form of psychotherapy is required; the patient needs an opportunity for exploration and clarification, and for gaining greater insight into the nature of his difficulties. Simply informing the patient that there is nothing wrong with him, or that he must pull himself together, is useless. Even telling the patient that his difficulties are psychological and indicating the emotional problems in his life is unlikely to be of benefit, because although he may acquiesce verbally, his emotional tension will not be thereby lessened.

A series of interviews, for which periods of at least half an hour or longer should be set aside, are needed when the patient is encouraged to talk about his difficulties. Initially, the discussions should be allowed to proceed in any direction the patient desires; subsequently, aspects of his problems which come to seem relevant may be suggested by the doctor as themes for more detailed discussion. The error that is commonly made with this form of psychotherapy is for the doctor to talk too much and give advice. In order that the patient may achieve a better knowledge of himself, it is essential that he should do most of the talking, the doctor saying little, but maintaining an attitude of interest and expectation. If the patient's flow of talk is arrested, encouragement can often be given, without diverting him from his present theme. Thus, if he says 'I wasn't able to cope at work', and then becomes silent, after giving him ample time to resume spontaneously, the doctor may say, 'You found the job too much for you?', which starts the patient off again. The effect of this approach is first that the patient feels better for having talked to someone about his troubles. A second effect is that frequently the patient comes to grasp more accurately the nature of his problems, and will, at that stage, often accept suggestions and interpretations which, if given earlier, would have been rejected. What emerges is that the patient is having difficulties with a person of importance to him: a spouse, a parent, or an employer, for example, and that he needs to improve his management of the relationship. He may be too dependent on his wife, too docile to his parent, or too subservient to his employer — in which case his interviews should encourage greater assertiveness.

When the psychological disorder takes the form of somatic symptoms and fear of bodily disease is prominent, it is not sufficient to tell the patient that there is no evidence of organic pathology. It is necessary to let him know that his distress and his symptoms are recognised as genuine and need exploration. It is often possible to use events in the patient's own experience to illustrate the influence of emotion on bodily functions. Many people can recognise what it feels like to be sick with excitement, to be aware of a pounding of the heart in moments of fear or to experience frequency of micturition when keyed up before an examination. Patients are further helped when they can go one stage further, to confront the painful situation and to master it, e.g. the patient can say to his employer that he considers he is being exploited and his abilities insufficiently recognised. When this is done, there is commonly an immediate, even if temporary, relief from the distressing symptom, together with a sense of accomplishment which encourages the patient to persevere with further efforts of self-discovery.

The use of drugs to obtain reduction of distressing mood disturbance is often a necessary preliminary to effective psychotherapy. A very anxious patient will not be able to concentrate sufficiently to benefit more than partially from clarification of conflicts discussed during an interview. Diazepam (6–40 mg/d) and chlordiazepoxide (10–60 mg/d) are effective anxiety-reducing drugs. The phenothiazines, though widely used (up to 150 mg/d), are more likely to give rise to lethargy or drowsiness but thioridazine, in the same dosage, can be of value when the patient is both fearful and restless.

In the treatment of all forms of neurotic illness it is important to decide what can best be done, within the limitations of resources for treatment and in the circumstances of each individual patient. The drugs specified above can be particularly helpful in tiding a neurotic patient with anxiety over an especially difficult period of subjective distress. They do not, however, do anything to resolve the causes of the patient's symptoms, and unless this is altered either through psychotherapy or through a significant change in personal circumstances, the symptoms will tend to recur and the patient may become dependent on the palliative drug.

Brief psychotherapy focuses upon recent events in the patient's personal experience and explores their emotional significance for him. By this method, many patients can be helped to reconstitute the way of life which, for the particular person, represents normal mental health.

Explorative psychotherapy, which calls on the patient to take stock of his relationships with people close to him and to modify some of his habitual patterns of behaviour towards them, is more time-consuming and aims to produce personality change as well as relief from the symptoms of the illness.

### Hysterical Psychoneurosis

Hysterical psychoneurosis is a protean group of disorders, common in all branches of medicine. Essentially a hysterical neurosis consists of the production of the symptoms or signs of a 'physical' illness by a patient for some personal purpose, without his being fully aware of his motive in doing so. Familiar examples are sudden 'blackouts' or 'loss of memory' by which a patient evades a particularly painful or humiliating occurrence.

**Aetiology.** Heredity is even less important in the development of hysterical neurosis than it is in anxiety neurosis, and plays but a minor role in its aetiology; the mode of transmission or the nature of what is transmitted is not known. Environment, by contrast, provides those situational factors which precipitate the development of hysterical symptoms. Lack of emotional security in the early years can encourage and prolong a state of child-like dependency. The lack of development of confidence to tackle practical difficulties makes a person rely on others to solve his problems and such a person may later react with hysterical illness. Gross hysterical symptoms occur frequently in association with educational and intellectual disadvantage, and are a particularly common occurrence in developing countries.

**Conversion Hysterical Neurosis.** This type of psychoneurosis includes the illnesses in which the patient presents with a physical symptom, such as sudden blindness, or paralysis of one or more limbs, or total loss of sensation in a part of the body. Neurological examination will often reveal that the disability does not correspond to the anatomical areas served by motor or sensory nerves: instead, the lesion illustrates the patient's own idea of what it is like to lose the power of the right hand, or to be unable to walk. In many cases, the patient has acquired a concept of a particular affliction as a result of seeing someone who was similarly handicapped. The form the symptom takes may be determined by identification with another person, as when the daughter, after her mother's death, develops the symptoms of her mother's last illness.

The grosser forms of conversion symptoms are not so common today as they were a generation ago, but still occur particularly commonly as a complication of injuries where a compensation award enters the picture. A striking feature of conversion hysterical neurosis is that although the patient may be quite severely incapacitated by the symptoms, he appears remarkably unconcerned about them. This is because the disability due to the illness has in fact intervened to remove a cause of anxiety, so that the patient feels strangely relieved, although he is not aware of the reason for his being so calm.

The list of conversion hysterical symptoms and signs is extensive, for there are few clinical features which may not be encountered in the many forms of this variable disorder. Some features, however, occur more commonly than others and may be arbitrarily divided into two groups, sensory and motor. *Sensory symptoms* may be of the special senses, such as blindness and deafness, or in the somatic sphere, when cutaneous and deep sensibility in their various forms are lost. The sensory loss does not obey anatomical or physiological laws but follows the patient's concept of disability. Cutaneous sensory loss may have a sharp horizontal upper margin on the limb. In monocular blindness, the patient may on occasion see with the 'blind' eye and the pupillary light reflex is preserved. There may also be subjective sensory symptoms such as headache, pain, tinnitus and so on.

*Motor symptoms* consist of aphonia, mutism and paralysis and rigidity of movements. Positive clinical features in the motor sphere consist of tremors, tics and explosive utterances, spasm of ocular muscles, and fits. These fits may vary from simply falling to the ground to bizarre attacks with wild movements of arms and legs. Carpopedal spasm and other manifestations of tetany may result from hysterical hyperventilation.

**Dissociative Hysterical Neurosis.** The second type of hysterical psychoneurosis includes the numerous altered states of awareness, such as faints, fits, amnesias, trances, twilight states and forms of multiple personality. A fugue state is one in which the patient wanders away from home in a condition of altered awareness. Hysterical stupor, when the patient lies motionless showing no reaction to the environment, is sometimes seen; in pseudodementia (seen on occasion in a prison setting) the patient behaves as if insane.

**Anorexia Nervosa.** In this condition, classified with the hysterical psychoneuroses, patients aim to become very slim and to stay so. Frequently preoccupied about food, the patient stubbornly seeks to lose weight. The determination to diet is a disorder of motivation. Exertion of the will, so that over-riding priority is given to becoming thin, is the chief feature of the disorder. It often follows teasing about being plump.

Young girls are mainly affected. If questioned suitably, they often reveal preoccupations (sometimes so distorted as to reach delusional proportions) relating to sex, sometimes following misinformation by parents; however, these girls also give evidence of great fear at growing up and accepting mature feminine responsibilities. They are often in a hostile relationship with their mothers. Frequently there have been upsetting life experiences, such as separation from or death of a parent. In addition to dread of sexual development, girls with anorexia nervosa often show athletic preoccupations and are overactive physically. Secondary gonadotrophic and ovarian hormone disturbances occur. Amenorrhoea at times precedes marked emaciation. The usual mood state is cheerful high spirits, but depression can occur. Sometimes eating orgies occur, after which the patient feels extremely guilty and in advanced stages of the disorder may induce vomiting. Those anorexics who in addition are vomiters and use purgation have a worse prognosis. Patients usually show unconcern about their physical deterioration and reject treatment, which often has to be very firmly advised and provided.

In-patient psychiatric treatment with psychotherapy to achieve emotional maturation is usually necessary, in addition to correction of the eating disorder.

**Diagnosis of Hysterical Psychoneurosis.** This can be the most difficult in medicine. Three steps are required: the first is to identify the psychoneurotic syndrome on the basis of its characteristic symptomatology, as described above. The second step to be taken should any doubt still exist is to demonstrate that there is no organic disease which can account for the symptoms and signs. Error in diagnosing hysterical psychoneurosis would be infrequent, however, if the diagnosis were not made until the third step was also taken: this consists of discovering what disappointment or setback preceded the development of symptoms. The precipitating cause of a hysterical illness is usually an emotionally charged experience or setback, the unpleasant consequences of which the patient cannot face, and so excludes it from consciousness and escapes from the situation by means of symptoms.

If evidence of previous hysterical breakdowns can be uncovered, the diagnosis is more secure. It should be kept in mind, however, that the stress of organic disease may provoke a superadded hysterical reaction in a person so disposed. An axiom worth remembering is that suspected hysterical neurosis appearing for the first time in a stable person in middle life has almost always an organic basis.

**Treatment** may be a difficult problem. Removal of a symptom can often be achieved by a prolonged interview in which intense persuasion is used; but if the precipitating situation is unaltered, relapse is usual. The method may be justified, however, in certain circumstances as when aphonia prevents discussion, or when loss of memory in hysterical amnesia prevents the patient from communicating his identity or revealing the events which precipitated his illness.

The principles described for psychotherapy in the treatment of anxiety neurosis are also relevant in hysterical psychoneurosis (p. 764). When hysterical personality disorder is also present, special aspects of management become necessary, as described on page 774.

## Obsessional Psychoneurosis

An *obsession* is a constantly recurring thought which the patient recognises as his own, but of which he tries to rid his mind because it is foolish or repugnant. In spite of his efforts to dismiss the thought, it persists in returning so that in the end he becomes tormented by it. A *compulsion* is a similarly insistent urge to perform, or to repeat, some act which the patient consciously repudiates as meaningless or troublesome; he struggles against the urge, but finds himself experiencing very acute anxiety, which is allayed only by giving in and performing the compulsive act.

Obsessive-compulsive symptoms may occur as episodes of illness in otherwise normal individuals. They may become aggravated during an episode of psychiatric illness. Sometimes obsessions and/or compulsions are the outstanding, if not the only, symptoms of which a patient complains. In this condition the patient, although perfectly lucid and in contact with the environment, may be severely handicapped by the unrelenting pressure of his unwelcome thoughts and impulses. The illness is also remarkable in that a person almost incapacitated by obsessional symptoms can appear normal to the external observer, until the appallingly repetitive thoughts are disclosed.

**Aetiology.** Obsessive-compulsive neurosis has an hereditary factor: one-third of the parents of obsessional patients and one-fifth of their siblings, have obsessional traits. Many observers believe that the meticulous, rigid routine imposed by such parents is more conducive to obsessional neurosis in the child than the hereditary endowment itself. Environmental factors, other than the influence of obsessive parents during the formative years, appear to contribute less to the causation of obsessional neurosis than is the case with the other syndromes of neurosis.

**Clinical Features.** Obsessions may be arbitrarily divided into ideas or images, impulses and ruminations. The *ideas* consist of thoughts, images (often obscene) and strings of words and phrases, which constantly recur to the patient despite resistance to them, and recognition that they are absurd and meaningless. The *impulses* are urges to some act such as killing offspring, or jumping under a train, or to less fearsome activities like laughing at sorrow or arranging objects in a certain set manner. Fears of some act may accompany impulses. A fear of knives develops from an impulse to use them for murderous ends. Likewise, a patient may not be troubled by obscene thoughts but rather by the fear that he may have such thoughts; he fills his mind with neutral thoughts lest obscenity should intrude. The idea representing an obsessive impulse keeps on invading the patient's consciousness. *Ruminations* comprise the practice of constantly turning over problems in the mind, seeking an answer to a question. Religious scruples are of this order, when the patient has repeatedly to examine and re-examine his conscience, uncertain as to whether he has offended or not.

These symptoms are often intermingled one with another, and may be of all degrees of intensity. Sometimes they are merely a nuisance, not interfering seriously with life, but preventing enjoyment and causing tension. In other cases they become so severe as to arrest all activity and make the ordinary daily round an impossible task. Thus a patient who was a house painter, stood for three hours, unable to paint a crack on the wall until he had the 'right' thoughts in his mind. Another patient, a housewife, spent all her time washing her hands for fear they should be contaminated, and so was unable to do her housework.

When the obsessions are severe they cause great anxiety and tension, the patients becoming increasingly agitated as they fight against the compulsion. In addition, they frequently become depressed, since life becomes so difficult and escape from the obsessions seems to be impossible. Suicide is, however, relatively uncommon except when depressive symptoms complicate the illness.

**Diagnosis** does not present great difficulty providing there is adherence to the exact criteria of the definition given above. There must be the feeling of compulsion and, most important, the patient must recognise it as senseless or absurd and resist it. Delusions are easily distinguished from obsessions: a patient does not feel the delusions are silly, but firmly believes in their truth. Similarly, such schizophrenic symptoms as feelings of compulsion or direction by some unknown force should not be confused with those of the obsessive-compulsive, who knows that the thoughts and impulses, however unwelcome, are his own thoughts and impulses. When the severity of such symptoms shows very marked fluctuation, a coexisting recurrent depressive illness should be suspected.

**Treatment.** The obsessional neurotic does not respond well to treatment, but often the condition is self-limiting, at least in its acute phases. The patient should be encouraged by being given the assurance that his doctor knows that his irrational, obscene or murderous thoughts are not indicative of his true nature, and that they are harmless. Behaviour therapy based on learning theory is sometimes helpful. He should be encouraged to avoid situations which foster the development of the obsessions and should diversify his interests as much as possible. The best antidote for obsessive ruminations is for the patient to keep at work, occupied with practical tasks which demand attention.

Severe obsessional symptoms may be helped by a tricyclic antidepressant drug. Clomipramine has been used, 75–450 mg daily in divided doses.

## Depressive Psychoneurosis

This type of depressive illness is at times also named '*reactive*'. Characteristically the morbidly depressed state comes on after a personal setback. This often takes the form of a loss of a person important to the patient, for example through death or separation as occurs with a divorce or a broken engagement. Careful exploration will show that the recent disappointment reflects one that occurred earlier in the patient's life. A typical example is the onset of depressive neurosis after a woman is left by her husband, and further interviewing discloses that she had lost a beloved father as a child. When the illness corresponds to an abnormal grief response after the death of a significant person, the term 'bereavement reaction' is sometimes used.

Only occasionally is psychiatric hospitalisation called for, the patient often responding well to out-patient psychotherapeutic interviews.

It may be confusing but it is nevertheless of the greatest importance to emphasise that admixtures of reactive and endogenous symptoms are extremely common. The clinical task is to scrutinise any case of depressive illness to determine the presence and amount of any component of 'endogenicity', i.e. so-called biological features including loss of energy, sleep disturbance, loss of appetite, constipation, impairment of libido, and — in severe cases — gross self-blame. In such mixed states antidepressant drugs are indicated, and good practice calls for a combined psychotherapeutic and pharmacological approach.

Admixtures of depressive symptoms with anxiety reaction occur frequently; some neurotically depressed patients are also hypochondriacal.

## Phobic Psychoneurosis

These widely prevalent illnesses consist of unjustified fear which is firmly related to a precise stimulus, either a place or an object. The patient may be appallingly terrified at being in a supermarket, a bus, an open space (*agoraphobia*), or a closed place (*claustrophobia*). Fear of flying can be a nuisance to a housewife and may deter the family from taking overseas holidays, a major handicap to a business executive, and an occupational disaster to a pilot or other member of air crew.

The phobic place or object can be so innocuous as to seem ridiculous, and dreading ridicule the patient may not be able to summon the courage to disclose the affliction to the doctor. Direct questioning may be needed to explore cues which are offered, such as a patient never coming unaccompanied to consult the doctor.

Phobias can at times be referred to parts of the body, hence the use at times of such terms as 'cardiac neurosis' and 'cancerophobia'.

Patients can be terrified that they may have an urge to urinate when a toilet may not be accessible; when afflicted with this syndrome, patients know exactly the locus of every public lavatory in their neighbourhood.

The subjective benefit to the patient of suffering from a phobic state (rather than, say, an anxiety reaction or an obsessional illness) is that life can be perfectly manageable as long as the phobic stimulus is avoided. A person with a dog phobia need only find a dogless route to work, if one exists.

Antianxiety medication can assist such patients greatly, in association with interviewing which encourages the patient to 'go against the phobia', to enter into as many social occasions as possible. A requisite of treatment is that the doctor should comprehend the terror experienced by the patient (often related to childhood traumatic experience) and avoid a belittling response even when the patient's fear is grotesquely unjustified. A form of treatment which has a high rate of success, *behaviour therapy*, is based on devising for the patient a hierarchy of experiences relating to the phobic object or situation, in which increasing exposure is gradually built up, always avoiding excessive anxiety. Someone with a dog phobia may look with the doctor or clinical psychologist at canine pictures, starting with a benign species and coming at length to an Alsatian; then real dogs can be introduced to the interview, first a docile, aged pet and perhaps later quite daunting beasts encountered on a walk can be approached with due circumspection.

## Personality Disorders

In every large community there are a number of people who do not conform to the prevailing norm. Statistically speaking, a person can be outside the range of normal either by being exceptionally gifted or by being so grossly underendowed as to be an eccentric or a social misfit; but it is the latter who are more likely to come to medical attention.

The personality disorders began to gain notice only late during the development of psychiatry as a medical discipline; they have been recognised increasingly as the out-patient responsibilities of psychiatrists have extended, and as psychiatric units have developed in general hospitals. The diagnostic differentiation between psychiatric illness and personality disorder is the more necessary because very often the two coexist. Indeed, clinical convention has it that hysterical psychoneurosis commonly supervenes in individuals with hysterical personality, obsessional neurosis in those with obsessional personality disorders, etc. In addition to their presentation with psychotic illnesses and psychoneuroses, people with abnormal personalities often appear clinically with psychosomatic disorders and may be chronic hospital attenders. Abnormal personalities may not enter the medical ambit at all, but be encountered in penal settings. Still others may continue unrecognised in the community and only escape anonymity when widespread screening of the population occurs, as in wartime when obligatory intake to the armed forces exposes all adults to clinical scrutiny.

The association between the different types of psychiatric illness and the various forms of abnormal personality is now recognised as a more complicated problem than the earlier statements of the position suggested.

The central feature of abnormal personality is some degree of persistent abnormality of behaviour which is frequently, but not necessarily, antisocial in its manifestations. The abnormality varies considerably in degree, ranging in severity from schizoid and hysterical people who are often valuable if somewhat unstable members of the community, to psychopaths who are socially destructive.

### Obsessional Personality Disorder

The obsessional person gives scant regard to the emotional aspects of a situation or an interaction. He is rigid rather than flexible, overattentive to details rather than to the wider scope of an event or encounter, and prefers to have everything predictable and orderly. He often appears officious, sometimes so pedantically that he can be comical, and not only controls himself excessively but also attempts to dominate others. He appears to behave in an excessively egotistical manner, and responds in an overriding way when involved in a venture calling for co-operation. He is overcareful, methodical, liking things cut-and-dried, concerned with neatness and orderliness. He can be very meticulous, punctual and overorganised, to the extent of becoming uncomfortable and even upset if his routines are disturbed by an unexpected development. He has a set of fixed standards and points of view, from which he can deviate only with great difficulty. He is uninfluenced, therefore, by the wishes, needs, opinions or views of other people.

The meticulousness and preservation of sameness extends to the person's mode of dress, which can be scrupulously neat. He can be overconscientious, paying greatly excessive attention to minutiae. He may work compulsively, and be unable to make use of opportunities for relaxation. Such a person, in consequence, can be of particular usefulness in a bureaucratic post calling for scrupulous concern with details. He may be highly obstinate when faced by any requirement that he should deviate from his straight and narrow path.

At times such a person appears to leave some loophole, so that the conformity, inhibition and rigidity is waived in some context or other. The precise, neat youngster, who must have everything in place, may for example permit himself to have his clothes cupboard in disorder, or may periodically forget thrift to overspend in a foolish self-indulgence which rationally is at odds with his habitual miserliness.

The gross form of the disorder is easy to recognise. The milder forms may be less obtrusive, and may be particularly evident only at times of pressure, as when an examination is looming for a youngster or when a house-proud woman has relatives coming to stay in her home.

## Schizoid Personality Disorder

The schizoid person is essentially solitary. He is aloof in his loneliness, detached and distant from other people. He has few close relationships, and may be much more preoccupied with some impersonal activity in the realms of electronics, physics, mathematics or engineering. Often the engrossing venture is a personal fad or invention, which may be of negligible application in ordinary life, but may be pursued with a single-minded devotion inappropriate to a mere hobby or interest.

Cold, quiet and shy, the person's abnormality may already have been apparent early in childhood, from an inability or disinclination to mix, and a preference for solitary pursuits. The lack of friendships may have been upsetting to the parents; as the person grows up, he can himself be distressed by his incapacity for any intimacy in his association with others.

The person may appear odd, eccentric, gawky, and in his awkward isolation may appear as a figure of fun. He may seem excessively secretive. Schizoid people are often solitary workers, who cannot function satisfactorily in a team. Bookish, reserved, out of touch with others, relatively blind to social cues, their personal lives may appear barren. However, this remote exterior may belie the strong emotions which some schizoid people cannot express. Others find a vehicle for their private feelings, and may keep a diary, or indulge in day-dreaming, or succeed in establishing some relationship in which the expression of emotion is allowed.

The schizoid person is at times mistrustful, seeing slights where none is intended. He is rigid and brittle. He has little empathy with other people, and so remains unaware of their intentions, feelings and wishes. When he attempts to appraise others intuitively, he is often wildly wrong, thereby complicating his already attenuated relationships. He can be made profoundly uncomfortable when well-meaning but misguided mentors or doctors attempt to have him mix more, or urge him to become intimate with another person, perhaps another isolate as lacking in interpersonal skills as himself.

Suspicion can become the prevailing response to others, the person believing that he is being exploited, misused or disparaged. Some clinicians would differentiate this development separately, diagnosing such a personality as *paranoid*.

## Hysterical Personality Disorder

People of this type can be identified on the basis of a constellation of behaviours: they seek to please and influence others; they crave attention; they are insincere; and they are given to excessive displays of emotion. They were often victims of inadequate maternal care in childhood.

An hysterical person appears to be exploitative, with an eye always on the other person. She talks for effect, not to convey any honestly felt intention. One feels her need for appreciation, and her readiness to express herself with that aim in view. She over-reacts in order to evoke a response from others.

Psychiatrists probably over-diagnose this type in abnormal women, attaching the label very much less often to men. The person is showy, histrionic in manner and dress, with a quality of spuriousness and exaggeration, even theatricality, in what she does. The exhibitionism appears intended to impress others, even to shock them. Speech is superficial, with plentiful hyperbole ('heavenly', 'ghastly'), which only heightens the effect of shallowness. Women of this type suffer from sexual timidity and frigidity, the more distressing to them because their frequently seductive manner and provocative dress invites advances with which they cannot cope; hysterical men also have difficulty in establishing a close relation with one woman, and may seek intimacy in a series of attachments of short duration.

## Sociopathy

The sociopath suffers from the most severe form of abnormal personality. Because of his serious defect in the capacity for feeling, he is often described as 'affectionless'. Lacking in conscience he has great difficulty in realising that other people are harmed when he behaves antisocially. Loveless, indifferent and destructive, he cannot form satisfactory relationships, and major failures repeatedly occur in his marriage, his work and his social life. He comes into conflict with the norms, customs and laws of his community, not learning from his failures, however catastrophic; already present from an early age, his social ineptitude is persistent, leading him chronically to be in trouble. Many sociopaths are superficially likeable and charming, and initially mislead well-meaning people whom they subsequently disappoint and mortify.

Impulsiveness is usually evident, the sociopath dismaying those associated with him by uncontrolled, often destructive outbursts in the absence of sufficient provocation. Such precipitate and deplorable action has been spoken of as 'short circuit reactions', to indicate that often the person is aware of the buildup to the outburst and will often admit that after the aggressive or destructive episode he feels calmer and relieved of tension.

The sociopath does not show ability to modify destructive behaviour reactions, or to learn from even drastic setbacks; he may be punished repeatedly for the same unacceptable behaviour, and yet continue it; the individual's antisocial patterns are often monotonously repetitive. Kleptomania, gambling or physical assaults may each be associated with excitement which the sociopath seeks and indulges repeatedly; the antisocial behaviour can be seriously destructive to others, as in cases of sadistic attacks on children or of fire-setting.

The lack of regard for the possible consequences of his actions is also impressive, the sociopath appearing not to care about the outcome, and scant in his consideration even of persons on whom his welfare depends. He disregards his obligations to others. The lack of concern amounts often to callousness. The Mental Health Acts in Britain allow for the compulsory hospitalisation of the 'seriously irresponsible' sociopath, and so does the legislation of many other countries.

His social relationships are shallow and transient. He is not loyal to individuals or to groups. He has poor judgement of situations, and often lies his way out of complications. He is indifferent to the welfare of others. He requires immediate satisfactions, not being able to postpone gratifications; he seeks instant excitement or relief of discomfort, and may misuse drugs or alcohol so that secondary addictions are common. Swindling and deception are frequent features.

Two types of sociopathy are distinguished:

*Aggressive Sociopath.* The hostility displayed in attacks on other people, damage to property, thefts and fraud may bring the sociopath to legal attention.

*Passive Sociopath.* A person of this type is seriously inadequate and cannot adapt to social requirements; he is chronically inept, passive and dependent. Many are placid and responsive; others are cold, withdrawn and apathetic. They may exist as aimless drifters, to be found in places where hobos congregate. Even if supported in a family or protective environment such as a half-way house or hostel, such people may be further incapacitated by the complications of drug addiction or alcoholism.

## Management Implications

The chief medical relevance of personality disorder, in terms of the doctor-patient relationship, is that patients respond to the clinician in accordance with their particular personality deviation. For this reason, diagnosis of the personality type permits the doctor to plan management realistically, so that he does not expect a degree of co-operativeness which the patient is not equipped to provide. In addition, he will be better able to predict the patient's pattern of behaviour in the future.

For example, the long-term managment of a patient with an hysterical personality disorder has much in common with that of a frightened or petulant child. It consists in convincing her that you are on her side, even while refusing to comply with some of her requests. Treating a patient with such a personality disorder is often a test of nerve; in the face of dramatic protestations and apparently alarming social crises, one must quietly but firmly insist upon facing the painful realities from which the hysteric has taken flight. If one has succeeded in gaining her confidence, helplessness and distress will sometimes disappear with dramatic suddenness, but all too often they are replaced by subsequent turmoil. The hysterical patient finds it difficult to abandon the defences against alarming feelings which she has been using since her early adolescence. In addition these patients are especially prone to develop an emotional dependence upon their doctor, which must be recognised and brought to their attention kindly but firmly. The family doctor can give helpful advice to other people in the patient's immediate environment, warning them that hysterical acting-out behaviour only becomes aggravated if too much attention is paid, and encouraging them to avoid entering into the patients' pattern of self deception. It is usually much easier for the onlookers than for the patient herself to see the real motivation of her symptoms, but of course, it is no use simply telling her — she has to discover for herself why she behaves in the way she does.

The achievement of a long-term cure of an hysterical personality disorder is a formidable task since it requires the patient to mature emotionally. Not surprisingly, both patients and their doctors often tacitly agree not to attempt it. Instead, the doctor may concentrate upon dealing with the most pressing difficulties of the patient's immediate predicament and may settle for her remaining a somewhat demanding and dependent patient. In that case, the goal for each consultation can be to ensure that the patient departs calmer and with more self-esteem than when she arrived. The doctor helps the patient discover some modifiable aspect in a problem which she had considered insoluble.

## Alcoholism and Drug Dependence

Addiction to alcohol or drugs represents a form of psychological dependence and indicates that the patient has been unable to attain adequate satisfaction or self-esteem in his personal life. Addictions to drugs and to alcohol are associated with a high risk of suicide. The underlying lack of self-confidence is often so deep-seated that prolonged treatment and rehabilitation is necessary once the drug or alcohol has been given up.

**Alcohol.** Alcoholics are often brought reluctantly to their doctor by close relatives who can see more clearly than the patient how seriously his life is being interfered with by his addiction. These unwilling patients are particularly difficult to treat; but the prospect is very different when the patient himself is distressed by his dependence and is anxious for change.

Alcoholism is a serious health problem in Britain, and more especially in Scotland. Mental disorders due to alcoholism are responsible for a quarter of male admissions to Scottish mental hospitals. It is an insidious condition, because the enjoyment of alcohol is socially accepted and even encouraged. The process by which an occasional drinker becomes an excessive drinker, and finally dependent on drink can be gradual; acquaintances, and even friends are reluctant to draw attention to a man's excessive drinking because the alcoholic is liable to fear being shunned and is liable to take offence. Here, however, doctors have a clear responsibility because often an intercurrent illness, chronic dyspepsia or haematemesis, or even a street accident will bring the patient to medical care, and a carefully taken history (especially if supplemented by information from others in the patient's family) will reveal the increasing dependence upon alcohol. Sometimes an unexpected hospital admission, interrupting a sustained high intake of spirits, results in the onset of *delirium tremens* which compels attention to the seriousness of the drinking problem. This acute confusional psychosis is characterised by gross peripheral tremors, great restlessness, confusion, misidentification of peopie and places and delusional ideas. These delusions may be agreeable but much more often they are threatening or even terrifying, especially when accompanied by hallucinatory visions. Because of these complications, hospital admission may be necessary when starting to treat an alcoholic.

The syndrome of alcoholism is characterised by: (1) a need for alcohol as for a drug, customary activities being difficult to perform without it; (2) taking of alcohol apart from social occasions; (3) tolerance, the person being able to drink increasing amounts without becoming incapacitated; (4) the abstinence response, i.e. unpleasant symptoms occurring as the blood alcohol level falls, e.g. tremor, sweating, wakefulness and tension; (5) loss of tolerance; becoming incapacitated before imbibing the amount of alcohol his system needs; (6) restitution, i.e. the rapid development of the entire syndrome after drinking is resumed following a period of abstinence.

*Treatment of Alcohol Addiction.* This consists initially of 'drying out', which often calls for hospital admission. Withdrawal symptoms can be controlled by phenothiazines, diazepam, haloperidol or chlormethiazole. The last is an hypnotic related to thiamin. It is probably the drug of choice in severe alcohol withdrawal syndromes including delirium tremens. In these circumstances it should not be used for longer than 1 week because of the danger of dependency. Vitamins B and C intravenously may also be of value.

The next phase of treatment, once the patient is abstinent, is to explore, by means of a series of interviews, the personal and other problems which require attention. Psychiatric assistance is needed if obvious psychological disorder is apparent once the drinking has stopped. Those abstinent alcoholics who consider themselves in danger of relapse can ensure their sobriety by taking disulfiram (0·5 g/d) or citrated calcium carbimide: when on these drugs, the patient will have an unpleasant reaction after taking only a small amount of alcohol.

The main requirement of treatment is that the alcoholic should become totally abstinent. Many alcoholics are active and valuable members of society and can maintain this necessary abstinence if given appropriate medical supervision.

**Morphine.** Dependence is seen in doctors, nurses, pharmacists and dentists, and at times in patients who become addicted through therapeutic use. The desired euphoric effect can be achieved by subcutaneous injection, but as tolerance grows intravenous injections are used. Hypodermic tattooing of the skin, thrombosed veins and pinpoint pupils are indications of the condition. Treatment, such as substitution with methadone, is best done at a centre with the necessary facilities.

**Heroin.** Dependence is increasing rapidly in incidence, and many addicts are young people. The drug has a marked euphoriant effect; it acts quickly and its desired action also dissipates quickly. The abstinence syndrome is particularly unpleasant. Many addicts cannot be cured, and their management then is by supplies of the smallest dose of the drug preventing the withdrawal symptoms, or by substitution of methadone in place of heroin.

**Cocaine.** Those addicted to cocaine take the drug in the form of snuff or intravenously. The most well-known toxic symptom is formication, the sensation of insects crawling under the skin. Use occurs mainly in those addicted also to heroin, the effect of cocaine alone being unsatisfactorily brief. Physical effects are anorexia, emaciation, nausea, insomnia and convulsions. By the Drug Addiction Act of 1968 issue of heroin and cocaine is limited in Britain to named doctors, usually psychiatrists in designated treatment centres.

**Lysergic Acid Diethylamide (LSD)** is used mainly by young people. Taken by mouth, it has dramatic effects lasting about 6 hours. Illusions occur, colour is intensified, mood changes include euphoria, awe or anxiety, a curious blurring between the individual and the environment is experienced, and phantasy thoughts, flight of ideas and delusions serve to heighten the mystical nature of the 'trip'. Physical dependence does not occur, but some users become psychologically dependent. Proponents of the drug as a 'mind expander' sometimes overlook the serious hazards; these include psychotic reactions with paranoid delusions which can last many weeks, and non-psychotic reactions chiefly terror; both can result in self-injury or suicide. A bad LSD experience can be cut short by chlorpromazine, used intramuscularly in severe cases.

**Cannabis** (hashish, marihuana, 'pot') is also used very commonly by the young, sometimes only a few times; there is no evidence that occasional use is harmful. At first the user feels 'high', and then drifts into a peaceful, drowsy state heightened by unusual mental images. Skin flushing, rapid pulse and dilated pupils may convey that a person has taken cannabis, usually by smoking a 'joint'. Many addicts use more than one drug. That physical dependence can occur is doubted, but marked psychological dependence is common.

**Barbiturate.** Many middle-aged or elderly women come to rely upon a nightly dose of sleeping tablets and some of them find that if they take two or three during the day, this helps to calm their nerves. Gradually, they begin to show the signs of chronic barbiturate over-dosage: slight ataxia, absent-mindedness amounting at times to confusion as to time and place, defective judgment, loss of emotional control, slurred speech and tremor of the fingers. A sudden cessation of barbiturates can be followed by a major epileptic fit. The withdrawal syndrome can be alarming, with headaches, insomnia and vomiting, and a delirious state with delusions. Small doses of barbiturates may need to be administered. A patient cured of one addiction, e.g. alcoholism, may start using another drug, e.g. barbiturate, which is erroneously regarded as innocuous.

**Amphetamine** formerly used in the treatment of obesity and still used for narcolepsy, soon came to be abused, particularly by teenagers, either alone or combined with barbiturate to provide a rapid lifting of the spirits and feeling of well-being. The use of amphetamine readily gives rise to a psychological dependency, when the daily dose taken can increase vastly, tolerance developing with continued use. The amphetamine addict has an impression of increased mental and physical drive and competence. There are also restlessness, irritability and excitability. Amphetamine can give rise also to an acute psychotic reaction with auditory and visual hallucinations and delusions of persecution. These features can be clinically indistinguishable from those of paranoid schizophrenia, but they clear up in about 3 weeks time after withdrawal of the drug. Since the Misuse of Drugs Act (1971) amphetamines are listed as controlled drugs in Britain, special regulations applying to prescribing. The drug is justified medically only in occasional cases of narcolepsy.

## Sexual Deviation

Sexual deviants are people who are unable to obtain physical and emotional satisfaction in normal sexual intercourse, but can do so only in ways which to a greater or lesser degree are socially condemned. Practices which alarm, threaten or injure other persons, such as exhibitionism, paedophilia (having sex with immature partners of either sex) or sadism (deriving sexual pleasure from inflicting pain) are still regarded as antisocial and are punishable by law. On the other hand, public opinon has become somewhat more tolerant of abnormal practices which do not interfere with other people. The change of opinion found expression in the Sexual Offences Act, 1967, which, for the first time in English history, excluded homosexual acts, carried out in private by consenting adults, from any legal sanction.

Most forms of deviant sexual behaviour, such as homosexuality, transvestism (deriving gratification from wearing the clothing of the opposite sex) and fetishism (when the person becomes sexually stimulated by parts of the body not usually experienced as erotogenic — e.g. the feet — or by articles of clothing or other objects) seem to be the result of distorted experiences at the stage of development when boys and girls learn their sexual role. These deviant forms of gratification often prove very resistant to change. If the patient suffers because of them — and many sexual deviants appear to be rather content with their lot — treatment often has to be limited to damping down the intensity of the sexual drive, e.g. by the administration of oestrogens to males or to helping the patient (and perhaps also the spouse) to accept the peculiarity.

## Psychosomatic Disorders

These are the physical illnesses which are caused in part by psychological factors or, when present, are maintained by psychological factors. Examples of such conditions are many cases of peptic ulcer, bronchial asthma, colitis and various forms of dermatitis. The implication of this term is that tension arising from a long-standing emotional conflict can induce changes in bodily function (e.g. excessive secretion of gastric juice; bronchospasm) which, when repeated over a period of time, can in turn lead to actual tissue damage.

For many years, attempts have been made to delineate particular personality types associated with different forms of psychosomatic illness. A review of this literature, however, fails to reveal a specific type of personality in relation to each of these disorders. Instead, psychosomatic subjects tend to be characterised by relatively constant emotional elements, the chief of which are dependency, anger, fear, which appear to be the most harmful when they are denied conscious expression. Repressed dependency needs have been particularly associated with peptic ulcer and ulcerative colitis, repressed anger with asthma and hypertension. Individual cases, however, when studied in depth, are not easily fitted into any common mould. Modern psychosomatic theory has, therefore, retreated to the more general observation that all psychosomatic patients have long-standing problems in the control of their own internal emotional homeostasis, and in the conduct of their relationships with people who matter in their private lives. It is probable that genetic factors, which have endowed some of us with a particularly vulnerable organ or organ system, will dictate both the occurrence of a psychosomatic illness (which often indeed coexists with neurotic symptoms) and the choice of the organ which is affected.

Treatment of the emotional disturbance and disregard of the local physical factors, or vice versa, will seldom lead to benefit for the patient, and an assessment must be made in each case of the relative importance of these two factors, so that whichever appears to have the greater aetiological significance can be the main target for therapy. The general practitioner is often in the best position to know the unrealised ambitions, the frustrations at work or at home, or the marital unhappiness which may form the background to the patient's illness. A knowledge of the family history may also reveal that hereditary predisposition plays a part in determining the physical form of the illness, as for example in migraine.

## Psychiatric Disorders in Relation to Age

The individual is confronted with new problems in adaptation at all the phases of major personality change, namely puberty, adolescence, pregnancy or following childbirth, at the menopause and on retirement. Mental disorders occur particularly at these times.

**Childhood.** Psychiatric disorder in children is now a major subspecialty of psychiatry. In childhood very significant phases in the development of personality are taking place; the child is at the mercy of the environment, utterly dependent on the adequacy of the parents and the provisions they make. In addition to behaviour disorders including untoward fear, aggressiveness, jealousy, stealing, school phobia and truancy, children require treatment for such distressing syndromes as enuresis, soiling (involuntary defecation), psychoneurotic illnesses, psychotic disorders including autism, and the handicaps such as stammering, dyslexia, extreme hyperactivity and organic brain damage.

The doctor responsible for the health of the child needs to collaborate closely with the child psychiatrist, with institutions which may be involved including the school, and with professional colleagues who contribute in any treatment, especially the clinical psychologist and the social worker. The parents must always be implicated clinically. The outcome of a programme of management often depends crucially on the comprehensiveness and adequacy of the co-operation between those involved.

**Adolescence.** Psychoses are rare until adolescence, when they increase in frequency; psychotic illnesses thereafter are increasingly common with advance of age. At adolescence, the period between puberty and young adulthood, the young person has to cope with more complex social involvement, sexual commitment and occupational challenge, while also separating from parents and detaching from their domestic arrangements. The personality changes of normal adolescence may be upsetting to some parents, teachers or other adults; a period of turmoil when the adolescent is aggressive, defiant or rebellious may precede the achievement of a stable adult personality. A previously polite child may become rude and sarcastic in the course of developing assertiveness and independence. Often the youngster surmounts troublesome behaviour if the family, school and community are understanding, encouraging and tolerant. But certain disturbances of adolescence require clinical attention. These include delinquent behaviour, deviant sexual practices with consequences which are harmful socially or damaging to the young person, inadequate school attainment, mood disturbance such as depression sometimes with attempts at suicide, withdrawal, social isolation and apathy, and, of course, bizarre behaviour with psychotic features such as delusions or hallucinations which may signal the onset of schizophrenic illness.

Adolescents can develop any of a range of psychiatric disorders, such as the adjustment reaction of adolescence, psychoneuroses, the functional psychoses, personality disorders, acute organic psychoses, drug and alcohol misuse and psychosomatic disorders.

**Adulthood.** Mental disorder may be associated with pregnancy or the puerperium. Puerperal psychoses may be schizophrenic in type or, more rarely, manic-depressive. Psychoneurotic illnesses also occur in the postpartum period.

The majority of patients receiving pyschiatric treatment are middle-aged. However, when the numbers of first hospital admissions are calculated in relation to the proportion of the general population in each group, the psychiatric admission rate to hospital rises steadily with increasing age, particularly after the sixth decade. In middle age, depressive psychosis is sometimes accompanied by intense anxiety, resulting in the syndrome of *agitated depressive psychosis*. The patient is characteristically restless, overwrought, hopeless, with extreme self-blame and low self-regard, and expressing nihilistic, guilty or hypochondriacal delusions. The previous personality in such patients was often characterised by over-conscientiousness or obsessionality.

Retirement from work can be a source of anxiety, especially for people who derived particular satisfaction, status, or esteem from working with others. Depressive illnesses with a sense of worthlessness or apathy can be a real burden for some at this stage of life. Women are often at risk in earlier middle life when their children leave home and make their separate existences, especially when mothering formed a predominant role in the woman's pattern of adjustment, unaccompanied by additional interests and commitments.

**The Elderly.** The care of the elderly plays an increasingly large part in contemporary society. Dementia has been discussed on page 756 but of great clinical importance is the fact that many elderly people with dementia can also become depressed. It is a most serious omission to fail to recognise this common illness in the elderly, who may be incapacitated by such superadded psychiatric disability, but become able to cope again when relieved of the morbid gloom and apathy by antidepressant therapy.

What is also not widely appreciated is the fact that episodes of neurotic illness, with anxiety states, phobias, hysterical symptoms or compulsions are also encountered in this age group, and are no less amenable to simple psychotherapy than at other ages. In the after-care of these older patients it is important to remember that social isolation is an important threat to their mental well-being. This becomes even more important when physical disability or deafness further restricts their opportunities of making contact with other people. Here voluntary agencies as well as local authority welfare and preventive services can do useful prophylactic work, but the family doctor is often in the best position to recognise when an ageing (and perhaps recently bereaved) patient is in special need of help.

Elderly patients easily develop delirium, and then adapt poorly to sudden changes of scene and bewildering happenings. It is helpful for them if they can be visited by only a few nurses and doctors who take pains to identify themselves; their sick-room should be well lit and they should be encouraged to keep a few treasured possessions on their bed-side table. Since patients with even very slight clouding of consciousness are prone to misunderstand what is happening round about them, any changes of routine or new procedures should be explained to them in advance, in simple terms and if necessary more than once.

## Conclusion

Psychiatric disorder can present diverse problems throughout an individual's life and also clinical challenges not only to psychiatrists but to all who practise medicine.

H. J. Walton

*Further reading:*

Forrest, A. D., Affleck, J. W. and Zealley, A. K. (eds) (1978) *Companion to Psychiatric Studies*, 2nd edn. Edinburgh: Churchill Livingstone. — A postgraduate textbook written by Edinburgh teachers.

Silverstone, T. & Turner, P. (1978) *Drug Treatment in Psychiatry*, 2nd edn. London: Routledge and Kegan Paul.

Slater, E. & Roth, M. (1970) *Clinical Psychiatry*, 3rd edn. London: Baillière, Tindall and Cassell. — An authoritative and comprehensive reference book.

Trethowen, W. H. (1979) *Psychiatry*, 4th edn. London: Baillière, Tindall. — A useful text for undergraduate students.

Walton, H. J. (1979) In *Clinical Examination*, ed. Macleod, J. 5th edn. Edinburgh: Churchill Livingstone.— For a detailed description of the psychiatric examination.

# 16. Acute Poisoning

Self-poisoning is a very common and urgent medical problem. The number of patients admitted to hospital because of it has increased steadily in Britain over the last 30 years, so much so that this type of behaviour has become endemic in our society. In England and Wales, there were 33 600 hospital admissions due to acute poisoning in 1962, whereas in recent years the figure has been well in excess of 100 000, representing 10 to 30% of all admissions to acute medical units in Britain with a general average of 15%. These hospital statistics are formidable, but the true incidence is probably much higher. Many symptomless children and up to 40% of adults who reach Accident and Emergency Departments may be sent home because the physical effects are mild. Many patients, estimated to be about 30%, are not even referred to hospital but are treated at home by their general practitioners. In Britain, therefore, it is more likely that the true incidence of poisonings is over 300 000 per annum.

The mortality due to acute poisoning in Britain has fallen in recent years but according to official statistics approximately 3500 deaths occur due to poisoning each year. It has been estimated, however, that about 80% of all deaths from acute poisoning occur outside hospital and so it is important that hospital statistics should not be considered alone as an index of the physical consequences of poisoning in the community. The fall in mortality has occurred, despite the increase in incidence, for two main reasons. Carbon monoxide poisoning has become rare since the relatively non-toxic natural gas replaced coal gas in domestic supplies, and prescriptions for barbiturates have been much reduced with the substitution of safer hypnotics such as benzodiazepines. Improved methods of treatment have also played their part, and in any good district hospital the mortality resulting from acute poisoning should be less than 1%. The major causes of death are now dextropropoxyphene, barbiturates, tricyclic antidepressants, salicylate and paracetamol. Perhaps as a result, there are two peaks in mortality; the first occurs in the 15 to 25 age group mainly from analgesics, and the second in patients over 65 due to barbiturates with, in addition, coexisting physical disease. At all ages the number of females who die tends to be greater than males, but this is probably a reflection of the fact that acute poisoning is commoner in women than in men. Among the 25 to 30 year olds, suicides constitute one in 10 of all deaths, and in doctors, death from acute poisoning is as common as death from carcinoma of the lung.

The problem of acute poisoning is not restricted to Britain but is experienced in all the developed and many developing countries of the world. In the United States of America five million poisonings occur every year and the number is increasing. Acute poisoning is the fourth most common cause of accidental death in that country and the reported mortality is over 5000 per annum. Poisoning is the most common medical emergency in paediatric hospitals. At all ages it accounts for 10% of all emergency home visits and 5 to 10% of adult medical admissions. In most European countries a similar problem exists, but direct comparison, especially in terms of mortality statistics, is difficult due to the wide variations in which deaths from poisoning are recorded and coded. Morbidity statistics are subject to even greater discrepancy and much more standardised information is required before the true international situation can be assessed.

This chapter deals with the clinical features, diagnosis and management of acute poisoning. Food poisoning is discussed on pages 57–59. Brief reference is made to industrial and agricultural poisons and to the effects of exposure to ionising radiation.

## Classification and Causes of Acute Poisoning

Acute poisoning can be accidental or intentional.

**Accidental Poisoning.** Death from accidental poisoning has increased almost three-fold in the past 30 years, women being more likely than men to die in this way. In Britain the mortality from this cause is approximately 15 per million population; in other European countries there is considerable variation. In Scandinavia, for example, the rate is about 20 per million. Except in children, it is doubtful if the official statistics reflect the true incidence of accidental poisoning. For example, it is difficult to believe the official figures that more adults die each year from accidental barbiturate poisoning than from suicidal poisoning by these drugs. Certification is often purposely made inaccurate to save family feelings.

SUBSTANCES INVOLVED IN ACCIDENTAL POISONING. Children are most frequently involved due to the careless storage of medicines and household products. Common causes include ingestion of medicine (e.g. aspirin, tricyclics, antihistamines or iron), a wide range of household substances (e.g. paraffin, detergents or bleach) weed killers (e.g. paraquat) and, rarely, poisonous berries. Inhalation of organic solvents (e.g. glues and cleaning fluids) and occasionally carbon monoxide from incomplete combustion due to faulty gas appliances or motor car exhaust pipes, also occurs.

**Intentional Poisoning.** This is due to a wide variety of causes ranging from a minority of patients who are determined on self-destruction, i.e. *suicidal poisoning*, to a large group who indulge in *self-poisoning* which some prefer to call *parasuicide*. The term *attempted suicide* is best discarded as it implies a motive to an act of self-administered poisoning, which is frequently incorrect. The majority of people who deliberately take poison do not wish to die; in fact, they often take positive precautions to ensure that help will be available. Self-poisoning is usually a conscious, often impulsive act undertaken to manipulate a situation or a person and secure redress of circumstances which have become intolerable. Frequently relatives and society rally to help and the situation which has caused so much distress is rectified. Mistakes, however, do occur through misjudgement of dosage or a lack of available help, and an act which was committed primarily to draw attention to a particular situation may end in death. Self-poisoning often occurs in a setting of poverty or alcoholism and with a background of a broken home in childhood. The alarming increase in the incidence of acute poisoning is largely due to self-poisoning which accounts for approximately 90% of all adult poisoned patients admitted to hospital. Such behaviour now constitutes a major social problem. This is the case particularly in areas of dense conurbation and is less marked in small towns and rural communities.

Homicidal poisoning, which is another form of intentional poisoning, is rarely encountered now in hospital practice.

SUBSTANCES AND METHODS USED IN INTENTIONAL POISONING. *Self-poisoning*. Perhaps the most important cause for the increase in self-poisoning is the ready availability of drugs in the community. There is no doubt that the dramatic increase in the frequency and size of individual prescriptions over the last 30 years in Britain, in the National Health Service, has tended to encourage the mistaken belief in the community that the taking of pills is the answer for all life's ailments. Almost any substance may be used for self-poisoning, but evidence of the importance of availability is the changing pattern of drugs taken in overdosage over the years. Ten years ago 60% of admissions were due to barbiturates and other hypnotics, notably methaqualone. As a result of campaigns and voluntary restrictions by doctors in prescribing, the incidence of these drugs in acute overdosage is now only 10%. In contrast, psychotropic drugs, especially sedatives and antidepressants, which are now commonly prescribed, are frequent causes of poisoning. Benzodiazepines account for 40% of poisonings and tricyclic antidepressants 13%. Salicylates and paracetamol each amount to 10%. A particularly alarming feature in recent years has been the progressive increase in incidence of acute overdosage with paracetamol in combination with dextropropoxyphene hydrochloride. This increase has paralleled a dramatic rise in prescribing of this analgesic and it is now the commonest cause of death due to poisoning in Britain.

Combinations of drugs are taken in about 40% of overdoses and alcohol is involved in 50% of poisonings in men and about 30% in women. These combinations may cause problems in assessment of the severity of poisoning and in treatment; chemical analysis also may be difficult.

*Suicide*. The methods adopted for deliberate self-destruction vary from country to country and between sexes. In Britain women most often use drugs with drowning second choice. Self-injury, such as hanging, is most common in men with drug overdosage second. In America, shooting is the first choice in males, but takes second place to drugs in women. For reasons stated, coal gas poisoning, which was previously common, now seldom occurs.

## Diagnosis of Acute Poisoning

**Information Service.** The impact made by poisoning on medical services has led to increasing demands for information regarding the toxicity of substances and drugs. In the last 25 years, therefore, there has been a proliferation of poisons information and poison control centres in many countries. Information can be obtained immediately on a 24-hour basis regarding the ingredients of a substance and the approximately fatal dose of a poison. In many of these centres the best method of treatment can be discussed with a physician trained in clinical toxicology. In order to provide as comprehensive, accurate and up-to-date information as possible with ready accessibility, much of the data has been computerised, especially in America where, in addition to regional centres, extremely comprehensive information may be obtained at national level.

**Clinical Features.** For the majority of poisons they are non-specific. Fortunately, the diagnosis is usually apparent from the history obtained from the patient, relatives or friends or on circumstantial grounds such as finding tablets beside the patient. Difficulty arises when there is no such information and the physician is faced with the diagnosis of the unconscious patient. It is helpful to remember that in the age group 15–40 acute poisoning is the commonest cause of unconsciousness in the absence of head injury. Pin-point pupils, vomiting and depressed respiration suggest overdosage of morphine and related alkaloids. In young people in particular, a history of marked and sometimes rapid changes in level of consciousness with associated respiratory and perhaps cardiac arrest is often associated with dextropropoxyphene poisoning, especially if taken with alcohol. Widely dilated pupils, bladder distension, absent bowel sounds, cardiac arrhythmias and pyramidal tract involvement characterise tricyclic antidepressant toxicity. Sweating, tinnitus, deafness and hyperventilation strongly suggest acute salicylate poisoning.

**Identification of Poisons.** More secure identification has now become possible by the marking of an increasing number of tablets and capsules with a code letter and number. Others can be recognised by their characteristic colour or shape. Coloured diagrams are available to aid this.

*Laboratory analysis.* The only conclusive identification of acute poisoning is laboratory analysis using specimens of blood, gastric aspirate or urine as appropriate. Simple, rapid screening methods using thin layer chromatography are available for approximately 90% of common poisonings and can be of considerable help to the clinician. Confirmatory and more precise quantitative measurement is usually done by gas chromatography which is sometimes combined with mass spectrometry. Simple clinical methods of analysis are available for salicylates and paracetamol. Although these analyses can be carried out, the results seldom influence treatment but may be of value for medico-legal purposes.

## General Therapeutic Measures

Treatment should not be delayed by spending excessive time in attempting to identify precisely the poison involved, since the essential immediate management of poisoning is dependent on the application of well-established basic therapeutic principles.

**Maintenance of respiration.** A clear airway is essential. This can be ensured by removal of dentures, vomitus, foreign bodies and excess mucus: the patient should be turned onto one side to prevent the tongue falling backwards and to avoid aspiration of vomitus and mucus. An oropharyngeal or cuffed endotracheal tube may have to be inserted to maintain a free airway. Artificial ventilation is required if respiration is depressed, using preferably the method of expired air resuscitation. Oxygen should be given through an oronasal mask. Prophylactic antibiotics to 'protect' the lungs are not recommended, but any infection which develops should be treated.

**Removal or Inactivation of the Poison.** It cannot be emphasised too strongly that it is very important that the poison must be eliminated as quickly as possible. The first-aid treatment is often the responsibility of the general practitioner in the patient's home while awaiting the arrival of an ambulance. Patients with gassing must be removed to fresh air as quickly as possible. When a liquid or solid poison is in contact with the patient's clothes these must be removed at once and any poison on the skin must be washed off to prevent absorption. When the poison has been swallowed conscious patients should be given activated charcoal prior to transfer to hospital. A decision as to whether emesis and gastric aspiration and lavage should also be undertaken will depend on three factors: (i) the substance ingested, (ii) the state of consciousness of the patient, and (iii) the length of time since the poison was ingested.

EMESIS; GASTRIC ASPIRATION AND LAVAGE (i) *Nature of substance ingested.* The only contraindication to inducing vomiting or passing a stomach tube is the knowledge that paraffin oil (kerosene) or other petroleum distillates have been swallowed, as the entry of even a small quantity of these substances into the lungs will lead to a severe pneumonia. Great care must be exercised in passing a stomach tube in corrosive poisoning, in alcoholics, in patients who have had gastric surgery and in the very young and elderly.

(ii) *Level of consciousness.* The second factor to be considered is the state of consciousness. Fully conscious patients should be made to vomit by giving syrup of ipecacuanha (15 ml followed by 200 ml of water) which is an effective emetic, especially in children. Its limitation is that there is an average delay in the onset of its action of about 18 minutes. When these measures are impracticable as in a hysterical patient, apomorphine hydrochloride (5 mg) may be given intramuscularly. It is a powerful emetic but unfortunately it can produce hypotension, shock and persistent vomiting. These effects can, however, be antagonised by administering naloxone 0·4 mg i.v., followed if necessary 3 minutes later by 0·8 mg i.v.

In a semiconscious patient emetics are to be avoided in view of the danger of aspiration pneumonia, but gastric aspiration and lavage can be employed provided the cough reflex is still present. In the deeply unconscious patient gastric lavage is particularly important, but, as the cough reflex may be absent, it is a highly dangerous procedure unless the lungs can be first protected by the insertion of a cuffed endotracheal tube.

(iii) *Time since ingestion.* If four hours have passed since ingestion very little or no recovery of the drug will be achieved by inducing vomiting or by gastric lavage. If it is known that the poison was taken less than four hours previously gastric aspiration and lavage must be done provided the factors already discussed have been considered. In salicylate poisoning, because of the almost inevitable pylorospasm which prevents the drug from leaving the stomach, it is not too late to undertake these procedures up to 24 hours after ingestion. In the case of tricyclic drugs a worthwhile recovery may be achieved up to 12 hours after ingestion.

*Technique of gastric aspiration and lavage.* With the foot of the bed raised about 0·5 m and the patient lying on the left side a wide-bore Jacques rubber stomach tube, English gauge 30, should be passed. A gag may be necessary to prevent biting on the tube. When the tube has been inserted, its position in the stomach is verified by aspiration of stomach contents or by blowing a little air through it and auscultating over the abdomen when a bubbling sound will be heard. Aspiration is best achieved by lowering the funnel to which the stomach tube is attached, to a level well below the patient's head. Aspiration is advisable prior to lavage as initial lavage will drive some of the stomach contents into the duodenum and promote absorption. When no further material can be aspirated, repeated careful lavage with tepid water should be undertaken, using the same apparatus and no more than 300 ml for each single washout. Lavage should be continued until the returning fluid is clear. Except in the specific instances given on page 787, little is achieved by employing lavage fluid other than water.

On occasions, after lavage, some further impairment of consciousness may occur; hence the value of leaving fluid in the stomach may be outweighed by the dangers of subsequent aspiration pneumonia if no cuffed endotracheal tube has been inserted. However, with this possibility in mind, the following may be left in the stomach after lavage: (i) 100 ml milk on account of its demulcent properties in corrosive poisoning; (ii) the chelating agent, desferrioxamine, in acute iron poisoning (p. 787).

It is frequently recommended that on completion of gastric lavage for salicylate poisoning a solution of sodium bicarbonate should be left in the stomach. This is not advisable. Although the bicarbonate counteracts irritation of the gastric mucosa and when absorbed may help to promote excretion of salicylate by rendering the urine alkaline, its presence in the stomach encourages further absorption of salicylate.

OTHER METHODS OF ELIMINATION OF THE POISON. If considerable absorption has occurred the patient may be gravely ill, hence measures to enhance elimination of the poison may be required. These can be carried out only in hospital because of the technical skill and special apparatus required; they include diuresis; forced diuresis (p. 789), peritoneal dialysis, haemodialysis, and exchange transfusion.

In recent years attempts have been made to develop safer ways of increasing removal of toxic substances from the body. The most promising of these is the use of haemoperfusion through ion-exchange resins or charcoal. An effective and safe technique is the use of charcoal coated with synthetic acrylic hydrogel. This offers a method of treatment which may be life-saving for some poisonings, such as medium- and short-acting barbiturates, for which previous techniques to increase elimination were unsuccessful. It is still not free from dangers and its use must be kept in perspective. Charcoal haemoperfusion, therefore, is indicated only in seriously ill patients in whom basic supportive therapy is inadequate.

ANTIDOTES. It is widely but erroneously believed that for each toxic substance there is a specific antidote. There are, in fact, no antidotes for the majority of substances producing poisoning. Certain pharmacological antagonists are, however, of value. Examples are naloxone (opiate poisoning), cobalt edetate (cyanide poisoning), desferrioxamine (iron poisoning) and n-acetylcysteine (paracetamol poisoning). Details of the use of these are given on pages 787 to 789.

**Treatment of Shock, Hypothermia and Convulsions.** *Shock*. The principles are described on page 167. The foot of the bed should be raised. Heat loss and sweating must be avoided. Oxygen should always be given.

*Hypothermia*. A rectal thermometer which records low temperatures is required for the accurate assessment of hypothermia. Since it reduces the oxygen demands of the tissues, hypothermia is not a deleterious feature unless the rectal temperature is below 35°C, when it may cause hypotension, sludging of the blood, confusion, coma and cardiac arrest.

The patient with hypothermia below 35°C should be rewarmed rapidly by external methods (e.g. a radiant heat cradle over the torso) and oxygen given. If there is hypotension or increased peripheral vascular resistance, warm fluids are administered intravenously. Metabolic acidosis is controlled by sodium bicarbonate (p. 141).

*Convulsions* should be controlled with diazepam (p. 679).

**Psychiatric Assessment.** As most instances of poisoning in adults are deliberate acts of self-poisoning it is very important that all patients, whether suffering from apparent accidental or intentional poisoning, should have a psychiatric assessment. Self-poisoning is often an important feature of various psychiatric disorders and of depression in particular. It is greatly to the benefit of the patient if the initial psychiatric interview takes place as soon as possible after the act before the patient and his relatives have time to discuss the event and thereafter present the same rationalised and often false picture. The incidence of repeated acts of self-poisoning has been shown clearly to be reduced by early psychiatric consultation.

## Notes on clinical features and treatment of poisoning by specific agents

The following descriptions are directed primarily towards adults. For children, appropriate adjustments in doses of drugs suggested in treatment regimens would require to be made.

**Amphetamine Group.** *Clinical features*. Alertness, excitement, tremor and insomnia are common. Confusion, aggressiveness, hallucinations and even homicidal tendencies may occur. Initial excitement may give way to lethargy and depression. Brisk reflexes, tachycardia and hypertension occur and nausea, vomiting, diarrhoea and abdominal colic, may be severe. In very heavy overdosage convulsions and deep unconsciousness are characteristic.

*Treatment*. 1. General measures. 2. Chlorpromazine 100 mg intramuscularly. 3. In severe poisoning, forced diuresis using intravenous ammonium chloride to make the urine acid.

**Barbiturates.** *Clinical features*. Absorption is unpredictable but drowsiness and coma develop rapidly. The duration of cerebral depression varies greatly with the type of barbiturate taken, the dose and the tolerance of the patient. In general a large dose of short- or medium-acting barbiturate causes more severe poisoning than long-acting phenobarbitone. Changes in the pupils and limb reflexes are very variable and are unreliable guides to the severity of the poisoning. Withdrawal features such as restlessness, insomnia, delirium and convulsions may occur. Ventilatory depression and hypotension may be severe. Hypothermia is common and if severe may be associated with renal failure. Bullous lesions occur in 6% of patients with acute barbiturate overdosage especially with short- or medium-acting drugs.

*Treatment*. 1. General measures with particular emphasis on respiratory and cardiovascular support. 2. When these measures fail, haemodialysis for phenobarbitone and barbitone, and charcoal haemoperfusion for short- and medium-acting barbiturates.

**Benzodiazepines.** *Clinical features*. Drowsiness, ataxia, dizziness, hypotension and ventilatory depression may all occur, but the toxic effects are usually surprisingly mild.

*Treatment*. General supportive treatment is adequate in almost all cases.

**Corrosives.** *Clinical features*. Stains and burns of the mouth and lips. Burns of fauces, abdominal pain and shock may result. Hepatic or renal damage occur.

*Treatment*. 1. General measures. 2. Gastric lavage with care. 3. Neutralise acid or alkali.

**Cyanides and Hydrocyanic Acid.** *Clinical features*. Odour of bitter almonds with shallow breathing; pink colour of skin and mucosae; widely dilated pupils and shock.

*Treatment*. This is very urgent. 1. General measures. 2. Cobalt edetate 300 mg in 20 ml intravenously over one minute. 3. If no recovery in the next minute, repeat 300 mg cobalt edetate. 4. If ingested, gastric lavage with 25% sodium thiosulphate. 5. Correct acidosis with intravenous sodium bicarbonate.

**Dinitro-ortho-cresol Weedkillers.** *Clinical features*. These may develop very rapidly. Yellow skin and burns of the lips and mouth. Anxiety, restlessness, fatigue, convulsions and coma. Tachypnoea, pulmonary oedema, hyperpyrexia and intense sweating are common. Acute renal and liver failure may result.

*Treatment*. 1. Wash exposed skin. 2. Sedation with chlorpromazine 100 mg intramuscularly. 3. General measures. 4. Tepid sponging to reduce temperature.

**Dextropropoxyphene.** See opium alkaloids.

**Domestic Bleach.** *Clinical features*. Local irritation if in contact with skin. If inhaled, cough and possible pulmonary oedema. If ingested, burning sensation of mouth and fauces. Nausea and vomiting.

*Treatment*. 1. Gastric lavage with 2·5% sodium thiosulphate or alternatively with milk. If severely ill sodium thiosulphate (1%) 250 ml intravenously.

**Iron Salts.** *Clinical features*. These are more severe in children but this poisoning is potentially dangerous at all ages. The poisoning occurs in three stages. The predominant initial features are epigastric pain, nausea and vomiting. Haematemesis is frequent and may cause shock. Respiration and pulse are rapid. These symptoms may settle after a few hours and there may then be a quiescent period lasting for up to several days, suggesting that all is well, but then frequent black and offensive stools may be passed, followed by acute encephalopathy and circulatory failure. Most deaths occur in this second stage, but even if the patient survives, acute liver and renal failure may develop later and both carry a high mortality.

*Treatment*. Speed is essential. 1. An intramuscular injection of 2 g desferrioxamine is given immediately. 2. Gastric lavage is performed with appropriate volumes of a solution of desferrioxamine (2 g) in 1 litre of warm water, following which 5 g of desferrioxamine in 100 ml of water or saline is left in the stomach. 3. This is followed by an intravenous infusion of desferrioxamine in saline, dextrose or blood. The amount should not exceed 15 mg/kg body weight/hour up to a maximum of 80 mg/kg in 24 hours. 4. Full supportive treatment for convulsions, shock, acidosis, blood loss and electrolyte disturbance is essential.

**Opium Alkaloids (Dextropropoxyphene).** *Clinical features*. Pinpoint pupils, pallor, nausea and vomiting, depressed respiration and coma are characteristic. These effects are potentiated by alcohol and when these are combined in acute overdosage sudden respiratory and cardiac arrest may occur even in previously healthy young people.

*Treatment*. 1. General measures. 2. If ingested gastric lavage with very dilute potassium permanganate – 1 in 10 000. 3. Naloxone 0·4 mg intravenously and 0·8 mg repeated intravenously three minutes later, if required. In heavy overdosage larger quantities may be necessary. The patient should be kept under close observation and naloxone repeated if required.

**Organophosphorus Compounds.** *Clinical features*. These insecticides are very toxic. Constricted pupils; cold perspiration; salivation, nausea, vomiting and diarrhoea; twitching, which may go on to convulsions; bradycardia; bronchospasm and pulmonary oedema.

*Treatment*. 1. Remove contaminated clothing and wash skin, but take care to wear protective gloves. 2. General measures. 3. Atropine 2 mg intravenously, but if cyanosis is present this must first be corrected by oxygen therapy. The atropine is repeated at 5 to 10 minute intervals to achieve full atropinisation and this is maintained for at least 2–3 days. 4. Pralidoxime should be given in addition to atropine in a dose of 30 mg/kg intravenously at a rate not exceeding 500 mg per minute and repeated every 30 minutes as necessary. More recently obidoxime 3 mg/kg body weight by intramuscular injection has been reported to be more effective than pralidoxime as it has a faster action and crosses the blood-brain barrier. When these anticholinesterases take effect the dosage of atropine should be reduced to avoid atropine toxicity.

**Paracetamol (Acetaminophen).** *Clinical features*. Nausea and vomiting initially, but at first symptoms are often non-specific. After 36 hours in severe poisoning (plasma paracetamol levels above 200 μg/ml at four hours after ingestion) more serious toxic effects may develop including hypotension, hypothermia, metabolic acidosis, hypoglycaemia, bleeding tendency and delirium. The main danger, however, is acute liver failure which tends to occur several days after ingestion and carries a high mortality.

*Treatment*. 1. General measures. 2. In moderate or severe poisoning (likely over 20 × 500 mg tablets) the liver damage may be prevented provided the following treatment is given within 12 hours of the poisoning. An initial dose of n-acetylcysteine 150 mg/kg is given intravenously over 15 minutes, followed by an infusion of 50 mg/kg in 500 ml 5% dextrose in 4, 8 and 8 hours (total 300 mg/kg in 20 hours). 3. Intravenous glucose may be required to correct hypoglycaemia.

**Paraffin and Petroleum Distillates.** *Clinical features*. Pallor; vomiting and diarrhoea; cough and dyspnoea.

*Treatment*. 1. Do not wash out stomach (p. 785). 2. Antibiotics if aspiration has occurred. 3. General measures.

**Salicylates.** *Clinical features*. Young children are much more susceptible to the toxic effects of salicylates than adults, particularly to the complex and altering metabolic disturbances which occur. Coma is common in children, in contrast to adults in whom coma is seen only in very severe poisoning. In adults, plasma salicylate levels above 3·6 mmol/*l* (50 mg/100 ml) indicate moderate or severe poisoning. In this situation, characteristic features are tinnitus, deafness and blurring of vision. Restlessness, sweating and increased metabolic rate also occur. Hyperventilation results in respiratory alkalosis. There may be vomiting and this, together with hyperventilation and profuse sweating, often results in severe dehydration. Hypokalaemia is common. The initial respiratory alkalosis is frequently followed by a metabolic acidosis, which may be severe, especially in children. Despite these formidable fluid, electrolyte and acid-base disturbances the patients may seem less ill than they really are. Marked acidosis should be regarded as a very serious feature as it may herald sudden respiratory or cardiac arrest.

*Treatment*. 1. General measures, but gastric aspiration and lavage should be done in all patients when practicable. 2. In moderate or severe poisoning *forced alkaline diuresis* should be given. The following should be mixed together and given intravenously at a rate of 2 litres hourly for 3 hours:

| | |
|---|---|
| Saline (0·9%) | 0·5 litre |
| Dextrose (5%) | 1 litre |
| Sodium bicarbonate (1·26%) | 0·5 litre |
| Potassium chloride | 3 g |

If this regimen of diuresis cannot be given because of renal or cardiac impairment, peritoneal dialysis or haemodialysis are effective. Careful monitoring of fluid replacement, electrolyte and acid-base status must be carried out during this treatment.

**Tricyclic Antidepressants.** *Clinical features*. These features appear one to two hours after ingestion, but seldom last longer than 18–24 hours. Dry mouth, dilated pupils, urinary retention and absent bowel sounds are common. Varying degrees of loss of consciousness result but deep coma is not common. Hallucinations and pressure of speech occur. Cardiac arrhythmias may be severe, especially in children, and hypotension may result. Torticollis and ataxia may be pronounced in children, but at all ages brisk reflexes are common and tonic-clonic movements occur. Ventilatory depression, on occasions, is severe.

*Treatment*. 1. General measures. 2. Gastric lavage is effective up to 12 hours after ingestion. 3. Supportive therapy is all that is required in the great majority of patients but, if inadequate, physostigmine salicylate (1–3 mg) by slow intravenous injection will abolish the central nervous system effects and some of the cardiac complications. If necessary, the injection may be repeated after 10 minutes. 4. Resistant arrhythmias may respond to 40 mEq sodium bicarbonate intravenously.

## Industrial and Agricultural Poisoning

Lead, cyanide (p. 787), mercury, beryllium (p. 293) and cadmium are potential causes of industrial poisoning. In agriculture many highly toxic weedkillers, including paraquat and the dinitro-ortho-cresol group, and organo-phosphorus insecticides have been developed in recent years. They have been responsible for only a small number of cases of acute poisoning in Britain owing to effective legislation for controlling their use. In some countries, however, they have caused many deaths.

## Exposure to Ionising Radiation

The use of nuclear radiation both for energy production and weapons raises the risk of a nuclear accident, either in peace or in war. There is much uninformed speculation about the effects of accidental exposure, some of it grossly exaggerated. No accident, however, can be treated lightly and the facts presented here, derived from the therapeutic use of ionising radiation and the effects of the atomic bombs dropped on Japanese cities, may provide some simple basic guidelines in the event of an accident.

Relatively high doses of radiation are tolerated when only part of the body is exposed but when the whole body is involved, tolerance is greatly reduced. Given time, the body is capable of repairing some of the damage done by radiation, provided it is not too severe. This forms the basis of the calculation of maximum permissible doses for workers employed in industrial projects in which radiation in one form or another is used. The therapeutic application of ionising radiation takes these factors carefully into account and also recognises the risk of inducing secondary malignancy. Since the majority of patients treated already has malignant disease, this risk is not generally regarded as a contra-indication.

When an industrial nuclear accident occurs it is vital that all personnel leave the scene of radioactivity as quickly as possible to minimise exposure. If accidental exposure occurs, it is essential to obtain as accurate as possible an estimate of the radiation dose received and this will usually require the expertise of medical physicists. Workers, who are likely to be exposed to radiation, generally carry monitoring badges from which the doses can be calculated. If the accidental dose is relatively small, all that may be required is to remove the person from risk of further exposure. When the dose received approaches the limits of what the body can tolerate, the immediate risks are to the haemopoietic and gastrointestinal systems and can be monitored by general medical review and blood counts. Nausea and vomiting occurring under two hours from the time of exposure carry a very grave prognosis and treatment is generally useless. In patients whose symptoms develop at a later stage, support may be given in a similar way as for acute myeloid leukaemia receiving ablative therapy. Bone marrow transplantation from a sibling should be considered if facilities are available. The patient should have tissue typing performed at the earliest opportunity before his or her cells disappear.

The effects of a major atomic explosion, as from an atomic bomb, depend on where the human being is in relation to the explosion. Many are killed outright. Immediate survivors may die sooner or later from burns, both from flash exposure or the fire storm that follows, from blast and crush injuries or from radiation sickness. Radiation damage is due firstly to the intense burst of neutrons emitted at the time of the explosion and thereafter to radioactive fallout, although this is small in bombs in which the fireball does not hit the ground. Within seven hours of such an explosion, the radiation from the fallout drops to 10% of what it was one hour after the explosion and after two days the radioactivity has reduced to 1%.

Survival from the effects of the Hiroshima bomb was 95% of those more than 2000 metres from the explosion, despite exposure to immediate radiation. There was virtually no fallout as the fireball did not reach the ground. There was a small but definite increase in both acute and chronic myeloid leukaemia in survivors; about 0·16% more of the population died than would have been expected. Fetuses and young children exposed at the time of the bomb showed abnormalities in some cases but subsequent survivors had normal healthy children with no increase in deformity. The incidence of other tumours in the exposed population has increased after a latent period of ten to fifteen years. These have occurred particularly in the thyroid, breast, lung, urinary tract and the haemopoietic systems. When last calculated in 1974, among a population of 54 000 exposed within 25 000 metres of the bomb, there was a total excess of death from malignant disease of 185 persons, or 0·4% of the population. Clearly the long-term effects of radiation are difficult to predict once exposure has occurred and the evidence from Hiroshima and Nagasaki is that the effect on survivors is less than was originally predicted, although the full score has yet to be counted.

The bombs used on the Japanese cities were small by modern standards. The scale of effects of the largest megaton bombs is not known but extrapolation from available evidence suggests that the population may be at risk up to 100 miles from the centre of the explosion in flat terrain. Hills and mountains may provide a degree of protection. Survivors who may benefit from medical treatment are likely to be so numerous as to overwhelm the medical and other services.

The need for prevention is obviously crucial and this responsibility involves every one of us.

ALEXANDER A. H. LAWSON

*Further reading:*

Matthew, H. & Lawson, A. A. H. (1979) *Treatment of Common Acute Poisonings*, 4th edn. Edinburgh: Churchill Livingstone.

# 17. Tropical Diseases and Helminthic Infections

In this chapter those diseases are described which are limited to the tropics or are commoner there than in temperate regions. Some, such as malaria and amoebiasis, are frequently seen in Britain in immigrants, visitors and returned travellers. As parasitic worms are prevalent in the tropics all common helminths are described, including the ubiquitous threadworm. A few conditions are also included which do not occur in the tropics but which are related to tropical infections and have not been described elsewhere in this book.

Before presenting individual diseases, consideration is given to the patterns of disease in tropical and developing countries, as they may differ materially from those encountered elsewhere. It will be seen that ill health in the tropics does not consist only of a battle between human hosts and pathogens. The difficult problem of how to raise the general standard of health in the tropics is discussed on page 897.

The diseases described in this chapter have been grouped according to the aetiological agents in the following manner:

*Protozoa, e.g.* malaria, amoebiasis, visceral leishmaniasis (kala azar), African trypanosomiasis (sleeping sickness).
*Bacteria*, e.g. leprosy, cholera, anthrax, plague.
*Spirochaetes*, e.g. yaws, relapsing fever, and *Spirillum*, i.e. rat-bite fever.
*Viruses*, e.g. yellow fever, dengue, rabies, Lassa fever, Ebola fever.
*Chlamydia*, e.g. lymphogranuloma venereum, trachoma.
*Rickettsiae*, e.g. typhus fevers, Q fever.
*Helminths:* (a) flukes, e.g. schistosomiasis.
(b) tapeworms, e.g. cysticercosis, hydatid disease.
(c) roundworms, e.g. threadworms, ascariasis, hookworms, filariae.
*Fungi*, e.g. histoplasmosis.
*Arthropods*, e.g. scabies.
*Snakes and aquatic animals*, e.g. adders, jelly fish.
*Vegetable toxins*, e.g. argemone poisoning.

Study of the diseases named above would give the British student a sound introduction to tropical medicine. The other conditions described in this chapter are especially relevant to students in other countries and should be considered by the British student as opportunity arises.

Specific measures for the prevention of each disease are emphasised. Tables of vaccinations and prophylactic measures advised for travellers are given on pages 893 and 894, and a map of the world (Fig. 17.1) indicates the main hazards to be encountered in different regions.

## PATTERNS OF DISEASE IN TROPICAL AND DEVELOPING COUNTRIES

Patients in the tropics suffer from disorders of all the major systems and psyche, as they do in temperate and developed countries. In tropical countries, however, the aetiological factors may be different, especially in the case of infectious disease which still represents the greatest problem. The genetic constitution of patients in many parts of the world makes them resistant to certain conditions and predisposes them to others. The battle against acute disease is often a single episode in a long campaign against chronic infection and malnutrition. Clinical patterns of illness in the tropics, therefore, differ in many ways from those in temperate zones. Although the principles of diagnosis and treatment will be the same, multiple pathologies and diagnoses are the rule rather than the exception and treatment may need to be modified in the light of the background factors. The preponderance of children in the tropics and the high incidence of diarrhoeal and parasitic disease and malnutrition creates special problems.

**The Background to Diseases in the Tropics.** *Genes and Race.* The best example of genetically determined disease is sickle-cell anaemia in which homozygous producers of haemoglobin S become anaemic and often die in infancy. The heterozygous carrier of haemoglobin S, on the other hand, is healthy and enjoys a measure of protection against the severe complications of malaria. Other examples of racially determined responses to disease are seen in leprosy, which is worse in Caucasians and Mongolians than in Negroes, and in tuberculosis, the pattern in Indians differing from that in Europeans.

*Nutrition and Agriculture.* The presence or absence of malnutrition depends on the availability of food, its cost and the correctness of its use. Traditional practices and taboos may limit the use of available food, e.g. the banning of eggs and milk in pregnancy. Malnutrition impairs both the cellular and humoral components of the immune reponse and predisposes children to infection which further drains the body's nutritional reserves and retards growth. Moderate degrees of undernutrition are much commoner than the gross malnutrition syndromes and may be overlooked.

Dietary toxins are found in some areas and produce conditions such as tropical spinal ataxia from cassava in Africa (p. 726), veno-occulsive liver disease from seneccio alkaloids in Jamaica and elsewhere (p. 411) and hepatoma from aflatoxin in badly stored nuts and cereals (p. 799).

*Infections.* Acute infectious diseases, especially malaria, measles and gastroenteritis, still account for the high infant mortality in some parts of the tropics where up to 40% of children die before the age of 5 years. Acute infections may precipitate the syndromes of malnutrition, which may then be complicated by further infection, for example measles leading to kwashiorkor and cancrum oris.

Many of the decimating diseases of the past are now controlled by vaccination (yellow fever), vector control (malaria and sleeping sickness) and general improvement of living standards (plague and relapsing fever), but in several instances control is imperfect and the disease reappears as, for example, malaria in the Indian subcontinent and relapsing fever among refugees. Other epidemic diseases such as cholera in Asia and meningococcal meningitis in Africa remain largely uncontrolled and still kill hundreds of thousands of people annually.

Chronic infections do serious damage to important organs, such as the liver or kidneys in schistosomiasis, the heart in trypanosomiasis cruzi (Chagas' disease), the lungs, bones and lymph nodes in tuberculosis, the bone marrow reserves of iron in ancylostomiasis, and of folate in malaria, the small bowel in strongyloidiasis and the muscles in leprosy. These organs may then fail prematurely if increased demand is imposed on them by work, pregnancy or additional disease. Such infections produce chronic ill health in millions of children and even more so in adults. Tuberculous lymphadenopathy is very common and may involve superficial nodes in all areas or be limited to deep nodes and then be a cause of undiagnosed fever. Very often the degree of suffering is not sufficient to take people to hospital, even if one is available, but the ceaseless pruritus and gradually failing vision of onchocerciasis, the persistent diarrhoea of schistosomiasis mansoni and the immobilising cellulitis of the guinea worm are other examples of conditions sufficiently debilitating to reduce performance, deepen poverty and lead to malnutrition. These chronic infectious diseases are enormous economic burdens on the nation as well as on the patient and the family.

*Epidemiological factors* determine the distribution, prevalence, incidence and endemicity of a disease, especially if it is infectious, and so alter its pattern in the community. Endemic malaria, poliomyelitis and viral hepatitis affect the indigenous children, who either die or become immune so that adults do not suffer from these diseases. Non-immune adults, such as tourists, invading soldiers or refugees are, however, fully susceptible unless specifically protected. Particular requirements of organisms, vectors, hosts or intermediate stages of parasites make rabies a sporadic disease, meningococcal meningitis a disease of the Sudan savanna, cholera a riverine disease, onchocerciasis a rural disease, Chagas a poverty disease, and hookworm primarily a farmer's disease. Cooking and eating habits determine the prevalence of paragonimiasis, clonorchiasis and tapeworm infection.

*Immunity and Autoimmunity.* The natural immunity of animals to some human infection such as smallpox, which has only man for its host, has enabled this disease to be abolished, whereas the eradication of yellow fever is prevented by the susceptibility of monkeys to it. Natural immunity of individuals may possibly explain why some people do not suffer certain infections, but immunity acquired in childhood is a more usual explanation. *Mycobacterium leprae*, for example, commonly causes subclinical but immunising infections in children living in an endemic area, so that clinical disease is seen mainly in teenagers and young adults in whom naturally acquired immunity has failed.

Most human infections are terminated or controlled by an efficient immune response. When the response is inefficient the organism multiplies unchecked, causing either death or chronic disease as in lepromatous leprosy or onchocerciasis. Immunity is usually accompanied by hypersensitivity, which often causes more damage than the organism itself, as in tuberculoid leprosy or hepatosplenic schistosomiasis. Sometimes the immune reponse seems to be inappropriate, as in the tropical splenomegaly syndrome of chronic malaria, or to be grossly exaggerated, as with the hyperglobulinaemia of trypanosomiasis. In sharp contrast with their prevalence in temperate countries, autoimmune diseases are relatively uncommon in the tropics.

*Variations within the Tropics.* As well as the gross but general differences between patterns of disease in tropical underdeveloped and temperate developed countries, there are many variations within the tropics. A certain condition may be present in only one climatic belt, continent or even community, but be very important there; examples are loiasis in the West African rain forest, Chagas' disease in South America and kuru among the Fore people of New Guinea. Individual infectious and parasitic diseases are considered later in the chapter; their distribution throughout the world is shown on a map in Figure 17.1.

## GEOGRAPHICAL INFLUENCES ON DISEASES OF THE MAIN SYSTEMS

### Cardiovascular Disease

Acclimatisation to a hot, humid environment demands a 20% increase in cardiac output and later an increase in plasma volume. A diseased heart is less able to

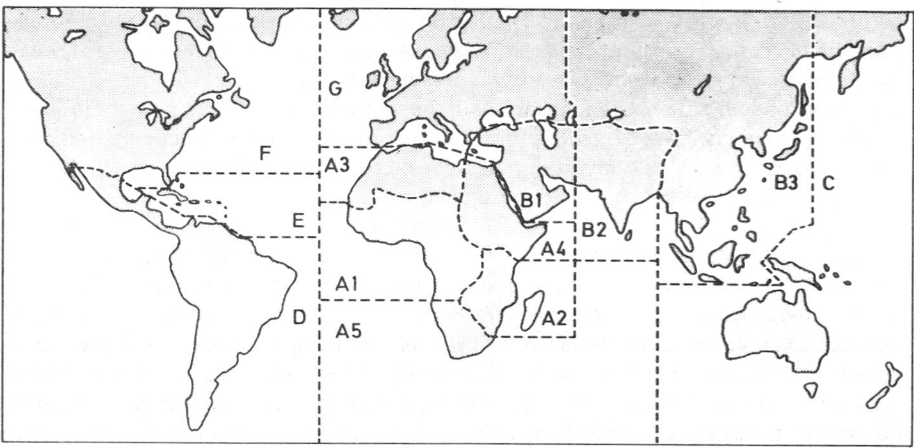


Fig. 17.1 Geographical distribution of disease (Based on information supplied by the Ross Institute of Tropical Hygiene, London)

| | Area | | | | | | | | | | | | |
|---|---|---|---|---|---|---|---|---|---|---|---|---|---|
| | Africa | | | | | Asia and Pacific | | | America | | | Europe | |
| Disease | A1 | A2 | A3 | A4 | A5 | B1 | B2 | B3 | C | D | E | F | G |
| Malaria | †† | †† | * | † | * | † | †† | †† | † | † | * | | |
| Schistosomiasis | † | † | * | †† | * | * | 1 | † | | † | * | | |
| Trypanosomiasis 2 | † | † | | * | * | | | | | † | | | |
| Leishmaniasis | * | 3,† | 3,* | † | * | † | † | * | | † | | | * |
| Cholera 4 | * | * | * | * | | * | †† | † | | | | | |
| Amoebiasis | † | † | † | † | † | † | †† | †† | † | †† | † | * | * |
| Typhoid fever | † | † | † | † | * | †† | †† | †† | * | † | † | * | * |
| Leprosy | †† | †† | † | †† | * | * | †† | †† | † | † | * | 5, | 5, |
| Onchocerciasis | †† | † | | † | | 6,* | * | | | 6,* | | | |
| Bancroftian | †† | †† | | † | | | † | †† | †† | † | * | | |
| and Brugia | | | | | | | | | | | | | |
| filariasis | †† | †† | | † | | | † | †† | †† | † | * | | |
| Paragonimiasis | * | | | | | | 7,* | †† | 7,* | | | | |
| Opisthorciasis and Clonorchiasis | | | | | | | | †† | † | | | | |

* endemic
† highly endemic
†† very highly endemic

1 Small foci in B2, near Bombay and Madras
2 Sleeping sickness in A, Chagas' disease in D
3 Visceral in A2, cutaneous in A3, both in other areas
4 Situation varies with gradual spread of seventh pandemic
5 Only a few small residual foci in F and G
6 Yemen only in B1, north of equator in D
7 Nepal and Ceylon in B2, Korea in C

acclimatise. The ECG pattern of normal individuals in Africa and other tropical countries commonly shows changes in the ST segments and T waves.

Rheumatic heart disease is worldwide, especially where there is overcrowding due to urbanisation and industrialisation. Endomyocardial fibrosis is just as important in children and young adults in parts of East and West Africa, Sri Lanka and Southern India, Brazil and Colombia. Cardiomyopathy is due to alcohol in parts of Africa and to thiamine deficiency in parts of South-east Asia and Southern Africa. In some countries congestive cardiomyopathy is a common cause of heart failure as is anaemia due to hookworms, sickle-cell disease or kwashiorkor.

Infective endocarditis is often secondary to skin sepsis but is no more common than in temperate climates whereas pericarditis is much more frequent and is usually either pyogenic or tuberculous. Chagas' disease, which accounts for 10% of all necropsies in Brazil, is an outstanding cause of myocarditis; other causes in the tropics are African trypanosomiasis, typhoid fever, diphtheria, rickettsial infections and acute schistosomiasis.

In some rural tropical communities blood pressure does not increase with age. The 'normal' blood pressure is usually lower than in temperate communities, essential hypertension is rare and pregnancy hypertension less common, but in other areas the opposite is true. Atherosclerotic and especially coronary heart disease is virtually unknown in many rural populations, whose plasma cholesterol levels are low and fibrinolytic activity high. Cor pulmonale is also rare in the tropics except where schistosomiasis is highly endemic.

Other forms of arterial disease are rare, but primary arteritis of the aorta, which can affect any of its major branches and of which the Takayasu syndrome is an example, is relatively common in Japan, South-east Asia and parts of Africa. In East and Central Africa an arteritis of unknown origin causes peripheral gangrene.

With the exception of tropical phlebitis, venous diseases such as haemorrhoids, varicose veins and deep vein thrombosis with its complication of pulmonary embolism are rare in the tropics.

**Tropical phlebitis** of uncertain origin occurs in tropical Africa. Vascular granulation tissue containing fibroblasts, endothelial cells and giant cells is laid down, especially in the middle coat of the vein, but extends outside the wall of the vein which becomes thrombosed. Splenic vein thrombosis may cause necrotic infarction and liquefaction in the spleen. When the affected vein is large, there will be pain along its course, followed by local swelling and congestion of distal veins and tissues. It may be possible to palpate the affected vein as a hard, cord-like structure. The patient is usually febrile. The venous lesion gradually resolves and the circulation is re-established. Treatment is symptomatic.

## Respiratory Disease

Acute respiratory infection is the commonest cause of childhood death all over the world, especially where measles is still prevalent. Most adult respiratory diseases in the tropics are also due to infection. Pneumococcal pneumonia and tuberculosis are commonest, followed by histoplasmosis in parts of South America, paragonimiasis in South-east Asia, filariasis (pulmonary eosinophilia) in India and the pulmonary complications of hepatic amoebiasis and schistosomiasis. Chronic bronchitis is rare in most rural areas, although common in North and Central India and parts of New Guinea where it is attributed to allergy to fungi growing in roof thatch. Asthma appears to be increasing in frequency in the tropics.

## Disease of the Alimentary Tract and Pancreas

Diarrhoea is the second commonest cause of death in childhood the world over and the most frequent in infancy in countries of poor hygiene if the mother is not breast feeding. In adults, infectious disorders are the most important causes of alimentary disease, especially acute gastroenteritis, giardiasis, typhoid and other salmonelloses, ileocaecal tuberculosis, amoebic and bacillary dysentery, schistosomiasis mansoni and, in some countries, tropical sprue (see below).

In underdeveloped countries the rural diet is rich in hand-milled grain fibre (bran) which is not only nutritious in vitamins, protein and iron and helps protect against deficiency diseases such as beriberi, but also makes a bulky soft stool which is passed two or three times daily. This bowel habit is associated with a virtual absence of appendicitis and diverticular disease. Other diseases which are rare in the tropics include Crohn's disease and ulcerative colitis. Cholecystitis is infrequent except as a complication from biliary flukes. The prevalence of peptic ulcers varies greatly between different regions; when it is high, gastric outlet obstruction is common. In certain parts of the tropics calcifying pancreatitis is common in children and young adults and may be related to protein deficiency associated with a highly alkaline vegetarian diet. In others it may be associated with alcohol.

## Tropical Sprue

Tropical sprue may be defined as malabsorption of two or more unrelated substances occurring in a patient in or from the tropics, in the absence of other intestinal disease or parasites. Its manifestations resemble those of coeliac disease.

**Aetiology** of sprue is unknown but its prevalence in certain well-defined tropical countries and indeed localities, and its epidemiological pattern, suggest that an infective agent may be involved initially. In established sprue the jejunal contents are grossly overpopulated with aerobic enterobacteria which seem to play a role in maintaining the disease. Sprue is not due to gluten or any other demonstrable sensitivity and there is usually no evidence of preceding malnutrition, but folate deficiency, as in pregnancy, may precipitate the disease. Not all cases necessarily have the same aetiology, which may account for occasional reports of sprue from Africa and elsewhere where the disease is not usually encountered. It occurs mainly in Asia, including Sri Lanka, Southern India, Malaysia, Indonesia, Hong Kong and China, some Caribbean Islands, Puerto Rico and parts of South America. Sprue is a problem mainly in European residents in Asia but also does occur in the indigenous tropical populations. It is common among travellers returning to Europe overland from India and Nepal.

**Pathology.** The changes closely resemble those of coeliac disease, although they tend to be less advanced. The jejunal villi are blunted or, rarely, absent and there is a subepithelial infiltration with plasma cells and lymphocytes. In severe cases the ileum is also affected. These changes are associated with malabsorption of fat, protein, carbohydrate and vitamins and the presence of diarrhoea which may lead to depletion of water, electrolytes, iron and calcium. A macrocytic anaemia is common with megaloblastic change in the bone marrow due to folate deficiency. Vitamin $B_{12}$ deficiency takes longer to develop and is encountered only in sprue of many months' duration.

Mild changes in the jejunal mucosa are common in asymptomatic indigenous peoples, without gross malabsorption, throughout the tropics (*tropical enteropathy*).

**Clinical Features.** Although the onset of sprue may be acute with explosive diarrhoea and occur within a few weeks of arrival in the tropics, it is more often insidious with increasing lassitude, mental apathy and depression, loss of weight, anorexia and flatulence. Remissions and relapses are a characteristic feature. In severe cases 10 stools or more may be passed daily, especially in the morning or during the night. Defaecation is urgent and often follows meals. The stool is bulky, frothy, pale and fatty, loose, foul-smelling and floats in the lavatory pan and is difficult to flush away. Vomiting may occur with nausea, abdominal distention and borborygmi. The tongue becomes sore, fiery red in colour, fissured and painful, and there may be difficulty in swallowing. As the disease progresses much weight is lost.

Continued malabsorption leads to specific malnutritional deficiencies; follicular keratosis (p. 101), angular stomatitis (vit. B), osteomalacia and tetany (vit. D), bleeding (vit. K) and hypoproteinaemic oedema, but peripheral neuropathy is rare. Loss of fluid and electrolytes causes dehydration, muscular weakness and cramps.

**Diagnosis.** The clinical features and the history of residence in an area noted for tropical sprue will suggest the correct diagnosis if care is taken to recognise the early and the mild cases as well as the late presentations. Evidence of malabsorption should be sought. Haematological changes start early; macrocytosis suggests folate deficiency and precedes the onset of frank megaloblastic anaemia. Serum and erythrocyte levels of folate are low. Anaemia may also be hypochromic from defective absorption of iron. Jejunal biopsy shows partial villous atrophy which is not specific for tropical sprue. Jejunal mucus and fluid is examined to exclude parasites. Barium meal and follow through examinations are necessary only to exclude other disease. Differential diagnosis is from other forms of steatorrhoea. Additional causes in the tropics are infections of the intestine with *Giardia intestinalis, Strongyloides stercoralis* or *Capillaria philippinensis*. Intestinal hurry as part of an allergic response in the early stages of ancylosotmiasis may suggest the onset of sprue. Early symptoms of sprue may erroneously be attributed to amoebiasis or neurosis.

**Treatment.** Rest in bed is required initially for the severely affected patient. Dehydration and potassium deficiency must be corrected. Tetracycline, 1 g daily in divided doses for 28 days, will usually eliminate the jejunal bacterial overpopulation, reduce diarrhoea and improve absorption. In addition folic acid, 5 mg daily (10 mg intramuscularly in severe cases), is given as this seems in many patients to improve absorption as well as to relieve symptoms due to folate deficiency. The jejunal mucosa soon returns to normal. Such a patient can continue to live in the tropics and remain well. It has not yet been established whether to give a small prophylactic dose of folic acid daily to prevent a relapse in patients remaining in the tropics or to administer folic acid only if a relapse occurs. Vitamin $B_{12}$ deficiency requires intramuscular injections of hydroxocobalamin, 1000 $\mu$g twice in 1 week, followed by a dose of 250 $\mu$g once a fortnight for 6 weeks in addition to folic acid. Anaemia is corrected and the danger of developing subacute combined degeneration of the spinal cord is avoided. Deficiencies of other vitamins and iron should be corrected. It is often helpful to give a multivitamin preparation containing 10 mg thiamin, 5 mg riboflavin and 50 mg nicotinamide twice daily for a few weeks.

Complicated diets are no longer advised but the diet initially should be bland and appetising, limited in fat and carbohydrate and high in protein. After recovery, the diet should contain meat, liver and green vegetables which are rich in folate. Folic acid supplements should be given to women who have had sprue should they become pregnant. Often, after apparently successful treatment, mild diarrhoea and flatulence may persist. These are usually due to secondary hypolactasia and respond to a lactose-free diet.

## Disease of the Liver, Kidney and Blood

*Liver disease* is a serious cause of disability and death throughout the tropics and subtropics. The microscopic structure of liver from a normal person in tropical Africa differs from that in a European. The hepatocytes are irregular in size and staining and frequently contain more than one nucleus. Portal tracts are infiltrated with mononuclear cells and a variable degree of fibrous tissue. Black pigment may be present in Kuppfer cells or portal tracts. These changes probably reflect the insults to which the liver is exposed in the tropics, including protein and vitamin malnutrition, alimentary infections and toxins, and systemic infections notably malaria and schistosomiasis. The effects of protozoal and helminthic infections on the liver are discussed on page 411.

In most areas where hygiene is poor, type A viral hepatitis is endemic and especially affects children. Cirrhosis of the liver and hepatoma are common in adults and a relationship has been postulated with hepatitis B virus which is extremely common in some parts of Africa where the prevalence exceeds 10% of the population. There is also increasing evidence incriminating aflatoxin isolated from badly stored groundnuts and grains as a cause of cirrhosis and hepatoma.

*Renal Disease.* Schistosomiasis haematobium, which is the commonest cause of haematuria in endemic areas, may grossly damage the bladder and ureters. Skin infection with streptococci is a frequent precursor of acute glomerulonephritis. Pyelonephritis is common and in males often follows a gonococcal stricture of the urethra. *Plasmodium malariae* is an important cause of the nephrotic syndrome in children. Lepromatous leprosy may also involve the kidneys. Bancroftian filariasis is a frequent cause of orchitis, epididymitis and hydrocele in endemic areas.

*Blood Disease.* In many tropical countries anaemia is common and often severe. This is largely explained by the high frequency of protozoal, helminthic and bacterial infections and the prevalence of malnutrition. It cannot be emphasised too strongly that the aetiology of anaemia in the tropics shows great variation from one country to another, and from one area to another, and effective management can only follow the clear appreciation of local patterns of disease, nutrition and social custom.

Ancylostomiasis is a major cause of iron deficiency anaemia. Although Addisonian pernicious anaemia occurs in all races, it is relatively uncommon in tropical countries where megaloblastic anaemia is much more frequently due to nutritional deficiency of folate or vitamin $B_{12}$.

The various types of haemolytic anaemia which occur in temperate climates are also encountered in tropical countries. Haemolytic anaemia in the tropics is frequently due to malaria. In addition two types of genetic abnormality resulting in haemolytic anaemia are also particularly common, namely deficiency of the enzyme glucose-6-phosphate dehydrogenase, and the haemoglobinopathies. Haemolysis also occurs in acute bartonellosis and may be caused by the venom of certain snakes.

## Metabolic, Endocrine and Connective Tissue Disorders

The prevalence of fluorosis is high in some areas (p. 97). Diabetes seems to be common throughout the tropics, but with few cardiovascular complications. The prevalence of other endocrine disorders is less certain.

Autoimmune disease is rare in most tropical countries. The incidence of dermatomyositis, scleroderma, lupus erythematosus and rheumatoid arthritis is low. Acute tropical polyarthritis, of obscure aetiology, is a common self-limiting disorder. Reiter's syndrome is frequent in Africa and causes much disability.

### Tropical Myositis

Painful tender muscles but without suppuration are a feature of several systemic infections, notably dengue fever, trypanosomiasis and relapsing fever, and are characteristic of trichinosis and cysticercosis.

The cause of suppurative myositis in the tropics is uncertain. Abscesses explored early are sterile but later culture of the pus usually yields *Staph. aureus*. Most cases occur in tropical Africa, South America and South Pacific Islands.

Pyomyositis starts with fever and painful induration of one or more of the large muscles, mostly in the lower limbs. The indurated area subsequently suppurates and a large abscess may form and be associated with a swinging temperature and leucocytosis. The affected area is swollen, hot and tender. When the pus is superficial, fluctuation can be detected.

Diagnosis is usually not difficult although meningitis or peritonitis may be simulated. The differential diagnosis includes Calabar swellings (p. 876), sparganosis (p. 867), scurvy and an underlying osteomyelitis. Staphylococcal pyaemia of other origin is characterised by numerous small abscesses. When an abscess has formed, it should be incised, the pus evacuated and antibiotics given.

## Neurological, Ophthalmic and Psychiatric Disease

Infections still cause much of the *neurological disease* throughout the tropics, e.g. pyogenic and tuberculous meningitis, rabies and arthropod-borne viral encephalitis, malaria, tetanus, poliomyelitis, cysticercosis and hydatid disease. Other examples are trypanosomiasis in Africa, bartonellosis and Chagas' disease in South America, and eosinophilic meningitis in the Far East. Leprosy is the commonest cause of peripheral neuritis in the world and Chagas' disease of systemic autonomic neuropathy. Tuberculoma is a frequent and amoebic abscess a rare cause of an intracranial space-occupying lesion. In some tropical communities cerebrovascular accidents and trauma are becoming the chief causes of neurological disease. Certain diseases, such as tabes dorsalis, multiple sclerosis, parkinsonism and vitamin $B_{12}$ neuropathy are rare.

There are several syndromes, due to dietary deficiencies or toxins, which are locally important. These include beriberi in the poorer areas of South-east Asia, Wernicke's encephalopathy among the Bantu in southern Africa and pellagra among maize eaters.

Tropical spinal ataxia may be caused by cyanide in undercooked cassava (p. 726). Causes of spastic paraplegia in the tropics include lathyrism in India and the horn of Africa, Burkitt's lymphoma in African adolescents, schistosomiasis in Africa and, commonest of all, spinal tuberculosis.

*Eye disease* is a major cause of suffering and poverty in the tropics; it often proceeds to blindness. The most frequent causes are neonatal ophthalmia, trachoma, onchocerciasis, malnutrition and leprosy.

The prevalence of *psychiatric diseases* in the tropics is similar to that in temperate countries, but some of the precipitating factors and symptom-complexes are different. Included among the causes of organic confusional states are alcoholism, meningitis, syphilis, malaria, trypanosomiasis and typhoid fever. Functional psychoses present in the same ways as in temperate countries, but acute emotional disturbances, especially in Africans, often present with schizophrenic features such as hallucinations and paranoia; the prognosis is, however, good. Fear, implanted by witchcraft, may have profound effects and, in addition, the subject may have been made to swallow potent poisonous charms. Neuroses are especially common in people from underdeveloped countries who are suddenly moved to a strange environment. Symptoms are often florid and usually hysterical, the patient having little understanding of their cause.

## Malignant Disease

Patterns of malignant disease vary greatly between different communities. Some tumours are rare — for example, carcinoma of the colon in Africa and Asia — and some extremely common locally. Hepatoma is frequent in parts of Africa and in the Singapore Chinese. Carcinoma of the mouth is the commonest cancer in India and Sri Lanka and carcinoma of the nasopharynx associated with the Epstein-Barr virus is frequent in Kenya and among Chinese in S. E. Asia.

*Kaposi's sarcoma*, or idiopathic multiple haemorrhagic sarcoma of the skin, is a multifocal malignancy composed of new blood vessels and large spindle cells. It presents as firm, bluish-brown nodules in the skin, usually on the limbs. Its incidence is high in parts of tropical Africa.

### Burkitt's Lymphoma

This tumour is uncommon outside the tropics. There is a relationship between its incidence and climatic factors (temperature and rainfall). It has been postulated that the Epstein-Barr virus, which can be isolated from all Burkitt's lymphomas, causes the malignant changes in children whose immune response has been temporarily depressed by malaria.

The tumour is a malignant lymphoma of a poorly differentiated lymphoblastic type. The histological pattern is of uniform masses of immature lymphoid cells, interspersed with many large clear histiocytes with poorly staining cytoplasm which create the typical 'starry sky' pattern.

**Clinical Features.** In Africa this tumour has a peak incidence between the ages of 4 and 8 years. Relatively few cases occur after puberty. The most frequent presenting feature is a tumour of the mandible or maxilla with loosening of teeth or exophthalmos due to invasion of the orbit. The eye may eventually be destroyed. All four quadrants of the jaw may be affected.

The second commonest clinical presentation is an abdominal tumour, usually caused by involvement of the kidneys, adrenals, ovaries, liver or abdominal lymph nodes. Involvement of the kidneys, adrenals and ovaries is often bilateral.

The third commonest presenting feature is paraplegia which is of sudden onset, flaccid from the outset and associated with incontinence of urine and faeces, without radiological evidence of vertebral collapse.

Other sites characteristically involved are the long bones of the limbs, the thyroid and salivary glands, the testes and the heart. Bilateral massive tumours of the breasts sometimes develop in young adult women. Spread to the bone marrow occurs relatively late in the disease. The rarity of peripheral lymphadenopathy is particularly characteristic.

**Treatment.** This tumour is unusually sensitive to a large range of cytotoxic drugs and to radiotherapy. As the tumour is probably always multifocal, systemic chemotherapy is preferred. The best results are obtained if the bulk of the tumour is first resected. Cyclophosphamide is given intramuscularly, 40 mg/kg body weight, every two weeks for 6 doses. Meningeal involvement is treated additionally with intrathecal methotrexate. Six year survival of 16–60% have been recorded depending on the stage of the disease.

# DISORDERS DUE TO CLIMATE

*Acclimatisation to Heat and Heat Injury; Exposure to Strong Sunlight; Solar Keratosis; Prickly Heat; Heat Exhaustion; Tropical Anhidrotic Asthenia; Heat Hyperpyrexia; Cold Injury; High Altitude Acclimatisation and Deterioration; Mountain Sickness.*

## Acclimatisation to Heat and Heat Injury

In cool climates heat production in the body is balanced by loss from the surface chiefly by radiation and convection. When the atmospheric temperature is above that of the body, evaporation of sweat is all-important in the maintenance of a stable body temperature, assisted to a minor degree by insensible loss through the skin and lungs.

Acclimatisation to heat is an essential preparation for workers exposed to excessive heat in certain industries in cool climates as well as for people who go to the tropics. This can be achieved by undertaking exercise daily under artificially produced or natural hot weather conditions for 10 to 14 days. The total volume of circulating fluid increases and is accommodated in the expanded vascular bed; this is accompanied by a diminished pulse rate and an increased cardiac output. Salt excretion by the kidneys and in sweat is reduced, mainly as a result of increased production of aldosterone. The sweat glands also become more active, responding more rapidly and efficiently to increases in body temperature; consequently the rise in body temperature in response to exercise diminishes. With these adjustments the individual is better able to work and remain well under conditions of high atmospheric temperature provided an adequate intake of water and salt is maintained.

Heat syncope (fainting, p. 146) occurs in people dressed in unsuitable clothes in a warm atmosphere with poor air circulation, at exercise or on suddenly standing up.

**Sunburn** is caused by exposure to ultraviolet light. The skin of those with fair complexions, green eyes and red hair is especially sensitive to strong sunlight. Natural tolerance to the sun may be won by gradual exposure which enables the skin to acquire protective pigmentation.

Short periods of unaccustomed strong sunlight produce only erythema and itchiness of the affected area of skin. Prolonged exposure causes acute pain, oedema, vesicles and bullae. These local changes are accompanied by malaise, headache and nausea. Severe cases may suffer from prostration and even acute circulatory failure. When a large area of skin has been damaged, this may interfere seriously with sweating and predispose to heat hyperpyrexia (p. 804).

No treatment is needed for mild sunburn, but for severe cases rest in bed in a cool room is required with sedatives to relieve the pain. Shock and dehydration must be corrected. Large blisters should be pricked. Calamine lotion containing 0·5% crystal violet should be applied to intact skin. Antihistamine drugs given by mouth help to relieve pruritus. Some protection is afforded by creams or lotions containing 5% para-aminobenzoic acid which absorbs ultraviolet light.

**Solar Keratosis.** After prolonged residence in the tropics atrophic patches are liable to develop on exposed parts of the body. The backs of the hands, the neck and the forehead are most commonly affected. These areas may later develop small patches of hyperkeratosis which occasionally progress to carcinoma. This process is most severe in albinos.

The skin should be protected as far as possible from the sunlight by clothing and creams. Hyperkeratotic areas can be removed by the application for one week of 5% fluorouracil ointment under an occlusive dressing.

**Prickly Heat.** *(Miliaria Rubra).* Many Europeans living in the tropics, especially when humidity is high, suffer from prickly heat. This arises from blockage of sweat ducts within the prickle cell layer of the epidermis so that sweat escapes into the epidermis and causes severe irritation. The lesions consist of numerous minute papules, surrounded by erythema, which become vesicular or pustular. The pus is sterile, although scratching may lead to secondary pyogenic infection. The lesions are most numerous in parts of the body in close contact with clothing.

The principles of treatment are to reduce sweating to a minimum and to overcome the blockage of the sweat ducts. If the patient can be transferred to a cool environment such as an air-conditioned room, the blocked ducts may become patent within a week or two. In severe cases it may be necessary to move to a cooler climate. Calamine lotion relieves the irritation.

In prevention, excessive washing and irritation from clothing should be avoided and a bland soap containing hexochlorophane used. Dusting powders should only be lightly applied. Clothing must be loose fitting, changed frequently and thoroughly rinsed after washing. Obese patients must lose weight. Curries, condiments and alcohol, which cause sweating, should be avoided.

**Tropical Anhidrotic Asthenia.** The majority of patients with this disorder have suffered from prickly heat which has left extensive areas of skin, especially on the trunk and limbs, incapable of sweating properly. The condition develops insidiously towards the end of the hot weather, with headache, giddiness, lack of energy, diminished sweating and often marked polyuria, the dilute urine containing chloride. Fever is common and hyperpyrexia may develop. The patient must live in a cool climate for several months until the skin has recovered and sweating has returned to normal.

**Heat exhaustion** is brought on by a period of great heat or by extra effort in hot weather, when the patient has not taken enough fluid and salt to balance the increased loss by sweating. The amount of fluid lost as sweat during a working spell in a hot environment may be as much as 6 to 8 litres and even in persons fully acclimatised to heat, this may entail a loss of approximately 2 g sodium chloride per litre of sweat. Ill-health, especially gastrointestinal disturbances with vomiting and diarrhoea, will increase the risk of heat exhaustion.

There are usually warnings which should be recognised. These include headache, giddiness, loss of appetite, nausea, cramps and irritability. Lack of thirst may disguise the severity of dehydration until tachycardia, hypotension and a cold clammy skin develop (the 'cold moist man', c.f. the hot dry man p. 804). A cool environment and cold drinks with added sodium chloride (10 g/*l*) are adequate for mild cases; others require intravenous rehydration. When heat exhaustion is not recognised and treated, the patient may pass into heat hyperpyrexia.

### Heat Hyperpyrexia (Heat Stroke)

This occurs in those exposed for considerable periods to unusually high environmental temperatures, independent of exposure to direct sunlight. Unacclimatised people are more liable to suffer, but a prolonged period of very high temperature may affect even those who are fully acclimatised, including local inhabitants. The disorder is always associated with cessation of sweating, and the rectal temperature may reach 42° to 43°C or even higher. Predisposing factors are those which interfere with the production and evaporation of sweat — unsuitable clothing, poor ventilation and heavy work in conditions of high temperature and humidity. Individuals with congenital absence of sweat glands, with cystic fibrosis or skin diseases are particularly vulnerable. Hyperpyrexia may follow heat exhaustion when dehydration leads to cessation of sweating.

**Pathological and Clinical Features.** The most important changes are in the central nervous system. There is general congestion of the brain with increased pressure of the cerebrospinal fluid. Microscopic examination may show degeneration of nerve cells, particularly in the hypothalamic region and base of the brain.

The onset is usually dramatic with no warning in a person who appears to be neither dehydrated nor deficient in salt, but who occasionally may have noticed that perspiration had become much less. The patient may have retired to rest feeling quite well and be found in coma a few hours later. Loss of consciousness is rapid and may be preceded by prodromal signs of cerebral irritation. On examination a dry burning skin is found (the 'hot dry man'). When the temperature reaches between 41° and 42°C unconsciousness supervenes and without treatment the patient dies. Hyperpyrexia may be complicated by acute circulatory failure, hypokalaemia, acute renal or hepatic failure and haemorrhage.

**Treatment.** The aim is to reduce the temperature as quickly as possible in order to prevent permanent damage to vital structures. This is done by spraying the naked patient with water or loosely wrapping him in a cool wet sheet and promoting evaporation by fanning, or by immersion in a bath of cold water. Parenteral antimalarial therapy (p. 810) should be given concurrently if malaria is a possibility. As the temperature falls, provided that the brain has not been irreparably damaged, consciousness returns. Cooling should be stopped when the rectal temperature has fallen to 39°C. The airway must be maintained and oxygen given. When return to consciousness is delayed, lumbar puncture and withdrawal of excess fluid may help. Intravenous hydrocortisone may be life saving in the presence of circulatory failure. Potassium deficiency should be corrected and severe haemorrhage controlled by blood transfusion. For the treatment of acute renal or hepatic failure see pages 448 and 399. During convalescence control of body temperature will remain unstable. With energetic treatment 90% of patients recover. When hyperpyrexia is secondary to heat exhaustion, dehydration is usually severe. Therefore, in addition to reducing the high temperature, adequate water and salt replacement is essential.

**Prevention of Ill-effects of Heat.** Careful selection should be made of those required to work under hot atmospheric conditions. General physical fitness, youth and mental stability are important. Fever, gastrointestinal disease, alcoholic excess and lack of sleep all predispose to ill-effects of heat. It is highly important that the skin should be healthy and that sweating should be normal.

When the atmospheric temperature is very high, leading to excessive sweating, even the fully acclimatised require to take extra fluid and salt. A daily intake of up to 15 litres of cool drinking water and 30 g of sodium chloride per person may be needed to prevent water and salt depletion. The extra salt is taken with food and in the drinking water, but it can, when necessary, be given in enteric coated tablets. A total of 30 g of sodium chloride is supplied by adding 3 flat teaspoonfuls of salt or 18 enteric coated tablets, each containing 650 mg of salt, to the normal daily intake of fluid and food.

In addition, everything possible should be done to improve working conditions by arranging for a free circulation of air and for a reduction of high temperature and excessive atmospheric humidity by air-conditioning. Clothing should be light and loose fitting. Hard or prolonged manual work should not be undertaken when atmospheric conditions are exceptionally unfavourable. Off-duty living conditions should be made as cool and comfortable as possible.

## Cold Injury

**Frostbite.** Dry cold, below 0°C, freezes poorly insulated tissues such as fingers, especially in people exercising at altitudes where oxygen demand is high and availability low. The warning sign is intense pain in fingers or feet. Superficial frostbite causes blistering of skin, and deep frostbite necrosis of tissues leading to gangrene. Frostbite is treated by rapidly rewarming the whole patient with good insulation and hot drinks, and by warming the affected part in water at 40°C.

**Accidental hypothermia** can be due to sudden immersion in a cold pond or sea, or to gradual but steady heat loss from exposure or from evaporation off the wet clothes of a poorly clad hill walker on a rainy day. The old and the sick become hypothermic if they are not well insulated at night. Clinical features and treatment are described on page 786.

## High Altitude Acclimatisation and Deterioration

The partial pressure of atmospheric oxygen decreases with altitude (p. 536). Physiological acclimatisation starts at about 7000 ft (2100 m) and most people feel the need to acclimatise by about 12 000 ft (3650 m). Pulmonary ventilation and perfusion increase, plasma volume decreases and renal excretion of bicarbonate increases. These and other changes serve to maintain arterial oxygen tension until erythrocyte production raises the haemoglobin and haematocrit. Above 14 000 ft (4270 m) heart rate and cardiac output increase and pulmonary artery pressure rises. Physically fit young people acclimatise best and do better with each ascent. Lowlanders, however, never attain the performance of highlanders. Lack of acclimatisation is shown by increased respiration, Cheyne-Stokes respiration, mild headache and irritability, easy fatiguability and sleeplessness.

Acclimatisation continues successfully up to 17 500 ft (5330 m) above which arterial oxygen saturation falls to 70% and physical performance starts to decline. Short bursts of work can be undertaken, but at the risk of the production of an exaggerated lactic acidosis. Prolonged residence above this height causes anorexia, weight loss, decreasing mental and physical capacity and increasing susceptibility to infection. There are no permanent human habitations above 15 000 ft (4575 m).

**Acute mountain sickness** is experienced by people who go up too high too quickly;

some suffer at 8000 ft (2440 m), others reach 19 000 ft (5795 m) without trouble. The earliest symptoms are headache, nausea and vomiting, followed by lassitude, muscle weakness, breathlessness, cyanosis, dizziness, rapid pulse and insomnia. The symptoms are probably due to intracellular oedema and may herald the onset of two severe, possibly fatal complications: pulmonary oedema (p. 145) and, less commonly, cerebral oedema. Paradoxically the robust young man is prone to pulmonary oedema, probably due to overconfidence. Cerebral oedema causes drowsiness, confusion, fits and coma. Its presence may be confirmed by the detection of papilloedema. Retinal haemorrhages also occur. These complications are prevented by ascending gradually and by acetazolamide. They are treated by descending rapidly and by giving oxygen. Frusemide (40–120 mg), or morphine (15 mg) is the treatment for pulmonary oedema, and dexamethasone (p. 684) for cerebral odema. Venous thromboses, which may lead to pulmonary embolism, may afflict the partially acclimatised; they are due to increased viscosity of blood and are prevented by adequate hydration and exercise.

**Chronic mountain sickness** is due to alveolar hypoventilation and chronic hypoxia and may affect highlanders as well as acclimatised lowlanders. It causes cyanosis, cardiac failure, pulmonary hypertension and neuropsychiatric symptoms. It is treated by taking the patient down to sea level.

*Further reading about disorders due to climate:*

Clark, E., *et al.* (1975) *Mountain Medicine and Physiology*. London: Alpine Club.
Edholm, O. G. & Bacharach, A. L. (1965) *Exploration Medicine*. Bristol: Wright.
Leithead, C. S. & Lind, A. R. (1964) *Heatstress and Heat Disorders*. London: Cassell.

## DISEASES DUE TO PROTOZOA

*Malaria; Amoebiasis; Giardiasis; Balantidiasis; Leishmaniasis; Trypanosomiasis; Toxoplasmosis*

### Malaria

Human malaria results from infection by *Plasmodium falciparum*, *P. vivax*, *P. ovale*, *P. malariae* and rarely other species. The infection may be acquired wherever there are human hosts carrying the parasites and a sufficiency of suitable anopheline mosquitoes, together with conditions of temperature and humidity which favour the development of the parasite in the mosquito. Malaria may also be transmitted by transfusion or inoculation of infected blood.

Malaria is endemic or sporadic throughout most of the tropics and sub-tropics below an altitude of 1500 m and excluding the Mediterranean littoral, the U.S.A. and Australia. One hundred million people are attacked annually of whom 1% die, mainly children.

As the result of WHO sponsored campaigns of prevention and more effective treatment, the incidence of malaria was greatly reduced in 1950–60 but since 1970 there has been a resurgence. Because of increased travel and neglect of chemoprophylaxis about 2000 cases are imported annually into Britain. Most are due to *P. vivax* from Asia. One in five, usually from Africa, is due to *P. falciparum* and of these 3% die because of late diagnosis.

**Pathogenesis.** The female anopheline mosquito becomes infected when it feeds on human blood containing gametocyctes, the sexual forms of the malarial parasite. The

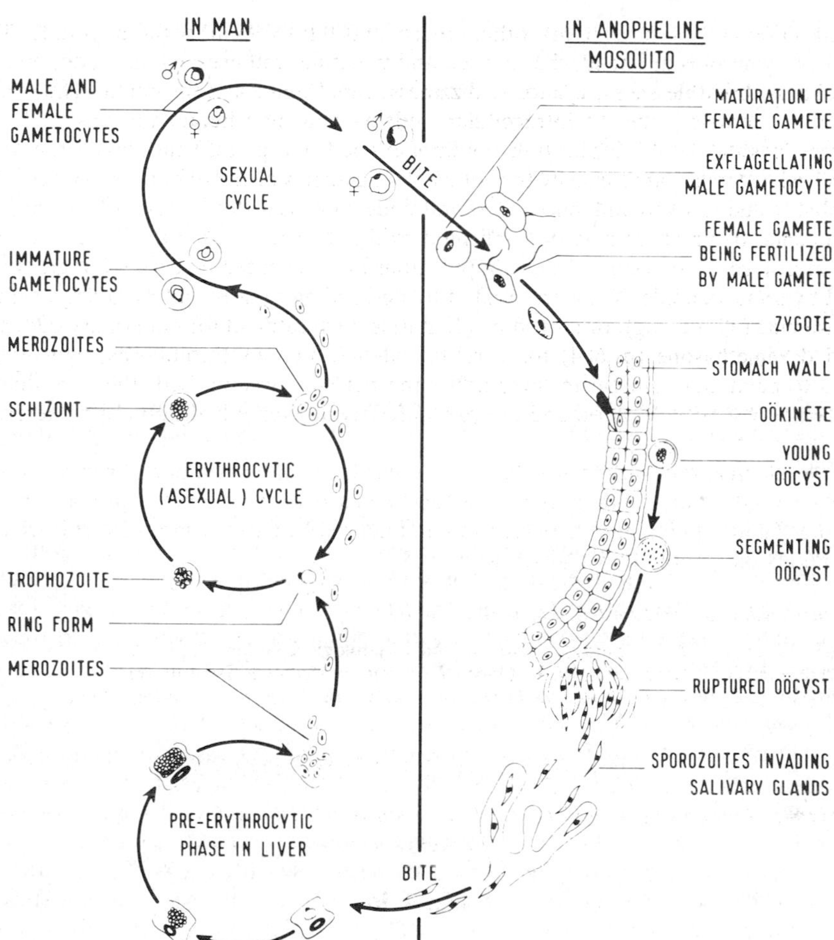


Fig. 17.2 Life cycle of malarial parasites. Adapted from Cruickshank, R. Duguid, J. P. Marmion, B. P. & Swain, R. H. A. (1973) *Medical Microbiology*. Edinburgh: Churchill Livingstone

further development and multiplication of the parasite is as shown in Figure 17.2. The development in the mosquito takes from 7–20 days. Sporozoites disappear from human blood within half an hour, but after 6½ days in *P. falciparum* malaria, 8½–11 days or occasionally longer for the other species, a greatly increased number of parasites, 'merozoites', leave the liver and invade red cells where further cycles of multiplication of parasites take place producing schizonts. Rupture of the schizont releases more merozoites into the blood and causes fever. *P. vivax*, *P. ovale* and *P. malariae* may also persist in the liver and only later invade the red cells. Each cycle in the red cells takes 48 hours in the case of *P. vivax* and *P. ovale* and results in a 'tertian' fever, the temperature rising on alternate days; *P. malariae* takes 72 hours resulting in a 'quartan' fever, while the cycle in *P. falciparum* takes rather less than 48 hours, is less well-synchronised and produces a more constant fever. Most anti-malarial drugs are effective chiefly in the asexual cycle in the red cells, hence *P. vivax*, *P. ovale*, and *P. malariae*, by persisting in the liver, may later cause relapses when they leave it and invade red cells. *P. falciparum* has no persistent exo-erythrocytic phase but recrudescences of fever may result from multiplication in the red cells of lingering parasites which have not been eliminated by inadequate treatment and immune processes.

Malaria is always accompanied by haemolysis and in a severe or prolonged attack anaemia may be profound. Haemolysis is most severe with *P. falciparum* which invades red cells of all ages. The other species invade only reticulocytes and infections remain lighter. Uninfected red cells are also destroyed by components of complement, activated in the circulation, adhering to them. Splenomegaly causes red cell sequestration with premature destruction and also haemodilution. Chronic malaria, especially during pregnancy, depletes folate stores. In *P. falciparum* malaria, red cells containing schizonts adhere to the lining of capillaries in brain, kidney, liver, lungs and gut. The vessels become congested and the organs anoxic. Rupture of schizonts liberates toxic and antigenic substances which cause further damage. Thus the main effects of malaria are haemolytic anaemia and, with *P. falciparum*, widespread organ damage.

**Clinical Features**. Malaria is first described as it occurs in the non-immune adult, falciparum malaria (see below) being the most dangerous form. The interval from the time of biting by the infected mosquito to the onset of detectable fever varies but is often about a week or 10 days for *P. falciparum* infections and somewhat longer for the other species. Occasionally an apparent primary attack of vivax malaria occurs months after the patient has left the tropics, and suppressive drugs may delay the onset for as long as a year after stopping the drug.

*P. vivax and P. ovale malaria*. In many cases the illness starts with a period of several days of continued fever before the development of classical bouts of fever on alternate days. The malarial paroxysm has three clinical stages: first a cold stage, followed by a hot stage, which ends in a sweating stage. In the cold stage or rigor the patient feels intensely cold and shivers, and frequently the teeth chatter. The temperature is already elevated and rapidly reaches its height, e.g. 40°C. Vomiting is often troublesome and headache severe. After half an hour or so, the hot stage is reached; the patient feels burning hot and may be delirious. After 1 to 6 hours, profuse perspiration starts, the temperature drops and the patient becomes comfortable, falls asleep and will feel reasonably well on the next day, but fever subsequently recurs on alternate days. Usually the spleen and, especially in children, the liver become palpable and tender, but the absence of detectable splenic enlargement does not exclude malaria. Herpes simplex, usually round the mouth, is a common accompaniment of malaria.

*P. malariae* malaria is usually associated with mild symptoms and bouts of fever every third day. With this infection parasitaemia may persist for many years without producing any symptoms.

*P. falciparum* infections are more dangerous than other forms of malaria. The onset, especially of primary attacks, is often insidious with malaise, headache and vomiting. Cough and mild diarrhoea are common. The fever has no particular pattern and does not usually rise quite so high as in the other forms. The cold, hot and sweating stages are seldom found. Jaundice is common, due to hepatitis and haemolysis. The liver and spleen enlarge and become tender. Anaemia develops rapidly. In uncomplicated cases only the ring stage of the parasites and later the gametocytes are found in the peripheral blood, whereas with the other species all stages of the parasites occur in the circulating blood. A patient with falciparum malaria, apparently not seriously ill, may suddenly develop serious complications. Children may die rapidly without any special symptoms other than fever. In pregnancy immunity is impaired, and abortion from parasitisation of the maternal side of the placenta is frequent. Congenital malaria is rare.

*Mixed infections* with more than one species of malaria parasite may occur.

COMPLICATIONS OF FALCIPARUM MALARIA. *Cerebral malaria* is the most urgent complication and is manifested either by the rapid development of coma, usually without localising signs, or by hyperpyrexia or acute mental changes. It is very rare for there to be an increase of cells in the cerebrospinal fluid.

*Blackwater Fever.* This is brought about by a rapid intravascular haemolysis and is invariably associated with a chronic falciparum malaria, most commonly in those who have taken antimalarial treatment irregularly. It is infrequent in indigenous races. The haemolysis may be quite unexpected and very extensive, destroying many uninfected as well as parasitised red cells. The attack may be provoked by administering quinine or by fatigue. The colour of the urine varies from dark red to almost black.

OTHER COMPLICATIONS. Impaired capillary function in the kidneys may produce acute renal failure and in the gastrointestinal tract vomiting or symptoms mimicking dysentery.

Relapses are characteristic of vivax, ovale and malariae infections. They seldom occur more than two years after the patient has left the malarious area but much longer intervals are recorded with *P. malariae.*

ENDEMIC MALARIA. The manifestations of malaria in unprotected indigenous residents show considerable variation according to the degree of endemicity, and the age of the patient and the development of immunity. In areas of hypoendemicity little immunity is acquired, epidemics of malaria are liable to occur and the disease does not differ materially from that in non-immunes. In mesoendemic areas malaria is frequent but only seasonal. Repeated infections lead to anaemia, considerable enlargement of spleen with the danger of its rupture from a minor blow, and chronic ill-health with bouts of fever. The growth and development of children may be retarded and *P. malariae* infections may cause immune-complex nephritis and the nephrotic syndrome. In hyperendemic areas malaria transmission takes place throughout the year, but with seasonal increases, and adults develop considerable immunity. Although they will have palpable spleens and occasional parasitaemia, malaria causes only occasional short bouts of fever. In holoendemic areas malarial transmission is intense throughout the year and adults do not suffer from the infection, a condition called 'premunity', and enlargement of the spleen does not usually persist. In hyperendemic and in holoendemic areas malaria takes a toll of older infants and young children. The regular taking of antimalarial drugs prevents the manifestations of chronic malaria but may impair the development of immunity. Individuals with the sickle-cell trait are less liable to develop the complications of falciparum malaria. People who have been subjected to splenectomy are especially liable to suffer severely from falciparum malaria because of impaired immune responses. They also become susceptible to species of *Babesia*, blood protozoa transmitted between animals by ticks.

TROPICAL SPLENOMEGALY SYNDROME. In some hyperendemic areas gross splenomegaly is associated with an exaggerated immune response to malaria and is seen, unexpectedly, in adults who have high antibody titres to malaria and low parasitaemias. The condition, which is commoner in females and in certain racial and family groups is characterised by enormous overproduction of IgM, levels reaching 3 to 20 times the local mean value. Much of the IgM is aggregated with other immunoglobulin or complement and precipitates in the cold, *in vitro*. The IgM aggregates are phagocytosed by reticuloendothelial cells in the spleen and liver, and the demonstration of this by immunofluorescence in a liver biopsy section is diagnostic. Light microscopy of the liver usually shows sinusoidal lymphocytosis. Anaemia and lymphocytosis can be confused with leukaemia. Portal hypertension may develop.

**Diagnosis.** If a febrile patient is in a malarious locality or has recently left such an area, malaria should be considered. Besides malaria there are many causes for acute febrile splenomegaly in the tropics. Gross enlargement of the spleen may also result from tuberculosis, visceral leishmaniasis, schistosomiasis mansoni and japonicum and chronic brucellosis as well as leukaemia and lymphoma. Well-stained blood films, thick and thin, should be examined and repeated if necessary. *P. falciparum* parasites may be very scanty, especially in those who have been partially treated. In semi-immunes in endemic areas malaria may co-exist with other diseases and not be the cause of the illness.

**Treatment.** GENERAL. The acutely ill patient should be put to bed and encouraged to drink fluid freely. Aspirin or paracetamol is useful for the relief of headache. When dehydration is marked and vomiting troublesome, intravenous fluids may be necessary.

SPECIFIC THERAPY OF THE ACUTE ATTACK. The drugs of choice are the 4-aminoquinolines, chloroquine or amodiaquine. The usual course of treatment is 600 mg of the effective base (4 tablets) followed by 300 mg base in six hours then 150 mg base twice daily for 3 to 7 more days. The initial dose for children is 5–10 mg/kg body weight. For semi-immunes a single dose is usually adequate. In areas of chloroquine resistance (most of S.E. Asia, Papua, parts of India and Bangladesh, the Kenya coast, Colombia and Venezuela) *P. falciparum* may respond poorly and quinine should be used to treat severe infections. Quinine dihydrochloride 650 mg three times daily for 2 days should be given by mouth, followed by a single dose of sulfadoxine 1·5 g combined with pyrimethamine 75 mg, i.e. 3 tablets of Fansidar.

*Treatment of Complicated P. falciparum Malaria.* Patients with 'cerebral malaria' or other severe manifestations are medical emergencies. The immediate administration of chloroquine or quinine is indicated, the drug being given very slowly preferably as an intravenous infusion over 1–4 hours to avoid peripheral circulatory failure or acute encephalopathy. Quinine is particularly indicated if a chloroquine-resistant infection is at all likely. The dose of chloroquine is 5 mg/kg body weight and of quinine 10 mg/kg body weight. The dose may be repeated three times at intervals of 8 hours. The drugs may instead be given intramuscularly but chloroquine may cause convulsions (especially in undernourished children) and quinine may cause necrosis; the hydrochloride is less irritant than the dihydrochloride. The results of prompt treatment are usually very gratifying. Dexamethasone (4 mg) is given if signs of cerebral oedema persist. If in the treatment of a comatose patient, return to consciousness is delayed, lumbar puncture is indicated to exclude coexisting bacterial meningitis. Oral treatment should replace parenteral as soon as the patient's condition allows.

*Treatment of Severe Anaemia and Blackwater Fever.* Severe anaemia requires transfusion with packed red cells. In blackwater fever prednisolone (20 mg) may prevent further haemolysis. If oliguria develops, frusemide or an infusion of mannitol may forestall renal failure. Rest, quiet and good nursing are essential. Fluids may be given orally. Intravenous fluid, if necessary, should be monitored by CVP (p. 167). Pulmonary oedema may develop and require urgent treatment.

TREATMENT OF TROPICAL SPLENOMEGALY SYNDROME. Splenomegaly and anaemia usually resolve over a period of months of continuous treatment with proguanil 100 mg daily, which should be continued for life to prevent relapse. Complicating folate deficiency is treated with folic acid 5 mg daily.

Malaria may complicate splenic enlargement associated with other disorders, such as chronic lymphatic leukaemia, and then treatment must be directed at all the conditions present.

RADICAL CURE OF MALARIA DUE TO *P. vivax*, *P. malariae* and *P. ovale*. While relapses can usually be prevented by taking one of the antimalarial drugs in suppressive doses over a period of months, radical cure can be ensured only by a course of one of the 8-aminoquinolines, which destroy these parasites in their exoerythrocytic phase in the liver, together with or following a course of chloroquine or amodiaquine. Primaquine given in a dose of 15 mg daily for 14 days produces a high percentage of cures. The patient must be under medical supervision for this period as haemolysis may develop in those who are G6PD deficient. Cyanosis due to the formation of methaemoglobin in the red cells is more common but not dangerous. Relapses after leaving endemic areas can be prevented by an alternative regime of 10 weekly doses of chloroquine, 300 mg base, with primaquine, 45 mg base (six tablets). Mild diarrhoea on the days of treatment is usually the only side-effect.

**Causal Prophylaxis and Suppression.** So far no drug is known which will destroy the sporozoites injected by the mosquito. Clinical attacks of malaria can, however, be prevented by drugs which attack the pre-erythrocytic form ('causal prophylaxis'), or by drugs which act on the parasite after it has entered the erythrocyte ('suppression'). The antifolates proguanil and pyrimethamine destroy the pre-erythrocytic stage of *P. falciparum*; they also act weakly on the asexual erythrocytic forms of all species of human malaria parasites. Consequently they protect against clinical attacks of malaria if started on entering a malarious region. These two drugs also inhibit further development of the falciparum gametocytes in the mosquito. Tables 17.1 and 17.2 give the recommended doses for protection of the non-immune. Resistance to the cheap and well tolerated drugs proguanil and pyrimethamine is increasing and frequently coincides with chloroquine resistance. Chloroquine must not be taken in too large a dose, or continuously as a prophylactic for over five years, as it may impair vision (p. 612).

**Prevention.** Control of anopheline mosquitoes, especially by the spraying of houses with residual insecticides, has greatly reduced or abolished the risk of malaria in many areas. However, unless eradication is complete, all visitors and non-immune residents should take regular prophylactic drugs as detailed above. Sleeping at night under a mosquito net or in a wire-screened and sprayed house, will give freedom from the nuisance of those mosquitoes which bite only in the dark and may also reduce the likelihood of acquiring other mosquito-borne infections.

*Further reading about malaria:*

Hall, A. P. (1977) The treatment of severe falciparum malaria. *Transactions of the Royal Society of Tropical Medicine and Hygiene*, **71**, 80.

Maegraith, B. G. (1974) Malaria. In *Medicine in the Tropics*, ed. Woodruff A. W. Ch. 2, pp. 27–73. Edinburgh: Churchill Livingstone.

Table 17.1 Prophylaxis of malaria

| Area | Antimalarial drugs | Adult prophylactic dose |
|---|---|---|
| Chloroquine resistance present | Pyrimethamine 12·5 mg plus diaminodiphenyl sulphone 100 mg (Maloprim)* | One tablet twice weekly |
| | OR | |
| | Pyrimethamine 25 mg plus sulphadoxine 500 mg (Fansidar)* | One tablet weekly |
| Chloroquine resistance absent | Chloroquine 100 mg, 150 mg or 300 mg of base | 300 mg weekly** |
| | OR | |
| | Proguanil 100 mg | 100–200 mg daily |
| | OR | |
| | Pyrimethamine 25 mg | 25 mg weekly |

*Chloroquine may be taken in addition where high *P. vivax* transmisson is present
** 600 mg weekly for the first six weeks has been advocated.

Table 17.2 Doses of antimalarials for children — where weight and age are both available, weight is preferable.

| Dose in relation to adult dose | Age range | Weight range |
|---|---|---|
| One-quarter | under 1 year | under 5 kg |
| One-half | 1–5 years | 5–20 kg |
| Three-quarters | 6–12 years | 20–40 kg |
| Adult dose | over 12 years | over 40 kg |

## Amoebiasis

Amoebiasis as described in this section is due to infection by *Entamoeba histolytica*. This potentially pathogenic amoeba is propagated between humans by its cysts, 10 microns or more in diameter. Another amoeba, *Ent. hartmanii*, is non-pathogenic, as is *Ent. coli* which is also harboured at times in the human intestine. In addition two amoebae of genera *Naegleria* and *Acanthamoeba* which inhabit polluted surface water and swimming pools all over the world are causes respectively of fulminating meningitis and granulomatous encephalitis.

**Pathogenesis.** Cysts of *Ent. histolytica* survive well outside the body and are ingested in water or uncooked food which has been contaminated by human faeces. In endemic areas lettuce is a common vehicle of infection. The disease is occasionally acquired in Britain. In the colon the vegetative trophozoite forms emerge from the cysts. While they remain free in the colon the condition is symptomless but under certain circumstances invasion and ulceration of the mucous membrane of the large bowel takes place causing the symptoms of amoebic dysentery. The lesions, which are usually maximal in the caecum but may be found as far down as the anal canal, are flask-shaped ulcers varying greatly in size and surrounded by healthy mucosa. Amoebae may find their way into a vein and be carried to the liver where they multiply and cause hepatocellular necrosis ('*amoebic abscess*'). The liquid contents at first have a characteristic pinkish colour which later may change to chocolate brown and finally to yellow or green. Amoebic ulcers only rarely penetrate through the muscular coat of the colon. A large vessel may sometimes be eroded, and severe intestinal haemorrhage result. A localised granuloma, '*amoeboma*', presenting as a palpable mass in the rectum or causing a filling defect in the colon on radiography, is a rare complication. Since it responds well to antiamoebic treatment it is important that it should not be mistaken for a carcinoma. Cysts may continue to be passed in the faeces when the disease is inactive.

**Clinical Features.** The incubation period varies from 2 weeks to many years, but is usually several months. *Intestinal amoebiasis*, or *amoebic dysentery* usually runs a chronic course with grumbling pains in the abdomen and two or more rather loose stools a day. Periods of diarrhoea alternating with constipation are a frequent feature. Mucus is usually passed, sometimes with streaks of blood, and the motions often have an offensive odour. On palpation of the abdomen there may be tenderness along the line of the colon, usually more marked over the caecum and pelvic colon. The right iliac pain may simulate acute appendicitis, and if an operation is performed the amoebae may cause ulceration of the wound and surrounding tissue. Perforation, when it occurs, is usually in the region of the caecum. Particularly in the aged, in the puerperium and with superadded pyogenic infection of the ulcers there may be more acute bowel symptoms, with very frequent motions and the passage of considerable quantities of blood and mucus, thus simulating bacillary dysentery or ulcerative colitis. Bacillary and amoebic dysentery may occur together, the bacillary infection probably lighting up latent amoebiasis.

*Hepatic amoebiasis* often occurs without a history of recent diarrhoea, and its possibility must be entertained in anyone who has lived in the tropics or subtropics. Early symptoms may be local discomfort only and malaise; later a swinging temperature, sweating and an enlarged tender liver, cough and pain in the right shoulder are characteristic, but symptoms may remain vague and signs minimal. In particular, the less common abscess in the left lobe may not be diagnosed. There is usually a moderate neutrophil leucocytosis and a raised diaphragm with diminished movement on the right side may be demonstrated. A large abscess may penetrate the diaphragm and rupture into the lung from where its contents may be coughed up. Rupture into the pleural cavity, the peritoneal cavity or pericardial sac is less common but more serious.

**Diagnosis.** The signs and symptoms of intestinal amoebiasis are often vague. A careful naked-eye inspection of a freshly passed motion should be made. Any exudate is examined at once under the microscope for motile trophozoites which are about 30 microns in diameter, with a clear ectoplasm and a granular endoplasm, and usually contain red blood cells. Pseudopodia containing clear ectoplasm are protruded and retracted. Movements cease very soon as the preparation cools. Macrophages are sometimes mistaken for amoebae. Sigmoidoscopy may reveal typical ulcers and a scraping should be examined for *Ent. histolytica*. In chronic amoebiasis several stools may need to be examined before cysts are found.

An amoebic abscess of the liver is suspected from the clinical and radiographic appearances. If the site of an hepatic abscess is not obvious clinically, radioisotope or ultrasonic scanning may be employed to demonstrate it. The fluid ('amoebic pus') from an abscess of the liver usually has a characteristic appearance, as described above, but only rarely contains free amoebae.

Antibodies are detectable by immunofluorescence in over 95% of cases of hepatic amoebiasis and intestinal amoeboma but in only about 60% of dysenteric amoebiasis. Precipitin tests are less sensitive but become negative in a few months after cure.

**Treatment and Prevention.** The symptoms of active intestinal amoebiasis are quickly controlled in all but the most severe cases by oral metronidazole, 800 mg three times daily for 5 days, tinidazole in single doses of 2 g orally daily for 3 days, or emetine hydrochloride 60 mg daily, subcutaneously for a few days. Furamide 500 mg should be given orally t.i.d. for 10 days after treatment by emetine. Four weeks after the course the patient should report for test of cure.

Early hepatic amoebiasis responds quickly to treatment by metronidazole, tinidazole or emetine as above, or to chloroquine 300 mg base b.d. for 2 days, followed by 150 mg b.d. for 14 days. Emetine should be followed by chloroquine and furamide to eliminate the intestinal infection. If the abscess is large or threatens to burst, or if the response to chemotherapy is not prompt, aspiration is also required and repeated if necessary. If culture of the 'pus' indicates that there is secondary bacterial infection, treatment will be required with an appropriate antibiotic. Rupture of an abscess into the pleural cavity, pericardial sac or peritoneal cavity necessitates immediate aspiration or surgical drainage. Small serous effusions resolve without drainage.

Personal precautions against contracting amoebiasis in the tropics and subtropics consist of not eating fresh uncooked vegetables or drinking unboiled water.

*Further reading about amoebiasis:*

Stamm, W. P. (1976) Amoebiasis: a neglected diagnosis. *Journal of the Royal College of Physicians of London,* **10**, 294–298.

## Giardiasis

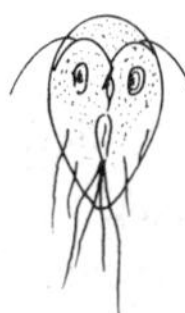

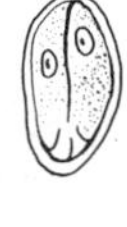

Fig. 17.3 *Giardia intestinalis*. Vegetative form (14 × 7μ); cystic form (8 × 12 μ)

Infection with the flagellate *Giardia intestinalis*, known also as *G. lamblia*, is worldwide but commoner in the tropics. It particularly affects children in endemic areas, tourists and patients in mental hospitals. The flagellates attach to the mucosa of the duodenum and jejunum and cause inflammation and partial villous atrophy. Recurrent attacks of urgent diarrhoea with abdominal discomfort and explosive loose pale stools are characteristic. There may be severe malabsorption. Lethargy, flatulence, abdominal distension, duodenal pain and nausea are frequent; vomiting may occur. Giardiasis is diagnosed by recognising the cysts in stools or the vegetative form in jejunal juice or mucus. Metronidazole 2 g as a single dose is given daily, after breakfast, for 3 days and the course should be repeated 1 week later. Patients should be warned not to drink alcohol nor drive a car or operate dangerous machinery while taking the drug. Children under 4 years are given one-quarter of the adult dose, from 4 to 8 years half the adult dose, preferably in a palatable suspension.

## Balantidiasis

*Balantidium coli* affects pigs in all countries and rarely infects pig farmers. This ciliate may cause local or extensive ulceration of the mucosa of the colon but often lives free in the lumen. Thus the infection may be symptom-free or frequent stools containing blood and mucus may be passed.

Therapeutic success may be obtained from tetracycline 500 mg four times daily for 10 days with the addition of ascorbic acid. Metronidazole, 1 g daily for 5 days, may be used but it is claimed that better results are achieved by nimorazole (Naxogin) 500 mg daily for 5 days.

## Leishmaniasis

This group of diseases is caused by protozoa of the genus *Leishmania*, conveyed to man by female sandflies in which the flagellate (promastigote) forms of leishmania develop. In man the leishmaniae are found in reticuloendothelial cells in oval forms known as amastigotes or Leishman-Donovan bodies (Fig. 17.4). Leishmaniasis may take the form of a generalised visceral infection, kala azar, or of a purely cutaneous infection, known in the Old World as oriental sore. In South America cutaneous leishmaniasis may remain confined to the skin or metastasise to the nose and mouth.

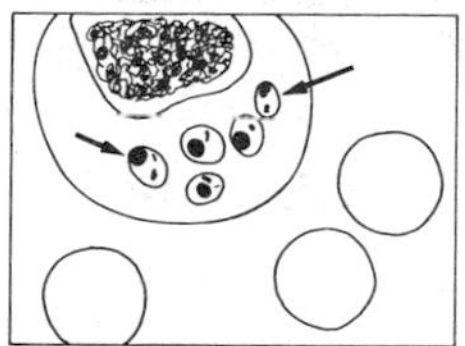

Fig. 17.4 *Leishmania donovani* amastigotes (L.D. bodies) in marrow smear

### Visceral Leishmaniasis (Kala Azar)

Kala azar is caused by *Leishmania donovani* and is prevalent in the Mediterranean and Red Sea littorals, where children are predominantly affected, Sudan, parts of East Africa, Asia Minor, mountainous regions of Southern Arabia, eastern parts of India, China and South America. In India, where the disease was epidemic, man appears to be the chief host but in many areas, including the Mediterranean area, dogs and foxes are the main reservoirs of infection. Here the disease is endemic and occurs chiefly in childhood or in tourists. In Africa various wild rodents provide the reservoir. Transmission, normally by sandflies, has also been reported to follow transfusion of infected blood.

**Pathology.** Multiplication, by simple fission, of leishmaniae takes place in reticulo-endothelial cells in various organs, especially the liver and spleen, which becomes greatly enlarged, and the bone marrow. There is usually a marked progressive granulocytopenia, the leucocyte count falling below $2{\cdot}0 \times 10^9/l$, and a slowly progressive anaemia. There is a great increase of gamma globulin which is mainly IgG. Successful chemotherapy reverses these changes; only rarely does appreciable fibrosis of the liver follow.

**Clinical Features.** The incubation period is usually about 1 or 2 months but up to 10 years has been recorded. The onset is usually insidious with a low grade fever, the patient remaining ambulant, or it may be abrupt with sweating and high intermittent fever, sometimes showing a double rise of temperature in the 24 hours. The spleen soon becomes enlarged, often massively. Hepatomegaly is less marked. If not treated, the patient will become anaemic and wasted, frequently with increased pigmentation especially on the face. Lymphadenopathy is common and rarely is the only clinical finding. After recovery dermal leishmaniasis sometimes develops. It may present first as hypopigmented or erythematous macules on any part of the body and later a nodular eruption may appear, especially on the face. In macular lesions intracellular amastigotes are scanty; in nodules they are more abundant.

Diagnosis is established by demonstrating the parasite in stained smears of aspirates of bone marrow, lymph node, spleen or liver, or by culture of these aspirates. Antibody is detected by immunofluorescence or complement-fixation early in the disease. The leishmanin skin test is negative.

**Treatment and Prevention.** The response to treatment varies with the geographical area in which the disease has been acquired. In Asia the disease is readily cured, but in the Sudan and East Africa it is more resistant. Sodium stibogluconate, a pentavalent antimony compound, gives good results. A solution containing 100 mg/ml is available for intravenous or intramuscular use. A suitable course of treatment for an adult is 10 mg/kg body weight i.v. daily for 10–20 days. Children are given relatively more, up to 20 mg/kg. The course may be repeated if necessary, after an interval of 14 days.

In some areas where the disease is resistant to antimony, pentamidine isethionate employed as in trypanosomiasis (p. 820) or amphotericin (p. 882) have been found effective but they are more toxic.

The results produced in each case must be assessed by careful observation of physical and laboratory findings, and treatment repeated as required. For the treatment of post-kala azar dermal leishmaniasis the same drugs are used as for visceral leishmaniasis but the response is slower, and intermittent treatment for months may be needed.

In an endemic area where they are the reservoir, infected or stray dogs should be destroyed. Sandflies should be combated (p. 846). Early diagnosis and treatment of human infections reduces the reservoir and controls epidemic kala azar in India. No vaccine is available.

### Cutaneous Leishmaniasis of the Old World (Oriental Sore)

Cutaneous leishmaniasis, which is caused by *Leishmania tropica* is a widespread zoonosis in the tropics and subtropics. It is conveyed from many different animals to man by sandflies. On inoculation the parasites are taken up by dermal histiocytes in which they multiply and around which lymphocytes and plasma cells accumulate.

With time, the histology becomes more tuberculoid and the overlying epidermis crusts and may ulcerate centrally. Healing is accompanied by subepidermal fibrosis.

**Clinical Features.** The incubation period is from 2 weeks to 5 or more years but usually is from 2 to 3 months. Lesions, single or multiple on exposed parts of the body, start as small red papules which increase in size and over which a crust may form. Tiny satellite papules are characteristic. Untreated the lesions will heal or will progress to form a rounded ulcer with well-defined indurated raised margins and a granulomatous base. Such a lesion may be up to 10 cm or more in diameter. A seropurulent discharge exudes which may dry and form an adherent scab. There is no pain or systemic disturbance. Sometimes, instead of an ulcer, a fungating nodular mass develops. Occasionally leishmaniae spread from the sore and give rise to nodules in the course of the lymphatics with enlargement of the related nodes. Untreated the ulcer lasts about a year. Healing produces a thin depressed, mottled scar. Cutaneous leishmaniasis may occur in a persistent relapsing form (leishmaniasis recidivans) having a histology indistinguishable from that of cutaneous tuberculosis.

Diffuse cutaneous leishmaniasis occurring in Ethiopia and Venezuela is probably attributable to a defective cell-mediated immune response to the parasite. The initial papule spreads locally and blood borne cutaneous lesions, which do not ulcerate, are widespread. The lesions contain numerous amastigotes within macrophages.

The appearance of a typical lesion in a patient from an endemic area suggests the diagnosis. Leishman-Donovan bodies can be demonstrated by inserting a dry needle into the margin of the ulcer, curetting the edge or making a skin slit smear (p. 827) and staining the material obtained with Giemsa's stain or culturing it. The Leishmanin skin test (p. 818) is positive except in diffuse cutaneous leishmaniasis. Serology is negative.

**Treatment and Prevention.** Unipolar coagulation diathermy has replaced earlier methods of inducing an inflammatory reaction to expedite cure. The local application of heat by infra-red, hot water or a thermostatically controlled pad at 40°C may accelerate healing.

When the lesions are multiple or in a disfiguring site it is better to treat the patient by parenteral injections of pentavalent antimony compounds such as sodium stibogluconate (p. 816)

Diffuse cutaneous leishmaniasis responds to antimonials in Venezuela but not in Ethiopia and tends to relapse. Cure may sometimes be achieved by a prolonged course of amphotericin (p. 882) or of pentamidine isethionate (p. 820) given once or twice weekly to minimise toxicity, weekly tests of the blood glucose being performed to detect the early signs of drug-induced diabetes.

In addition to those prophylactic measures described under visceral leishmaniasis against animals and sandflies, a lasting immunity can be achieved by deliberate inoculation of a living culture of *L. tropica* on the upper arm, which produces a typical sore but protects against a subsequent, possibly disfiguring, lesion.

### Cutaneous Leishmaniasis of the New World

In South and Central America, cutaneous leishmaniasis is endemic and mostly caused by *L. braziliensis* and *L. mexicana*. They occur in hot, moist, forest regions and are conveyed to man from a variety of rodents by several species of sandflies. The disease can be separated into three types. *L. mexicana* is responsible for chicleros ulcer, the self-healing sores of Mexico, Guatemala and Honduras, and for some of the sores in the north of South America, including diffuse cutaneous leishmaniasis. *L. braziliensis* extends widely from the Amazon basin as far as Paraguay and Costa Rica and is responsible for self-healing sores and for 'espundia'. A third variety of the disease occurring in the Peruvian Andes is known as 'uta' and is caused by *L. peruviana*, dogs providing the reservoir.

**Pathological and Clinical Features.** The microscopic appearances of the skin lesions may be similar to oriental sore but are not always characteristic. The mucocutaneous lesions begin as a perivascular infiltration; later endarteritis may lead to destruction of the surrounding tissues (see below). Lesions of *L. mexicana* and *L. peruviana* closely resemble those of *L. tropica*, but lesions on the pinna of the ear are common and are chronic and destructive. The primary lesions of *L. braziliensis* are similar but in some areas up to 80% develop 'espundia' i.e. metastatic lesions in the mucosa of the nose or mouth.

Mucosal lesions either accompany the skin lesions or appear some years later. The nasal mucosa becomes congested and later all tissues of the nose ulcerate except for the bone. The lips, soft palate and fauces may be invaded and destroyed leading to terrible suffering and deformity. Secondary bacterial infection is a common aggravating factor.

Diagnosis depends on the history and clinical appearance, confirmed by demonstration of the protozoon in smears, culture or histological section. As parasites are not easily found the Leishmanin test is of value. In this an antigen prepared from a culture of leishmaniae is used and 0·1 ml of this is injected intradermally. A positive case will show erythema and induration at the site of the injection after 48 hours.

**Treatment.** Purely cutaneous disease may be successfully treated by sodium stibogluconate given as recommended for visceral leishmaniasis (p. 816) but in established espundia amphotericin (p. 882) may be necessary.

## African Trypanosomiasis (Sleeping Sickness)

African sleeping sickness is caused by trypanosomes conveyed to man by the bites of infected tsetse flies of either sex. The disease is naturally acquired only in Africa between 12°N and 25°S. Two trypanosomes affect man, *Trypanosoma* (*Trypanozoon*) *brucei gambiense* conveyed by *Glossina palpalis* and *G. tachinoides* and *T.(T.)b.rhodesiense* transmitted by *G. morsitans*, *G. pallidipes*, *G. swynnertoni* and *G. palpalis*. Gambiense trypanosomiasis has a wide distribution in West and Central Africa reaching to Uganda and Kenya; rhodesiense trypanosomiasis is found in parts of East and Central Africa. In West Africa trypanosomiasis is mainly at the riverside, where the fly rests in the shade of trees. Animal reservoirs of *T.(T)b.gambiense* have not been identified although pigs may harbour it. *T.(T.)b.rhodesiense* has a large reservoir in numerous wild animals and transmission takes place in the shade of woods bordering grasslands. Devastating epidemics of both types have occurred. Trypanosomiasis of cattle, caused mainly by *T.(T.)b.brucei*, is also widespread and seriously reduces grazing land and the production of meat and milk.

**Pathological and Clinical Features.** Only a low percentage of tsetse flies are infected. A bite by a tsetse fly is painful and commonly becomes inflamed but, if trypanosomes are introduced, the site of the bite may again become painful and swollen about 10 days later, ('trypanosomal chancre') and the regional lymph nodes enlarge. Within 2 to 3 weeks of infection the trypanosomes invade the blood stream. In gambiense infections the disease usually runs a slow course over months or years with irregular bouts of fever and enlargement of lymph nodes. These are characteristically firm, discrete, rubbery and painless and are particularly prominent in the posterior triangle of the neck. Sometimes during these early weeks transient circinate erythematous eruptions can be seen and there is tachycardia. The spleen and liver may become palpable. After some months, in the absence of treatment, the central nervous system is invaded. This is shown clinically by headaches and changed behaviour, insomnia by night and sleepiness by day, mental confusion and eventually tremors, pareses, wasting from inanition, coma and death. The histological changes in the brain are similar to those found in viral encephalitis but trypanosomes are scattered in the substance of the brain and large mononuclear (morula) cells are found whose cytoplasm is eosinophilic and contains globules of IgM.

In rhodesiense infections fever is higher and more constant than in gambiense infections, so that within a few weeks the patient is usually severely ill and may have developed pleural effusions and signs of myocarditis or hepatitis. Enlargement of lymph nodes is usually less than in gambiense infections. The clinical manifestations of involvement of the nervous system may not be obvious but within a few weeks of infection the cerebrospinal fluid will be abnormal and in the untreated case death ensues from toxaemia or heart failure. If the illness is less acute, drowsiness, tremors, and coma may be prominent.

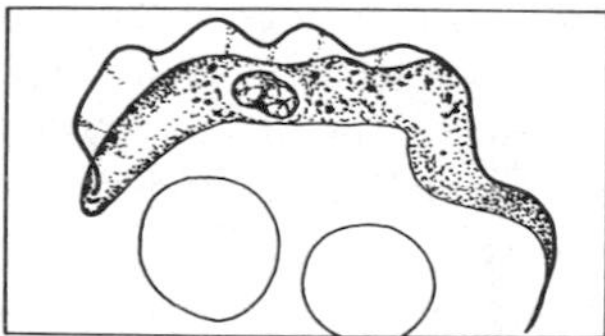

Fig. 17.5 Trypanosome in blood film

**Diagnosis.** In any febrile patient from an endemic area trypanosomiasis should be considered. In rhodesiense infections the trypanosomes can often be detected by microscopic examination of a wet blood film in which agitation of red cells by the trypanosomes is seen. Thick and thin blood films stained as for the detection of malaria, will reveal trypanosomes (Fig. 17.5). In the earliest stages of gambiense infections the trypanosomes may be seen in the blood or from puncture of the primary lesion but it is usually easier to demonstrate them by puncture of a lymph node. Using a medium sized dry needle, the node, held between finger and thumb, is punctured and the node moved on the needle and the material aspirated and examined in a similar way to the blood. Concentration methods include microhaematocrit, buffy coat microscopy and miniature anion exchange chromotography. Animal inoculation is sometimes used for the detection of rhodesiense infections. Serological tests are also employed. If the central nervous system is affected the cell count and protein content of the cerebrospinal fluid are increased and the glucose diminished and sometimes trypanosomes may be found by centrifugation. Except in cases with undoubted established neurological abnormalities, lumbar puncture should be deferred until the first dose of a trypanocidal drug has been given. This will reduce the risk of implantation of trypanosomes into the cerebrospinal fluid by the lumbar puncture needle.

Very high levels of serum IgM or the presence of IgM in the cerebrospinal fluid are suggestive of trypanosomiasis.

**Treatment.** If treatment is begun early, before the brain has been invaded, the prognosis is good. For this purpose either suramin or pentamidine isethionate may be used, the latter being employed only for gambiense infections. After the nervous system is affected an arsenical will be required to penetrate into the brain.

*Suramin* is usually given intravenously. An initial trial dose of 200 mg is given to test for sensitivity. This is followed on the next day by 1 g dissolved in 10 ml of distilled water repeated at intervals of 3 to 5 days to a total dosage of 5 to 10 g. Children are given doses according to weight. Toxic effects include dermatitis, nausea, vomiting, peripheral neuritis and nephritis. The urine should be examined before each injection and the drug temporarily discontinued if red cells and casts appear.

*Pentamidine isethionate* is less toxic than suramin. It is rather painful when administered intramuscularly but intravenous administration causes profound hypotension. The intramuscular dose is 3 to 5 mg/kg body weight to a maximum of 250 mg dissolved in 5 ml distilled water, on alternate days for 10 injections.

*Melarsoprol* is a chemical combination of the trivalent melarsan oxide and dimercaprol. It is presented as a 3·6% w/v solution in glycolpropylene and is administered intravenously. It has proved highly efficacious in advanced rhodesiense infections, which were formerly fatal, and for other resistant and relapsing cases. The main danger is encephalopathy due to a Jarisch-Herxheimer reaction following the death of many trypanosomes and encephalopathy due to arsenic which kills 10% of cases. Before commencing treatment with melarsoprol the patient's general condition may be improved by a few preliminary injections of suramin. The initial dose of melarsoprol is assessed on the patient's general condition rather than on the weight. Patients who are severely ill may only tolerate 0·5 ml and the initial dose must never exceed 2 ml. Further injections are given on the second and third days. The maximum dose is 3·6 mg/kg body weight, i.e. 5 ml for a man of 50 kg. There then follows a rest period of 1 to 2 weeks followed by a second series of three injections. If the initial dose was very small, additional courses may be required during the next 4 or 5 weeks. The total dosage aimed at is 30 ml.

*Nitrofurazone* is liable to produce haemolytic anaemia in those whose red cells are deficient in G6PD and peripheral neuritis, but it has been used successfully in cerebral trypanosomiasis in a dose of 10 mg/kg body weight t.i.d. for 10 days.

**Prevention.** Against *T.(T.)b.gambiense* a single intramuscular injection of 250 mg pentamidine gives protection for six months because of the slow excretion of the drug. As the protection against *T.(T.)b.rhodesiense* is less sure and shorter in duration, chemoprophylaxis is not advised in rhodesiense areas. In such areas it is safer to have no protection but to ensure early recognition of the 'trypanosomal chancre' and to have the blood examined whenever there is any fever. In endemic gambiense areas various measures may be taken against tsetse flies and field teams detect and treat early human infections. In rhodesiense areas control is more difficult.

## American Trypanosomiasis (Chagas' Disease)

The cause of Chagas' disease is *Trypanosoma* (*Schizotrypanum*) *cruzi* transmitted to man from the faeces of a reduviid bug in which the trypanosomes have a cycle of development before becoming infective to man. The bugs are liable to fly down from the ceilings of primitive houses on to the faces of those sleeping below. Infected faeces from the bug are rubbed in through the conjunctiva, mucosa of mouth or nose or through an abrasion of the skin. Dogs and cats are the sources of infection for bugs in houses although in nature opposums and armadillos are commonly infected. Acute illness has also followed transfusion of infected blood.

The trypanosomes travel by the blood stream and develop into amastigote forms in the tissues. These multiply in many sites, e.g., in the myocardium causing pseudocysts, in the muscle fibres, and also in the nervous system, giving rise to the changes described below. Chagas' disease occurs widely in South and Central America.

**Clinical Features.** The entrance of *T.(S.) cruzi* through an abrasion produces a dusky-red firm swelling with enlargement of regional lymph nodes. A conjunctival lesion, though less common, is more characteristic; the unilateral firm reddish swelling of the lids may close the eye and constitutes 'Romana's sign'. Young children are most commonly affected. Evidence of a generalised infection soon appears, with fever, generalised lymphadenopathy and enlargement of the spleen and liver. Neurological features include insomnia, personality changes and signs of meningo-encephalitis. Most survive but may later develop features of the chronic infection. Indeed in most cases the early infection is silent. Only infants die readily from the acute infection, death being caused in the first few days of the illness by encephalitis or a few weeks later by myocarditis or overwhelming infection. Chronic infections frequently damage Auerbach's plexus with resulting dilatation of various parts of the alimentary canal, especially the colon and oesophagus. Dilatation of the bile ducts and bronchi are also recognised sequelae. Invasion of the myocardium causes a cardiomyopathy characterised by cardiac dilatation, arrhythmias, partial or complete heart block and sudden death.

**Diagnosis.** In the acute illness *T.(S.) cruzi* may be seen in a blood film; in chronic disease it may be recovered by xenodiagnosis. In the latter method infection-free, laboratory-bred, reduviid bugs are fed on the patient and subsequently the hind gut or faeces of the bug are examined for parasites. Complement-fixation and fluorescent antibody tests are positive in 95% of cases.

**Treatment and Prevention.** Nifurtimox, a nitrofurantoin, given orally, is used in treatment. The dosage, which has to be carefully supervised to minimise toxicity while preserving parasiticidal activity, is: under 10 years, 15–20 mg/kg body weight and 10–17 years, 12·5–15 mg/kg for 90 days; over 17 years, 8–10 mg/kg for 120 days. Cure rates of 80% in acute disease and 90% in chronic disease are obtained. Temporary side-effects include anorexia, nausea, vomiting and epigastric pain; insomnia, headache, vertigo and excitability; myalgia and arthralgia.

Preventive measures include improved housing and destruction of reduviid bugs by spraying of houses with lindane (gamma BHC).

## Toxoplasmosis

Toxoplasmosis is caused by *Toxoplasma gondii*, a small protozoon. It is probable that human infection after birth results from the ingestion of cysts excreted in the faeces of infected cats. Transmission from a mother infected during pregnancy to the fetus causes congenital toxoplasmosis. Human toxoplasmosis is worldwide.

**Pathology.** In the congenital form the organism is widespread in the central nervous system, eyes, heart, lungs and adrenals. If the infant survives, the parasite soon disappears from most organs except the central nervous system and retina. The brain shows large areas of necrosis with cyst formation and patchy calcification; the spinal cord may be similarly affected. In the acquired disease the organism commonly invades lymph nodes and spleen and less commonly liver and myocardium.

**Clinical Features.** The manifestations in congenital infections are mainly cerebral. There may be hydrocephalus or microcephaly associated with convulsions, tremors or paralysis with resultant contractures. Radiological examination may show patches of calcification in the brain. Microphthalmos, nystagmus and chorioretinitis are common. The cerebrospinal fluid is often xanthochromic with increased protein and mononuclear cells. An enlarged liver, jaundice, diminished thrombocytes and purpura may also be found. Congenital infections are usually fatal, and if the child survives it is usually gravely incapacitated.

Many acquired infections are symptomless. In the acute form there may be pneumonia with fever, cough, generalised aches and pains, profound malaise, a maculopapular rash and rarely jaundice and myocarditis. In the more chronic infections, often afebrile, there may be only enlargement of the lymph nodes with a lymphocytosis showing atypical mononuclear cells similar to those present in infectious mononucleosis. Toxoplasmosis is recognised as a cause of chorioretinitis and uveitis in adults.

**Diagnosis.** In congenital toxoplasmosis the neurological signs and symptoms suggest the diagnosis. The mothers from whom the infection is transmitted have symptomless infections. Serological tests are of value. Antibodies detectable by fluorescence or the dye test appear early in the disease and persist for years. Complement fixing antibodies are late to appear and decline more quickly. A rise in titre indicates acute infection. Antibodies may not be detectable in adult ocular toxoplasmosis. Biopsy material from a lymph node may be inoculated into a laboratory animal, or show characteristic histological changes.

**Treatment.** A combination of a sulphonamide 1 g 6-hourly and pyrimethamine 25 mg daily for 2 weeks should be administered in all active cases. If this fails tetracycline (250 mg 6 hourly) is given for four weeks. For uveitis and choroidoretinitis corticosteroids are given in addition.

## DISEASES DUE TO BACTERIA, SPIROCHAETES AND SPIRILLA

1. *Bacteria; Granuloma inguinale*; *Bartonellosis*; *Melioidosis*; *Leprosy*; *Mycobacterial Ulcer*; *Cholera*; *Anthrax*; *Plague*; *Tularaemia*; *Chancroid*.
2. *Spirochaetes*; *Yaws*; *Endemic (non-veneral) Syphilis*; *Pinta*; *Relapsing Fevers*.
3. *Spirilla and Streptobacillus*; *Rat-bite Fever(s)*.
4. *Mixed spirochaetal and bacterial*; *Tropical Ulcer*; *Cancrum Oris*.

## 1. Diseases due to Bacteria

### Granuloma Inguinale

Granuloma inguinale is a widely spread venereal disease due to *Donovania granulomatis*, characterised by intracellular Donovan bodies, 1 to 2 microns in size, demonstrable in the endothelial and mononuclear cells of the lesion.

**Pathological and Clinical Features.** The incubation period varies from a few days to 3 months. The primary lesion is a small nodule or papule in the skin or mucous membrane of the external genitalia, which progresses to form a superficial serpiginous ulcer spreading peripherally. Autoinfection of an opposing surface also extends the spread to warm areas of the body, particularly the flexures of the thighs, the perineum and gluteal cleft. The face and mucous membrane of the mouth may also be affected. Untreated, the lesions may continue for years, spreading at the periphery and leaving an unhealthy scarred area which tends to break down.

Fibrosis may lead to scarring and stenosis of the urethra, anus or vagina. The lymph nodes, however, are not affected, and constitutional symptoms are slight or absent. A few cases of generalised infection have been reported.

The detection of Donovan bodies in stained smears of deep scrapings is diagnostic.

**Treatment.** Streptomycin 1 g daily for 7 to 14 days intramuscularly or tetracycline 500 mg 6 hourly for 10 days orally is the treatment of choice. Surgery may be needed to alleviate the effects of scarring.

### Bartonellosis

*(Carrión's Disease, Oroya Fever, Verruga Peruana)*

This disease is caused by *Bartonella bacilliformis*, transmitted by sandflies. It is prevalent in narrow hot valleys on the western slopes of the Andes at heights between 2000 and 10 000 ft (600–3000 m), in Peru, Ecuador, Bolivia, Colombia and Chile.

**Pathological and Clinical Features.** In the acute form of the disease, Oroya fever, there is severe haemolysis. Bartonellae are present in large numbers in the erythrocytes and also in the endothelial cells lining small blood vessels. In the later stage of the disease, verruga peruana, cutaneous nodules form, microscopically resembling haemangiomas but containing scanty bartonellae in the endothelial cells.

After an incubation period of 14 to 21 days fever and haemolysis develop suddenly, accompanied by pains in muscles and joints, nausea, vomiting and diarrhoea, delirium or coma. The spleen and liver are enlarged and tender. Untreated the mortality in the acute form of the disease, especially prevalent in children, is over 90%. Secondary infection by salmonellae is a frequent cause of death.

The cutaneous form, verruga peruana, usually follows 30 to 40 days later. The eruption consists of crops of cherry-red haemangioma-like cutaneous nodules 2 to 10 mm in diameter. They are distributed peripherally on the head and limbs and occasionally on the mucosa of the mouth and pharynx and heal in 2 to 3 months.

The diagnosis is confirmed by the demonstration of bartonellae in the erythrocytes, blood cultures or skin lesions.

**Treatment and Prevention.** In the early febrile stage penicillin, streptomycin or tetracycline for five days give good results. Blood transfusions, fluids and electrolytes may be urgently required. The use of insecticides, insect repellants and sleeping under fine mesh nets are advisable for personal protection.

## Melioidosis

Melioidosis is caused by *Pseudomonas pseudomallei*, a mico-organism closely related to *Ps. mallei*, the cause of glanders, which is a rare disease of horses and grooms. *Ps. pseudomallei* is found in puddles following recent rain which indicates it may be saprophytic in nature. Observations suggest that many infections are acquired through abrasions of the skin. Diabetics and patients with severe burns are particularly vulnerable to infection.

The disease is commonest in the Far East and S.E. Asia and occurs rarely in India, Africa, Australia and America.

**Pathological and Clinical Features.** A bacteraemia is followed by the formation of abscesses in the lungs, liver and spleen. In the majority there are high fever, prostration and signs of pneumonia, with enlargement of the liver and spleen and sometimes dysenteric symptoms. A chest radiograph resembles that of acute caseous tuberculosis. In more chronic forms multiple abscesses also recur in subcutaneous tissue and bone.

Culture of blood, sputum or pus may yield *Ps. pseudomallei*. Except in fulminating infections, antibodies, which are common also to those produced in glanders, may be detected by agglutination and complement-fixation tests. A haemagglutination test is more sensitive and is specific for *Ps. pseudomallei*.

**Treatment.** In acute cases prompt treatment, without waiting for cultural confirmation, with tetracycline 3 g daily and chloramphenicol 3 g daily, in divided doses, is life-saving. Treatment is maintained for weeks or months until cavities have healed.

## Leprosy

Leprosy is a chronic granulomatous disease caused by *Mycobacterium leprae*, an acid- and alcohol-fast bacillus which has a very slow multiplication time of 21 days. It is one of the most seriously disabling and economically important diseases of the world and it is estimated that 20 million people are affected. Growth of *Myco. leprae* in artificial media has not yet been achieved but thymectomised and irradiated mice, and the armadillo, are proving useful models of the disease. Local multiplication of the organism in the foot-pads of mice is proving a most useful technique for demonstrating the identity and viability of *Myco. leprae* and the existence of drug-resistant strains, for the screening of drugs and for studying vaccines. The most important mode of spread of *Myco. leprae* is by droplets from the sneezes of lepromatous patients whose nasal mucosa is heavily infected. It is not certain whether the organism enters by inhalation or through the skin. The incubation period is usually between 2 and 5 years.

The disease is common in tropical Asia, the Far East, tropical Africa, Central and South America, and in some Pacific Islands. It is still endemic in southern Europe, North Africa and the Middle East.

**Pathology.** The organisms show a predilection for nerve tissue, skin and the mucosa of the upper respiratory tract. The reaction of the host to their presence varies widely. The early infection, usually transient and self-healing, is called '*indeterminate*'. The histological appearances in it are non-specific. If the infection does not heal it develops into one of the determinate types, whose features reflect the balance between the host cell-mediated immune response and bacillary multiplication.

In *tuberculoid leprosy* there is a marked tuberculoid response, indicative of vigorous cell-mediated immunity, around nerves, sweat glands and hair follicles. Caseation does not occur except occasionally in a nerve. Organisms are scanty, and found mainly in the vicinty of terminal nerve endings in the dermis. They are seen only after prolonged search or by the use of concentration techniques. Tuberculoid leprosy is probably non-infective.

In *lepromatous leprosy*, the infective form of the disease, organisms are present in great abundance in the dermis, eventually replacing the normal architecture. They are mainly grouped in 'globi', which are large macrophages, often showing foamy degeneration, containing 50 or more organisms, and found in nerve tissue, the erectores pilorum muscles and the endothelial cells of blood vessels but rarely in the cells of the epidermis itself. They are carried in the blood stream to the peripheral nerves, eye, and mucosa of the nose and upper respiratory tract, the testes and small muscles and bones of the hands, feet and face, in which they multiply.. Nephritis and amyloidosis are common late complications.

In lepromatous leprosy there is no cell-mediated immunity to *Myco. leprae*; the lepromin test is negative and *in vitro* tests of cellular hypersensitivity are negative.

Between these two 'polar' types of leprosy, there is a spectrum of manifestations grouped under the terms '*borderline*' or '*dimorphous*'. The host reaction varies from the near-lepromatous to the near-tuberculoid; it may alter also from time to time in the same patient. *Myco. leprae* are demonstrable in varying numbers. The differing tissue reponse is usually paralleled by the reaction in the lepromin test which after 4 weeks determines sensitivity to an intradermal injection of a sterilised extract of lepromatous tissue. Positive reactions are obtained in tuberculoid leprosy, negative responses in lepromatous leprosy and negative or weak positive responses in borderline leprosy. This test is of no value in establishing the diagnosis of leprosy since positive results are also found in many normal people, but it is useful in helping to classify the disease.

Leprosy may result in severe peripheral neuropathy and its sequelae. The principal mixed nerve trunks of the limbs and face may be severely damaged in their superficial course due to cellular reaction to degenerating leprosy bacilli, rather than to the presence of living organisms.

Any determinate form of leprosy may undergo an acute exacerbation or *reaction* which is caused by an episode of acute allergic inflammation. In lepromatous disease the reaction, *lepra reaction type 2*, is due to vasculitis which follows the deposition of immune complexes. In borderline and tuberculoid disease the reaction, *lepra reaction type 1*, is due to a sudden increase in cellular hypersensitivity. Borderline reactions are often accompanied by a shift in the patient's disease in the spectrum, either towards the tuberculoid pole (upgrading) or towards the lepromatous pole (downgrading).

**Clinical Features.** The disease usually becomes manifest insidiously. The most common first symptom is a small but persistent area of impaired sensation or numbness. In other cases the first noticeable feature may be macules, which are usually hypopigmented and erythematous. The disease may also present acutely, in reaction, with neuritis, iritis or erythema nodosum leprosum.

The macule of *indeterminate leprosy* is an inconspicuous lesion 2 to 3 cm in diameter, situated anywhere on the body, exhibiting slight pigmentary and sensory changes. This lesion usually heals spontaneously.

*Tuberculoid* leprosy is characterised by one or a few solitary lesions in skin and peripheral nerves. Skin lesions are macular or raised as plaques or as rings whose flat centres indicate central healing. The lesion is hypopigmented in dark skins, coppery in pale skins, with a well-defined margin. Its surface is dry, often scaly, and usually anaesthetic unless the lesion is on the face. Lesions are of almost any size and occur anywhere on the body, especially on outer surfaces of arms, legs or buttocks. The nerve twig supplying the skin lesion or a large peripheral nerve at one of the sites of predilection may be enlarged e.g. the ulnar nerve above the elbow, the median above the elbow or at the wrist, radial at the wrist, common peroneal in the popliteal fossa, posterior tibial around the medial malleolus, and great auricular across the sterno-mastoid muscle.

The main complications of tuberculoid leprosy follow from nerve damage. Sensory loss permits trauma from pressure, friction, burns and cuts, the effects of which are intensified if there are abnormal pressures from contractures following muscular paralysis. Autonomic nerve damage causes dry skin which cracks easily and heals slowly. Secondary bacterial infection in an anaesthetic, unprotected limb leads to cellulitis, osteomyelitis and gross tissue destruction which produces the deformities with which the disease is still, so unnecessarily, associated. Paralyses result in claw hand and dropped foot from damage respectively to the ulnar and peroneal nerves. A combination of fifth and seventh cranial nerve damage exposes an anaesthetic cornea to trauma and sepsis, so the eye easily becomes blind.

Tuberculoid leprosy tends spontaneously to heal slowly, often without residual disability. Sometimes its course is punctuated by a reaction and occasionally it down-grades into the borderline part of the spectrum.

*Lepromatous* lesions of the skin are described as they progress from early to late, as being macular, infiltrative, diffuse or nodular. Lepromatous macules are numerous, hypopigmented and erythematous. They differ from tuberculoid macules in that they are small, widely scattered on the body, usually symmetrically, and with margins that merge imperceptibly with normal skin. Sensation in them is not impaired. They are often inconspicuous except to the trained eye. As the disease advances, the macular lesions become infiltrated and succulent; in advanced lepromatous leprosy nodular lesions appear, especially on the ears and face, and eyebrows are lost. A less common manifestation of lepromatous leprosy is diffuse symmetrical thickening of the skin, often with thickened lobes of the ear, producing the 'leonine facies'.

Clinical evidence of nerve damage appears relatively late in lepromatous leprosy. Anaesthesia and anhidrosis are first detected in the dorsal aspects of the forearms and lower legs, later in a 'glove and stocking' distribution and eventually over the trunk and face, although the palms, soles, axillae and groins may be spared. Muscular weakness results from bacillary infiltration as well as from nerve damage.

The testes may be destroyed and gynaecomastia ensue. The mucous membranes of the nose, mouth and trachea may ulcerate; necrosis of the cartilage and bones may result in late deformities of the phalanges and of nose and oral cavity and loss of the upper incisor teeth. Adjacent lesions may spread into the eye but, more commonly, this is infected through the blood stream. The most frequent lesions in the eye are miliary lepromata on the iris and superficial punctuate keratitis.

*Borderline or dimorphous leprosy* may present with lesions intermediate in character between lepromatous and tuberculoid, or as a mixture of them. Skin lesions are often bizarre. The eyes and nose are spared. Nerve lesions are more numerous than in tuberculoid disease. Borderline disease is immunologically unstable. If the patient's defences succeed in controlling the infection, the disease will upgrade to tuberculoid and heal, but with severe residual disability. If the defences fail the disease downgrades to lepromatous and the complications of extensive bacillary multiplication are added to those of widespread nerve damage. In either event the patient is liable to undergo reactions.

*Reactions.* Untreated lepromatous leprosy gradually gets worse. Reactions may be defined as episodes of acute inflammation in pre-existing lesions of leprosy. Sometimes a reaction is the first clinical manifestation of the disease. One-half of patients with lepromatous leprosy and one-quarter with borderline lepromatous disease will be likely to suffer *type 2 lepra reactions* at some time during the course of their disease, most commonly in their second year of treatment. These reactions are characterised by fever and the appearance of crops of painful roseolar papules or nodules, called erythema nodosum leprosum, which may necrose and discharge sterile pus, before subsiding. In addition deeper subcutaneous nodules, iritis, orchitis, lymphadenitis, nerve pain and tenderness, and oedema of hands and feet may develop. Such reactions may threaten eyes and nerves and a succession of them may be extremely debilitating.

*Type 1 lepra reactions* in borderline disease are especially common in patients near the tuberculoid pole. They occur spontaneously or may be precipitated by treatment. Skin and nerve lesions become acutely inflamed, painful and tender. Nerve function is rapidly lost, irretrievably so unless the reaction is promptly treated. Rarely lesions in the skin ulcerate and nerves caseate.

**Diagnosis.** Leprosy at or near the lepromatous pole is diagnosed by demonstration of *Myco. leprae* in material obtained by a skin-slit smear. The skin over a lesion and of each ear lobe is pinched between finger and thumb to expel blood, incised with the point of a scalpel and the exposed dermis scraped with the flat of the blade. The tissue juice obtained is smeared on a microscope slide and stained by a modified Ziehl-Neelsen's method. Nasal mucus may also contain the organisms in lepromatous leprosy and this is a good indication of infectivity. *Myco. leprae* are less readily demonstrable in skin smears in borderline disease and are undetectable in tuberculoid disease.

In borderline, and especially tuberculoid disease, the cardinal signs of leprosy are enlarged nerves and anaesthesia. Nerves are usually enlarged at sites of predilection asymmetrically and irregularly: they may be tender. Loss or diminution of sensation, or misreference (the inability to locate accurately the site stimulated) may be detected in a skin lesion or in the distribution of a large peripheral nerve. Biopsy of skin or nerve is seldom necessary.

There are virtually no other diseases with enlarged peripheral nerves; familial hypertrophic neuritis and primary amyloidosis are rare. A peripheral nerve may become thickened by a neuroma or as the result of trauma. Sometimes leprosy presents as a mono- or polyneuritis without skin lesions.

**Treatment** of leprosy lasts for years, even life. The physician must gain the patient's confidence. The patient must understand the disease and its complications, comply and persevere in the treatment and learn to look after anaesthetic limbs, control fear and cope with any stigma that exists in the community. Admission to hospital for a few days is useful to establish rapport and start education.

SPECIFIC CHEMOTHERAPY. The essential features of the available drugs are given in Table 17.3.

Patients with multi-bacillary disease (lepromatous and borderline lepromatous) are

Table 17.3 Main features of drugs available to treat leprosy

| Drug | Dose (mg) | Peak Serum level × MIC | Serum level MIC:days | Bactericidal activity |
|---|---|---|---|---|
| Dapsone | 100 | 100–500 | 4–12 | + |
| Acedapsone | 225 | 16 | 200 | – |
| Rifampicin | 600 | 30 | 1 | +++ |
| Clofazimine | 100 | (Stored in R.E. cells, possible depot) | | ? |
| Ethionamide | 500 | 60 | 1 | ++ |
| Thiacetazone | 150 | 8 | 1 | – |

preferably isolated until they are rendered non-infectious by a few days treatment with rifampicin. Ideally initial treatment should be with three drugs to prevent the emergence of dapsone resistance: rifampicin for six weeks, clofazimine for two years and dapsone for life. Many countries cannot afford rifampicin but even two days treatment will kill over 99% *Myco. leprae* and may prevent dapsone resistance. A cheap alternative is thiacetazone but it is a weak drug and there is cross resistance with ethionamide. The dose of dapsone in children is 2 mg/kg/d.

In many countries where leprosy is endemic clinics are held weekly by paramedical staff and a supervised dose of 300 mg dapsone is given. Toxic effects are rare but include haemolytic anaemia and psychosis. If they develop dapsone is temporarily withheld and resumed at half dosage.

Patients with paucibacillary disease (indeterminate, tuberculoid and borderline tuberculoid) should be treated with dapsone alone for 2, 5 and 7–10 years respectively.

Dapsone resistance is emerging in up to 15% of lepromatous patients treated, often intermittently or in low dosage, for 10–20 years with dapsone alone. It presents as the re-emergence of solitary nodules or as a more generalised relapse. Resistance is confirmed by mouse footpad inoculation, or by supervised full dose dapsone treatment. It is treated either by clofazimine alone, to which no resistance has yet appeared, or by combined treatment with daily ethionamide and rifampicin given on the first two days of each month. Clofazimine is a red-brown dye and gradually colours the skin and all bodily secretions and is therefore not always acceptable to a pale skinned patient. It does however reduce the incidence of lepra reaction type 2.

TREATMENT OF REACTIONS. *Type 1 lepra reactions*, in borderline or tuberculoid disease, causing pain or tenderness in nerves are treated with corticosteroids, such as prednisolone in a dose of 40–80 mg initially, followed by 20 mg daily for a few days until the inflammation is settling, then tailing off the drug over several weeks. Mild reactions, limited to skin lesions, are treated with aspirin 600 mg and chloroquine 150 mg base three times daily or an organic trivalent antimonial, such as stibophen in a dose of 2 ml intramuscularly on alternate days for six doses. Treatment with dapsone is continued.

*Type 2 lepra reactions* in lepromatous patients respond rapidly to thalidomide in a dose of 100 mg four times daily. This drug must never be given to premenopausal women because of its disastrous teratogenic effects. If thalidomide is contraindicated, the other anti-inflammatory drugs are used; reactions threatening nerve damage or extensive skin ulceration or orchitis require systemic corticosteroids. Iritis is a dangerous complication and can usually be managed by local measures, namely the instillation of 1% hydrocortisone drops or ointment (or the subconjunctival injection of a depot preparation of methyl prednisolone), and the twice daily instillation of 1% atropine drops.

MANAGEMENT OF NERVE DAMAGE. In the event of acute paralysis complicating reactional neuritis, the affected limb is splinted, exercised passively each day until function begins to return when active exercises can be added. A patient with an anaesthetic limb must be taught to accept the limitations it imposes, to adjust life accordingly, to inspect that limb daily for trauma or infection and to learn how not to damage it. Tarsorrhaphy helps protect an exposed anaesthetic cornea. Secondary sepsis is treated with appropriate antibiotics and osteomyelitis and its sequelae are managed in the most conservative manner possible. Patients with plantar ulcers are confined to bed, or given crutches or a walking plaster until healing is complete. Shoes must fit and protect anaesthetic feet against trauma and must be made specially if there is added deformity.

**Prevention and Control.** In endemic areas the disease is commonest among intimate contacts of patients, and children and young adults are especially susceptible. *Myco. leprae* is easily spread and two-thirds of contacts undergo subclinical immunising infections within 2 years of regular exposure. Of the small proportion of contacts (about 1%) that develop clinical disease only about 2% will be lepromatous. It is at the moment impossible to identify this small group at risk and logical prophylaxis is impossible. No specific vaccine is available. BCG is of some value, especially in Africa, and should be given to all child contacts of lepromatous patients. Dapsone, in a dose of 5 mg daily, may be given for 2 years to infant contacts of lepromatous patients. Neither measure is a substitute for 6 monthly examination of contacts.

Mass prophylaxis is impossible, but mass treatment and follow-up of all cases identified during a population survey reduces deformity and lowers the incidence of leprosy. With improvement of socioeconomic conditions the disease tends to disappear. The rapid spread of dapsone resistance poses a great problem to existing control schemes.

*Further reading about leprosy:*

Browne, S. G. (1979) *Leprosy in the Bible*, 3rd edn. London: Christian Medical Fellowship.

Bryceson, A. D. M. & Pfaltzgraff, R. E. (1979) *Leprosy for Students of Medicine*, 2nd edn. Edinburgh: Churchill Livingstone.

## Mycobacterial Ulcer

This condition, first accurately described in Australia and New Guinea, later named Buruli ulcer from its frequency in the Nile valley of Uganda, is caused by *Mycobacterium ulcerans*. The epidemiology is unknown. It begins as a single small subcutaneous nodule situated commonly on the leg or forearm. The skin over the centre of the nodule ulcerates and, untreated, the ulcer extends to involve a progressively larger area. Histologically there is much necrosis of subcutaneous fat and *Myco. ulcerans* are abundant in the necrotic tissue in the base of the ulcer.

If suspected before ulceration, the nodule should be excised and healing readily follows. Ulcers require to be excised and skin grafted. Antimycobacterial chemotherapy is disappointing.

## Cholera

Cholera, an acute disease of the gastrointestinal tract, is caused by the contamination of food or drink by strains of *Vibrio cholerae*. There are different serotypes named Inaba, Ogawa, Hikojima and also the biotype El Tor (serotype Ogawa), which since 1961 has become widespread throughout the Far and Near East. It appears to be displacing the classical *V. cholerae* from most areas and since 1970 has caused recurrent outbreaks in Africa. Sporadic infections imported by travellers have appeared in European countries, including Britain, and infection from eating shell-fish has been proved. Formerly thought to be of low pathogenicity, its virulence is now found to be equal to that of other strains. These disease-producing vibrios have to be distinguished from the many non-pathogenic cholera-like vibrios. The most important endemic foci of cholera are in the lower reaches of the Ganges and Brahmaputra rivers. *Vibrio cholerae* usually disappear from the stools of patients within a few days but exceptionally they may persist up to a month after the acute attack and El Tor vibrios rarely continue to be excreted for years. The disease appears to be maintained in endemic areas by very mild infections in a population with a considerable resistance to it.

**Pathology.** Cholera vibrios multiply in the lumen of the small bowel and are non-invasive. They secrete a powerful exotoxin (enterotoxin) which stimulates the adenyl cyclase-adenosine monophosphate pathway of the mucosa, resulting in an outpouring of normal alkaline, small bowel fluid. Severe dehydration follows rapidly even though absorption of fluid by the bowel is hardly impaired. There may be acidosis and depletion of sodium and potassium with attendant complications, of which renal failure is the most important.

**Clinical Features.** After an incubation period of a few hours to 5 days severe diarrhoea without pain or colic, followed by vomiting, usually begins suddenly. Fluid gushes effortlessly from the bowel and stomach. After the faecal contents of the gut have been evacuated the typical 'rice-water' material is passed. This consists of clear fluid with flecks of mucus. In severe cases an enormous quantity of fluid and electrolytes is rapidly lost. This soon leads to intense dehydration with agonising muscular cramps. The skin becomes cold, clammy and wrinkled and the eyes sunken. The blood pressure falls, the pulse becomes imperceptible, and the urine output falls. The patient, however, usually remains mentally clear. Unless fluid and electrolytes are replaced the patient may die from acute circulatory failure within a few hours. With proper treatment, however, improvement is rapid. Rarely anuria persists and may lead to death.

Although this is the classical picture of cholera, the majority of infections cause only a mild illness with slight diarrhoea. Occasionally a very intense illness, 'cholera sicca', occurs in which the patient is overwhelmed by the infection and the rapid loss of fluid into the dilated bowel kills the patient before typical gastrointestinal symptoms appear.

In children under 12 years of age the mortality is higher (15 to 17%) than in adults (4 to 6%). Pulmonary oedema, febrile reactions to therapy, pyrexial convulsions and encephalopathy, tetany, meteorism, hypoglycaemia, hypernatraemia, acidosis and water retention and frequently malnutrition are believed to be the adverse factors in paediatric practice.

**Diagnosis.** During a cholera epidemic the diagnosis is usually easy. It is, however, important that an atypical case should be recognised early so that the outbreak may be brought rapidly under control. Microscopic examination of the stool may detect the characteristic movement of the cholera vibrio. Culture of the stool or a rectal swab is used to isolate and identify the organism. Other diseases such as acute bacillary dysentery, viral enteritis, *P. falciparum* malaria, food poisoning, including *Vibrio parahaemolyticus* infections from eating infected shell fish and certain chemical poisons may produce symptoms like those of cholera. Cholera is notifiable under the International Health Regulations.

**Treatment.** The chief aim in treatment is to maintain the circulation and prevent renal failure by replacement of water and electrolytes; the earlier this is started, the better is the prognosis. A quick clinical assessment of the patient's state of dehydration is made from the appearance of the patient, the pulse, blood pressure and skin turgor. In severe cases or when there is vomiting, fluids are given intravenously. A large needle is plunged into a large vein (the femoral vein can always be quickly found) and the fluid is run in as fast as possible until pulse and blood pressure return. The rest of the estimated deficit is replaced more slowly. If intravenous fluids or apparatus are unavailable, a nasogastric tube is passed and fluid is poured in remorselessly. Vomiting usually stops once the patient is rehydrated and fluid should then be given orally every hour. Patients can be made to drink up to 500 ml hourly. The quantity of fluid required is calculated every 8 hours from the output of urine, stool, vomit and estimated insensible loss which may be as much as 5 litres in 24 hours in a hot humid climate. Total fluid requirements can be in excess of 50 litres over a period of 2 to 5 days. Accurate records are essential and are greatly facilitated by the use of a 'cholera cot' which has a reinforced hole under the patient's buttocks beneath which a graded bucket is placed. The ideal solutions are shown in Table 17.4.

Table 17.4 Ideal solutions for treatment of cholera

| Intravenous | | | Oral | |
|---|---|---|---|---|
| | g/*l* | mmol/*l* | | g/*l* |
| Sodium chloride | 5 | Na 133<br>Cl 98 | Commercial salt (NaCl) | 4·2 |
| Potassium chloride | 1 | K 98<br>Cl 98 | Potassium chloride<br>or citrate | 1·8<br>2·7 |
| Sodium bicarbonate | 4 | $HCO_3$ 48 | Sodium bicarbonate | 4 |
| | | | Glucose | 20 |

Other satisfactory fluids include Ringer lactate (B.P.) or Hartman's solution and Darrow's solution, in which case supplements of potassium are given as 10 mmol/*l* of intravenous fluid or 2–4 g potassium chloride or citrate three times daily by mouth. Isotonic saline is better than nothing but every 2 litres should be alternated with 1 litre of isotonic sodium lactate (18·7 g/*l*) or bicarbonate (14 g/*l*) and added potassium. The presence of glucose in the oral fluid has been shown to promote electrolyte absorption.

The use of correct fluids for replacement has done away with the need for estimation of plasma electrolytes or specific gravity. In children, the elderly, the anaemic and those with underlying heart disease overvigorous intravenous rehydration readily causes pulmonary oedema. Children require most careful attention to fluid balance.

Ringer lactate is the fluid of choice and it is important that the oral fluid contain glucose. Renal failure is managed in the usual way (p. 448).

Three days' treatment with tetracycline 250 mg 6 hourly or furazolidine in a single dose of 400 mg reduces the duration of excretion of vibrios and the total volume of fluid needed for replacement.

**Prevention and Control.** Personal prophylaxis means strict personal hygiene. Water for drinking should come from a clean piped supply or be boiled. Flies must not be allowed access to food. Vaccination with a killed suspension of *V. cholerae* is given in two doses of 0·5 and 1·0 ml 1 to 4 weeks apart but it should not be relied upon to give full protection.

In an epidemic, control of water sources and of population movement are most important. Mass vaccination with a single dose of vaccine and mass treatment with tetracycline are valuable. Disinfection of infective discharges and soiled clothing, the therapeutic use of tetracycline and scrupulous hand washing by medical attendants reduces the danger of spread from treatment centres. It is an international requirement for travellers passing through endemic zones to be in possession of a certificate of vaccination (Table 17.10).

## Anthrax

Anthrax is a disease of domestic animals which become infected by inhaling or ingesting spores of *Bacillus anthracis* passed in faeces. Grazing lands remain infective for years. In man anthrax is an occupational disease of farmers, butchers and dealers in hides, animal hair and wool and handlers of bone meal from endemic areas. In primitive conditions, where skins are used as sleeping mats, for clothing or for carrying water, and where diseased cattle are eaten, anthrax is endemic.

**Pathology.** The primary lesion in man may be in the skin, nares, pharynx, larynx, lung or intestinal tract, from any of which sites the infection may spread to lymph nodes and lead to a bacteraemia and infection of spleen, lungs, meninges and brain. The microscopical changes are those of haemorrhagic inflammation with areas of necrosis and interstitial oedema. There is a neutrophil leucocytosis of the blood and infiltration in the tissues without abscess formation.

**Clinical Features.** The incubation period is usually 1 to 3 days. When the infection is acquired from a skin or hide or from handling or slaughtering an animal, a cutaneous lesion indicates the portal of entry. This usually takes the form of a 'malignant pustule' on an exposed part of the body, commonly the face. It begins as an itching papule which enlarges and forms a vesicle filled with serosanguineous fluid surrounded by gross oedema. The lesion is relatively painless and accompanied by slight enlargement of regional lymph nodes. The vesicle dries up to form a thick black 'eschar' surrounded by blebs. Occasionally there are multiple lesions. In endemic areas patients may exhibit only slight constitutional symptoms and little oedema but in non-immune persons high fever and toxaemia are usual and if the sufferer is not energetically treated an overwhelming bacteraemia may prove fatal. Occasionally there may be no localised pustule but only oedema.

When infected meat is eaten, an ulcer with much surrounding oedema may be seen in the pharynx or more commonly the infection causes a severe gastroenteritis which frequently terminates fatally. Some people, usually of an older age, escape unscathed after eating infected meat, presumably because of previously acquired immunity.

Those who acquire the infection by inhalation, 'wool-sorters' disease', may develop an acute laryngitis or a virulent haemorrhagic bronchopneumonia. Anthrax may also present as meningitis.

**Diagnosis.** The appearance of a cutaneous lesion and the environmental and occupational history should suggest the diagnosis. A stained smear of fluid taken from the edge of a malignant pustule demonstrates the organism, which may be confirmed in an atypical case by culture and pathogenicity tests in mice, rabbits or guinea-pigs. *B. anthracis* is also recoverable from laryngeal and pulmonary anthrax and from the CSF in meningitis. If a group of people who have feasted on an animal which has sickened and died are taken abruptly ill with fulminating gastroenteritis, anthrax should be suspected.

Post-mortem examination is not to be lightly undertaken because of the risk of spreading the infection. *B. anthracis* may be cultured from the faeces. Suspected animal products can be investigated by the use of anthrax immune serum.

**Treatment and Prevention.** Effective treatment consists of giving penicillin to which *B. anthracis* is usually susceptible or tetracycline in combination with streptomycin, in full doses, for 3 to 5 days. In the presence of urgent symptoms, if an anti-anthrax serum of known potency is available, it should be administered intravenously, in a dose not exceeding 50 ml.

The disease is controlled in cattle by slaughter and deep burial of the diseased animal, by the administration of prophylactic antiserum to healthy animals at risk and by annual immunisation with attenuated cultures. Imports from endemic areas should be subject to strict control and sterilisation. A vaccine is used to protect laboratory workers.

## Plague

Plague has been a recurrent scourge of man from ancient times and earned the name of the Black Death. Now it is limited to rodents in the wild with occasional sporadic human cases or local outbreaks. The causative organism, *Yersinia pestis*, is a small bipolar staining Gram-negative bacillus. It is spread between rodents by their fleas and if domestic rats become infected then infected fleas leaving a dead rat may bite and infect man. In the late stages of human plague *Y. pestis* may be expectorated and inter-human spread by droplets, 'pneumonic plague', may result. This condition can also be caused by the accidental inhalation of a laboratory culture or by hunters inhaling dust containing viable organisms from infected wild rodents or fleas. Recent outbreaks have predominantly been in Vietnam and East Africa with sporadic cases in U.S.A. and elsewhere.

**Pathology.** Rarely a vesicle with surrounding cellulitis is evident at the site of the flea-bite. The more usual initial lesion is acute haemorrhagic inflammation in and around the lymph nodes regional to the site of entry of the organisms. Signs of a haemorrhagic septicaemia are seen in all fatal cases, with subpericardial and meningeal haemorrhages. There may be haemorrhagic foci of consolidation in the lungs, enlargement of lymph nodes and spleen and multiple small necrotic foci in the liver. In some severe cases there may be little or no swelling of regional lymph nodes; these are the cases clinically presenting as 'septicaemic plague'. In deaths from 'pneumonic plague' the findings are those of acute congestion in one or more lobes of the lungs and evidence of generalised haemorrhagic septicaemia. Patients suffering from pneumonic plague treated with antibiotics may develop pulmonary abscesses. *Y. pestis* are numerous in all affected organs.

**Clinical Features.** The incubation period is short, 3 to 6 days, but less in pneumonic plague.

*Bubonic Plague.* The onset is usually sudden with a rigor, high fever, dry skin and severe headache. Soon aching and then also swelling at the site of the affected lymph nodes begin. The most common site of the bubo, made up of the swollen lymph nodes and surrounding tissue, is one groin but, according to the site of the biting by the flea, the bubo may instead be axillary, cervical, epitrochlear or popliteal. Some cases are relatively mild but in the majority signs of toxaemia rapidly increase, with a rapid pulse, dilated heart and mental confusion. The spleen is usually palpable.

*Septicaemic Plague.* Those not exhibiting a bubo usually, but not invariably, deteriorate rapidly. Pneumonia and expectoration of blood-stained sputum containing *Y. pestis* may complicate bubonic or septicaemic plague.

*Pneumonic Plague.* The onset is very sudden with cough and dyspnoea. The patient soon expectorates copious blood-stained frothy, highly infective sputum, becomes cyanosed and rapidly deteriorates. Radiographs of the lung show a lobar opacity.

**Diagnosis.** Early diagnosis is urgent. A report of deaths among rats or of human infection should alert all medical personnel. Staining a smear of an aspirate from a bubo with methylene blue will show the characteristic organisms. For confirmation the aspirate or blood can be cultured. A leucocytosis distinguishes septicaemic plague from typhoid fever; blood culture is usually necessary to establish the diagnosis although occasionally the organisms can be seen in a stained blood film. The sputum of a patient with pneumonic plague contains *Y. pestis*. Serological tests show increasing titres of antibodies in convalescence. Plague is notifiable under the International Health Regulations.

**Treatment.** Streptomycin is the drug of choice in the treatment of bubonic plague. The first dose should be 1 g intramuscularly, followed by 500 mg every 6 hours until the temperature has been normal for 24 hours, after which 1 g should be given daily for a further 6 days. Tetracycline has proved to be almost as effective as streptomycin; the initial dose should be given intravenously. The adult oral dose is 1 g every 6 hours for 48 hours or longer, depending on the response. After improvement the dose is reduced to 2 g daily and continued for a further 14 days. The bubo should not be incised unless rupture is imminent. With antibiotic treatment it is uncommon for suppuration of buboes and ulceration to develop. In pneumonic or severe septicaemic plague a combination of tetracycline and streptomycin is administered, intravenously if necessary, or co-trimoxazole in full doses. Full recovery from pneumonic plague may be assisted by postural drainage of lung abscesses.

**Prevention.** Prophylaxis against bubonic and septicaemic plague largely depends on preventing biting by fleas carrying plague. Rats should be prevented access to food. Powders containing 1·5% Dieldrin or 2% Aldrin applied to floors and blown into rat holes kill all the fleas and remain active for 9 to 12 weeks.

For personal protection there are two main types of vaccine, the killed vaccine given in two or three doses, and one containing live avirulent organisms requiring one dose only. Both vaccines cause fever. Booster doses are required after 3 to 6 months. Vaccines are of proved value only in the prevention of flea-borne plague.

In an outbreak unvaccinated contacts and all contacts of pneumonic plague should be protected by tetracycline or by intramuscular streptomycin, 1 g daily, or a sulphonamide such as sulphadimidine 3 to 6 g daily for a week. Patients expectorating *Y. pestis* should be isolated and those attending them should wear masks, protective gowns and gloves.

*Further reading about plague:*

WHO (1970) Expert Committee on Plague 4th report TRS W 477. Geneva.
Ziegler, P. (1969) *The Black Death*. London: Collins.

## Tularaemia

Tularaemia is an infection due to *Yersinia tularensis* transmitted to mammals and birds by the bites of infected blood-sucking flies and ticks. Man may be accidentally infected in a laboratory or while skinning infected wild rabbits or hares. In Norway lemmings are another source. The micro-organisms enter through dermal abrasions, the conjunctiva or mouth. Contaminated water, infected meat and the bites of infected arthropods are less common sources of human infection.

The disease is found in the Americas, Japan, the USSR, and most European countries.

**Pathological and Clinical Features.** Focal areas of necrosis occur especially in lymph nodes, spleen, liver, kidneys and lungs. There may be cutaneous, oral or ophthalmic lesions when infection is by these routes.

The incubation period is from 1 to 10 days. There is a sudden onset of high fever followed by sweating and prostration. After some early remission of the fever, the temperature rises again after a few days and remains elevated for 10 to 15 days but in severe infections there may be no early remission and the fever may last continuously for 3 or 4 weeks. There is a moderate neutrophil leucocytosis. The spleen is sometimes palpable. About 2 days after the onset a lesion develops in the conjunctiva of one eye or in the skin at the portal of entry. Such a site is swollen and painful and accompanied by enlargement of the regional lymph nodes. When the mouth has been the portal of entry a buccal ulcer or inflamed tonsils may be found. Pleuropulmonary and pericardial inflammatory lesions result from inhalation of the organisms or from haematogenous spread. Lymph nodes may remain enlarged for months.

The organism may be isolated by repeated blood culture or guinea-pig inoculation. An intradermal test using killed *Y. tularensis* may be positive as early as the third day and positive agglutination and complement-fixation tests after 10 to 12 days. Antibodies produced by brucellae may also agglutinate suspensions of *Y. tularensis*.

**Treatment and Prevention.** Intramuscular streptomycin 1 g daily for 7 days or tetracycline 250 mg 6 hourly for 2 weeks is usually curative. Masks should be worn in the laboratory and gloves should be used when skinning rabbits and hares in endemic areas. Adequate cooking renders infected meat safe for eating.

## Chancroid (Soft Sore)

This is an important and common venereal disease of the tropics, presenting usually in males since the condition in females is asymptomatic, and difficult to recognise.

The causative organism, *Haemophilus ducreyi*, a Gram-negative bacillus, is 1 to 2 microns in length and is seen in pairs, chains or arranged like fish in shoals. Invasion of the lesions by pyogenic organisms is common.

**Clinical Features.** The incubation period is usually 2 to 3 days. The initial lesion is a small red papule on the mucous or skin surfaces of the genitalia or on the surrounding skin. In a few days painful necrosis, ulceration and purulent discharge appear, and a well-demarcated surrounding zone of erythema develops. Frequently the lesions are multiple from auto-inoculation and are seen in all stages of development. The inguinal lymph nodes may enlarge, soften and suppurate. Malaise and fever may accompany the local signs.

**Diagnosis.** Differentiation is required from syphilis, lymphogranuloma venereum, granuloma inguinale and genital herpes. Scraping or aspiration of material from the lesion may reveal the *Haemophilus* which is, however, often overgrown by secondary invaders. Aspiration of a lymph node may be more successful. Autoinoculation of fluid from the lesion on the scarified forearm produces a swelling in which biopsy will demonstrate a recognisable histology. A skin test using a commercial vaccine (e.g. Dmelcos) is also available.

**Treatment.** It is important not to mask or miss associated syphilis; therefore only local cleansing with saline should be undertaken and an oral sulphonamide administered until four dark-ground examinations have failed to reveal *Treponema pallidum*. Thereafter excellent results will be obtained with tetracycline. Serological tests to exclude latent syphilis should be carried out 3 months after the completion of the course of treatment.

## 2. Diseases due to Spirochaetes

### Yaws

Yaws is a granulomatous disease mainly involving the skin and bones and caused by *Treponema pertenue*, morphologically indistinguishable from the causative organisms of syphilis and pinta. The three infections induce similar serological changes and possibly some degree of cross immunity. Organisms are transmitted by bodily contact from a patient with infectious yaws through minor abrasions of the skin of another person, usually a child. Infection is most likely to take place in huts at night when the temperature and humidity are high and families use communal sleeping mats.

Yaws is still to be found among backward indigenous people. Areas of infection exist in Mexico, Panama, the Northern parts of South America, West Indies, Central, East and West Africa, the Pacific Islands, Malaysia, Burma, Thailand (uncommonly in India and Sri Lanka), and also in Indonesia and the Far East, including China where it extends into temperate zones. The mass campaigns by WHO in 1950–1960 treated over 60 million people and eradicated yaws from many areas.

**Pathology.** At the site of the inoculation a proliferative granuloma develops containing numerous treponemes. This primary lesion is followed by eruptions, the most characteristic being multiple papillomatous lesions of the skin with a histology similar to the primary lesion. In addition there may be hypertrophic periosteal lesions of many bones with underlying cortical rarefaction. All these lesions of 'early yaws' heal without appreciable scarring or deformity unless there has been secondary infection. After a variable interval 'late yaws' may develop, characterised by destructive lesions which closely resemble the gummata of tertiary syphilis and which heal with much scarring and deformity.

**Clinical Features.** The incubation period is 3 to 4 weeks. The primary lesion or 'mother yaw' is usually on the leg or buttocks. The secondary eruption usually follows a few weeks or months later, sometimes before the primary lesion has healed. The most typical are the so-called papillomata, often very numerous, consisting of exuberant tissue covered with a whitish-yellow exudate, and more prolific in the moist flexures and around the mouth. There may be successive crops of lesions. The subject, usually a child, may remain active and unconcerned except for the irritation of the sores and from the flies which they attract. These lesions are highly contagious. Sometimes a pathologically similar lesion erupts through the palm or sole, when walking becomes painful. The resultant gait has given rise to the description, 'wet crab yaws'. The bones of all the fingers distal to the carpus, except the terminal phalanges, particularly in children, may rarify and be surrounded by periosteal deposits. There may be a swelling of a long bone and also of the nasal bones (goundou). The distorted tibia may remain as the 'sabre tibia' but most of the lesions of early yaws will eventually subside. Healing is much more rapid after the administration of penicillin.

*Latent yaws*. Following the spontaneous resolution of 'early yaws' serological changes may persist, to be followed by further manifestations of 'early yaws' or, after an interval of as much as 5 to 10 years, by the tertiary lesions of 'late yaws'.

*Late yaws*. Solitary or multiple nodular lesions develop. They ulcerate and spread superficially and also, in places, penetrate deeply into the underlying tissue. In this way gross disfigurement may be caused with distressing ulceration and deformity. The lesions tend to heal with scarring in one part while the ulcer is extending in another. In addition, in radiographs, localised areas of rarefaction may be shown in long bones with surrounding periostitis. Clinically these present as localised swellings of bones over which tissue may ulcerate giving a picture resembling the gummatous ulceration of tertiary syphilis. Lesions in the hand, skull, nose and palate are common. Gross mutilation making the nose and mouth one open cavity ('gangosa') is one of the most tragic results still compatible with life. Other late lesions include hyperkeratosis with fissuring of the palms and soles 'dry crab yaws', hydrarthrosis, bursitis and juxta-articular nodules consisting of painless, firm, subcutaneous fibrous deposits about the elbows, hips and knees.

Unlike tertiary syphilis, yaws does not affect the internal viscera or the cardiovascular and nervous systems.

**Treatment and Prevention.** Long-acting penicillin is highly effective. Very good results follow the intramuscular administration of 750 mg of procaine penicillin on two occasions at an interval of 1 week. Tetracycline 1 to 2 g daily for 5 days is as successful as penicillin.

With improved housing and increased cleanliness the disease disappears. In few fields of medicine have chemotherapy and improved hygiene achieved such dramatic success as in yaws.

## Endemic (Non-venereal) Syphilis

In certain tropical countries, where lack of hygiene prevails, this treponematosis occurs as a family disease. The causative organisms are regarded as modified strains of *Treponema pallidum*, with which they are morphologically identical but biologically distinct.

Congenital infections are extremely rare and sexual transmission unusual. The common mode of infection is through an abrasion, the disease being transmitted from one child to another and occasionally from a child to a parent. Sometimes it spreads in a closed community by the use of common drinking vessels and possibly mechanically by flies. The poor social conditions in which the disease prevails are similar to those where yaws is found but the clinical lesions resemble those of juvenile syphilis.

In contrast to venereal syphilis the primary lesion is rarely seen, except when a child has inoculated the nipple of the mother during suckling, in which case the lesion presents as an ulcerative papule without regional adenitis. The secondary and tertiary lesions include all the common types of skin and bone manifestations of syphilis but the typical papillomatous lesions of yaws are infrequent. 'Mucous patches' in the mouth, due to superficial ulceration, are common and are often the first sign of endemic syphilis. Visceral and neurological lesions are absent or rare. Serological tests give identical results with venereal syphilis and yaws.

The disease responds to treatment by penicillin in the same way as venereal syphilis (p. 66). In the social conditions in which it is found the treatment of choice is usually a long-acting penicillin. Prevention depends on the development of improved social and economic conditions and the mass treatment of affected communities with penicillin.

## Pinta

Pinta is a clinical and geographic variant of endemic syphilis caused by the related organism *Treponema carateum*. It is endemic in localised areas in Central and South America and in some West Indian and South Pacific Islands.

The incubation period is 14 to 20 days. There is a primary scaly papular lesion on an exposed part, usually the leg. The lesion enlarges slowly, up to 10 cm in diameter and is surrounded by smaller papules. Regional lymph nodes enlarge and like the primary lesion contain treponemes. The second stage is manifest 5 to 12 months later and consists of a generalised eruption of macules and miliary papules, 'pintids', pinkish and slightly scaly. Most of these heal but others coalesce and form hyperpigmented patches, commonly on the face and exposed parts. The secondary lesions may persist for years and may be accompanied by hyperkeratosis of palms and soles. In the tertiary stage the affected patches become atrophic and depigmented. In the second and tertiary stages there are serological changes closely resembling those of syphilis but no effective cross immunity.

Treatment is by a long-acting penicillin (p. 73).

## The Relapsing Fevers

The relapsing fevers are a group of diseases due to infections by spirochaetes of the genus *Borrelia* transmitted by lice or soft (*Argasid*) ticks. The louse-borne *Borrelia recurrentis* infects only man and is not transmitted from a louse to its progeny. This disease appears in epidemics particularly during wars or famine when refugees are crowded together in conditions under which infestation with the human body-louse is frequent and an infected louse is introduced. It may accompany louse-borne typhus. The disease is endemic in Ethiopia from where recently recorded epidemics have probably arisen. Epidemics occur in hot as well as in cold climates.

*Bór. duttoni*, the cause of tick-borne relapsing fever, is transmitted by various species of the genus *Ornithodoros*. Ticks live for years and once infected remain so for life and convey the infection to the offspring. Tick-borne relapsing fever is thus an endemic disease.

## Louse-borne Relapsing Fever

Lice cause itching. Borreliae are liberated from the infected louse when it is crushed during scratching which also inoculates the borreliae into the skin.

**Pathology.** The borreliae multiply in the blood, where they are abundant in the febrile phases, and invade most tissues especially the liver, spleen and meninges. Hepatitis causing jaundice is frequent in severe infections and there may be petechial haemorrhages in the skin, mucous membranes and serous surfaces of internal organs.

In the pyrexial phases free borreliae are demonstrable lying between red cells in a blood film. Thrombocytopenia is marked and liver function is impaired. The urine frequently contains protein and sometimes there is frank haematuria.

**Clinical Features.** After an incubation period varying from 2 to 12 days there is a sudden onset of fever. The temperature rises to 39·5° to 40·5°C and is accompanied by a rapid pulse, headache, generalised aching, injected conjuctivae and frequently a petechial rash, epistaxis and herpes labialis. As the disease progresses, the liver and spleen frequently become tender and palpable and jaundice is common. There may be severe serosal and intestinal haemorrhage. Mental confusion and meningism may occur. The fever ends by crisis between the fourth and tenth day, often associated with profuse sweating, hypotension, circulatory and cardiac failure. There may be no further fever but, in a proportion of cases, after an afebrile period of about 7 days there may be one or more relapses which are usually milder and less prolonged. In the absence of specific treatment mortality may be as high as 40%, especially among the elderly and malnourished.

The organisms are demonstrated in the blood during fever either by dark ground illumination of a wet film or by staining thick and thin films.

**Treatment and Prevention.** The problems of treatment are to minimise the severe Jarisch-Herxheimer reaction which inevitably follows successful chemotherapy and to prevent relapses. The safest treatment is with procaine penicillin 200 mg intramuscularly followed the next day by 0·5 g tetracycline. Tetracycline alone is effective and prevents relapse, but gives rise to a worse reaction. Doxycycline, 200 mg once by mouth, as an alternative to tetracycline has the advantage of being curative also for typhus, which often accompanies epidemics of relapsing fever.

Treatment is followed within a half to 3 hours by a chill or rigor, a brisk rise of temperature to 40–42°C, tachypnoea, tachycardia and often cough, confusion, distress, delirium and, occasionally, convulsions and coma. This phase is rapidly followed by profound hypotension and vasodilatation which may last from 8–12 hours and may be complicated by cardiac failure. The patient must be confined strictly to bed for 48 hours after treatment, carefully observed and managed as complications demand.

Tepid sponging for fever over 41°C, careful attention to hydration, preferably by oral fluids, and prompt treatment of cardiac failure are required.

The patient and his clothing and all contacts must be freed from lice as in epidemic typhus (p. 857).

### Tick-borne Relapsing Fever

This disease, due to *Borrelia duttoni*, is conveyed by a variety of soft ticks and its endemicity is governed by the presence of the vector. In the Mediterranean area *Ornithodoros tholozani* is responsible; in the Middle East, Iran, Afghanistan and India and in the New World there are other vectors. These ticks can become infected from rodents or bats as well as by congenital transmission and man is only an incidental host. In Central and East Africa, however, *O. moubata* is the vector and man is probably the only important mammalian host. The disease in these areas is thus confined to old camp sites, old houses and their immediate surroundings, infested with *O. moubata* infected from man or by congenital transmission. *O. moubata* lives in dried mud floors and the cracks of the walls of huts plastered with mud.

The pathological changes resemble those of louse-borne relapsing fever but with late neurological lesions.

**Clinical Features.** These are similar to those of louse-borne relapsing fever. The febrile bouts, although severe, last usually only for 3 to 5 days, and the apyrexial periods may also be shorter. Relapses are, however, more frequent and may be as numerous as 10. Iritis and neurological complications, including cranial nerve palsies, optic atrophy, localised palsies and spastic paraplegia, may develop during these later relapses.

The methods used in diagnosis are similar to those for louse-borne relapsing fever. *Bor. duttoni* are, however, scantier in the peripheral blood but laboratory animals are readily infected.

**Treatment and Prevention.** As many strains are resistant to penicillin, tetracycline 1 g daily for 7 days is given and the course repeated after an interval of a week. Except for the Jarisch-Herxheimer reaction, good results follow a single dose of 200 mg doxycycline. Ticks can be killed by lindane (gamma BHC) applied to the inside of the walls, floors and across the entrance to houses.

## 3. Other Infections

*(Spirilla and Streptobacillus; Mixed spirochaetal and bacterial)*

### Rat-bite Fevers

There are two rat-bite fevers, one caused by *Spirillum minus*, the other by *Streptobacillus moniliformis*. The latter in addition to being transmitted by a rat-bite has also occurred as an epidemic due to infected milk (Haverhill fever) and in other cases also there has been no known contact with rats or mice. Both infections are worldwide in distribution.

**Pathological and Clinical Features.** The manifestations of both fevers are very similar. In *Sp. minus* infection (Sodoku) the wound usually heals. After 5 to 21 days it suddenly becomes inflamed, indurated, purplish and painful; it may ulcerate and is accompanied by lymphangitis, regional lymphadenitis, leucocytosis, splenomegaly and fever. After a week the local and general reactions subside but recur after a further few days. Periods of fever lasting 24 to 48 hours are followed by a rapid fall of temperature and, without treatment, febrile bouts may continue to recur for weeks and the patient becomes anaemic. A macular or maculopapular dusky red rash, sparse over the trunk and extremities, appears during the febrile phases.

In streptobacillus fever the incubation period is 1 to 5 days. The bite usually heals well but occasionally an abscess forms in the wound. Regional lymphadenopathy is not marked. The general symptoms resemble those of *Sp. minus* infections but there is frequently painful arthritis and it is unusual to have recurrences of fever after the initial bout which only lasts 48 to 72 hours. Sometimes painful swollen joints may be accompanied by a remittent fever suggesting sepsis.

**Diagnosis and Treatment.** *Sp. minus* can be demonstrated in the exudate from the inflamed bite or in fluid aspirated from a lymph node, either by examination under darkground illumination or by inoculation intraperitoneally into an uninfected mouse. Blood inoculated into mice or guinea-pigs will yield *Sp. minus* in the peritoneal fluid 5 to 14 days later. There are serological cross reactions with syphilis. In *Strep. moniliformis* infections specific seroagglutinins are demonstrable after 10 days. A titre of 1 in 80 or a rising titre is considered diagnostic but the serological tests for syphilis are negative. The organism can be recovered from the blood or, more easily, from an effusion into an inflamed joint. Both infections are readily cured by penicillin, streptomycin or tetracycline.

## Tropical Ulcer

Tropical ulcer is a specific infection with *Borrelia vincenti* and *Fusobacterium fusiforme* occuring especially in adolescent males. Minor injury in the presence of undernourishment, poor hygiene and debilitating disease are predisposing factors.

**Pathological and Clinical Features.** The initial lesion of a tropical ulcer is a bleb filled with sanguineous fluid. It may be painful and itchy with some constitutional upset. Soon the bleb ruptures, and a green-grey moist slough is exposed which rapidly spreads in the skin and subcutaneous tissue up to a diameter of 5 cm or more. In a few days these tissues slough and liquefy releasing an offensive discharge. After about a week there is usually no further spread and the necrotic tissue separates, exposing an ulcer. In a chronic ulcer the edges are raised and slope sharply. The damage may be limited to the skin and superficial fascia, but in severe cases deep structures, e.g. tendons, nerves, blood vessels and periosteum, may be invaded. Bone is rarely affected. Tropical ulcers generally affect the parts of the body exposed to trauma, especially the lower third of the leg and the foot. The ulcer is usually solitary.

General constitutional effects of a tropical ulcer are slight, and adenitis is not found except as a result of secondary infection.

The ulcer heals slowly with a tissue-paper-like scar which breaks down easily. Big ulcers lead to scarring and deformity. Epitheloma usually of relatively low malignancy sometimes arises in the edge of a chronic tropical ulcer.

**Treatment and Prevention.** Rest in bed with elevation of the affected part and a generous diet with adequate proteins are important. Local treatment consists in thorough cleansing of the ulcer with hypertonic magnesium sulphate. Procaine penicillin 300 mg i.m., metronidazole 400 mg t.i.d., or tetracycline 2 g daily for 7 days gives good results. Chronic ulcers are excised and grafted. Ulcers over 5 cm diameter also need grafting.

Where tropical ulcers are a risk, abrasions should be cleansed and covered. The provision of a good diet, washing facilities and a first-aid service have abolished tropical ulcers from labour forces on well-run estates.

### Cancrum Oris

Cancrum oris is now rarely observed except in poorly nourished children in the tropics. It is characteristically preceded by an infective illness, especially a severe attack of measles. The pathology is that of a rapidly developing gangrene, beginning inside the mouth and penetrating through the lips and cheek resulting in severe disfigurement. Untreated it frequently causes death. However, with or without treatment, gangrene becomes demarcated and ulceration follows. *F. fusiforme* and *Bor. vincenti* are frequently found in the ulcer.

Penicillin or sulphonamides arrest the infection but do not prevent gangrene of already diseased tissue. The gangrenous area is cleansed with antiseptics. Parenteral fluids, usually including blood are needed. Food and vitamins are best supplied through a nasogastric tube. Subsequently skilled plastic surgery may do much to overcome the hideous defects. Prevention depends on improved nutrition and hygiene in the community and on control of acute infectious diseases.

## DISEASES DUE TO VIRUSES, CHLAMYDIA AND RICKETTSIAE

1. *Viral: Yellow Fever; Dengue; Sandfly Fever; Rift Valley Fever; Kyasanur Forest Disease; Japanese B Encephalitis; Rabies; Lassa Fever; Ebola Fever.*
2. *Chlamydial: Lymphogranuloma Venereum; Trachoma.*
3. *Rickettsial: Typhus fevers; Q Fever; Rickettsialpox; Trench Fever.*

### 1. Diseases due to Viruses

There is a vast number of diseases in the tropics due to viruses. Many are cosmopolitan, like rabies and diseases transmitted by faecal contamination such as poliomyelitis and infective hepatitis and by droplets as in measles and influenza. In addition a large number of viruses pathogenic to man are arthropod-borne, known by the abbreviation 'arboviruses'. The majority give rise to a febrile illness of brief duration, following which there is partial or complete immunity against further attacks. Some, in the non-immune, may be neurotropic, giving rise to encephalitis of varying severity. Others, notably yellow fever, may show viscerotropic activity.

*Arboviruses* are divided into groups on the basis of their antigenic behaviour:

*Group A* causes Eastern, Western and Venezuelan equine encephalitis and Chikungunya, O'nyong-nyong and Semiliki Forest fevers. All these are conveyed by mosquitoes.

*Group B* causes yellow fever, dengue, Japanese B encephalitis, West Nile, St Louis and Murray Valley fevers conveyed by mosquitoes, and also causes Kyasanur Forest disease, diphasic meningoencephalitis, Russian spring-summer fever, louping-ill and Omsk haemorrhagic fever, conveyed by ticks.

*Group C* is limited to South America.

The remaining arboviruses, including those causing sandfly fever, are placed in a number of small groups or are at present ungrouped.

There are over 80 arboviruses known to affect man. Within each group viruses produce common and specific antibodies. Common antibodies produced in response to one virus may protect against others of that group. Although the clinical manifestations in an endemic area may be sufficiently characteristic for a fairly reliable diagnosis to be made of such diseases as dengue, sandfly fever and Kyasanur Forest disease, a certain diagnosis rests upon the isolation of the virus in the early stage of the disease by inoculation of laboratory animals or fertile eggs, or by the demonstration of a significant increase in titre of antibodies in sera taken during and after the illness.

Specimens of blood and serum are sent on ice to a specialised laboratory. The identification of the virus may be a laborious and lengthy procedure but may prove to be of extreme importance, as for example, when the outbreak of Kyasanur Forest disease was differentiated from yellow fever.

Prevention of diseases due to arboviruses at present rests mainly on the control of the vectors, but efficient vaccines against yellow fever and Kyasanur Forest disease are available.

## Yellow Fever

The arbovirus of yellow fever is transmitted to monkeys and man by the bite of an infected *Aedes* mosquito. The virus is in man's blood for 2 days before the onset of fever, for the first 4 days of the fever and exceptionally for longer. The mosquito becomes infective for man 10 to 20 days after ingesting blood containing the virus and remains infective for its life which may be as long as 7 months.

In the forests the virus is conveyed between monkeys by mosquitoes living among the tree tops causing high mortality in monkeys. Man becomes infected by felling trees and being bitten by the mosquitoes. In Africa the mosquito *Anopheles africanus* is the reservoir of infection and transmits the virus to monkeys which develop only transient infections. They may raid plantations near to forests and *Aedes simpsoni*, present in these rural areas, may become infected by biting the monkeys and later infect man. In urban areas the disease is limited to human beings, the virus being conveyed from man to man by *Aedes aegypti* which breeds in small collections of water in the vicinity of human dwellings. Urban yellow fever is endemic especially in Western and Central Africa, but the areas where it is a risk are much more extensive, stretching from the Atlantic Coast south of the Sahara to the Red Sea and Indian Ocean, and south to Angola and Zambia. Yellow fever is also endemic in the jungles of Panama and South America with the exception of Uruguay and Chile. Life-long immunity is conferred by the disease and babies born to immune mothers are protected for 2 to 4 months. The infrequency of overt disease among indigenous people in endemic areas and the results of serological studies suggest that many people acquire immunity from subclinical infections with this and other related arboviruses.

**Pathology.** The main lesions are found in the liver and kidneys but haemorrhages take place into many organs. If the disease has not been rapidly fatal the tissues will be jaundiced. Liver cell necrosis and fatty degeneration are widespread but maximal in the mid-zonal region. Characteristic inclusions, 'Councilman bodies' (p. 392) and 'Torres bodies', are usual. The kidney shows acute tubular necrosis and subcapsular haemorrhages.

**Clinical Features.** The incubation period is from 3 to 6 days. A mild attack consists of a short fever accompanied by proteinuria, with little or no jaundice. The classical attack falls into three phases: the initial fever, a period of calm and a subsequent period of reaction or intoxication. In very severe attacks there is no calm period. Viral activity ceases at the end of the first stage, the pathology and clinical features of the third stage being the result of hepatic and renal dysfunction which are the usual causes of death in yellow fever. The onset of the fever is sudden, sometimes with a rigor. The fever is highest on the first day and then declines. There are severe supraorbital headaches, backache and pains in bones. The face is flushed, the conjunctivae injected and the tongue is coated and its edges are red. The patient becomes prostrated; vomiting may be pronounced and the vomit may contain bile or altered blood. If vomiting persists the prognosis is grave. There is increasing epigastric pain, mental irritability and photophobia. The pulse rate falls more quickly than the temperature, and bradycardia is marked by the third day. This disproportion between pulse and temperature is very characteristic (Faget's sign). There is a persistent leucopenia. The urine contains protein in increasing quantities and, later, casts appear and the volume decreases. At the end of four days the temperature reaches normal and the second stage, the period of calm, is reached. Recovery may now take place without further fever and there is no residual damage.

In more serious cases the third stage, of intoxication, follows after a few hours, the temperature rising but the pulse still remaining slow. Jaundice becomes pronounced and the liver palpable and tender. The urine contains bilirubin and red cell casts. There is bleeding, sometimes profuse, from gums, nose, stomach, intestine and urinary tract; petechiae, conjunctival haemorrhages and ecchymoses in the skin may appear. The patient remains mentally clear and anxious until near death, which is only briefly preceded by coma. The pulse rate increases rapidly in the late stages. In fulminating infections the patient dies within a few days of the onset. Death rarely occurs in those who survive for 12 days. In some outbreaks meningo-encephalitis has been a prominent feature.

**Diagnosis and Treatment.** In an endemic area fever, leucopenia and proteinuria with or without jaundice should suggest the possibility of yellow fever. Viruses may be isolated from the blood in the first few days. There will be a rising titre of antibodies. In fatal cases retrospective diagnosis by histological examination of the liver is important on public health grounds. The disease is notifiable under the International Health Regulations. There is no specific treatment. The patient should be nursed under a mosquito net for the first 4 days of the illness because the blood is infectious. Dehydration should be corrected by intravenous glucose saline and blood transfusions should be given if blood loss is severe. Acute renal failure is treated as described on page 448.

**Prevention.** A single vaccination with the 17 D nonpathogenic strain of virus, available at internationally recognised centres, gives full protection for at least 10 years, the period of validity of the vaccination certificate. Ten days after vaccination adequate antibodies are present in the blood and the certificate of vaccination becomes valid. The vaccine does not produce appreciable side-effects in adults, unless they are allergic to egg protein, when desensitisation may be necessary. Vaccination is not recommended in children under 9 months of age because of a slight risk of encephalitis. No ill-effects have as yet been observed from vaccination during pregnancy.

Only travellers possessing valid certificates of vaccination against yellow fever are allowed to proceed from an endemic area to 'receptive areas', by which is meant countries free from the disease but in which the potential vectors exist. In this way the disease has not yet entered Asia. As an additional precaution mosquito control of airports should be maintained. The urban disease can be eradicated by the abolition of the breeding places of *Aedes aegypti*, by the use of residual insecticides in houses and by mass vaccination in endemic areas. If susceptible mosquitoes are present and the virus persists in forests humans living near are at risk.

## Dengue

Six antigenic variants of dengue virus have been described. It is transmitted to man by mosquitoes, chiefly *Aedes aegypti*. Man is infective to the vector 18 hours before the temperature rises and for at least 3 days after the onset of symptoms. The mosquito can transmit the disease 8 to 12 days after feeding on a patient suffering from dengue and remains infective for life.

The disease is a risk in many tropical and subtropical countries, especially in coastal areas. It is most prevalent during the hot season when the mosquitoes are numerous. One attack usually gives immunity for about 9 months and after several attacks a considerable degree of permanent immunity is attained. Some cross-immunity exists between dengue and other members of the B group of arboviruses, including the virus of yellow fever.

**Clinical Features.** The incubation period is usually 5 to 6 days. The disease varies considerably in its severity. It may be a sharp illness with marked constitutional symptoms and signs lasting for 7 to 10 days or a milder disease resembling sandfly fever. Subclinical infections are common. A prodrome of malaise and headache for 2 days may precede the acute onset, characterised by fever and intense backache and generalised pains especially severe in the orbital and periarticular areas. Painful movement of the eyes, photophobia, conjunctival injection and lachrymation, nausea, vomiting, anorexia, prostration, insomnia and depression are often features of the disease. In severe cases the temperature may remain elevated for 7 to 8 days. An afebrile interval lasting 24 to 48 hours may intervene at the end of the third day when symptoms subside temporarily, to be followed with a recurrence of symptoms and a further febrile period of a day or two ('saddleback fever'). There is bradycardia, cervical lymphadenopathy and leucopenia.

A rash may appear, especially during the second febrile period. It is morbilliform but the colour resembles that of scarlet fever. It usually begins on the dorsum of the hands and feet and spreads up the arms and thighs to the trunk. After the temperature has fallen, depression and prostration often persist.

Since 1956 there has been a series of outbreaks of dengue in South-East Asia, sometimes in association with the Chikungunya virus, in which the disease has been complicated by shock and haemorrhage, with a variable mortality among indigenous children, but reaching 10% of those ill enough to be admitted to hospital. The condition is sometimes called *dengue haemorrhagic fever*. There is an increase of IgE in the serum. Disseminated intravascular coagulation and complement activation which leads to vascular damage are thought to be triggered by hypersensitivity to the virus.

Diagnosis is usually easy in an endemic area when a patient has the characteristic symptoms and signs. However, mild cases may resemble other viral diseases and a severe attack may be mistaken for anicteric yellow fever, but the absence of urinary changes will help to differentiate it. The virus can be recovered from the blood and antibody titres rise.

**Treatment and Prevention.** There is no specific treatment. The severe pains can be relieved by aspirin or paracetamol, but occasionally opiates are required. Blood transfusions and corticosteroids are indicated in the haemorrhagic varieties.

The patient is nursed under a mosquito net. Breeding places of *Aedes* mosquitoes should be abolished and the adults destroyed by insecticides.

### Sandfly Fever

This fever is caused by a small group of closely related arboviruses transmitted by the sandfly *Phlebotomus papatasii* and by other species of this genus. No animal reservoir is known. Man is infective to the vector for 24 hours before and for 24 hours after the onset of the fever. The sandfly can transmit the disease about 7 days after biting an infected person and remains infective for life.

This infection is endemic around the Mediterranean and eastwards into India, Burma and China, especially during the hot dry season. One attack confers immunity for only a few months, so repeated infections are necessary to maintain protection. There is no cross-immunity between dengue and sandfly fever.

**Clinical Features.** After an incubation period, usually of 3 to 4 days, the onset is sudden with a rapid rise of temperature. The symptoms and signs are very similar to those of dengue (p. 845). The fever, however, is usually of shorter duration, up to 3 days, and there is no rash.

In an endemic area the general course of the illness suggests the diagnosis, but a blood film should always be examined to exclude malaria. The virus can be recovered from the blood and antibodies detected.

**Treatment and Prevention.** Treatment is on the same lines as for dengue.

Sandflies are extremely sensitive to insecticides and combined with the use of repellants useful protection is obtained. The ordinary mosquito net sprayed with an insecticide will keep out the tiny sandfly.

### Rift Valley Fever

This disease is caused by a virus which normally infects sheep and goats in East and South Africa. It is usually conveyed by a culicine mosquito, especially *Culex pipiens*. Cattle and other domestic animals may act as amplifying hosts. Sporadic infections have followed direct contact with infected meat and from inhalation. In 1975 an outbreak occurred in South Africa with 12 cases of encephalitis, 4 fatal. Since 1977 there have been large outbreaks in Egypt with four clinical types; uncomplicated fever resembling dengue fever, or fever with retinal changes, with haemorrhages and jaundice or with meningo-encephalitis. Deaths occurred among the latter two groups. There is no specific treatment.

## Kyasanur Forest Disease

The arbovirus responsible for this disease caused a fatal epizootic in monkeys in Mysore State. The vectors are hard (*Ixodid*) ticks, increased numbers of which had been introduced by the grazing of cattle in the area. Human disease, first encountered in 1957, is of great interest as it was at first feared to be an outbreak of yellow fever in Asia and illustrates how changing pastoral activities may lead to unexpected outbreaks of human disease.

The chief pathological lesions are found in the liver and kidneys.

The disease in man may be mild with only a short febrile attack or it may be a severe illness with fever lasting for over a week with great prostration and generalised pains in muscles. Mucosal surfaces may bleed. Some patients may relapse after 9 to 21 days with fever, jaundice and meningism. In fatal cases death is usually due to liver failure.

The patient requires careful nursing; no specific treatment is known. A vaccine has been prepared.

## Japanese B Encephalitis

This arbovirus is transmitted to man by the bites of infected culicine mosquitoes which have fed on infected animals or birds, notably nestling herons. Pigs and other domestic animals are important sources of infection acting chiefly as amplifiers of the virus brought to them by mosquitoes. The virus is widespread in the Pacific Islands from Japan to Guam, in the Philippines, Taiwan, Borneo, Malaysia and Singapore. Devastating epidemics, with a high mortality rate, have occurred. In endemic areas, serological surveys indicate a high incidence of subclinical infection and only sporadic cases may be encountered. Inflammatory and degenerative changes are found in the brain.

**Clinical Features.** Many infections are subclinical but overt disease may occur at any age, although children are particularly susceptible. With the development of encephalitis the patient experiences a very severe headache, fever, often with rigors, and vomiting. The physical signs in severe cases are neck rigidity, congestion of the optic fundi, imperfectly reacting pupils, muscular twitching and tremors; and, in severe cases, progressive coma, muscular rigidity and cranial nerve palsies. The cerebrospinal fluid is under raised pressure and an increase of cells and protein appears within several days. The acute illness may last from a few days to 2 weeks or longer. Convalescence is prolonged and tedious. Persistent neurological damage is a feature only in children and after prolonged illness in adults. The mortality rate in overt disease varies from 15 to 40%.

The virus has only rarely been recovered from the blood or cerebrospinal fluid but in fatal cases may sometimes be obtained from the brain. Increasing titres of specific antibodies in the blood is the usual basis for diagnosis.

**Treatment and Prevention.** There is no specific treatment and the value of corticosteroids has not yet been established. Skilled nursing and aids for the patient in coma, may be life-saving. The elimination of breeding places of the vector mosquitoes, the control of piggeries, and the use of insecticides, where practicable, should be instituted. There is no vaccine available.

## Rabies

Rabies is caused by a bullet-shaped member of the rhabdoviruses. The virus, which causes an encephalitis, affects a wide range of animals and is conveyed by bites and licks on abrasions or on intact mucous membranes. Transmission by droplets in confined spaces has also been demonstrated. In Europe the maintenance host is the fox and in recent years the disease has spread from Poland westwards through Germany and has progressively penetrated through France. Man is most frequently infected from dogs but cats and other animals may be responsible. In the U.S.A. skunks are an important host and may infect man, while in Central and South America vampire bats also cause death of domestic animals and occasionally man. Insectivorous bats only rarely convey the infection.

**Pathological and Clinical Features.** The incubation period, during which the virus is spreading centripetally along axons to the brain, varies in man from a minimum of 9 days to many months but is usually between 4 and 8 weeks. Severe bites, especially if on the head or neck are associated with short incubation periods. Although only a proportion of people inoculated with the virus develop the disease, once it is manifest it is almost invariably fatal. At the onset there may be insidious fever and a return of pain or paraesthesia at the site of the bite. After a prodromal period of from 1 to 10 days, during which anxiety may be increasingly evident, the characteristic fear of water, responsible for the alternative name of 'hydrophobia', becomes evident in many cases. Although the patient is thirsty, attempts at drinking provoke violent contractions of the diaphragm and other inspiratory muscles and thereafter the sight or even the sound of water may precipitate these distressing spasms and attacks of panic. Delusions and hallucinations may develop accompanied by spitting, biting and maniacal behaviour, with lucid intervals in which the patient is acutely anxious. Sedatives may considerably modify this ordeal. Cranial nerve lesions develop and terminal hyperpyrexia is common. Death ensues, usually within a week from the onset of symptoms.

In a small proportion of cases there is an ascending paralysis without mental excitement and these patients survive, on average, 12 days. This type is particularly associated with bites from vampire bats.

During life the diagnosis is usually made solely on clinical grounds but rapid immunofluorescent techniques to detect antigen in corneal impression smears or skin biopsies have been successfully employed.

**Treatment.** Three cases of probable rabies have survived. Intensive care is needed with facilities to control cardiac and respiratory failure. Usually only palliative treatment is possible once symptoms have appeared. The patient should be heavily sedated with diazepam 10 mg 4–6 hourly, supplemented by chlorpromazine 50–100 mg, if necessary. A gastrostomy is the kindest way to give fluids and food. Particularly if there is doubt as to the diagnosis or if the patient has previously received a course of prophylactic vaccine the possibility of recovery should be entertained.

**Prevention.** *Pre-exposure prophylaxis* is required by those who handle professionally potentially infected animals, those who work with rabies virus in laboratories and those who live at special risk in rabies endemic areas. Protection is afforded by two intradermal injections of 0·1 ml human diploid cell strain vaccine, given four weeks apart, followed by yearly boosters.

*Post-exposure prophylaxis.* The wound should be thoroughly cleansed, preferably with a quaternary ammonium detergent or soap, surgically debrided and left unsutured. Rabies can usually be prevented if treatment is started within a day or two of biting. Delayed treatment may still be of value. For maximum protection hyperimmune serum and vaccine are required. The biting animal should be confined, if possible. If it is healthy after five days, it does not have rabies and treatment is stopped. If it dies, or is killed, the brain is examined by immunofluorescence for Negri bodies. If positive, or if the animal escapes, treatment is continued.

The safest antirabies antiserum is human rabies immune globulin. The dose is 20 i.u./kg body weight, once. Half is infiltrated around the bite and half is given intramuscularly at a different site from the vaccine. The dose of hyperimmune animal serum is 40 i.u./kg body weight. Hypersensitivity reactions, including systemic anaphylaxis are common. The safest vaccine, free of complications, is human diploid cell strain vaccine. 1·0 ml is given intramuscularly on days 0, 3, 7, 14, 30 and 90. Of the older vaccines, the Semple-type, containing killed virus, is potent and widely available. It causes a serious neuro-paralytic accident in one in 1600 recipients. The dose is 5 ml subcutaneously into the anterior abdominal wall, daily for 14 days, with boosters 10, 20 and 90 days later. The duck embryo vaccine is safer (one accident in 30 000) but less reliably potent. Where human products are not available and when risk of rabies is slight (licks on the skin, scratches or abrasions, or minor bites of covered arms or legs) it may be justifiable to delay starting treatment up to 5 days while observing the confined animal or awaiting examination of its brain.

Human rabies is an infrequent disease even in endemic areas. Its fearful manifestations, however, justify stringent attempts being made to prevent its spread. In endemic areas household dogs should have a yearly dose of a Flury canine (live) vaccine, and stray dogs killed. Importation of all animals into uninfected countries should be strictly controlled, with isolation in quarantine for a minimum of 6 months. Vigilance and appropriate measures of control over infected maintenance hosts, such as the fox, are urgently required where areas of endemicity are extending.

*Further reading about rabies:*

Symposium on Rabies (1976) *Transactions of the Royal Society of Tropical Medicine and Hygiene*, **70**, 175–205.

WHO Expert Committee on Rabies (1973) *Technical Report Series*. World Health Organization, **523**, 6th report.

## Lassa Fever

This disease, first observed in 1969, is due to an arenavirus, a group which also includes the viruses responsible for Argentine and Bolivian haemorrhagic fevers. Recognised outbreaks have so far been limited to subsaharan West Africa. The natural reservoir is the multi-mammate rat and spread is probably through urine. The mode of human infection is unknown but case to case transmission in hospital occurs through direct inoculation and possibly inhalation.

**Clinical Features.** The disease has the general features of a viral infection, high fever, intercostal myalgia, bradycardia, a low blood pressure and leucopenia. Adherent yellow exudates on the pharynx are particularly characteristic. The fever lasts between 7 and 17 days. In severe cases liver failure, shock and electrolyte imbalance develop. Mortality rates of overt infections have varied from 36% to 52% but mild and subclinical infections also occur.

The virus has been isolated in special laboratories from serum, pharynx, pleural exudate and urine but diagnosis will usually be established from 'paired sera', the later specimens being taken 6–8 weeks after the onset of infection. The diagnosis should be considered in Britain in patients presenting with fever within 10 days of leaving West Africa.

**Treatment and Prevention.** Strict isolation and general supportive measures, preferably in a special unit, are required. There is no proved specific therapeutic measure. The administration of convalescent immune plasma has been followed by recovery and is therefore recommended for prophylaxis after accidental exposure to infection.

### Ebola Fever

In Marburg, West Germany, in 1967 a severe infectious illness broke out among laboratory workers who had handled tissues from a batch of green monkeys imported from Uganda. In 1976 outbreaks of the disease occurred in Sudan and Zaïre from a focus on the Ebola River. The viruses causing these two outbreaks have a unique identical structure but are antigenetically distinct. Sporadic cases have occurred elsewhere in Africa. The natural animal reservoir of these viruses is not known nor is the usual mode of spread, but man-to-man transmission can take place. In these outbreaks the mortality has varied from 25% of treated patients to over 90% in the untreated, but successive human passage seems to reduce virulence.

After an incubation period of 5 to 9 days, the illness presents suddenly with fever, severe myalgia and diarrhoea. By the fourth or fifth day the fauces become inflamed and a bright red, follicular rash appears on the extensor surfaces of the limbs; it spreads to the trunk and face, becomes maculopapular and finally confluent and livid. There may be lymphadenopathy. About the sixth day, in severe cases, bleeding associated with thrombocytopenia starts usually in the gastrointestinal tract. The virus also attacks the brain, kidneys and lungs. Fatal complications, often between the sixth and tenth days of the illness, include haemorrhage, secondary infection, encephalitis, renal failure and pneumonia.

Treatment consists of supportive measures, replacement of blood and the management of complications. Immune plasma may be beneficial if given at an early stage. No vaccine is available.

### Haemorrhagic Fever with Renal Syndrome

This disease, formerly called epidemic haemorrhagic fever, is attributable to a virus, although confirmation of its successful isolation is still awaited. Outbreaks occurred in Manchuria and Korea and a similar disease has been reported from Scandinavia and the U.S.S.R. There is a close association with small mammals, in particular bank voles, and it has been established that man becomes infected by droplets without the intervention of an arthropod vector.

The main changes arise from increased capillary fragility. Thus there are widespread internal haemorrhages and leakage of plasma.

**Clinical Features.** After an incubation period of 12 to 16 days there is a sudden onset of high fever. After about 5 days the temperature falls, and the second or toxic stage begins; haemorrhages now take place into the skin and from mucous membranes. The urine contains red cells, casts and a large amount of protein. Anuria may threaten. The leucocyte count, low in the early stages, rises, at first with primitive granulocytes and later with primitive lymphocytes, resembling leukaemia. The platelet count is diminished and there is a prolonged bleeding time. Death may ensue in this stage but in favourable cases convalescence begins towards the end of the second week, with a plentiful flow of urine of low specific gravity, free from protein and casts. Full recovery is usual but very slow and polyuria may continue for some months.

In an endemic area the diagnosis is suggested by the characteristic clinical signs and the successive changes in the blood.

**Treatment.** The disease is managed symptomatically. Oliguria and anuria are treated as advised for acute renal failure (p. 448).

## 2. Diseases due to Chlamydia

### Lymphogranuloma Venereum

Lymphogranuloma venereum is caused by a member of the genus *Chlamydia* which also includes the causative organisms of psittacosis-ornithosis (p. 244) and trachoma. The disease is sexually transmitted and is widely distributed in the tropics, especially in seaports. The primary herpetiform lesion is small and very superficial. The infection passes from the primary lesion to the regional lymph nodes and there forms a granuloma with necrosis, abscess formation and surrounding fibrosis.

**Clinical Features.** An evanescent genital lesion appears 1 to 4 weeks after infection. The draining lymph node and then other local nodes enlarge and become matted together, tender and adherent to the deep tissues and overlying skin. There may be fever and loss of weight. Thick glairy fluid is eventually discharged through the skin by numerous small sinuses. Healing is very slow and often associated with marked scarring. The infection may spread to the other groin and to pelvic lymph nodes.

Sinus formation from pelvic nodes damages surrounding structures with extremely serious and disabling results. Fistulae may form between the rectum, vagina and urethra, and ulcerative proctitis may cause stricture of the rectum. In the female obstruction to the lymphatics may lead to elephantiasis of the external genitalia, a condition called 'esthiomene'.

It is not normally possible to demonstrate the organism. Immunodiagnosis is by a complement fixation test.

**Treatment.** Rest in bed is important. Many cases respond well to 4 g sulphadimidine daily in divided dose for 14 days. Alternatively tetracycline 2 g daily for 14 days may be used. Chronic cases require much longer chemotherapy. Inguinal nodes may require aspiration but should not be incised. When extensive sinuses have formed, complete excision of the mass of inguinal nodes may be required. Severe pelvic complications and rectal stricture require surgery.

### Trachoma

Trachoma is a specific communicable keratoconjunctivitis caused by *Chlamydia trachomatis* and characterised by follicles, papillary hyperplasia, pannus and, in its later stages, cicatrisation. Transmission is usually by contact or from fomites in unhygienic surroundings and some infections occur during birth from infected genital passages.

Vast numbers of people suffer from trachoma in the hot dry dusty areas of the subtropics and tropics but it is also present in Southern Europe, and among immigrants in Britain. The disease varies markedly in incidence and in severity in different geographical areas. In endemic areas the disease is commonest in children.

**Pathology.** The infection lasts for years, may be latent over long periods and may recrudesce. The conjunctiva of the upper lid is first affected with combined vascularisation and cellular infiltration, pannus, spreading to the upper cornea and later to other areas producing corneal opacity and impairment of vision. Cicatricial deformity of the upper tarsal plate is an early feature.

**Clinical Features.** The onset is usually insidious and infection may not be apparent to the patient. Early symptoms include conjunctival irritation, watering, stickiness and blepharospasm. In underdeveloped areas, unless discovered on surveys, the condition may not be reported until vision begins to fail.

The ophthalmic appearances are described in 4 stages (WHO):

*Stage I.* Immature follicles are seen on the upper tarsal conjunctiva including the central area and early corneal changes are usually present.

*Stage II.* Well developed mature soft follicles are present with papillary hyperplasia. Pannus and corneal infiltrates extend from the upper limbus.

*Stage III.* Some or all of the signs of stage II exist with scarring developing, usually from necrosis of follicles.

*Stage IV.* The follicles and infiltrates of stage III have been replaced by scar tissue and the disease is no longer infectious although further changes in the scars may follow. The degree of scarring varies from minimal involvement to trichiasis, entropion, corneal opacities and gross impairment of vision.

Trachoma may also present as an acute ophthalmia neonatorum with secondary bacterial infection.

The early follicles of trachoma are characteristic, but clinical differentiation from conjunctivitis due to other viruses may be difficult at this stage. Intracellular inclusions may be demonstrated in conjunctival scrapings by staining with iodine or immunofluorescence. Chlamydia may be isolated in chick embryo or cell culture.

**Treatment and Prevention.** Local ophthalmic ointment or oily drops of 1–3% tetracycline may be used twice daily for 3 months. In mass therapy in endemic areas such topical application twice daily for 3 to 6 consecutive days each month for 6 months has given good results. An oral sulphonamide daily for 3 weeks is a useful addition to treatment. Deformity and scarring of the lids, corneal opacities, ulceration and scarring require surgical treatment, after control of local infection.

Personal and family cleanliness should be improved. Proper care of the eyes of newborn and young children is essential. The finding of a case, particularly in a child, should lead to examination of the whole family. Population surveys should lead to discovery and treatment of asymptomatic infections. Trachoma clinics are required in areas of high endemicity.

## 3. Diseases due to Rickettsiae

Rickettsiae are natural inhabitants of the cells of the intestinal canal of arthropods. Some species may parasitise higher mammals including man. Rickettsiae are intermediate between viruses and bacteria and require living cells for their multiplication. Infection is usually conveyed to man through the skin from excreta of the arthropods but the saliva of some biting vectors is infected. Transovarian infection in arthropods to the next generation occurs in ticks and mites, which serve as reservoirs as well as vectors of infection.

**Pathological and Clinical Features.** In man rickettsiae multiply in vascular endothelial cells especially of capillaries and other small vessels, producing lesions in the skin, central nervous system, heart, lungs, kidneys and skeletal muscles. Endothelial proliferation, associated with a perivascular reaction (nodules of Fraenkel) may cause thromboses and small haemorrhages. In epidemic typhus the brain and in scrub typhus the cardiovascular system and lungs are particularly attacked.

The rash in epidemic, endemic and scrub typhus is at first central, but in tick typhus it starts peripherally. In Q fever only a sparse rash is occasionally seen. An eschar is often found in tick and scrub typhus and in rickettsialpox, but not in epidemic and endemic typhus or in Q fever. An eschar is a necrotic sore, often scabbed, at the site of the bite and is due to vasculitis following immunological recognition of the inoculated organism. Regional lymph nodes often enlarge. The common clinical findings in this group of diseases are fever, severe prostration, mental disturbance and often a rash.

**Diagnosis.** The Weil-Felix reaction, which is the non-specific agglutination by the patient's serum of the strains of organisms Proteus OX 19 or OXK, helps in the differentiation of human infections (Table 17.5). A fourfold rise in titre is diagnostic.

Species specific antibodies may be detected by complement fixation, microagglutination and fluorescence in specialised laboratories. Rickettsiae may be isolated from the blood in the first week of illness by intraperitoneal inoculation into male guinea pigs, mice or voles.

## Epidemic Typhus Fever

Louse-borne or epidemic typhus is caused by *R. prowazeki* and is transmitted by infected faeces from the human body louse, usually through scratching the skin, or sometimes by inhalation. Patients suffering from epidemic typhus infect the lice, and these leave when the patient is febrile. In conditions of overcrowding the disease spreads rapidly. During interepidemic periods the disease may be maintained by inapparent or latent cases or perhaps by infected fleas and rats.

Table 17.5 Weil-Felix reaction

| Disease | Vector | Weil-Felix Reaction | |
|---|---|---|---|
| | | OX 19 | OXK |
| Epidemic typhus | Louse | +++ | negative |
| Endemic typhus | Flea from rat | +++ | negative |
| Rocky Mountain spotted fever | Tick | + | negative |
| Other forms of tick typhus | Tick | + | variable |
| Scrub typhus | Larval mite | negative | +++ |
| Q (Query) fever | None or tick | negative | negative |
| Rickettsialpox | Mite from mouse | negative | negative |
| Trench fever | Louse | negative | negative |

Although rickettsialpox and trench fever have not been found in the tropics they are included here to complete the group.

**Clinical Features.** The incubation period is usually 12 to 14 days. There may be a few days of malaise but the onset is more often sudden with rigors, fever, frontal headaches, pains in the back and limbs, constipation and bronchitis. The face is flushed and cyanotic, eyes congested, and the patient soon becomes dull and confused.

The rash appears on the fourth to the sixth day and often resembles measles. In its early stages it disappears on pressure but soon becomes petechial with subcutaneous mottling. It appears first on the anterior folds of the axillae, sides of the abdomen or back of hands, thence on the trunk and forearms. The neck and face are seldom affected.

During the second week symptoms increase in severity. Sordes collect on the lips, and the tongue, dry and brown, becomes shrunken and tremulous. The spleen becomes palpable, the pulse feeble and the patient stuporous and delirious. If the patient recovers, the temperature falls rapidly at the end of the second week and convalescence ensues. In fatal cases the patient usually dies in the second week from general toxaemia, cardiac or renal failure or pneumonia.

Common complications are bronchopneumonia, parotitis, venous thrombosis and gangrene of fingers, toes, nose or genitalia. In endemic areas, e.g. Ethiopia, indigenous people may suffer relatively mildly. A mild relapse (Brill's disease) may occur after many years.

**Diagnosis and Treatment.** The clinical features are diagnostic when there is an epidemic of the disease but in mild cases may be much less distinctive. Laboratory aids to diagnosis are discussed on page 853 and treatment on page 856.

## Endemic Typhus Fever

Flea-borne or 'endemic' typhus caused by *R. mooseri* is endemic world-wide. Man is infected when, by scratching, he introduces the faeces or contents of a crushed flea which has fed on an infected rat. The incubation period is 8 to 14 days. The symptoms resemble those of a mild louse-borne typhus. The rash may be scanty and transient. Diagnosis is discussed on page 853 and treatment on page 856.

## Tick-borne Typhus Fevers

### Rocky Mountain Spotted Fever

The causal organism, *R. rickettsi* is transferred by the bite of hard (*Ixodid*) ticks which carry the infection to rodents and dogs and on occasion to man. It is widely distributed in western and south-eastern states of the U.S.A. and also in South America. The pathological changes are similar to those in epidemic typhus. Haemorrhages and gangrene of the genitalia, ears and digits are more common.

**Clinical Features.** The incubation period is about 7 days. There may be an eschar at the site of the bite, with enlargement of the regional lymph nodes. Symptoms closely resemble those of louse-borne typhus. The rash appears about the third or fourth day, at first like measles, but in a few hours the typical maculopapular eruption develops. Each day it becomes more distinct and papular and finally petechial. The rash first appears on the wrists, forearms and ankles, spreads in 24 to 48 hours to the back, limbs and chest and lastly to the abdomen where it is least pronounced. The fully developed rash often affects also the palms, soles and face. Petechiae may appear in crops. Cutaneous and subcutaneous haemorrhages of considerable size may appear in severe cases. The liver and spleen become palpable. Complications are as in louse-borne typhus. Untreated, the course of the disease may be mild or rapidly fatal.

**Diagnosis and Treatment.** There may be a history of a bite by a tick. The character of the rash, appearing first at the periphery, is helpful. Laboratory aids to diagnosis are discussed on page 853 and treatment on page 856.

### Other Forms of Tick-borne Typhus Fever

The causal agents of African tick-borne typhus are *R. conori* and a substrain *R. conori pijperi.* They cause typhus in South and East Africa, the reservoir hosts being dogs and rodents. 'Fièvre boutonneuse' of the Mediterranean is similar, as is also the infection in Queensland where *R. australis* is the causal organism. Infected hard ticks may be picked up by walking on grasslands, or dogs may bring the ticks into the house. An eschar and lymphadenitis are usual. A maculopapular rash may cover the trunk and limbs and affects the palms and soles but may be scanty. There may be delirium and meningeal signs in severe infections but recovery is the rule except in the debilitated. There are no haemorrhages into the skin.

## Scrub Typhus Fever

Mite-borne or 'scrub' typhus is caused by *R. tsutsugamushi* transmitted by the bite of infective larval trombiculid mites. It occurs in the Far East, Assam, Burma, Pakistan, India, Indonesia, S. Pacific Islands and Queensland.

**Pathological and Clinical Features.** The pathology is similar to that of louse-borne typhus, but lesions in the lungs are more prominent. In most cases one or more eschars develop, surrounded by an area of cellulitis and enlargement of regional lymph nodes. The incubation period is about 9 days.

The onset of symptoms is usually sudden with headache, often retro-orbital, fever, malaise, weakness and cough, occasionally with diarrhoea. The conjunctivae become injected. In severe cases the general symptoms increase, with apathy and prostration. An erythematous maculopapular rash often appears on about the fifth to the seventh day and spreads to the trunk, face and limbs including the palms and soles with generalised painless lymphadenopathy. The rash fades by the fourteenth day. The temperature rises rapidly and continues as a remittent fever with sweating until it falls by lysis about the twelfth to the eighteenth day. In severe cases the patient is prostrate with cough, pneumonia, confusion and deafness. Cardiac failure, renal failure and haemorrhage may develop. Convalescence is often slow and tachycardia may persist for some weeks.

**Diagnosis and Treatment.** In endemic areas diagnosis is often possible on the clinical findings. Laboratory aids to diagnosis are discussed on page 853 and treatment on page 856.

## Q (Query) Fever

This disease occurs throughout the world and its causative organism, *Coxiella burneti*, differs sufficiently from other rickettsiae to be placed in a separate genus.

Ticks of several genera are vectors and these convey the organisms between many wild animals and to large domestic animals. These organisms are resistant to drying and so lend themselves to dissemination by air. Man becomes infected by inhaling or ingesting infected dust, rarely, if ever, by the bite of a tick. Dried genital discharges, milk and urine from infected animals appear to be important sources of infection amongst meat handlers and agricultural workers. Infected straw and other packing material have also been incriminated.

**Clinical Features.** The incubation period is 7 to 14 days. The onset is sudden with fever, sweating and malaise, cough, retro-orbital pain and anorexia. The temperature rises from 39° to 40·5°C with daily remissions, to fall to normal after 4 to 15 days. The pulse is slow, prostration often marked, and a cough is often present about the fifth or sixth day with scanty sputum, occasionally bloodstained. Pains in the chest are frequent, but physical signs are minimal. The spleen is sometimes palpable and occasionally a sparse rash is present. Radiographs usually show patchy homogeneous ground-glass areas of consolidation, single or multiple, usually towards the base of the lungs. These usually resolve in about 10 days. With the fall of temperature convalescence is usually rapid and complete. Hepatitis, encephalitis and myocarditis are occasional complications. *C. burneti* is an uncommon but serious cause of infective endocarditis (p. 181).

**Diagnosis and Treatment.** The clinical symptoms resemble those of viral pneumonia or of septicaemia. Laboratory aids to diagnosis are discussed on page 853 and treatment below.

## Rickettsialpox

This disease is due to *R. akari*, transmitted from the domestic mouse by a mite. It appears to be restricted to New York and Philadelphia where mice are now adapted to live in communal rubbish chutes of apartment houses.

The illness starts with a papule, which develops into an eschar, and is followed a week later by the sudden onset of fever, sweating, backache and a rash, maculopapular at first but which soon vesiculates and crusts, healing without scarring.

## Trench Fever

Trench fever is caused by *R. quintana* and is spread to man by louse faeces. It was prevalent in the First World War among troops in the trenches and again in the Second World War in the USSR. The disease is otherwise rare.

The incubation period is 10 to 20 days. The onset is sudden with headache, severe pains in trunk and limbs. The temperature rises sharply and remains raised for 5 to 7 days. The initial illness is like a mild case of typhus fever but febrile relapses are common, usually at intervals of 5 to 6 days and may be debilitating.

## Treatment of the Rickettsial Diseases

*Antibiotics.* The various fevers due to rickettsiae vary greatly in severity but respond to tetracycline and chloramphenicol. Tetracycline is given in a dose of 250 mg 4 times daily. In severe infections the dose is 500 mg 4 times daily for the first 3 days. The fever usually settles within 2 or 3 days. As there is a tendency to relapse tetracycline should be continued for 5 to 7 days after the patient is afebrile. In endemic areas good results have been obtained in louse-borne typhus by a single dose of 100 mg doxycycline. Erythromycin 500 mg 4 times daily is also effective for Q fever.

*General Management.* Patients suffering from louse- or flea-borne typhus are a danger to others unless they have been disinfested.

When the temperature is high, i.e. over 41°C, tepid sponging gives great comfort. If headache is intense and fails to respond to aspirin or codeine, lumbar puncture should be performed to relieve the increased intracranial pressure and to detect any concomitant bacterial meningitis. Delirium may need to be controlled by sedatives while awaiting the effects of specific chemotherapy. Pneumonia may be a serious feature in scrub typhus and oxygen may be needed. Convalescence is usually protracted especially in older people.

**Prevention.** For louse- and flea-borne typhus and in trench fever steps should be taken to get rid of all lice and fleas and their faeces. An insecticide powder can be insufflated into the undergarments of those at risk without their undressing. 5% carboxyl or 0·5% malathion are replacing 2% gamma-benzene hexachloride and DDT to which lice are becoming resistant. Residual insecticide powder on floors and bedding prevents fleas hatching. To prevent flea-borne typhus, food stores and granaries should be protected from rats. Rats and their fleas must be destroyed.

Attendants on patients with louse-borne typhus should wear protective clothing smeared with an insect repellent such as dimethylphthalate (DMP). The patient should be washed, and an insecticide applied all over, especially to the hairy parts. Clothing should be disinfested with insecticide, or sterilized in a domestic tumble drier or autoclaved.

To guard against tick-borne typhus, dogs should be regularly disinfested of ticks with forceps and should not be allowed to sleep in bedrooms. Protection of the legs when walking through grasslands may reduce the risk of picking up infected ticks. The early removal of ticks and cleansing the site of the bite are also important. Floors of log cabins in the U.S.A. should be creosoted annually.

Mite-borne typhus is acquired when man enters scrub country in endemic areas. Protection against the larval mite can be secured by wearing suitable clothing, the inside of which has been smeared once a week with a mite-repellent such as DMP. Mites can be destroyed by aerial spraying of infected areas with Aldrin or Dieldrin, repeated every 3 months.

*Active Immunisation.* Those likely to be at risk can be protected by vaccines prepared from killed cultures of *R. prowazeki*, *R. mooseri* or *R. rickettsi* cultured in eggs. Three doses each of 1 ml should be given subcutaneously at intervals of 7 to 10 days and booster doses of 1 ml should be given at 6-monthly intervals or yearly. No protective vaccine is available against mite-borne typhus.

## DISEASES DUE TO HELMINTHS

Infections caused by the commoner helminths, or worms, are described in this section, grouped according to the three zoological classes which parasitise man: (1) trematodes or flukes, (2) cestodes or tapeworms and (3) nematodes or roundworms. Much morbidity is caused in the tropics by helminths, many of which may be found in people even years after leaving the tropics.

The only prevalent parasitic helminth of humans in Britain is the nematode *En-*

*terobius (Oxyuris) vermicularis* or threadworm. Other worms which may be acquired in Britain include the roundworms, *Ascaris lumbricoides, Toxocara canis, Trichuris trichiura* (whipworm) and *Trichinella spiralis*. *Taenia saginata* (beef tapeworm), *Echinococcus granulosus* causing hydatid disease and *Fasciola hepatica*, an endemic fluke infecting sheep, are occasionally acquired in Britain.

Helminths invading tissues usually provoke an eosinophilia. A creeping eruption, or 'larva migrans', is caused when the larva of *Ancylostoma braziliense* travels in the skin and similar but more quickly moving lesions, 'larva currens', are caused by *Strongyloides stercoralis*. Visceral larva migrans is associated with *Toxocara canis*. Adult *Loa loa* and the larvae of *Gnathostoma spinigerum* provoke allergic swellings.

## 1. Diseases due to Trematodes (Flukes)

*Schistosomiasis; Paragonimiasis; Liver Flukes; Fasciolopsiasis*

### Schistosomiasis (Bilharziasis)

Schistosomiasis was endemic in ancient Egypt (1250 B.C.) but became a serious problem in the nineteenth century after perennial irrigation was instituted. It is one of the most important causes of morbidity in the tropics and is being spread by irrigation schemes.

There are three species of the genus *Schistosoma* which commonly cause disease in man, *S. haematobium, S. mansoni* and *S. japonicum*. *S. haematobium* was discovered by Theodor Bilharz in Cairo in 1861 and the genus is sometimes called *Bilharzia* and the disease bilharziasis. The ovum is passed in the urine or faeces and gains access to fresh water where the ciliated miracidium inside it is liberated and enters its intermediate host, a certain species of fresh water snails, in which it multiplies. Large numbers of fork-tailed cercariae are then liberated into the water where they may survive for 2 to 3 days. Cercariae can penetrate the skin if there is only a thin film of water next to it, or the mucous membrane of the mouth of their definitive host, man. They transform into schistosomulae and moult as they pass through the lungs, diaphragm and liver to the portal vein where they mature. The male worm is up to 20 mm in length and the more slender cylindrical female, usually enfolded longitudinally by the male, is rather longer (Fig. 17.6). Within 4 to 6 weeks of infection they migrate to the venules draining the pelvic viscera where the females deposit their ova. The eggs of *S. haematobium* pass mainly through the walls of the bladder and rectum. The eggs of *S. mansoni* and *S. japonicum* pass mainly through the lower bowel wall.

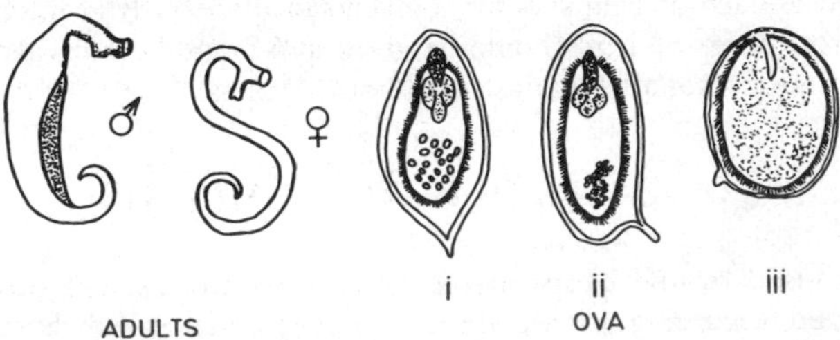


Fig. 17.6 Schistosoma. i. *S. haematobium*, ii. *S. mansoni*, iii. *S. japonicum* (80–160 × 50–70$\mu$)

**Pathology.** Penetration of the skin by the cercariae may produce a papular eruption which may later become vesicular. A similar cutaneous eruption may follow invasion of the skin by cercariae of non-human schistosomes. During the migration of the immature schistosomes, transitory lesions may be produced, including areas of pneumonia. At this stage there is usually an eosinophilia but the count falls progressively after the disease is established. In a heavy schistosomal infection ova may be found widely distributed in many tissues, but each species has a special territory for maximum egg deposition (see below). After the egg has escaped from the vein, a granuloma forms around it consisting of epithelioid cells, fibroblasts and giant cells surrounded by a zone of plasma cells and eosinophils. When the egg is near a mucosal surface, aided by the cytolytic enzyme excreted by the miracidium, it may be discharged into the bowel or bladder. If, however, the ovum is retained in the tissues the miracidium soon dies and the egg then either disintegrates or becomes calcified, and fibrous tissue forms at the site. The degree of fibrosis depends on the intensity of the infection and the frequency of re-infection. In endemic areas the immune response to an established infection may limit re-infections.

**Clinical Features of the Early Infection.** Occasionally there may be itching at the site of cercarial penetration, lasting 1–2 days. After a symptom-free period of 3 to 5 weeks allergic manifestations may develop such as urticaria, eosinophilia, fever, aches in the muscles, abdominal pain, splenomegaly, headaches, cough and sweating. Patches of pneumonia may be present. These allergic phenomena (*Katayama syndrome*) may be severe in infections with *S. mansoni* and *S. japonicum* but are rare with *S. haematobium*. After 1 or 2 weeks these features subside and for 2 or 3 months there may be no further symptoms until the deposition of eggs causes fresh ones to develop. The symptoms then depend on the intensity of the infection and the species of the infecting schistosome.

Diagnosis and treatment are discussed on page 861.

## Schistosoma haematobium

This species of schistosome affects mainly the urinary bladder, ureters and genitalia. The egg is easily recognised by its terminal spine. Man is the only natural host. *S. haematobium* is highly endemic in Egypt, the east coast of Africa and the adjacent islands and occurs throughout most of Africa, in Iran, Iraq, Syria, Yemen, South Arabia, Lebanon and Israel. It also occurs in Turkey, Cyprus and in solitary foci in Portugal and the Maharashtra State of India.

**Pathology.** The early changes are hyperaemia and petechiae of the bladder mucosa, followed by papilloma formation, ulceration and fibrosis. Calcification of ova produces, in intense infections, sandy patches at the base of the bladder. The lower third of the ureter is liable to fibrosis, calcification, dilatation with reflux, or stenosis. The capacity of the bladder decreases. Hydronephrosis and renal failure follow, often complicated by secondary bacterial infection of the urinary tract and the formation of calculi and sometimes amyloid disease. Squamous cell carcinoma of the bladder in relatively young males is of common occurrence in some areas of high endemicity of *S. haematobium*. Egg deposition may damage the urethra, with sinus formation, the seminal vesicles, vagina, cervix, Fallopian tubes and rectum. Deposition of ova in the pulmonary arterioles may lead to pulmonary hypertension and cor pulmonale. These lung changes are especially frequent in combined infections with *S. haematobium* and *S. mansoni*. Discrete granulomas in the lung may be large enough to be visible radiologically. Ova may also be carried to the central nervous system, skin and elsewhere.

**Clinical Features.** The characteristic early localising symptom is usually painless, terminal haematuria with or without frequency of micturition. Frequency of micturition follows when the disease is long established, due largely to the contracted fibrosed or calcified bladder. Pain is often felt in the iliac fossa or in the loin, passing down to the groin. In advanced cases pyelonephritis, hydronephrosis or pyonephrosis may be accompanied by hypertension or uraemia. Disease of the seminal vesicles may lead to haemospermia. Females may be sterile and schistosomal lesions of the cervix may be mistaken for carcinoma. Intestinal symptoms may result from lesions in the bowel wall.

The severity of *S. haematobium* infection varies greatly, and many with light infections suffer a minimum of discomfort. However, as the adult worms can live for 20 years or more and progressive lesions may develop, treatment should always be given, unless contraindicated by renal failure.

### Schistosoma mansoni

This species of schistosome affects particularly the large bowel. Man is the only natural host of importance although the infection is also found in baboons. *S. mansoni* is endemic in the Nile Delta and Libya, Southern Sudan, East Africa continuing as far south as the Transvaal and in West Africa from Senegal and Gambia to Cameroun, throughout Zaïre and also Arabia. It is also found in South America in Venezuela, Brazil and in the West Indian Islands of the lesser Antilles, Puerto Rico and Dominica.

**Pathology.** The early lesions are congestion and petechiae of the large bowel mucosa, followed by papillomas, which become pedunculated, and fibrosis. The rectum is first and most affected but later the whole colon may be involved. Occasionally a segment of bowel becomes thickened and stenosed but malignant change is not a feature.

Granulomatous hepatitis, in response to eggs deposited in the liver, causes hepatomegaly and mild splenomegaly. In heavy infections, periportal fibrosis (pipe stem cirrhosis) is followed by portal hypertension and massive splenomegaly, oesophageal varices and ascites. The portal shunt provided by these varices enables ova to reach the lungs and cause pulmonary granulomas, fibrosis, gross pulmonary hypertension and right ventricular failure. Ectopic deposition of ova into the central nervous system is commoner than with *S. haematobium*.

**Clinical Features** The early manifestations are described on page 859. The characteristic symptoms of local disease begin two months or longer after infection. They may be slight or consist of abdominal pain and frequent stools which contain blood stained mucus. With severe advanced disease increased discomfort from rectal polypi may be experienced. The early hepatomegaly is reversible but portal hypertension may cause fatal haematemesis or progressive ascites. Jaundice and hepatic failure is uncommon. Paraplegia rarely occurs from migrating worms, being more commonly due to a granuloma compressing the cord. *S. mansoni* infections predispose to the carrier state of *Salm. typhi*.

## Schistosoma japonicum

*S. japonicum* infects particularly the portal drainage of the small intestine and upper part of the large bowel. The adult worm parasitises, in addition to man, the dog, rat, field mouse, water buffalo, ox, cat, pig, horse and sheep. *S. japonicum* is prevalent in the Yangtse-Kiang basin in China where the infection is a major public health problem. It also has a focal distribution in Japan and occurs in the Philippines, Celebes, Laos, Thailand, Vietnam and the Shan States of Burma.

**Pathology and Clinical Features**. The histopathology of *S. japonicum* is similar to that of *S. mansoni* but as this worm produces more eggs the lesions tend to be more extensive and widespread. The small intestine and upper part of the large bowel are most affected, and hepatic fibrosis with splenic enlargement is usual. Deposition of eggs in the central nervous system, especially in the brain, causes symptoms of cerebral irritation or compression in about 5% of infections. The clinical features of schistosomiasis due to *S. japonicum* resemble those of very severe infection with *S. mansoni*. Evidence of cerebral involvement includes Jacksonian epilepsy, hemiplegia, blindness and terminal coma. Paraplegia from compression of the cord may also occur. The morbidity and mortality rate in *S. japonicum* infections is greater than from either of the other species.

## Diagnosis of Schistosomiasis

A history of residence in an endemic area with symptoms as described will indicate the need for a careful investigation. In *S. haematobium* infection the terminal spined egg can usually be found by microscopical examination of urine, especially of a late morning specimen. The eggs may also be found by microscopic examination of the stools or of a fragment of unstained rectal mucosa removed through a proctoscope. In a case of some duration a radiograph may show calcification in the wall of the bladder while intravenous urography may show stenosis or dilatation of the ureters, reduction in capacity of the bladder, or hydronephrosis. Such changes are found commonly in endemic areas and have been shown to be frequent even in children, in whom large intravesical granulomas are common. In a heavy infection with *S. mansoni* or *S. japonicum* the characteristic egg can usually be found in the stool. When, however, the infection is light it may be necessary to repeat the examinations over a number of days. Cystoscopy or sigmoidoscopy may enable the diagnosis to be made from the macroscopic appearance. Otherwise biopsy specimens should be removed and examined for ova. Serological tests (complement fixation or immuno-fluorescence) are being increasingly used to reveal evidence of infection, past or present.

The bowel symptoms and barium enema appearances of *S. mansoni* and *S. japonicum* infection may be very like those associated with intestinal amoebiasis or with a neoplasm of the large bowel, so steps should be taken to exclude these. There may also be concomitant bacillary dysentery.

## Treatment of Schistosomiasis

The object of specific treatment is the killing of the adult schistosomes or, failing this, at least a significant reduction in egg laying. The latter is still of considerable value to the individual patient and in mass treatments of a community the spread of infection by snails is reduced. Even in endemic areas reinfection is not inevitable. In the presence of extensive liver damage no drug is safe and established portal hypertension will not be improved by chemotherapy.

*Niridazole*, 25 mg/kg body weight daily, orally in 3 divided doses, for 7 days is highly effective in haematobium schistosomiasis but rather less so in mansoni schistosomiasis. The drug colours the urine brown but the only serious occasional side effect is a temporary psychosis, especially liable to occur if the liver is diseased.

*Stibocaptate*, a combination of a trivalent antimony compound and dimercaprol, is given intramuscularly in a dose of 8 mg/kg body weight daily, on alternate days or spaced as tolerated, for a total of 5 doses. It is rather more effective than niridazole and dimercaprol reduces the toxic effects of antimony (see below).

*Hycanthone* in a single dose of 1·5 mg/kg body weight gives good results. The drug sometimes causes vomiting but it is dangerous to administer a phenothiazine because of the synergistic toxic effects of the drugs on the liver.

*Oxamniquine* orally in a dose of 10 mg/kg body weight b.d. for two days is now regarded as the best treatment for *S. mansoni. Praziquantel* (not yet generally available) in a single oral dose of 50 mg/kg body weight promises to be highly effective for schistosomiasis haematobium and mansoni and reasonably good for japonicum.

*Sodium antimonyl tartrate* was for many years the standard drug and is still used for japonicum schistosomiasis. For other infections it is no longer indicated because of the need for caution in its intravenous administration and its occasional dangerous cardiotoxicity. The total dose required is 2 g given at 18 or more separate injections spaced over 3 to 6 weeks as tolerated, beginning with a dose of 30 mg and gradually increasing to 120 mg each.

*Surgical aid* may be required to deal with residual lesions but large vesical granulomas usually respond well to chemotherapy. In cases of chronic *S. haematobium* infection, ureteric stricture and the small fibrotic urinary bladder may require plastic procedures. For rectal papillomas removal by diathermy or by other means may give the patient considerable relief. Granulomatous masses in the brain or spinal cord may call for neurosurgery if the manifestations do not yield to chemotherapy. For portal hypertension a portocaval shunt may have to be considered.

**Prevention**. This presents great difficulties, and so far no really satisfactory means of controlling schistosomiasis has been established. If the ova of the schistosome in the urine or faeces are not allowed to contaminate fresh water containing the required snail host, then the life cycle is terminated.

The provision of latrines and of a safe water supply remains a major problem in rural areas throughout the tropics. In the case of *S. japonicum*, moreover, there are so many hosts besides man that the proper use of latrines would be of little avail. Mass treatment of the population helps against *S. haematobium* and *S. mansoni* but this method has so far had little success against *S. japonicum*.

Attack on the intermediate host, the snail, presents many difficulties and has not on its own proved successful on any scale.

*Personal Protection*. Contact with infected water must be avoided. Accidental immersion or contact should be followed by a shower and vigorous towelling. Storage of water, free of snails, for three days will usually kill cercariae.

## Paragonimiasis (Endemic Haemoptysis)

There are several species of the flukes of the genus *Paragonimus* which may affect man, the commonest being *P. westermani*. The adult worms measuring 10 × 6 mm live in small cysts in the lung and elsewhere. If a pulmonary cyst ruptures, the sputum of the patient contains ova, some of which may be expectorated and the others swallowed and passed in the faeces. From these eggs the larval worms emerge in water and seek the first intermediate host, a freshwater snail. Larvae emerging from the snail enter freshwater crabs or crayfish. If man or certain other mammals eat these crustacea raw or inadequately cooked, infection takes place. Human infections are most frequent in the Far East but there are also endemic foci in South America, Cameroun, Nigeria, Somalia and India.

**Pathological and Clinical Features**. The adults lie in cysts up to 1 cm in diameter, containing reddish brown fluid, situated chiefly in the lung. There are seldom more than 20 such cysts present. In heavy infections cysts may also be present in the pleural or peritoneal cavities, in the brain, muscles, skin or elsewhere.

The first symptoms are slight fever, cough and the expectoration of sputum streaked with blood. Occasionally there are bouts of frank haemoptysis with severe pain in the chest. Increasing signs in the chest may simulate pneumonia or pulmonary tuberculosis which frequently co-exists. When the parasites lodge in the abdomen there may be symptoms of enteritis or hepatitis. If they settle in the abdominal wall they may produce sinuses with a discharge through the skin. Development in the central nervous system may cause signs of cerebral irritation, encephalitis or myelitis. The disease may be very chronic and the adult worms may survive for 20 years.

Ova may be found on microscopic examination of the faeces, sputum, or a discharge. The radiological appearances of affected lungs are variable but the lesions are usually situated close to the pleural surfaces. Extrapulmonary lesions are diagnosed in life by biopsy.

**Treatment and Prevention**. Antibiotics are useful to combat secondary pyogenic infections. The specific drug is bithionol given in a dose of 50 mg/kg body weight daily in three divided doses on alternate days. In all, 10 to 15 days of treatment are required and the results are encouraging. Lesions localised to or maximal in one lobe of a lung may be treated surgically.

In an endemic area crab or crayfish should not be eaten unless adequately cooked. Immersion of crustaceans in wine or brine does not kill the parasites.

## Liver Flukes

Table 17.6 sets out the main features of the diseases caused by flukes which infect the bile ducts of man (p. 864).

## Fasciolopsiasis

*Fasciolopsis buski* is the largest fluke to infect man. The adults, 2–7·5 cm long, inhabit the small intestine of man, pigs and dogs. It is common in Central and S. China and among Chinese in S.E. Asia. The infection is spread from ova passed in the faeces into water. The intermediate hosts are snails. Man becomes infected by ingesting metacercariae encysted on water plants, particularly when he uses his teeth to peel them.

Light infections are symptomless. Heavy infections give rise to epigastric pain and loose motions. Very heavy infections may be fatal. The diagnosis is made by detecting ova or adult worms in the faeces. Tetrachloroethylene as prescribed for hookworms

Table 17.6 Diseases caused by flukes in the bile ducts

| Disease | Clonorchiasis | Opisthorciasis | Fascioliasis |
|---|---|---|---|
| Parasite | *Clonorchis sinensis* | *Opisthorcis felineus* | *Fasciola hepatica* |
| Other mammalian hosts | Dogs, cats, pigs | Dogs, cats, foxes, pigs | Sheep, cattle |
| Mode of spread | Ova in faeces into water | As for *C. sinensis* | Ova in faeces on to wet pasture |
| 1st intermediate host | Snails | Snails | Snails |
| 2nd intermediate host | Freshwater fish | Freshwater fish | Nil (encysts on vegetation) |
| Geographical distribution | Far East, esp. S. China | Far East, esp. N.E. Thailand | Cosmopolitan incl. Britain |
| Pathology | *Esch. coli* cholangitis, liver abscesses, biliary carcinoma | As for *C. sinensis* | Toxaemia, cholangitis, eosinophilia |
| Symptoms | Often symptom-free, recurrent jaundice | As for *C. sinensis* | Obscure fever, tender liver, may be ectopic subcut. fluke |
| Diagnosis | Ova in stool or duodenal aspirate | As for *C. sinensis* | As for *C. sinensis* also immunofluorescence |
| Prevention | Cook fish | Cook fish | Avoid contaminated watercress |
| Treatment | Hexachloroparaxylol 300 mg/kg daily for 3 days | As for *C. sinensis* | Bithionol 30 mg/kg daily for 10–15 days |
| | or Niclofolan 2 mg/kg body weight repeated after 2 days | | |

(p. 870) is effective treatment. Prevention is by the proper disposal of faeces. Edible water plants can be made safe by immersing them in boiling water.

## 2. Diseases due to Cestodes (Tapeworms)

*Taenia saginata; Taenia solium and Cysticercosis; Echinococcus granulosus; Multiceps multiceps; Diphyllobothrium latum; Diphyllobothrium mansoni; Dipylidium caninum; Hymenolepis nana*

Cestodes are ribbon-shaped worms which inhabit the human intestinal tract. They have no alimentary system and absorb nutrients through the surface. The anterior end, or scolex, is provided with suckers for attachment to the host. From the scolex arises a series of progressively developing segments, the proglottides, which when shed may continue to show active movements for some time. Cross-fertilisation takes place between segments. Ova, present in large numbers in mature proglottides, remain viable for weeks and during this period they may be consumed by the intermediate host. The larvae liberated from the ova pass into the tissues of the intermediate host, and the human disease is acquired by eating undercooked beef infected with *Cysticercus bovis*, the larval stage of *Taenia saginata* (beef tapeworm), undercooked pork containing *Cysticercus cellulosae*, the larval stage of *T. solium* (pork tapeworm), or undercooked freshwater fish containing larvae of *Diphyllobothrium latum* (fish tapeworm). Usually only one adult tapeworm is present but up to 10 have been reported. The adult worm produces little or no intestinal upset in human beings, but knowledge of its presence, by noting segments from it in the faeces or on underclothing, may distress the patient. The life-cycles of *Diphyllobothrium mansoni, Dipylidium caninum and Hymenolepis nana* are different (p. 867).

### Taenia saginata

This worm may be several metres long. The scolex, the size of a pin head, has four suckers; mature segments 1·3 cm × 1 cm, contain a central-stemmed uterus with 15 to 20 lateral branches which are easily seen if the segments are left in water for 24 hours (Fig. 17.7). The ova of both *T. saginata* and *T. solium* are spherical and indistinguishable microscopically. The thick outer shell has radial striations and the ovum contains six hooklets.

Infection with *T. saginata* occurs in all parts of the world, including Britain. The patient usually notices segments on underclothing or in stools. The segments should be identified. Ova may also be found in the stool.

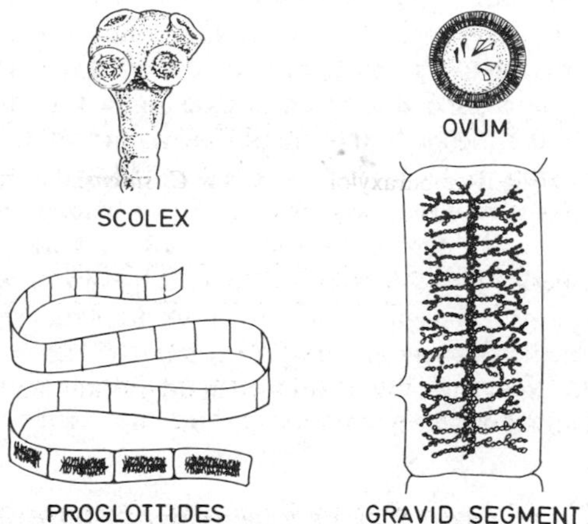


Fig. 17.7 *Taenia saginata* (Ova 30–40$\mu$)

**Treatment and Prevention**. Before any food is taken in the morning, niclosamide, 2 tablets of the drug, each containing 0·5 g, are chewed and swallowed with a little water. One hour later a further 2 tablets are similarly taken. There are no side-effects and the worm is usually destroyed. Prevention depends on efficient meat inspection or the thorough cooking of beef.

### Taenia solium and Cysticercosis

*T. solium*, the pork tapeworm, was formerly cosmopolitan in distribution but is now rare except in Central Europe, Ethiopia, South Africa and in parts of Asia. It is not so large as *T. saginata*, and the uterus usually has less than 14 lateral branches. The scolex has, in addition to suckers, two circular rows of hooklets anterior to the suckers. The adult worm is found only in man following the eating of undercooked pork containing cysticerci.

*Human cysticercosis* results from ova being swallowed or gaining access to the human stomach by regurgitation from the intestine harbouring an adult worm. In the stomach the larvae are liberated from the eggs, penetrate the intestinal mucosa and are carried to many parts of the body where they develop and form cysticerci. The most common locations are the subcutaneous tissue and skeletal muscles; when superficially placed they can be palpated under the skin or mucosa as pea-like ovoid bodies. Here they cause few or no symptons; however cysts may also develop in the brain. About 5 years later the larvae die; in the brain the tissue reaction may cause epileptic fits, obscure neurological disorders, personality changes and occasionally internal hydrocephalus. After death of the larvae in muscles the cysts calcify and this enables them to be recognised radiologically. In the brain, however, much less calcification takes place and in this situation calcified larvae are only occasionally demonstrated radiologically. Epileptic fits starting in adult life should suggest the possibility of cysticercosis if the patient has lived in an endemic area. The subcutaneous tissue should be palpated and radiological examination of the skeletal muscles for calcified cysts must be made and repeated after intervals of 6 months if at first negative.

Less than 14 lateral branches of the uterus is characteristic of *T. solium* but a more certain differentiation from *T. saginata* can be made by enzyme electrophoresis.

**Treatment and Prevention**. *T. solium* can be destroyed by niclosamide (p. 865).

Treatment of cysticercosis of the brain is essentially the same as for idiopathic epilepsy; sedatives and anticonvulsants should be given to tide the patient over the period until the reaction in the brain has subsided. Most patients treated on these lines make a good recovery. Operative intervention is seldom indicated.

Prevention of *T. solium* infection consists in cooking pork well before eating it. Cysticercosis is avoided if food is not contaminated by ova or segments and if there is no regurgitation of gravid segments or ova into the stomach as may occur from vomiting in a patient harbouring an adult *T. solium*. Great care must be taken by nurses and others to avoid ingesting ova from hands contaminated by attending to a patient harbouring an adult worm.

### Echinococcus granulosus (Taenia echinococcus) and Hydatid Disease

This is the smallest tapeworm of medical importance. The larval stage, a hydatid cyst, occurs in sheep, cattle and other animals, including camels. Dogs, by ingesting these cysts, are the most important definitive hosts and a man, after handling a dog, may swallow ova excreted by the dog. The embryo is liberated from the ovum in the small intestine and gains access to the blood stream; it develops most frequently in the liver. The resultant cyst grows very slowly. It may calcify or may rupture giving rise to multiple cysts. A variant, *E. multilocularis*, causes a similar but more severe infection, 'alveococcosis' which invades the liver like cancer.

In man a hydatid cyst is typically acquired in childhood and it may, after growing for some years, cause pressure symptons. These will vary, depending on the organ or tissue involved. In nearly 75 % of patients with hydatid disease the right lobe of the liver is invaded and contains a single cyst. In others a cyst may be found in lung, brain, orbit or elsewhere. The diagnosis depends on the clinical, radiological, and ultrasound findings in a patient who has lived in close contact with dogs. Intradermal (Casoni), complement-fixation, and immunofluorescent tests usually give support to the diagnosis.

**Treatment** of hydatid disease is surgical. Great care is taken to avoid spillage and cavities are sterilised with 2% formalin, 0·5% silver nitrate or 30% sodium chloride. Treatment of multiple cysts, which are causing symptoms, by fluormebendazole, 2 g daily for 10–12 months is, at present, being evaluated.

*Further reading about treatment of hydatid cysts:*

Saidi, P. & Nazarian, I. (1971). Surgical treatment of hydatid cysts. *New England Journal of Medicine*, **284**, 1346.

## Other Tapeworms

**Multiceps multiceps.** This tapeworm of dogs occurring in sheep grazing areas of East and Southern Africa has a similar life cycle to *Echinococcus granulosus*. Only its larval stage, *Coenurus serialis* is known in man. It is liable to cause a space occupying cyst in the brain, especially in the posterior fossa.

**Diphyllobothrium latum** is relatively common in Finland and the Scandinavian countries but is also acquired from rivers and lakes of many other countries, including some in Africa and Asia. The ova are excreted in the faeces of an infected man or other fish-eating animal. The larval stages take place first in a small freshwater crustacean, *Cyclops* or *Diaptomus* which in turn is swallowed by a fish. The infections are usually symptomless. Occasionally there are signs of allergy and in a small percentage of cases a megaloblastic anaemia develops, the worm competing with the host for vitamin $B_{12}$. The diagnosis is made by finding ova in the stool and treatment is by niclosamide as for *T. saginata.*

**Diphyllobothrium mansoni (Spirometra erinacei).** The adult worms are harboured by cats and dogs. The second larval stage, a sparganum, is occasionally found in the subcutaneous tissues of man. The Masai in East Africa probably become infected by ingestion of the first intermediate host, a *Cyclops*, from well water and the patient presents with a painful swelling usually in the lower limbs. In the Far East ocular *sparganosis* arises from the migration of a sparganum from a split frog applied as a traditional poultice. Sparganosis also occurs in the U.S.A. Surgical removal is required. The exact species can be established only by feeding the removed sparganum to an uninfected cat or dog.

**Dipylidium caninum** is a short tapeworm of dogs and cats. The ova are passed in the faeces and the larva has to undergo development in a flea or louse before being swallowed by the definitive host. Children are occasionally infected by picking up and ingesting an infected flea from a dog. The diagnosis is made by finding segments or ova in the stools. Treatment, in appropriate doses for a child, is by niclosamide as for *T. saginata*.

**Hymenolepis nana.** This dwarf tapeworm is unusual in not requiring an intermediate host. It is a common infection in children living in insanitary conditions in the tropics and subtropics. Apart from an eosinophilia, no signs or symptoms are present except in the presence of numerous worms, when enteritis and allergic phenomena may be encountered. The diagnosis is made by recognising the ova in the faeces. Treatment is by niclosamide as for *T. saginata*.

## 3. Diseases due to Nematodes (Roundworms)

*Enterobius vermicularis; Ascaris lumbricoides; Toxocara canis; Ancylostomiasis; Larva Migrans; Strongyloidiasis; Filariasis; (Bancroftian filariasis, Brugia filariasis, Loiasis, Onchocerciasis, etc.) Dracontiasis; Oesophagostomiasis; Angiostrongylus; Trichuris trichiura; Trichinella spiralis; Capillariasis; Gnathostomiasis; Anisakiasis*

### Enterobius vermicularis (Threadworm)

This helminth is common throughout the world, including Britain. It affects children especially. The sexes are separate, the male being 2–5 mm long and the female 8–13 mm (Fig. 17.8). After the ova are swallowed, development takes place in the small intestine, but the adult worms are found chiefly in the colon.

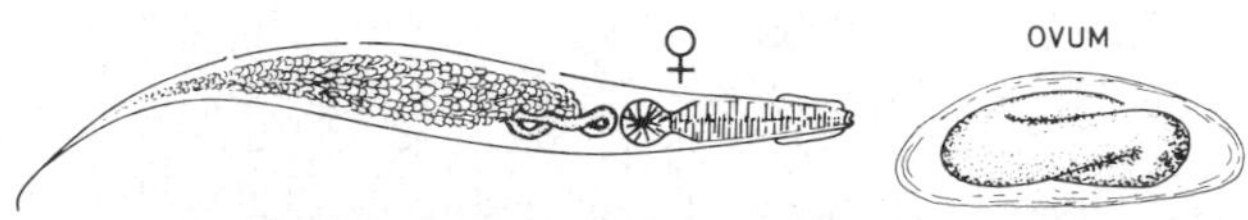


Fig. 17.8 *Enterobius vermicularis* (Ova 55 × 25μ)

The gravid female worm lays fully developed ova around the anal orifice, and her movements in this region are responsible for intense itching, especially at night. The ova are often carried to the mouth on the fingers of the child and so reinfection takes place. In female patients the genitalia may be invaded. The adult worms may be seen moving on the buttocks or in the stool. Ova are detected by applying the adhesive surface of cellophane tape to the perianal skin in the morning. This is then examined on a glass slide under the microscope.

**Treatment**. Piperazine salts are effective remedies administered with senna. The adult dose is 10 g of the combined preparation containing 4 g of piperazine phosphate; children under 6 years are given 5–7·5 g. The drug is taken in a single dose but should be repeated if the infection persists. Other effective anthelmintics are viprynium embonate, mebendazole and pyrantel embonate. Success is more likely to be achieved if the whole family is treated simultaneously, particularly as symptomless infections may be present in adults. Prevention of reinfection is most important. Nails should be kept short, biting of nails forbidden and the hands washed carefully, especially before meals.

### Ascaris lumbricoides ('Roundworm')

This is a large, pale yellow roundworm 20–35 cm long, something like an earthworm, but not segmented. The sexes are separate and ova are passed in the faeces.

Man is infected by ingesting food contaminated with ova containing developed embryos. The larvae escape from the ova in the duodenum and find their way to the lungs where they develop further. After invading the alveoli they then ascend the bronchi and trachea and are swallowed, thus entering the small intestine where they reach maturity. In heavy infections, such as occur in the tropics, migration of many larvae through the lung may cause pulmonary eosinophilia (p. 273 – Löffler's syn-

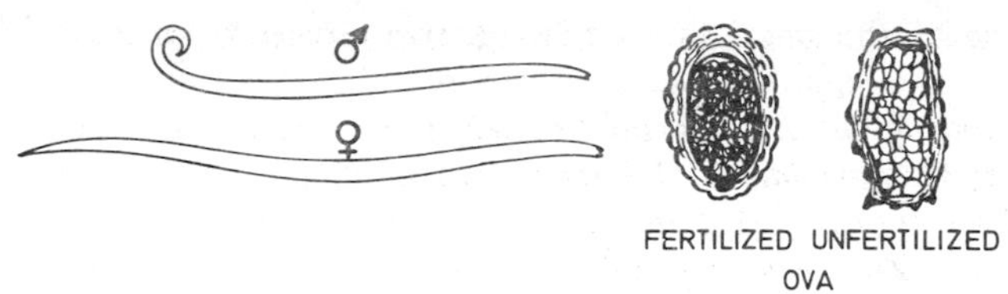


Fig. 17.9 *Ascaris lumbricoides* (Ova 60 × 45$\mu$ fertilised; 90 × 40$\mu$ unfertilised)

drome). Symptoms due to adult worms may be absent or consist of nausea, colicky abdominal pain and irregular motions. Sometimes a worm is vomited or passed *per rectum*. In children with severe infections a tangled mass of worms may cause intestinal obstruction. Many worms competing with the host for nourishment may contribute to malnutrition. Other complications include blockage of the bile or pancreatic duct and obstruction of the appendix by adult worms. The diagnosis is made by finding ova in the faeces or by observing an adult worm (Fig. 17.9). A solely male infection is usually revealed only after the giving of an anthelmintic to a patient with an unexplained eosinophilia. Occasionally the worms are demonstrated radiographically by barium.

**Treatment**. Piperazine salts are easily administered and effective and should be given as recommended for threadworms. Levamisole in a single adult dose of 120 mg (40 mg up to age 3 years) is an effective alternative. If intestinal obstruction threatens, levamisole is given in small divided doses. If obstruction is severe and fails to respond to nasogastric suction and sedation, surgery is required, when the worms are 'milked' past the obstruction, or removed by enterostomy. If the gut is gangrenous resection is necessary.

## Toxocara canis

This is a common intestinal ascarid of dogs. The eggs are passed in the animal's faeces. Children who are in close contact with infected puppies are particularly liable to ingest ova of *Toxocara canis*. Larvae, liberated in the stomach, then migrate through the body and may cause allergic phenomena such as asthma, eosinophilia and also splenomegaly ('visceral larva migrans'). The worms do not usually mature in the human host. Occasionally a granuloma develops around a dead larva in the eye, resembling a neoplasm and causes an obstruction to vision. Serology may aid diagnosis.

The larval worms can be killed by diethylcarbamazine (9–12 mg/kg body weight daily for 3 weeks). Granulomas may require surgical treatment.

## Ancylostomiasis (Hookworm Infection)

Ancylostomiasis is caused by parasitisation of the small intestine with *Ancylostoma duodenale* or *Necator americanus*. The adult hookworm is a greyish-white nematode about 1 cm long (Fig. 17.10) which lives, often in large numbers, in the duodenum and upper jejenum. The egg is thin-shelled and oval, and when passed in the faeces 2 to 8 lobes may be seen in the yolk. In warm moist soil the larvae develop and reach the filariform infective stage. On coming in contact with human skin they penetrate it and are carried to the lungs. After entering the alveoli they ascend the bronchi, are swallowed and develop in the small intestine, reaching maturity in 4 to 7 weeks after infection. The larvae may also enter through the mucous membrane of the mouth. Man is the only host.

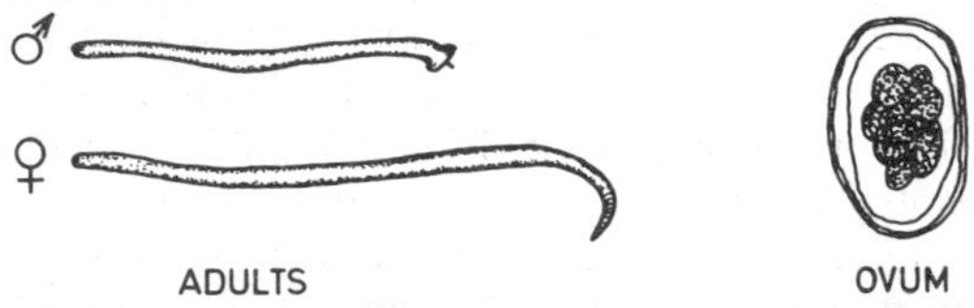


Fig. 17.10 *Ancylostoma duodenale* (Ova 60 × 40$\mu$)

Hookworm infection is widespread under insanitary conditions in the tropics and subtropics and occurs in certain mines in Europe. *A. duodenale* is endemic in the Far East and Mediterranean coastal regions and is also present in Africa. *N. americanus* is endemic in West, East and Central Africa and Central and South America as well as in the Far East.

**Pathology**. At the site of entry the larvae may cause allergic inflammation. When infection is heavy, reaction to the passage through the lungs may cause a patchy inflammation accompanied by eosinophilia. In the small intestine the worms attach themselves to the mucosa by their buccal capsule and withdraw blood. The mean daily loss of blood from one *A. duodenale* is 0·15 ml and for *N. americanus* 0·03 ml. The degree of iron and protein deficiency which develops depends not only on the load of worms but also on the nutrition of the patient and especially on the stores of iron, so that in a light infection there may be no anaemia. In the early stage of infection a considerable eosinophilia commonly occurs.

**Clinical Features**. In a well nourished person with a light established infection there may be no symptoms. At the time of infection hookworm dermatitis (ground itch) may be experienced, usually on the feet. An itchy erythema appears first and soon develops through papules and vesicles to the pustular stage. In a heavy infection the passage of the larvae through the lungs causes a paroxysmal cough with blood-stained sputum, associated with patchy pulmonary consolidation (an example of Löffler's syndrome). When the worms have reached the small intestine, vomiting and epigastric pain, like that of a duodenal ulcer, may ensue. Sometimes frequent loose stools are passed, the condition then resembling early sprue or giardiasis. In the undernourished, especially when there is a heavy infection and in children a severe iron deficiency anaemia and hypoproteinaemia may develop with a puffy face, peripheral oedema or ascites, tachycardia, breathlessness and signs of cardiac failure. In children mental and physical development may be retarded.

**Diagnosis**. The characteristic egg can be recognised in the stool. The oedema with anaemia has to be differentiated from that due to kwashiorkor, heart failure or nephritis. If hookworms are present in numbers sufficient to cause anaemia, tests of the stool for occult blood will be positive and ova will be present in large numbers.

**Treatment and Prevention**. Specific medication should be given early in the morning when the patient has fasted overnight. A well-established drug is tetrachloroethylene which is given orally. The dose is 0·1 ml/kg body weight with a maximum of 4 ml. The drug has usually to be given on two or more occasions not more frequently than on alternate days. Tetrachloroethylene rapidly deteriorates in warm climates and so must be stored in a cool dark place.

Bephenium hydroxynaphthoate, containing 2·5 g base, as a single dose, is an alternative drug with few side-effects. No preparation or purgation is required. It is more expensive than tetrachloroethylene and is not as effective for *N. americanus* as for *A. duodenale*. Levamisole in a single dose of 3 tablets each of 40 mg after a light breakfast, is moderately effective against *A. duodenale* but less so against *N. americanus*, and is an alternative. Mebendazole, bitoscanate and pyrantel pamoate are also used. Mebendazole, 100 mg b.d. orally for three days, is effective against the soil transmitted helminths, *Ascaris,* hookworms, *Strongyloides* and *Trichuris* which may be simultaneously harboured. However, the safety of mebendazole has recently been questioned and a modification, fluormebendazole, has been recommened in its place.

Anaemia associated with hookworm infection responds well to oral iron. When it is severe enough to cause heart failure blood should be transfused slowly, with frusemide 20 mg in each unit.

The community should be educated in the use of properly constructed latrines. Mass treatment of the entire population may help bring the disease under control but can be costly. Nutrition should be improved; wearing shoes should be encouraged.

## Hookworms causing Larva Migrans

*Ancylostoma braziliense and A. caninum* are intestinal parasites of dogs with a similar life cycle to *A. duodenale*, but in man they cause a creeping eruption or cutaneous larva migrans. The larva burrows between the corium and stratum granulosum and progresses irregularly at about 1 cm in 24 hours. The skin at the advancing end is erythematous and the older part of the burrow discoloured and scaly. The patient experiences considerable discomfort from itching. The larva may remain active for some weeks or months. Treatment is topical. One 0·5 g tablet of thiabendazole is ground into 5 g petroleum jelly and rubbed in twice daily. Symptoms are relieved and the larva dies in a day or two. Oral thiabendazole is seldom required.

## Strongyloidiasis

*Strongyloides stercoralis* is a very small nematode (2 mm x 40 microns) which parasitises the mucosa of the upper part of the small intestine in large numbers. The eggs hatch in the bowel and appear in the faeces as rhabditiform larvae which in moist soil moult and become the infective filariform larvae. These, on entering the tissues of man, undergo a development cycle similar to that of hookworms but the female worms burrow into the mucosa and submucosa. In the intestine a few rhabditiform larvae develop into filariform larvae which may then penetrate the mucosa or the perianal skin and lead to auto-infection and a very persistent infection still seen in some ex-prisoners of the Second World War. Man is the chief natural host, but dogs and cats may also be infected.

Strongyloidiasis is worldwide in the tropics and subtropics and is especially prevalent in the Far East.

**Pathology**. There may be a dermatitis at the time of entry of the larval worms. In the intestine the female worm burrows into the mucosa and sets up an inflammatory reaction; with very heavy infections the mucosa may be severely damaged leading to malabsorption. Granulomatous changes, necrosis, and even perforation and peritonitis may also occur. Eosinophilia commonly persists. Actively motile larvae are passed in the faeces. Immunosuppression due to disease or drugs such as corticosteroids, may lead to fatal systemic strongyloidiasis.

**Clinical Features.** An itch may be produced during invasion of the skin. With slight infections there will be no intestinal symptoms, but in more severe cases abdominal pain and diarrhoea may be produced, which is on occasion severe. Urticaria, anaemia, weakness and emaciation may also be present as well as signs of malabsorption, ileus or volvulus. Penetration of the skin about the anus or the intestinal wall by filariform larvae may lead to extremely itchy, linear, urticarial weals. These usually subside in a few hours but tend to keep on recurring. The eruptions may extend 3 or 4 cm in an hour. This rapid progress has led to the term 'larva currens' being used rather than 'larva migrans' or creeping eruption. In addition there are frequently urticarial weals or less well defined areas of erythema. These skin lesions may persist for years without there being any intestinal symptoms.

Systemic strongyloidiasis causes diarrhoea and pneumonia and is rapidly fatal unless diagnosed and promptly treated.

**Diagnosis and Treatment.** Motile rhabditiform larvae can be seen on microscopic examination of the faeces and occasionally in the sputum, urine or bile. Excretion of them is intermittent so repeated examinations may be necessary. In ancylostomiasis, ova, not larvae, are found in a fresh stool. Filarial serology is positive in 15% of patients.

Thiabendazole given orally in a dose of 25 mg/kg body weight twice daily for 2 to 4 days, according to its tolerance, produces a high percentage of cures. Urticaria may recur and a second similar course of thiabendazole may be required.

## Filariases

A number of different nematodes of the family *Filariidae* affect man. The adults are thin worms varying from 2 to 50 cm in length and the larvae or microfilariae are easily visible under the low power of the microscope. The mature females are viviparous. The adults of the species *Wuchereria bancrofti* and *Brugia malayi* inhabit and tend to block lymphatic vessels. Adult filariae of the species *Loa loa* wander in the subcutaneous tissue and cause 'Calabar' swellings. The adults of *Onchocerca volvulus* may be surrounded by fibrous tissue in subcutaneous nodules but it is their larvae which cause a dermatosis and sometimes serious lesions in the eye. The larvae of *Dipetalonema streptocerca* may produce a similar but milder dermatosis but *Dipetalonema perstans* and *Mansonella ozzardi*, the larvae of which circulate in the blood, are non-pathogenic. The microfilariae have distinguishing morphological appearances (Fig. 17.11). It should be noted that the microfilariae of *Wuchereria*, *Brugia* and *Loa* are sheathed, the remainder unsheathed. Filarial infections are commonly associated with a marked eosinophilia.

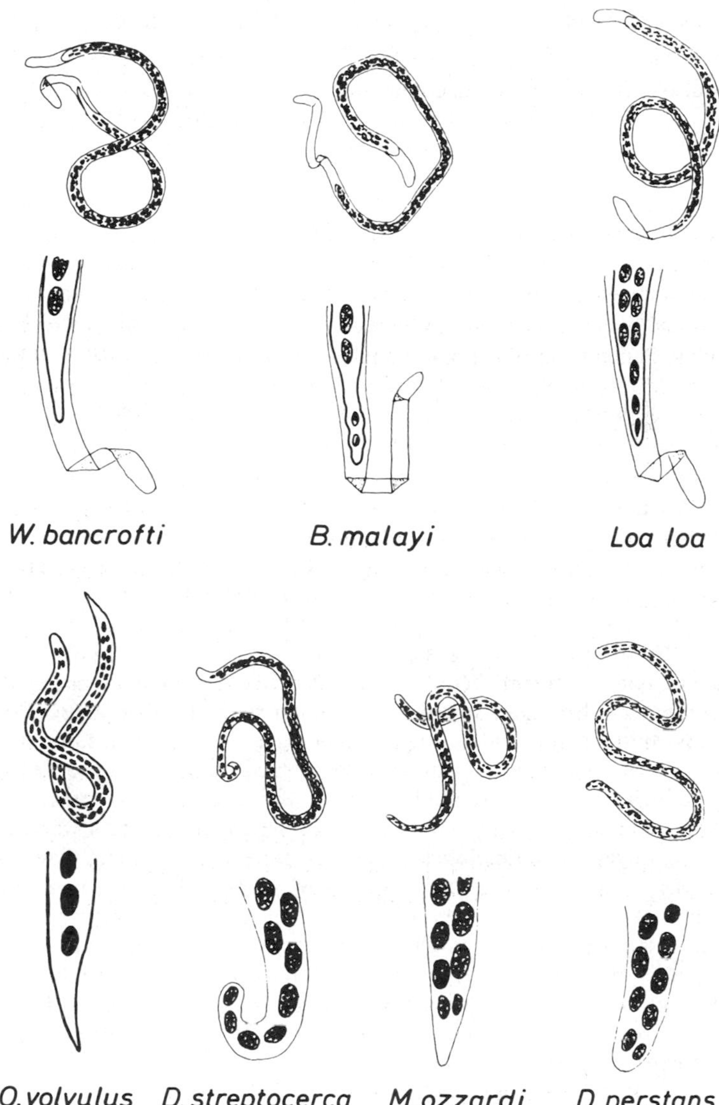


Fig. 17.11 Microfilariae (170–320 × 3–10 μ)
Second and fourth rows show tails (greatly enlarged).

## Bancroftian Filariasis

*Wuchereria bancrofti* is conveyed to man by the bites of infected mosquitoes of a number of different species, the most common being *Culex fatigans*. The adult worms, 4 to 10 cm in length, live in the lymphatics of man, and the females produce microfilariae which at night circulate in large numbers in the peripheral blood. In the mosquito the microfilaria develop and enlarge and the surviving few are able to infect man when the mosquito again bites. As *Culex fatigans* bites at night the nocturnal periodicity of the microfilariae, first demonstrated by Manson in 1877, facilitates the spread of the infection. In some of the Pacific islands there is a non-periodic strain of *W. bancrofti* maintained by mosquitoes which bite in the day-time. When not circulating in the peripheral blood, the microfilariae are chiefly in the capillaries in the lungs. The infection is widespread in tropical Africa, the North African coast, coastal areas of Asia, Indonesia and Northern Australia, South Pacific Islands, West Indies and also in North and South America.

**Pathology.** The microfilariae do not harm the human host. Light infections may remain symptomless but are likely to be associated with an eosinophilia. In more intense and repeated infections the presence of mature worms in the lymphatic vessels and nodes leads to allergic inflammation around the lymphatics and to temporary lymphatic obstruction. Eventually, after repeated attacks, in some of which secondary bacterial infections may play a part, permanent obstruction of a main lymphatic trunk may be produced. Lymphatics rupture and lymph spills into tissues. Progressive enlargement of the limb or region below the obstruction then follows with thickening and fibrosis of the tissues.

**Clinical Features.** After an incubation period of not less than 3 months the first manifestations are bouts of fever accompanied by pain and tenderness along the course of inflamed lymphatic vessels over which there is cutaneous erythema. In addition there may be some scattered urticaria. Inflammation of the spermatic cord, epididymitis and orchitis may be caused by lymphangitis. After a few days the fever abates and the symptoms and signs subside. Further attacks are likely to follow and temporary oedema from obstructed lymphatics tends to become more persistent, and some enlargement of regional lymph nodes may remain. The lymphatics draining the lower limbs, the scrotum and the upper limbs are those most frequently affected, mainly or only on one side, and often accompanied by the formation of superficial lymph varices and the production of hydroceles. Progressive enlargement, coarsening, corrugation and fissuring of the skin and subcutaneous tissue, with warty superficial excrescences, develops gradually until a leg resembles that of an elephant. The name 'elephantiasis' is thus applied to this condition which may also occur in an upper limb, the scrotum, vulva or breast. The scrotum may reach an enormous size. Obstruction of the abdominal or thoracic lymphatics may lead to chyluria, chylous ascites or a chylous pleural effusion. The interval between infection and the onset of elephantiasis is usually not less than 10 years, after which the condition tends to be slowly but remorselessly progressive. Gross elephantiasis develops only in association with repeated infection in highly endemic areas.

**Diagnosis.** In the earliest stages of lymphangitis the diagnosis is made on clinical grounds, supported usually by an eosinophilia and sometimes by a positive complement-fixation or intradermal test. After about a year from the time of infection microfilariae appear in the blood at night and can be seen moving in a wet blood film or a sample of lysed blood passed through a microfilter and identified after staining. They are usually present in hydrocele fluid which may on occasion yield an adult filaria. With the establishment of permanent elephantiasis it becomes unusual for microfilariae to reach the blood stream and eventually the adult worms may die but the lymphatics remain obstructed. Shadows of calcified filariae may sometimes be demonstrable by radiography. An initial exaggeration of symptoms following the administration of the specific drug, diethylcarbamazine, is indicative of a filarial infection.

*Non-filarial elephantiasis,* usually affecting only one lower limb, occurs in certain geographical areas which are free from filariasis. It is attributable to damage to lymphatics by silicates absorbed from soil derived from volcanic rocks.

*Immunodiagnosis*. Indirect fluorescence detects antibody in over 95% of active cases and 70% of established elephantiasis. Cross reactions occur in 15% of cases of strongyloidiasis and 5% of other intestinal nematodes. The test becomes negative 1–2 years after cure. Complement fixation is rather less specific and sensitive. Intradermal tests of immediate hypersensitivity are positive and persist for life. None of these tests distinguishes between the different filarial infections.

**Treatment.** Diethylcarbamazine, given orally, has a rapid destructive effect on microfilariae and a slower action against adult filariae. The dosage is up to 9 to 12 mg/kg body weight daily in three divided doses for 21 days. The full dosage should, however, only be reached slowly, starting with 50 mg (one tablet) and doubling daily if no untoward allergic responses ensue. This course may be repeated twice at intervals of 4 to 6 weeks. To control allergic phenomena antihistamines or corticosteroids may be required. In established elephantiasis plastic surgery, preferably after preliminary radiological investigation of the lymphatics, is indicated. Great relief may be obtained by removal of excess tissue but recurrences are probable unless new lymphatic drainage is established. Tight bandaging, or bed rest with suspension or raising of the affected part or the nightly use of pneumatic stockings, may control the swelling to some extent.

**Prevention.** In endemic areas treatment of the whole population with diethylcarbamazine, 100 mg for adults (50 mg for children) three times daily for 7 days, has reduced but not eliminated the infection. Children are given such a course on starting and just before leaving school. This mass treatment should be combined with control of the vector by insecticides. Personal protection is obtained by the wearing of protective clothing and the use of insect repellants. Where the vector is a night-biting mosquito wire-screening of the house or the use of mosquito nets prevent infection. Early chemotherapy prevents later elephantiasis.

### Brugia Filariasis

*Brugia malayi* resembles *W. bancrofti* closely. The microfilariae usually exhibit nocturnal periodicity but a semiperiodic form, which may affect man, commonly infects animals. A similar filaria, *Brugia pahangi*, is found chiefly in animals but has been transmitted to man. It, or a similar filaria, may be responsible for some cases of tropical pulmonary eosinophilia (p. 274). The vectors of *B. malayi* are mosquitoes mostly belonging to the genus *Mansonioides*. *B. malayi* is found in Indonesia, Borneo, Malaysia, Vietnam, South China, South India and Sri Lanka. A distinct, closely related, species, *B. timori* occurs in Timor.

The pathology, clinical manifestations, treatment and personal prophylaxis are the same as those recorded for *W. bancrofti* except that elephantiasis is usually limited to the legs. A selective weed-killer, phenoxylene, has been used with success to rid ponds of the water hyacinth upon which the larvae of *Mansonioides* are dependent.

### Loiasis

Loiasis is caused by infection with the filaria *Loa loa*. The adults, 3 to 7 cm × 0·4 mm, parasitise chiefly the subcutaneous tissue of man. The larval microfilariae circulate harmlessly in the peripheral blood in the day-time. The vector is *Chrysops*, a day biting, forest dwelling, fly.

**Pathology.** The adult worms move about in the subcutaneous tissues and other interstitial planes. Usually there is little evidence, apart from an eosinophilia, of a reaction of the host's tissues but from time to time a short-lived oedematous swelling (a 'Calabar' swelling) is produced, presumably around an adult worm. Heavy infections may rarely cause encephalitis, especially when treated.

**Clinical Features.** The incubation period is commonly over a year but is often as short as 3 months. The infection is often symptomless. The first sign is usually a Calabar swelling. This is an irritating tense localised swelling which is painful if it is near a joint. The swelling is generally on a limb; it measures a few centimetres in diameter but sometimes is more diffuse and extensive. It usually disappears after a few days but may persist for 2 or 3 weeks. A succession of such swellings may appear at irregular intervals, often in near-by sites. Sometimes there is some urticaria and pruritus elsewhere. Occasionally a worm may be distinctly seen wriggling under the skin, especially of an eyelid and may cross the eye under the conjunctiva, taking many minutes to do so. When an adult worm is moving in retro-orbital tissues, severe unilateral headache resembling migraine is experienced.

The crossing of the eye by a worm or it penetrating the skin or characteristic Calabar swellings in one who has resided in an endemic area enable a clinical diagnosis to be made. This will usually be supported by an eosinophilia. The demonstration of microfilariae of *Loa loa* in the blood (or the recovery of an adult from the skin or eye) establishes the diagnosis. The filarial indirect fluorescent antibody test is positive in 95% of cases, complement fixation in 80% and the intradermal test is usually positive (p. 875). Occasionally a calcified dead worm may be seen on a radiograph.

**Treatment and Prevention.** Diethylcarbamazine (p. 875) gradually increased to a dose of 9 to 12 mg/kg body weight daily and continued at that dosage for 21 days is curative. Treatment may precipitate a severe reaction characterised by fever, malaise, joint and muscle pain and rarely encephalitis.

Protection is afforded by siting houses away from trees and by having dwellings wire-screened against the fly. Protective clothing and repellents are also useful. Mud flats where *Chrysops* is breeding should be treated with Dieldrin or other chemicals to destroy the larvae and pupae. Treatment of the population with diethylcarbamazine will diminish the infective rate of the potential vector.

### Onchocerciasis (River Blindness)

Onchocerciasis is the result of infection by the filaria *Onchocerca volvulus*. Although only about 0·3 mm in diameter, the adult female may be as long as 50 cm, the male being much shorter. The infection is conveyed by flies of the genus *Simulium* which inflict a painful bite. In West Africa the vector is *S. damnosum*, in northern Nigeria also *S. bovis* and in East Africa and Zaïre *S. neavei*. The flies breed in rapidly flowing well aerated water, the larvae being attached to submerged vegetation and rocks. The larvae of *S. neavei* may be attached to crabs and mayfly nymphs. Adult flies bite during the day-time both inside and outside houses. Man is the only known definitive host.

Onchocerciasis is endemic in well defined areas throughout tropical Africa, in Southern Arabia and also in South Mexico and Guatemala. It is estimated that over 20 million people are infected. In parts of West and Central Africa it affects the whole adult population and blindness rates of 10% are common, reaching 35% in some parts of Ghana. Because of onchocerciasis huge tracts of fertile land lie virtually untilled.

**Pathology.** Infective larvae of *O. volvulus* are introduced into the skin by the bite of an infected *Simulium*. The worms mature in 2 to 4 months and live for up to 17 years in small colonies in subcutaneous and connective tissue. At sites of trauma, over bony prominences and around joints, fibrosis may form nodules around adult worms which otherwise cause no direct damage. In these nodules, in the tissues around, and widely distributed in the skin, innumerable microfilariae, discharged by the female *O. volvulus*, move actively and may invade the anterior part of the eye. Live microfilariae elicit little tissue reaction, but dead microfilariae may cause severe allergic inflammation leading to hyaline necrosis and loss of collagen and elastin. In the eye, death of microfilariae causes conjunctivitis, sclerosing keratitis with pannus formation, iritis which may lead to glaucoma and cataract and, in some parts of Africa, choroidoretinitis and optic neuritis.

**Clinical Features.** The infection may remain symptomless for months or years. The first symptom is usually itching at first localised to one quadrant of the body and later becoming generalised and involving the eyes. In Europeans evanescent oedema of part or all of a limb is an early sign, followed by papular urticaria spreading gradually from the site of infection. This is difficult to see on dark skins in which the commonest signs are papules excoriated by scratching, spotty hyperpigmentation from resolving inflammation and more chronic changes of a rough, thickened skin or inelastic wrinkled skin. Superficial lymph nodes enlarge and may hang down in folds of loose skin at the groins. Hydrocele, femoral hernias and scrotal elephantiasis occur. In chronic infections, firm subcutaneous nodules (onchocercomas) are palpable, one or more cm in diameter.

Eye disease is commonest in some highly endemic areas and is associated with chronic heavy infections and nodules on the head. Early manifestations include itching, lachrymation, conjunctival injection and evidence of the features listed under pathology. Classically, 'snow flake' deposits are seen in the edges of the cornea.

**Diagnosis.** The finding of nodules or characteristic lesions of the skin or eyes, in a patient from an endemic area, associated with eosinophilia, is suggestive. Aggravation of the dermatosis after treatment with diethylcarbamazine supports the diagnosis. A certain diagnosis may be made by removal of a nodule and the demonstration of adult worms and unsheathed microfilariae within it. A skin snip or shaving, repeated if necessary from calf, buttock and shoulder is placed in saline under a cover slip on a microscope slide and examined after one hour. In all but the lightest infections microfilariae are seen wriggling free. Microfilariae can also sometimes be seen moving in the anterior chamber of the eye examined with a slit-lamp or identified in a conjunctival snip. Filarial antibodies may be detected by immunofluorescence in 95% of cases and by complement fixation in 50%. The intradermal test is usually positive.

**Treatment and Prevention.** Any nodules detected should be removed.

Diethylcarbamazine (p. 875) rapidly kills the microfilariae and this causes an allergic reaction for the first few days of treatment. The itch increases, eye lesions are aggravated and there may be accompanying fever with pain in the joints. Other reactions include hypotension and respiratory distress. Only a small dose should be given initially, 25 mg on the first day, this being gradually increased as the drug is tolerated until, if possible, a dose of 12 mg/kg body weight is reached. This dose should be continued for 21 days. An antihistamine, such as chlorpheniramine maleate, may alleviate mild reactions but corticosteroids, locally as drops to the eyes and systemically, are needed to control severe reactions. Ideally the patient should be in bed for the first 24 hours of treatment.

Adult worms are killed by suramin (p. 820), the intervals between intravenous injections of 1 g should be 5 to 7 days and the maximum total dose 6 g. In endemic areas where reinfection is inevitable, and in patients with little or no eye involvement, repeated courses of diethylcarbamazine or long-term suppression with 50 mg daily may be preferred to the potential toxicity of suramin.

Mass treatment is impossible at present. The fly can be destroyed in its larval stage by the application of insecticide to streams or the adult flies can be attacked by spraying vegetation near streams. Dimethylphthalate applied to skin or clothing will repel simulia for several hours. Long trousers or skirts and sleeves discourage the fly from biting.

## Other Filariases

**Dipetalonema streptocerca.** Microfilariae and adult worms of this parasite have been identified in the skin of man and chimpanzees in Ghana, Cameroun and Zaïre. The intermediate host and vector is the midge *Culicoides grahami*. The microfilariae may produce a mild dermatosis of the trunk, usually less irritating than the dermatosis of onchocerciasis. This filariasis also responds to a course of diethylcarbamazine.

**Dipetalonema perstans** is a filarial parasite of man which is usually non-pathogenic. In endemic areas microfilariae of *D. perstans* are commonly found in the peripheral blood in which they circulate both by day and night. The adults inhabit chiefly the retroperitoneal and perirenal tissues and have been found in the pericardial sac. The intermediate hosts and vectors are the midges *Culicoides austeni* and *C. grahami*. This filaria is found throughout equatorial Africa as far south as Zambia, also in Trinidad and parts of northern and eastern South America.

*D. perstans* has never been shown to cause disease but it may be responsible for a persistent eosinophilia and occasional allergic manifestations. *D. perstans* is resistant to diethylcarbamazine and the infection may persist for many years.

**Mansonella ozzardi.** This filaria of man is non-pathogenic and is found in the West Indies and central and northern parts of South America. The adults inhabit the mesentery and subperitoneal tissues. The microfilariae circulate in the blood. The intermediate hosts are species of *Culicoides*. Diethylcarbamazine is ineffective.

**Tropical pulmonary eosinophilia** is attributable to an infection with a filarial worm such as *Dirofilaria* or *Brugia pahangi*, which is unable to mature in man. Alternatively it may be an unusual host reaction to the microfilariae of *Wuchereria bancrofti* or *Brugia malayi*. The disease is found in many tropical regions including India, Sri Lanka, Malaysia, China, Philippines, Australia, South America and uncommonly in Africa. Clinical features are discussed on page 274. It is successfully treated by diethylcarbamazine 12 mg/kg body weight daily for 10 days.

## Dracontiasis (Guinea Worm Infection)

The female *Dracunculus medinensis*, which measures over a metre in length, 0·9 to 1·7 mm in diameter, lives in the interstitial and subcutaneous tissues of man. The male worm, which is rarely seen, is only 2·5 cm long and dies earlier. Man is infected by ingesting a small crustacean, *Cyclops*, which inhabits the bottom of wells and ponds and which contains the infective larval stage of the worm. When the cyclops is ingested by man the mature larvae penetrate the intestinal wall and migrate through the connective tissue of the host. After 9 to 18 months the fully mature female seeks the surface of the skin where a vesicle is raised, soon ruptures and exposes the anterior end of the worm. The distended uterus then ruptures and discharges its larvae externally. The worm is attracted to the surface by cooling, hence the larvae are likely to be expelled into water and complete the life cycle. Man is the most important host but *D. medinensis* has been found in dogs and cats.

The disease can be extremely disabling and is especially liable to affect farmers at the beginning of the rains and thus seriously interfere with planting. It is found in West, Central and East Africa, the Sudan, Arabia, Iran, Turkey, Pakistan, Central India, Burma, the Caribbean Islands and the northern parts of South America.

**Clinical Features.** When mature the adult may sometimes be felt beneath the skin. Some hours before the head of the worm emerges from the skin there is usually some local redness and tenderness. There may also be general allergic symptoms, erythema, giant urticaria, nausea, vomiting and diarrhoea. These symptoms usually subside as soon as the vesicle has ruptured and the larvae begin to be discharged. This is usually complete in 3 to 4 weeks, after which the worm is often spontaneously extruded and healing takes place. The vesicle commonly appears in the lower part of the leg or in any area which has been kept moist and relatively cool. If the worm dies or is broken during extraction there will be a marked allergic inflammation. The patient is immobilised by pain and swelling. Secondary infection is common and causes severe cellulitis, septicaemia, aseptic or pyogenic arthritis. Tetanus is a well recognised complication. Multiple infections may occur and reactions around aberrant worms may cause serious lesions, exceptionally spinal cord compression.

Diagnosis is usually easy from the appearance of a vesicle, the protrusion of a worm and the recognition of the discharged larvae. A radiograph occasionally shows calcified worms.

**Treatment and Prevention.** Traditionally the protruding worm has been extracted by winding it out gently over several days on a sterile match stick. Niridazole in doses of 25 mg/kg body weight daily in 2 divided doses for 10 days may reduce inflammation and aid the extraction of the worm. Antibiotics and prophylaxis of tetanus are required for secondary infection.

The provision of a satisfactory water supply would eradicate the infection. Where this is impracticable, wells and ponds may be protected or treated chemically.

## Other Round Worms

**Oesophagostomiasis.** Species of the genus *Oesophagostomum*, a nematode related to hookworms, may cause a granuloma of the wall of the small intestine resembling a neoplasm. It has been reported chiefly from Uganda and is diagnosed at laparotomy.

**Angiostrongylus.** *A. cantonensis*, a nematode affecting the lungs of rodents, has a larval stage in molluscs and freshwater shrimps. In the Far East and the Pacific, where infected crustacea are eaten or infected slugs on vegetables are inadvertently swallowed, the larvae may cause a serious eosinophilic meningitis and immature worms may be found in the cerebrospinal fluid. Thiabendazole is effective but patients often recover spontaneously.

**Trichuris trichiura (Whipworm).** Under unhygienic conditions infections with whipworm are common and they are occasionally acquired in rural districts in Britain. Man is the only host. The ova are passed in stools and infection takes place by the ingestion of earth or food contaminated with ova which have become infective after lying for 3 weeks or more in moist soil. The adult worm is 3–5 cm long and has a coiled anterior end resmbling a whip (Fig. 17.12). Whipworms inhabit chiefly the caecum but occasionally also the lower ileum, appendix and colon. There are usually no symptoms, but intense infections in children may cause persistent diarrhoea or rectal prolapse. The diagnosis is readily made by identifying ova in faeces. In heavy infections adult whipworms are found in the anal canal. Treatment is by oral mebendazole in doses of 100 mg twice daily for 3 days, preceded by loperamide but the safety of mebendazole has been questioned (p. 871).

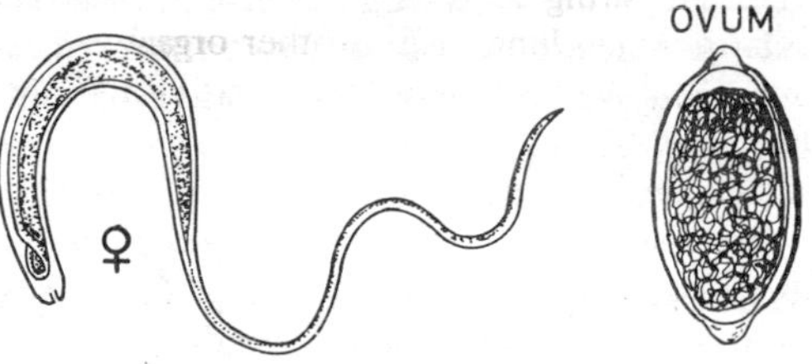


Fig. 17.12 *Trichuris trichiura* (Ova 50 × 22 μ)

**Trichinella spiralis.** This parasite of rats and pigs is transmitted to man by eating partially cooked infected pork, usually as sausage or ham. Symptoms result from invasion of the body by larvae produced by the adult female worm in the small intestine and from their encystment in striated muscles. Outbreaks have occurred in Britain as well as in other countries where pork is eaten. Polar bear meat is another source.

The clinical course of trichinosis depends largely on the number of larvae. If there are only a few worms present there may be no symptoms but many worms may cause nausea and diarrhoea 24 to 48 hours after the infected meal. Soon, however, these symptoms are overshadowed by those associated with larval invasion, namely fever and oedema of the face, eyelids and conjunctivae. Invasion of the diaphragm may lead to pain, cough and dyspnoea; involvement of the muscles of the limbs, chest and mouth causes stiffness, pain and tenderness in the affected muscle groups. Pyrexia may reach 40°C with daily remissions. Larval migration may cause acute myocarditis and encephalitis. An eosinophilia is usually found after the second week. An intense infection may prove fatal, but in those who survive complete recovery is the rule.

It is not uncommon for a group of persons who have eaten infected pork from a common source to develop symptoms about the same time. When suspected, biopsy from the deltoid or gastrocnemius after the third week of symptoms may reveal encysted larvae. Precipitin and intradermal tests are also helpful.

Thiabendazole (50 mg/kg body weight) on two successive days, acting as a larvicide may relieve muscle pain. Given early in the infection it may kill adult worms in the gut. Corticosteroids are given to control the serious effects of acute inflammation.

**Capillariasis.** Infection with *C. phillippinensis* suddenly appeared as an epidemic in the Philippines in the 1960s and in Thailand. Adult worms 2–4 mm long invade the jejunal mucosa, causing abdominal pain with severe diarrhoea and malabsorption. Eggs resembling those of *Trichuris* are passed in the faeces and a salt water fish may be an intermediate host. Untreated, mortality is high, but thiabendazole (p. 872) given for up to one month is effective.

**Gnathostomiasis.** *G. spinigerum* is a nematode of dogs and cats. In the Far East the third stage larva is acquired by man eating inadequately cooked infected fish or by swallowing water containing infected *Cyclops*. The immature worm usually migrates to the subcutaneous tissue where it causes recurrent swellings. The geographical distribution of this infection distinguishes it from loiasis in which similar 'Calabar' swellings are a feature. The full grown adult worm, which may be as long as 3 cm, may develop in man. When the worm, usually single, is visible through the skin it can be removed surgically. During migration in the deeper tissues the worm may cause injury to the brain, kidney, lung, eye or other organs. Eosinophilia is usually pronounced. Diagnosis is easy when the adult worm is visible. Otherwise serological tests are performed. Treatment is not satisfactory but some success has been obtained with bithionol used as for paragonimiasis.

**Anisakiasis (Herring Worm Disease).** *A. marina* is an ascarid which parasitises herrings and other marine animals. Human infections occur in Holland and Japan from the consumption of raw herrings. An eosinophilic granuloma forms in the intestine and may give rise to colic, fever and intestinal obstruction. An indirect haemagglutination test has been used for diagnosis. Surgery may be required.

## DISEASES DUE TO FUNGI (MYCOSES)

*Histoplasmosis; Mycetoma; Blastomycosis; Chromoblastomycosis; Sporotrichosis; Cryptococcosis; Coccidioidomycosis; Paracoccidiodomycosis; Rhinosporidiosis; Superficial Mycoses*

### Histoplasmosis

Histoplasmosis is caused by *Histoplasma capsulatum (Darling)* which is a yeast in its parasitic phase but is a filamentous fungus of soil at other times. A variant, *Histoplasma duboisii*, is found in parts of tropical Africa (p. 883). The spores of *Histoplasma* remain viable for years in the soil and infection is by inhalation of infected dust. Occasionally infection passes through the buccal or intestinal mucosa or through the skin. The disease attacks dogs, rats and mice, and the fungus multiplies in soil enriched by the droppings of chickens, pigeons and bats. The infection is thus a hazard for explorers of caves.

### HISTOPLASMA CAPSULATUM

This is found in all parts of the United States of America, especially in the East Central States, and less commonly in Latin America from Mexico to Argentina, in Europe, North, South and East Africa, Nigeria, Malaysia, Indonesia and Australia.

**Pathological and Clinical Features.** The parasite in its yeast phase multiplies mainly in reticulo-endothelial cells and produces areas of necrosis in which the parasites may abound. From these foci the blood stream may be invaded leading to metastatic lesions in the liver, spleen and lymph nodes. Pulmonary histoplasmosis may produce pathological changes similar to those of tuberculosis.

Probably 90 % of pulmonary infections are benign producing no symptoms, but more severe infections may closely simulate pulmonary tuberculosis, including the production of a primary complex with enlarged satellite lymph nodes, multiple small discrete lesions and occasionally cavitation. Healed lesions may calcify. Lesions of the skin or mucosa may be found on the rare occasions when infection has entered that way and are common in disseminated histoplasmosis which is characterised by enlargement of the liver, spleen and lymph nodes, irregular pyrexia, anaemia and leucopenia. Addison's disease may be produced by caseation in the adrenals. Endocarditis is rare. When the mucosa of the mouth and gastrointestinal tract become infected, the predominant symptoms may be vomiting and diarrhoea. Occasionally the central nervous system is invaded. The severity of the symptoms of histoplasmosis varies from, in the majority of cases, a slight fever of short duration, like influenza, to a severe and prolonged pyrexial illness which ultimately proves fatal.

**Diagnosis.** In an area where the disease occurs, histoplasmosis should be suspected in every obscure infection in which there are pulmonary signs or where there are enlarged lymph nodes with or without hepatosplenomegaly. Tissue is obtained by biopsy for impression smear, histology, culture and animal inoculation. Radiological examination in long standing cases may show calcified lesions in the lungs, spleen or other organs. In the more acute phases of the disease single or multiple soft pulmonary shadows with enlarged tracheo-bronchial nodes may be seen. Delayed hypersensitivity to the intradermal injection of histoplasmin is present in patients with either active or healed infections but is usually negative in the rapidly progressive form of the disease. Complement fixing antibodies are detected within 3 weeks of the onset of an acute primary infection and increase in titre as the disease progresses. Precipitating antibodies may also be detected.

**Treatment.** Specific treatment with amphotericin is indicated only in severe infections. The dosage is 0·5 mg/kg body weight, in 500 ml of 5% glucose given intraveneously over a 6-hour period, gradually increasing to a maximum of 1·0 mg/kg body weight. Treatment is given on alternate days. If badly tolerated, the dosage may have to be reduced. Side-effects are malaise, anorexia, nausea, fever, headache and venous thrombosis. These may be controlled to a considerable extent by the addition of 10 mg prednisolone to the intravenous solution. Plasma urea rises and haemoglobin falls during treatment, but later return to normal. Amphotericin may have to be continued for up to a month or longer, depending on the clinical response. Recovery from generalised histoplasmosis is rare.

### Histoplasma duboisii

*Histoplasma duboisii*, the fungus of African histoplasmosis, is considerably larger than the classical *H. capsulatum*. It is found in Ghana, Uganda, Nigeria, Senegal, Sudan and Zaïre.

This disease differs in several ways from *H. capsulatum* infection. The bones, skin, lymph nodes and liver develop granulomatous lesions or cold abscesses resembling tuberculosis, but the lungs are seldom involved. The visceral form with liver and splenic invasion is often fatal, while ulcerative skin lesions and bone abscesses follow a more benign course.

Radiological examination may show rounded foci of bone destruction sometimes associated with abscess formation. Multiple lesions of the ribs are common and the bones of the limbs may also be involved. Diagnosis is by isolation of the fungus. Immunodiagnostic tests are helpful.

The disease is treated in the same way as *H. capsulatum* infections. A solitary lesion in bone may require only local surgical treatment.

## Mycetoma (Madura Foot)

Mycetoma, in this restricted sense, is a chronic fungal infection of the deep soft tissues and bones, most commonly of the limbs, but also of the abdominal or chest wall or head. It is produced by members of two groups of organisms classified as *Eumycetes* and aerobic *Actinomycetes*. A feature common to both groups is the formation by the fungus of grains, with characteristic colours, ranging from 60 microns to 3 mm in diameter. The incidence appears to be related to climate, being especially high when an arid hot season ends in rains. The more common species of fungi causing mycetoma, as defined above, are shown in Table 17.7. The fungus can be identified by the microscopic appearances of the tissue and grains and confirmed by culture. Antibodies can usually be demonstrated by precipitation.

**Pathological and Clinical Features**. The lesions may occur in any part of the body but as the fungus is usually introduced by a thorn they are more common in the foot and leg in those who walk bare-footed. At the site of implantation the mycetoma begins as a painless swelling which grows and spreads inexorably within the soft tissues causing swelling and eventually penetrates bones. The histology is that of a chronic granuloma with a fibrous stroma and cyst-like spaces in which lie the characteristic grains. Nodules develop under the epidermis and these rupture revealing sinuses through which mucopus containing the coloured grains is discharged. Some sinuses may heal with scarring while fresh sinuses appear elsewhere. There is little pain and usually no fever, but progressive disability. Secondary pyogenic infection does not usually penetrate far down the sinuses, possibly because of antibiotic activity of the fungi.

Although pigment may be carried to regional lymph nodes, it is exceptional for the fungus to reach the nodes unless there has been surgical interference. When the lesion is in the scalp, the skull may be affected but the dura mater appears to be an effective barrier. Apart from involvement of bones by a spreading mycetoma, intraosseous lesions may be found in the metaphysis of a long bone, especially at the upper end of the tibia and sometimes there may be an encapsulated periosteal mass.

*Nocardia brasiliensis* often affects the skin of the back. It is seldom localised and may spread widely.

Table 17.7 Fungi causing mycetoma

| Species | Type of Grains |
|---|---|
| Eumycetoma | |
| *Madurella mycetoma* | brown or black (big) |
| *Madurella grisea* | black or brown (big) |
| *Exophiala jeanselmei* | black |
| *Petriellidium boydii* | white or yellow (big) |
| *Acremonium* spp. | white or yellow |
| Actinomycetoma | |
| *Actinomadura madurae* | white, yellow, red (big) |
| *A. pelletieri* | red (small) |
| *Streptomyces somaliensis* | white or yellow (big) |
| *Nocardia brasiliensis* | white, yellow (microscopic) |

**Treatment**. The difference between *Eumycetes* and *Actinomycetes* is crucial in that there is no drug of proven efficacy for the former. Sporadic successes with griseofulvin against *Eumycetes* have been reported, but the results have been mostly disappointing and up to the present eumycetoma requires to be surgically removed. It has a strong tendency to recur locally unless the excision has been adequate or the amputation high enough. The treatment of actinomycetoma is more hopeful. It is treated with oral rifampicin (4 mg/kg body weight daily) or streptomycin (14 mg/kg daily i.m. daily) plus oral dapsone (1·5 mg/kg b.d.) or oral co-trimoxazole for 4–24 months. *Nocardia* infection may respond to dapsone alone. *In vitro* sensitivities should be carried out for each isolate. Precipitating antibodies disappear if treatment is successful.

## Other Mycoses

**Blastomycosis.** *North American blastomycosis* is caused by *Blastomyces dermatitidis.* It also occurs in Africa. This infection may give rise to cutaneous lesions, especially of the face. Systemic infection begins in the lungs and mediastinal lymph nodes and resembles pulmonary tuberculosis. Bones, the central nervous system and the genito-urinary tract may also be affected. Parenteral treatment with amphotericin (p. 882) has achieved much success. Co-trimoxazole may also be effective.

**Chromoblastomycosis** *(Mossy Foot)*. True mossy foot is an infection due to one of several pigmented fungi and is to be distinguished from the warty excrescences which accompany the chronic lymphatic obstruction of elephantiasis and also from mycetoma.

These fungi are acquired on splinters from decaying timber and give rise to a warty condition of the foot and also rarely affect the face, and upper limbs. The diagnosis is confirmed by the recognition of dark brown spheroid bodies 4 to 8 microns in diameter in biopsy specimens or by culture.

Treatment is oral 5-fluorocytosine 30–50 mg/kg body weight 6 hourly for several months. Blood levels are monitored, especially when renal function is poor. In stubborn cases amphotericin is added (p. 882).

**Sporotrichosis** is caused by *Sporothrix schenckii.* The infection occurs throughout the world and is prevalent in Central and Southern Africa. It causes swellings resembling gummata or a chancroid type of ulcer and affected lymphatic vessels may be thickened and palpable as a chain of nodules. Uncommonly dissemination takes place into lungs, bones, the central nervous system and elsewhere. The fungus can be cultured from discharges or biopsy material.

Potassium iodide up to 10 g daily should be given orally until some time after apparent clinical cure. Widely disseminated infections respond to amphotericin.

**Cryptococcosis** is caused by *Cryptococcus neoformans*. Its distribution is worldwide. It causes local gummatous-like tumours and granulomatous lesions of the lung, bones, brain and meninges. The cerebrospinal fluid often contains the fungus when the nervous system is affected. The diagnosis is made by culture or recognition of spores in the cerebrospinal fluid, biopsy and serological detection of antigen.

Amphotericin should be given intravenously and, in disease of the nervous system, intrathecally or 5-fluorocytosine orally (p. 884). Surgical removal of local pulmonary lesions may be necessary. Recovery may be monitored by fall in antigen titre.

**Coccidioidomycosis** is caused by *Coccidioides immitis*. This infection is found in Southern United States, and in Central and South America. The disease is acquired by inhalation. In 40% of cases it affects the lungs, lymph nodes and skin. Rarely it may be carried by the blood stream to the bones, adrenals, meninges and other organs. In 60% of cases the infection is asymptomatic. Infections, including subclinical attacks, are followed by immunity.

The fungi grow readily on culture media but as they are highly infective, diagnostic investigations are usually limited to intradermal, complement-fixation and precipitin tests.

Some localised pulmonary lesions can be successfully treated by surgery. Amphotericin may be beneficial and miconazole shows promise.

**Paracoccidiodomycosis** is caused by *Paracoccicidiodes brasiliensis* and occurs in South America. Mucocutaneous lesions occur early. Involvement of lymphatic nodes and the lungs is prominent and the gastrointestinal tract may also be attacked. Prolonged treatment with oral sulphonamides and amphotericin may be curative. The imidazoles, miconazole and ketoconazole are showing promise.

**Rhinosporidiosis** is caused by *Rhinosporidium seeberi* and occurs in South America, India, Sri Lanka, and East Africa. This organism forms a cyst which on rupture discharges spores which spread by lymphatics to connective tissue. It produces polypi in the nose and localised swellings on the cheek and elsewhere. The characteristic sporangia and spores are recognised histologically. The organism has not yet been cultured. Treatment is surgical.

**Superficial mycoses** are cosmopolitan and include *Tinea versicolor* and dermatophytosis (ringworm infection). *Tinea imbricata*, characterised by multiple concentric rings, is a common cause of severe pruritus in some Pacific Islands and in South East Asia. It responds to griseofulvin.

Infection of the scalp by *Trichophyton schoenleinii* produces a mass of creamy white material with an offensive odour, the lesion being known as favus. It is treated by epilation and powerful topical fungicides or griseofulvin.

# DISEASES DUE TO ARTHROPODS

*Infections Conveyed by Arthropods; Crab Louse Infestation; Scabies; Tick Paralysis; Tungiasis; Spider Bite; Scorpion and Bee Stings; Myiasis; Porocephalosis*

In addition to the diseases in which arthropods act as vectors and which are summarised in Table 17.8, there are conditions due directly to arthropods.

**The crab louse,** *Phthirius pubis,* infests the pubic hair, other hairy parts, the eyelashes and the hair above the brow of children, causing itching. Gammabenzene hexachloride 1% should be applied to the body and liquid paraffin to the eyelashes.

**Scabies** is due to the mite *Acarus scabei*; it is common in the tropics but may be mimicked by onchocerciasis. It causes itching, initially between the fingers or on the buttocks or penis where the mite burrows, and later all over the body. Scabies is treated by a single application of gammabenzene hexachloride 1% to the whole body below the neck or by three daily applications of benzyl benzoate 15%.

**Tick paralysis** is due to venom in the saliva of certain hard ticks, when such a tick remains attached to the head or neck for some days causing a flaccid paralysis and failure of respiration. If the tick is removed in time, recovery ensues.

**Tungiasis** (Jiggers) is due to infestation with *Tunga penetrans* (the chigoe or jigger flea). It is widespread in tropical America and Africa. Man and pigs are important

Table 17.8 Infections conveyed by arthropods

| Name | Genus | Disease |
|---|---|---|
| House fly | *Musca* | Dysenteries, enteric fevers, salmonelloses, ?cholera, ?trachoma, ?tropical ulcer. |
| Horse fly | *Tabanidae* | ?anthrax, tularaemia |
| Oscinid fly | *Hippelates* | ?yaws, streptococcal dermatitis and nephritis |
| Tsetse fly | *Glossina* | African trypanosomiasis |
| Mosquito | *Anopheles* | Malaria, some arboviruses, Bancroftian and Brugia filariasis in some areas. |
| | *Aedes* | Yellow fever, dengue, and other arboviruses. |
| | *Culex* | Bancroftian and Brugia filariasis, Japanese B encephalitis and other arboviruses |
| Black fly | *Simulium* | Onchocerciasis. |
| Midges | *Culicoides* | *Dipetolema perstans*, *D. streptocerca*, *Mansonella ozzardi*. |
| Soft ticks | *Ornithodoros* | Tick-borne relapsing fever |
| Hard ticks | (*Ixodidae*), *Riphecephalus* etc. | Some typhus fevers, ?Q fever, Kyasanur Forest disease, tularaemia. |
| Sandflies | *Phelbotomus* | Leishmaniases, sandfly fever, bartonellosis. |
| Lice | *Pediculus* | Epidemic typhus fever, louse-borne relapsing fever, trench fever, *Dipylidium caninum*. |
| Mites | *Leptotrombidium* | Scrub typhus fever |
| | *Allodermanyssus* | Rickettsialpox |
| Winged Bug | *Triatoma* | Chagas' disease. |
| Fleas | *Xenopsylla* | Plague, endemic typhus fever. |
| | *Ctenocephalides* | *Dipylidium caninum*. |

hosts. The pregnant female flea burrows into the skin about the toes and soles and grows as large as a pea, packed with eggs which are subsequently discharged on to the surface. The burrows irritate and become inflamed but the chief danger is from secondary pyogenic infection or tetanus. The chigoe and egg sac should be removed with a sterile needle and a mild antiseptic ointment applied. Massive infestations, such as may be seen in neglected children and in senile persons, may be treated by immersing the feet in an aqueous solution containing benzene hexachloride 5% and cetrimide 0·8%.

**Spider Bite.** Most spiders have poison glands to kill their prey. Only two genera have enough venom to harm man. *Latrodectus* species are widespread in warm climates, including the Mediterranean basin and Central Europe but the most dangerous *L. mactans*, the 'Black Widow' is tropical. The females are black or brown, 40 mm long with a coloured 'hour glass' marking on the ventral surface of the abdomen; they are shy, inhabiting burrows, dark corners of sheds and privies and bite only if disturbed. The bite site burns, and cramping muscular pain spreads over the body, simulating an acute abdomen or tetanus. The patient is nauseated, sweaty and restless and may become shocked. Mortality exceeds 5%. Specific antivenom is helpful, if available. Intravenous injection of 10 ml calcium gluconate 100 g/*l* and hot baths relieve muscle pain.

The hairy brown spider, *Loxosceles*, of Central and Southern America lives among furniture in houses and stores. Its bite causes pain, erythema, swelling and extensive local necrosis. Antihistamines and corticosteroids are said to be helpful.

**Scorpion Stings.** There are many genera of scorpions found in the tropics and subtropics. Paired poison glands are situated in the terminal segment of the flexible jointed tail which is curved dorsally over the scorpion's body before striking.

There is a single puncture wound at the site of the sting. Intense local pain is felt immediately, and a red oedematous weal, sometimes haemorrhagic, soon appears. Children particularly show severe general symptoms which include, sweating, salivation, nausea, vomiting and depression of respiration and may die. From S. India and Jordan occasional deaths of adults also are reported in whom there is evidence of disseminated intravascular coagulation. In Trinidad stings of the scorpion, *Tityus trinitatis*, frequently cause acute pancreatitis from which recovery is usual.

Pain can be relieved by immersing the part in water as hot as the patient can tolerate, or by the local injection of xylocaine. If antivenom is available a child should be given 5 ml of the serum intramuscularly. When required, treatment for shock or disseminated intravascular coagulation is given.

**Bee stings** are always painful and in those who have become sensitised anaphylaxis may result in rapid death. In the majority of fatal cases there has been a severe reaction to a bee sting on an earlier occasion. Desensitisation may be practised with some degree of success. Emergency treatment of anaphylactic shock consists of 0.5 ml of adrenaline injection given intramuscularly followed by an intravenous injection of hydrocortisone hemisuccinate 100 mg. An allergic individual should learn to carry adrenaline ready for immediate self-injection. Less severe symptoms may be relieved by an antihistamine. Severe envenomation from multiple stings causes shock, local tissue necrosis, intravascular haemolysis and acute nephritis. As they continue to release venom the 'stingers' of the bees should be removed from the skin by scraping with the blade of a knife.

**Myiasis** is an infestation of various tissues of man by the larvae of flies.

CUTANEOUS MYIASIS. A common cause of cutaneous myiasis is *Cordylobia anthropophaga* (Tumbu fly) which lays its eggs on laundry spread on grass. The larvae penetrate the skin and produce lesions like boils with central orifices through which they breathe. On reaching maturity they emerge.

Another cause is *Dermatobia hominis* which deposits its eggs on the ventral surface of the abdomen of other *Diptera*, especially mosquitoes. When the mosquito bites man or other animals, the warmth of the body stimulates the emergence of the larva. It burrows through the mosquito-made wound into the subcutaneous tissue and grows. A drop of thick oil, such as liquid paraffin, usually brings a larva out in search of air and facilitates its removal. Occasionally the common warble fly (*Hypoderma bovis*) may infest man. *Auchmeromyia luteola*, the Congo floor maggot, imbibes blood through the skin, dropping off when disturbed.

MYIASIS OF WOUNDS, SORES AND CAVITIES. The larvae of many flies including *Callitrogra hominivorax* (Screw worm), *Wohlfahrtia, Calliphora, Lucilia, Sarcophaga* and *Fannia* may infest necrotic tissue in open wounds or ulcers and occasionally invade living tissue. *Chrysomya bezziana* is found in Africa, India and South Vietnam. It may penetrate the nasal sinuses and cause great destruction. *Wohlfahrtia magnifica* is the only specific myiasis-producing fly known to infest man in Europe. The application of 10% chloroform in a light vegetable oil is the treatment of choice for infested wounds.

INTESTINAL MYIASIS. In the tropics especially, vague digestive disturbances or abdominal cramps with diarrhoea and vomiting may be caused by dipterous larvae in the intestinal canal. The eggs or larvae are ingested with food, but it is also possible for flies to deposit eggs on the skin around the anus whence the larvae may crawl into the rectum, vagina or even up the urethra and reach the bladder. Species of the genera *Fannia* and *Sarcophaga* are most frequently encountered. When larvae are swallowed they are passed in the stool or vomited. Occasionally larvae of *Aphiochaeta* or *Megaselia* may pupate in the bowel and live flies escape from the anus with the stool. An aperient is usually all the treatment that is required.

AURAL AND NASAL MYIASIS. When there is an aural discharge, *Callitrogra hominivorax, Sarcophaga, Calliphora* and *Fannia* may be attracted to the ear and aural myiasis result. The nasal cavities and eyes may also be infested, and serious destruction result. Instillation of 10% chloroform in a light oil kills the larvae.

OCULAR MYIASIS. The maggot of *Oestrus ovis* sometimes infests the human eye. The egg may be deposited in the eye of someone tending sheep. A stinging sensation is felt, followed, as the larvae develops, by severe pain in the eye. A drop of cocaine is required so that the lids can be opened to allow extraction of the maggot.

**Porocephalosis** means invasion of the body by 'tongue worms', degenerate arthropods of which *Armillifer armillatus*, *A. moniliformis* and *Linguatula serrata* occur in man. Adult *Armillifer* parasitise the trachea and bronchi of snakes. Man is infected by ingesting ova on uncooked vegetables or by eating undercooked snakes. The condition is usually symptomless in man but calcified nymphs may be seen in radiographs of the chest and abdomen.

Halzoun is the name given in the Middle East to a form of acute dysphagia and laryngeal obstruction from pharyngitis and oedema of the larynx. It is due to the ingestion of nymphs of *Linguatula serrata* in undercooked liver and lymph nodes of sheep and goats. Foxes and dogs are the definitive hosts. Antihistamines and a local anaesthetic spray are suggested for treatment.

# DISEASES DUE TO VENOMOUS SNAKES AND AQUATIC ANIMALS

*Snake Bite; Aquatic Animals as Vectors of Helminths; Jellyfish Stings; Stings from Cone Shells; Stinging Fish; Poisonous Fish*

## Snake Bite

Poisonous snakes belong to five families:

1. *Colubridae*, many of which are non-poisonous, include the Opisthoglypha which are poisonous but only rarely dangerous to man because the grooved fangs are the most posterior teeth in the upper jaw. Examples are tree snakes.
2. *Elapidae* have forward grooved fangs which are fixed in the upper jaw below or in front of the eyes. The nostrils are lateral and there are large scales over the head. The family includes cobras, kraits and mambas.
3. *Hydrophidae* are poisonous sea-snakes; they have an eel-shaped tail and rather flattened body. Sea-snakes are found along the shores of the Indian and Pacific oceans and are mostly poisonous. The most common dangerous species is *Enhydrina schistosa*. *Laticauda colubrina*, the banded sea snake or 'coral snake' is poisonous but not aggressive.
4. *Viperidae* are true vipers, including Russell viper and adders. At rest the long canalised fangs lie along the palate pointing posteriorly but during the act of biting they are rotated forward.
5. *Crotalidae* include the pit viper (pit between the nose and the eye) and the rattlesnake.

**Pathology.** The venoms of *Viperidae* and *Crotalidae* are cytolytic and haemolytic causing swelling and necrosis of tissues spreading from the site of the bite, often with some intravascular haemolysis, or else they cause disseminated intravascular coagulation and haemorrhages. The venoms of most *Elapidae* are powerfully neurotoxic, but that of the Asian cobras (*Naja* spp.) is also cytolytic. The venoms of the spitting cobra, (*Naja nigricollis*) and of the *Colubridae* are cytolytic. *Hydrophidae* venom contains a myotoxin which causes necrosis of muscle.

**Clinical Features.** It is estimated that less than half of those bitten by a potentially lethal snake develop systemic poisoning, but the victim is nearly always acutely anxious. The important signs of systemic envenomation are for *Viperidae* and *Crotalidae*, hypotension, blood-stained sputum and, later, non-clotting blood, for *Elapidae*, ptosis and glossopharyngeal palsy and for *Hydrophidae*, general myalgia and, later, brown or red urine from myoglobinuria.

Bites of *Viperidae* and *Crotalidae* and the Asian cobras give rise to severe pain and early swelling locally and oozing of blood-stained serum from the fang punctures. In severe poisoning extensive swelling of the limb may ensue with discolouration and blistering followed by superficial necrosis and sloughing. Secondary bacterial sepsis is uncommon unless meddlesome incisions have been made or dressings applied prior to sloughing. Systemic involvement exceptionally leads to rapid cardiovascular shock but, more commonly, to bleeding from the lung and into tissues with the danger of death from anaemia or heart failure. In the majority slow healing of the bitten part ensues.

The neurological effects of envenomation from *Elapidae* are usually manifest within 2 hours (exceptionally up to 10 hours) of the bite. They consist of drooping eyelids, incoordinate speech, unsteady gait and difficulty in respiration, progressing in the untreated to generalised paralysis. There may be little, if any, swelling at the site of the bite.

Fishermen dragging nets ashore in muddy water, at or near a river mouth, are the usual victims of bites by *Hydrophidae*. Bathers and paddlers are seldom attacked. The bite on ankle, foot, wrist or hand is felt as a sharp prick but thereafter is painless, inconspicuous and without local swelling. Symptoms of envenomation appear within 1 hour and consist of pain and stiffness, initially in the muscles of the neck, back and proximal parts of the limbs but rapidly becoming generalised. Passive movements provoke intense pain. Later, in severe poisoning, trismus, ptosis and external ophthalmoplegia may appear. Three to six hours after the onset of poisoning, the urine contains myoglobin and protein. Death may result from extensive paresis leading to respiratory failure or from renal failure. If poisoning is less severe, the victim survives but muscle weakness may persist for months.

**Treatment.** The following first-aid measures can be carried out by untrained personnel. First determine, if possible, whether the bite is of a poisonous snake by killing, examining and retaining the snake, if it can be done safely, and by searching the bite for fang punctures. Reassure the patient and give a mild sedative. Keep the patient at rest and apply a constricting ligature such as a handkerchief above the wound sufficiently firmly to retard the flow in the veins but not to stop the arterial circulation. The ligature must be released for 1 minute in every 30. Venom on the surface of the wound should be wiped away gently with a cloth or washed away with water. The bitten part should be immobilised as for a fracture.

The further treatment depends on the type of venomous snake.

In Britain the only naturally occurring poisonous snake is the adder, *Vipera berus*. If there is a swelling surrounding the bite the victim should be closely observed in hosptial for 24 hours, but usually no specific treatment is indicated. If, however, there is persistent or recurrent hypotension, or rarely haemorrhages, it will be necessary to give an infusion of the specific Zagreb antivenom. The contents of 2 ampoules are given in isotonic saline during 20 to 30 minutes and repeated if there is by then no clinical improvement. Adrenaline must be ready in case of anaphylaxis.

In other countries if there is evidence of systemic envenomation from a land snake or if local swelling is marked or spreading up the tissue, specific or polyvalent antiserum should be given in an intravenous infusion. Except in extreme urgency, 0·2 ml of the antiserum should be injected subcutaneously to test for serum sensitivity and the patient observed for 15 minutes. If a severe reaction occurs desensitisation is attempted by giving repeated small doses subcutaneously. Information accompanying antivenom is often incorrect. Usually 100 ml (e.g. 10 ampoules) diluted in 200 to 300 ml isotonic saline should be infused. In severe neurotoxic poisoning, this should be repeated within 1 hour, if improvement is not manifest. If blood remains incoagulable, antivenom is repeated every 6 hours. If the antivenom was appropriate for the species of snake involved the effects on systemic manifestations are dramatically beneficial. No dressing should be applied to the bitten part and unless there are signs of systemic poisoning it is doubtful if antivenom is of material value.

Those bitten by sea-snakes should be given similar first-aid treatment, being kept at rest and transported by stretcher to hospital. If more than 1 hour elapses after the bite without the appearance of signs of toxicity only reassurance is required. If there is clear evidence of systemic poisoning specific antiserum should be given intravenously, preferably after testing for anaphylaxis. Acute renal failure may be treated successfully by renal dialysis.

*General measures.* Shock should be combated by rest, warmth and fluid by mouth or intravenously, and blood should be transfused when indicated. Respiratory weakness following an elapine bite will benefit from oxygen and respiratory paralysis by mouth-to-mouth breathing or by the intratracheal method. Bacterial infection is more likely in *Viperidae* and *Crotalidae* bites, and here penicillin, tetanus toxoid or antitoxin and anti-gas gangrene serum may be advisable.

## Diseases due to Aquatic Animals

Aquatic animals may act as vectors of helminths (Table 17.9), cause stings or be poisonous to eat.

**Jellyfish Stings.** Various jellyfishes, notably the Portuguese man-of-war, *Physalia*, cause lesions in the skin and general reactions in man. The long filamentous tentacles hanging from its under surface contain glands which release a toxin when they come in contact with the human skin, producing linear reddish-brown weals. Excruciating local pain is felt, and general symptoms may follow, including profuse sweating and severe griping abdominal pains. Very occasionally a patient dies within a short time of being stung by a jellyfish, in which case one of the *Cubomedusae* (sea-wasps or box-jellies), *Chironex fleckeri* or *Chiropsalmus quadrigatus* is probably responsible.

'Irukandji stings' affects bathers in the sea off N.E. Australia at certain seasons. They are caused by minute Carybdeid (simple sea-wasps). Acute poisoning develops in a few minutes characterised by violent abdominal and generalised pains, vomiting and prostration. The victim appears seriously ill for a few days but always recovers.

*Treatment.* Methylated spirits or other alcohol should be applied to the stung parts. Dry sand or powder should then be applied and the tentacles and slime scraped off. Resuscitation may be required. An antivenom for sea-wasp stings is available in Australia.

Table 17.9 Aquatic animals as vectors of helminths

| Aquatic animal | | Helminth |
|---|---|---|
| *Intermediate host* | | |
| Snails | | *Schistosoma* spp. |
| *1st host* | *2nd host* | |
| Snails | Fish | *Clonorchis sinensis* |
| Snails | Fish | *Opisthorchis felineus* |
| Snails | Nil | *Fasciola hepatica* |
| Snails | Crabs, crayfish | *Paragonimus* spp. |
| Cyclops, Diaptomus | Fish | *Diphyllobothrium latum* |
| Cyclops, Diaptomus | Fish | *Gnathostoma spinigerum* |
| Cyclops, Diaptomus | Nil or frogs | *Diphyllobothrium mansoni* |
| Cyclops, Diaptomus | Nil | *Dracunculus medinensis* |
| Molluscs, Shrimps etc. | Nil | *Angiostrongylus cantonensis* |

**Stings from Cone Shells (Conidae).** There are many varieties of cone shells. The occupant is often poisonous and can give a sting causing death by respiratory paralysis.

**Stinging Fish.** The stonefish (*Synanceja trachynis*) is the most deadly of the stinging fish and it can easily be mistaken for a piece of coral. Along its back are 13 large spines each containing paired poison sacks. The poison causes great pain and swelling at the sites of the stings and may cause death from respiratory paralysis. The poison is destroyed by the application of hot water and an antivenom is available in Australia.

**Poisonous Fish.** *Ciguatera* poisoning arises from ingesting a heat stable toxin present in numerous species of carnivorous fish whose prey have fed on blue-green algae on coral reefs. Nausea, vomiting, paraesthesiae, muscle weakness and respiratory paralysis are the main symptoms.

*Scombroid* poisoning results from the ingestion of histamine, broken down from histidine in decomposing mackerel or tuna.

*Tetraodon* poisoning results from eating puffer fish and other spiny fish which are inherently poisonous.

*Further reading about venomous snakes and aquatic animals:*

Reid, H. A. (1974) In *Medicine in the Tropics*, ed. Woodruff, A. W. Ch. 33, pp. 541–548. Edinburgh: Churchill Livingstone.

## DISEASES DUE TO VEGETABLE TOXINS

The deleterious effects produced by the ingestion of aflatoxin (p. 799), unripe cassava (p. 727) and bush teas (p. 411) have been mentioned. In addition, argemone and ackee poisoning merit consideration.

### Epidemic Dropsy (Argemone Poisoning)

This disease is due to the use of mustard oil contaminated with the seeds of a poppy weed, *Argemone mexicana* which grows commonly in mustard crops and contains a toxic alkaloid, sanguinarine. This substance interferes with the oxidation of pyruvic acid, which accumulates in the blood and tissues of the patient. Epidemic dropsy occurs in groups of people partaking of the same food, especially curried rice prepared with contaminated mustard oil. It occurs in India, especially in Bengal, Bihar, Orissa, Madhya Pradesh and Uttar Pradesh. Cases have also been noted among Indian expatriates in Fiji.

**Pathology.** There is dilatation of the smaller arterioles and of capillaries, especially those of the skin, heart muscle and uveal tract. New blood vessels in the deeper layers of the skin and mucosa may form haemangiomas.

**Clinical Features.** The onset may be gradual or acute. Nausea, vomiting and diarrhoea often precede the onset of the oedema of the legs and feet and are accompanied by symptoms and signs of cardiac failure which may be fatal, and fever. An erythematous mottling of the skin may follow the oedema, and haemangiomatous tumours up to 1 cm in diameter may appear in the skin or mucosal surfaces. Glaucoma is a serious complication.

**Treatment and Prevention.** Cardiac failure is treated in the usual way. A high protein diet must be given and all contaminated mustard oil excluded. Improvement is often slow. Glaucoma may require surgery.

Steps should be taken to prevent contamination of mustard crops with the weed *A. mexicana*. A test can be carried out to detect this contaminant in mustard oil.

### Vomiting Sickness of Jamaica (Ackee Poisoning)

This illness occurs in young undernourished children who eat unripe fruit of a common West Indian and South American tree, *Blighia sapida* which contains a water-soluble toxin, which blocks gluconeogenesis in the liver. The first symptom is vomiting, followed by drowsiness, convulsions, coma and marked hypoglycaemia. If started early, continuous intravenous glucose can bring about recovery. Without treatment the mortality rate is high.

## Advice to Travellers

A pamphlet, *Notice to Travellers*, published by Her Majesty's Stationery Office, London, gives a list of vaccinations currently obligatory for travellers. Much useful advice may be found in *Preservation of Health in Warm Climates*, The Ross Institute, London and in *Travel Medicine* by Turner, A.C. Edinburgh: Churchill Livingstone, from which Tables 17.10 and 17.11 are taken. In addition, it is very important that all visitors to the tropics and subtropics should take prophylactic antimalarial drugs regularly from the day before travel and continue until 4 weeks after returning to a non-malarious area. Details are given on page 812. Neglect of this advice has been responsible for fatalities. Yellow fever vaccination is available at recognised centres in Britain, see *Notice to Travellers*.

A map illustrating the distribution of disease is shown in Figure 17.1.

Global aspects of the prevention of disease and the promotion of health are discussed in the next chapter.

A. D. M. BRYCESON
F. J. WRIGHT

Table 17.10 Immunisations required under International Health Regulations

| Where required | Validity | Minimum age | Other comments |
|---|---|---|---|
| *Cholera*<br>Always entering and *transitting* Pakistan, India, Burma, Also some other countries in Middle and Far East and Africa | After 6 days for 6 months | Usually 1 year. However some countries no minimum age limit or less than 1 year | A few countries require 2 injections at 1 week interval |
| *Yellow Fever*<br>Central Africa 15°N to 10°S. Central America, northern border of Panama State to 15°S but including Bolivia and excluding part of eastern Brazil and Panama Canal | After 10 days for 10 years | Usually 1 year. A few countries have no minimum age limit or less than 1 year | Not at same time as polio vaccine. |

Table 17.11 Medically recommended immunisations

| Inoculation | Where advised | Course programme | Validity | Minimum age advised | Other comments |
|---|---|---|---|---|---|
| Typhoid Paratyphoid (TAB) | Everywhere except Northern Europe | Intradermal injection.4–6 weeks between 1st and 2nd, 6–12 months between 2nd and 3rd | Booster injection every 3 years | 2 years | Can be combined with tetanus as TABT |
| Tetanus | Everywhere | Frequency as above but subcutaneously. Combined with TAB: frequency as above but intradermally | Booster injection every 3–5 years | NIL | Can be combined with TAB as TABT |
| Poliomyelitis | Everywhere | 3 oral doses of attenuated virus at monthly intervals | 1 Booster dose every 5 years; if over 5 years 2 doses are recommended | NIL | If same time as yellow fever use subcut. dead vaccine |
| Plague | Vietnam, Laos, Khmer Republic, Ethiopia. Possibly Pakistan and India. | 2 injections at 10–20 day intervals, 3rd 6 months later | 6 months | 1 year | Preferably not at same time as TAB and typhus |
| Typhus | Vietnam, Laos, Khmer Republic, Ethiopia. Possibly Pakistan and India. Essential for overlanders | 2 injections at 7–10 day intervals. 3rd 6 months later | 1 year | 1 year | Preferably not at same time as TAB and plague |
| Gamma Globulin for type A Hepatitis | Countries where sanitation is poor | 1 injection | 4–6 months | 10 years | Necessity for repetition after 6 months is arguable |

Malarial prophylaxis, see page 812.

*Further reading about parasitology and tropical diseases:*

Standard textbooks:
Craig, C. F. & Faust, E. C. (1970) *Clinical Parasitology*, 8th edn. Philadelphia: Lea & Febriger.
Jelliffe, D. B. & Stanfield, J. P. (eds.) (1978) *Diseases of Children in the Subtropics and Tropics*, 3rd edn. London: Arnold.
Wilcocks, C. & Manson-Bahr, P.E.C. (1972) *Manson's Tropical Diseases*, 17th edn. London: Ballière, Tindall and Cassell.
Woodruff, A. W. (1974) *Medicine in the Tropics.* Edinburgh: Churchill Livingstone.

# 18. Promotion of Health and Prevention of Disease

**In Tropical and Developing Countries.** A survey of patterns of disease in the tropics and developing countries was made on pages 792 to 806 and methods of prevention of individual diseases have been discussed. The promotion of health and the prevention of disease is, however, related to fundamental principles sometimes far removed from medical therapeutics and prophylactic measures for individual diseases.

Whereas obesity is a major problem in affluent communities, undernutrition and malnutrition are dominant in underdeveloped countries. Adequate nutrition depends primarily on preserving the fertility of the soil and making good use of its vegetable products and, if customs permit, of the animals which are themselves dependent on the vegetation. Preservation or construction of water supplies is also a fundamental need and afforestation and contour terracing may help to prevent the land becoming denuded by floods. Only if a poor country can become richer, can sustained improvement in health be expected. More efficient agriculture and animal husbandry will tend to lead to improved health and economy; further progress may follow the utilization of mineral resources and the development of productive industries and tourism. Much help has been given in starting these processes by outside agencies but in order that lasting benefit should accrue it must be accompanied by better education. It is of paramount importance that the people concerned must themselves be fully convinced of the value and practicability of the projects and desire their benefits. Progress may be slow when improvements in health necessitate changes in food habits and other traditional practices, and will be maintained only when projects become an integral part of the development programme of the country and are operated largely by local personnel. Training of local nationals is, therefore, essential.

Increases in food supplies may be outstripped by increases in population. Family planning is, thus, a priority in many developing countries and emphasis should be laid both on the successful bringing up of healthy children and on the reduction of the population growth. Any progress can be vitiated by war or other political disturbance, hence the preservation of peace and law and order are crucial. Alcoholism is an enemy too little recognised in underdeveloped countries. It affects people in all socio-economic groups and causes a disproportionate number of deaths from road accidents, frequently of those people whom a country can least afford to lose.

It will be clear that the medical practitioner's role in these measures will be chiefly that of an informed adviser. The relative values to community health of money spent, for example, on improved schooling as compared with eradication of malaria may be very difficult to assess, yet governments with limited resources have frequently to decide between such priorities. It has been shown in some areas that the provision of a protected water supply is the most economical way of improving health. Irrigation schemes may be essential to increase the areas of fertile land but expert advice may be required to prevent the spread thereby of malaria, schistosomiasis and onchocerciasis. The eradication of onchocerciasis and animal trypanosomiasis would lead, but at great expense, to the conversion of vast tracts of unused fertile land to pastoral and agricultural use.

In developing countries the provision of curative measures, which may also be important factors in prevention, involves the same principles as in affluent societies but their application is modified by the limitations of available finance and personnel. Priority should be given to measures which will improve the health and prospects of children and wage earners. In order to reach the scattered rural population a chain of health centres, under 5-year-old clinics and peripheral aid posts have proved of great value. At the health centres maternity and child welfare have priority and at all levels health education is actively pursued. Breast feeding of all children for at least the first 6 months should be the rule and importation of expensive foreign baby foods should be kept to a minimum. Immunisation of children and, in the case of tetanus, of expectant mothers also, may do much to reduce mortality rates. Domiciliary visits from the centres increase the contact with outlying homesteads. The vulnerability of small children to gastroenteritis underlines the importance of education in cleanliness and the provision of pure water supplies, but may also necessitate the provision of local facilities for rapid rehydration.

Making the best use of medical auxiliaries is essential if the health services are to be made widely available. Peripheral clinics have to be related to district and central hospitals from which some degree of supervision can be exercised and to which patients can be referred if transport is available. Minimal curative medicine is carried out at the peripheral clinics, but preventive measures must be seen to be related to curative medicine, otherwise little support for them will be forthcoming. The provision of specialised care, even in the central hospitals, should not be out of proportion to the general standard of medical care and medical education should include experience in both categories. Political pressure to divert effort and money into prestige units should be resisted.

**In Disaster Situations**. If earthquakes, floods, drought or other disasters strike an area, help from outside is urgently needed to maintain food supplies and to prevent the spread of disease from sudden impairment of hygiene. When the disaster is war, a nuclear accident (p. 790), earthquakes or volcanic eruptions it may be difficult and dangerous to get supplies to the stricken areas. Failure of food and medicines to reach the people is often more the result of disorganization than unavailability of supplies that can be flown in from international donors. Relief agencies from different countries often try to operate without adequate communication with local community leaders or one another. Governments in countries where famine is recurrent should have civil servants permanently employed in keeping plans for famine relief up to date.

**In Developed Countries**. The term 'developed' is used to denote wealthy communities, mainly industrial. It is not intended to imply that the acquisition of more material possessions is necessarily a desirable goal or that the way of life in developed societies does not contain defects, some of which are deleterious to health.

National and local government bodies assume the responsibility for ensuring the availability of adequate food supplies, education, housing, health services and the prevention of environmental pollution but the family doctor plays an important role in encouraging people to make full use of preventive services. Genetic counselling, immunisation programmes and the early recognition and treatment of disease, the provision of iron and folic acid for expectant mothers, vitamins C and D for young children and financially subsidised school meals do much to ensure a good beginning in the building of a healthy nation. Where local mineral deficiencies exist, fluoridation of water to prevent dental caries and iodized salt to prevent goitre have proved their value.

The medical profession must continue to seek improvement in the working conditions in mines and factories, to identify industrial hazards and to draw attention to the special needs of persons in stressful occupations or doing repetitive work on mass production assembly lines.

Screening for disease can be carried out readily by the family doctor and can be supplemented by the use of mass miniature chest radiography. Malignant disease of the breast, cervix and uterus can be detected at a very early stage, if apparently healthy young women are examined regularly. For those in the middle years of life, medical reviews, at intervals of no longer than 2 years, facilitate the early recognition of disease such as hypertension, diabetes and malignancy.

The needs of the elderly must be met by prophylactic measures such as the use of vitamins C and D, the assessment and treatment of the multiple disabilities frequently overlooked in this age group, social support and community services for the isolated and the provision of suitable accommodation for those requiring continuing care.

For patients of all ages it is the doctor's duty to encourage healthy living habits in matters such as exercise and diet with emphasis on an energy value appropriate to the needs of the individual, moderation in the intake of saturated fat and an ample content of dietary fibre.

The *dietary guidelines* in Scandinavia for the general public were introduced in 1968 and have since been followed, with local modifications, in several major industrial countries: 'The supply of calories (energy) in the diet should in many cases be reduced to prevent overweight. The total consumption of fat should be reduced from 40% (the present figure) to between 25 and 35% of energy. The use of saturated fat should be reduced and consumption of polyunsaturated fats increased (p. 903). Consumption of sugar and sugar-rich products should be reduced. The consumption of vegetables, fruit, potatoes, skimmed milk, fish, lean meat and cereal products should be increased.

From the medical and nutritional standpoint the importance of taking regular exercise from an early age for all those who have mainly sedentary occupations should also be emphasized.'

Food additives are rightly kept under regular and careful review by responsible governments.

There must be a constant awareness of the dangers of tobacco smoking, of excessive consumption of alcohol and of the abuse of drugs by patients and their over prescription by doctors. Much can be done to promote mental health by doctors listening attentively to patients and thus helping individuals to contend with their problems while also detecting those at risk from psychiatric disturbances. There is increasing evidence that good mental health retards physical deterioration in mid-life. A religious belief may be essential for full health.

In all communities, there should be continuing demands for improvement in housing standards and in food hygiene. In many societies the morbidity and mortality from road traffic accidents is rapidly increasing and is related to the abuse of alcohol and psychotropic drugs. In urban areas there are growing problems in regard to corruption, crime, violence, baby and wife battering, rape and drug abuse. But there are much greater hazards. Man has now the capacity to destroy himself not only with nuclear weapons but by using up the natural resources of the planet so fast and by polluting the environment so thoroughly that he is in danger of precipitating his own doom. Everyone, especially doctors, economists, agriculturists and statesmen, is involved in this challenge and the response to it is vital.

JOHN MACLEOD
A. S. TRUSWELL
F. J. WRIGHT

*Further reading about the promotion of health and prevention of disease:*

Davey, T. H. & Wilson, T. (1971) *Davey and Lightbody's Control of Disease in the Tropics,* 4th edn. London: H. K. Lewis.

Davidson, Sir Stanley, Passmore, R., Brock, J. F. and Truswell, A. S., (1979) *Human Nutrition and Dietetics*, 7th edn. Edinburgh: Churchill Livingstone.

Djukanovic, V. & Mach, E. P. (eds.) (1975) *Alternative Approaches to Meeting Basic Health Needs in Developing Countries. A Joint UNICEF/WHO Study*. Geneva: WHO.—Barefoot doctors. etc.—practical approaches to providing health care in rural areas of developing countries.

Howe, G. M. & Lorraine, J. A. (eds.) (1980) *Environmental Medicine*, 2nd edn. London: Heinemann.—Wide-ranging reviews by experts on environmental and social threats to health.

King, M. (1966) *Medical Care in Developing Countries*. Nairobi: Oxford Press.

Morley, D. (1973) *Paediatric Priorities in the Developing World*—Obtainable at low cost from Institute of Child Health, 30 Guildford Street, London WC1.

Ninth Report of the Joint FAO/WHO Expert Committee on Nutrition (1976) *Food and Nutrition Strategies in National Development*. WHO Tech. Rep. Ser. No. 584. Geneva.

# 19. Appendices

## Diets

The diet sheets that follow have been constructed to illustrate the quantitative and qualitative aspects of diets required for the treatment of obesity and diabetes mellitus. The quantities given in a standard diet sheet will obviously require some modification in relation to the size, age, sex, and occupation of the patient. In the dietetic treatment of most diseases it is unnecessary to weigh accurately the amounts of the different foods eaten. Under these circumstances sufficient accuracy will be secured by the use of household measures as illustrated in Diet 1 and by the terms 'small', 'medium' or 'large' helping for meat, fish or chicken. A small helping weighs approximately 1 to 2 oz (30–60 g), a medium helping 2 to 3 oz (60–90 g) and a large helping 4 oz (120 g) or more.

The qualitative content of the diet, i.e. the actual food consumed, will vary widely. The examples detailed here are suitable for persons whose food habits are those of the Western world. If they are to be effective therapeutically, diet prescriptions must be carefully adapted to take account of national, cultural and local eating habits.

The subcommittee on Metrication of the British National Committee for Nutritional Sciences of the Royal Society recommended in 1972 that kilojoules should be used in place of kilocalories. 1 kcal = 4·184 kJ, so that the calorie conversion factors (heat of combustion; available energy) for carbohydrate, fat, protein and alcohol are 16, 37, 17 and 29 kJ/g. Useful practical approximations are: 950 kcal = 4000 kJ; 1450 kcal = 6000 kJ; 2850 kcal = 12000 kJ

### 1. Low Energy (Calorie) Diet

suitable for adults with obesity with or without diabetes

Approximately: Protein 60 g. Carbohydrate 100 g. Fat 40 g. Energy 1000 kcal (4184 kJ)

*Early morning* — Cup of tea, milk from allowance,* if desired.

*Breakfast* — 1 egg or 1 oz (30 g) grilled lean bacon (2 rashers) *or* cold ham *or* breakfast fish.
2/3 oz (20 g) white or brown bread, *or* exchange, with butter from allowance.*
Tea or coffee, with milk from allowance.

*Mid-morning* — Tea or coffee, with milk from allowance, or 'free' drink from Group A3.
1 cream cracker or water biscuit.

*Mid-day meal* — Clear soup, tomato juice or grapefruit, if desired.
Small helping, 2 oz (60 g) lean meat, ham, poultry, game or offal *or* 3 oz (90 g) white fish (steamed, baked or grilled) *or* 2 eggs *or* 1½ oz (45 g) cheese.
Salad or vegetables from Group A1 as desired.
1 1/3 oz (40 g) bread (white or brown) *or* exchange, with butter from allowance if desired.
1 portion of fruit from bread exchange list below.
Tea or coffee with milk from allowance.

*Mid-afternoon* — 2/3 oz (20 g) white or brown bread, *or* exchange, with butter from allowance.

| | |
|---|---|
| *Evening Meal* | Clear soup, meat or yeast extracts, tomato juice or grapefruit, if desired.<br>Small helping, 2 oz (60 g) lean meat, ham, poultry, game or offal *or* 3 oz (90 g) white fish (steamed, baked or grilled) *or* 1 egg *or* 1½ oz (45 g) cheese.<br>Salad or vegetables from Group A1 as desired.<br>1⅓ oz (40 g) bread (white or brown) *or* exchange, with butter from allowance if desired.<br>1 portion of fruit from list below.<br>Tea or coffee with milk from allowance. |
| *Before bed* | Tea or coffee with milk from allowance.<br>1 cream cracker or water biscuit |
| **Allowance for day:* | ⅓ pint milk (200 ml) with the cream poured off the top.<br>½ oz (15 g) butter or margarine. |

*Exchanges for ⅔ oz (20 g) bread (½ slice from a large cut loaf):*

| | |
|---|---|
| 2 cream crackers | 1 potato (the size of a hen's egg) |
| 1½ of any crispbread. | 1 portion of fruit (from list below) |
| 2 water biscuits | |
| 1 oatcake | |

*Exchanges for 1⅓ oz (40 g) bread (1 slice from a large cut loaf):*

| | |
|---|---|
| 4 cream crackers | 2 potatoes |
| 3 Ryvita | 4 water biscuits |
| 2 oatcakes | |

*Fruit list*: 1 medium apple, 1 orange, 1 pear, 1 small banana, 10 grapes.

## GROUP A: FOODS WHICH MAY BE TAKEN AS DESIRED

1. *Vegetables*

Artichoke, asparagus, aubergine, French beans, runner beans, broccoli, Brussels sprouts, cabbage, carrots, cauliflower, celeriac, celery, chicory, courgette, cucumber, endive, leeks, lettuce, mushrooms, mustard and cress, onions, parsley, pumpkin, radishes, salsify, seakale, spinach, swede, tomatoes, turnip, turnip tops, vegetable marrow, watercress.

2. *Fruits* (stewed without sugar, or raw)

Gooseberries, grapefruit, lemon, melons (cantaloupe, water or honeydew), rhubarb, blackcurrants, red currants, blackberries, strawberries and raspberries.

3. *Drinks*

Water, soda water, tea or coffee (without milk or sugar) lemon juice, tomato juice, diabetic fruit squash, Marmite, Bovril, Oxo, clear soup (chicken or beef cubes may be used).

4. *Miscellaneous*

Saxine, saccharine or any proprietary sweetening agents except Sucron and sorbitol. Salt, pepper, mustard, vinegar, herbs, spices, gelatine, Worcester Sauce, flavourings and colourings may be used.

## GROUP B: FOODS TO BE AVOIDED

Sugar (brown or white), glucose, sorbitol.
Sweets, toffees, chocolates, cornflour, custard powder.
Jam, marmalade, lemon curd, syrup, honey, treacle.
Tinned, frozen or bottled fruits.
Dried fruits, e.g. dates, figs, prunes, apricots, sultanas, currants, raisins, bananas, grapes.
Cakes, buns, pastries, pies, steamed or milk puddings.
Sweet or chocolate biscuits, scones.
Cereals, e.g. rice, sago, macaroni, barley, spaghetti, etc.
Breakfast cereal, porridge.

Cocoa, Ovaltine, Horlicks, etc.
Ice cream, fresh or synthetic cream. Table jelly.
Evaporated or condensed milk.
Peas, parsnips, beetroot, sweetcorn, haricot beans, butter beans, broad beans, lentils.
Nuts.
Salad cream, salad dressing, mayonnaise.
Tomato and brown sauce or any thickened sauce.
Sweet pickles and chutney.
Thickened soups, gravies, Bisto.
Alcoholic drinks, e.g. beer, wine, sherry, spirits.
Sweetened fruit juices, fruit squash, Coca Cola and other sweet, fizzy, 'soft drinks'.
Lemonades, Lucozade, Ribena.
Starch-reduced products, 'diabetic' foodstuffs.
Sausages.
*All Fried Foods.*

All foods must be served without thickened gravies and sauces. All foods may be baked, grilled, boiled or steamed—*but not fried.*

## 2. Measured Diabetic Diet

METHOD OF CONSTRUCTING A DIET RESTRICTED IN CARBOHYDRATE CONTAINING APPROXIMATELY 1800 KCAL (7560 KJ) WITH 210 G CARBOHYDRATE 80 G PROTEIN AND 70 G FAT SUITABLE FOR ADULTS WITH DIABETES MELLITUS

Use is made of the Atwater calorie conversion factors of 4, 4 and 9 kcal/g for carbohydrate, protein and fat respectively. Each *carbohydrate exchange* contains approximately 10 g carbohydrate, 1·5 g protein and 0·3 g fat. Calorie value is about 50 (equivalent to $^2/_3$ oz bread).

Each *protein exchange* contains approximately 7 g protein and 5 g fat. Calorie value is about 70 (equivalent to 1 oz meat).

Each *fat exchange* contains approximately 12 g fat and almost no carbohydrate or protein. Calorie value is about 110 (equivalent to $^1/_2$ oz butter). One pint of milk contains approximately 30 g carbohydrate, 18 g protein and 24 g fat. Calorie value is about 410.

In practice, for quick construction of a diabetic diet it is usually only necessary to work in terms of grams of carbohydrate and total calories. Thus, a diet prescription for 210 g carbohydrate, 1800 kcal would be calculated as follows:

1. The daily intake of carbohydrate (210 g) represents 21 carbohydrate exchanges.
2. The daily allowance of milk is decided, either on the basis of the patient's food habits, or on his special requirements. In this example it is $^2/_3$ pint (400 ml), which contains 2 carbohydrate exchanges, leaving 19 for distribution throughout the day.
3. The daily allowance of protein is then decided. Five protein exchanges will provide 350 kcal.
4. The calories allocated so far amount to 1580; a further 220 kcal are needed to bring the total up to 1800 kcal. This must be provided by fat. As one fat exchange provides 110 kcal, two are needed.

| Exchanges | Grams of carbohydrate | kcal |
|---|---|---|
| $^2/_3$ pint milk (400 ml) = 2 carbohydrate exchange | 20 | 280 |
| 19 carbohydrate exchanges | 190 | 950 |
| 5 protein exchanges | — | 350 |
| Total | 210 | 1580 |
| 2 fat exchanges | — | 220 |
| GRAND TOTAL | 210 | 1800 |

5. Finally, the exchanges (21 carbohydrate, 5 protein and 2 fat) are distributed throughout the day according to the eating habits and daily routine of the patient.

*Useful CHO exchanges*
Each item on this list = 1 CHO exchange (10g CHO):
1/2 slice bread from a large loaf, 1 large digestive biscuit, 2 Rich Tea biscuits, 2 cream crackers, 2 heaped teaspoons Ovaltine or Horlicks, 8 tablespoons natural unsweetened orange juice or grapefruit juice, 1 medium sized eating apple or orange, 10 grapes, 1 small banana, 1/3 pint milk, 1 teacup cooked porridge, 1 teacup of cream or tinned soup, 2/3 teacup cornflakes, 1 small packet of crisps.

## 3. Unmeasured Diabetic Diet

Patients who are unable to measure their diet or for whom this is unnecessary, are given a list of foods which are grouped into three categories.

I. *Foods to be avoided altogether:*

1. Sugar, glucose, jam, marmalade, honey, syrup, treacle, tinned fruits, sweets, chocolate, lemonade, glucose drinks, proprietary milk preparations and similar foods which are sweetened with sugar.
2. Cakes, sweet biscuits, chocolate biscuits, pies, puddings, thick sauces.
3. Alcoholic drinks unless permission has been given by the doctor.

II. *Foods to be eaten in moderation only:*

1. Breads of all kinds (including so-called 'slimming' and 'starch-reduced' breads, brown or white, plain or toasted).
2. Rolls, scones, biscuits and crispbreads.
3. Potatoes, peas and baked beans.
4. Breakfast cereals and porridge.
5. All fresh or dried fruit.
6. Macaroni, spaghetti, custard and foods with much flour.
7. Thick soups.
8. Diabetic foods.
9. Milk.

III. *Foods to be eaten as desired:*

1. All meats, fish, eggs.
2. Cheese.
3. Clear soups or meat extracts, tomato or lemon juice.
4. Tea or coffee.
5. Cabbage, Brussels sprouts, broccoli, cauliflower, spinach, turnip, runner or French beans, onions, leeks or mushrooms, lettuce, cucumber, tomatoes, spring onions, radishes, mustard and cress, asparagus, parsley, rhubarb.
6. Herbs, spices, salt, pepper and mustard.
7. Saccharine preparations for sweetening.

For overweight diabetics butter, margarine, fatty and dried foods must be restricted.

## 4. Fat-Modified Diet

Low in saturated fats and cholesterol with increased amounts of polyunsaturated fat.

*Foods to be avoided:*

Butter and hydrogenated margarines. Use polyunsaturated margarine, e.g. 'Flora'.
Lard, suet, shortenings and cakes, biscuits and pastries made with these.
Fatty meat and visible fat on meat. Meat pieces, sausages and luncheon meats.
Whole milk and cream.
Chocolate, ice cream (except water ices). Cheese, except low fat cottage cheese.
Coconut, coconut oil and 'Coffee mate'.
Eggs—no more than 1 to 2 egg yolks per week, including that used in cooking.
Organ meats—liver, kidneys and brain.
Shellfish and fish roes.
Fried foods unless fried in polyunsaturated oil (like sunflower or corn oil).
Potato crisps and most nuts.

Gravy unless made with polyunsaturated oil, and tinned soups.
Salad dressing unless made with polyunsaturated oil.

*Use:*
Polyunsaturated margarine, e.g. Flora instead of butter.
Polyunsaturated oil, e.g. Sunflower or corn oil in place of lard.

*Further reading about dietetics and additional diets:*

Davidson, Sir Stanley, Passmore, R., Brock, J. F. & Truswell, A. S. (1979) *Human Nutrition and Dietetics*, 7th edn. Edinburgh: Churchill Livingstone.

## Desirable Weights

TABLE 19.1

WEIGHTS FOR AGE: BIRTH TO 5 YEARS, SEXES COMBINED[1]

| | WEIGHT (kg) | | | | WEIGHT (kg) | | |
|---|---|---|---|---|---|---|---|
| Age (months) | Standard[2] | 80% Std | 60% Std | Age (months) | Standard[2] | 80% Std | 60% Std |
| 0 | 3.4 | 2.7 | 2.0 | | | | |
| 1 | 4.3 | 3.4 | 2.5 | 31 | 13.7 | 11.0 | 8.2 |
| 2 | 5.0 | 4.0 | 2.9 | 32 | 13.8 | 11.1 | 8.3 |
| 3 | 5.7 | 4.5 | 3.4 | 33 | 14.0 | 11.2 | 8.4 |
| 4 | 6.3 | 5.0 | 3.8 | 34 | 14.2 | 11.3 | 8.5 |
| 5 | 6.9 | 5.5 | 4.2 | 35 | 14.4 | 11.5 | 8.6 |
| 6 | 7.4 | 5.9 | 4.5 | 36 | 14.5 | 11.6 | 8.7 |
| 7 | 8.0 | 6.3 | 4.9 | 37 | 14.7 | 11.8 | 8.8 |
| 8 | 8.4 | 6.7 | 5.1 | 38 | 14.85 | 11.9 | 8.9 |
| 9 | 8.9 | 7.1 | 5.3 | 39 | 15.0 | 12.05 | 9.0 |
| 10 | 9.3 | 7.4 | 5.5 | 40 | 15.2 | 12.2 | 9.1 |
| 11 | 9.6 | 7.7 | 5.8 | 41 | 15.35 | 12.3 | 9.2 |
| 12 | 9.9 | 7.9 | 6.0 | 42 | 15.5 | 12.4 | 9.3 |
| 13 | 10.2 | 8.1 | 6.2 | 43 | 15.7 | 12.6 | 9.4 |
| 14 | 10.4 | 8.3 | 6.3 | 44 | 15.85 | 12.7 | 9.5 |
| 15 | 10.6 | 8.5 | 6.4 | 45 | 16.0 | 12.9 | 9.6 |
| 16 | 10.8 | 8.7 | 6.6 | 46 | 16.2 | 12.95 | 9.7 |
| 17 | 11.0 | 8.9 | 6.7 | 47 | 16.35 | 13.1 | 9.8 |
| 18 | 11.3 | 9.0 | 6.8 | 48 | 16.5 | 13.2 | 9.9 |
| 19 | 11.5 | 9.2 | 7.0 | 49 | 16.65 | 13.35 | 10.0 |
| 20 | 11.7 | 9.4 | 7.1 | 50 | 16.8 | 13.5 | 10.1 |
| 21 | 11.9 | 9.6 | 7.2 | 51 | 16.95 | 13.65 | 10.2 |
| 22 | 12.05 | 9.7 | 7.3 | 52 | 17.1 | 13.8 | 10.3 |
| 23 | 12.2 | 9.8 | 7.4 | 53 | 17.25 | 13.9 | 10.4 |
| 24 | 12.4 | 9.9 | 7.5 | 54 | 17.4 | 14.0 | 10.5 |
| 25 | 12.6 | 10.1 | 7.6 | 55 | 17.6 | 14.2 | 10.6 |
| 26 | 12.7 | 10.3 | 7.7 | 56 | 17.7 | 14.3 | 10.7 |
| 27 | 12.9 | 10.5 | 7.8 | 57 | 17.9 | 14.4 | 10.75 |
| 28 | 13.1 | 10.6 | 7.9 | 58 | 18.05 | 14.5 | 10.8 |
| 29 | 13.3 | 10.7 | 8.0 | 59 | 18.25 | 14.6 | 10.9 |
| 30 | 13.5 | 10.8 | 8.1 | 60 | 18.4 | 14.7 | 11.0 |

[1]Based on table by Jelliffe (1966).
[2]Boston standards (Stuart & Stevenson, 1959), taking mean of boys and girls. Boys are 0.05 to 0.15 kg heavier and girls 0.05 to 0.15 kg lighter.

## TABLE 19.2

## DESIRABLE WEIGHTS OF ADULTS
According to height and frame

| Height without shoes (approximate equivalents) | | | Desirable weight in kilograms and pounds (in indoor clothing), ages 25 and over | | | | | |
|---|---|---|---|---|---|---|---|---|
| metres | ft | in | Small frame kg | Small frame lb | Medium frame kg | Medium frame lb | Large frame kg | Large frame lb |
| **Men** | | | | | | | | |
| 1.550 | 5 | 1 | 50.8–54.4 | 112–120 | 53.5–58.5 | 118–129 | 57.2–64 | 126–141 |
| 1.575 | 5 | 2 | 52.2–55.8 | 115–123 | 54.9–60.3 | 121–133 | 58.5–65.3 | 129–144 |
| 1.600 | 5 | 3 | 53.5–57.2 | 118–126 | 56.2–61.7 | 124–136 | 59.9–67.1 | 132–148 |
| 1.625 | 5 | 4 | 54.9–58.5 | 121–129 | 57.6–63 | 127.139 | 61.2–68.9 | 135–152 |
| 1.650 | 5 | 5 | 56.2–60.3 | 124–133 | 59 –64.9 | 130–143 | 62.6–70.8 | 138–156 |
| 1.675 | 5 | 6 | 58.1–62.1 | 128–137 | 60.8–66.7 | 134–147 | 64.4–73 | 142–161 |
| 1.700 | 5 | 7 | 59.9–64 | 132–141 | 62.6–68.9 | 138–152 | 66.7–75.3 | 147–166 |
| 1.725 | 5 | 8 | 61.7–65.8 | 136–145 | 64.4–70.8 | 142–156 | 68.5–77.1 | 151–170 |
| 1.750 | 5 | 9 | 63.5–68 | 140–150 | 66.2–72.6 | 146–160 | 70.3–78.9 | 155–174 |
| 1.775 | 5 | 10 | 65.3–69.9 | 144–154 | 68 –74.8 | 150–165 | 72.1–81.2 | 159–179 |
| 1.800 | 5 | 11 | 67.1–71.7 | 148–158 | 69.9–77.1 | 154–170 | 74.4–83.5 | 164–184 |
| 1.825 | 6 | 0 | 68.9–73.5 | 152–162 | 71.7–79.4 | 158–175 | 76.2–85.7 | 169–189 |
| 1.850 | 6 | 1 | 70.8–75.7 | 156–167 | 73.5–81.6 | 162–180 | 78.5–88 | 173–194 |
| 1.875 | 6 | 2 | 72.6–77.6 | 160–171 | 75.7–83.9 | 167–185 | 80.7–90.3 | 178–199 |
| 1.900 | 6 | 3 | 74.4–79.4 | 164–175 | 78.0–86.2 | 172–190 | 82.6–92.5 | 182–204 |
| **Women** | | | | | | | | |
| 1.425 | 4 | 8 | 41.7–44.5 | 92–98 | 43.5–48.5 | 96–107 | 47.2–54 | 104–119 |
| 1.450 | 4 | 9 | 42.6–45.8 | 94–101 | 44.5–49.9 | 98–110 | 48.1–55.3 | 106–122 |
| 1.475 | 4 | 10 | 43.5–47.2 | 96–104 | 45.8–51.3 | 101–113 | 49.4–56.7 | 109–125 |
| 1.500 | 4 | 11 | 44.9–48.5 | 99–107 | 47.2–52.6 | 104–116 | 50.8–58.1 | 112–128 |
| 1.525 | 5 | 0 | 46.3–49.9 | 102–110 | 48.5–54 | 107–119 | 52.2–59.4 | 115–131 |
| 1.550 | 5 | 1 | 47.6–51.3 | 105–113 | 49.9–55.3 | 110–122 | 53.5–60.8 | 118–134 |
| 1.575 | 5 | 2 | 49 –52.6 | 108–116 | 51.3–57.2 | 113–126 | 54.9–62.6 | 121–138 |
| 1.600 | 5 | 3 | 50.3–54 | 111–119 | 52.6–59 | 116–130 | 56.7–64.4 | 125–142 |
| 1.625 | 5 | 4 | 51.7–55.8 | 114–123 | 54.4–61.2 | 120–135 | 58.5–66.2 | 129–146 |
| 1.650 | 5 | 5 | 53.5–57.7 | 118–127 | 56.2–63 | 124–139 | 60.3–68 | 133–150 |
| 1.675 | 5 | 6 | 55.3–59.4 | 122–131 | 58.1–64.9 | 128–143 | 62.1–69.9 | 137–154 |
| 1.700 | 5 | 7 | 57.2–61.2 | 126–135 | 59.9–66.7 | 132–147 | 64 –71.7 | 141–158 |
| 1.725 | 5 | 8 | 59 –63.5 | 130–140 | 61.7–68.5 | 136–151 | 65.8–73.9 | 145–163 |
| 1.750 | 5 | 9 | 60.8–65.3 | 134–144 | 63.5–70.3 | 140–155 | 67.6–76.2 | 149–168 |
| 1.775 | 5 | 10 | 62.6–67.1 | 138–148 | 65.3–72.1 | 144–159 | 69.4–78.5 | 153–173 |

Based on weights of insured persons in the United States associated with lowest mortality (*Statist. Bull. Metrop. Life Insur. Co.*, 40, Nov.–Dec. 1959).

# Notes on International System of Units (SI Units)

*Examples of Basic SI Units*

| | |
|---|---|
| Length | metre (m) |
| Mass | kilogram (kg) |
| Amount of substance | mole (mol) |
| Energy | joule (J) |
| Pressure | pascal (pa) |

*Examples of Decimal Multiples and Submultiples of SI Units*

| *Factor* | *Name* | *Symbol* |
|---|---|---|
| $10^6$ | mega- | M |
| $10^3$ | kilo- | k |
| $10^{-1}$ | deci- | d |
| $10^{-2}$ | centi- | c |
| $10^{-3}$ | milli- | m |
| $10^{-6}$ | micro- | $\mu$ |
| $10^{-9}$ | nano- | n |
| $10^{-12}$ | pico- | p |
| $10^{-15}$ | femto- | f |

*Volume*. The basic SI unit of volume is the cubic metre (1000 litre). Because of its convenience the litre is used as the unit of volume in laboratory work.

*Amount of Substance ('Molar') Concentration* (e.g., mol/*l*, μmol/*l*) is used for substances of defined chemical composition. It replaces equivalent concentration (mEq/*l*), which is not part of the SI system, for reporting measurements of sodium, potassium, chloride and bicarbonate (the numerical value of these four measurements is unchanged because the ions are univalent).

*Mass Concentration* (e.g. g/*l*. μ/*l*) is used for all protein measurements, for substances which do not have a sufficiently well defined composition and for serum vitamin $B_{12}$ and folate measurements. The numerical value in SI units will change by a factor of 10 in those instances previously expressed in terms of 100 ml.

Haemoglobin is an exception. It is agreed internationally that in the meantime haemoglobin should continue to be expressed in terms of g/dl.

SI units are not employed for enzymes nor usually for immunoglobulins.

# Biochemical Values

Approximate adult ranges

| | B = Whole Blood<br>P = Plasma<br>S = Serum | SI Units | Other Units |
|---|---|---|---|
| P | Alanine aminotransferase (ALT) (glutamate-pyruvate transaminase: GPT) | | 3–30 units/*l* |
| B | Ammonium | 23–47 μmol/*l* | 40–80 μg/100 ml |
| P | Amylase | | 150–340 units/*l*<br>80–180 Somogyi/100 ml |
| P | Aspartate aminotransferase AST. (glutamate–oxaloacetic transaminase GOT) | | 5–40 units/*l* |
| P | Bicarbonate | 24–32 mmol/*l* | 24–32 mEq/*l* |
| P | Bilirubin (total) | 5–17 μmol/*l* | 0.3–1.0 mg/100 ml |
| S | Caeruloplasmin | 0.3–0.6g/*l* | 30–60 mg/100 ml |
| P | Calcium (total) | 2.12–2.62 mmol/*l* | 8.5–10.5 mg/100 ml |
| B | Carbon dioxide ($P_{CO_2}$) | 4.8–6.0 kPa | 36–45 mm Hg |
| P | β-Carotene | 0.9–5.6 μmol/*l* | 50–300 μg/100 ml |
| P | Chloride | 95–105 mmol/*l* | 95–105 mEq/*l* |
| P | Cholesterol | 3.6–7.8 mmol/*l* | 140–300 mg/100 ml |
| S | Copper | 13–24 μmol/*l* | 80–150 μg/100 ml |
| P | Cortisol | 220–720 nmol/*l* | 8–26 μg/100 ml |

| | B = Whole Blood<br>P = Plasma<br>S = Serum | SI Units | Other Units |
|---|---|---|---|
| P | Creatinine | 62–124 μmol/*l* | 0.7–1.4 mg/100 ml |
| P | Ethanol, marked intoxication | 65–87 mmol/*l* | 0.3–0.4g/100 ml |
| | alcoholic stupor | 87–109 mmol/*l* | 0.4–0.5g/100 ml |
| | alcoholic coma | > 109 mmol/*l* | > 0.5g/100 ml |
| P | Fibrinogen | 1.5–4.0 g/*l* | 150–400 mg/100 ml |
| P | γ - glutamyl transferase (γ - GT) | | 6–28 units/*l* (male<br>4–18 units/*l* (female) |
| B | Glucose (fasting) | <5.5 mmol/*l* | <100mg/100 ml |
| P | Haptoglobins (Hb binding) | 0.3–2.0 g/*l* | 30–200 mg/100 ml |
| P | Iron | 14–29 μmol/*l* | 80–160 μg/100 ml |
| P | Total iron binding capacity (as iron) | 45–72 μmol/*l* | 250–400 μg/100 ml |
| B | Lactate | 0.4–1.4 mmol/*l* | 3.6–13.0 mg/100 ml |
| P | Lactate dehydrogenase (LD) | | 120–365 units/*l* |
| B | Lead | 0.5–1.9 μmol/*l* | 10–40 μg/100 ml |
| P | Lipids (total) | 4.0–10.0 g/*l* | 400–1,000 mg/100 ml |
| P | Magnesium | 0.7–1.0 mmol/*l* | 1.8–2.4 mg/100 ml |
| P | Osmolality | 285–295 mmol/kg | 285–295 mosm/kg |
| B | Oxygen ($Po_2$) | 11–13 kPa | 83–98 mm Hg |
| P | Phosphatase, acid | | > 8.2 units/*l* |
| | prostatic | | > 7.2 units/*l* |
| P | Phosphatase, alkaline | | 21–100 units/*l*<br>3–13 K-A units |
| P | Phosphate (as inorganic P) | 0.8–1.4 mmol/*l* | 2.5–4.5 mg/100 ml |
| P | Potassium | 3.8–5.0 mmol/*l* | 3.8–5.0 mEq/*l* |
| S | Proteins–total | 62–82 g/*l* | 6.2–8.2g/100 ml |
| | –albumin | 36–52 g/*l* | 3.6–5.2g/100 ml |
| | —globulins | 24–37 g/*l* | 2.4–3.7 g/100 ml |
| B | Pyruvate | 45–80 μmol/*l* | 0.4–0.7 mg/100 ml |
| P | Sodium | 136–148 mmol/*l* | 136–148 mEq/*l* |
| P | Thyroxine | 244–465 nmol/*l* | 3.1–5.9 μg/100 ml |
| P | Transferrin | 1.2–2 g/l | 120–200 mg/100 ml |
| P | Triglyceride (as triolein) | 0.28–1.69 mmol/*l* | 25–150 mg/100 ml |
| P | Urate | 0.12–0.42 mmol/*l* | 2–7 mg/100 ml |
| P | Urea | 2.5–6.6 mmol/*l* | 15–40 mg/100 ml |
| P | Vitamin A | 0.7–1.7 μmol/*l* | 20–50 μg/100 ml |

*Note:* HORMONES. As levels may vary with the method used and with factors such as age, sex and stress, the reference values should be obtained from the laboratory carrying out the estimations.

## Haematolgical Values

| | S.I. Units | Other Units |
|---|---|---|
| Bleeding time (Ivy) | Up to 11 min | |
| Blood volume | | |
| Red cell mass, men | 30 ± 5 ml/kg | |
| women | 25 ± 5 ml/kg | |
| Plasma volume (both sexes) | 45 ± 5 ml/kg | |
| Total blood volume, men | 75 ± 10 ml/kg | |
| women | 70 ± 10 ml/kg | |
| Folate – serum | 2 –20 μg/*l* | 2 – 20 ng/ml |
| red cell | > 100 μg/*l* | > 100 ng/ml |
| Haemoglobin, men | 13 – 18 g/d*l* | 13 – 18 g/100 ml |
| women | 11.5 – 16.5 g/d*l* | 11.5 – 16.5 g/100 ml |
| Leucocytes – adults | 4.0 – 11.0 x $10^9$/*l* | 4000 – 11000/μ*l* 4.0 – 11.0 x $10^3$/$mm^3$ |
| Differential white cell count | | |
| Neutrophil granulocytes | 2.5–7.5 x $10^9$/*l* | 40–75% |
| Lymphocytes | 1.0 – 3.5 x $10^9$/*l* | 20 – 45% |
| Monocytes | 0.2 – 0.8 x $10^9$/*l* | 2 – 10% |
| Eosinophil granulocytes | 0.04 – 0.4 x $10^9$/*l* | 1 – 6% |
| Basophil granulocytes | 0.01 – 0.1 x $10^9$/*l* | 0 – 1% |
| Mean corpuscular haemoglobin (MCH) | 27–32 pg | 27–32 μμg |
| Mean corpuscular haemoglobin concentration (MCHC) | 30 – 35 g/d*l* | 30 – 35% |
| Mean corpuscular volume (MCV) | 78 – 98 fl. | 78 – 98 $\mu^3$ or $\mu m^3$ |
| Packed cell volume (PCV) or | | |
| haemotocrit, men | 0.40 – 0.54 l/*l* | 40 – 54% |
| women | 0.37 – 0.47 1/*l* | 37 – 47% |
| Platelets | 150 – 400 x $10^9$/*l* | 150 000 – 400 000/μ*l* or / $mm^3$ |
| Red cell count, men | 4.5 – 6.5 x $10^{12}$/*l* | 4.5 – 6.5 x $10^6$/μ*l* or mm |
| women | 3.8 – 5.8 x $10^{12}$/*l* | 3.8 – 5.8 x $10^6$/μ*l* or mm |
| Red cell life span (mean) | 120 days | |
| Red cell life span T½ ($^{51}$Cr) | 25 – 35 days. | |
| Reticulocytes (adults) | 10 x 100 x $10^9$/*l* | 0.2 – 2% |
| Vitamin $B_{12}$ (in serum as cyanocobalamin) | 160 – 925 ng/*l* | 160 – 925 pg/*l* or μμg/*l* |

## Drug Nomenclature and Prescription

In this book the names that have been given for drugs have almost invariably been those approved for use in Britain. These are devised or selected by the British Pharmacopoeia Commission and published by the Health Ministers at regular intervals. It must be realised, however, that many countries have their national non-proprietary names, and that the World Health Organisation also has its own list. Usually these various names are similar, but there are significant differences, for example, paracetamol (B.P.) is listed as acetaminophen in the United States Pharmacopoeia. Proprietary names are given in this book only in exceptional circumstances, but can usually be found in the British National Formulary, the Data Sheet Compendium and as an addendum to some textbooks. There may be many totally different names for the same substance and this can cause confusion.

Abbreviations used in relationship to the administration of drugs are i.m. (intramuscular injection) i.v. (intravenous injection), s.c. (subcutaneous injection), b.d. (twice daily) and t.i.d. (thrice daily).Polypharmacy should be avoided if possible, one reason being the danger of interactions between drugs. Moreover, patient compliance (i.e. the taking of medicines as prescribed) is improved if the instructions are simple and specific, especially for the elderly. The dosage given is a guide for use in adults of average build and should be checked against that in a national formulary or in the manufacturer's instructions. It is particularly important to confirm that a dosage given in mg/kg body weight is, indeed, correct, and great care must be taken to ensure that no error occurs in the quantity of a drug prescribed for an infant or child.

Some drugs, e.g. in the chemotherapy of malignant disease, are prescribed in weight of drug per square metre of body surface. With the use of a nomogram, the body surface area can be calculated from the height in centimetres and the weight in kilograms.

*Standard reference books*:

Approved Names (1977) British Pharmacopoeia Commission. London: Her Majesty's Stationery Office.

British National Formulary (1981) The British Medical Association and The Pharmaceutical Society of Great Britain, London.

Martindale – The Extra Pharmacopoeia (1977) 27th edn. London: The Pharmaceutical Press.

*Further reading about drugs*:

Girdwood, R. H. (ed.) (1979) *Clinical Pharmacology*, 24th edn. London: Baillière Tindall.

# Index

## A

# B

# C

# D

# E

# F

## G

## H

## I

## J

## K



## L

## M

## N

## O

# P

## Q



## R

# S

# T

## U

# V

## W



## X



## Y



## Z